Techniques in Hand Surgery

Techniques in Hand Surgery

■

Editor

WILLIAM F. BLAIR, MD

Professor, Division of Hand Surgery
Department of Orthopaedics
University of Iowa
Iowa City, Iowa

■

Associate Editor

CURTIS M. STEYERS, MD
Professor, Division of Hand and Microsurgery
Department of Orthopaedics
University of Iowa
Iowa City, Iowa

Illustrations by
Bernie Kida, MFA, CMI
Medical Creative Services
Scottish Rite Medical Center
Atlanta, Georgia

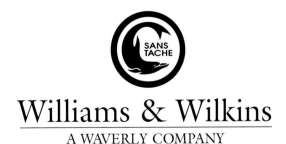

Williams & Wilkins

A WAVERLY COMPANY

BALTIMORE • PHILADELPHIA • LONDON • PARIS • BANGKOK
BUENOS AIRES • HONG KONG • MUNICH • SYDNEY • TOKYO • WROCLAW

1996

Editor: Darlene Cooke
Managing Editor: Fran Klass
Production Manager: Laurie Forsyth
Book Project Editor: Robert D. Magee
Designer: Cathy Cotter
Typesetter: Maryland Composition
Printer: Quebecor
Binder: Quebecor

ISBN 0-683-00842-0

Accurate indications, adverse reactions, and dosage schedules for drugs are provided in this book, but it is possible that they may change. The reader is urged to review the package information data of the manufacturers of the medications mentioned.

Printed in the United States of America

Library of Congress Cataloging in Publication Data

Techniques in hand surgery / editor, William F. Blair; associate
   editor, Curtis M. Steyers.
      p.   cm.
   Includes bibliographical references and index.
   ISBN 0-683-00842-0
   1. Hand—Surgery.   I. Blair, William F.   II. Steyers, Curtis M.
   [DNLM: 1. Hand—surgery.   2. Surgery, Operative—methods.   WE 830
T256 1996]
RD559.T435   1996
617.5′75059—dc20
DNLM/DLC
for Library of Congress   95-7309
                                                             CIP

The Publishers have made every effort to trace the copyright holders for borrowed material. If they have inadvertently overlooked any, they will be pleased to make the necessary arrangements at the first opportunity

96 97 98 99
1 2 3 4 5 6 7 8 9 10

■ PREFACE

The education of developing young hand surgeons and the continuing education of experienced hand surgeons are vitally important processes. A quality educational experience should provide basic science and clinical knowledge, a clear understanding of indications for operative intervention, mastery of operative techniques, and realistic concepts about outcomes. These concepts form the basis of responsible and effective clinical decisions.

The process of mastering basic techniques in hand surgery can be compromised if resource material is not conveniently organized or readily available. *Techniques in Hand Surgery* brings together, in one reference, detailed descriptions of the most important and widely used operations in hand surgery. The contributors, all knowledgeable and authoritative hand surgeons, describe the operations in a consistent chapter format that is intended to facilitate ready access to essential information. The text emphasizes precise descriptions of the recommended operative techniques, and the key features of the techniques are carefully and fully illustrated.

A section in each chapter on the History of the Technique implies that surgical technique in hand surgery is a dynamic process, that it is evolving. I welcome not only my colleagues' scholarly critique of this text, but their future modifications of and contributions to the technical aspects of hand surgery.

■ *ACKNOWLEDGMENTS*

Although this text represents my own considerable commitment, the contributors clearly deserve the highest of credits. They are expert in their fields; they have unique developmental and practical experience with the operations they have described. I was and remain impressed with their willingness to participate in this project, their dedication, the time and energy they devoted to their work, and the quality of their chapters.

The completion of a project of this magnitude requires both artistic and technical support. Mr. Bernie Kida was as pleasant to work with as he is gifted in the art of medical illustration. The publisher's editoral staff were always encouraging yet professional; I appreciate their trust in my scholarly vision. Pivotal to the success of this project was the completion of considerable correspondence, the organization of records and manuscripts, effective communications, and many manuscript revisions, all done by or under the guidance of Gloria Yorek, my secretary. Loyalty, affability, and patience have no price.

All who have participated in writing and producing this hand surgery text have been notably accepting and understanding of my editorial direction and standards. I remain sincerely appreciative of their generous support.

■ CONTRIBUTORS

Brian D. Adams, MD
Associate Professor
Division of Hand and Microsurgery
Department of Orhopaedic Surgery
University of Iowa
Iowa City, Iowa

John M. Agee, MD
Director, Hand Biomechanics Lab, Inc.
Sacramento, California

Edward E. Almquist, MD
Clinical Professor, Department of Orthopaedics
University of Washington
Seattle Hand Surgery Group
Seattle, Washington

Peter C. Amadio, MD
Professor of Orthopaedic Surgery
Consultant in Hand Surgery
Mayo Clinic
Rochester, Minnesota

Dennis J. Andersen, MD
Fellow, Hand and Microsurgery
Department of Orthopaedic Surgery
University of Iowa
Iowa City, Iowa

Steven D. Antrobus, MD
Department of Plastic & Reconstructive
    Surgery
University of Texas Southwestern
Dallas, Texas

Duffield Ashmead, IV, MD
Assistant Clinical Professor
University of Connecticut
Farmington, Connecticut

Robert L. Bass, MD
Hand Surgery Associates
Denver, Colorado

Jeffrey Bechler, MD
San Diego, California

Robert Beckenbaugh, MD
Professor of Orthopaedics
Consultant in Hand Surgery
Mayo Foundation, Mayo Graduate School of
    Medicine
Mayo Clinic
Rochester, Minnesota

Mark R. Belsky, MD
Associate Clinical Professor of Orthopaedic
    Surgery
Tufts University School of Medicine
Chief Orthopaedic Surgery
Newton Wellesley Hospital
Newton, Massachusetts

Robert J. Belsole, MD
Professor, Orthopaedic Surgery
Director, Division Orthopaedic Surgery and
    Hand Surgery
University South Florida College of Medicine
Tampa, Florida

Michel Y. Benoit, MD
Assistant Professor
Department of Orthopaedics & Rehabilitation
McClure Musculoskeletal Research Center
The University of Vermont College of
    Medicine
Burlington, Vermont

Peter E. Bentivegna, MD
Former Fellow
University of Utah Hand/Microsurgery
    Service
Attending Surgeon
Cape Cod Hospital
Hyannis, Massachusetts

Richard A. Berger, MD, PhD
Associate Professor and Consultant of
    Orthopaedic Surgery and Anatomy
Mayo Clinic and Mayo Foundation
Rochester, Minnesota

Anders Berggren, MD, PhD
Associate Professor of Plastic Surgery
Faculty of Health Sciences
University of Linkoping
SWEDEN

Paul A. Binhammer, MD
Lecturer, University of Toronto Faculty of
    Medicine
Division of Plastic Surgery
Sunnybrook Health Science Center
Toronto, Ontario, CANADA

Allen T. Bishop, MD
Associate Professor of Orthopaedic Surgery
Mayo Medical School
Consultant in Hand & Microsurgery
Department of Orthopedics
Mayo Clinic
Rochester, Minnesota

William F. Blair, MD
Professor, Division of Hand and Microsurgery
Department of Orthopaedics
University of Iowa Hospitals and Clinics
Iowa City, Iowa

Leonard S. Bodell, MD
Adjunct Associate Professor
Arizona State University/BioEngineering
Tempe, Arizona
Adjunct Research Scientist
Harrington Foundation
Phoenix, Arizona

John T. Bolger, MD
Clinical Instructor in Orthopaedic Surgery
Medical College of Wisconsin
Milwaukee, Wisconsin
Attending Orthopaedic Hand Surgeon
Waukesha Memorial Hospital
Waukesha, Wisconsin

Forst E. Brown, MD
Professor & Chairman
Section of Plastic Surgery
Dartmouth - Hitchcock Medical Center
Lebanon, New Hampshire

Mary Lynn Brown, MD
Matthews Orthopaedic Clinic
Orlando, Florida

Richard A. Brown, MD
Assistant Clinical Professor
Department of Orthopaedics
School of Medicine
University of California, San Diego
San Diego, California
San Diego Orthopaedic Medical Group, Inc.
La Jolla, California

Robert H. Brumfield, Jr., MD
Clinical Associate Professor
Department of Orthopaedic Surgery
University of Southern California School of
    Medicine
Consultant, Arthritis Service
Rancho Los Amigo Medical Center
Downey, California

Dieter Buck-Gramcko, MD
Associate Professor for Hand Surgery
University of Hamburg
Chief, Unit for Hand Surgery
Children's Hospital Wilhelmstift
Hamburg, GERMANY

Richard J. Burton, MD
Professor and Chairman, Department of
    Orthopaedics
University of Rochester Medical Center
Rochester, New York

Edward R. Calkins, MD
Director, Fallon Clinic Hand Center
Worcester, Massachusetts

Phyllis Chang, MD, FACS
Assistant Professor
Department of Surgery, Division of Plastic
    Surgery
Division of Hand and Microsurgery
Department of Orthopaedic Surgery
Department of Otolaryngology, Head and
    Neck Surgery
University of Iowa Hospitals
Iowa City, Iowa

Larry K. Chidgey, MD
Associate Professor
Department of Orthopaedics
University of Florida
Gainesville, Florida

James C. Y. Chow, MD
Clinical Assistant Professor
Southern Illinois University School of Medicine
Springfield, Illinois
Orthopaedic Clinic of Mt. Vernon
Orthopaedic Research Foundation of Southern
    Illinois
Mt. Vernon, Illinois

Mark S. Cohen, MD
Assistant Professor
Director, Hand and Elbow Program
Rush-Presbyterian-St. Lukes Medical Center
Chicago, Illinois

Myles J. Cohen, MD
Assistant Professor, Department of Surgery
University of Southern California School of
    Medicine
Chief of Surgery
Cedar Sinai Medical Center
Los Angeles, California

Don A. Coleman, MD
Associate Professor
Department of Orthopaedics
University of Utah Health Science Center
Salt Lake City, Utah

Paul A. Cook, MD
Division of Orthopaedic Surgery
The Ohio State University Hospital
Columbus, Ohio

Albert E. Cram, MD
Professor and Director
Section of Plastic and Reconstructive Surgery
University of Iowa Hospitals and Clinics
Iowa City, Iowa

A. George Dass, MD
Assistant Clinical Professor, Department of
  Surgery
College of Human Medicine, Michigan State
  University
McLaren Regional Medical Center
Flint, Michigan

Thomas F. De Bartolo, MD
Attending Hand/Orthopaedic Surgeon
Mason City Clinic
Medical Director Upper Extremity Industrial
  Medicine Clinic
North Iowa Mercy Health Center
Mason City, Iowa

Gregory G. Degnan, MD
Assistant Professor of Orthopaedic Surgery
University of Virginia Health Science Center
Assistant Professor of Surgery
Uniformed Services University of Health
  Sciences
Charlottesville, Virginia

Edward Diao, MD
Assistant Professor, Department of
  Orthopaedic Surgery
Chief, Hand and Microvascular Surgery
  Service
University of California, San Francisco
Attending Surgeon
University of California Medical Center
UCSF/Mount Zion Medical Center
San Francisco General Hospital
San Francisco, California

James R. Doyle, MD
Professor and Chairman
Division of Orthopaedics
Department of Surgery
John A. Burns School of Medicine
University of Hawaii
Honolulu, Hawaii

Gregory J. Dray, MD
Active Medical Staff
St. Joseph's Hospital
Memorial Mission Hospital
Asheville, North Carolina

John J. Drewniany, MD
Private Practice
Hand Surgery
Jacksonville Hand Associates
Jacksonville, Florida

John Wight Duram, MD
Private Practice
Hand and Orthopaedic Surgery
Flagstaff, Arizona

Richard G. Eaton, MD
Chief, Hand Surgery Service
Department of Orthopedic Surgery
St. Luke's/Roosevelt Hospital Center
Professor of Clinical Orthopedic Surgery
Columbia University
College of Physicians and Surgeons
New York, New York

Bradford W. Edgerton, MD
Clinic Associate Professor (Plastic Surgery)
Hand Fellowship Director
University of Southern California
Los Angeles, California

Lee E. Edstrom, MD
Surgeon-in-Chief, Department of Plastic
  Surgery
Rhode Island Hospital
Associate Professor, Chief and Program
  Director
Division of Plastic Surgery
Brown University
Providence, Rhode Island

Fredrik AF Ekenstam, MD, PhD
Associate Professor
Department of Plastic and Hand Surgery
University Hospital
Uppsal, SWEDEN

Anton J. Fakhouri, MD
Clinical Associate Professor
University of Illinois
College of Medicine
Oak Lawn, Illinois

Robert Falender, MD
Medial Arts Orthopaedics
St. Francis Hospital & Health Centers
Beech Grove, Indiana

John F. Fatti, MD
Assistant Chairman, Department of
    Orthopaedics
Crouse Irving Memorial Hospital
Clinical Assistant Professor
State University Hospital Health Science
    Center
Syracuse, New York

Donald C. Ferlic, MD
Associate Clinical Professor
University of Colorado Health Science Ctr.
Denver, Colorado

Diego L. Fernandez, MD
Associate Professor of Orthopaedic Surgery
Department of Orthopaedic Surgery
Lindenhof Hospital
Berne, SWITZERLAND

Teri S. Formanek, MD
Iowa Medical Center
Cedar Rapids, Iowa

Robert J. Foster, MD
Associate Clinical Professor of Orthopaedics
University of Colorado Health Sciences Center
Denver, Colorado
Active Staff
St. Francis Hospital and Memorial Hospital
Colorado Springs, Colorado

Guy D. Foulkes, MD
Clinical Instructor in Orthopaedic Surgery
University of California at Los Angeles
Consulting Specialist
Olive View Medical Center
Sylmar, California

Joel L. Frazier, MD
Assistant Professor of Surgery
Division of Orthopaedics
Ohio State University
Columbus, Ohio

Alan E. Freeland, MD
Professor and Chief, Hand Surgery
Department of Orthopaedic Surgery
University of Mississippi Medical Center
Jackson, Mississippi

Gary K. Frykman, MD
Clinical Professor, Orthopaedic Surgery
Loma Linda University School of Medicine
Chief of Hand Service
Jerry L. Pettis Memorial Veteran's Hospital
Loma Linda, California

Marc Garcia-Elias, MD, PhD
Chief Section, Hand Surgery
Hospital General De Catalunya
Hand Surgeon
Institute Kaplan
Barcelona, SPAIN

William B. Geissler, MD
Associate Professor, Orthopaedic Surgery
University of Mississippi Medical Center
Jackson, Mississippi

Richard H. Gelberman, MD
Reynolds Professor and Chairman,
    Orthopaedic Surgery
Washington University School of Medicine
St. Louis, Missouri

Harris Gellman, MD
Professor, Orthopaedic Surgery & Plastic
    Surgery
University of Arkansas School of Medicine
Little Rock, Arkansas

Steven Z. Glickel, MD
Assistant Clinical Professor of Orthopaedic
    Surgery
Columbia University, College of Physicians &
    Surgeons
Associate Director, Hand Surgery Service
Chief, Hand Surgery Clinic
St. Luke's-Roosevelt Hospital and Center
New York, New York

James L. Gluck, MD
Kansas Orthopaedic Center
Wichita, Kansas

Leonard Gordon, MD
Attending Surgeon and Director of
Microsurgical Reasearch Laboratory
California Pacific Medical Center
Associate Professor of Anatomy &
    Orthopaedic Surgery
University of California
San Francisco, California

Marc E. Gottlieb, MD
Chief of Surgery, Healthwest Regional Medical
    Center
Assistant Professor of Plastic Surgery
Mayo Clinic
Phoenix, Arizona

Thomas L. Greene, MD
Florida Orthopaedic Institute
Tampa, Florida

Jack L. Greider, Jr. MD
Clinical Assistant Professor
Department of Orthopaedic Surgery
University of Florida
Jacksonville, Florida

O. Allen Guinn, III, MD
Connecticut Combined Hand Surgery
 Fellowship
Hartford, Connecticut

Amit Gupta, MD
Clinical Instructor, Department of
 Orthopaedics
University of Louisville
Louisville, Kentucky

Lars Hagberg, MD, PhD
Department of Hand Surgery
Lund University
Malmo University Hospital
Malmo, SWEDEN

Charles Hamlin, MD
Assistant Clinical Professor
University of Colorado School of Health
 Sciences
Denver, Colorado

Douglas P. Hanel, MD
Associate Professor
Hand and Microvascular Surgery
University of Washington
Seattle, Washington

Jayaram S. Hariharan, MD
Fellow, Hand and Microvascular Surgery
 Service
Department of Orthopaedic Surgery
University of California @ San Francisco
San Francisco, California

Hill Hastings, II, MD
Clinical Associate Professor
Department of Orthopaedic Surgery
Indiana University Medical Center and
The Indiana Hand Center
Indianapolis, Indiana

Vincente R. Hentz, MD
Professor of Functional Restoration
(Hand Surgery)
Stanford University School of Medicine
Stanford, California

Lawrence Colwyn Hurst, MD
Professor and Acting Chairman
Department of Orthopaedics
Chief, Division of Hand Surgery
University Hand Center at Stony Brook
Setauket, New York

Richard S. Idler, MD
Clinical Assistant Professor of Orthopaedic
 Surgery
Indiana University School of Medicine
Assistant Clinical Professor of Plastic Surgery
University of Kentucky Medical School
Louisville, Kentucky

Joesph E. Imbriglia, MD
Professor of Orthopaedic Surgery
Medical College of Pennsylvania-Hahnemann
 University
Philadelphia, Pennsylvania
Chief, Division of Hand Surgery
Allegheny General Hospital
Pittsburgh, Pennsylvania

Michael E. Jabaley, MD
Clinical Professor of Orthopaedic & Plastic
 Surgery
Department of Surgery
University of Mississippi Medical Center
Jackson, Mississippi

Michael Jablon, MD
Assistant Clinical Professor of Orthopaedics
University of Illinois
Director of Hand Surgery
Michael Reese Hospital
Chicago, Illinois

Peter J.L. Jebson, MD
Fellow Associate, Division of Hand and
 Microvascular Surgery
Department of Orthopaedic Surgery
University of Iowa Hospitals and Clinics
Iowa City, Iowa

Charles D. Jennings, MD
Great Falls Orthopaedic Associates
Great Falls, Montana

Michael L. Jones, MD
Clinical Professor
University of Texas Health Science Center at
 San Antonio
San Antonio, Texas

Neil Ford Jones, MD
Professor and Chief of Hand Surgery
UCLA Medical Center
University of California at Los Angeles
Los Angeles, California

Jesse B. Jupiter, MD
Director, Orthopaedic Hand Service
Visiting Orthopaedic Surgeon
Massachusetts General Hospital
Associate Professor Orthopaedic Surgery
Harvard Medical School
Boston, Massachusetts

Julie A. Katarincic, MD
Instructor in Orthopaedic Surgery
Mayo Medical School
Senior Associate Consultant, Orthopaedic
    Surgery,
Surgery of the Hand
Mayo Clinic and Mayo Foundation
Rochester, Minnesota

Jefferson J. Kaye, MD
Chairman, Department of Orthopaedic Surgery
Ochsner Clinic & Alton Ochsner Medical
    Foundation
Associate Professor of Orthopaedic Surgery
Tulane University School of Medicine
New Orleans, Lousiana

Thomas R. Kiefhaber, MD
Assistant Professor
Department of Orthopaedics
University of Cincinnati
Cincinnati, Ohio

William B. Kleinman, MD
Clinical Professor of Orthopaedic Surgery
Indiana University School of Medicine
Director, Congenital Upper Limb Deformity
    Clinic
The James Whitcomb Riley Hospital for
    Children
Indiana University Medical Center
Senior Attending Hand Surgeon
The Indiana Hand Center
Indianapolis, Indiana

Raymond Kobus, MD
Clinical Instructor, Department of Orthopaedic
    Surgery
The Ohio State University Hospitals
Columbus, Ohio

L. Andrew Koman, MD
Professor, Department of Orthopaedic Surgery
Wake Forest University
North Carolina Baptist Hospital Medical
    Center
Winston-Salem, North Carolina

Gary R. Kuzma, MD
Hand Center of Greensboro
Clinical Assistant Professor
Department Orthopedic Surgery
Bowman Gray School of Medicine
Winston-Salem, North Carolina

David M. Lamey, MD
Fellow in Hand Surgery
Roosevelt Hospital
New York, New York

Lewis B. Lane, MD
Clinical Associate Professor of Surgery
    (Orthopaedics)
Cornell University Medical College
Attending, Hand Service
Hospital for Special Surgery
New York, New York
Chief Hand Surgery and Associate Chief
    Orthopaedic Surgery
North Shore University Hospital
Manhasset, New York

Joseph P. Leddy, MD
Clinical Professor
Chief, Section of Hand Surgery
Division of Orthopaedic Surgery
Department of Surgery
UMDNJ - Robert Wood Johnson Medical
    School
New Brunswick, New Jersey

David M. Lichtman, MC
John Dunn Professor of Hand and Upper
    Extremity Surgery
Baylor College of Medicine
Houston, Texas

Terry R. Light, MD
Dr. William M. Scholl Professor & Chairman
Department of Orthopaedic Surgery
Loyola University Chicago Stritch School of
    Medicine
Attending Surgeon
Shriners Hospital
Chicago Unit
Chicago, Illinois

Henry H. Lin, MD
Associated Orthopaedic Specialists P.S.
Spokane, Washington

Ronald L. Linschoid, MD
Professor of Orthopaedic Surgery
Mayo Medical School
Consultant Emeritus
Department of Orthopaedics
Mayo Clinic
Rochester, Minnesota

Graham D. Lister, MD, PhD
Professor of Surgery
Department of Orthopaedic Surgery
University of Utah
Salt Lake City, Utah
Department of Plastic Surgery and Burns
University of LJUBLJANA, Slovenia
Slovenia

Timothy S. Loth, MD
Hand Department
Iowa Medical Clinic P.C.
Cedar Rapids, Iowa

Gary M. Lourie, MD
Assistant Director of Hand Clinic
Scottish Rite Children's Medical Center
Clinical Assistant Professor of Orthopaedics
Emory University School Of Medicine
Atlanta, Georgia

Dean S. Louis, MD
Professor of Surgery
University of Michigan Medical Center
Chief, Orthopaedic Hand Service
University of Michigan Hospitals
Ann Arbor, Michigan

John D. Lubahn, MD
Chairman, Department of Orthopaedics
Hamot Medical Center
Regional Campus Medical College of
    Pennsylvania
Instructor in Orthopaedics
Shriners Hospital for Crippled Children
Instructor in Orthopaedics
Saint Vincent Health Center
Erie, Pennsylvania

Lawrence M. Lubbers, MD
Senior Attending Staff
Riverside Methodist Hospital
Director of the Microsurgery Lab
Clinical Associate Professor
The Ohio State University
Columbus, Ohio

George L. Lucas, MD
Professor & Chairman
Division of Orthopaedic Surgery
University of Kansas-Wichita
Hand Surgeon-The Wichita Clinic
Wichita, Kansas

Ronald J. Mann, MD
Professor Orthopaedic Surgery (Retired)
Hand Surgery, University of Utah Medical
    School
Indialantic, Florida

Paul R. Manske, MD
Fred C. Reynolds Professor Orthopaedic
    Surgery
Washington, University
Director, Hand Clinic,
St. Louis Shriners Hospital
St. Louis, Missouri

Daniel P. Mass, MD
Professor of Clinical Surgery
Section of Orthopaedic Surgery &
    Rehabilitation Medicine
University of Chicago
Chicago, Illinois

Gail F. Mattson-Gates, MD
Clinical Assistant Professor (Plastic Surgery)
University of Southern California
Los Angeles, California

Edward C. McElfresh, MD
Chief Orthopaedics, Minneapolis VAMC
Associate Professor, Dept. of Orthopaedics
University of Minnesota Medical School
Minneapolis, Minnesota

John A. McFadden II, MD
Assistant Professor
Department of Orthopaedic Surgery and
    Division of Plastic Surgery
Medical University of South Carolina
Charleston, South Carolina

Roy A. Meals, MD
Associate Clinical Professor
Department of Orthopaedic Surgery
University of California at Los Angeles
Los Angeles, California

Charles P. Melone, Jr., MD
Clinical Professor, Orthopaedic Surgery
Director Orthopaedic Hand Surgery
New York University Medical Center
New York, New York

Lewis H. Millender, MD
Clinical Professor Orthopaedic Surgery
Tufts Medical School
Director Occupational Medicine Program
New England Baptist Hospital
Boston, Massachusetts

Moheb S. Moneim, MD
Professor & Chairman, Department of
    Orthopaedics & Rehabilitation
Chief, Div. of Hand Surgery, Dept. of
    Orthopaedics & Rehabilitation
University of New Mexico Health Sciences
    Center
Albuquerque, New Mexico

Owen J. Moy, MD
Assistant Professor of Orthopaedic Surgery
State University of New York at Buffalo
School of Biomedical Sciences
Hand Center of Western New York
Millard Fillmore Hospitals
Buffalo, New York

Edward A. Nalebuff, MD
Clinical Professor of Orthopaedic Surgery
Tufts University School of Medicine
Chief of Hand Surgery
New England Baptist Hospital
Boston, Massachusetts

David L. Nelson, MD
Practice of Hand Surgery
Greenbrae, California

Mary Lynn Newport, MD
Assistant Professor, Department of
    Orthopaedic Surgery
University of Connecticut Health Center
Farmington, Connecticut
Chief Hand Clinic
Hartford Hospital
Hartford, Connecticut

Nina Njus, MD,
Clinical Instructor
Northeast Ohio Univ. College of Medicine
Rootstown, Ohio

George E. Omer, Jr., MD
Professor and Chairman Emeritus
Department of Orthopaedics and
    Rehabilitation
University of New Mexico
Albuquerque, New Mexico

Lewis H. Oster, Jr., MD
Hand Surgery Associate
Denver, Colorado

Professor Leif T. Ostrup
Professor of Plastic Surgery
University Hospital
Linkoping, SWEDEN

Andrew K. Palmer, MD
Director of Hand Surgery
Professor of Orthopaedic Surgery
SUNY Health Science Center at Syracuse
Syracuse, New York

Bruce G. Peat, MD
Consultant Plastic and Hand Surgeon
Middlemore Hospital
Auckland, New Zealand

Martin A. Posner, MD
Associate Clinical Professor of Orthopaedics
Mt. Sinai School of Medicine
Chief of Hand Services
Hospital for Joint Diseases
Lenox Hill Hospital
Director Emanuel B. Kaplan Fellowship in
    Hand Surgery
Hospital for Joint Diseases
New York, New York

Matthew D. Putnam, MD
Assistant Professor of Orthopaedics
Department of Orthopaedics
University of Minnesota
Minneapolis, Minnesota

Michael E. Rettig, MD
Clinical Instructor
Department of Orthopaedic Surgery
New York University Medical Center
New York, New York

Rod J. Rohrich, MD
Professor and Chairman, Division of Plastic
    Surgery
University of Texas Southwestern Medical
    Center
Crystal Charity Ball Distinguished Chair in
    Plastic Surgury
Chairman, Parkland Memorial Hospital (For
    Plastic Surgery)
Chairman, Veterans Affairs Medical Center
    (For Plastic Surgery)
Chairman, Zale Lipshy University Hospital
    (For Plastic Surgery)
Chairman, Children's Medical Center (For
    Plastic Surgery)
Dallas, Texas

Mitchell B. Rotman, MD
Assistant Professor
Department of Orthopaedic Surgery
Hand and Microvascular Surgery
St. Louis University Health Science Center
St. Louis, Missouri

Richard A. Ruffin, MD
Orthopaedic Association
Hand Surgery Division
Oklahoma City, Oklahoma

Robert C. Russell, MD
Professor of Surgery and Director of the
    Microsurgery Research Unit
Hospital Affiliations:
Memorial Medical Center
St. John's Hospital
Chairman, Department of Plastic Surgery
Southern Illinois University School of Medicine
Springfield, Illinois

Miguel J. Saldana, MD
Assistant Professor Surgery
USUHS
Bethesda, Maryland

Robert R. Schenck, MD
Director, Section of Hand Surgery
Associate Professor
Department of Plastic and Orthopaedic
    Surgery
Rush-Presbyterian-St. Luke's Medical Center
Chicago, Illinois

William H. Seitz, Jr., MD
Head of Hand and Upper Extremity Surgery
  Clinics
The Mt. Sinai Medical Center
Assistant Clinical Professor of Orthopaedic
  Surgery
Case Western Reserve University School of
  Medicine
Cleveland, Ohio

Walter Short, MD
Assistant Professor of Orthopaedic Surgery
State University of New York Health Science
  Center
Syracuse, New York

Barry P. Simmons, MD
Associate Professor of Orthopaedic Surgery
Harvard Medical School
Chief, Hand & Upper Extremity Service
Brigham & Women's Hospital
Boston, Massachusetts

David J. Smith, Jr., MD
Professor of Surgery
Associate Chairman, Department of Surgery
Section Head of Plastic and Reconstructive
  Surgery
University of Michigan Medical Center
Ann Arbor, Michigan

Brett J. Snyder, MD
Chief Resident, Division of Plastic and
  Reconstructive Surgery
Stanford University Hospital
Stanford, California

Osamu Soejima, MD
Assistant Professor and Chief, Hand Surgery
  Service
Department of Orthopaedic Surgery
Fukuoka University School of Medicine
Fukuoka, JAPAN

Peter J. Stern, MD
Norman S. & Elizabeth C.A. Hill Professor and
  Chairman
University of Cincinnati College of Medicine
Department of Orthopaedic Surgery
Cincinnati, Ohio

Curtis M. Steyers, MD
Professor, Department of Orthopaedic Surgery
Division of Hand and Microsurgery
University of Iowa
Iowa City, Iowa

Edward A. Stokel, MD
Private Practice of Hand Surgery
John Muir Medical Center
Walnut Creek, California

William M. Swartz, MD
Associate Clinical Professor
University of Pittsburgh
Pittsburgh, Pennsylvania

Robert M. Szabo, MD
Professor of Orthopaedics and Surgery
University of California Davis School of
  Medicine
Chief of Hand and Microvascular Surgery
Department of Orthopaedics
Sacramento, California

Julio Taleisnik, MD
Clinical Professor of Surgery (Orthopaedic)
University of California, Irvine
Orange, California

Andrew L. Terrono, MD
Assistant Clinical Professor
Department of Orthopaedics
Tuft University
New England Baptist Hospital
Boston, Massachusetts

Lacy E. Thornburg, MD
St. Vincent Hand Fellow
The Indiana Hand Center
Indianapolis, Indiana

Jeffrey J. Tiedeman, MD
Clinical Instructor
University of Nebraska Medical Center
Department of Orthopaedics
Omaha, Nebraska

Matthew M. Tomaino, MD
Assistant Professor
Department of Orthopaedic Surgery
Chief, Microvascular Surgery
Division of Hand and Upper Extremity
  Surgery
University of Pittsburgh
Pittsburgh, Pennsylvania

Thomas Earl Trumble, MD
Associate Professor
Chief of Hand and Microvascular Surgery
Department of Orthopaedics
University of Washington
Seattle, Washington

Richard L. Uhl, MD
Associate Professor of Surgery
Chief, Section of Hand Surgery
Division of Orthopaedics
Albany Medical College
Albany, New York

James W. Vahey, MD
Private Practice
Orthopaedic Specialists of Nevada
Las Vegas, NV

Stanley M. Valnicek, MD
Assistant Clinical Professor of Plastic Surgery
University of Saskatchewan
Saskatoon, Saskatchewan, CANADA

Steven F. Viegas, MD
Professor of Orthopaedic Surgery & Anatomy
   and Neurosciences
Chief, Division of Hand Surgery
Department of Orthopaedic Surgery &
   Rehabilitation Services
The University of Texas Medical Branch
Galveston, Texas

H. Kirk Watson, MD
Director, Connecticut Combined Hand Surgery
   Fellowship
Hartford, Connecticut
Chief, Hand Surgery, Newington Children's
   Hospital
Newington, Connecticut
Clinical Professor, University of Connecticut
Farmington, Connecticut
Associate Professor, University of
   Massachusetts
Worchester, Massachusetts
Assistant Clinical Professor, Yale New Haven
   Medical School
New Haven, Connecticut

Marwan A. Wehbe, MD
Medical Director, Pennsylvania Hand Center
Bryn Mawr, Pennsylvania
Clinical Associate Professor of Orthopaedic
   Surgery
Thomas Jefferson University
Philadelphia, Pennsylvania
Attending Orthopedist and Hand Surgeon
Bryn Mawr Hospital
Bryn Mawr, Pennsylvania

Arnold-Peter C. Weiss, MD
Associate Professor
Division of Hand, Upper Extremity &
   Microvascular Surgery
Department of Orthopaedics
Brown University School of Medicine
Rhode Island Hospital
Providence, Rhode Island

Dale R. Wheeler, MD
Clinical Assistant Professor
Department of Orthopaedics
Division of Hand Surgery
School of Medicine & Biomedical Science
State University of New York at Buffalo
Buffalo, New York

E.F. Shaw Wilgis, MD
Associate Professor of Plastic & Orthopaedic
   Surgery
The Johns Hopkins Hospitals
Chief, Division of Hand Surgery
Director of the Raymond Curtis Hand Center
Union Memorial Hospital
Baltimore, Maryland

Thomas W. Wolff, MD
Assistant Clinical Professor of Orthopaedic
   Surgery
University of Louisville School of Medicine
Louisville, Kentucky

Phillip E. Wright, MD
Chief, Hand Surgery
Regional Medical Center at Memphis
Director Hand Surgery Fellowship
Campbell Clinic
University of Tennessee
Associate Professor, Orthopaedic Surgery
Campbell Clinic, University of Tennesse
Germantown, Tennessee

Norman P. Zemel, MD
Clinical Associate Professor
Department of Orthopaedics
University of Southern California School of
   Medicine,
Los Angeles, California
Associate, Kerlan-Jobe Clinic
Inglewood, California

Richard Zienowicz, MD
Assistant Professor of Plastic Surgery
Brown University
Chief of Plastic Surgery
Providence VA Medical Center
Attending Surgeon
Rhode Island Hospital
Providence, Rhode Island

CONTENTS

SECTION ONE: TRAUMA

Part II: Ligament Reconstruction

Part III: Tendon Reconstruction

Part IV: Tendon Transfers in Rheumatoid Arthritis

Trauma

PART

I

*Skin Coverage and
Nail Repair*

1

ALBERT E. CRAM

Split-Thickness Skin Grafts

Soft tissue defects fall into two basic categories when considering strategies for closure: those that can be closed primarily and those that cannot. Wounds of the hand that cannot be closed primarily because of their size and location may be closed by a variety of techniques, including closure by split-thickness skin graft. The concept of transplanting partial-thickness skin seems so simple; Reverdin[8] first described the technique in France, and Pollock[6] popularized it in England in the latter part of the nineteenth century.[8,6] The technical skills required to apply this modality successfully can be acquired easily using the gas and electric dermatomes available in the modern operating suite. Success with this technique of wound closure generally depends more on judgment, case selection, and adherence to basic principles than on development of particular operative skills.

Split-thickness skin grafts involve the transfer of the epithelium and a portion of the dermis from a chosen donor site to an open wound bed. These tissue transfers most commonly are autogenous in nature, but also could be either allograft or Xenograft if only temporary closure is needed. Thickness of the graft may vary and can usually be chosen and controlled by the surgeon. Unfortunately, even the thickest split-thickness graft cannot approach the durability of normal palmar skin, and when placed on the palmar surface, such grafts never achieve the stability of the glabrous skin in relation to the underlying bony structure.

Graft thickness has a significant effect on the amount of contraction that the graft undergoes after graft take. Thin grafts produce more rapid healing and generally less disfigurement at the donor site than do thick split-thickness grafts. The thinner the graft in relation to total skin thickness at the donor site, the greater the degree of contraction on the wound bed.[7] Graft contraction is never desirable but is especially devastating when it occurs across flexor surfaces such as the palmar surface of the fingers.[7] Such contraction across joints will result in clinically significant contracture with loss of hand function. Splinting and very aggressive hand physical therapy can ameliorate contractures to some degree, but thin grafts in palmar surface applications will produce mediocre results at best.

All donor sites are at risk for development of hypertrophic scars, and even thin grafts usually will result in permanent color change at the donor site. Skin accessories such as hair follicles and glandular elements are seldom included in the graft due to their superficial depth, and when present as in thicker grafts, may not survive. This skin lacks the elastin fibers seen in normal skin and tends to be dry and prone to injury. Fresh skin graft must be protected from excess sunlight and from any significant trauma until it reaches maturity approximately 6 to 18 months after transfer.

A number of factors will exert some effect on skin graft take. There must be adequate blood supply in the recipient site. Split-thickness skin will survive on periosteum but will not survive over bone denuded of periosteum. Where only small sections of denuded bone are present, split-thickness skin may survive if there is good blood supply to the graft on each side of the defect and the distance to be bridged is small. Paratenon also will support a skin graft, while tendon stripped of its paratenon will not. Wherever there is significant denuded bone or tendon, split-thickness skin graft will not provide good coverage and other techniques should be chosen.

Infection at the recipient site usually will prevent graft survival. Robson and Krizek have shown that the presence of 10^5 bacteria per gram of tissue is associated with a high incidence of graft failure.[9] Wounds may appear quite clean clinically and still carry bacterial counts at this level and higher. Some organisms such as the Streptococcal species that have very potent fibrinolytic activity may produce graft failures at levels below a 10^5 concentration.

The thickness of the skin graft in relation to the total skin thickness available at the donor site also will affect the development of scar at the donor site.[1] Even very thin grafts usually produce some permanent visible change in the donor site skin. Donor sites usually follow a course of excessive erythematous coloration early after harvest with gradual fading to a hue lighter than surrounding normal skin. Deep split-thickness donor sites often will remain in the erythematous phase for a number of months and may show significant scar hypertrophy. These wounds may become infected, and in cases where infection is severe may convert to full-thickness skin loss, ultimately requiring split-thickness skin graft closure themselves. If placed across joints, these donor site complications could lead to contracture, so care in the planning of donor sites is an obvious priority.

■ INDICATIONS AND CONTRAINDICATIONS

Wound closure in the hand should follow the same basic principles that are applied to all wound closure. The wound must be analyzed for extent of injury with special attention to possible damage to the critical deep structures. The method of wound closure chosen will depend on whether there is too much tissue missing to allow safe primary closure. Heavy contamination, significant undermining with vascular compromise, or avulsion of significant amounts of skin and subcutaneous tissue often produce a wound that can only be closed by a distant pedicle flap (such as the groin flap), a free flap, or by a split-thickness skin graft (Figs. 1-1 and 1-2). Where possible, missing tissue should be replaced by like tissue. Split-thickness skin graft can only replace the missing dermis and epidermis, but often this will be adequate to restore hand function.

Wound closure by use of split-thickness skin graft in isolated hand injuries offers the advantage of easily accessible donor sites. Where the hand injury is part of a massive body surface area burn, donor site availability may be limited, but the hands would be very high on the priority list for coverage in this circumstance. The skin is easy to apply to the wound, and postoperative management is straightforward.

■ FIGURE 1–1
The patient (a 19-year-old man) had his hand caught in a heated press. The dorsal skin was crushed and burned.

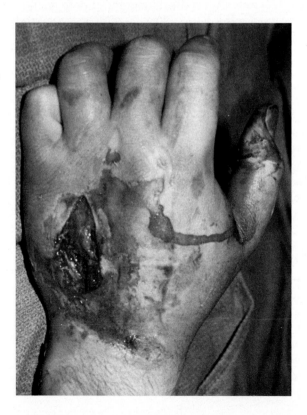

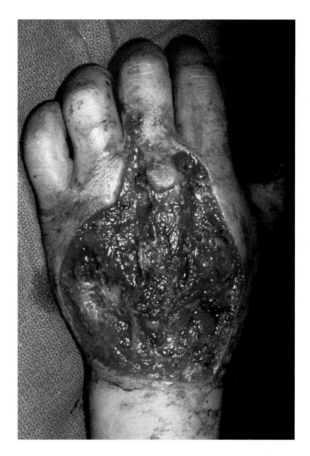

After debridement and the formation of granulation tissue, the bed is ready to receive a split-thickness skin graft.

Split-thickness grafts usually can provide adequate coverage and reasonably good function for dorsal hand injuries. On the fingers, split-thickness skin grafts are used to fill the defect left at the donor site of cross finger flaps. Split-thickness grafts also are used to cover large donor defects used for hand reconstruction such as the radial forearm free flap.

The major contraindication to the use of split-thickness skin graft for wound closure is the lack of an adequate recipient bed. This condition exists primarily when the wound bed has large areas of exposed bone or tendon without periosteum or peritenon. Massive contamination is a relative contraindication to autograft closure, but often the wound can be adequately prepared by debridement and pressure lavage techniques. At times, temporary coverage with Xenograft is appropriate in such circumstances.[2] Relative contraindications to the use of split-thickness skin graft in closure of hand wounds include the need for more durable coverage where other closure techniques would produce a better long-term functional result. There are situations in palmar injury, such as burns or deep abrasion injuries, in which split-thickness skin graft provides the best coverage; when such wounds are small, a local flap often will provide more durable coverage.

Anesthesia must be provided at both the recipient site and the donor site. Where these sites are anatomically adjacent (e.g., when the forearm is used as a donor site), a regional technique such as an axillary block will meet the patient's needs. If the donor site is distant, such as the hip, then it often is simpler to provide a general anesthetic. It is possible to provide a local anesthetic field block at the donor site, but I recommend this only for small donor sites.

Donor Site Preparation   When a graft is being harvested from the forearm of the injured hand, the usual surgical preparation encompasses the donor site. A wet shave of the

■ SURGICAL TECHNIQUES

proposed donor site just before surgical preparation is necessary if there is a large amount of hair at the donor site. If the donor site is distant from the recipient bed, then the patient must be positioned to provide access to the chosen site and the donor field, and should be prepared and draped at the same time as the hand. Any effective antibacterial preparation solution is satisfactory. After the wound is prepared and draped, it can be covered with a sterile towel until it is time to harvest the graft. If an iodine-based preparation solution is used, I recommend washing away the solution with normal saline just before graft harvest.

Graft Harvest   The method chosen for split-thickness skin graft harvest will vary with the needs of the recipient site and the equipment available to the surgeon. A variety of free hand dermatomes are available and can serve quite well where a small graft is all that is required.[4] These knives can deliver good quality skin in the hands of an experienced surgeon and many, such as the Goullian dermatome (Fig. 1–3), have guards that limit the depth of cut, making them safer for those with less experience.[4] The guard device can be damaged if not handled properly, so one must always check the guard to blade depth visually before using the device. The larger freehand blades such as the Watkins knife (Fig. 1–3) are capable of taking much larger grafts but safe use requires supervised experience and much practice to get high-quality skin and produce a satisfactory appearance at the donor site.

Drum dermatomes, such as the Reese dermatome, generally are the most reliable at producing consistent and accurate donor skin thickness.[10] Their use requires skill that can only be acquired with practice, and in inexperienced hands the device can be dangerous to the surgeon and to the patient. Operating room personnel who set up this equipment also must be quite familiar with the procedures required.[10] In general, the newer gas- and electric-powered dermatomes have replaced the freehand and drum dermatomes.

Electric- and gas pressure-driven dermatomes are reliable, and their use is easily taught. These devices (Fig. 1–4) can be set for a variety of depths and widths and if properly set up can provide very high-quality split-thickness skin graft. Most of these devices are limited to approximately 4 inches of maximum width, but this should suffice for the majority of hand grafts. Depth usually can be varied between 0.002 inch to approximately 0.030 inch. This versatility is useful, but the accuracy of some models may deteriorate because of repeated handling or because of wear of parts as the device ages.

Having chosen the nitrogen-powered dermatome, the depth must be set. In most cases

■ FIGURE 1–3
A hand-held Goullian dermatome (the small upper handle) has a guard to limit the depth of the harvested graft. The larger Watson knife is useful for larger graft harvest but requires experience.

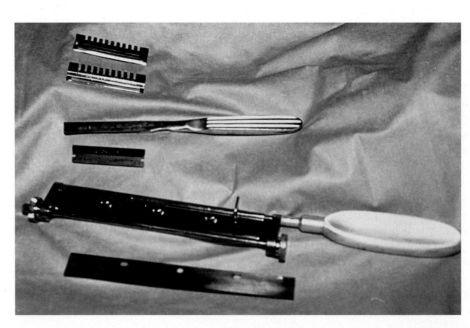

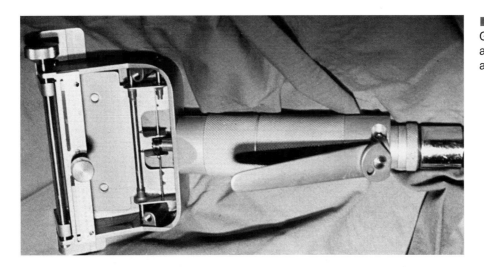

Gas-driven dermatomes are adjustable and reliable.

where we are applying graft to the dorsum of the hand, a depth of 0.012-inch is advised. Grafts for the palm can be thicker, but this increases the risk of hypertrophic scar at the donor site. I then rinse the donor site with a saline-soaked lap pad to remove any residual antiseptic. Some might advise the application of mineral oil to the surface of the donor site at this point but I find that I can take excellent grafts using only the saline-soaked lap pad just before the dermatome pass.

The dermatome is applied firmly to the donor site and traction applied proximally and distally by the surgeon and the assistant. The surgeon will generally do best if the dermatome is in the dominant hand and traction is applied at the distal end of the dermatome pass while the assistant applies traction at the proximal end.

Graft harvest usually is carried out after the recipient site has been prepared by debridement. This allows an accurate assessment of the required amount of donor skin. It is recommended that the graft harvest team change to fresh gloves to avoid bringing contamination from the wound to the harvest site. The harvested skin can either be taken directly to the recipient site and applied or it may be stored on saline-moistened sponges until the recipient site is ready for graft application. A final recipient bed inspection to ensure hemostasis is indicated because an expanding hematoma beneath the graft can lead to graft loss.

Split-thickness graft may be applied as sheet graft or as an expanded graft. Donor site availability and the ordinarily small surface area requirements in hand surgery seldom create an absolute need for expansion of the donor skin. Nevertheless, use of "pie crusted" skin graft has become almost routine. After harvest, donor skin may be passed through a Tanner mesh device (Fig. 1–5) or similar commercially available skin expanders to lacerate the skin at close intervals.[11] A 1 to 1.5 mesh pattern is most commonly used. This skin can then be applied in an expanded or unexpanded mode depending on the surface area needs at the recipient site. The interstices created by the meshing device allow the escape of blood or serum from the interface between the recipient bed and the graft during the first few hours after the dressings have been applied.[11] The potential improvement in graft take must be balanced against the diamond-shaped scar pattern that is inherent to the healing of mesh grafted skin. Where cosmesis is of paramount concern to the patient, the use of unmeshed skin is recommended. Where graft take and function are the primary concern, I invariably use skin meshed at a 1 to 1.5 ratio. Larger mesh ratios are available, but their use is not recommended in the hand.

Graft Immobilization   Grafts placed on an adequate recipient bed must be fixed in place on the bed if they are to become vascularized. Any technique that prevents movement between the graft and its recipient bed will succeed. In the hand, all techniques should include immobilization of the hand, preferably in a position of function for at least 96

■ FIGURE 1–5
A meshing device may
be used to expand the
skin to facilitate wound
coverage and drainage.

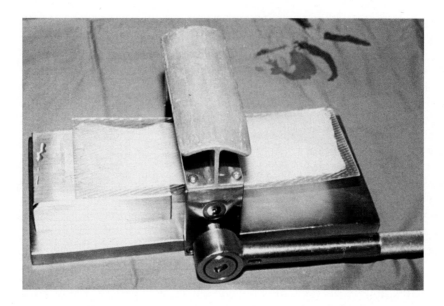

hours. The graft must be held to the bed by staples, sutures, dressings, or a combination of these. At the intact skin margins of small grafts, I often place a series of 4-0 silk sutures around the periphery and tie the long end of these sutures over a cotton ball bolus dressing. This stint dressing technique can be used on wounds as large as the entire dorsum of the hand. The pressure provided by the stint helps to promote hemostasis. The only disadvantage of this method of fixation is the inability to visualize the graft until the stint is removed. I remove the stints on the fifth postoperative day.

An alternative method of graft fixation is to apply a nylon net dressing over the graft after placing staples or chromic sutures at the periphery. The nylon net can be sutured peripheral to the graft in a manner that applies gentle pressure to the grafted area, unless the graft is on a concave surface such as the palm. When using this technique, it is possible to remove dressings placed over the nylon net to inspect the graft at any point in time during the postoperative period. I usually reserve this technique for larger grafts and prefer the stint dressing technique described above for grafts smaller than 4 cm in diameter. I use the stint technique almost exclusively in those rare occasions when split-thickness grafts are required in the palm.

Before placement of the cotton balls or other stint material, the wound is covered with an occlusive dressing. I prefer Xeroform gauze, but Vaseline gauze would work as well. I use the same dressing over the nylon net followed by a bulky dressing when not using the stint technique. Elastic bandages are applied as the final layer, and the recipient site is elevated above heart level for the first 96 hours.

Donor Site Management The skin graft donor site represents the equivalent of a partial-thickness burn injury. The patient often will identify the donor site as his or her most painful wound. Donor site healing will take place by epithelial migration from the hair follicles and glandular structures in the donor site. Wounds taken at 0.012 to 0.015 inch thickness will normally be re-epithelialized in 7 to 10 days. I prefer the use of Xeroform gauze applied to the donor site at the time of harvest. A layer of nonstick dressing such as Telfa is applied over the Xeroform, followed by a bulky dressing and Curlix wrap held in place with an elastic bandage. Forty-eight hours postoperatively, the dressing may be removed down to the Xeroform gauze, which is left in place. The dressing will then separate spontaneously as the donor site re-epithelializes. As an alternative, the donor site may be dressed with a totally occlusive dressing such as Op Site. This may improve patient comfort but in my experience the Xeroform technique is less prone to complications. If the donor site becomes infected, it can convert to a full-thickness wound. If the wound develops any signs of infection during the postoperative period, topical antimicrobial treatment should begin at once.

Split-thickness skin graft is initially held to the wound bed by some form of dressing. Within hours of the operation, a fibrin "glue" is in place and will hold the split-thickness skin graft to the bed.[3] This tenuous biologic bond is not strong enough to withstand any significant shearing forces, so in the early postoperative period the patient is dependent on the mechanical forces exerted by the dressing that is placed over the graft. Lack of attention to this critical dressing is a common cause of graft loss. Between 72 and 96 hours, if the graft position relative to the wound bed has been maintained and if the blood supply was adequate and the bacterial counts were low, there should be true graft take with the development of circulation and enough collagen formation to allow safe dressing removal.

The presence of expanding hematoma or seroma accumulation in the very early postoperative period can result in hydraulic separation of the graft from the wound bed and may prevent graft survival.[5] The need for hemostasis in the recipient bed is obvious, and some combination of pressure over the graft or a mechanism for fluid egress helps to prevent graft loss. The use of expanded skin or application of a "pie crusting" technique along with rigorously applied dressings usually succeeds in preventing graft loss from hematomas. Dressings may be of many types, from nylon net to a tie over stint dressing, but the important principle is the prevention of motion at the graft–recipient bed interface until biologic graft adherence has been achieved.

Situations may arise that would make temporary closure of the wound desirable. Where the degree of contamination is significant or the delay between injury and treatment or the quality of the wound bed makes immediate flap closure appear risky, a temporary wound closure with Xenograft may be a wise choice. Porcine Xenograft is available commercially and has a long shelf life. A questionable wound can be closed with the Xenograft and this biologic dressing changed at 1- to 5-day intervals until the graft exhibits adherence to the wound bed.[2] Porcine graft will not survive but adherence due to the fibrin glue between the Xenograft and wound bed usually indicates a blood supply and bacterial balance that would support permanent closure. When quantitative culture techniques are not available, this technique provides good clinical evidence that the wound has less than 10^5 bacteria per gram of tissue. Human allograft skin often was used for this same indication in the past, but the possible transmission of HIV and other viral agents has significantly inhibited the use of cadaver skin in non–life-threatening situations. Techniques involving the transfer of thin sheets of cultured epithelium have little practical value in hand surgery.

■ TECHNICAL ALTERNATIVES

Dressing removal at the fifth postoperative day should be viewed as a part of the operative procedure and approached with the same attention to detail. Both the physician and the patient should be positioned for comfort during the procedure. In the case of children, it may be necessary to provide pharmacologic sedation if parental presence and reassurance fail to produce adequate cooperation. The bond between the graft and its host bed may be incomplete in some areas and will be tenuous throughout. Often the cotton balls of a stint must be soaked thoroughly with saline and allowed to loosen over time before an attempt is made to pull them free. It is preferable to pull at a 180° angle rather than perpendicular to the graft surface if the bottom layer of gauze is still adherent to the graft. A careful and patient approach usually will minimize graft trauma and allow safe dressing removal. In the majority of cases, the wounds may be left open after dressing removal on the fifth postoperative day. If there has been some graft loss, it may be necessary to provide for Xeroform or other dressing changes depending on the physician preference for dressing materials on open wounds.

Rehabilitation should begin as soon as it is apparent that graft survival has occurred. Usually an active range of motion program can begin on the fifth postoperative day, if the skin graft is the only consideration. If there are grafts across joints and contracture could be a problem, the patient may require splinting in the position of function when

■ REHABILITATION

■ FIGURE 1–6
The use of an unmeshed graft on the hand of the same 19-year-old man provided quality coverage that is aesthetically pleasing.

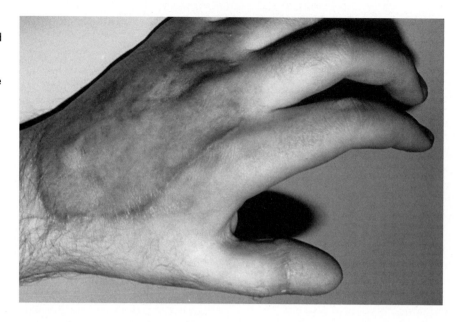

not actively engaged in range of motion activities. Patients with burned hands often require splints at night for several months after skin grafting. Therapists need to exercise some caution in manipulating immature grafts during passive range of motion activities.

■ OUTCOMES

Split-thickness skin graft can provide coverage in cases of soft tissue deficit in hand injuries (Fig. 1–6). The technique is useful for both temporary and permanent coverage where primary closure is not possible and more durable closure such as flaps of various types are not possible. Where the wound bed has an adequate blood supply and the bacterial count is less than 10^5, split-thickness skin graft can almost always provide wound closure. The primary technical requirements are adequate debridement of the wound and hemostasis. The graft–wound bed interface must be immobile for the first 96 hours. Prevention of contractures is the primary postoperative concern, and as always rehabilitation is dependent on knowledgeable therapists and a compliant patient.

References

1. Barker DE: Skin thickness in the human. Plast Reconstr Surg, 1951; 7:115–116.
2. Bromberg BE, Song C, Mohn MP: The use of pigskin as a temporary biologic dressing. Plast Reconstr Surg, 1965; 36:80–90.
3. Burleson R, Eiseman B. Nature of the bond between partial-thickness skin and wound granulations. Surgery, 1972; 72:315–322.
4. Goulian D: A new economical dermatome. Plast Reconstr Surg, 1968; 42:85–86.
5. Littlewood AHM: Seroma: An unrecognized cause of failure of split-thickness skin grafts. Br J Plast Surg, 1960; 13:42–46.
6. Pollock GD: Cases of skin grafting and skin transplantation. Trans Clin Soc London, 1871; 4:37–41.
7. Ragnell A: The secondary contracting tendency of free skin grafts. Br J Plast Surg, 1953; 5:6–24.
8. Reverdin JL: Greffe Epidermique. Bull Soc Imp Chir (Paris), 1869; 10:483–511.
9. Robson MC, Krizek TJ: Predicting skin graft survival. J Trauma, 1973; 13:213–217.
10. Rudolph R: Reese Dermatome In: Rudolph R, Fisher JC, Ninnemann JL (eds): Skin Grafting. Boston: Little, Brown and Company, 1979:46–47.
11. Tanner JC, Shea PC Jr., Bradley WH: Two years experience with mesh grafting. Am J Surg, 1966; 111:543–547.

ROBERT R. SCHENCK

2

Full Thickness Skin Grafts to the Hand

The goal of reconstruction for loss of skin coverage in the hand is to provide stable, painless, well-padded coverage with adequate sensory function and acceptable appearance. In 1984, I published the results of hypothenar full-thickness skin grafts for skin coverage in the hand.[10] Split-thickness hypothenar grafts[9] and full-thickness skin grafts from the plantar area of the foot[7,11] and other sources had been previously reported. Although full-thickness hypothenar skin grafts had been used to replace unsatisfactory results of previous grafting,[4] these grafts otherwise had been largely ignored.

In my clinical practice, I had discovered that split-thickness skin grafts were frequently hypersensitive, often did not stand up to the rigors of daily wear and tear on the fingertips, and at times were cosmetically unsuitable. The problem with cosmesis was frequently found in individuals with increased skin pigmentation, in whom the split-thickness grafts from areas other than the palm or sole were applied to the palmar surfaces of the digits or hand. Full-thickness skin grafts from non-palmar/plantar areas were little better. Also, full-thickness skin grafts from the plantar areas resulted in a foot wound that gave problems with ambulation during donor-site healing. The hypothenar area of the hand had none of these disadvantages and thus became a preferred source for grafts to the digits and hand.

Loss of skin from the palmar aspect of the fingers and hand is the prime indication for the use of full-thickness skin grafts, although dorsal defects, particularly of the fingers, can also be effectively managed by this method. Larger defects (greater than 2.5 × 8.0 cm), such as those from avulsion wounds of the dorsum of the hand, may require full-thickness skin grafts from a larger donor area (e.g., the groin area, lateral or cephalad to perineal hair).[2,3] Burn wounds, tangentially excised, may be better served at least initially with split-thickness skin grafts, either solid or meshed.[6] Exposed tendon, nerve, or bone should not be permanently covered by skin grafts alone and require local or distant flap coverage. A relative contraindication for full-thickness skin grafts, at least initially, is severe contamination as from agricultural accidents.

Full-thickness skin grafts can be obtained from the hypothenar area using regional or local anesthesia. A block of the ulnar nerve suffices for both donor and recipient areas when only the small finger is involved. For other fingers or larger areas, a total wrist block or an axillary block is sufficient. Alternatively, local infiltration can be used separately for the hypothenar donor area and a digital block used for the involved finger.

If the fingertip has been amputated, any projecting bone of the distal phalanx is rongeured to a level slightly shorter than that of the surrounding soft tissue. An ellipse is drawn with methylene blue on the hypothenar area of the hand, so that the dorsal limit of the ellipse is placed at the juncture of palmar skin and dorsal skin (Fig. 2–1) A change in the character or color of the skin indicates this dorsal limit. In an adult, the hypothenar area can provide donor skin measuring 2 to 2.5 cm in width and 6 to 8 cm in length. The skin is taken as a full-thickness skin graft, leaving behind as much fat and subcutaneous tissue as possible. The graft may be grasped at each corner with a delicate hemostat, and the inverted skin may then be draped over the surgeon's index finger. Thorough defatting is accomplished with a pair of slightly curved scissors. The defatting must be meticulous

■ HISTORY OF THE TECHNIQUE

■ INDICATIONS AND CONTRAINDICATIONS

■ SURGICAL TECHNIQUES

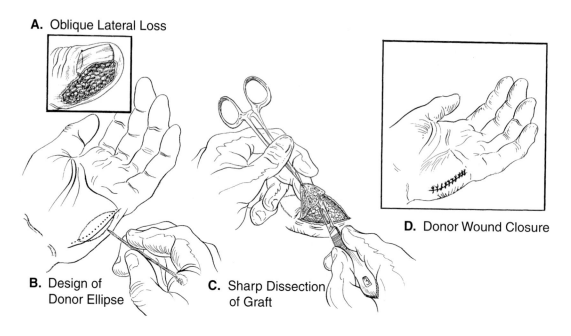

A. Oblique Lateral Loss

B. Design of Donor Ellipse

C. Sharp Dissection of Graft

D. Donor Wound Closure

■ FIGURE 2–1

A, Oblique lateral loss of tissue is one appropriate use for the hypothenar full-thicknesss skin graft. **B**, The longitudinal axis of the donor ellipse closely parallels the midlateral axis of the hand. **C**, The full-thickness skin ellipse is placed on traction and sharply dissected, leaving the graft dermis as free as possible of subcutaneous fat. **D**, The donor wound is closed using 3-0 Nylon sutures. (From Schenck RR: Fingertip Injuries. In: March JL (ed): Current Therapy in Plastic and Reconstructive Surgery: Trunk and Extremities, Philadelphia: B.C. Decker, Inc., 1989. Reproduced by permission of Mosby-Year Book Inc., St. Louis.)

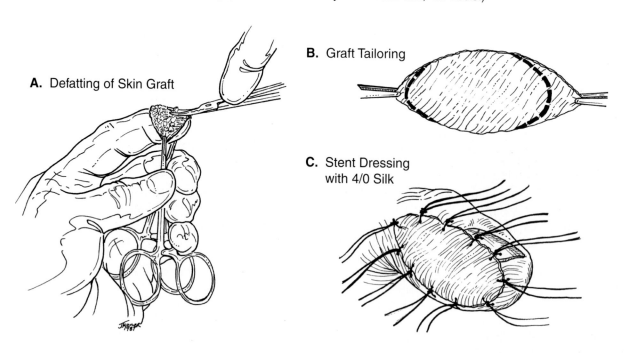

A. Defatting of Skin Graft

B. Graft Tailoring

C. Stent Dressing with 4/0 Silk

■ FIGURE 2–2

A, The inverted skin graft is held by two hemostats draped over a finger and defatted with the use of the convexity of a pair of fine scissors. **B**, The graft is tailored to exactly match the size of skin loss. **C**, The skin graft is secured with 4-0 silk sutures that will be tied over the dressing bolus. (From Schenck RR: Fingertip Injuries. In: March JL (ed): Current Therapy in Plastic and Reconstructive Surgery: Trunk and Extremities, Philadelphia: B.C. Decker, Inc., 1989. Reproduced by permission of Mosby-Year Book, Inc., St. Louis.)

Figure 3.

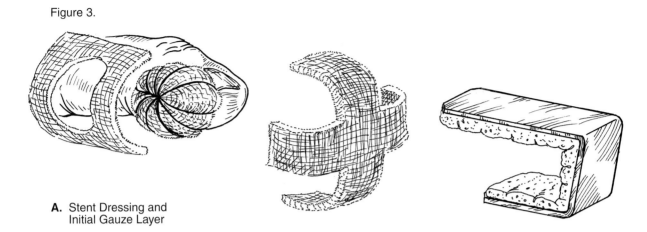

A. Stent Dressing and
Initial Gauze Layer

B. Cruciate Gauze Dressing   **C.** Padded Aluminum Splint

■ FIGURE 2–3
A, The initial gauze layers are cut out to fit around the stent dressing. **B**, A cruciate gauze
dressing covers all sides of the digit. **C**, A foam-padded aluminum splint is secured by 1″ elastic tape. (From Schenck RR: Fingertip Injuries. In: March JL (ed): Current Therapy in Plastic
and Reconstructive Surgery: Trunk and Extremities, Philadelphia: B.C. Decker, Inc., 1989. Reproduced by permission of Mosby-Year Book, Inc., St. Louis.)

to allow later ingrowth of capillaries to ensure viability (or *take*) of the skin graft
(Fig. 2–2).

The graft is tailored to match the area of skin loss and sutured in place with 4-0 silk
sutures. The ends of the silk sutures are left long and are then tied over a stent dressing
(Fig. 2–3). Silk does not slip as easily during the tying process and thus assists in setting
proper tension on the dressing. This tension ensures that the sutures are tied securely
enough to provide complete contact of the dressing on the graft to prevent its movement,
yet not so tightly that the surrounding tissues are distorted or their circulation compromised. The dressing consists of a layer of Xeroflow or Xeroform (Sherwood Medical Indus-
tries, St. Louis, MO) to prevent adherence to the graft, followed by a saline-moistened
gauze that is cut to conform exactly to the shape of the graft, and then one or two more
layers of dry gauze. All of this is secured by the silk sutures when they are tied. This type
of dressing prevents movement of the graft on its bed and helps to prevent hematoma
formation under the graft. Movement of the graft on its bed or separation of the graft
from the bed by fluid reduces graft take.

The donor area is closed, without undermining, with 3-0 nylon sutures, which are left
in place for 3 weeks. This period allows complete healing of the donor site, which is always
closed with some degree of tension.

Further gauze dressings are then applied around the bolus dressing, and the digit (or
entire hand if necessary) is immobilized. The digits are immobilized with an aluminum–foam splint and the hand with a plaster splint secured with dressing material, bias-
cut stockinet, and Elastoplast (Beiersdorf, Inc., Norwalk, CT) tape.

Postoperatively, the grafted area is left undisturbed for 10 to 14 days to allow secure
adherence of the skin graft. The bolus dressing, when properly applied, ensures healing;
inspecting the skin graft margins in the interim provides no additional benefit.

Relatively large areas can be treated in this way, using the hypothenar areas of both
hands, if necessary (Figs. 2-4, 2-5, 2-6, and 2-7). The functional and cosmetic results are
satisfying for both patient and surgeon.

■ FIGURE 2–4
This 37-year-old man lost
significant areas of pal-
mar skin from his thumb
and index fingers in an
industial accident. Local
flaps would have been in-
adequate and distant
flaps too bulky, leaving
skin grafting as the logical alternative.

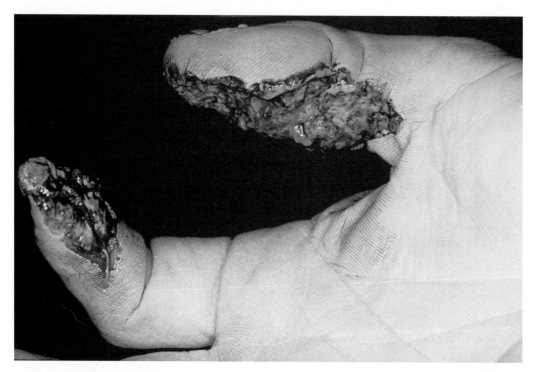

■ FIGURE 2–5
The right hypothenar
area provided donor skin
measuring 6.5 × 2.5 cm
for the right thumb defect
and a smaller area, 2.0
× 2.5 cm, was obtained
from the left hypothenar
area to cover the index
finger.

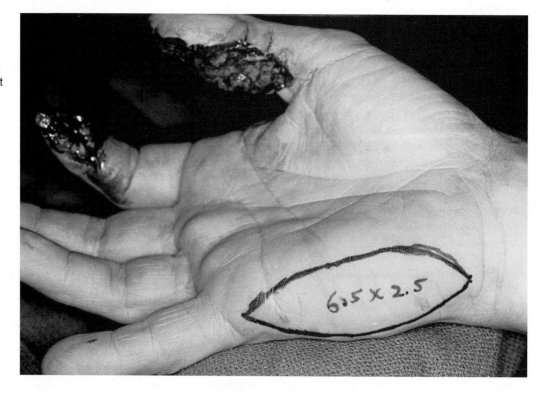

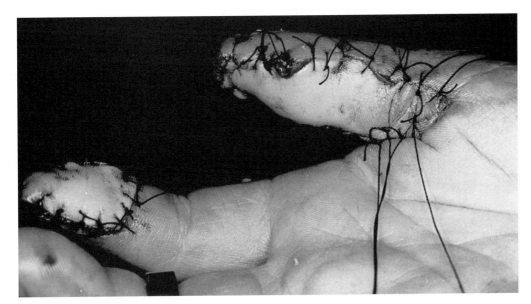

■ FIGURE 2–6
The skin grafts have been placed on the wounds and are secured with 4-0 silk sutures. Vaseline-impregnated gauze is used for the first layer of dressing, followed by moist and then dry layers of gauze cut to conform to the graft dimensions and secured by the tie-over silk sutures.

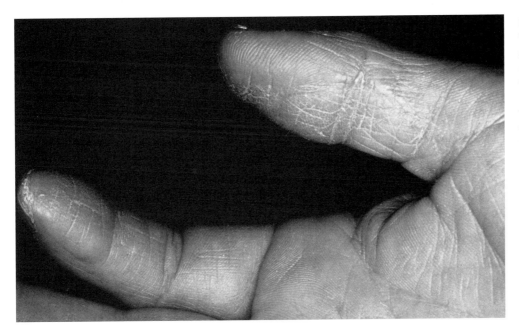

■ FIGURE 2–7
The final result, shown at 8 months, reveals excellent cosmetic and functional results. The thumb had 9 mm and the index finger 7 mm two-point discrimination. Note that even the flexor crease has been restored at the interphalangeal joint area of the thumb.

■ TECHNICAL ALTERNATIVES

The V-Y flap remains an excellent coverage method in situations wherein enough volar skin is left.[1] Palmar skin from the thenar crease area[5] has a disadvantage because it may produce a scar in the center of the palm.

If full-thickness skin is needed in an area larger than can be provided by the use of bilateral hypothenar areas, full-thickness skin can be obtained from the groin areas, lateral or cephalad to the hairy perineal area.

Two common errors are to either incompletely defat the graft or to improperly immobilize the skin graft. Both jeopardize the take of the skin graft. Proper immobilization includes the use of a stent or tie-over dressing, protecting the finger or hand with a splint, and applying a sling to elevate the hand at heart level.

Care should be taken to not remove the donor site sutures too early, which may allow partial dehiscence of the donor area and delayed healing. A common error is to place the donor area on the palmar aspect of the hypothenar eminence rather than on the ulnar border of the palm. This makes closure more difficult and results in a scar that is more visible and potentially sensitive when grasping. When properly placed, the hypothenar full-thickness skin graft donor site is well hidden and asymptomatic. Another error is to take racially pigmented skin from a distant site and place it on the palmar aspect of the fingers or hand; the resulting cosmesis is unacceptable. The hypothenar skin matches the adjacent area of the recipient wound so well that it may later be difficult to discern the exact margins of the graft.

■ REHABILITATION

After the initial dressing removal in 10 to 14 days, the graft may need to be lightly redressed and protected for a week. Graft take is manifest by normal coloration of the skin and lack of serous drainage, either around the margins of the graft or between the dermis and epidermis. If the graft take is secure, therapy may be begun immediately. The correct time to begin therapy is a clinical decision made for each individual patient. Only rarely is a desensitization program of the grafted area needed. No specific therapy is needed for the donor area after suture removal at 21 days.

■ OUTCOMES

The skin of the palm differs from the hair-bearing skin of the rest of the body in several ways. Palmar skin has a thick epidermis, with a particularly thick layer of keratin on its outer surface. Pigment cells containing melanin are few, and sebaceous glands are absent. In addition, connective tissue is more compact and therefore less elastic. These characteristics allow greater resistance to pressure, friction, and trauma.

Replacement of this specialized skin with full-thickness skin from the hypothenar area provides skin that has these qualities and appearance. Napier[8] emphasized that the quality of return of sensibility in the grafted area is related to the nature of the grafted skin because the pattern of the nerve plexus just below the basal layer of the epidermis is responsible for the extent and quality of its re-innervation.

In the group that I reported in 1984[10] of 25 cases of hyothenar full-thickness skin grafts to the fingertips, 86% achieved excellent or good two-point discrimination, a result probably partly due to the quality of the grafted skin. All patients could differentiate between coarse and smooth surfaces with their reconstructed digits. After 1 year, none complained of hypersensitivity to touch. Twenty-three digits had an excellent cosmetic result, three digits were rated acceptable, and none were poor.

The full-thickness skin graft is an excellent method of reconstruction for loss of skin of the hand. The hypothenar area is an easily accessible donor area and provides skin that closely matches the original skin's cosmesis and function.

References

1. Atasoy E, Iokimidis E, Kasdan MI, Kutz JE, Kleinert HE: Reconstruction of the amputated fingertip with a triangular volar flap. J Bone Joint Surg (Am), 1970; 52:921–926.
2. Evans DM: The Management of the Skin in Injuries of the Hand. In: Lamb DW, Hooper G, Kuczynski K (eds): The Practice of Hand Surgery, 2nd Ed, Oxford: Blackwell Scientific Publications, 1989:121–147.
3. Hurwitz DJ, White WL: Application of glove design in resurfacing the dorsum of the hand. Plast Reconstr Surg, 1978; 62:385–389.
4. Lie MK, Margargle RK, Posch JL: Free full-thickness skin graft from the palm to cover defects of the fingers. J Bone Joint Surg (Am), 1970; 52:559–561.
5. Mack GR, Nevaiser RJ, Wilson JN: Free palmar skin grafts for resurfacing digital defects. J Hand Surg, 1981; 6:565–567.
6. MacMillan BG: The use of mesh grafting in treating burns. Surg Clin North Am, 1970; 50: 1347–1359.
7. Micks JE, Wilson JN: Full-thickness sole-skin grafts for resurfacing the hand. J Bone Joint Surg (Am), 1967; 49:1128–1134.
8. Napier JR: The return of pain sensibility in full-thickness skin grafts. Brain, 1952; 75:147–166.
9. Patton HS: Split skin graft from hypothenar area for fingertip avulsions. Plast Reconstr Surg, 1969; 43:426–429.
10. Schenck RR, Cheema TA: Hypothenar skin grafts for fingertip reconstruction. J Hand Surg, 1984; 9A:750–753.
11. Webster JP: Skin graft for hairless areas of hands and feet. Plast Reconstr Surg, 1955; 15: 83–101.

3

V-Y Closure Fingertip Injuries

The goals of surgical management of the fingertip injury are to provide the following: nearly normal sensibility, a nontender fingertip, maximum length, appropriate nail appearance and support, normal joint movement, and the best cosmesis possible. V-Y advancement flaps can achieve these goals. The two basic types of V-Y advancement flaps used for fingertip injuries are the lateral flap and the volar flap. The lateral flap was introduced by Kutler[9] in 1944 and the technique was revised by Fisher[3] in 1967. The volar flap was first described by Tranquilli-Leali[12] in 1935 and was made popular by Atasoy and coworkers[1] in 1970. Variations on these have followed.[7,11] Before the introduction of these V-Y flaps, fingertip injuries were allowed to heal by secondary intention or were closed by volar flap advancement over a shortened phalanx, by skin grafts, or by pedicle flaps. Kutler[9] cited the advantages of his technique over the older methods. His procedure obviated the necessity of shortening the finger by ¾ to 1 inch to allow closure. He considered his technique to be less complex than skin grafts and the previously described pedicle flaps. Also, he believed his technique provided a nontender smooth fingertip, rather than the sensitive irregular one that followed granulation and closure by secondary intention. Atasoy and coworkers[1] considered their technique to provide even better sensation than that of Kutler.

■ HISTORY OF THE TECHNIQUE

The choice of technique for repairing fingertip amputations or avulsions should be determined by the type of injury, the anticipated functional result of the closure used, the potential complications, and the complexity of the procedure. Healing of the small wound (less than 1 cm) by secondary intention (contraction and epithelization) provides excellent results, with nearly normal sensation, minimal scarring and tenderness, and excellent function. Cold sensitivity usually occurs but this appears to be related to the injury itself. Skin grafts are simpler to perform than flaps but do not provide appropriate sensory organs (e.g., Meissner's corpuscles) to ensure good sensory return. Moreover, skin grafts can not be used to cover exposed bone. The V-Y flap can close the traumatic wound with tissue similar in type to that destroyed or amputated. Exposed bone is covered with a flap that provides padding and that should reduce tip tenderness and provide nail support. Because the V-Y flap has normal to nearly normal sensation, it is of particular value in covering wounds that involve contact areas.

■ INDICATIONS AND CONTRAINDICATIONS

The technique of V-Y closure has as its principle the mobilization of a vascularized and sensate flap of skin and subcutaneous tissue. The flap is released from its fibrous attachments to the bone and tendon sheath, and the digital neurovascular structures are stretched to allow the flap to advance sufficiently to close the traumatic defect. This requires a knowledge of the local anatomy, judgement in planning the flap, and skill in its execution. Indeed, a lack of knowledge of the local anatomy is a contraindication to use of the V-Y flap. In a symposium on fingertip injuries, Flatt[4] stated, "These are very seductive flaps that appear to be simple when seen in a diagram . . . [but] these flaps require a tremendous amount of judgement to get good results." This opinion is shared by many hand surgeons.

Both the lateral and volar V-Y flap are indicated for transverse or slightly dorsal oblique wounds in which bone is exposed. The wound resulting from an oblique transverse amputation can be closed by asymmetrically placed lateral flaps. V-Y flaps are not indicated when there is a less than 1-cm loss of soft tissue without exposed bone or usually when the wound is oriented in a volar oblique direction but Furlow's[7] modification of the volar flap can be used for some volar oblique wounds. Larger wounds (larger than 1 cm) obviate the use of V-Y flaps because their excursion is limited. The volar flap is easier to perform than the lateral flap but probably has a greater incidence of altered tip sensation, a flattened tip, and palmar-curved nail.

Kutler-Type Lateral V-Y Flaps   Kutler[9,10] was the first to describe the use of flaps (6 to 8 mm long) from the lateral side of the digit to close tip-amputation defects. These flaps comprise the tissue that forms the "dog ears" during direct closure. The anatomy of the soft tissue in this area determines the technique for flap mobilization and advancement.

Digital anesthesia is obtained with a metacarpal block; I routinely use lidocaine without epinephrine. After surgical preparation and saline irrigation, the injured finger is exsanguinated with a Penrose drain or Tournicot. A forearm or upper-arm tourniquet can be used when multiple fingers are involved or when regional anesthesia is employed. Debridement of devitalized tissue and foreign material is necessary to produce a surgically clean wound. It may be necessary to debride or smooth the exposed bone.

The lateral flaps are drawn following the recommendations of Shepard.[11] The proposed dorsal incision is described from the amputation site 1 to 2 mm lateral to the nail fold and is continued proximally in a straight line midway between the palmar and dorsal surfaces of the bone (Fig. 3–1). The length of the incision should be about twice the width of the flap, which in the adult male is usually 6 to 7 mm. The proposed lower oblique incision is drawn from the palmar edge of the amputation to join the proximal extent of the dorsal incision. The dorsal incision is carried through skin and subcutaneous tissues down to the periosteum distally and the collateral ligament proximally.

It is important to recall the pertinent anatomy of this area. The fibrous bands that connect the dermis to the periosteum are thicker laterally and dorsally and are relatively thin on the palmar side. The neurovascular bundles and adipose tissue are more prominent in the palmar pad than dorsally and laterally. Mobilization of these Kutler-type flaps is usually restricted dorsally, whereas the innervation and blood supply is primarily palmar. Adequate advancement of the flaps requires the complete release of the dorsal–lateral fibrous bands. Therefore, the fibrous bands connecting the flap to the periosteum are divided from a dorsal approach down to the level of the palmar incision (Fig. 3–2). The palmar incision is made through skin only. While tension is placed on the distal aspect of the flap with a skin hook, gentle scissors dissection of the fibrous septa encountered in the palmar wound is performed. The septa can be palpated with the tips of the scissors and then divided to release the flap (Fig. 3–3). The two flaps can then be advanced toward and sutured to the other and to the distal aspect of the nail bed (Fig. 3–4). Interrupted nonabsorbable sutures [e.g., 5-0 Prolene (Ethicon, Inc., Somerville, NJ) are preferable]. The flaps can be advanced up to 10 mm. If there is too much tension on the flaps, a small amount of bone can be removed with a rongeur. It also may be necessary to excise a small amount of fat at the suture line. The apex of the "V" is then closed to form a "Y" using interrupted skin sutures. Before the dressing is applied, the tourniquet is released and the viability of the flaps is confirmed. When there is any question regarding the circulation of the flaps, sutures should be cut and the flaps allowed to return to their resting position. Hemostasis should be ensured, warm saline-soaked sponges placed on the fingertip, further bone resected, and another attempt made to advance the flaps. When this is unsuccessful, it is preferable to use another technique for closure rather than to leave vascularly impaired flaps covering the tip.

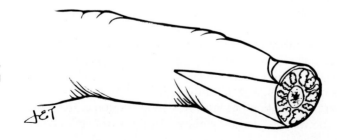

■ FIGURE 3–1
Drawing for lateral V-Y flap. The dorsal incision is lateral to the nail fold, extends proximally along the midline of the bone.

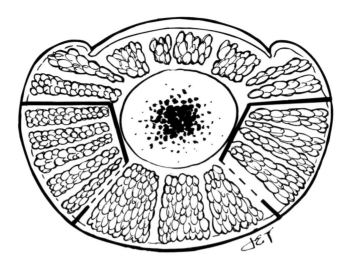

■ FIGURE 3-2
Solid lines indicate sharp and complete dissection. Dotted lines indicate locations of scissor dissection to free septa.

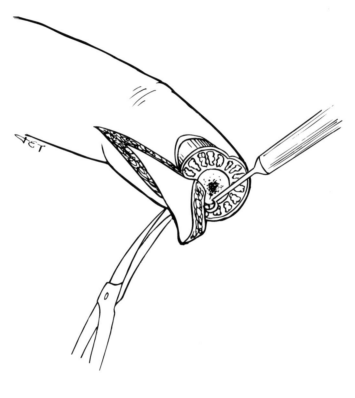

■ FIGURE 3-3
Flap is freed by gentle scissor dissection of the fibrous septum.

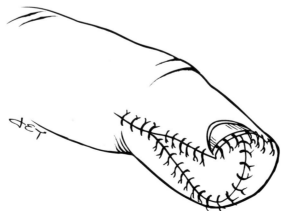

■ FIGURE 3-4
The two lateral flaps have been sutured in the midline and to the nail bed with interrupted sutures.

The wound is then covered with a nonadherent strip, such as Xeroform (Kendall Sherwood, Mansfield, MA), and a light absorbent dressing. It is advisable to protect the fingertip with a metal or plastic splint. I frequently apply an antibiotic ointment to the junction of the nail bed and flaps. Prolonged postoperative analgesia is provided by an additional metacarpal block using bupivacaine. Perioperative antibiotics are used in the following situations: when there has been a significant crush component to the injury, when the wound has been contaminated, or when there has been a delay in closure (more than 4 hours).

The patient is instructed that it is mandatory to keep the hand elevated for at least 48 hours; a sling may be used. After that time, the dressing can be reduced to a small adhesive bandage and active motion is encouraged. A protective splint can still be used. This program should begin within the first few days after injury. A formal physical therapy referral and program is usually unnecessary but instructions for soaks and active and passive range-of-motion exercises are provided in the clinic. Sutures are removed 10 to 14 days after surgery.

Volar V-Y Advancement Flaps   The volar V-Y flap, which has been popularized by Atasoy and coworkers,[1] is based on the same principle of advancement of similar sensate and vascularized skin to cover an amputation stump. The flap is freed of its fibrous attachments to the periosteum and tendon sheath and the neurovascular bundle is stretched to allow sufficient advancement (about 10 mm).

As with the lateral flap, anesthesia is obtained with a lidocaine metacarpal block, later supplemented with bupivacaine. A surgically clean wound is obtained with debridement and saline irrigation. Tourniquet control is indicated. A pattern of the defect is then prepared and transferred onto the palmar skin proximal to the defect. I prefer to draw the skin pattern 1 mm larger than the measured defect. The proposed palmar skin incisions are marked from the lateral edges of the amputation site to enclose the skin pattern and are continued proximally and obliquely to meet in the midline of the finger, usually at the distal finger crease. This creates a triangular flap (Fig. 3–5). The oblique incisions are about 1.5 times the width of the flap. The skin is incised through dermis only (Fig. 3–6). The flap is then elevated from a distal approach. The fibrous septa connecting the flap to the underlying periosteum and tendon sheath are divided under direct vision. The tip of the dissecting scissors is then used to bluntly dissect and divide the Grayson's and Cleland's ligaments that surround the neurovascular bundles and connect the flap to the surrounding tissues. A skin hook is used to exert traction on the distal aspect of the flap during this dissection (Fig. 3–7). Mobilization of the flap must be sufficient to allow advancement, without tension, of the flap to the nail bed; 10 mm advancement can be expected. The bipolar cautery is preferred for hemostasis. The flap is sutured to the nail

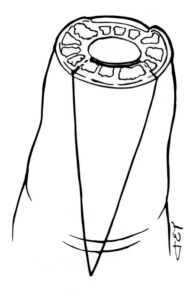

■ FIGURE 3–5
The volar flap is drawn to provide sufficient area of the skin flap to cover the amputation stump.

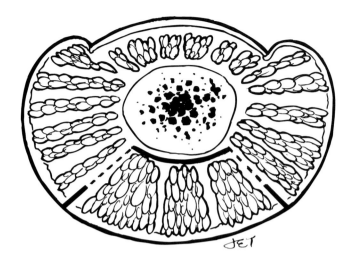

■ FIGURE 3–6
Solid lines indicate the complete dissection of the flap from the periosteum and the flexor sheath. The dotted lines indicate the area for scissors dissection of the septa to free the flap and its neurovascular bundles.

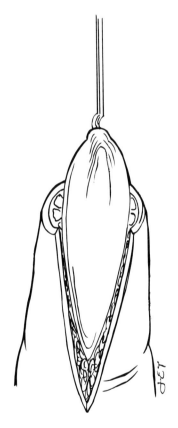

■ FIGURE 3–7
Flap is advanced distally after freeing fibrous connections.

bed with nonabsorbable sutures such as 5-0 Prolene or nylon. The apex of the "V" is closed in a similar manner with interrupted sutures (Fig. 3–8). The sutures should be kept close to the skin edge to reduce interference with the vascular supply. The tourniquet is then deflated or removed to check the flap's blood supply. Antibiotic ointment is applied to the skin edge, followed by a nonadherent strip, a light absorbent dressing, and a protective tip splint. Antibiotic use is comparable to that with the Kutler flaps. Hand elevation for at least the first 2 days is critical; a sling may be used.

As with the lateral flaps, dressings should be changed within several days and active exercises should be instituted. Sutures are removed in 10 to 14 days. A protective splint for the tip may be necessary for several weeks. The patient can be expected to return to work by 1 month if there are no complications.

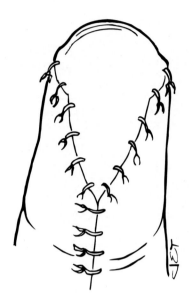

■ FIGURE 3–8
Donor site of the flap is closed and the flap approximated to the nail bed with interrupted sutures.

■ TECHNICAL
ALTERNATIVES

The principal problem with the lateral flap technique is the difficulty in mobilization of the flaps. When the vascular supply is injured, flap necrosis follows. Shepard[11] reported no incidence of flap necrosis in his series of 37 patients but Freiberg and Manktelow[6] reported two cases in a series of 22 patients. Flap necrosis has also been reported by Haddad.[8] Because of the concern with flap circulation, some authors recommend limiting the length of the pedicle to reduce tension and the resulting vasoconstriction (Haddad recommends $\frac{1}{4}$ to $\frac{3}{8}$ inches; Freiberg and Manktelow recommend up to $\frac{1}{2}$inch). Excess tension on the flap may cause wound dehiscence. Infection may be a problem; therefore, early postinjury follow-up is important.

Adequate mobilization of the volar flap is the principal technical problem with this technique, and a flattened appearance of the tip may occur. Also, the volar oblique amputation running from palmar-proximal to dorsal-distal presents a challenge for closure with local flaps. Furlow's[7] modification of the Atasoy-Kleinert flap[1] provides a solution, however. Furlow recommends suturing the two distal lateral points of elevated flap together in the midline, then advancing this "cup" flap to the edge of the nail bed.[7]

■ OUTCOMES

Because the lateral flaps provide a thick fatty pedicle over the stump, curvature of the nail over the reconstructed fingertip is not as common as with other techniques. Sensation is usually good and patients are able to return to work in most cases by 1 month after injury. Frandsen,[5] however, reported an average time off work of 61 days for his patients who had Kutler-type flaps. Cold intolerance, hypersensitivity, and paresthesia are experiences by more than 50% of patients[5] but may subside over time.

Although Atasoy and coworkers[1] reported that 56 of 61 patients with volar flaps had normal sensation and motion, other studies have indicated a high percentage of patients with hypesthesia, dysesthesia, and cold intolerance.[2,5,13] A decrease in sensibility was noted in 20 patients followed by Tupper and Miller[13] for an average of 5.9 years. The average difference in two-point discrimination between the injured and contralateral fingertips was 2.75 mm, and in von Frey monofilament discrimination was 0.6. Frandsen[5] reported an average return to work of 29 days for the patients in his study.

Every surgeon performing hand surgery for traumatic conditions should be familiar with the technique of V-Y advancement flaps as described here. In selected cases, this use of sensate local tissue provides excellent cover of the amputated tip and eliminates the need for marked shortening of the amputation stump. Attention to detail is critical to achieving success.

References

1. Atasoy E, Ioakimidis E, Kasdan ML, Kutz JE, Kleinert HE: Reconstruction of the amputated finger tip with a triangular volar flap. J Bone Joint Surg, 1970; 52A:921–926.
2. Conolly WB, Goulsten E: Problems of digital amputations: a clinical review of 260 patients and 301 amputations. Aust NZ J Surg, 1973; 43:118–123.
3. Fisher RH: The Kutler method of repair of fingertip amputations. J Bone Joint Surg, 1967; 49A:317–321.
4. Flatt A: Symposium: fingertip injuries; with Howard FM, Murray JF, Newmeyer WL. Contemp Orthop, 1986; 13:81–82.
5. Frandsen PA: A V-Y plasty as treatment of fingertip amputations. Acta Orthop Scand, 1978; 49:255–259.
6. Freiberg A, Manktelow R: The Kutler repair of fingertip amputations. Plast Reconstr Surg, 1972; 50:371–375.
7. Furlow LT Jr: V-Y "cup" flap for volar oblique amputation of fingers. J Hand Surg, 1984; 9B: 253–256.
8. Haddad RJ: The Kutler repair of fingertip amputations. South Med J, 1968; 61:1264–1267.
9. Kutler W: A method for repair of finger amputation. Ohio State Med J, 1944; 40:126.
10. Kutler W: A new method for fingertip amputation. JAMA, 1947; 133:29.
11. Shepard GH: The use of lateral V-Y advancement flaps for fingertip reconstruction. J Hand Surg, 1983; 8A:254–259.
12. Tranquilli-Leali E.: Ricostruzione dell'apice delle falangi ingueali mediante autoplastica volare peduncolata per scorrimento. Infortun Traum Lav, 1935; 1:186.
13. Tupper J, Miller G: Sensitivity following volar V-Y plasty for fingertip amputations. J Hand Surg, 1985; 10B:183–184.

RICHARD J.
ZIENOWICZ
LEE E. EDSTROM

4

Transposition Flaps

■ HISTORY OF THE TECHNIQUE

The unique anatomic characteristics of the skin and soft tissues of the hand require careful consideration in choosing flap type and design. Transposition flaps are one of the three types of local flaps of great importance to the hand surgeon. They are arguably the most common type of local flap used on the hand.[4] There is frequent confusion in terminology applied to transposition, rotation, and advancement flaps. Certainly, variants of the three flaps have been used for centuries. McGregor in 1960 defined a flap that moves soft tissue laterally into a defect as a transposed flap.[9] Milford in 1971 borrowed McGregor's diagram and changed the name to transposition flap.[10] Lister has contributed to a better understanding of this subject and the reader is strongly encouraged to review his writings.[6-8] Specifically, he 1) clarified the ambiguity in definitions of the three types of local flaps, 2) appropriately recognized the rhomboid and Z-plasty flaps as true transposition flaps, 3) devised a useful classification system, and 4) demonstrated applications of this reasoning in representative clinical cases.

A transposition flap is raised from its bed and moved laterally either to an immediately adjacent defect or over a peninsula of intervening skin.[7] They are most commonly random pattern flaps, deriving their circulation from the subdermal plexus, and occasionally axial pattern flaps, with a demonstrated axial blood supply. Generally, a 1:1 length-to-width ratio in flap design is considered to be safe; higher ratios, although often entirely viable, require superior vascularity and minimal tension when inset.

■ INDICATIONS AND CONTRAINDICATIONS

Lister described two basic types of random pattern transposition flaps.[7,8] A type I flap involves transposition, which leaves a secondary defect requiring a skin graft. The classic "dorsal rotation flap" described by Lister for thumb web-space contractures is actually a type I transposition flap. This type of flap is especially useful on the dorsum of the hand and is indicated when sufficient dorsal skin remains available after acute injury that leaves tendons exposed and in need of expedient coverage. It is contraindicated in the context of uncertain vascularity of the involved tissues.

Figure 4–1 demonstrates a wound that is indicated for transposition flap closure. It occurred after injury by a power auger, causing metacarpal fractures and extensor communis avulsions to the index and long fingers. The dorsal skin became necrotic, leaving underlying hardware exposed after debridement. The defect should be considered according to the hand position that enlarges it most (i.e., full flexion or extension, according to the wound location). The area of greatest tissue availability is chosen and a type I transposition flap is drawn adjacent to the defect in an area in which vascular integrity is not in question (Fig. 4–2).

■ SURGICAL TECHNIQUES

These procedures are typically rapidly executed by the experienced surgeon under tourniquet control. Bier block regional anesthesia can be used but local anesthesia (1% lidocaine) most often suffices nicely and has clear advantages that will be described. Epinephrine is not used so that the surgeon may assess hemostasis with more certainty later in the operation. Exsanguination is performed by elevating the extremity for about 30 seconds and inflating a proximal arm tourniquet to 100 mm above systolic pressure. This limited exsanguination allows the surgeon to better identify blood vessels that, given their location, need to be selectively sacrificed or preserved. Cutaneous nerves are also more easily differentiated from vessels and their preservation enhanced. The flap is raised immediately above the extensor retinaculum or more distally, the paratenon—cautiously preserving

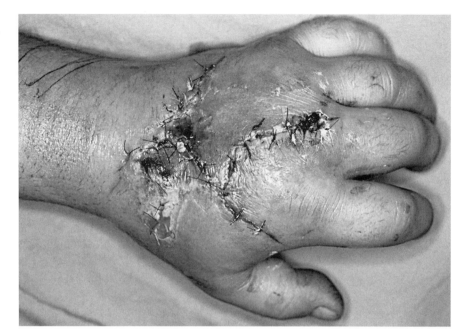

■ FIGURE 4–1
Provisional closure of extensive avulsion injury to dorsum of hand, with accompanying extensor communis and indicis proprius transections and index and long finger metacarpal fractures, which have been repaired with plates and screws.

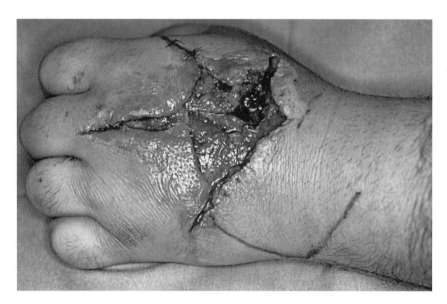

■ FIGURE 4–2
Debridement of necrotic tissues has been performed and type I transposition flap is designed. Exposed hardware is seen in the base of the wound.

this important layer that will support a skin graft if necessary. After complete exsanguination, this layer appears as a transparent glistening film over the underlying tendons. With limited exsanguination, minuscule widely dispersed blood vessels can also be appreciated. The flap is then generously undermined, along with the borders of the existing defect. The tourniquet, which has ordinarily been inflated about 10 minutes during flap elevation, is deflated for 3 seconds and then reinflated, permitting easy visualization of small vessels requiring coagulation. This process is repeated until hemostasis is achieved; finally, the tourniquet is left deflated while the flap is inset. Adequate hemostasis cannot be overemphasized because these small local flaps are intolerant of underlying hematoma for two reasons. First, pressure-induced occlusion of their random blood supply can occur and second, the delayed effect of ferric oxide free radicals on the microcirculation as the heme moiety is metabolized can ultimately lead to vascular thrombosis.[1] Inset (Fig. 4–3) is performed with nonabsorbable 5-0 suture and buried 5-0 absorbable dermal sutures. The absorbable dermal sutures allow earlier removal of skin sutures, thus minimizing suture-

■ FIGURE 4–3
Flap has been trans-
posed and inset and
donor site covered with
split-thickness skin graft.

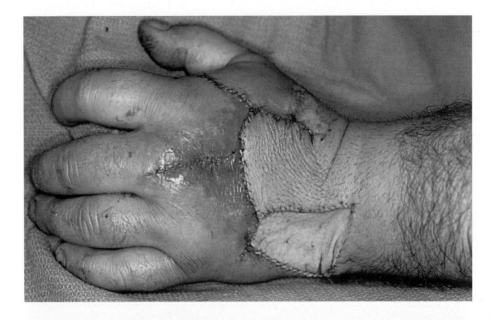

■ FIGURE 4–4
Wound seen 3 months
later. Fractures and ten-
don repairs have healed
uneventfully.

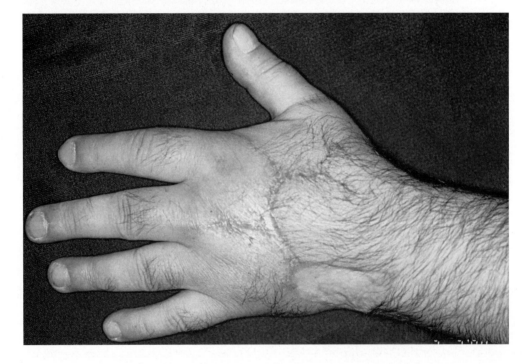

tract scarring. A split-thickness skin graft is harvested from the superior lateral thigh with an electric Padgett dermatome at a depth of 0.012 inches. It is then "pie-crusted" with small perforations with a No. 11 scalpel to allow egress of blood and serum and sutured into place with 5-0 plain gut. Xeroform and normal saline–soaked cotton balls are then applied. Because of the laxity of the dorsal hand skin, significant dog ear resection is usually not necessary. If necessary, the resected tissue should not contribute to the vascular supply of the transposed flap. The hand is then wrapped with gauze dressing and a dorsiflexion splint applied to eliminate tension, which could lead to vascular compromise of the flap. Limited active range of motion is permitted at 1 week but the splint is reapplied at bedtime for an additional week. Sutures are removed at 7 to 10 days. Figure 4–4 shows the result at 1 month postoperatively.

    Type II flaps allow direct closure of their donor defect after transposition. A Z-plasty, which has ubiquitous applications in the hand and elsewhere, is classified under this type. It transposes two similarly sized flaps, leaving no donor defect, and its practical value lies in scar lengthening. The rhomboid flap, with its precise geometric design, is most frequently associated with the names of Limberg and Dufourmentel.[2,5,6] Both effect closure of a rhomboid-shaped defect, which may occasionally occur spontaneously as the result of trauma or disease. More often, the surgeon adjusts a circular defect by minor excision to conform to the transposed rhomboid-shaped flap. The rhomboid shape described in these flaps is typically comprised of alternating 60 and 120° angles.

The surgeon using this type of flap can theoretically design any of four different flaps, based on a given rhomboid defect (Fig. 4–5). Flexibility in flap design when creating the defect and choosing its orientation is limited by existing skin tension and potential skin compliance adjacent to the defect. One must judge the area of greatest laxity, allowing easiest approximation of the pivot point of the flap (A1) to a point adjacent to a diagonal drawn to the opposite far corner of the flap (A) (Fig. 4–5). Figure 4–6 represents a well-differentiated squamous cell carcinoma (and cutaneous horn), with planned excision according to the optimal recruitment of skin for a tensionless closure (Fig. 4–7). The flap is raised using the same technique already described. The flap is undermined at its base and pivot point (A1). Point A1 is approximated to point A, resulting in a linear lateral closure, thus avoiding the need for a skin graft (Fig. 4–8). A 6-week postoperative result demonstrates the superior aesthetic result versus that which would have occurred with a traditional skin graft (Fig. 4–9).

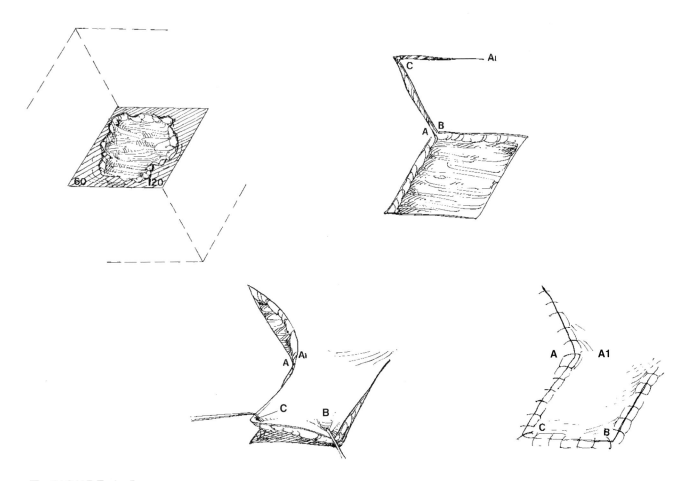

■ FIGURE 4–5
Limberg flap options (compare with Fig. 4-7).

■ FIGURE 4-6
Well-differentiated squamous cell carcinoma with cutaneous horn.

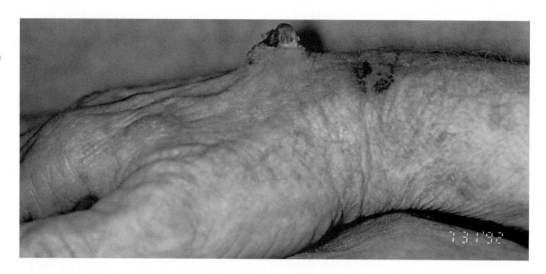

■ FIGURE 4-7
Limberg flap designed. Ability to close point *A* to *A1* determines optimal location.

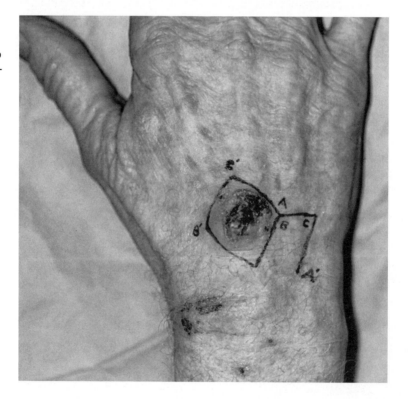

Axial pattern flaps such as the flag flap originally described by Vilain are based on an extension of the dorsal digital artery, which can arise from either the proximal digital, dorsal interosseous, or metacarpal artery.[3,8,11] This transposition flap requires skin graft closure of the donor site. Figure 4–10 demonstrates use of the axial transposition flap to close a defect on an adjacent finger dorsum. In other regions, this is often referred to as a banner flap because of its characteristic shape. The required amount of tissue is outlined and an extension included to allow closure without a dog ear (this tissue is discarded). The flap is elevated immediately above the paratenon layer, transposed, and closed in the manner previously described (Fig. 4–11). The donor site also closes as a straight line. One month follow-up shows slight hypertrophy in the web space, which has disappeared with time (Fig. 4–12).

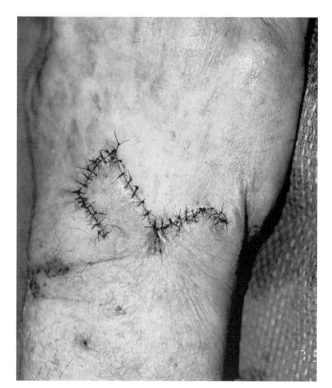

■ FIGURE 4–8
Flap transposed and donor site closed primarily (conferring type II designation).

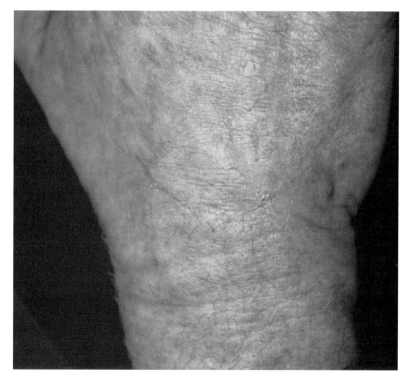

■ FIGURE 4–9
Six-week postoperative result.

■ FIGURE 4–10
Type II axial pattern flap
designed to cover adja-
cent phalanx.

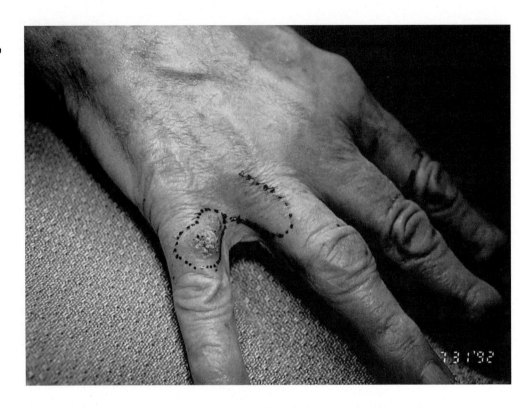

■ FIGURE 4–11
Flap transposed and
inset.

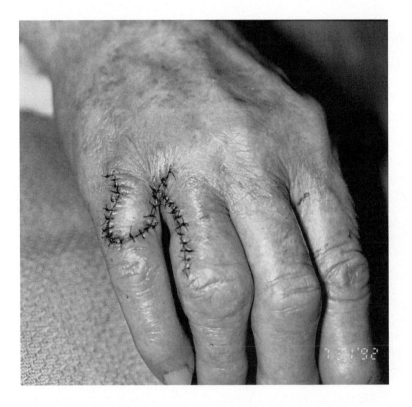

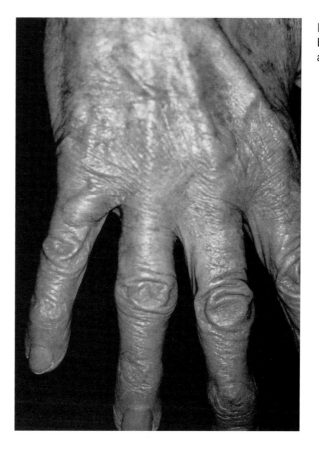

■ FIGURE 4–12
Early postoperative result at 1 month.

All flap complications invariably result from an insult to flap perfusion. Inadequate length-to-width ratio, excessive tension of closure, compression—either external (from splint, dressing, or patient position) or internal (from hematoma or infection)—leads to vascular compromise.

    ■ TECHNICAL ALTERNATIVES

The greatest pitfall to an unsuccessful outcome is underestimating the flap size necessary to fill the involved defect. Most fresh wounds appear larger than the actual original soft-tissue loss because of recoil of the margins from inherent elasticity. This permits the surgeon to use a moderately smaller flap design if he can demonstrate adequate mobility of the tissue abutting the defect. In an area such as the palm, wherein the viscoelasticity of the skin is minimized by its thickness, one should be more generous in estimating flap size than on the dorsum, with its thinner, more mobile, and more distensible skin. A maneuver that can often help when excessive tension occurs because of size underestimate or poor tissue compliance is called the back-cut. This cut is placed at the pivot point and angled across the flap base. It permits further movement of the tip of the flap along its line of tension at the potential expense of flap vascularity.

One cannot overestimate the value of a well-executed postoperative dressing. The skin grafted donor site requires gentle compression, which must not be transmitted to the transposition flap. Normal saline–soaked cotton balls provide a superbly conforming bolster, which when combined with an appropriate splint provides sufficient immobilization to allow good graft establishment while preventing further undue flap tension. Elevation in a foam block, such as a Carter pillow, prevents inadvertent flap compression and shearing forces generated by the patient. Lastly, drains do not prevent hematoma formation, so that it behooves the surgeon to obtain adequate hemostasis before closure. Gradual progressive tourniquet release, with inspection and control, can obviate most surgical hematomas.

■ REHABILITATION

Generally, most transposition flaps, even those accompanied by a skin graft (type I flaps), require strict immobilization for 7 to 10 days, at which time gentle active range-of-motion exercises can be initiated. When the flaps are designed to allow postoperative splinting in the resting position, recovery is usually straightforward. Hand therapy may be required for extenuating circumstances, such as prolonged immobilization for tendon or bone healing. Ordinarily, supervision by a hand therapist is unnecessary if healing has occurred per primum and the patient is motivated; if this is questionable, early supervised active range-of-motion exercises should be employed.

■ OUTCOMES

The final clinical result is typically highly satisfying to both patient and surgeon. When cosmetic improvement of scarred areas is later desired, tissue expansion of the flap and adjacent areas can be performed to permit skin-graft excision. Myriad other possibilities clinically continue to arise for the use of highly dependable, functional, and often remarkably aesthetic transposition flaps.

References

1. Angel MF: The etiologic role of free radicals in hematoma induced flap necrosis. Plast Reconstr Surg, 1986; 77:795–803.
2. Dufourmentel C: Le fermeture des pertes de substance cutanee limitees "Le lambeau de rotation en L pour losange" dit "L.L.L." Ann Chir Plast, 1962; 7:61.
3. Iselin F: The flag flap. Plast Reconstr Surg, 1973; 52:374–377.
4. Lesavoy M: Local Incisions and Flap Coverage. In: McCarthy JG, May JW, Littler JW (eds): Plastic Surgery, Philadelphia: WB Saunders, 1990:4441–4458.
5. Limberg AA: Mathematical principles of local plastic procedures on the surface of the human body. Leningrad: Government Publishing House for medical literature; 1946. (Megdiz).
6. Lister GD, Gibson T: Closure of rhomboid skin defects: the flaps of Limberg and Dufourmentel. Br J Plast Surg, 1972; 25:300–314.
7. Lister GD: The theory of the transposition flap and its practical application in the hand. Clin Plast Surg, 1981: 8:115–128.
8. Lister GD: Skin Flaps. In: Green DP (ed): Operative Hand Surgery, New York: Churchill Livingstone, 1988:1839–1933.
9. McGregor IA: Fundamental Techniques of Plastic Surgery and Their Surgical Applications. Edinburgh: E&S Livingstone, Ltd., 1960:130–134.
10. Milford L: The Hand. St Louis: CV Mosby, 1971: 16–17.
11. Vilain R, Dupuis JF: Use of the flag flap for coverage of a small area on a finger and the palm. Plast Reconstr Surg, 1973; 52:397–401.

5

Rotation Flaps of the Hand

The challenge of reconstructive surgery is to replace lost tissue with tissue of similar texture, quality, and functional characteristics. This is possible with tissue from local or distant sites. These reconstructive techniques utilize V-Y advancement, transposition, and cross-finger and neurovascular island flaps.[1–8] Local rotation flaps have evolved through a variety of surgical techniques and can be an excellent method for selected clinical problems.[2,3,5–7]

To achieve the best outcomes, it is important to understand the principles of flap design.[2,3,5,6] These principles are well-discussed by Lister[6] and are reemphasized here. Rotation flaps are random pattern flaps in which the incision developing the flap is sutured to itself in a staggered fashion to close both the donor and recipient sites with the same piece of tissue. Because the same piece of skin is advanced and used to close both defects, the pliability of the skin is paramount. Unlike many areas of the body, there is a shortage of available skin with which to work on the hand. The skin that is available is highly specialized from one area to the next, and use of skin from one area to cover another may severely impair function of the hand. There are two specific types of skin with which to work: dorsal and palmar. Generally, dorsal skin is more extensible, nonglabrous, hirsute, thin, and movable with respect to underlying structures. In contrast, palmar skin has specialized glabrous epithelium that is immobile with respect to underlying structures. It has a high density of specialized sensory receptors and a relatively thick subcuticular layer, in addition to exceedingly poor mobility. Of these two types of available skin, the dorsal skin is much more amenable to rotation flaps; therefore, dorsal defects lend themselves more readily to this type of closure. Rotation flaps have been reported for the palmar surface[2,3,5] but in many circumstances, they are less desirable than other methods of reconstruction.

The usual indications for rotation flap closure of the hand or fingers are small to medium-sized dorsal defects that cannot or should not be closed primarily because of the size of the defect or compromise of function that would occur with primary closure (Fig. 5-1). The tissue surrounding both the defect and the proposed flap should be uninjured. Elevation and transfer of the flap should not compromise hand function. Injury of the structures beneath the proposed donor or recipient sites does not preclude use of the rotational flap as long as the vascular supply of the flap is intact. Relative contraindications include patients with severe peripheral arterial disease, smokers, and patients with conditions of sympathetic over-activity.

Closure of hand defects may be performed under local, regional, or general anesthesia if care is taken not to compromise the vascular supply of the flap with large volumes of local anesthetic or anesthetics containing epinephrine. Normally, the procedure may be effectively accomplished under regional anesthesia, with tourniquet control of bleeding and with the aid of loupe magnification.

The first step is to ensure that the full extent of the defect is known by careful inspection followed by debridement of all nonviable tissue. Once the full extent of the defect is known, an estimate of the available tissue for transfer can be made. In obtaining this estimate, it is important to place the hand in both flexed and extended postures to appreciate how little "extra" tissue is available. By definition, a rotation flap borders the defect

■ HISTORY OF THE TECHNIQUE

■ INDICATIONS AND CONTRAINDICATIONS

■ SURGICAL TECHNIQUE

A skin defect after resection of a squamous cell carcinoma on the dorsum of the hand.

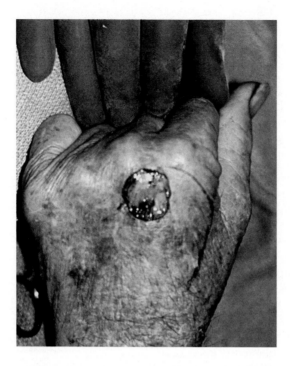

and is developed by extending arcs from the defect in a radial direction. The base or bases of the flap may be in any direction, but are commonly directed proximally or distally. It is not unusual to need one proximally based flap and one distally based flap opposite the other to close a moderately sized defect.

Estimates of Lister's "line of maximal extensibility"[6] can be made by distracting the sides of the defect with skin hooks across the defect to determine which direction of pull affords the greatest defect coverage. Again, it is important to perform this maneuver with the hand in both extended (the normal surgical position) and flexed positions. Otherwise, the limitation of the flap will not be fully recognized, leading to loss of a portion of the flap (which is usually the most important part of the flap) or loss of function of the hand (usually a loss of flexion of the fingers). Classically, proximally based flaps are the most commonly used; however, Quaba and Davidson[7] have challenged this practice, arguing that the main arterial supply to the skin of the dorsum of the hand comes from perforators of the deep and superficial arches at the level of the metacarpophalangeal joints. A third source of arterial supply is the dorsal carpal arch at the level of the base of the metacarpals. Once the line of maximal extensibility has been determined (this line typically runs medially and laterally to the axial line of the hand), one or more flaps are designed.

The flaps are developed in a relatively avascular plane below the superficial veins but superficial to the underlying cutaneous nerves. The flaps should not be grasped with forceps, but carefully manipulated with skin hooks to prevent crushing the tissue. The sutures along the line of maximal tension should be placed initially. This permits the surgeon an opportunity to evaluate the function of the hand with the flaps in place and determine whether there is too much tension on the flaps or if hand function is compromised. When too much tension is noted, adjustments are made to alleviate the tension. These adjustments can be made in one or more ways:

1. Making the flap wider. By extending the arc of the flap and doubling the width of the flap, the tension along the critical line can be reduced by fifty percent. If the width is tripled, the tension is reduced to thirty-three percent. Therefore, it is wise to design flaps as wide as possible to reduce tension across the suture line.
2. Making the flap longer. The same principle applies if the arc is extended laterally or in a proximal and distal direction. The limitation of this maneuver is that the distal end of the flap is at greater jeopardy as the length to width ratio exceeds 1:1.

3. Making an extension cut along the side of the flap opposite the defect. This maneuver has the same effect as lengthening the flap and the same limitation regarding the length to width ratio, but is helpful in areas where the defect is located distally and no lengthening of the flap is possible.
4. Making a back cut. This maneuver releases tension along the critical line without lengthening the flap or extending it. This narrows the flap base and is limited by the same length to width consideration as other maneuvers.

Once the flap is developed and transposed, the skin is closed in a single layer with interrupted sutures, utilizing non-absorbable suture material (Fig. 5–2). The interrupted suture allows the surgeon to make adjustments to the flap easily during closure. The tourniquet is deflated after skin closure to assess the vascularity of the flap before dressing application. Local anesthetic without epinephrine may be used for pain control around the operative site and may have some beneficial effect on the flap. Dressings that keep the flap moist are applied, (e.g., Adaptic, Bacitracin ointment) and the surgical site is covered with gauze and a loosely fitted elastic bandage.

■ TECHNICAL ALTERNATIVES

Rotation flaps have limited use in hand surgery and must be carefully planned. The main advantage of this flap is that it is readily available and matches the characteristics of the tissue that has been lost. Alternatives include primary closure; other types of local flaps, including transposition flaps and pedicle flaps, and distant flaps. Foremost in the surgeon's mind should be preservation of hand function.

The most common pitfall with rotation flaps is the unrealistic expectation of what the flap can cover while preserving hand function. Loss of a portion of the flap can have serious consequences and the surgeon should consider contingencies such as other available local or distant flaps before beginning the rotation flap. The quality of the surrounding skin, the pathological process responsible for the defect, and the surgeon's experience must also be considered. Once the flap has been started, the surgeon should be flexible and adjust the operative plan if circumstances warrant. If it becomes obvious that the original operative plan is inadequate, the surgeon might need to extend or lengthen the flap, use a back cut, or develop a second opposing rotation flap. These contingencies should be discussed with patients preoperatively. Pressing forward with an inadequate initial plan only complicates the situation and is not in the patient's or physician's best interest.

■ OUTCOMES

In discussions of their experiences with rotation flaps of the hand, authors generally describe effective coverage and aesthetically acceptable results (Fig. 5–3). Because the

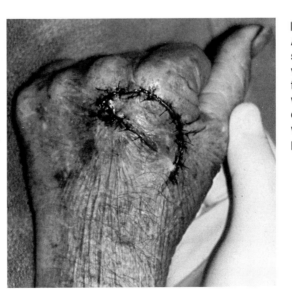

■ FIGURE 5–2
A rotation flap was designed, elevated and advanced to close the defect. Note that a back cut was necessary to achieve closure intra-operatively with the hand in a flexed position.

■ FIGURE 5–3
The flap has healed and
a full range of finger flexion was preserved.

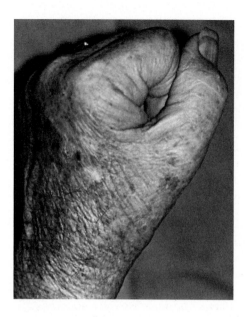

indications for the operation and the nature of the procedure are variable, the results are difficult to quantitate or assess in objective terms. When appropriately indicated and carefully performed, I find rotation flaps to be a predictable and valuable technique in reconstructive hand surgery.

References

1. Dap F, Dautel G, Voche P, Thomas C, Marle M: The posterior interosseous flap in primary repair of hand injuries. A review of 23 cases. J Hand Surg, 1993; 18B:437–445.
2. Furnas DW: Z-plasties and related procedures for the hand and upper limb. Hand Clinics, 1985; 1:649–665.
3. Gilbert DA: An overview of flaps for hands and forearm reconstruction. Clin Plas Surg, 1981; 8:129–139.
4. Kleinman WB, Putnam MD: Microvascular free-tissue transfers to the hand and upper extremity. Hand Clinics, 1989; 5:423–444.
5. Lane CS, Kuschner SH: A technique for planning skin flaps in the hand. J Hand Surg, 1992; 17A:1162–1163.
6. Lister GD: Local flaps to the hand. Hand Clinics, 1985; 1:621–640.
7. Quaba, AA. Distally based dorsal hand flap. Br J Plas Surg, 1990; 43:28–39.
8. Upton J, Havlik RJ, Khouri RK: Refinement in hand coverage with microvascular free flaps. Clin Plas Surg, 1992; 19:841–857.

ROD J. ROHRICH,
STEVE D. ANTROBUS

6

Volar Advancement Flaps

The principle of volar flap advancement in the reconstruction of fingertip injuries was first described by Moberg[10] in 1964. The volar flap as initially described was intended for use in the thumb. The flap was raised through bilateral mid-axial incisions and it included both neurovascular pedicles. This volar advancement flap was the first flap to succeed in restoring normal sensation to the skin over the digits. In addition, the flap provided durable full-thickness soft-tissue coverage, with minimal donor site morbidity, and it preserved digital length.

Use of the advancement flap was extended to include fingertip amputations by Snow[15] in 1967. Amputations through the distal phalanx of the index finger were successfully repaired, with restoration of normal sensibility. Digital length, which in the past had been sacrificed to achieve primary closure, was preserved. O'Brien[11] in 1968 described a proximal transverse skin incision across the base of the flap, creating a homodigital bipedicle island flap. This innovation allowed greater advancement, making it possible to cover terminal defects of 1.5 cm or more.

As the technique came into popular use, several surgeons described their successful experiences with the flap in both thumb tip and fingertip reconstruction, including Keim and Grantham[7] in 1969 and Posner and Smith[12] in 1971. More extensive use of the flap in fingertip reconstruction began to reveal potential complications, namely dorsal skin necrosis. Shaw[14] in 1974, referring to the vascular anatomy of the distal phalanx described by Flint,[5] emphasized the importance of preserving distal dorsal blood supply. Although the independent dorsal blood supply to the thumb decreases the risk to the dorsal skin, the technique of completely elevating the volar flap risks vascular compromise of the distal dorsal skin in the fingers. Shaw suggested that this potential complication could be avoided by careful preservation of the perforating vessels, which branch off from the volar digital arteries and course into the dorsal aspect of the fingers.

The value of the volar advancement flap in delayed reconstruction of thumb tip injuries was emphasized by Millender, Albin, and Nalebuff[9] in 1973. In their series, the volar advancement flap was successful in restoring padded sensitive skin to old injuries that had resulted in insensible skin over the pinch surface, painful neuromas of the tip, and atrophic insensitive scars.

Further technical refinements of the procedure by Macht and Watson[8] in 1980 minimized potential complications of the volar advancement flap and established the flap as being safe and effective for repair of both fingertip and thumb tip injuries.

Fingertip injuries are some of the most common traumatic injuries in the United States.[1] There is no uniform agreement about the optimum technique for each type of injury. This is reflected by the large variety of reconstructive options available to the surgeon. The options range from allowing healing by secondary intention to the use of complex microsurgical free flaps. One should assess each injury on an individual basis, considering the patient's age, hand dominance, occupation, and potential future hand use, in addition to the relative importance of the injured digit and the overall functional status of the other digits and the other hand.

The volar advancement flap has many advantages over alternative local, regional, and distal flaps. These include 1) immediate restoration of essentially normal sensation, 2) preservation of length, 3) low morbidity of the donor site, 4) single-stage procedure, 5)

■ HISTORY OF THE TECHNIQUE

■ INDICATIONS AND CONTRAINDICATIONS

■ FIGURE 6–1
The angle and level of fingertip amputation determines the most appropriate closure. The volar advancement flap is particularly applicable to the oblique volar tip amputation (angle 2).

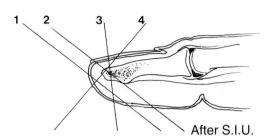

After S.I.U.

restoration of pulp contour and character, 6) relatively short rehabilitation, 7) simultaneous use in multiple digits, 8) use in both primary and secondary reconstruction, and 9) no requirement of cortical relearning.

The volar advancement flap is of great value in the reconstruction of digital tip amputations. This is particularly true of injuries of the thumb and index finger, in which both pulp sensibility and preservation of digital length are essential. The fine prehensile function of these two digits requires nearly normal sensation. In addition to restoring normal sensation, the flap provides full-thickness coverage, preserves critical digital length, and avoids painful scars on opposing pulp surfaces.

The level and angle of the amputation are important factors in the selection of reconstructive techniques. Superficial tip amputations without major skin loss or exposed bone heal by secondary intention with good results (Fig. 6–1, angle 1). Transverse guillotine amputations and dorsally directed amputations with exposed bone (Fig. 6–1, angles 3 and 4) may be closed with local V-Y advancement flaps when sufficient local tissue is available. The volar advancement flap is particularly applicable to oblique volar tip amputations (Fig. 6–1, angle 2). Volar tissue defects larger than dime size on the fingers or quarter size on the thumb may require reconstructive techniques more complex than the volar advancement flap.

The volar advancement flap is ideally suited for reconstruction of oblique volar thumb tip injuries. The shorter length of the thumb and the independent dorsal blood supply decrease the risk of flexion contracture or dorsal skin loss. In addition, the Dellon[3] modification of the Moberg flap allows coverage of tissue defects of up to 3 cm. Although the volar flap has been described for use in all five digits, it has been suggested that better functional results may be achieved with regional flaps in the three ulnar fingers, in which sensitivity is of secondary importance.[4] These regional flaps, including the standard cross-finger flap, the side cross-finger flap, the thenar flap, and the thenar-crease flap, result in poor sensitivity but provide satisfactory tissue coverage. Use of the volar advancement flap is often limited by the quantity of skin available for advancement. In certain cases, staging of the advancement can be used to provide additional length.[8]

In addition to its use in acute reconstruction of thumb tip and fingertip injuries, the volar advancement flap is a valuable technique in secondary reconstruction of old injuries or revision of failed primary procedures.[9] Furthermore, in an acute crush injury of a thumb tip or fingertip, a primary skin graft followed by a delayed volar advancement flap in 10 to 12 weeks may be preferable to primary reconstruction.[9]

■ SURGICAL TECHNIQUES

The volar advancement flap is best performed in the operating suite using a regional block. Our preference is a wrist or axillary block. It is imperative to perform a meticulous sensory examination of the injured digits before anesthesia. After standard preparation and draping techniques, the arm is exsanguinated using an Esmarch's tourniquet, and a pneumatic pressure cuff is placed on the upper arm and inflated to 250 mm Hg of mercury to maintain a bloodless field.

Careful debridement of skin and scar tissue is performed, with removal of bone fragments and conservative trimming of sharp bony edges. When resecting anesthetic scars in delayed reconstructions, a 2-mm distal rim is left in place to facilitate closure. When tissue viability is questionable, the tourniquet may be temporarily released to assess tissue perfusion. Nail injuries may be severe enough to require ablation. Even a deformed nail is often useful in picking up small objects and should be preserved if possible. This is particularly true of the thumb nail, and the nail can always be removed later if necessary.

A thorough understanding of the vascular anatomy of the distal digits is required for successful application of the volar flap. The vascular supply of the thumb tip differs from that of the other digits. The dorsalis pollicis arteries branch from the first dorsal metacarpal artery and supply the length of the dorsal thumb. Therefore, disruption of its volar blood supply rarely leads to vascular compromise of the dorsal tip. In contrast, the terminal branches of the dorsal digital arteries in the fingers of the hand are small and do not reach the distal phalanx. Communicating vessels from the proper digital arteries supply the dorsum of the fingers distal to the termination of the dorsal vessels (Fig. 6–2). Most of the distal dorsal blood supply of the fingers is supplied by the volar vasculature.

Elevation of a volar flap in the fingers without preservation of the distal perforators risks vascular compromise of the dorsal tip and subsequent necrosis. Therefore, the volar advancement flap is of special value in the thumb, in which the procedure is particularly safe, and in the index finger, in which the importance of sensitivity outweighs the relative risk of dorsal skin necrosis.

The initial skin incisions are made on both the radial and ulnar mid-axial lines. These incisions, placed along the dorsal aspect of the flexion creases, remain dorsal to the neurovascular bundles (Fig. 6–3).

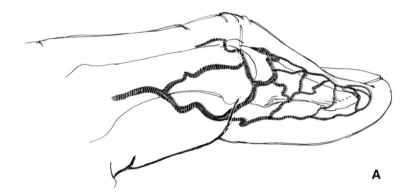

A

■ FIGURE 6–2
A and **B**, Communicating vessels from the proper digital arteries supply the dorsum of the fingers distal to the termination of the dorsal vessels.

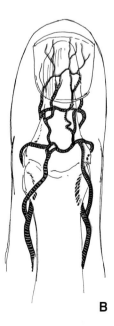

B

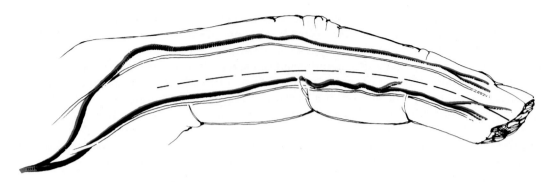

■ FIGURE 6–3
Radial and ulnar mid-axial skin incisions, placed along the dorsal aspect of the flexion creases, remain dorsal to the neurovascular bundles.

For distal tip amputations, the initial incisions should extend to the proximal interphalangeal flexion crease of the fingers or to the base of the proximal phalanx of the thumb. This initial incision can be extended as far proximally as the web space of the fingers. On the thumb, the incision can extend onto the thenar eminence, as described by Dellon[3] (Fig. 6–4).

In this modification, care must be taken during flap elevation on the ulnar side of the thumb because the entrance of the princeps pollicis artery is variable. The radial and ulnar defects created by the distal advancement of the flap are closed by two additional local rotation flaps. These scars follow the natural lines of the hand.

A careful spreading dissection technique is used to partially elevate the flap. The volar flap, including the neurovascular bundle, is not cut free but is gradually separated until the bridging tissues allow sufficient advancement for tip coverage (Fig. 6–5). Dissection proceeds just volar to the flexor tendon sheath and care must be taken not to enter or damage the sheath. Particular care is also taken to identify and preserve the dorsal blood supply that is provided by the perforating vessels. These vessels originate from the digital arteries and are distributed at an angle dorsally and distally. Thus, as the flap and neurovascular bundles are advanced distally, the perforating vessels rotate at their origin and may be maintained intact.

Magnifying loops and meticulous technique are required for safe elevation of the flap. Flexion of the digit shortens the required distance for flap advancement and decreases the amount of flap mobilization required. The digit is periodically flexed during the operation to judge the adequacy of mobilization. Dissection is continued proximally until a tension-free closure is possible.

Various options are available for treatment of the base of the flap. If adequate mobilization is obtained, allowing tip coverage of the flexed finger, the base may be left intact (Fig. 6–6A). Leaving the base intact allows about 1 cm of advancement. A transverse incision placed at the flap base, with care taken to spare the neurovascular bundle, can achieve about 1.5 cm of advancement.[11] The resulting defect is filled with a full-thickness skin graft (Fig. 6–6B). House[6] and Chase[2] recommend bilateral Z-plasties of the proximal mid-axial incisions to gain lateral advancement of the flap. A V-to-Y advancement of the base of the flap allows advancement of the entire flap and obviates the need for additional skin grafting (Fig. 6–6C).

If sufficient advancement cannot be obtained, the procedure may be staged. The remaining distal defect may be grafted and the procedure repeated in 6 months.[8]

After mobilization of the flap, the digit is flexed 30 to 45° in the metacarpophalangeal and interphalangeal joints, and the flap is sewn into place. If the volar flap blanches, further proximal dissection may be needed. The distal portion of the flap often must be contoured to avoid a squared-off tip. This can be achieved by excising small triangles of tissue on the radial and ulnar aspect of the flap tip. This avoids scarring of the middle of

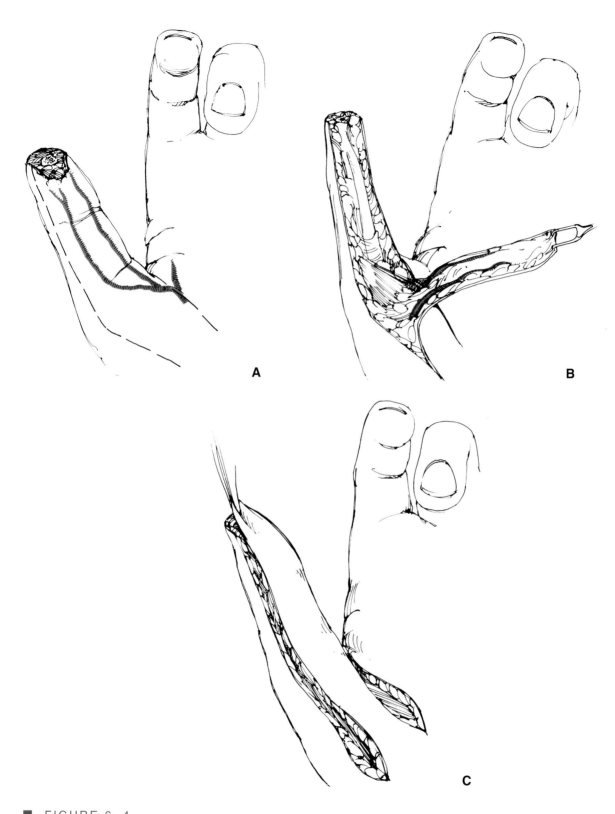

■ FIGURE 6–4

A through **C**, In the thumb, the incisions can extend proximally on the thenar eminence.

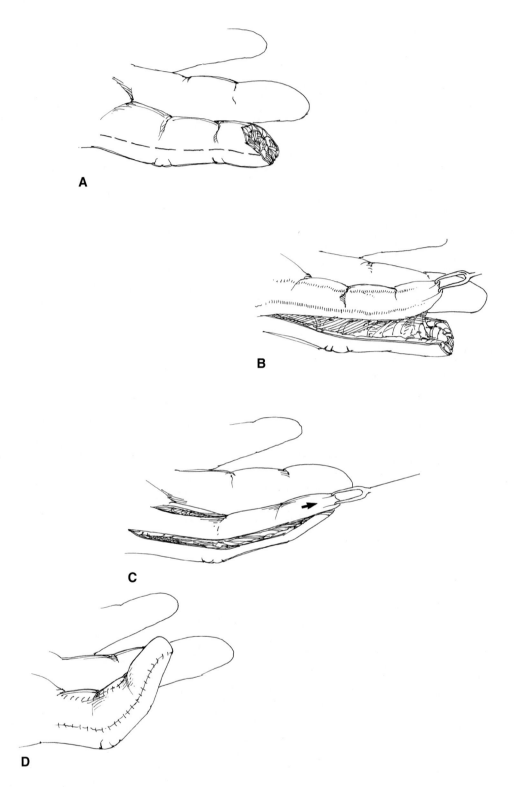

■ FIGURE 6–5

A through D, The volar flap with the neurovascular bundles is gradually mobilized to allow sufficient advancement for tip coverage.

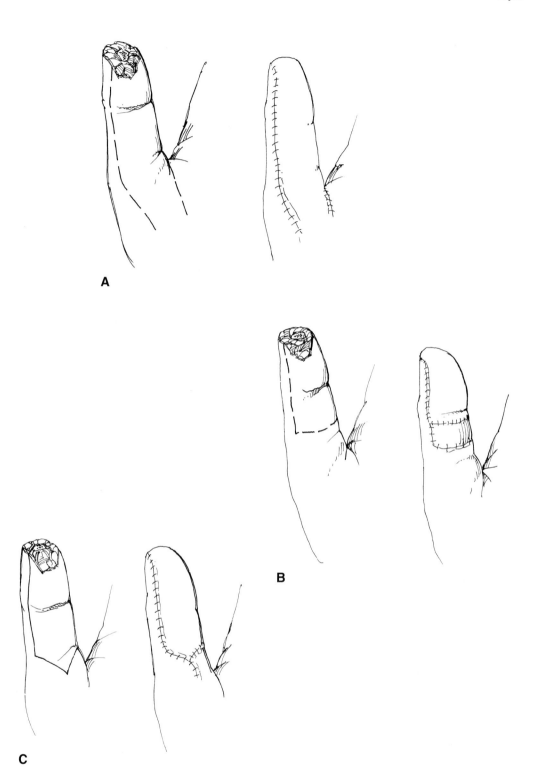

A

B

C

■ FIGURE 6–6
A through **C**, The base
of the advanced flap can
be left intact (**A**), released transversely, sparing the neurovascular
bundle and deep veins,
and skin grafted (**B**), or
advanced using the V-to-
Y technique (**C**).

the volar tip and allows the flap to more closely approximate the cut edge of the nail bed
and sides of the digit. When possible, the flap is attached directly to the nail through
needle holes made in the nail. Simple interrupted sutures are used to close the wound.
Slight diagonal placement of the sutures allows the flap to be gradually advanced distally
during closure. After the flap is securely sutured into place, the digit is splinted in a flexed
position.

■ TECHNICAL
ALTERNATIVES

Many technical alternatives to the volar advancement flap are available, each with its own advantages and disadvantages. These include 1) scar formation with secondary wound healing, 2) full- or split-thickness skin grafting, 3) volar or lateral V-Y advancements, 4) cross-finger flaps, 5) regional pedicle flaps, 6) local rotational flaps, 7) neurovascular island flaps, and 8) microsurgical free flaps.

The widely used V-Y flaps are useful procedures. Their use, however, is limited to transverse or slightly oblique amputations having adequate marginal skin. Only moderate advancement is possible (0.4 to 0.5 cm) and these flaps have a high incidence of persistent hypersensitivity.

Cross-finger flaps and thenar flaps provide protective sensibility and adequate soft-tissue coverage and have a role in reconstruction of digits in which sensibility is of secondary importance. The disadvantages of these flaps include donor-site morbidity, joint stiffness, and the two-stage nature of the procedures.

Complex digital injuries involving severe pulp loss may require microsurgical replacement of composite tissues. These techniques yield functional results comparable with full-thickness skin grafts in lesser injuries and sensory return equal to that achieved by conventional means.[13] The disadvantages include the complexity of the procedures and donor-site morbidity.

Because the volar advancement procedure involves significant dissection near the neurovascular bundle, injury to these structures, with resultant loss of the volar flap, is a potential pitfall. Complications related to volar flap loss have not been reported, however.

Minor complications such as epidermal inclusion cysts, symptomatic neuromata, nail deformities, and symptomatic nail scars occur occasionally and may require reoperation.

■ REHABILITATION

The patient may be discharged home within 24 hours postoperatively. The splint and wires are removed in 10 days, at which time mobilization is begun. Progressive exercises, including both active and passive extension, are used to regain full range of motion and to correct flexion deformity. The elastic nature of the tissue allows postoperative stretching to correct the flexion contracture. Interphalangeal joint flexion contractures can be expected to improve within a few weeks.

■ OUTCOMES

The greatest advantage of the volar advancement flap is the consistent restoration of normal or nearly normal sensibility to injured terminal digits. In several reported series involving a total of 134 digits, including both thumb tip and fingertip injuries and both primary and secondary reconstruction, sensibility was returned to normal or within 2 mm of the contralateral values in almost every case.[4,7-9,12]

The potential complications of the volar advancement flap include dorsal skin necrosis, dysesthesia or altered sensation, flexion contracture, and loss of the flap. Dorsal skin necrosis is a potential complication when using the flap in fingertip reconstruction. This can be avoided, however, by careful preservation of the bridging vessels. In the series of Macht and Watson[8] involving 69 digits (including 29 fingers), dorsal tip or flap necrosis was not observed. Superficial blistering of the dorsal skin of the finger may occur but usually heals spontaneously.

A 50% incidence of residual pain and local tenderness has been reported in one series of patients followed-up 6 months postoperatively.[4] This has not been a universal finding, however, and most patients return to work in about 6 weeks, without significant sensory impairment. Clinically significant flexion contracture has not been reported as being a problem. Macht and Watson[8] reported full range of motion or less than 5° of extension loss in all digits that were normal before surgery. A decrease or loss of the hyperextendability of the interphalangeal joint of the thumb is routinely observed but does not represent functional impairment.

The many advantages of the volar advancement flap and its relatively low incidence of complications make it a valuable technique in terminal digital reconstruction.

References

1. Centers for Disease Control: Occupational finger injuries—United States. 1982. MMWR, 1983: 33:589–591.
2. Chase RA: Skin and Soft Tissue. Atlas of Hand Surgery, Vol 2, Philadelphia, WB Saunders Co, 1984, p. 15.
3. Dellon AL: The extended palmar advancement flap. J Hand Surg, 1983; 8:190–194.
4. DeSmet L, Kinnen L, Moermans JP, Ceuterick P, Van Wetter P: Fingertip amputations: distal or advancement flaps. Acta Orthop Belg, 1989; 55:177–182.
5. Flint MH: Some observations on the vascular supply of the nail bed and terminal segments of the finger. Br J Plast Surg, 1956; 8:186–195.
6. House JH: Modification of volar advancement flap. American Society for Surgery of the Hand Newsletter. No. 1982:14, February, 1982 p. 14.
7. Keim HA, Grantham SA: Volar flap advancement for thumb and fingertip injuries. Clin Orthop, 1969; 66:109–112.
8. Macht SD, Watson HK: The Moberg volar advancement flap for digital reconstruction. J Hand Surg, 1980; 5:372–376.
9. Millender LH, Albin RE, Nalebuff EA: Delayed volar advancement flap for thumb tip injuries. Plast Reconstr Surg, 1973; 52:635–639.
10. Moberg E: Aspects of sensation in reconstructive surgery of the upper extremity. J Bone Joint Surg, 1964; 46A: 817–825.
11. O'Brien B: Neurovascular island pedicle flaps for terminal amputations and digital scars. Br J Plast Surg, 1968; 21: 258–261.
12. Posner MA, Smith RJ: The advancement pedicle for thumb injuries. J Bone Joint Surg, 1971; 53A:1618–1621.
13. Rose EH, Norris MS, Kowalski TA: Microsurgical management of complex fingertip injuries: comparison to conventional skin grafting. J Reconstr Microsurg, 1988; 4:89–98.
14. Shaw MH: Neurovascular island pedicled flaps for terminal scars—a hazard. Br J Plast Surg, 1974; 24:161–165.
15. Snow JW: Use of a volar flap for repair of fingertip amputations. Plast Reconstr Surg, 1967; 40:163–168.

EDWARD R. CALKINS
DAVID J. SMITH, JR.

7

The Cross-Finger Flap

■ HISTORY OF THE TECHNIQUE

The technique of the cross-finger flap permits the transfer of a delayed skin flap from the dorsum of an adjacent finger to the palmar or dorsal side of the injured finger. It was developed for coverage of wounds having exposed tendon or bone or extensive loss of the fibrofatty tissues on the palmar side of the finger.[5,26] Before its development, such palmar and dorsal finger injuries were managed with cross-arm flaps, thoracic or abdominal flaps, or amputation; for fingertip injuries having exposed bone, the wounds were allowed to close secondarily or were covered with thenar flaps, or the finger was shortened and the soft tissues closed.[9,26] The cross-arm, thoracic, or abdominal flaps are cumbersome for patients, and children are nearly impossible to immobilize during the delay period. The tissue these flaps provide is bulky and poorly matched for the hand. Thenar flaps notoriously leave persistently painful scars that restrict the activities of manual laborers. Digital amputation or shortening can affect agility, strength, and aesthetic form.

In 1950, Gurdin and Pangman made the first written report on experience with the cross-finger flap.[9] Cronin published a more extensive report in 1951 and claimed priority by referring in that paper to a 1949 scientific exhibit in which he presented the procedure.[5] In 1951, Tempest presented an exhaustive paper concerning the coverage of fingertip injuries with the flap, which was published the following year.[26] Other authors have described various modifications of the procedure for use in special circumstances. Several groups have described a radial-innervated index finger–based flap for coverage of the thumb tip;[1,3,7,11,18,24] others have described an innervated cross-finger flap for the other fingers.[2,4] A de-epithelialized cross-finger flap has been described for coverage an of adjacent finger dorsal wound.[22,23]

■ INDICATIONS AND CONTRAINDICATIONS

The cross-finger pedicle flap was primarily developed for the closure of palmar finger wounds that could not be satisfactorily closed by simpler means, such as skin graft or Z-plasty. It is a reliable method for replacing lost or severely scarred skin and subcutaneous tissue. The flap is particularly well suited for coverage of wounds having exposed tendon or bone. It may be used for coverage of the acute injury site[6,8] or for coverage after secondary reconstruction.[6] In either situation, the wound must be adequately prepared by appropriate debridement and bacterial control. Examples of indications for its use include 1) coverage of the soft-tissue deficit resulting from flexor tenolysis and proximal interphalangeal joint capsulotomy for a severe flexion contracture; 2) replacement of badly scarred soft-tissue over the palmar aspect of the finger in preparation for later staged flexor tendon grafting; 3) acute coverage of an exposed, injured flexor tendon after an avulsion injury of the palmar skin and fat of the finger; and 4) coverage of a severe "knuckle" abrasion, with loss of dorsal skin, subcutaneous fat, extensor mechanism, and an open proximal interphalangeal joint.

Because it provides padded but thin coverage, the cross-finger flap may also be indicated for closure of fingertip and pulp injuries.[5,13–15,23,26,27] The flap provides one method of preserving digital length, particularly in oblique injuries having significant pulp loss. Reports on the quality of sensory recovery in the flap vary and are discussed further under "Outcomes." Some authors have recommended direct re-innervation of the flap by transferring a dorsal digital nerve with the flap and performing a microneurorrhaphy with a terminal branch of the digital nerve of the injured finger.[2,4] The index, middle, or ring finger could be the donor for innervated resurfacing of the thumb tip using this method.

A dorsal digital branch of the radial cutaneous nerve can be elevated from an index finger–based cross-finger flap and transposed to the ulnar side of the thumb for immediate restoration of sensation.[1,3,7,11,18,24] This procedure requires cortical reorganization for correct sensory perception. Also, the presence of the intact sensory axons in the flap may inhibit neurotization or suppress axonal activity within the flap by the median-derived thumb digital nerves.[16,19,21,28]

In addition to providing coverage for palmar digital injuries, a laterally based dorsal flap can be de-epithelialized, then turned over onto an open wound having exposed extensor mechanism or bone or having an open joint on the adjacent finger.[22] The donor site and the flap are both grafted. This flap has also been used as a vascularized vein-graft carrier.[17] A proximally or distally based transposition flap can also be designed for coverage of extensor surface wounds.[5,6]

Horn warns that use of the flap in patients who have arthritis or Dupuytren's disease might result in persistent stiffness.[10] As long as the surgeon and patient recognize the risk and act to minimize its impact, we believe that the cross-finger flap could be used in carefully selected patients who have arthritis or Dupuytren's disease. There may be an increased risk of flap infarction in patients having vasospastic syndromes and in those having diabetes mellitus.[10,13] We use the flap in patients having diabetes mellitus who have no evidence of vascular insufficiency or peripheral neuropathy in the hand. Caution should be used in older patients, in whom irreversible joint stiffness may follow;[14] one group has denied the procedure to patients older than 45, but they do not divide the pedicle until 21 days.[12] Exercising care in the design and elevation of the flap and dividing the pedicle within 2 weeks extends the age range well beyond 45 years.[13,15] Although some argue against the use of the cross-finger flap in younger children,[14] we and others believe that with adequate immobilization using either a long-arm cast or Kirschner wire fixation, no lower age limit exists.[27]

Patients with fingertip injuries and a more proximal nerve or soft-tissue injury of the finger have a markedly reduced rate of sensory return to a cross-finger flap.[15] These patients' fingertip wounds may be more suitably closed by another method. A shortened digit may be preferable to an insensate or hyperesthetic tip. Closure by secondary intention has a major role in many fingertip injuries.

■ SURGICAL TECHNIQUES

The anesthetic method should be determined by the predicted length of the procedure and by whether procedures are necessary in areas other than the affected upper extremity. In most cases, a Bier block or an axillary block is appropriate. For the appropriately selected patient, the procedure can even be performed under digital block. Children should be operated on under general anesthesia.

The procedure must be performed using tourniquet control and the aid of magnifying loupes. Meticulous hemostasis must be maintained with bipolar cautery. The flap should be handled with delicate skin hooks only.

The surgeon should concentrate first on the wound to be covered. The acute wound should be irrigated and debrided of any devitalized tissue or foreign material. The chronic wound should be restored to its acute state. Elevate and freshen the wound margins and excise or incise contracted scar tissue to restore the wound to its original dimensions. Excise wounds such that the longitudinal borders of the flap will cross any joints in a zigzag fashion; this reduces the chance of subsequent scar contracture over the joint. Make a template of the wound with a piece of glove paper or a foil suture package.

The cross-finger flap is most often described as a laterally based flap raised over the dorsal aspect of the middle phalanx. A cross-finger flap can also be proximally or distally based, and it can be elevated from the dorsal or lateral surface of the finger. It also can be raised over the proximal or middle phalanx.[6,23,26] This description, however, concentrates on the classically described laterally based flap (Fig. 7–1A through C); the principles discussed here can be applied to various forms of the flap. Selection of the flap design is based on the location and configuration of the wound.

Choose the finger adjacent to the injured finger that is easiest to position as the flap donor. Use the template to select the optimal location and orientation of the flap, then

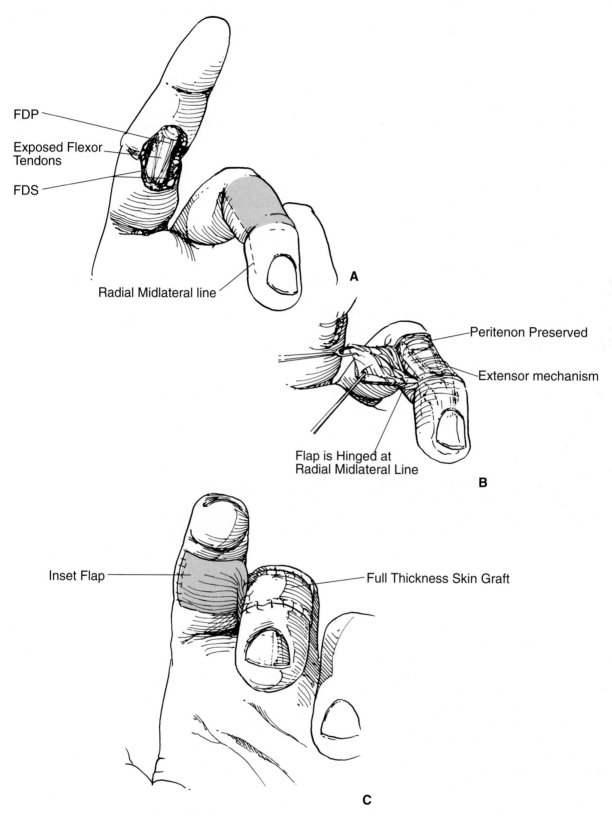

FDP

Exposed Flexor Tendons

FDS

Radial Midlateral line

A

Peritenon Preserved

Extensor mechanism

Flap is Hinged at Radial Midlateral Line

B

Inset Flap

Full Thickness Skin Graft

C

■ FIGURE 7–1

A, The exposed flexor tendons of the index finger require coverage with well-vascularized pliable soft tissue. For wound coverage, the classic cross-finger flap is outlined over the dorsal surface of the middle-finger middle phalanx. Basing the flap more proximally permits easier insetting and immobilization; it also lessens the chance of a postoperative proximal interphalangeal joint contracture of the middle finger. This could be raised as an "aesthetic unit" between the proximal and distal extensor creases of the middle-finger proximal interphalangeal joint. **B,** The flap is raised with its distal edge at the ulnar mid-lateral line, and it is hinged at the radial midlateral line. The paratenon overlying the extensor mechanism is carefully preserved. **C,** Because this wound involves a joint surface, the wound is debrided back to the mid-lateral line on each side to prevent flexion contracture of the longitudinal scars. The flap is inset and the donor site covered with a full-thickness skin graft.

outline the template over the dorsum of the adjacent finger. Usually, a laterally based flap is raised over the dorsum of the middle phalanx. The template outline is oriented so that it can be easily transposed to the wound when the flap is raised. The flap margins are drawn to incorporate the template outline. Position the hinge at precisely the mid-lateral line on the side of the finger adjacent to the wounded finger. Position the distal margin at precisely the mid-lateral line on the opposite side. The transverse margins of the flap are ideally situated just distal to the proximal interphalangeal joint and just proximal to the distal interphalangeal joint. Skin grafting of this entire "aesthetic unit" of the finger yields a cosmetic result that is superior to grafting of a smaller area. If necessary to provide adequate tissue, however, the proximal transverse margin can be moved farther proximally to incorporate the skin over the proximal interphalangeal joint and the proximal phalanx.[6]

Make incisions through the skin and subcutaneous tissues. Extend the incision down to the paratenon overlying the extensor mechanism. This layer must be preserved. Elevate the flap between the paratenon and the subcutaneous tissue, beginning at the mid-lateral incision and progressing toward the opposite mid-lateral hinge. Avoid injury to the under-surface of the dorsal veins as you elevate the flap. When an innervated flap is planned, be sure to isolate and raise a segment of the dorsal cutaneous nerve branch proximal to its entry into the proximal flap margin (Fig. 7–2).

The skin is anchored to the finger by multiple ligamentous fibers. When the flap extends over the proximal interphalangeal joint, the surgeon must cut the peritendinous fibers that bind the skin to the extensor mechanism. To each lateral side of the extensor mechanism, cutaneous extensions of the oblique retinacular ligament, the transverse retinacular ligament and the lateral band must be cut. Near the base of the flap, Cleland's cutaneous ligaments must be cut to provide full mobility to the flap.

With the flap completely elevated, release the tourniquet and obtain hemostasis. Next,

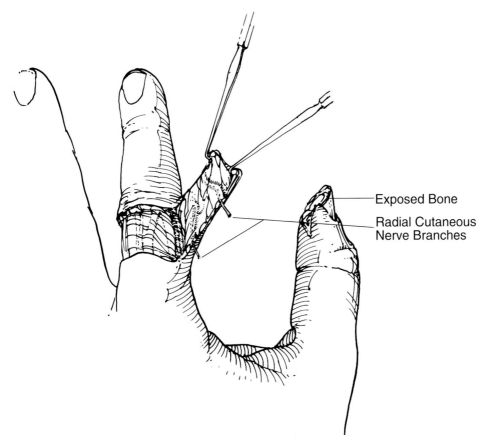

Exposed Bone

Radial Cutaneous
Nerve Branches

■ FIGURE 7–2
The thumb has an extensive, oblique pulp amputation, with bone exposed over the ulnar and palmar surfaces. This has resulted in a critical loss of sensory surface. A radially based cross-finger flap is raised over the proximal phalanx of the index finger. Two branches of the radial cutaneous nerve are isolated proximal to the proximal margin and divided. Under the operating microscope, these are coapted to distal branches or fascicles of the thumb ulnar digital nerve.

provisionally inset it to the wound on the adjacent finger. Trim the flap concentrically with the wound margins; be sure to leave additional skin outside the original template outline to allow tension-free closure. Inset the flap with interrupted fine nylon sutures.

Obtain a full-thickness skin graft from the ipsilateral antecubital fossa or medial arm. We find that these sites provide a good color match. Some prefer to obtain the graft from the groin but this darker skin results in an unattractive color mismatch. Meticulously defat the skin. Suture it into place over the flap donor site and the flap hinge with fine chromic gut sutures. Some secure the graft with a bolster. We find that a well-contoured wet cotton dressing provides more reliable and even pressure application and superior protection from shear.

Dress the wounds with a nonadherent porous fabric [e.g., Nterface (Winfield Labs, Richardson, TX)]. Be sure to place cotton or another soft absorbent material between all the fingers to prevent maceration. Pad the fingers and palm with cotton. Moisten the cotton and contour it over the skin-graft site. Secure this in place with cast padding, and apply a palmar splint. We immobilize the hand in the intrinsic-plus position, with some necessary modification to prevent tension on the flap. Wrap the splint with 4-inch bias-cut stockinet. In children, additional immobilization is necessary. We use a long-arm cast, with the elbow flexed 90°. Others use Kirschner wires drilled transversely from the proximal to the middle phalanx of the tethered fingers. Instruct the patient to keep the hand elevated above their heart.

The flap is divided after a 10- to 14-day delay. Longer delays are unnecessary and contribute to finger stiffness. Flap division should also be performed in the operating room to allow elevation of the wound margin and meticulous insetting of the divided flap edge. In adults, the procedure can be performed with digital blockade anesthesia; children should receive general anesthesia. Cover the wounds with only a light nonadherent dressing that does not interfere with motion.

Dorsal finger wounds can be covered with proximally or distally based cross-finger flaps or with a de-epithelialized laterally based, turn-over, cross-finger flap. When performing a de-epithelialized cross-finger flap, try to raise the epithelium and some dermis in a single piece, so that it can be replaced on the donor or recipient digit. Cover the remaining defect with a full-thickness skin graft.

■ TECHNICAL
ALTERNATIVES

For fingertip injuries, alternative methods of treatment include healing by secondary intention, bone shortening and primary closure, skin grafts, V-Y flaps, volar advancement flaps, palmar flaps, distant pedicle flaps, composite grafting, microneurovascular replantation, and microneurovascular toe pulp or onycho-osteocutaneous transfer. More proximal wounds that are not amenable to primary closure or skin grafting may be closed with V-Y flaps, neurovascular island flaps, distant pedicle flaps, or several forms of microvascular free-tissue transfer.

Several technical errors may result in an unsatisfactory outcome. These can occur at each stage of the operation, including wound-site preparation, flap design, flap elevation and insetting, and flap division. Such errors may produce immediate consequences, such as flap necrosis, or late consequences, such as joint contracture.

Failure to excise a wound overlying a joint in a zigzag fashion or back to the mid-lateral line results in placement of the longitudinal margins of the flap over the joint. This results in contracture of the scar between the flap and the native skin. Secondary release of such a contracture can be exceedingly difficult.

Failure to use a wound template and to carefully orient and design the flap can result in a flap that simply does not reach all of the wound margins. This can be avoided by transposing the wound template between the wound and the donor sites. If the template does not reach, neither will the flap.

It is critical to maintain a wide base (the hinge) when designing this random-pattern flap. Designs that require back-cuts or a tapered hinge greatly increase the risk of flap necrosis. For the same reason, the surgeon must prevent tension or torquing across the flap base.

Raise the flap as an aesthetic unit whenever possible. Full-thickness skin grafts placed over complete aesthetic units usually result in remarkably inconspicuous donor sites. Conversely, a skin graft placed over a segment of the aesthetic unit is invariably ugly.

Be careful not to divide the delayed flap too closely to the recipient side. The flap is usually bulky and stiff from edema at this stage. The surgeon needs a generous margin on the flap to inset its proximal longitudinal border. An insufficient margin may result in an incompletely covered wound or in a longitudinal scar over a joint.

Postoperative rehabilitation, including the home program, should be discussed with the patient preoperatively. When possible, the patient should also meet the hand therapist preoperatively. If other injuries do not contraindicate it, the patient should begin a hand therapy program immediately after the second stage of the procedure. Initial activities should include active and passive range of motion and edema control. Patients who have had a sensory index to thumb cross-finger flap should begin a sensory re-education program. Later, patients require instruction in scar massage; some may need pressure garments fitted if hypertrophic scarring develops. Patients also need assistance in a desensitization program.

■ REHABILITATION

There is little disagreement that given a well-designed and carefully inset flap and skin graft, this technique provides a satisfactory aesthetic result.[12,15] In lightly pigmented patients, it provides an excellent color match; however, in deeply pigmented patients it may result in a patchwork-quilt effect. It provides a durable and reliable surface for the finger.[12] Hyperesthesia of the flap rarely occurs. Sensory return and restoration of full joint mobility are less reliable, however.

■ OUTCOMES

Most patients who undergo a noninnervated cross-finger flap have return of protective sensation (8 mm two-point discrimination)[20] but the sensation in the flap remains less than that in normal pulp. The two-point discrimination distance in the flap is about twice that in normal pulp.[25] The return of sensation is best and most predictable in younger patients (younger than 20).[15,20] In patients older than 40, only about half regain protective sensation.[15] The potential for sensory return is significantly compromised by seroma or infection beneath the flap during early healing.[15] Bacterial control of the wound and meticulous operative technique are critical to the immediate and long-range outcome of the procedure.

Patients who are without concomitant finger injuries, who have a minimum delay before pedicle division, and who begin range-of-motion therapy immediately after the second-stage procedure usually regain full joint motion.[13,15] This is true even in older patients. Early flap division and a routine well-organized postoperative hand therapy program are the variables that the surgeon can readily influence to improve range-of-motion outcome.

Patients who work at manual labor can return to work after an average of about 70 days;[13] there are some patients who require more time to return to work, particularly those having associated injuries. People with physically sedentary jobs may return to work earlier.

References

1. Adamson JE, Horton C, Crawford H: Sensory rehabilitation of the injured thumb. Plast Reconstr Surg, 1967; 40:53–57.
2. Berger A, Meissl G: Innervated skin grafts and flaps for restoration of sensation to anesthetic areas. Chir Plastica (Berlin), 1975; 3:33–37.
3. Bralliar F, Horner RL: Sensory cross-finger pedicle graft. J Bone Joint Surg, 1969; 51A: 1264–1268.
4. Cohen BE, Cronin ED: An innervated cross-finger flap for fingertip reconstruction. Plast Reconstr Surg, 1983; 72:688–697.
5. Cronin TD: The cross finger flap: a new method of repair. Am Surg, 1951; 17:419–425.
6. Curtis RM: Cross-finger pedicle flap in hand surgery. Ann Surg, 1957; 145:650–655.

7. Gaul JS Jr: Radial-innervated cross-finger flap from index to provide sensory pulp to injured thumb. J Bone Joint Surg, 1969; 51A:1257–1263.
8. Gault DT, Quaba AA: The role of cross-finger flaps in the primary management of untidy flexor tendon injuries. J Hand Surg, 1988; 13B:62–65.
9. Gurdin M, Pangman WJ: The repair of surface defects of fingers by transdigital flaps. Plast Reconstr Surg, 1950; 5:368–371.
10. Horn JS: The use of full thickness skin flaps in the reconstruction of injured fingers. Plast Reconstr Surg, 1951; 7:463–481.
11. Holevich J: A new method of restoring sensibility to the thumb. J Bone Joint Surg, 1963; 45B: 496–502.
12. Johnson RK, Iverson RE: Cross-finger pedicle flaps in hand surgery. J Bone Joint Surg, 1971; 53A:913–919.
13. Kappel DA, Burech JG: The cross-finger flap: an established reconstructive procedure. Hand Clin, 1985; 1:677–683.
14. Kislov R, Kelly AP Jr: Cross-finger flaps in digital injuries, with notes on Kirschner wire fixation. Plast Reconstr Surg, 1960; 25:312–322.
15. Kleinert HE, McAlister CG, MacDonald CJ, Kutz JE: A critical evaluation of cross finger flaps. J Trauma, 1974; 14:756–763.
16. Lo Y-J, Poo M-M: Activity-dependent synaptic competition in vitro: heterosynaptic suppression of developing synapses. Science, 1991; 254:1019–1022.
17. Martin DL, Kaplan IB, Kleinert JM: Use of a reverse cross-finger flap as a vascularized vein graft carrier in ring avulsion injuries. J Hand Surg, 1990; 15A:1555–159.
18. Miura T: Thumb reconstruction using radial-innervated cross-finger pedicle graft. J Bone Joint Surg, 1973; 55A:563–569.
19. Murphy RK, Lemeere CA: Competition controls the growth of an identified axonal arborization. Science, 1984; 224:1352–1355.
20. Nicolai JPA, Hentenaar G: Sensation in cross-finger flaps. Hand, 1981; 13:12–16.
21. Riddle DR, Hughes SE, Belczynski CR, DeSibour CL, Oakley B: Inhibitory interactions among rodent taste axons. Brain Res, 1990; 533:113–124.
22. Robbins TH: The use of de-epithelialised cross-finger flaps for dorsal finger defects. Br J Plast Surg, 1985; 38:407–409.
23. Russell RC, Van Beek AL, Wavak P, Zook EG: Alternative hand flaps for amputations and digital defects. J Hand Surg, 1981; 6:399–405.
24. Rybka FJ, Pratt FE: Thumb reconstruction with a sensory flap from the dorsum of the index finger. Plast Reconstr Surg, 1979; 64:141–144.
25. Smith JR, Bom AF: An evaluation of fingertip reconstruction by cross-finger and palmar flap. Plast Reconstr Surg, 1965; 35:409–418.
26. Tempest MN: Cross-finger flaps in the treatment of injuries to the finger tip. Plast Reconstr Surg, 1952; 9:205–222.
27. Thomson HG, Sorokolit WT: The cross-finger flap in children: a follow-up study. Plast Reconstr Surg, 1967; 39:482–487.
28. Walker MA, Hurley CB, May JW Jr: Radial nerve cross-finger flap differential nerve contribution in thumb reconstruction. J Hand Surg, 1986; 11A:881–887.

8

Thenar Flaps

Reconstruction of a distal volar index finger soft tissue defect with exposed profundus tendon using a flap from the thenar eminence was first described by Gatewood[6] in a 1926 case report in the *Journal of the American Medical Association.* Interestingly, Gatewood was a Chicago general surgeon who had only one name. He described a "horseshoe shaped flap," which was ulnarly based and elevated off the thenar eminence. It was "planned so that when reflected, the blood supply would be interfered with as little as possible." He did not mention what he did with the donor site defect, which apparently was allowed to heal by secondary intention.

A number of other closure options were advocated in the literature after 1926, including full-thickness Wolfe grafts by O'Malley[13] in 1934, lateral V-Y advancement flaps by Kutler[9] in 1947, local cross finger pedicle flaps from the dorsal surface of an adjacent digit by Gurdin[7] in 1950 and Cronin[3] in 1951. The thenar flap was again rediscovered by Adrian Flatt[4,5] in 1955, and the technique more fully detailed in a 1957 article in the *British Journal of Bone and Joint Surgery.* Dr. Flatt initially described the technique as a "palmar flap" in 1955 but changed the name to a "thenar flap" in his 1957 description of the technique. He described a proximally based thenar flap, which "should not be more than twice it's width," that was elevated off the thenar eminence with "about two thirds of the thickness of the subcutaneous fat carried on the flap." The rest was left behind as a bed for a split-thickness skin graft from the forearm that he used to close the palmar donor site. Flatt advised against flexing the injured digit too far into the palm, elevating the flap too much toward the ulnar side of the hand, dividing the flap too early before adequate revascularization had occurred or too late leading to stiffness of the reconstructed digit.

Barton,[2] in 1975, presented a modification of the technique similar to the original description by Gatewood, using an ulnarly based square shaped flap but elevated from closer to the metacarpophalangeal (MP) joint flexion crease. This was said to require "slightly less flexion" of the injured digit and was "easier to apply the split thickness graft to the donor area."

In 1976, Smith and Albin[16] described an alternative donor site closure method for the thenar flap using an H-shaped incision over the thenar eminence. Proximally and distally based flaps were elevated and advanced toward each other to cover the fingertip, which was immobilized for 14 to 17 days. The proximal flap was then detached proximally and the distal flap was detached from the finger. The divided proximal flap was then sutured to the volar edge of the fingertip defect to close the finger, and the detached distal flap was advanced proximally to close the donor defect in the palm. This technique avoided a palmar skin graft and the "risk of painful scarring."

Most recently, in 1993, with the advent of microsurgery, Kemei and co-authors[8] in Japan described two cases of fingertip reconstruction using a free thenar flap based on the superficial palmar branch of the radial artery and the palmar cutaneous branch of the median nerve. The flap vessel is identified before elevation with a Doppler flow probe, and the donor site can be closed primarily. This flap has the advantage of a primary nerve repair to one of the cut digital nerves of the injured digit and has the potential for improved sensibility. The disadvantage is the exacting technique necessary to dissect and repair the 1 mm superficial palmar branch of the radial artery, its vena comitans and the palmar cutaneous branch of the median nerve.

■ HISTORY OF THE TECHNIQUE

Traumatic amputation of a fingertip is the most commonly seen upper extremity injury. A number of closure options have been reported in the literature, including skin grafts,[10,13,14] local V-Y advancement flaps,[1,9,14] volar advancement flaps,[11,12,14] or cross finger flaps from the dorsal or lateral surface of an adjacent digit.[3,7,14,15,17] Another option for fingertip closure is a flap elevated from the palm of the hand, either from the thenar eminence, the mid-palm, the MP joint flexion crease or the hypothenar eminence. The injured digit must be flexed into the palm, and, therefore, these flaps are best suited for younger patients with supple digits—especially children. They are best used for traumatic amputations of the fingertip that are angled volarly with exposure of the tuft of the distal phalanx. The amount of soft tissue loss in the digit is critical in determining whether a palmar flap should be used for fingertip reconstruction. A defect that involves two thirds of the volar soft tissue pad or less is ideally suited for a palmar flap. A smaller tip defect can be closed with an MP flexion crease flap. A defect that involves the entire volar surface of the digit is probably better treated by using a cross finger flap. Digits that have sustained multiple tissue injuries with fractures or divided digital arteries, nerves, or tendons are less suitable for closure of fingertip defects using a palmar flap because prolonged stiffness may result from immobilization of the digit in the palm.

The sensory receptor sites present in glabrous skin, namely Pacinian and Meisners corpuscles and Merkel cell neurite discs, are present only in glabrous skin making it the preferred tissue for fingertip reconstruction. Elderly patients or those with systemic disease resulting in digital stiffness such as arthritis or Dupuytren's contracture are usually not candidates for the prolonged immobilization required with a palmar flap. Patients with decreased peripheral blood flow such as those with collagen vascular disease or diabetes mellitus also are poor candidates for pedicle flap closure of fingertip injuries.

Palmar flaps are best done using an arm or forearm tourniquet and general or regional block anesthesia. The injured digit must be thoroughly debrided of macerated or severely contaminated tissue before proceeding with flap closure. I use a hand-held spray bottle to thoroughly irrigate the fingertip wound before and after the skin edges and subcutaneous tissue are carefully debrided with iris scissors before flap coverage. The tuft of the distal phalanx also may require some debridement to the level of the remaining dorsal nailbed. The injured digit is then flexed into the palm to determine the best location and type of palmar flap that can be used for fingertip closure.

The best option for closure of a fingertip amputation on a radial digit is to elevate a flap from the MP joint flexion crease of the thumb.[14,15] The donor site is clearly visible in most individuals; it is the skin between the two creases formed by flexing the MP joint of the thumb or finger. The flap is radially based and elevated to a width of 1 to 2 cm (Fig. 8–1A). It can be extended to a length of 3 to 4 cm around the base of the thumb (Fig. 8–1B). The distal end of the flap is tapered to facilitate primary donor site closure (Fig. 8–1C). It is elevated at the level of the flexor pollicis longus tendon and the neurovascular bundles, which should be identified, protected, and left in place. This flap is best used for distal tip loss and does not provide as much tissue volume as is possible with standard palmar flaps. The flap easily reaches the index and long fingertips and in some patients the ring and small digits. The donor site is closed primarily by flexing the thumb at the MP joint and avoids a palmar scar (Fig. 8–1D). The injured digit also is held in less flexion than is required for a palmar flap, decreasing the chances of residual digital stiffness. The thumb regains full extension after healing and the donor site is nearly invisible. All thenar flaps require the digit to be immobilized with a splint for 12 to 18 days using a dorsal plaster or thermoplastic splint.

A standard thenar or hypothenar flap is done by flexing the injured fingertip into the palm, and the dimensions of the flap are determined by the size and shape of the fingertip defect. A proximal or distally based thenar flap, slightly larger than the fingertip defect is elevated at the level of the muscle fascia (Fig. 8–2A). The finger is flexed into the palm to rest in a relaxed position. The corner of the digital defect can be sutured to the edge of the donor defect in the palm with a 4-0 nylon suture to reduce tension on the flap (Fig.

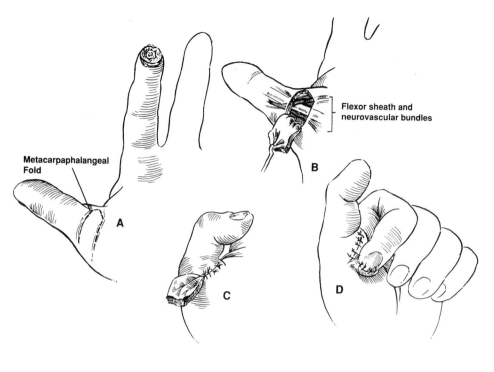

■ FIGURE 8–1
A, A radially based flap is outlined in the metacarpophalangeal flexion crease of the thumb. **B,** The flap is elevated at the level of the flexor pollicis longus tendon, exposing the digital nerves and arteries. **C,** The donor site is closed primarily by slight flexion of the thumb at the MP joint. **D,** The flap is sutured across the defect on the injured finger, which is held in less flexion than with standard palmar flaps.

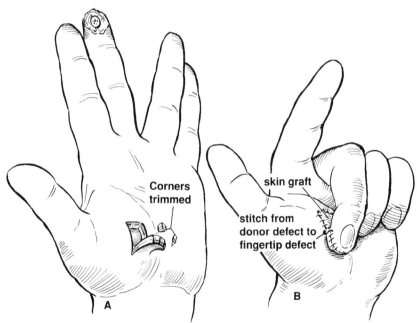

■ FIGURE 8–2
A, A standard thenar flap is proximally based and elevated at the level of the thenar muscle fascia. The flap tip can be trimmed to fit the exact contour of the defect on the tip of the injured finger. **B,** The finger is flexed into the palm and the donor site is closed with a skin graft.

8–2B). The flap is sutured to the tip defect with 5-0 nylon sutures, and the donor site is closed with a split-thickness skin graft from the hypothenar eminence or a full-thickness skin graft from the wrist or groin. The tourniquet is released and the blood supply to the flap determined by observation. To preserve adequate blood supply, the base of the flap must not be excessively kinked or folded. A similar flap can be elevated from the hypothenar eminence to close digital defects on the ulnar digits.

An H-shaped incision to raise the donor flap was described by Smith and Albin.[16] This technique can be improved by using the entire proximally based flap to cover the fingertip defect at the first surgery. The distally based flap is advanced proximally to close the donor defect by excising small Burrows triangles from the edges of the advancement flap

■ FIGURE 8-3
A, A modification of the technique described by Smith and Albin is to incise two flaps in an H shape with small Burrows triangles cut at the base of the distal flap. **B,** The proximal flap is turned in a standard fashion to cover the fingertip while the distal flap is advanced proximally to close the donor defect at one operation.

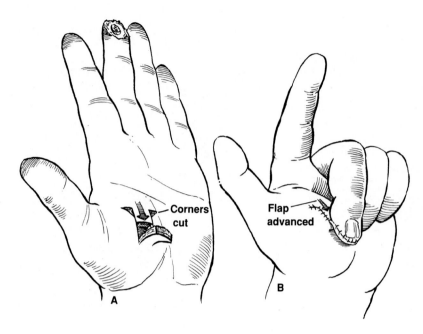

■ FIGURE 8-4
A, A modification of the thenar technique described by Swartz, especially good for ulnar digits, is a proximally based flap elevated from the thenar eminence flexion crease in the palm. **B,** The donor site is closed primarily by adducting the thumb.

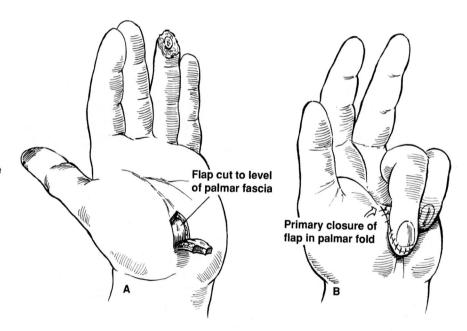

to facilitate proximal movement and primary donor site closure (Fig. 8–3A). More of the proximal flap can be attached to the fingertip, increasing the area of inset and improving the chances of revascularization (Fig. 8–3B).

Swartz (personal communication) uses a modification of the thenar flap for ulnar digits by elevating a proximally based palmar flap from the thenar crease area (Fig. 8–4A). This flap is planned in a similar fashion by flexing the injured digit into the center of the palm. The flap is designed to a maximum width of 2 cm along the thenar crease and is tapered distally. It is elevated at the level of the palmar fascia including the skin and palmar fat. The palmar skin edges are undermined slightly allowing the donor site to be closed primarily by slightly adducting the thumb (Fig. 8–4B).

■ TECHNICAL
ALTERNATIVES

The tourniquet should always be released to be sure the attached flap has sufficient blood supply. All thenar flaps from any location in the palm have the disadvantage of leaving a scar or skin graft in the palm, which, on rare occasions, can be symptomatic, especially in patients who use their hands for laboring activities. The authors preference for fingertip closure from the palm is an MP joint flap.

The MP flexion crease flap has the disadvantage of providing less volume of tissue than is possible with standard thenar flaps. Injury to the digital arteries and nerves of the thumb are possible if careful dissection of the flap is not performed at the level of the flexor pollicis tendon sheath.

The advantages of the MP joint flexion crease flap are that less flexion is required to inset the injured digit into the flap and the donor site is virtually invisible as a straight line over the volar surface of the MP joint of the thumb.

All thenar flaps require immobilization of the digit for 12 to 18 days, using a dorsal plaster or thermoplastic splint. Early active and passive range of motion is encouraged after the flap is divided and inset to prevent digital stiffness and to restore full thumb motion. Hand therapy to restore motion is especially important in all patients. All thenar flaps provide digital resurfacing with glabrous skin, which may regain better sensibility and function than nonglabrous skin from dorsal cross finger flaps. Patients may later require sensory reorientation and desensitization instruction for painful scars. Scar massage and pressure garments are used when necessary.

■ REHABILITATION

In my practice, patients who have undergone fingertip reconstruction using palmar or thenar crease flaps have regained good sensibility in the flap that is less than normal but appears to be greater than is achieved in standard cross finger flaps. Glabrous skin fingertip reconstructions usually provide stable soft tissue coverage, which permits individuals who perform manual labor to return to work. Some residual digital stiffness has been observed in older patients, especially males with thick heavy hands. Other types of digital reconstruction may be less likely to cause stiffness. Complications from the procedure are infrequent if care is taken to provide precise surgical technique and gentle handling of tissue.

■ OUTCOMES

References

1. Atasoy E, Ioakimidis E, Kasdan ML, Kutz JE, Kleinert HE: Reconstruction of the amputated finger tip with a triangular volar flap: a new surgical procedure. J Bone Joint Surg, 1970; 52A: 921–926.
2. Barton NJ: A modified thenar flap. Hand, 1975; 7:150–151.
3. Cronin TD: The cross finger flap: a new method of repair. Am Surg, 1951; 17:419–425.
4. Flatt AE: Minor hand injuries with bone joint surgery. J Bone Joint Surg, 1955; 37B:117–125.
5. Flatt AE: The thenar flap. J Bone Joint Surg, 1957; 39B:80–85.
6. Gatewood: A plastic repair of finger defects without hospitalization. JAMA, 1926; 87:1479.
7. Gurdin M, Pangman WJ: The repair of surface defects of fingers by transdigital flaps. Plast Reconst Surg, 1951; 7:463–481.
8. Kamei K, Ide Y, Kimura T: A new free thenar flap. Plast Reconstr Surg, 1993; 92:1380–1384.
9. Kutler W: A new method for finger tip amputation. JAMA, 1947; 133:29–30.
10. Mandal AC: Thiersch grafts for lesions of the finger tip. Acta Chirg Scand, 1965; 129:325–332.
11. Moberg E: Aspects of sensation in reconstructive surgery of the upper extremity. J Bone Joint Surg, 1964; 46A:817–825.
12. O'Brien B: Neurovascular island pedicle flaps for terminal amputations and digital scars. Br J Plast Surg, 1968; 21:258–261.
13. O'Malley TS: Full thickness skin grafts in finger amputations. Wis Med J, 1934; 33:337–340.
14. Russell RC, Casas LA: Management of fingertip injuries. Clin Plast Surg, 1989; 16:3, 405–425.
15. Russell RC, VanBeek AC, Wavak P, et al: Alternative hand flaps for amputations and digital defects. J Hand Surg, 1981; 6:399–405.
16. Smith RJ, Albin R: Thenar "H-flap" for fingertip injuries. J Trauma, 1976; 16:778–781.
17. Tempest MN: Cross-finger flaps in the treatment of injuries to the finger tip. Plast Reconstr Surg, 1952; 9:205–222.

DON A. COLEMAN
STAN M. VALNICEK

9

Neurovascular Island Flaps

■ HISTORY OF THE
TECHNIQUE

Loss of sensation to the thumb pad can be a significant functional deficit because of the thumb's pivotal role in fine pinch and grasp activities. Normal pinch and grasp require intact sensation and the ability to discriminate objects held in the hand without visual input (tactile gnosis) as described by Moberg.[9] This function is impaired when there is loss of sensibility or loss of soft tissue, including sensory end organs in the thumb pad. When sensibility cannot be restored by nerve repair or reconstruction or when sensibility and padding are required, transfer of local innervated skin is indicated to restore function.

The concept of neurovascular island flaps for thumb reconstruction is based on Bunnel's[1] application of digit transfer on a neurovascular pedicle in 1928 and was first proposed by Moberg[9] in 1955. It was performed by Littler in 1956, and the first series standardizing the technique were reported by Littler[7] in 1960 and Tubiana and Duparc[15] in 1961. In 1964, Hueston[4] called the transfer of a sensory island of skin to an anesthetic area of the hand the most important development in hand surgery in the previous decade. Hueston extended the flap to include the whole territory of the palmar digital nerve, including the dorsal sensory branch, to allow thumb and first web reconstruction with flaps up to 6 × 2 to 3 cm in size. In 1968, Eaton[2] investigated the anatomy of the neurovascular pedicle and clarified the relation between the draining veins and the artery and nerve. Since that time, several authors have described refinement of clinical technique and indications and improved understanding of the complications and shortcomings.[3,5,10–12,14]

■ INDICATIONS AND
CONTRAINDICATIONS

Indications for neurovascular island flaps are: poor thumb pulp sensation after thumb replantation or osteoplastic reconstruction, large pulp defects where skeletal length is to be maintained and sensation is important, and irreversible loss of median nerve sensibility that cannot be reconstructed with standard nerve grafting techniques.[6,14] Most neurovascular island flaps are used in a reconstructive setting. Lister[6] has proposed immediate use for acute thumb pulp loss if three criteria are met: the pulp loss is the major injury, it is a recent and clean wound, and the surgeon is experienced in the technique. Care must be taken to ensure that flow exists to the relevant vessels irrespective of the timing of the reconstruction. Preoperative angiography or Doppler flow testing can help with this evaluation.

Neurovascular island flaps have several advantages. They transfer sensation to an anaesthetic region, including not only pressure, light touch, and movement but also tactile gnosis. The composition and distribution of sensory end organs in the island flap is a close match to the thumb pad. If proximal thenar digital nerve integrity exists, then neurorrhaphy to the donor digital nerve of the island flap can provide restoration of the original cortical pattern of sensibility. The island flap can reconstruct a larger area than the Moberg local advancement flap and does not require the microvascular expertise necessary for a toe pulp free tissue transfer. Neurovascular island flaps also can increase the vascularity of the recipient area with improvement of cold intolerance and wound healing. Finally, the transfer can provide durable cornified sweat-producing skin that improves tactile adhesion and usability.

Absolute contraindications for use of neurovascular island flaps are trauma to the palm or vascular pedicle, or presence of peripheral vascular disease. Relative contraindications are the presence of diabetes or connective tissue disease, absence of normal sensation in the donor skin, and lack of useful motion in the hand for grip or pinch.

The choice of a donor site depends on the nature of the neurologic deficit as well as the amount of innervated tissue required. The ulnar aspect of the ring finger is used most commonly and can be taken with the radial side of the small finger on the common digital nerve to reconstruct the first web space in addition to the thumb. The ulnar side of the long finger and radial side of the ring finger are both noncontact sides and provide longer arcs of pedicle rotation. They do require some intact median nerve sensation as opposed to flaps from the fourth web space. An ideal although rarely encountered donor site is well innervated and perfused skin from otherwise damaged fingers that are to be amputated.

The margins of the defect are marked out, and a pattern is transferred to the selected donor digit. In designing the flap on the donor digit, the distal incision should be 3 to 4 mm proximal to the midline of the nail plate. The standard margins of the flap are the palmar and lateral midlines of the finger. One may include skin dorsal to the lateral midline if the dorsal sensory branch of the digital nerve also is included. The proximal end should take into account the desired size of the flap as dictated by the recipient site pattern, and can be extended anywhere from the middle phalanx to a point that includes the entire web space. In acute injuries, the flap should be smaller to correct for the retracted skin edges at the recipient site.

Proximal to the flap, a midlateral incision is marked out to the base of the digit. This is extended to the midpalm with a zig-zag incision to allow exposure of the neurovascular pedicle. The recipient defect should be outlined but not incised until the island flap is raised and shown to be viable (Fig. 9–1).

Careful dissection is required to preserve the viability of the island flap and protect the deep structures. Knowledge of the relation of the neurovascular bundle to the flexor sheath and Grayson's ligaments is imperative. The dorsal sensory branch of the digital nerve must be identified and preserved to prevent loss of dorsal sensation and neuroma formation. One may wish to include this branch in the island flap if the posterior skin margin is posterior to the midlateral line. The communicating arterial branch to the deep arch usually joins the common digital artery at its bifurcation and must be carefully ligated. In tunneling the island flap across the palm, one must identify and protect the neurovascular bundles to the intervening digits.

The operation can be done under local anesthesia, but regional or general anesthesia are preferred. All dissection is performed under loupe magnification and tourniquet control. Incisions on the donor digit are designed as described previously. Sullivan and co-authors[5]

■ SURGICAL TECHNIQUES

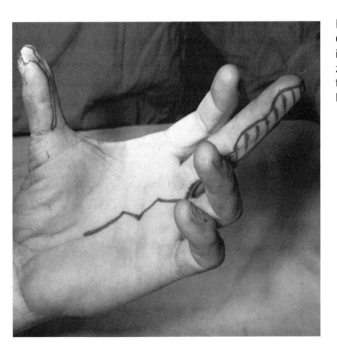

■ FIGURE 9–1
Outline of thumb defect, island flap, and proximal zig-zag incision. (All photos courtesy of Graham D. Lister, M.D.)

reported a 7% (3 of 41) incidence of the common digital artery to the ring-little web arising from the deep arch and thus having an inadequate arc of rotation for transfer. Exposure is therefore begun in the palm proximal to the donor web space to confirm the origin of the common digital artery from the superficial arch. The island flap is then incised and elevated from distal to proximal, and a generous cuff of subcutaneous tissue is left around the pedicle to preserve venous drainage (Fig. 9–2). The proper digital artery to the adjacent finger is ligated unless the flap includes the entire web (Fig. 9–3). The communicating branch to the palmar metacarpal artery of the deep arch is ligated next. The proper digital nerve is now dissected free of the dorsal sensory branch and the nerve to the adjacent digit down to the level of the superficial arch (Fig. 9–4). Risk exists that the digital artery may be kinked by the adjacent digital nerve (Figs. 9-5 and 9-6).[6] The dorsal sensory branch may be included as mentioned previously. At this point, the arc of rotation of the island flap must be determined. Mobilization must be continued until the flap can reach the abducted extended thumb pad without tension. A tunnel is fashioned from the palmar incision to the thumb defect. The tunnel should be in the plane below the superficial palmar fascia just distal to the transverse carpal ligament, and be brought out on the radial side of the first web (Fig. 9–7). Now the tourniquet can be released to obtain hemostasis and ascertain the viability of the flap. If the flap is robust, the excision of the thumb defect can proceed. The skin margins of the recipient site are undermined slightly to accept the flap. Extension of the thumb incision onto the first web may facilitate tunneling. If the skin quality of the excised segment is adequate, it may be used to skin graft the donor site. The tunnel should be assessed to confirm it is sufficient to easily accept the flap. The overlying skin may need to be released completely. Stay sutures are placed on either side of the flap to maintain its orientation during passage. One must avoid torsion, tension, and

■ FIGURE 9–2
Generous cuff of subcutaneous tissue left to preserve venous drainage.

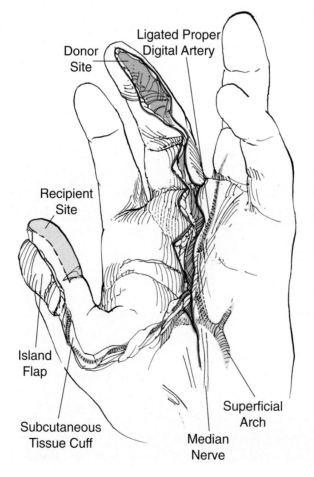

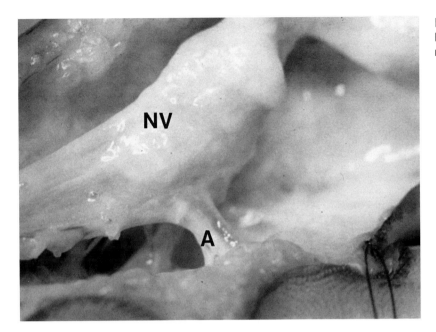

Proper digital artery to ring finger.

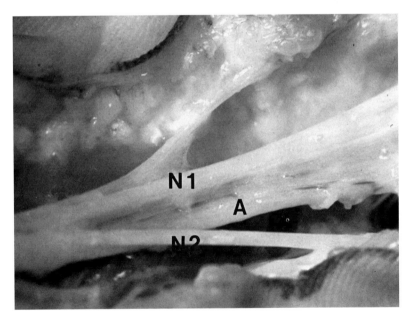

The common digital nerve split to the level of the superficial palmar arch.

kinking.[15] The flap may now be sutured in place loosely with nonabsorbable interrupted sutures. Tension should be assessed with the thumb in maximal abduction and extension. The remaining wounds can now be closed after re-exsanguinating the arm and inflating the tourniquet. The donor finger is closed with a full thickness skin graft with a tie-over dressing (Fig. 9–8).

The extremity is placed in a well padded dressing and protective splint with the hand in the position of safety. The thumb is maximally extended and abducted to allow healing and adhesion formation to the neurovascular bundle at full excursion. However, the surgeon must be careful to avoid excessive traction, which will cause vascular compromise. The tie-over on the donor finger is removed after 1 to 2 weeks. The recipient site should be inspected regularly in the first 48 hours for signs of ischemia or venous congestion. Tight bandages and thumb position may need to be altered.

■ FIGURE 9–5
Flap artery may be kinked by the proper digital nerve to the ring finger.

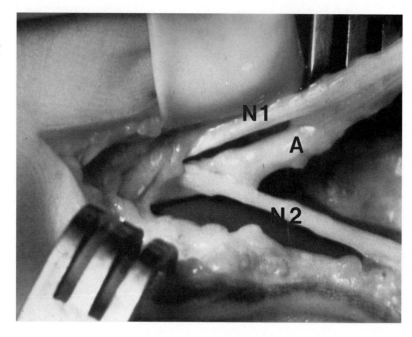

■ FIGURE 9–6
Flap being passed under proper digital nerve to ring finger.

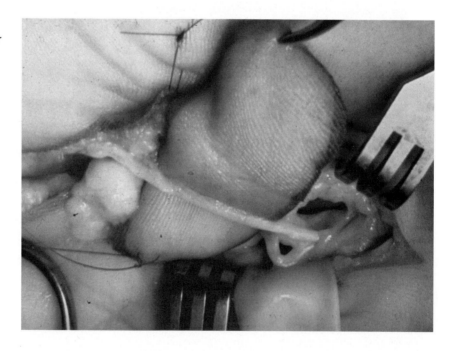

■ TECHNICAL ALTERNATIVES

    There are several reconstructive alternatives that must be considered in the preoperative planning. The palmar advancement flap, as described by Moberg, and the thenar and hypothenar flaps can be used to reconstruct isolated full-thickness thumb tip defects. They are ideal for smaller and more distal defects because of their lesser technical difficulty, but, because of their design, they can lead to joint flexion contracture. A radial innervated dorsal transposition flap from the index finger or thumb is useful for first web or thumb pad reconstruction in combined median and ulnar nerve injuries. These flaps are more limited in their excursion than the island flap and do not provide as close a match in terms of skin type and sensory receptor distribution. A free neurovascular island flap from the great toe may be connected to the median nerve proximal to the zone of injury to restore the appropriate sensory distribution and provide good skin cover over smaller

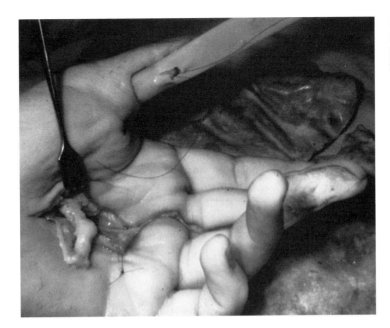

■ FIGURE 9–7
Flap being passed from palm to radial aspect of thumb.

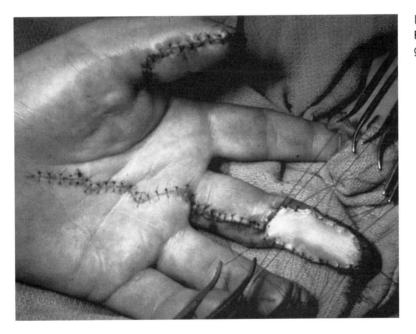

■ FIGURE 9–8
Flap in place with skin graft on donor site.

defects. This technique is dependent on intact proximal nerves and vessels as well as microsurgical expertise.

There are several pitfalls associated with neurovascular island flaps. Poor sensory outcome can be minimized by preferential use of the most distal portion of the donor finger skin, preserving as much subcutaneous tissue on the neurovascular pedicle as possible, avoidance of tension and kinking in the pedicle and inclusion of the dorsal sensory branch of the digital nerve if the posterior margin of the donor skin island is posterior to the midaxial lines as espoused by Markley.[8] Proper planning with meticulous technique using loupe magnification and tourniquet hemostasis is essential.[15] Omer and co-authors[11] and Krag and Rasmussen[5] have noted a progressive postoperative decrease in sensibility as measured by two-point discrimination to the level of protective sensation only. Thompson[14] and Henderson and Campbell Reid[3] believe that this deterioration can be prevented by careful attention to the technical details of the procedure. Hyperesthesia is not uncommon and may be caused by local nerve regeneration. Murray and co-authors[16] and Tubiana[15] caution against performing the procedure in patients with pre-existing causalgia. Cortical retraining is often incomplete, especially in adults. Omer and co-authors[11] have shown that sensory perception eventually localizes to both the donor and recipient sites. Although this has not reduced the functionality of the transposed sensation to the thumb, it can be prevented if the donor nerve is sectioned and connected to any available thenar digital nerves. Finally, flexion contracture of the donor digit may occur after surgery. This is dependent on the size of the donor defect and the quality of "take" of the skin graft. It is minimized by careful attention to hemostasis and graft immobilization and usually resolves within 1 year after surgery with passive stretching exercises.[6,12]

■ REHABILITATION

After 5 to 7 days, the initial dressing and plaster splint are removed. Gentle range of motion exercises are begun by the hand therapist. For the next 2 weeks, the patient wears a custom-molded orthoplastic protective splint for the donor finger and thumb when not in therapy. The splint is applied on the palmar surface from the forearm to the fingertips and allows healing to proceed with the interphalangeal joints straight and the thumb abducted and extended to minimize contracture. The metacarpophalangeal joints are flexed almost 90°, and the wrist is slightly extended. After 2 weeks, the tie-over dressing on the donor site and the sutures at the recipient site are removed. Rehabilitation by the therapist is directed at maintaining motion in the donor and recipient fingers, minimizing hypersensitivity, and improving the level of corticosensory re-education. Exercises include active and passive range of motion in both digits as well as massage and other desensitization techniques. Corticosensory re-education is difficult to achieve in adults. Nevertheless, patients should practice manipulating objects to improve their conscious sensory representation and tactile gnosis. Formal therapy continues until the patients are capable of doing their exercises on their own at home or have plateaued in terms of their progress. Patients can begin restricted activities at 3 weeks with no heavy lifting or strenuous use of the hand. Full activity is usually permitted by 6 to 8 weeks depending on the degree of healing.

■ OUTCOMES

There are several studies demonstrating the long-term outcome of neurovascular island flaps. In combining the results of the series, many patients experienced some difficulty with hyperesthesia (23%) and cold intolerance (32%). These symptoms are generally mild and restricted to the donor site, although recipient site hypersensitivity has been reported.[10] The recent series of Henderson and Campbell Reid,[3] Stice and Wood,[12] and Thompson[14] have shown that proper attention to detail in the technique can lead to good sensibility with no deterioration over time. The majority of patients are able to return to work and to integrate the reconstructed thumb into the full range of daily activities. The degree of corticosensory re-education seems low in the adult population, but undoubtedly this did not detract from the usefulness of this technique. With proper patient selection, planning, execution, and rehabilitation, this is still a very useful technique in the armamentarium of the reconstructive hand surgeon.

References

1. Bunnell S. Digit transfer by neurovascular pedicle. J Bone Joint Surg, 1952; 34A:722–774.
2. Eaton RG. The digital neurovascular bundle, a microanatomic study of its contents. Clin Orthop, 1968; 61:176–185.
3. Henderson HP, Campbell Reid DA. Long term follow-up of neurovascular island flaps. Hand, 1980; 12:113–122.
4. Hueston J. The extended neurovascular island flap. Br J Plast Surg, 1965; 18:304–305.
5. Krag C, Rasmussen K. The neurovascular island flap for defective sensibility of the thumb. J Bone Joint Surg, 1975; 57B:495–499.
6. Lister G. Skin flaps. In: Green DP (ed): Operative Hand Surgery, 2nd Ed, New York: Churchill Livingstone, 1988:1773–1779.
7. Littler JW. Neurovascular skin island transfer in reconstructive hand surgery. Trans Scand Intl Congress Soc Plast Surg, 1960; 175–179.

8. Markley JM Jr. The preservation of close two-point discrimination in the interdigital transfer of neurovascular island flaps. Plast Reconstr Surg, 1977; 59:812–816.

9. Moberg E. Discussion of Brooks D. Nerve grafting in orthopedic surgery. J Bone Joint Surg, 1955; 37A:305–326.

10. Murray JF, Ord JVR, Gavelin GE. The neurovascular island pedicle flap. An assessment of late results in sixteen cases. J Bone Joint Surg, 1967; 49A:1285–1297.

11. Omer GE Jr, Day DJ, Ratliff H, Lambert P. Neurovascular cutaneous island pedicles for deficient median nerve sensibility. J Bone Joint Surg, 1970; 52A:1181–1192.

12. Stice C, Wood MD. Neurovascular island skin flaps in the hand: Functional and sensibility evaluations. Microsurgery, 1987; 8:162–167.

13. Sullivan JG, Kelleher JC, Baibak GJ, Dean RK, Pinkner LD. The primary application of an island pedicle flap in thumb and index finger injuries. Plast Reconstr Surg, 1967; 39:488–492.

14. Thompson JS. Reconstruction of the insensate thumb bony neurovascular island transfer. Hand Clinics, 1992; 8:99–105.

15. Tubiana R, Duparc J. Restoration of sensibility in the hand by neurovascular skin island transfer. J Bone Joint Surg, 1961; 43B:474–480.

10

Radial Forearm Flap

■ HISTORY OF THE TECHNIQUE

The radial forearm flap was described as a free flap by Song and others at Ba-da-Chu Hospital in the People's Republic of China where it was first performed in 1978.[10] News of this flap reached the Western literature in 1981[7] and the possibility of using this flap as a distally based flap was quickly recognized. In 1981, Stock and coworkers described a distally based reversed-flow radial forearm flap.[12] Two years later, Biemer and Stock also described the inclusion of part of the radius in an osteocutaneous forearm flap.[1] Since that time, the popularity of this flap has become widespread. Based on the radial artery distally, this fasciocutaneous flap has enjoyed wide application for reconstruction of upper extremity defects.[6] Subsequent investigations into the blood supply of the forearm have demonstrated that in addition to the forearm skin, a variety of composite flaps (including portions of the radius, the palmaris longus muscle and tendon, the superficial branch of the radial nerve, and fascia-only forearm flaps) can be transferred on this blood supply.[3,14] Tissues from the volar forearm that are carried in this pedicle flap provide a variety of solutions for reconstruction of complex hand injuries.

■ INDICATIONS AND CONTRAINDICATIONS

Radial Forearm Fasciocutaneous Flap The primary indication for using a distally based radial forearm pedicle flap is to provide coverage of dorsal or palmar degloving injuries in which deeper structures are exposed (Fig. 10–1). The volar forearm skin provides an excellent substitute for soft tissue of the hand and digits. The skin is thin and often hairless and has a suitable texture for hand resurfacing. Unlike other fasciocutaneous flaps (notably, the lateral arm flap, the scapular flap, and the groin flap), the volar forearm flap includes less subcutaneous fat. Additionally, should sensation be required, the cutaneous nerves of the forearm can be anastomosed to suitable recipient nerves, providing sensory restoration with an average two-point discrimination of 36 mm.[13] The advantage of this flap, compared with standard flaps such as the pedicle groin flap, is that the entire reconstruction can be completed in the same injured extremity in one step under regional anesthesia. When the flap is based distally as a pedicle flap, microsurgical techniques are not required and the operation is relatively quick. In addition, the arm may be elevated postoperatively, avoiding the dependent position that is required with the groin flap.

Osteocutaneous Radial Forearm Flap Indications for using the radiovolar cortex of the distal radius in conjunction with the volar forearm skin are segmental bone loss of the metacarpals, digits, or both, in which vascularized bone and overlying soft-tissue coverage are required for successful reconstruction.[13] This flap has been used successfully for thumb reconstruction, using the radial bone to replace the thumb metacarpal, phalanges, or both.[1] The thin forearm skin contours nicely around the phalanx and additional tissues can be provided as needed for complex reconstruction, including tendons, nerves, and the radial artery itself, using a flow-through design.

The radial forearm fascia alone provides a highly vascularized gliding tissue to wrap around severely scarred tissue beds wherein nerve or tendon grafting is required.

Radial volar forearm flaps, either the fasciocutaneous or osteocutaneous types, are contraindicated when the vascular integrity of the hand is compromised or when blood flow through the ulnar artery does not perfuse the radial digits. This can occur as a result of a previous ulnar artery injury or an incomplete superficial palmar arch. Before use of this flap, a timed Allen's test is used to assess cross-perfusion with the ulnar artery circulation

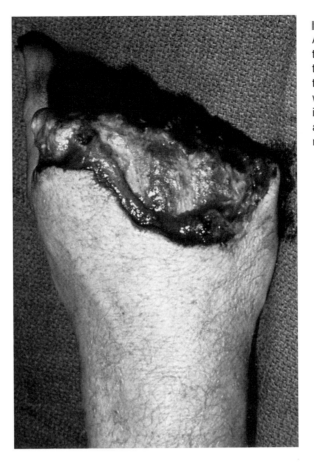

■ FIGURE 10–1
A 35 year-old farmer sustained a traumatic amputation of four fingers. Extensive soft-tissue loss with exposed metacarpals is an indication for coverage with a distally based radial arm flap.

(or interosseous circulation). Failure to identify the absence of cross-perfusion, present in about 15% of patients, can lead to inadequate circulation to the flap or more importantly, critically diminished blood flow to the hand. Jones and O'Brien reported acute hand ischemia when this flap was used under these adverse anatomic circumstances.[8] An equivocal Allen's test necessitates further evaluation of the forearm circulation. Although arteriography gives the most detailed information, noninvasive Doppler ultrasound studies can confirm patent vessels.

In young patients, hypertrophic scars or unsightly skin grafts can occur at the radial forearm flap donor site. Significant concern about the cosmetic appearance of a skin graft on the volar forearm donor defect is a relative contraindication because less conspicuous donor sites are available. In my opinion, the most aesthetic donor sites for resurfacing the dorsum of the hand remain the temporoparietal fascia flap and the groin flap.

The volar forearm skin can be transferred either as a distally based pedicle flap or as a proximally based free flap. When the former is used, the venous return for this flap is retrograde.[9] Connections between the two venae comitans permit reverse flow, bypassing the valves or rendering them incompetent.[8] To preserve these venous channels when elevating the flap, the adventitia and other perivascular tissues are left undisturbed. If the flap is elevated on its proximal blood supply, either the superficial veins or the venae comitans can be used. The size of flap that can be transferred encompasses virtually the entire volar forearm,[5,11] extending dorsally about a third of the circumference on the radial border. The flap is not usually raised past the mid-lateral line, so that dorsal skin can be used to cover the radial nerve in the closure.

The distally based radial forearm flap can be elevated with or without tourniquet control under regional or general anesthesia. I prefer to elevate this flap without the tourniquet, thereby permitting accurate hemostasis and identification of small vessels that aid in pre-

■ SURGICAL TECHNIQUES

serving the cutaneous circulation. The skin flap is outlined, based on a thin foam pattern of the defect in the hand. The rotation point of the flap is at the proximal wrist crease, and sufficient vascular pedicle must be included in the design to permit rotation into the injury site (Fig. 10–2). Distal defects, particularly in the fingers, require several centimeters of vascular pedicle, whereas dorsum of the hand or palmar defects require a shorter pedicle. If the flap is designed to reach the dorsum of the hand, additional pedicle length can be gained by dissecting the vessels as far distally as the snuffbox. This moves the pivot or rotation point distally. Should nerve reconstruction be required, orientation of the cutaneous nerves of the forearm to the desired recipient nerves should be considered. This kind of reconstruction is complex and requires accurate preoperative planning (Fig. 10–3).

■ FIGURE 10–2
Vascular anatomy and design of the retrograde radial forearm flap. The venae comitans of the radial artery permit retrograde venous return by interconnecting vessels. The point of rotation is at the proximal wrist crease. Large flaps, encompassing the entire volar forearm, may be transferred to the hand.

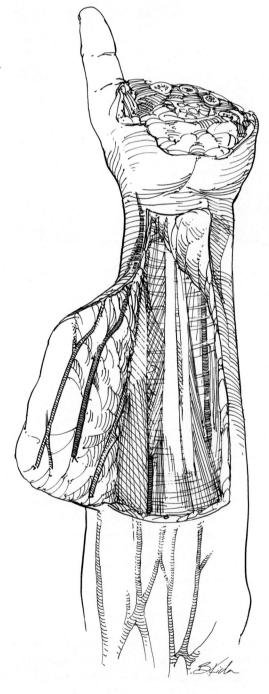

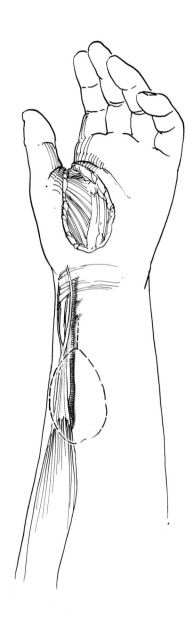

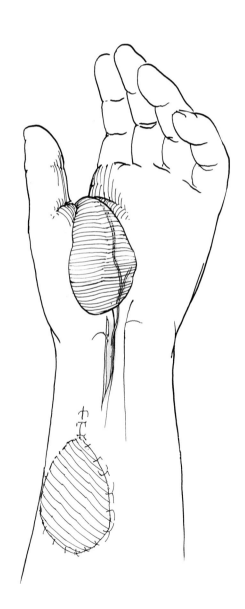

■ FIGURE 10–3
A plan for orienting nerve repairs, using a distally-based forearm flap. The cutaneous nerves of the forearm may be used to provide sensibility to the palmar or dorsal surface of the hand. On the palmar surface, the flap should be routed dorsal to the thumb, so that the nerve repairs align themselves proximally.

The incision should encompass the skin, subcutaneous tissue, and the volar forearm fascia. Under loupe magnification, the fascia–skin unit is elevated from the flexor carpi ulnaris muscle medially, and the flexor carpi radialis muscle laterally to the intermuscular septum, where the radial artery lies just radial to the flexor carpi radialis tendon. It is easier to begin the dissection in the distal forearm, where the artery is readily palpated and identified. It is crucial that the mesentery of vessels emanating from the radial artery be kept in continuity with the flap. It is easy to separate the artery from the overlying flap early in the dissection without realizing it. Once the relation of artery to mesentery is established, confidence in the dissection is gained. As the flap is elevated in the forearm, vessels to the underlying muscles, particularly the flexor pollicis longus muscle and brachioradialis muscles, require bipolar coagulation. As the dissection proceeds proximally, the radial artery is considerably deeper and its vascular mesentery is more pronounced. The key to the dissection remains staying beneath the forearm fascia. After the entire flap has been elevated, the radial artery is dissected proximal to the flap and as far as its junction with the brachial artery if necessary. A nontraumatic clamp is placed on the artery proximally to assess retrograde blood flow. If a tourniquet is used during the dissection, the tourniquet is released and the quality of flap bleeding and hand perfusion is assessed. The flap edges should bleed briskly and capillary refill should be readily apparent. Finally, the proximal radial artery and venae comitans are ligated and divided and the flap allowed to perfuse on its distally based radial artery pedicle.

Frequently, these flaps are somewhat congested early on, particularly when the hand has been allowed to rest in a dependent position. This congestion is probably due to the altered venous return in the distally based flap or, in smaller flaps, to the failure to include a sufficient venous outflow in the flap design. Should this congestion be significant and worrisome, the vein should be anastomosed with a vein graft to a regional vein for additional venous outflow. Usually, this maneuver is not required.

A nonmeshed split-thickness skin graft is then placed over the donor site soon after the flap is elevated. A nonadherent gauze is placed on the skin graft and a firm circumferential dressing applied. A tie-over dressing is not used on convex surfaces such as the forearm. The dressing is changed at 5 days and the splint reapplied for a total of 2 weeks. The hand is then placed in a volar splint extending to the fingertips for 5 days; digital motion is then permitted. Postoperative care includes elevation of the extremity for 7 to 10 days.

■ TECHNICAL ALTERNATIVES

Other possible donor sites for resurfacing the hand include the posterior interosseous artery pedicle flap, the lateral arm free flap, and the temporoparietal fascia free flap, all of which have their particular advantages. The posterior interosseous artery flap provides a suitably sized flap for hand reconstruction, avoids sacrificing a major artery, and does not require microsurgical techniques. The lateral arm free flap is a good alternative but is somewhat thicker than the radial forearm flap and requires experience with microvascular techniques. The temporoparietal fascia free flap provides fascia only and requires a skin graft on top of the fascia. For resurfacing the dorsum of the hand and digits, the temporoparietal fascia flap is usually my first choice.

■ REHABILITATION

The radial forearm donor site requires little specific rehabilitation once wound healing has occurred. Flexor tendon gliding occurs with active exercise beginning at 2 weeks and the cessation of splinting. Hypertrophic scarring may be controlled by a compression garment or elastic wrap. Silicone sheeting combined with compression has been reported to flatten thickened scars. Should the skin graft prove undesirable for cosmesis, serial excisions or tissue expansion followed by graft excision can be performed.

■ OUTCOMES

Several authors have reported prolonged cold intolerance when this reconstructive technique has been used.[2,4,15] It is difficult to assess the role of the flap in this cold intolerance because most patients who sustain severe hand injuries have cold intolerance even without such a flap. Nevertheless, depriving the hand of a significant blood supply along its radial border may be a contributing factor to this recognized problem. These same authors state, however, that after two winters this complication has usually diminished or disappeared.

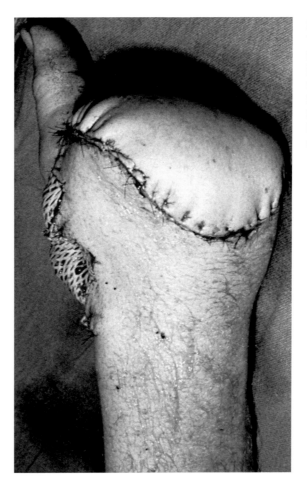

■ FIGURE 10–4
Two weeks postoperatively, the flap in the farmer's hand remains mildly swollen but the distal metacarpals and palm are well covered by durable full-thickness skin and subcutaneous tissue.

The most serious complication of using this flap is failure to recognize those patients (about 15%) who do not have vascular connections between the ulnar and radial circulation. The timed Allen's test is used to document this cross-over blood supply; when this is inconclusive, an arteriogram is warranted. Although it is not necessary to reconstruct the radial artery when this flap is used as a distally based flap, in the circumstance that the blood flow to the hand is in jeopardy, reconstruction of the radial artery with a saphenous vein graft must be given serious consideration.[8]

The distally based radial forearm flap is reliable; the vessels are large and readily dissected. Skin quality is appropriate for hand applications and provides protective sensibility when a sensory nerve repair is included in the flap design. In my experience, the donor site is well tolerated in older patients (patients older than 50) and probably should not be used in younger patients (patients younger than 25) because of unsightly scarring.

In summary, the distally based radial forearm flap is an effective technique for providing soft tissues to the hand and fingers (Fig. 10–4). Its judicious use permits one-stage reconstruction of soft-tissue defects without the need for microsurgery. Proper patient selection and attention to the details of donor-site care minimize the risks of significant complications.

References

1. Biemer E, Stock W: Total thumb reconstruction: a one stage reconstruction using an osteocutaneous forearm flap. Br J Plast Surg, 1983; 36:52–55.
2. Boorman JG, Brown JA, Sykes PJ: Morbidity in the forearm donor area. Br J Plast Surg, 1987; 40:207–212.

3. Cormack GC, Duncan MJ, Lamberty BGH: The blood supply of the bone component of the compound osteocutaneous radial artery forearm flap—an anatomical study. Br J Plast Surg, 1986; 39:173–175.

4. Fenton DM, Roberts JO: Improving the donor site of the radial artery flap. Br J Plast Surg, 1985; 38:504–505.

5. Foucher G, Citron N, Hoang P. Technique and Applications of the Forearm Flap in Surgery of the Hand: A Report on 33 Cases. In: Urbaniak JR (ed): Microsurgery for Major Limb Reconstruction, St. Louis: C.V. Mosby Company, 1987:256–263.

6. Foucher G, VanGenechten MM, et al: A compound radial artery forearm flap in hand surgery: an original modification of the Chinese forearm flap. Br J Plast Surg, 1984; 37: 139–148.

7. Guo F, et al: Forearm free skin flap transplantation. Natl Med J China, 1981; 61:139.

8. Jones BM, O'Brien CJ: Acute ischemia of the hand resulting from elevation of a radial forearm flap. Br J Plast Surg, 1985; 38:396–397.

9. Lin S, Lai C, Chiu C: Venous drainage in the reverse forearm flap. Plast Reconstr Surg, 1984; 74:508–512.

10. Song R, Gao Y, Song Y, et al: The forearm flap. Clin Plast Surg, 1982; 9:21–26.

11. Soutar D, Tanner N: The radial forearm flap in the management of soft tissue injuries of the hand. Br J Plast Surg, 1984; 37:18–26.

12. Stock W, Muhlbauer W, Biemer E: Der neurovaskuläre Unterarm-Insel-Lappen. Z Plast Chir, 1981; 5:158.

13. Swartz WM: Restoration of sensibility in mutilating hand injuries. Clin Plast Surg, 1989; 16: 515–529.

14. Timmons MJ: The vascular basis of the radial forearm flap. Plast Reconstr Surg 1986; 77: 80–92.

15. Timmons MJ, Missooten FEM, et al: Complications of radial forearm donor sites. Br J Plast Surg 1986; 39:176–178.

BRUCE G. PEAT
GRAHAM D. LISTER

11

Groin Flaps

The importance of an axial blood supply to pedicled skin flaps from the groin area was first recognized by John Wood in 1863[1] and further described by Shaw and Payne in 1946.[11] Both of the flaps described by these authors incorporated the superficial inferior epigastric artery (SIEA). Modern use of the "groin flap" was popularized by McGregor and Jackson in 1972,[9] basing the axis of the flap on the superficial circumflex iliac artery (SCIA). The anatomic basis of the flap[13] (Fig. 11–1) and its application to hand reconstruction have been described, especially by McGregor and Jackson[9] and Lister and coworkers.[8]

Superficial skin loss in the hand can be repaired by skin grafting, whereas small areas of deeper skin loss can be reconstructed using local rotation or transposition flaps. The treatment of more extensive deep soft-tissue defects exposing tendon, nerve, or bone requires regional flaps in the form of reversed forearm flaps, distant pedicle flaps, or free flaps. Of the pedicle flaps, the axial groin flap is the most versatile and popular. The multistage pedicle groin flap is preferred by some[3] and is indicated in all cases in which the skin of the pedicle will certainly be used on the hand (e.g., to cover a later toe transfer; Fig. 11–2C and D).

The groin flap is contraindicated in the older-than-50 age group because of the complication of joint stiffness. It is also contraindicated in young children, who are not capable of participating in postoperative flap care and pedicle monitoring.

Under general anesthesia, the anterior superior iliac spine (ASIS), pubic bone, inguinal ligament, and origin of the femoral artery are marked on the skin. The SCIA arises from the femoral artery 2.5 cm below the inguinal ligament and is present in 96% of patients.[6] Passing laterally parallel to the inguinal ligament, the SCIA lies initially deep to the deep fascia. At the medial border of the sartorius muscle, a deep muscular branch is given off. The superficial main artery passes through the deep fascia as it crosses sartorius, continues laterally, and divides into three small branches at a point 2.5 cm below the ASIS.[13] The flap is well drained by superficial and deep veins passing to the femoral triangle.[10]

Careful consideration is given to the approach of the flap to the recipient defect on the hand. The length and orientation of the pedicle should be designed to allow maximal tension-free insetting of the flap, avoidance of pedicle kinking, freedom of joint motion, and positioning of the patient for comfort. Because the groin flap contains more subcutaneous fat than the hand and often passes over a convex hand surface, the groin flap should be larger than the hand defect. The exact dimensions of the flap depend on the thickness of the subcutaneous fat but the size should enable tension-free insetting.

The pattern of the hand defect is then placed on the skin immediately inferior and posterior to the ASIS. An outline of the pattern is marked on the skin to represent the pedicle. The flap may be extended beyond the ASIS with a 1:1 length-to-breadth ratio. Medial to this pattern, the pedicle of the flap (which will be tubed later) is outlined with its axis centered on the SCIA. The pedicle should be designed at least 6 cm wide to include the variations in origin of the vessel.[6] Tubing of the flap pedicle is preferred and in many patients, the thickness of subcutaneous fat necessitates a wider pedicle. Groin donor defects up to 12 cm in width may be closed directly, aided by hip flexion, whereas larger donor sites must be skin grafted.

When raising the flap (Fig. 11–1), the entire margin is first incised down to the superficial surface of the deep fascia. The distal edge of the flap is raised by using a scalpel to incise

■ HISTORY OF THE TECHNIQUE

■ INDICATIONS AND CONTRAINDICATIONS

■ SURGICAL TECHNIQUES

■ FIGURE 11–1
Groin flap. The groin flap
is based on the superfi-
cial circumflex iliac artery
(SCIA), which runs paral-
lel to and about 1 inch inferior to the inguinal ligament. It emerges through
the deep fascia as it
crosses the sartorius and
branches at the level of
the anterior superior iliac
spine. When the flap is
raised, the lateral femoral
cutaneous nerve should
be preserved or in cer-
tain cases (see text), divided and repaired. The
fascia that is divided at
the lateral margin of the
sartorius muscle can be
seen.

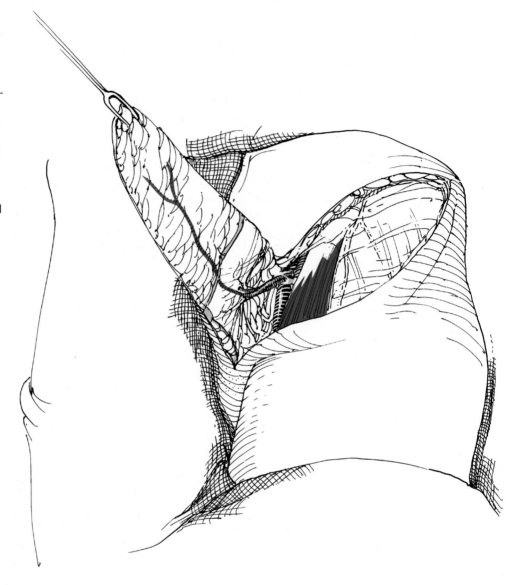

the subcutaneous plane to the ASIS, preserving the deep fascia intact. The inferior incision
is deepened through the deep fascia to reveal the tensor muscle of the fascia lata and the
sartorius muscle. The fascia is divided at the lateral border of sartorius muscle, parallel
to the muscle fibers, from inferior to superior for the entire width of the flap. As the flap
is elevated from the deep fascia covering the tensor muscle of the fascia lata laterally and
from muscle fibers of the sartorius muscle medially, the SCIA is seen in the deep fascia
as it is lifted off the sartorius muscle. While retracting the flap caudally, the incision in
the sartorius fascia is turned medially at its upper extent, just below the ASIS and inguinal
ligament. Here the lateral cutaneous nerve of the thigh is encountered, and care should
be taken to preserve it. Occasionally, branches of the nerve pass superficially to the SCIA;
these must be divided, passed deep to the vessel, and repaired. While elevating the flap,
the fascia is carefully dissected off the sartorius muscle to its medial border. The superficial
inferior epigastric artery may be encountered along the superior border of the flap medial

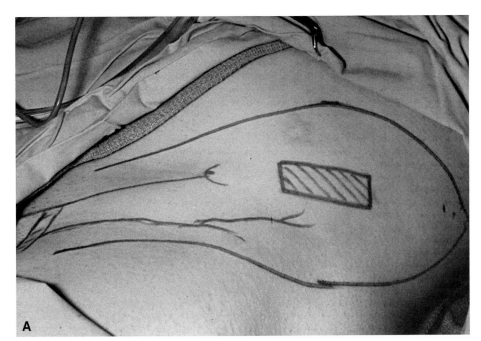

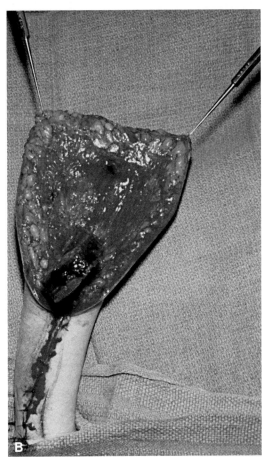

■ FIGURE 11–2
Groin flap with iliac crest.
A, The groin flap has
been marked following
the inguinal ligament and
the expected course of
the superficial circumflex
iliac artery. **B**, A bloc of
iliac crest has been taken
with the groin flap and is
bleeding well in the distal
portion of the tube.

■ FIGURE 11–2
(continued)
C and **D**, A long tube pedicle was retained to provide all cover necessary for transfer of a toe to the finger position.

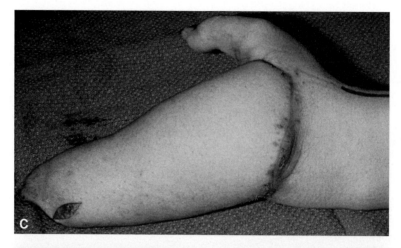

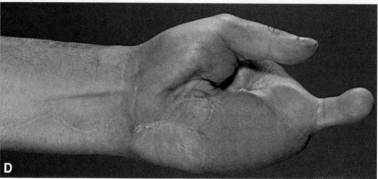

to the ASIS. When present, it provides a useful anatomic landmark to the location of the SCIA because in 50% of cases, the two vessels have a common origin from the femoral artery. The dissection usually stops at the medial border of sartorius muscle but if a longer pedicle is required or if the flap is intended for the contralateral hand, the deep muscle branch is divided and the SCIA freed to its origin. To facilitate contouring, subcutaneous fat can be liberally trimmed from the random portion of the flap and from the margins of the axial portion of the flap, provided that the deep fascia is not transgressed.

The groin defect is closed in two layers, commencing laterally and aided by hip flexion. The pedicle is then tubed, commencing medially with a single layer of interrupted sutures. The tubing process should be carried a little farther than appears necessary because once the flap is sutured to the hand, it is easier to remove than to insert tube stitches.

The hand is brought to and placed under the flap in the previously planned position. The flap is sutured to the hand, commencing at the more distal margin and then proceeding alternately around both sides of the flap, placing sufficient stretch on the flap to achieve evenly matched edges.

After insetting the flap, the limb should be immobilized for 1 to 2 days by taping it to the abdomen and back. Sufficient padding should be placed beneath the hand and arm to prevent kinks in the tube. All restraints are then removed and the patient is given responsibility for the flap. Clear instructions should be given to avoid kinkinq of the pedicle. The patient should be instructed to exercise every waking hour, taking the elbow through 0 to 90° motion by a combination of shoulder and back movements. All joints distal to the elbow must be taken through a full range of motion. Rigid external fixation of the upper limb to the pelvis has not been necessary and may restrict range-of-motion exercises. Although this regime may be followed by the older child, it is not advocated for the younger child, in whom a free groin flap may be a better clinical option.

The optimum time to divide the pedicle varies. In ideal circumstances, with primary healing of a nearly circumferentially inset flap to an unscarred bed, division and tension-

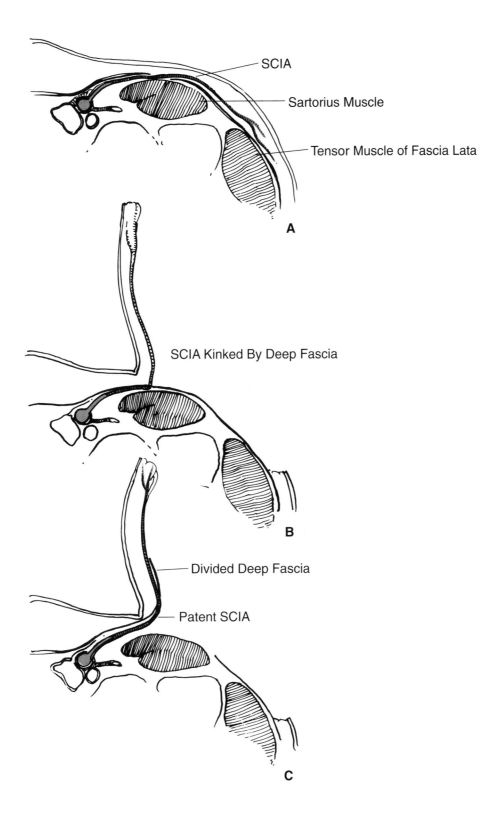

SCIA

Sartorius Muscle

Tensor Muscle of Fascia Lata

A

SCIA Kinked By Deep Fascia

B

Divided Deep Fascia

Patent SCIA

C

■ FIGURE 11–3

A, In cross-sectional diagram, the course of the superficial circumflex iliac artery is shown. The *black line* represents the deep fascia; the superficial circumflex iliac artery pierces that fascia. **B**, If the flap is raised without dividing the fascia, the vessel is restrained and kinked by that deep fascia, reducing significantly the blood flow to the flap. **C**, If the fascia is divided as recommended at the lateral margin of the sartorius, this kink in the vessel is eliminated.

free insetting may be completed at 3 weeks. The ability of the flap to survive can be predicted by clamping the pedicle for half an hour with a Penrose drain and clinically assessing perfusion of the flap. In less than ideal circumstances, a delay procedure should be performed. This procedure is performed under local anesthesia by incising halfway around the tube pedicle and dividing all deep soft tissue in the pedicle. The wound is then sutured and the flap divided completely 1 week later.[7,14] Insetting of the flap at the time of pedicle division should be postponed for a week if back bleeding from the flap on the hand is poor, to avoid marginal flap necrosis.

■ TECHNICAL ALTERNATIVES

Variations of the groin flap include a composite osteocutaneous flap, including vascularized iliac bone[2] (Fig. 11–2A and B), and a Y-shaped combined hypogastric and groin flap used to resurface the dorsal and palmar surfaces of the hand.[12]

The hypogastric flap based on the SIEA is an acceptable alternative pedicle flap. Where thin pedicle skin is required, as in thumb reconstruction, the random-pattern infraclavicular flap is superior to the groin flap, although it is cosmetically unacceptable in women.

The free flap offers distinct advantages over the pedicled flap in many cases. Although a more complex initial operation, a free flap can be tailored more precisely than a pedicle flap, possibly entailing less hospitalization and lower costs, and has the advantage of a permanent blood supply. It is therefore the cover of choice for large, deep defects. A preference for free-tissue transfer also exists when severe scarring or radiotherapy damage to the hand precludes adequate neurovascularization of a groin flap.

The major pitfalls in the use of the groin flap are 1) failure to divide the deep fascia, which results in kinking of the pedicle vessel and necrosis of the flap (Fig. 11–3); 2) making the flap too narrow, yet persisting with tubing; 3) kinking the pedicle either by poorly contouring the flap to the hand or inadequate postoperative care; 4) undermining the margins of the secondary defect before closure, predisposing to hematoma in the groin; 5) premature removal of the sutures in the secondary defect because of erythema (which should be ignored because it is due to tension), creating a wound similar to a decubitus and almost as difficult to treat; 6) dividing the flap without a preliminary delay when the marginal wound is not soundly healed or the skin of the tube is required on the hand; and 7) using the flap in obese patients.

■ REHABILITATION

The sutures are removed from the hand 2 weeks postoperatively. If the hip was flexed to facilitate closure, the patient is instructed to gradually allow the hip to extend to neutral over a 2-week period. The sutures are removed from the groin 3 weeks postoperatively.

Promptly after the detachment and inset of the flap, the patient's rehabilitation needs are assessed. The range of motion of all upper extremity joints, including the shoulder, are measured and strength testing of all muscle groups is completed. Under the supervision of a hand therapist, active and passive range-of-motion exercises and strengthening exercises are started. The program is monitored at weekly intervals for 3 weeks and then modified, depending on pre-existing conditions, ancillary procedures, and patient progress.

■ OUTCOMES

Graff and Biemer[5] reported a 13% incidence of marginal necrosis plus an incidence of wound infection, seromas, and deep vein thrombosis of 10% each. Freedlander[4] and coworkers reported a 17% incidence of infection and a 20% incidence of partial flap necrosis in 73 groin flaps, with one mortality from a pulmonary embolus. These reports are at odds with the experience of the senior author, who has encountered complications in less than 5% of a series that commenced when he assisted McGregor with the first groin flaps raised. The complete survival of the groin flap can usually be predicted with sufficient confidence that reconstruction, including joint replacement and tendon graft, can be performed at the time of flap application.

References

1. Boo-Chai K: John Wood and his contributions to plastic surgery: the first groin flap. Br J Plast Surg, 1977; 30:9–13.
2. Button M, Stone EJ: Segmental bony reconstruction of the thumb by composite groin flap: a case report. J Hand Surg, 1980; 5:488–491.
3. Chow JA, Bilos ZJ, et al: The groin flap in reparative surgery of the hand. Plast Reconstr Surg, 1986; 77:421–426.
4. Freedlander B, Dickson WA, McGrouther DA: The present role of the groin flap in hand trauma in the light of a long-term review. J Hand Surg, 1986; 11B:197–190.

5. Graf P, Biemer E: Morbidity of the groin flap transfer; are we getting something for nothing? Br J Plast Surg, 1992; 45:86–88.

6. Katai K, Kido H, Numaguchi Y: Angiography of the iliofemoral arteriovenous system supplying free groin flaps and free hypogastric flaps. Plast Reconstr Surg, 1979; 63:671–679.

7. Lister GD: Skin flaps in operative surgery. In: Green DP (ed): 3rd Ed, New York: Churchill Livingstone, 1993:1741–1822.

8. Lister GD, McGregor IA, Jackson IT: The groin flap in hand injuries. Injury, 1973; 6:229–239.

9. McGregor IA, Jackson IT: The groin flap. Br J Plast Surg, 1972; 25:3–16.

10. Penteado CV: Venous drainage of the groin flap. Plast Reconstr Surg, 1982; 71:678–684.

11. Shaw DT, Payne RC: One-stage tubed abdominal flaps. Surg Gynecol Obstet, 1946; 83:205–209.

12. Smith PJ: The Y-shaped hypogastric-groin flap. Hand, 1982; 14:263–270.

13. Smith PJ, Foley B, McGregor IA, Jackson IT: The anatomical basis of the groin flap. Plast Reconstr Surg, 1972; 49:41–47.

14. Wray RC, Wise DM, Young VL, Weeks PM: The groin flap in severe hand injuries. Ann Plast Surg, 1982; 9:459–462.

12

Nail Bed Repair

■ HISTORY OF THE TECHNIQUE

An individual's nails often reveal their normal day by day activities and contribute significantly to first impressions. An examination of the nail bed can also give insight into the general state of health. A normal-appearing nail is critical in maintaining aesthetics as well as function.

Historically, an injured nail bed was treated by debridement followed by dressings to allow healing by secondary intention. In 1955, Flatt observed that this "conservative" treatment produced distorted nails and sensitive scarred fingertips.[5] In his report and in one in 1946 by Hanrahan,[7] fingertips with partially or completely destroyed nail beds were covered by split-thickness skin grafts. During the same period, Swanker[18] (1947) suggested using nail grafts from other digits or toes. McCash[12] (1955) reported that his preference was to use partial grafts from the great toe, including nail bed and matrix, as suggested by Sheehan[17] in 1929, but he also included the germinal matrix. In 1957, Schiller[16] urged replacing the avulsed nail whenever possible because it provided a protective dressing for the wounded nail bed, a natural splint for phalangeal fractures, and a smooth surface to aid the regrowth of the new nail and facilitate the repositioning of the avulsed matrix. Kleinert and coworkers[8] in 1967 classified nail bed injuries and developed step-by-step principles of treatment that included using an intermediate dermal graft.

In the 1980s, further improvement in nail injury treatment was attempted using reverse dermal grafts,[2] silver-impregnated porcine xenografts,[4] and free nail bed grafts,[9,15] with fairly good results.

Immediate proper repair of the damaged nail bed was advocated as early as 1955 by Flatt[5] and in 1967 by Kleinert and coworkers.[8] In 1984, Zook[23] published his extensive studies of 299 nail injuries treated over 5.5 years, and primary repair of nail bed injuries became the standard treatment, replacing the earlier technique of debridement followed by dressings. Primary repair can be by either direct suturing or the use of partial-thickness nail grafts but it is essential that the repair be made properly at the time of injury to prevent deformity.[22] This principle of primary repair is presented as my recommended technique in management of nail bed injuries.

■ INDICATIONS AND CONTRAINDICATIONS

The most frequent cause of nail deformity is a missed injury to the nail bed.[23] The best results are to be gained with careful attention to detail and proper treatment at the time of acute injury. In a nail injury, missing a nail bed laceration leads to deformity of the nail, which is not easily corrected, even with the best of reconstructive techniques. Therefore, it cannot be emphasized enough that accurate approximation of the nail matrix at the initial treatment is critical to achieving a normal-appearing nail.

The indication for exploration of the nail bed includes history of significant blunt trauma to the nail or associated trauma to the fingertips. A hematoma larger than 25% of the surface of the nail may indicate an underlying injury, enough to disrupt nail bed blood vessels. Therefore, the nail should be removed and the nail bed explored for injury. Radiographs should be obtained to rule out the presence of a phalangeal fracture.

In addition to subungual hematoma, acute nail bed injuries may be classified as 1) laceration of the nail and underlying nail bed; 2) crushing-laceration injuries, resulting in stellate or complex lacerations of the nail bed; 3) avulsions of the nail such that the nail comes to lie dorsal to the eponychial fold, with or without a distal phalangeal fracture; and 4) complex injuries, with loss of the nail bed.

Although the type of treatment of nail bed injuries depends on the classification and severity of the injury, each type of nail bed injury should be repaired immediately unless there is a concomitant life-threatening injury requiring immediate attention. In such situations, the nail bed repair can be delayed 10 to 14 days, although results may be compromised.

The nail bed, or plate, is composed of the dorsal nail, the intermediate nail, and the ventral nail. The intermediate nail is the main mass of the nail and extends from a point immediately distal to the insertion of the extensor tendon to the distal lunula. The intermediate nail, or germinal matrix, is formed from the ventral floor and lateral walls of the nail fold and is intimately related to the dorsal periosteum of the distal phalanx. The germinal matrix is primarily responsible for the growth of new nail. The distal edge of the germinal matrix is marked by the moon-shaped lunula, located just distal to the cuticle, which is opaque because of incompletely cornified nail. The ventral nail, or sterile matrix, extends from the distal edge of the lunula to the edge of the fingertip. Lastly, the dorsal nail is produced by the dorsal roof of the nail fold (Fig. 12–1).[20,21,24]

■ SURGICAL TECHNIQUES

Subungual Hematomas   One of the most common causes of nail injury is blunt trauma. When trauma disrupts blood vessels in the nail matrix, a collection of blood forms under the nail plate. Unless there is a tear in the nail to provide drainage for the accumulated blood, pressure from the hematoma can cause severe pain. Quick relief can be provided by draining the hematoma through a hole in the nail.

Small hematomas can be drained without anesthetic but aseptic technique should be practiced. A traditional method of treatment is to heat the straight edge of a paper clip with a lighted alcohol wick until red hot, then evacuate the hematoma by creating a drainage hole through the nail. Care must be taken that a large enough hole is made; otherwise, the underlying fluid can be seared and the hole plugged.[13] In many emergency rooms, an alternative method is to use a hand-held battery-powered cautery, such as the Concept (Largo, FL) cautery. The cautery is sterile, disposable, and avoids the risk of an open flame. Whatever instrument is used to trephine the nail plate, care should be taken to avoid injuring the underlying nail bed.

When a larger hematoma (more than 25% of the surface of the nail) is present, there is a high likelihood of an underlying injury to the matrix. To explore the nail bed, a digital block of local anesthetic (lidocaine) is used. A quarter-inch Penrose drain is used as a tourniquet at the base of the finger. A useful technique in the emergency room is to prepare and anesthetize the injured finger and place a sterile glove onto the patient's hand; make an opening at the tip of the glove overlying the injured digit and roll the rubber down to the base of the finger to create a digital tourniquet and surrounding sterile field. The nail should be carefully and completely removed to inspect the underlying matrix and to evacuate the hematoma (Fig. 12–2)

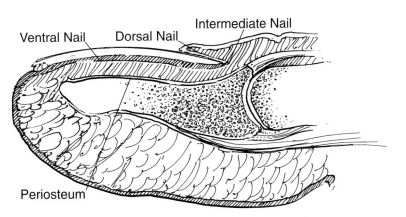

Ventral Nail   Dorsal Nail   Intermediate Nail

Periosteum

■ FIGURE 12–1
The anatomy of the nail bed in sagittal section.

Lacerations of the Nail and Nail Bed   Simple lacerations of the nail bed may be fixed by direct approximation of nail bed edges, using a digital block with lidocaine and a Penrose or glove tourniquet. Generally, the entire nail should be removed to adequately inspect and repair the nail bed (Fig. 12–3A).[1] Occasionally, when the injury is far distal, partial nail removal may be sufficient for exposure of the laceration.

   To help align the nail bed fragments, one side of the cuticle (eponychium) should be

■ FIGURE 12–2
When a hematoma is larger than 25% of the surface of the nail from significant trauma, the nail should be removed to adequately examine the underlying nail bed and to evacuate the hematoma.

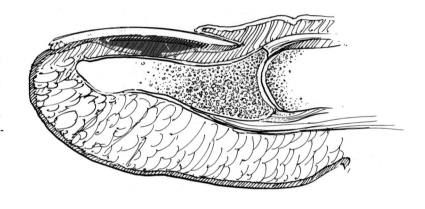

■ FIGURE 12–3
A, The nail is completely removed, exposing the nail bed injury. **B**, Suture of the cuticle (eponychium) helps to align the repair; 7-0 absorbable chromic or Vicryl sutures are used to repair the nail bed. **C**, Splinting of the repaired nail bed is accomplished by securing the nail beneath eponychial fold with suture or tapes.

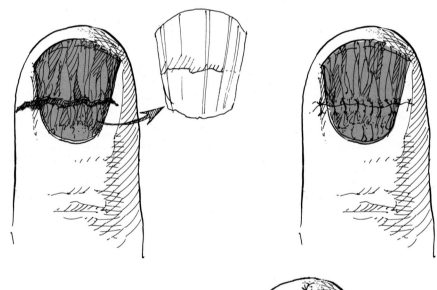

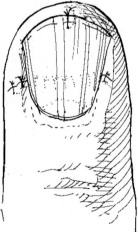

sutured first with 5-0 nylon. In children, absorbable 5-0 chromic catgut should be used to avoid traumatic suture removal. The nail bed tissue is delicate and friable. Spatulated ophthalmic needles on 6-0 chromic or 6-0 Vicryl (Ethicon, Somerville, NJ) suture are especially useful (Fig. 12–3B). Special care must be taken to avoid tearing the nail bed by following the curve of the needle when passing a suture. Loupe magnification also enhances the accuracy of the repair.

If the nail is available, it should be replaced after repair of the nail bed. Replacing the nail protects and splints the wounded fingertip and helps to shape the healing nail bed (Fig. 3C).[16,22] When the nail is missing, Xeroform (Sherwood Medical, St. Louis, MO) or Adaptic (Johnson and Johnson, Arlington, TX) can be used to cover the nail bed and to keep the nail fold open, preventing adhesions. Artificial nail splints have also been made with polypropylene[11] and metal foil from Xeroform or suture packages.[3]

Stellate Lacerations When a widely distributed force injures the nail, a stellate "bursting" lesion may result. There may also be associated distal phalanx fractures. When treating stellate lacerations, it is important to try to approximate as many of the fragments of the nail bed as possible. Individual or loose tissue should be minimally debrided and whenever possible secured as free grafts. The goal is to recreate a foundation or flat "scaffold" for adherence of the regenerating nail.

Associated distal phalanx fractures must be anatomically reduced and fixed with a small K-wire to avoid persistent nail bed deformity. Nondisplaced phalangeal fractures may be adequately splinted by replacement of the nail.

Avulsions of the Nail Bed With complex avulsion injuries, a portion of the sterile matrix (ventral nail) is missing. When the missing portion is attached to the avulsed portion of the nail, best results can be obtained if the nail portion with the nail matrix can be incorporated into the repair (Fig. 12–4A). Holes must be predrilled into the nail plate or a 2-mm rim of the avulsed nail trimmed off to allow sutures to be placed within the nail bed. One should avoid trying to completely separate the matrix from the avulsed nail because maceration of this delicate tissue may occur (Fig. 12–4B).

Complex Injuries With Partial Loss of the Nail Bed If the avulsed nail fragment is missing, the defect can be covered with a split-thickness skin graft or a reverse dermal graft. More extensive repairs using split-thickness grafts of an adjacent nail,[18] a nail bed taken from a toe,[12] or porcine xenografts[4] have been reported to give good results. Zook found that if a split-thickness nail graft cannot be obtained from the undamaged portion

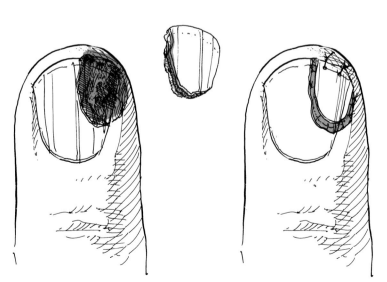

■ FIGURE 12–4
A, When a portion of the sterile matrix is detached after an avulsion injury, nail matrix can be incorporated into the repair. **B**, Two millimeters of avulsed nail has been trimmed away to allow direct suturing of the nail bed.

of the injured nail, a split-thickness nail graft from the large toe is necessary to obtain a large enough graft.[22]

The split-thickness nail graft is harvested from the large toe under tourniquet using a No. 20 or No. 10 blade, making sure that only translucent tissue is removed from the recipient site. The split-thickness nail graft is then sewn into the fingernail defect with 6-0 chromic catgut or Vicryl sutures. Once again, to prevent tearing of this delicate tissue, the curve of the needle must be followed with each pass of the suture.

In each type of acute injury, after repair, the wound is dressed with Bacitracin (E. Fougera & Co., Melville, NY) ointment and Xeroform petrolatum gauze that has been cut to conform to the shape of the nail. The native nail may be carefully placed under the eponychium to prevent adhesions and to splint nondisplaced fractures. As an option, to secure the nail, proximal or distal sutures of 4-0 Prolene (Ethicon, Somerville, NJ) may be placed through predrilled holes in the nail but care must be taken not to injure the germinal matrix. When the native nail is missing, suture foil may be cut in the shape of the nail and used to splint the eponychium and protect the nail bed repair. A bulky dressing and volar alumafoam aluminum splint completes the necessary dressing. The extremity should be elevated for the first week postoperatively to minimize swelling.

■ TECHNICAL ALTERNATIVES

Although most nail bed injuries require immediate suture or grafting, some clean partial fingertip amputations may be an exception. In these cases, a perfectly normal nail eventually forms if sufficient germinal nail matrix and fingertip soft-tissue are present and not injured.[10]

The major pitfall in management of nail bed injuries, however, remains the missed diagnosis, with resulting deformity of the nail. Other technical problems can complicate the treatment of nail bed injury. Subungual hematomas can become infected after drainage if aseptic technique is not used or if the patient contaminates the injured nail. In the lacerated nail, with nail still attached on one or both sides of the laceration, there is a temptation to suture just the nail together. This results in a less than perfect approximation of the underlying nail bed and should not be attempted. In the presence of a fracture of of the distal phalanx, an anatomic reduction is critical before nail bed repair. Because of the intimate relation of the nail bed to the periosteum, an offset in the dorsal cortex makes anatomic nail bed repair impossible. Also, any small fragments of bone should be carefully identified and removed before nail bed repair. When the nail is replaced after nail bed repair, there is a tendency for the nail to displace out of the eponychial fold, distorting the repaired nail bed. This can be prevented by either suturing or taping the nail in place.

■ REHABILITATION

The first postoperative dressing may be changed in 5 to 10 days, leaving the Xeroform gauze intact if it is adherent to the nail bed. Thereafter, application of Bacitracin ointment with dry sterile dressings once a day is recommended. Skin sutures are removed in 7 to 10 days but the absorbable sutures on the nail bed are left intact unless tissue reaction, with significant inflammation, occurs.

The nail bed usually becomes hard and nontender about 10 days after injury and dressings are no longer required.[13] After 2 weeks, the nail bed is sufficiently healed for the nail to be removed.[6]

The new nail grows in over a 3- to 6-month period.[6,8,13,14] It may be prudent to inform the patient of the normal range of healing time and also that persistent nail deformity may occur, requiring secondary reconstruction.[19]

If a phalangeal fracture is present, after removal of the K-wire a four-pronged padded aluminum splint may be useful. Protective distal interphalangeal joint splinting may continue for 3 to 6 weeks, with encouragement of proximal interphalangeal joint motion.

Activities of daily living may commence immediately after surgery but elevation of the extremity is recommended for at least 1 week. The patient should be reminded not to jostle the dressing, which may lead to shearing of delicate nail bed tissue. Return to work 7 to 10 days after surgery is possible if protection of the affected extremity can be continued. For those individuals performing bimanual labor or having more extensive injuries, a minimum of 3 to 6 weeks recovery time is advised.

An excellent result, as defined by Zook,[23] is a normal-appearing nail that is identical to the opposite nail. This is the expected result after repair of simple lacerations of the nail bed. Complex stellate lacerations and injury to the germinal matrix may show variable results, particularly when there is soft-tissue loss. These range from very good (the repaired nail exhibiting one minor variation from identical to the opposite nail), good (two minor variations), fair (three minor or one major variation), to poor (more than three minor or one major variation).[23] Major variations from normal include split nails, nails with less than two thirds adherence, and a rough nail surface.[23] Minor variations from normal include variations in nail shape, longitudinal ribs, transverse grooves, changes in the eponychium, a slightly rough nail surface, and two thirds or more adherence but less than full adherence. Out of the above, nonadherence of the nail is the most common nail deformity after nail bed injury.[24,25]

■ OUTCOMES

These secondary deformities, whether major or minor, may become a source of great distress to patients because of recurrent trauma, pain, or disfigurement. Therefore, whenever possible, primary repair of the nail bed should be attempted at the time of acute injury.

References

1. Beasley RW: Fingernail injuries. J Hand Surg, 1983; 8:784–785.
2. Clayburgh RH, Wood MB, Cooney WP: Nail bed repair and reconstruction by reverse dermal grafts. J Hand Surg, 1983; 8:594–599.
3. Cohen MS, Hennrikus WL, Botte MJ: A dressing for repair of acute nail bed injury. Orthop Rev, 1990; 19:882–884.
4. Ersek RA, Gadaria U, Denton DR: Nail bed avulsions treated with porcine xenografts. J Hand Surg, 1985; 10A:152–153.
5. Flatt AE: Nailbed injuries. Br J Plast Surg, 1955; 8:38–43.
6. Flatt AE: In: The Care of Minor Hand Injuries, 4th Ed, St. Louis: CV Mosby Co, 1979.
7. Hanrahan EM: The split thickness skin graft as a cover following removal of a fingernail. Surgery, 1946; 20:398–400.
8. Kleinert HK, Putcha SM, Ashbell TS, Kutz JE: The deformed nail, a frequent result of failure to repair nail bed injuries. J Trauma, 1967; 7:177–190.
9. Koshima I, Soeda S, Takase T, et al: Free vascularized nail graft. J Hand Surg, 1988; 13:29–32.
10. Ogo K: Does the nail bed really regenerate? Plast Reconstr Surg, 1987; 80:445–447.
11. Ogunro EO: External fixation of injured nail bed with the INRO surgical nail splint. J Hand Surg, 1989; 14A:236–241.
12. McCash CR: Free nail grafting. Br J Plast Surg, 1955; 8:19–33.
13. Newmeyer WL, Kilgore ES: Common injuries of the fingernail and nail bed. Am Fam Physician, 1977;16:93–95.
14. Rosenthal EA: Treatment of fingertip and nail bed injuries. Orthop Clin North Am, 1983; 14:675–697.
15. Saita H, Suzuki Y, Fujino K, Tajima T: Free nail bed graft for treatment of nail bed injuries of the hand. J Hand Surg, 1983; 8:171–178.
16. Schiller C: Nail replacement in finger tip injuries. Plast Reconstr Surg, 1957; 19:521–530.
17. Sheehan JE: Replacement of thumb nail. JAMA, 1929; 92:1253–1255.
18. Swanker WA: Reconstructive surgery of the injured nail. Am J Surg, 1947; 74:341–345.
19. Van Beek AL, Kassan MA, Adson MH, Dale V: Management of acute fingernail injuries. Hand Clin North Am, 1990; 6:23–35.
20. Zook EG, Van Beek AL, Russell RC, et al: Anatomy and physiology of the perionychium: a review of the literature and anatomic study. J Hand Surg, 1980; 5:528–536.
21. Zook EG: The perionychium: anatomy, physiology, and care of injuries. Clin Plast Surg, 1981; 8:21–31.
22. Zook EG: Injuries of the Fingernail. In: Green DP (ed): Operative Hand Surgery, New York: Churchhill Livingstone, 1982:895–914.
23. Zook EG, Guy RJ, Russel RC: A study of nail bed injuries: cause, treatment, and prognosis. J Hand Surg, 1984; 9A:247–252.
24. Zook EG: Anatomy and physiology of the perionychium. Hand Clin North Am, 1990; 6:1–8.
25. Zook EG: Reconstruction of a functional and esthetic nail. Hand Clin North Am, 1990; 6:59–68.

PART
II

Tendon Repairs

13

Extensor Tendon Repairs in Zones 1–2

Dorsal tendon injuries located at the distal interphalangeal (DIP) joint are classified as zone 1 injuries, and those at the middle phalanx are in zone 2.[18] The most frequent cause of zone 1 extensor tendon injury is acute, forceful hyperextension or hyperflexion while the digit is extended. The resulting closed disruption of the extensor tendon over the DIP joint produces a characteristic extensor lag called mallet or drop finger.[3]

Historically, both the DIP and proximal interphalangeal (PIP) joints were maintained in full extension for the treatment of a closed mallet deformity.[8] Smillie[14] immobilized the DIP joint in slight hyperextension and the PIP joint in 60° of flexion with a plaster cast. Subsequently, Kaplan[6] suggested that the PIP joint did not need to be flexed, as the extensor apparatus is moderately lax over all three finger joints while the DIP joint is held in extension. In 1969, Stack[15] reported good results in a 12-year experience using a specialized molded plastic splint, which allowed for PIP joint motion while extending the DIP joint.

Splinting is quite effective for closed tendon ruptures of the distal phalanx. However, there is some controversy over indications for operative treatment, when mallet finger is associated with intra-articular fracture or dislocation.

Closed Injuries   Zone 1 extensor tendon injuries should be addressed in a timely fashion. A persistent inability to extend the DIP joint creates an imbalance of the extensor tendon system. This may result in hyperextension of the PIP joint and flexion of the metacarpophalangeal (MP) joint (swan neck deformity).

Injuries associated with mallet finger deformity may range from pure tendon rupture, to tendon rupture with a chip fracture, to tendon rupture with a fracture of the base of the distal phalanx. When a large fracture fragment (over 30% of the articular surface) is present, there also may be palmar subluxation of the distal phalanx (Fig. 13–1, types A through E).

Forceful hyperflexion usually results in pure tendon ruptures (type A) or tendon ruptures with a small bone fracture (type B). These ruptures can be treated by static splints or, in special circumstances, with K-wire fixation, maintaining the distal joint in extension for 6 to 8 weeks.

Acute hyperextension often causes a significant fracture of the distal phalanx. If the fracture measures one third or greater of the articular surface (types C and D), is widely displaced, or leads to palmar subluxation of the distal phalanx (type E), splinting may not be adequate treatment. Several authors[3,6,9,11,16] have recommended that these injuries be treated primarily as a fracture, with open reduction and K-wire fixation. All authors have commented on the technical difficulty of open treatment.

Conversely, Wehbé and Schneider[19] compared outcomes of operation versus splinting in the treatment of mallet finger in 160 patients and found that surgery had no advantages, but it resulted in a higher rate of morbidity than did splinting. Even in cases of mallet finger with an associated large fracture or palmar subluxation of the distal phalanx, remodeling of the joint was observed, with an acceptable outcome after splinting alone.

I recommend closed treatment of mallet deformities with splinting whenever possible. Even in the presence of a good-sized dorsal fracture fragment (up to 30% of the articular

■ HISTORY OF THE TECHNIQUE

■ INDICATIONS AND CONTRAINDICATIONS

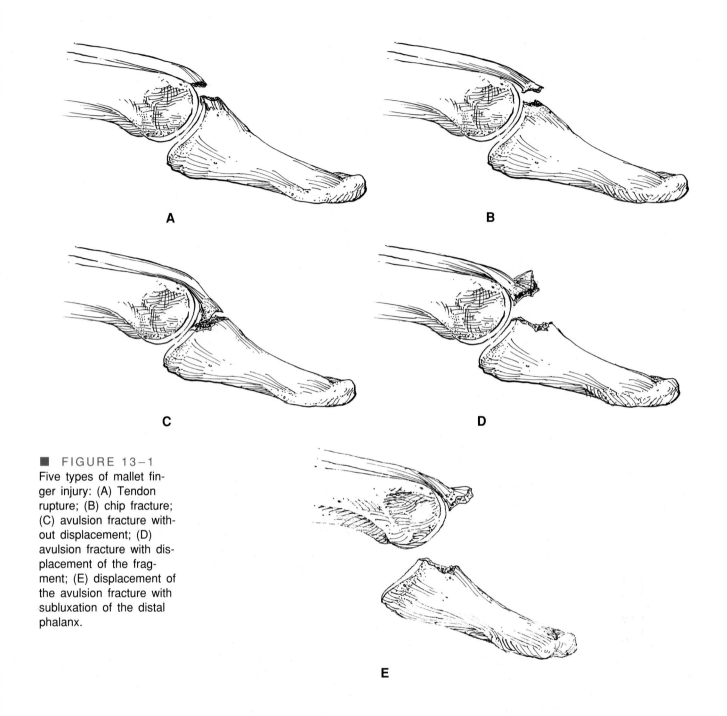

■ FIGURE 13–1
Five types of mallet finger injury: (A) Tendon rupture; (B) chip fracture; (C) avulsion fracture without displacement; (D) avulsion fracture with displacement of the fragment; (E) displacement of the avulsion fracture with subluxation of the distal phalanx.

surface) and palmar subluxation of the distal phalanx, it may be worthwhile to undertake a trial of nonoperative management.

Surgical management, including K-wire placement, is reserved for patients with special job requirements. Certain health professionals, such as dentists and surgeons, may be especially hindered at work by trying to place a glove over such splints, and a 0.035 or 0.045 K-wire with the end cut off beneath the skin provides an alternative treatment.

Open Injuries   Open injuries of zone 1 tendons with lacerations at or near the DIP joint have potential for contamination. Undetected partial lacerations may progress to complete rupture of the conjoint tendon. Treatment should include careful irrigation and inspection of the joint, followed by direct tendon repair. If there is any question regarding the viability of soft tissue coverage over the distal phalanx, open tendon repair should be delayed.

Highly contaminated injuries such as human bites should have aggressive wound care and debridement, followed by delayed repair.

Rupture of the extensor tendon at the level of the middle phalanx (zone 2) may be caused by laceration, crush, avulsion, or deep abrasion to the digit. In complex trauma, repair of nerves or flexor tendons may have higher priority, precluding immediate repair of the extensor tendon. When extensor tendon lacerations are repaired within 10 to 14 days of injury, the results are the same as an immediate repair.[5]

Finally, when there is extensive injury to both joint and tendon at the same level, arthrodesis of the DIP joint at 15° of flexion may offer the best functional outcome.[5,16]

The terminal extensor tendon represents the distal extension of the merged lateral bands that insert on the dorsal base of the distal phalanx. The more central fibers of the tendon are bordered by the distal extensions of the oblique retinacular ligaments that insert on the lateral base of the distal phalanx adjacent to the terminal tendon.[20] At the level of the middle phalanx (zone 2), the extensor apparatus is oriented about the dorsal one half of the digit. Here, the lateral bands, which are distal continuations of the intrinsic muscles, change from a volar-lateral location into a dorsal site, blending with fibers from the central slip on the dorsal surface to form the conjoint tendon.[6]

■ SURGICAL TECHNIQUES

Closed Injuries   The initial treatment of closed extensor tendon injuries at the DIP joint is splinting, for 6 to 8 weeks. The readily available Stack splint (Link America, Inc., East Hanover, NJ)[15] is applied with tape to maintain the DIP joint in slight hyperextension. The proper size splint should be selected so that the proximal portion of the splint can be secured to the dorsum of the middle phalanx, while the distal fingertip rests within the tip of the splint. The fit should be snug but not too tight. If the splint is removed for hand-washing, care must be taken to maintain the distal joint in neutral position at all times.

Alternative splints have been recommended, including alumifoam padded dorsal splints and adaptations of the Stack splint. A plaster of Paris cast remains a viable option for the patient if there is a question of compliance.

Open Injuries   Wound exploration of open zone 1 injuries should be done in a bloodless field, using aseptic technique. The majority of simple skin and tendon lacerations may be treated by local infiltration or dorsal finger block using 1% lidocaine, without vasoconstrictors. Partial or complete lacerations of the extensor tendon over the DIP joint are repaired with nonabsorbable figure-of-eight 5-0 sutures. The tendon itself may be dissected and repaired as an isolated layer, or alternatively, to avoid additional dissection, skin and tendon may be sutured closed as a single layer[3] (Fig. 13–2).

Some intact extensor tissue will invariably be found in simple lacerations in zone 2, as the extensor tendon surrounds the dorsal one half of the middle phalanx. Passive extension of the DIP joint facilitates retrieval and approximation of the cut tendon ends. Repair can be performed using nonabsorbable figure-of-eight 5-0 sutures, burying the knots on the volar surface. I prefer closing the skin in a separate layer, but simultaneous suture of extensor tendon with dorsal skin has been described.[3]

In the case of missing extensor tissue, or extreme contamination, it is better to allow secondary healing than to attempt primary suturing of extensor tendon ends under tension. This allows the residual intact portion of extensor tendon to assume normal resting tension.[1] When soft tissue is missing, in the presence of significant contamination, initial debridement can be carried out, with temporary coverage of the middle phalanx with xenograft (pigskin), or allograft (cadaver skin).[5] The biologic dressing is changed every 48 hours. Tissue adhesion is a reliable sign that bacterial control has been achieved, and secondary soft tissue reconstruction may be performed.

■ TECHNICAL ALTERNATIVES

Complications of closed treatment of zone 1 injury include: pressure ulcers of the skin, full-thickness skin necrosis, a persistent palpable bump on dorsum of the finger, displace-

A and B, Simultaneous suture of a lacerated extensor tendon, incorporating the dorsal skin, using a running, simple technique. Sutures are removed in 10 to 12 days, but continuous splinting maintaining the DIP joint in extension for 6 weeks is required.

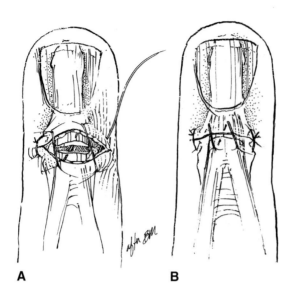

A   **B**

ment of the fracture fragment, and a persistent extensor tendon lag.[13,17] After study of skin vascularity at the level of the DIP joint, Rayan and Mullins[13] recommended that the involved finger be hyperextended to the point of skin blanching, and then the DIP joint extended only 50% of that degree when splinting to avoid skin pressure complications. There are two techniques[7] that may avoid skin necrosis and enhance compliance: one is to dispense three types of splints, which the patient alternates weekly, thus relieving specific pressure points. The other is to fashion a low-profile splint using 1-inch Coban wrap, followed by a paper clip taped to the dorsum of the DIP joint (which can be bent for slight hyperextention of the distal joint), followed by another layer of Coban wrap. Care should be taken not to excessively hyperextend the digit, to avoid dorsal skin necrosis. In addition, if there is a sizable dorsal fracture fragment, hyperextension will have a tendency to displace the fracture.[2]

Complications of open treatment of zone 1 injury include: deep infection, joint incongruity, nail deformity, sutures cutting through thin skin, malunion of the fracture, fixation or hardware failure, and joint stiffness with limited extensor and flexor limitation.[12,17,19]

■ REHABILITATION

The duration of splinting is adapted to the severity of injury. In zone 1 extensor tendon injury, whether treatment is closed or open, continuous extension of the DIP joint must be maintained for 6 weeks. If extensor lag is still present when the patient is re-examined, another 6 weeks of splinting is initiated. After the initial period of continuous splinting (minimum of 6 weeks), when full DIP extension is achieved, careful, gentle active flexion may be initiated, with the patient removing the splint only for range of motion exercises. In the first week of mobilization, active extension should be encouraged, and flexion of the DIP joint limited to 20° to 25°. In the second week, flexion of the distal joint is advanced to 35° provided there is no extensor lag.[4] After these first 8 weeks of splinting, the splint should be worn at night only for an additional 2 to 4 weeks. Proximal interphalangeal joint motion is encouraged from the time of initial repair, while the DIP joint is immobilized.

Following repair of zone 2 extensor tendon lacerations, a static volar splint with the MP and interphalangeal joints in neutral position is maintained for 3 to 4 weeks, followed by protected, range of motion exercises. If a zone 2 laceration is accompanied by associated injuries, consideration should be given to dynamic extension orthotics. When soft tissue stabilization has been achieved, usually within 1 to 5 days of surgery, a splint that passively extends the fingers, but allows the patient to actively flex the MP joints through an arc of motion is applied.[1] Patients are encouraged to perform these motions for 5 minutes each hour. Dynamic splinting is continued for 5 to 6 weeks after surgery.

Splinting of closed zone 1 extensor tendon injury has been quite successful, even when diagnosis is delayed beyond the acute phase of trauma.[12] Stern compared the complication rate of operative and nonoperative treatment of mallet finger. Although there was a 45% complication rate in 84 digits that were splinted, the complications were mostly skin related, and usually transient. In contrast, 53% of the 45 surgically treated digits developed complications, with three quarters of the complications still present after 3 years. Also, the splinted group had an average of 15° more flexion than had those treated surgically.[17]

In a long-term follow-up of repaired extensor tendons, Newport and co-authors[10] examined 12 tendons repaired in zone 1. Only 5 of 12 were excellent or good, and 7 of 12 were fair or poor. All 6 tendons repaired surgically in zone 2 were deemed fair. They concluded that extensor injuries with associated injuries do more poorly than extensor tendon injuries without associated injuries, and perhaps loss of active flexion is often underestimated.

Wehbé compared the results of operative and nonoperative treatment in 160 patients with mallet deformity. Twenty-one patients had associated mallet fractures. Surgical treatment offered no advantage over nonoperative treatment and had a greater rate of morbidity. Even patients with persistent palmar subluxation of the distal phalanx were shown to remodel the phalanx, with good outcomes.[19]

The results of these studies suggest that, whenever possible, closed treatment of zone 1 extensor injuries should be attempted. Following open repair of zone 1 or 2 extensor tendons, careful rehabilitation is necessary to optimize final motion.

■ OUTCOMES

References

1. Blair WF, Steyers CM: Extensor tendon injuries. Orthop Clin N Am, 1992; 23:141–148.
2. Blue AI, Spira M, Hardy SB: Repair of extensor tendon injuries of the hand. Am J Surg, 1976; 132:1–132.
3. Doyle JR: Extensor tendons—acute injuries. In: Green DP (ed): Operative Hand Surgery, 2nd Ed, New York: Churchill Livingstone, 1988:2045–2072.
4. Evans RB: Therapeutic management of extensor tendon injuries. In: Hunter JM, Schneider LH, Mackin EJ, Bell J (eds): Rehabilitation of the Hand, 3rd Ed, St. Louis: Mosby, 1990: 492–511.
5. Elliott RA Jr: Extensor tendon repair. In: McCarthy JG (ed): Plastic Surgery, Philadelphia: W. B. Saunders, 1990:4565–4594.
6. Kaplan EB: Anatomy, injuries and treatment of the extensor apparatus of the hand and fingers. Clin Orthop, 1959; 13:24–41.
7. Kasdan ML, Amadio PC, Bowers WH (eds): Technical Tips for Hand Surgery, St. Louis: Mosby, 1994:4–5.
8. Lewin P: A simple splint for baseball finger. JAMA, 1925; 85:1059.
9. Luban JD: Mallet finger fractures: A comparison of open and closed technique. J Hand Surg, 1989; 14A:394–396.
10. Newport ML, Blair WF, Steyers CM: Long-term results of extensor tendon repair. J Hand Surg, 1990; 15A:961–966.
11. Niechajev IA: Conservative and operative treatment of mallet finger. Plast Reconstr Surg, 1985; 76:580–585.
12. Patel MR, Shekhar SD, Bassini-Lipson L: Conservative management of chronic mallet finger. J Hand Surg, 1986; 11A:570–573.
13. Rayan GM, Mullins PT: Skin necrosis complicating mallet finger splinting and vascularity of the distal interphalangeal joint overlaying skin. J Hand Surg, 1987; 12A:548–552.
14. Smillie IS: Mallet finger. Br J Surg, 1937; 24:439–445.
15. Stack HG: Mallet Finger. Hand, 1969; 1:83–89.
16. Stark HH, Boyes JH, Wilson JN: Mallet finger. J Bone Joint Surg, 1962; 44A:1061–1068.
17. Stern PI, Kastrup JJ: Complications and prognosis of treatment of mallet finger. J Hand Surg, 1988; 13A:3–334.
18. Verdan CE: Primary and secondary repair of flexor and extensor tendon injuries. In: Flynn JE (ed): Hand Surgery, 2nd Ed, Baltimore: Williams & Wilkins, 1975:146–147.
19. Wehbé MA, Schneider LH: Mallet Fractures. J Bone Joint Surg, 1984; 66:658–669.
20. Zancolli E: Structural and Dynamic Basis of Hand Surgery, Philadelphia: J. B. Lippincott, 1968:105–106.

DENNIS J. ANDERSEN

14

Extensor Tendon Repairs in Zones 3–4

■ HISTORY OF THE TECHNIQUE

Injuries to the extensor tendons of the hand are problems commonly seen by hand surgeons. The exposure of the dorsum of the hand and fingers during active use, combined with the superficial nature of the extensor tendons, makes them particularly vulnerable to damage from mild to severe trauma.[14]

The relative simplicity of repairing the extensor tendons is equally well known.[5,10] Ease of exposure,[6,10] superficial location,[10,17] looseness of the overlying skin, lack of retraction of cut tendon ends,[6] and the ability to use simple suture techniques[5] all contribute to the cavalier attitude with which these injuries are sometimes approached. Likewise, the presumption that a persistent extensor lag or weakness is less detrimental overall than flexor dysfunction[2,17] may lead to the mistaken notion that extensor injuries are benign and undeserving of our clinical research focus.

While many authors have made casual mention of our limited appreciation for extensor injuries,[2–4,6,9–11,13,14,17] only recently have studies focused on this issue.[4,14] Newport and co-workers showed that the number of good or excellent results may be as low as 64%, and injuries that occur within extensor zones III and IV faired the worst in terms of overall motion.[14] Loss of flexion was both more frequent and more severe than was loss of extension; simultaneous fracture, dislocation, or injury to the joint capsule or flexor tendon predictably made the results even worse.[4,14]

The anatomy of extensor zones III and IV offers explanations that account for the difficulties encountered in treating injuries at this level.[5] The same superficial location that allows for easy repair also predisposes to adhesions between the tendon and subcutaneous tissue at the repair site.[2,6,13] Absence of a fibrous digital sheath, as in flexor tendons, enhances this predisposition.[5,8] In addition, only 2 to 3 mm of tendon excursion occurs at the level of the proximal phalanx during active finger motion,[8,13,14] while it has been suggested that 3 to 5 mm of excursion during tendon healing is necessary to prevent such adhesions.[7,14] Lovett has also stated that loss of 2 mm of extensor excursion at the proximal interphalangeal (PIP) joint level results in 50 percent loss of digital motion.[13]

The limited excursion of the tendon makes the balance between motions of the central tendon and the lateral bands very susceptible to any change in length,[9,14] whether it occurs from lengthening due to stretching of the intervening scar or from iatrogenic shortening during suturing. Suturing of the damaged tendon itself may be difficult because of the thinness of the tendon in zones III and IV.[2,9] Also, because of the paucity of soft tissue protection, concomitant injuries to the proximal phalanx and PIP joint are quite frequent.[2,9] Finally, the need to splint in extension may contribute to ultimate loss of flexion.[14]

Despite all the potential hurdles and the numerous advances in the treatment of digital flexor injuries, surgical techniques in the repair of acute zone III and IV extensor injuries have remained essentially unchanged for several decades.[1,2,5,6,8–10,14,17] Effort has been more active in rehabilitation of extensor tendons following repair. Yet, even though recent experience with dynamic splinting has shown some cause for optimism, it does not appear to offer much advantage in injuries in zones III or IV.[3,7,8,11]

Clearly, extensor tendon injuries should not be taken lightly. Attention must particularly be devoted to the precision of surgical repair, as little margin exists for tendon adhesion or alteration in length before adverse consequences are seen in function.

Extensor tendon injuries in zones III and IV occur by laceration or rupture.[10] Pain usually accompanies the injury, along with difficulty achieving full extension of the finger. Diagnosis in open injuries is often obvious, with lacerated tendon end directly visualized within the wound. Closed injuries or lacerations with small skin wounds, however, can be much more subtle. If the disruption involves the central tendon alone, as is frequently the case, extension of the PIP joint is still possible through the lateral bands.[5]

Suspicion of an acute extensor tendon injury should occur in any patient with a swollen, tender PIP joint.[5,13] Digital block anesthesia can assist during physical examination.[9] Although full passive extension of the PIP joint may be possible, a 15–20 degree loss of active extension with the wrist and metacarpophalangeal (MP) joints fully flexed may occur with an acute injury.[5] Terminal extension is also likely to be weak in an acute injury, so testing active extension against resistance is helpful.[8,13] Boyes diagnosed central tendon injuries acutely by holding the PIP joint in full extension and noting the amount of passive flexion of the DIP joint.[5] He noted that with increased tension on the lateral bands, distal interphalangeal (DIP) joint flexion is reduced.

Open lacerations are likely to enter the joint in zone III or involve periosteal damage in zone IV,[3,7] and they therefore require urgent cleansing and appropriate antibiotics. Primary operative repair is usually recommended at the same time.[2,10,13,17] Operative repair has also been recommended in cases of avulsion of the central tendon insertion along with a bony fragment, or when rupture is associated with dislocation of the PIP joint.[17]

Partial lacerations often occur in zone IV, where the curvature of the underlying bone protects the lateral aspects of the dorsal apparatus.[5] Such partial lacerations may occur with relatively normal motion, but pain with active extension is likely. If doubt regarding the integrity of the extensor remains after thorough examination, extension of the wound following adequate anesthesia for direct visualization of the tendon is necessary.[5]

Associated injuries are common and must be addressed along with the tendon. Fractures are evaluated with appropriate radiographic studies and rigidly fixed. Open injuries over the PIP joint require thorough irrigation and closure of the capsule. Skin grafting or flap coverage with secondary tendon reconstruction may be necessary in cases of soft tissue loss overlying the tendon.[5] Alternatively, with extensive intra-articular injury or full thickness tissue loss including the tendon (ie. burns or abrasions), PIP fusion may be considered.[6,9]

Closed avulsion injuries occur commonly over the PIP joint in zone III, and usually involve only the central tendon near its insertion. These tendon disruptions can usually be treated adequately with splint immobilization for 5–6 weeks.[2,5,10,17] Splinting of the PIP joint alone in full extension, while allowing flexion of the DIP joint, helps to draw the tendon ends together, thus maintaining the normal length relationships between the central tendon and the lateral bands.[10] Some authors have recommended a transarticular K-wire as a more secure way of holding the PIP joint extended,[2,6,17] however, adjustable splinting allows controlled correction of any developing flexion deformity.[5] Splinting and protected motion in partial lacerations is normally sufficient, but delayed rupture, usually at 10–14 days, can occur. They are treated as closed injuries.[6]

Approximately 10–21 days after an acute injury that has been untreated, a characteristic boutonnière deformity may be noted,[5] because of unopposed superficialis flexion of the PIP joint,[17] volar migration of the lateral bands,[2,10,17] and increased extension force directed at the DIP joint.[2,17]

Treatment of older injuries with established boutonnière deformity remains controversial. Elliott felt that the elongated central tendon and volar subluxation of the lateral bands in any injury more than 12–14 days old made this deformity resistant to splinting alone.[6] Weakness and inability to flex the DIP joint results in significant disability.[13] He proposed mobilization of the lateral bands and anatomic surgical repair.[6] However, others have found closed splinting more predictable in both early boutonnière deformities, as well as those over 6 months duration.[5,9]

The ability to perform primary repair depends on the state of the superficial soft tissue.[17] Under favorable conditions, primary repair allows restoration of normal anatomy. How-

■ INDICATIONS AND
CONTRAINDICATIONS

ever, priority must be given to skin cover, flexor tendons, neurovascular structures, and bone.[6] Severe injury to these structures may require postoperative management that is unfavorable to the extensor mechanism. For example, the need for early mobilization of flexor tendons or fixation of joints in flexion to protect nerve repairs may interfere with the postoperative splinting required for extensor healing and rehabilitation. Under such conditions, one may be well-advised to appropriately treat such a priority defect, and plan extensor reconstruction secondarily.[6]

■ SURGICAL TECHNIQUES

At the time of the initial assessment of any open laceration, the primary focus should be on the prevention of infection.[5,17] Thorough irrigation and debridement of all wounds is therefore mandatory. Elliott advised immediate repair only within the first six hours after injury, with wound care, antibiotic, and secondary repair thereafter.[6] However this rigid time frame seems quite arbitrary. If the level of contamination and the condition of the soft tissue cover permit immediate wound closure, and no priority injury is present to obviate proper splinting, then primary repair of the extensor mechanism should be performed.

Simple lacerations in zones III and IV can often be treated adequately under local anesthesia. However, regional or general anesthesia would be a more appropriate choice for those injuries that involve skin or tendon loss, open fractures, or open joints. Tourniquet control of bleeding and extension of the wound through longitudinal midlateral or curved dorsal incisions are often necessary to ensure sufficient exposure and access to injured structures. Regional or general anesthesia allows better patient tolerance of tourniquets, and necessary repairs can be performed under more relaxed conditions.

In zone III, the skin laceration is usually transverse, and the PIP joint is often exposed.[2,9] A short longitudinal extension of the wound helps to increase exposure and access to the joint for irrigation. The central slip is usually involved in dorsal lacerations,[2] with or without injury to the lateral bands. Retraction of the cut tendon ends is minimal,[6] and detailed dissection to identify each individual component of the extensor mechanism is unnecessary.[5] If sufficient tendon remains attached distally at the bony insertion, a primary repair is performed of the tendon and dorsal capsule using 4-0 or 5-0 nonabsorbable suture.[6] Buried figure-of-eight technique is usually adequate, with care to avoid bunching of the tendon (Fig. 14–1). The original length of the tendon should be restored as closely as possible. Repair of lacerated lateral bands is also performed using buried, interrupted suture.[17] Reconstruction of the triangular ligament by means of a few sutures reapproximating the distal portions of the lateral tendons may also help to keep them from subluxating volarly.[17]

If the central tendon is lacerated at or close to its insertion into the base of the middle phalanx, primary tendon repair may be impossible. In this circumstance, a simple suture technique may be used to reattach the tendon to bone using a nonabsorbable suture (Fig. 14–2).[12] Alternatively, a Bunnel type weave can be placed to firmly grasp the tendon end, with the suture then being passed through a transverse drill hole to secure the tendon to the base of the middle phalanx (Fig. 14–3).[5]

In zone IV, the lateral bands lie volar to the dorsal cortex of the proximal phalanx and, therefore, are relatively protected, while the central tendon remains vulnerable.[5] The main goal of primary repair in complete lacerations is to restore the proper length relationships between these structures. Exposure and repair of the tendon is performed as described for zone III lacerations. Wound extension, as necessary, and minimal subcutaneous dissection are performed to identified the tendon ends.[6] An effort should be made to cover any exposed bone with periosteum, as this may minimize the adherence of tendon to bone.[10] Figure-of-eight, non-absorbable suture is used to gently bring the tendon ends into reapproximation without bunching. If involved, lateral bands are sutured separately.[5]

In both zone III and IV injuries, the PIP joint should be maintained in full extension for six weeks.[5,6,8,10,13] This allows for maintenance of the proper length relationships of the extensor components until healing is established. This is most reliably accomplished with a percutaneous K-wire inserted obliquely across the PIP joint to fix it in this position.[6,10,13]

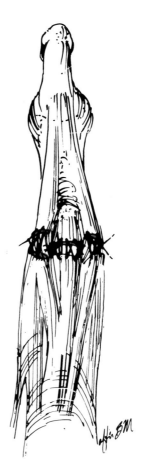

■ FIGURE 14–1
Primary repair of extensor tendon in zone III using figure-of-eight suture technique.

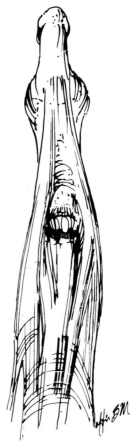

■ FIGURE 14–2
Direct repair of extensor tendon to bone, using drill holes in the base of the middle phalanx.[12]

■ FIGURE 14–3
Direct repair of extensor
tendon to bone, using a
Bunnell suture and a
transverse drill hole
through the base of the
middle phalanx.

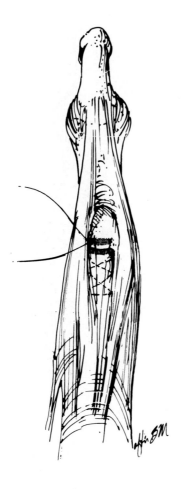

Skin is closed as a separate layer with 5-0 or 6-0 nylon. A non-adherent gauze dressing
and light plaster hand splint is applied, leaving the DIP joint free to move.

■ TECHNICAL
ALTERNATIVES

    While repair of extensor lacerations over the PIP joint using buried sutures is technically
quite simple, some authors have advocated using a vertical figure-of-eight technique, to
bring the tendon, capsule, and skin together via a single suture. Indeed, in simple lacerations, just about any method by which the tendon ends can be brought together will
succeed.[5]

    In more complex injuries involving loss of tendon substance, however, a much more
difficult situation is posed, as primary tendon repair is either impossible, or would result
in an unacceptable amount of shortening. One method described by Aiche and co-workers
can be used to overcome this dilemma when the injury is to the central slip only.[1,5,9]
Following identification and dissection of the lateral bands on both sides, each is split
longitudinally a distance of two centimeters. The resulting two slips from each lateral
band are left attached at their ends. The central halves are then brought together in the
midline over the lacerated central tendon and sutured side to side to reinforce this structure
(Fig. 14–4). In essence, a new central tendon is constructed using the central half of each
lateral band.

    If the loss involves the lateral bands as well as the central tendon, Snow described a
technique whereby a distally based, retrograde flap is made from the proximal portion
of the central tendon and used to bridge the gap (Fig. 14–5).[5,9,16]

    Difficulty in direct repair secondary to frayed tendon ends may be encountered in zone
IV, as well. One must avoid the tendency to draw the distant tendons together, as significant shortening may result.[13] Shortening may occur, as well, from carelessly placed sutures
that needlessly bunch the tendon.[9]

    In addition, although sufficient exposure is necessary to adequately perform a repair,

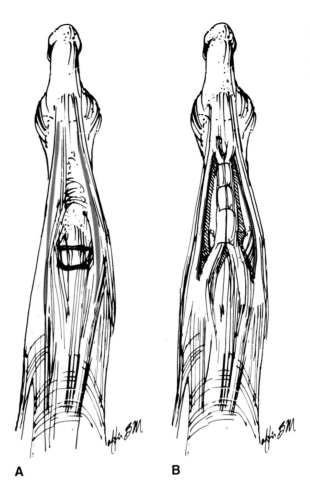

■ FIGURE 14–4
Aiche[1] technique for mobilization of the lateral
bands. A) The lateral
bands are split in longitudinal fashion, and the medial halves are sutured together and to the capsule
in the midline. B) The lateral halves are left undisturbed.

A   **B**

unnecessarily extensive dissection around the extensor tendon may add to the natural tendency to form adhesions, especially in zone IV.[6]

■ REHABILITATION

Postoperatively, the patient is maintained in a bulky, plaster-reinforced dressing, with the wrist held in neutral, the MP joints at 20 degrees of flexion, and the interphalangeal (IP) joints fully extended.[5,10] Elevation of the extremity is encouraged. At two weeks, the splint is discontinued, and sutures are removed. Active DIP joint flexion is encouraged immediately,[6,8,9] if the injury was isolated to the central tendon. If the lateral bands were involved, it will be necessary to immobilize the DIP joint in extension for four weeks.[8]

The transarticular K-wire is removed at five to six weeks, and active exercises are instituted.[8,13] Initially, the MP joint should be held manually in flexion as active PIP extension is performed, to more effectively transmit extensor force to this joint.[8] Between exercise sessions, the PIP joint is maintained in full extension by a static splint for 2 more weeks.[8,13] Dynamic flexion splinting may be added to the regimen in cases where recovery of flexion is slow,[8,13] however, one must be cautious to avoid creating an extensor lag. Joint blocking techniques are utilized, and active resistive exercises are incorporated at 9 to 10 weeks.[8] Some authors have recommended internal splinting for only 4 weeks in patients over 45 years of age and the advancement of the mobilization program by one week.[6,13]

If an extensor lag of greater than 20° develops at any time during mobilization, static splinting should be resumed full time for another two weeks. If a lag develops during dynamic flexion, alternating dynamic flexion and extension splinting may be used. Only when full PIP extension is easily held should extension splinting be discontinued altogether.[13]

In reliable patients, a transartricular K-wire may not be necessary, as an externally applied splint can be equally effective at holding the PIP joint in full extension.[5] Usually,

■ FIGURE 14−5
Snow[16] technique for reconstructing the extensor
mechanism in situations
of substance loss. A) A
retrograde flap from the
central slip is used to
reinforce the area of re-
pair. B) The proximal de-
fect is closed side-to-
side.

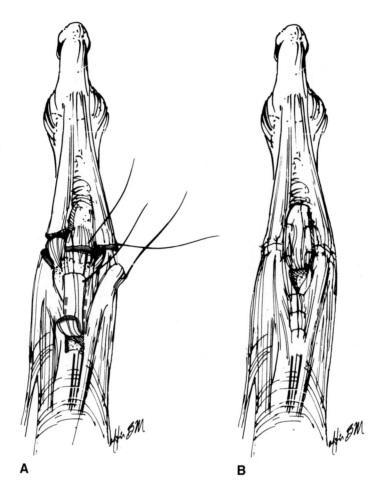

A   **B**

only the PIP joint needs to be immobilized in the splint during rehabilitation.[8] Frequent adjustments of the splint may be necessary.

Edema can be controlled using Coban wraps. Early scar management consists of massage, with or without the use of silicone elastomer pressure molds.[8]

Recent efforts in the use of early controlled motion with dynamic splintage in extensor injuries have offered some encouraging results in lesions proximal to the MP joints.[3,4,7,8] However, this method may have less applicability in zones III and IV, where overall tendon excursion is only 2−3 mm, and rehabilitation appears to focus more on overcoming joint stiffness rather than tendon glide.[7,8]

■ OUTCOMES

Although traditionally simple extensor lacerations are expected to do well, a recent retrospective analysis has shown that as few as 64% of all extensor injuries, and less than 50% of zone III and IV injuries, will achieve a good or excellent result (defined by extensor lag of less than 10° and total loss of flexion of less than 20°).[14] Loss of motion is probably the area of greatest concern, and injuries within zones III and IV have the worst prognosis overall, both in terms of extensor lag and loss of flexion.[13,14] Diminished flexion may, in fact, be more of a problem, both in prevalence and degree.[4,14] In Newport's study, 71% lost flexion at the PIP, while 35% lost extension. Extensor lag at the DIP joint was also noted to occur in zone III and IV injuries.[14]

Possible explanations for the poor recovery of motion are many: the anatomic complexity of the extensor apparatus,[2,10] the delicate balance between the intrinsic and extrinsic forces,[9,17] the poor quality of the tendon[10] and repair techniques,[3,15] the close proximity to the bone[10] and subcutaneous tissue overlying the proximal phalanx leading to adhesion formation,[17] and the propensity for associated injuries.[9,14]

Associated injuries (fracture dislocation, joint capsule, or flexor tendon damage) occurred 64% of the time in Newport's study, and were shown to worsen the prognosis.[14] Patients with a fracture had 50% good or excellent results compared to 64% in isolated lacerations. This is likely due to both the injury itself and the necessary immobilization. Joint dislocation has a similar effect on prognosis, although joint capsule disruption without dislocation does not necessarily affect the overall result. Combinations of associated injuries had the worst effect on overall prognosis (33% good or excellent).[14]

On the other hand, total active motion and grip strength were not adversely affected by associated injuries to any significant degree. Total active motion remained 80–90% and grip strength 95% of normal. Likewise, 95% of the patients were pleased with their functional result, and only 10% had to change jobs or hobbies.[14]

The one co-variable that is difficult to evaluate experimentally is patient motivation. Few surgeons can deny treating the occasional individual with a markedly complex injury who ultimately achieves a remarkable result, or, conversely, one in which a simple laceration yields considerable impairment. Intelligence and motivation of the patient, it would seem, can have as much influence on the outcome as the experience and ability of the surgeon.[6]

It is clear that extensor tendon injuries do pose greater difficulty than is generally appreciated. Attention to the details involved in each injury is a must. Yet, despite the many areas of concern, good results can be attained in zones III and IV. As more research better defines the role of each component involved in extensor injuries, it is hoped that improvement in overall results will follow. Although it is conceivable that improvements in surgical technique may be seen, it is likely that the most significant advances in the near future will be made in the area of rehabilitation.

References

1. Aiche A, Barskey AJ, Weiner DL: Prevention of boutonnière deformity. Plast Reconstr Surg, 1979; 46:164–167.
2. Blue AI, Spira M, Hardy SB: Repair of extensor tendon injuries of the hand. Am J Surg, 1976; 132:128–132.
3. Browne EZ, Ribik CA: Early dynamic splinting for extensor tendon injuries. J Hand Surg, 1989; 14A:72–76.
4. Chow JA, Dovelle S, Thomes J, Callahan D: Post-operative management of repair of extensor tendons of the hand-dynamic versus static splinting. Orthop Trans 1987; 11:258–259.
5. Doyle JR: Extensor tendons—acute injuries. In: Green DP, ed. Operative Hand Surgery, 3rd ed, New York: Churchill Livingstone, 1993:1925–1954.
6. Elliott RA: Injuries to the extensor mechanism of the hand. Orthop Clin North Am, 1970; 1: 335–354.
7. Evans RB, Burkhalter WE: A study of the dynamic anatomy of extensor tendons and implications for treatment. J Hand Surg, 1986; 11A:774–779.
8. Evans RB: Therapeutic management of extensor tendon injuries. Hand Clin, 1986; 2:157–169.
9. Froehlich JA, Akelman E, Herndon JH: Extensor tendon injuries at the proximal interphalangeal joint. Hand Clin, 1988; 4:25–37.
10. Herndon JH: Tendon injuries—extensor surface. Emerg Med Clin North Am, 1985; 3: 333–340.
11. Hung LK, Chan A, Chang J, Tsang A, Leung PC: Early controlled active mobilization with dynamic splintage for treatment of extensor tendon injuries. J Hand Surg, 1990; 15A:251–257.
12. Kaplan EB: Anatomy, injuries, and treatment of the extensor apparatus of the hand and the digits. Clin Orthop, 1959; 13:24–41.
13. Lovett WL, McCalla MA: Management and rehabilitation of extensor tendon injuries. Orthop Clin North Am, 1983; 14:811–826.
14. Newport ML, Blair WF, Steyers CM: Long-term results of extensor tendon repair. J Hand Surg, 1990; 15A:961–966.
15. Newport ML, Williams CD: Biomechanical characteristics of extensor tendon suture techniques. J Hand Surg, 1992; 17A:1117–1123.
16. Snow JW: Use of a retrograde tendon flap in repairing severed extensor tendon in the PIP join area. Plast Reconstr Surg, 1973; 51:555–558.
17. Tubiana R: Surgical repair of the extensor apparatus of the finger. Surg Clin North Am, 1968; 48:1015–1031.

MARY LYNN
NEWPORT

15

Extensor Tendon Repairs in Zones 5–6

■ HISTORY OF THE
TECHNIQUE

The tendons in zones 5 and 6 are the most commonly injured extensor tendons.[9] The exposed nature of the dorsum of the hand and proximity of the extensors to the metacarpo-phalangeal (MP) joint make these areas particularly vulnerable. Extensor tendon injuries, although common, seldom receive the careful attention given flexor tendon injuries, and the ease of exposure in all zones makes it inviting to care for many extensor tendon lacerations in the emergency department. Well-respected authors[3,12] have warned against such a cavalier attitude, and recent evidence has shown that there can be significant problems after repair of even "simple" extensor lacerations.[9,11] Although the number of clinical studies examining extensor tendon lacerations is relatively small, they show that when carefully evaluated, these injuries may have only 60% good or excellent results.

Whereas sophistication toward flexor repair has blossomed in past years, sophistication toward extensor repair has lagged far behind. Recently, however, that has changed markedly with a surge of research concentrating on quality operative results for extensor injuries and innovative postoperative programs.[1,2,5,6,11] Although static splinting remains the most frequently used postoperative routine, Evans and Burkhalter in 1986 were the first to show that extensor repair could be significantly improved using a different approach.[5] They combined the well-known postoperative dynamic splint used for rheumatoid MP joint reconstruction with the Kleinert principle of rubber band–mediated tendon gliding in a dynamic extensor outrigger. Their assumption was that such dynamic splinting, especially when compared with static splinting, improved results by decreasing adhesion formation. Initial investigation of the biomechanics of extensor repair by Newport and coworkers[9] has shown, however, that adhesion formation—at first hypothesized to be the major contributor to poor results—is perhaps only one factor. Typical repair techniques used today significantly shorten the extensor tendon by bunching the ends, and such shortening contributes biomechanically to decrease MP and proximal interphalangeal (PIP) joint motion.[11] In addition, the mattress and figure-of-eight techniques, often used in extensor repair, are weaker in strength and poorer in biomechanical characteristics than the modified Kessler and modified Bunnell techniques and may not be capable of withstanding the forces that may occur during dynamic splinting.[11]

It is clear that only a basic understanding of extensor tendon repair exists, both in terms of clinical results and in biomechanical factors. It is also clear that this state of affairs has been recognized and is currently being addressed. There is no doubt that the accepted standard of care for extensor injuries will continue to evolve and improve in the near future.

■ INDICATIONS AND
CONTRAINDICATIONS

Extensor tendons in zones 5 and 6 are injured through laceration, avulsion, or rupture. Diagnosis of injury includes pain with or inability to fully extend the finger. Because extensor tendon ends seldom lay or stay in direct apposition, intervention in the form of direct repair is usually necessary.

The diagnosis of central extensor tendon injury in zones 5 and 6 is generally not difficult. The patient is unable to actively extend the MP joint or joints and there is an obvious wound on the dorsum of the hand. Careful testing for MP joint extension should be performed because interphalangeal joint extension, which occurs by the intrinsic musculature, may be misinterpreted as extrinsic extensor integrity. With the wrist held in neutral position, the patient should be asked to fully extend the MP joints while keeping the interphalangeal joints in extension throughout. Yet another diagnostic maneuver is necessary to ensure that MP joint extension of an affected finger is not being produced by an adjacent intact junctura tendinum. This can occur when the tendon laceration is proximal to the junctura and the MP joint is extended through a junctura attached to an intact tendon. This maneuver consists of flexing all MP joints and individually extending each finger, keeping the remaining MP joints in flexion. This counteracts any extension that might be mediated through an intact junctura. Extension of each MP joint against gentle resistance should also be performed to help delineate any partial laceration of the extensor tendon. When a partial laceration is present, extension is either incomplete or painful. An incomplete laceration must be diagnosed and appropriately treated to prevent later rupture. After a thorough examination, if doubt still exists concerning the integrity of an extensor tendon, direct visualization is necessary through the wound or by longitudinally extending the wound and inspecting the tendon. This must be performed with adequate anesthesia, hemostasis, and lighting.

Zones 5 and 6 injuries are often associated with other injuries to the hand, including joint capsule damage, fractures, tendon loss, and skin loss. The first priority in such complex injuries is thorough debridement of foreign material and nonviable tissue after tetanus prophylaxis. Fractures should be stabilized as rigidly as possible to allow dynamic splinting postoperatively when other conditions permit. Soft-tissue coverage can often be managed by mobilizing the pliant skin on the dorsum of the hand but when this is not possible, other options must be considered. The radial artery forearm flap (Chinese flap) is an excellent, relatively simple way to cover the dorsum of the hand when the injury has been confined to that area. Other options include pedicle flaps from the groin or chest or microvascular free flaps from the lateral arm or dorsum of the foot, all of which have indications that are better discussed elsewhere. Split-thickness skin grafting can be performed when the paratenon of the extensor tendons is intact; however, the aforementioned flaps provide more durable coverage and allow better tendon gliding.

For complex injuries that can be adequately debrided, all reconstruction can be performed in one or two stages, with final skin coverage performed at the second sitting, 1 to 2 days after initial injury. When the wound is contaminated, sequential debridements are necessary before finally addressing bone, tendon, and skin elements. Bone loss should be managed initially with wire spacers or with plate and screws. Tendons should be repaired after bony length has been restored but before secondary bone grafting. Tendons can be kept moist with proper dressings and frequent debridements until final repair can be performed. Only in cases of significant (greater than 1 cm) extensor tendon loss should primary tendon repair not be performed. In those circumstances, adequate wound debridement and skeletal fixation should be followed with skin coverage and short intercalary extensor tendon grafts for smaller wounds or silicone tendon rods in a staged reconstruction for severe loss.

In most circumstances, lacerations in zone 5 can be treated similarly to those in zone 6, except that the underlying MP joint capsule is often injured. It is imperative in the emergency department to ascertain the integrity of the joint, either through careful inspection of the wound or by injecting the joint with saline or methylene blue in an area away from the laceration under aseptic conditions. This method should detect even small tears in the capsule as the saline or dye seeps into the wound. When the joint capsule has been breached, joint irrigation and debridement should take precedence, and the patient taken emergently to the operating room.

Closed rupture of the central tendon in zone 5 or 6 is rare but rupture of the sagittal bands holding the tendon in place over the MP joint in zone 5 is not. This occurs after a blow to the hand or forcible extension or flexion of the MP joint. The middle finger is most commonly involved, and the rupture is most often on the radial side. This allows dislocation of the central tendon ulnarly into the metacarpal valley, with resultant ulnar deviation of the finger and inability to actively extend the MP joint. These patients are often able to hold the MP joint extended strongly against resistance after the finger is passively extended but are unable to initiate extension. Ulnar-sided ruptures are uncommon but have been reported.[7] Acute injuries (within hours) may be considered for conservative treatment with a splint holding the MP joint in neutral deviation and 0° flexion. To insure that the sagittal fibers are adequately apposed and the tendon properly centered over the MP joint, operative treatment provides a more reliable outcome.

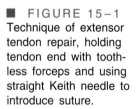

■ SURGICAL TECHNIQUES

Once an extensor tendon injury has been identified, wounds that are not contaminated and in which no capsular damage is present can be treated with irrigation and loose skin closure, splinting, and semi-elective surgical repair. Contaminated wounds, open fractures, or open joints with extensor injury should be treated emergently. Depending on the extent of the injury, intravenous regional, axillary, or scalene block is the anesthetic technique of choice unless prohibited by other factors. A tourniquet is recommended to help obtain the best possible visualization of the wound. Under most conditions, all structures can and should be repaired at the initial surgical procedure. If the initial wound allows adequate assessment of injuries and adequate access to injured structures, it is not extended. When adequate visualization or access is not possible, the wound should be extended longitudinally in line with the affected finger, converting horizontal lacerations into zigzag exposures as necessary.

In zone 6, the areolar tissue surrounding the extensor tendon is gently dissected, so that the lacerated tendon ends are freely mobile and easily handled. Although seldom needed because extensors do not tend to retract significantly, as do flexor tendons, a Keith needle can be used to transfix the tendon proximally, distally, or both to keep the ends easily accessible within the wound. Suturing of the tendon itself is often difficult and frustrating. Extensor tendons are flat and thin, fray easily, and tend to overlap when sutured. I prefer to use forceps without teeth and hold the tendon end perpendicular to its axis (Fig. 15–1). A curved needle can be used but a straight needle makes it easier to introduce the suture into the free tendon end, which may be trimmed slightly if necessary. The needle is introduced into the mid-substance of the free end to obtain an adequate purchase in the thin, flat extensor tendon. Generally, the suture should be introduced into the direct center of the tendon and advanced for a length of about 1.5 cm before exiting the side of the tendon for the horizontal component of the modified Bunnell technique. One study has shown

■ FIGURE 15–1
Technique of extensor tendon repair, holding tendon end with toothless forceps and using straight Keith needle to introduce suture.

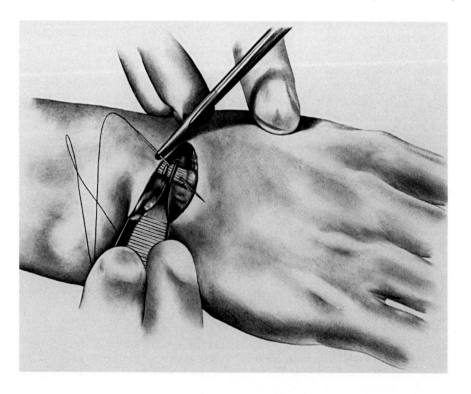

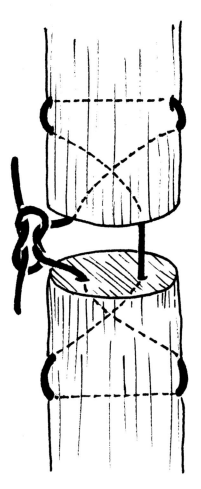

■ FIGURE 15–2
Modified suture technique
of Bunnell.

that the Kleinert modification of the Bunnell technique (Fig. 15–2) is the strongest available technique for extensor repair in zone 6 and produces the least shortening of the tendon and least loss of finger range of motion in a cadaver model.[11] Suture material should be of monofilament synthetic substance stout enough to hold securely (e.g., 4-0 Prolene) [Ethicon, Somerville, NJ]. One suture per tendon is all that is necessary; no further repair or tidying of tendon ends is desirable or possible. The tourniquet should be deflated before closure if extensive dissection has been performed and hemostasis obtained by electrocautery. In clean wounds, the skin is closed with fine nonabsorbable sutures, such as 5-0 nylon in a horizontal mattress.

A similar approach is taken with extensor tendon lacerations in zone 5. If the injury includes laceration of the MP joint capsule, the joint is thoroughly irrigated and inspected for damage. This is performed by flexing the joint and retracting the lacerated capsule radially and ulnarly. The lacerated tendon can usually be retracted proximally or distally to allow visualization. If the capsule laceration is too small to allow adequate inspection and irrigation, it should be extended longitudinally just enough to accommodate visualization. The capsule should be loosely closed with fine absorbable sutures (4-0 Vicryl) [Ethicon, Somerville, NJ] over a passive drain. Transverse injuries may also damage the sagittal bands of the extensor mechanism. When this has occurred, each sagittal band should be accurately reapproximated with fine absorbable interrupted sutures (5-0 Vicryl), with care taken to center the extensor tendon accurately over the joint.

In severely contaminated wounds, such as a human bite or a farm injury, thorough irrigation and debridement should follow appropriate antibiotic administration. A culture should also be obtained after debridement. The joint capsule should not be closed but packed open with fine mesh gauze. The gauze also holds the skin open. Both wounds should be allowed to close by secondary intention only.

Sagittal band rupture in zone 5 generally requires surgical reapproximation. This is performed with regional anesthesia under tourniquet control. A 4- to 5-cm long incision centered over the MP joint is taken through the fine areolar tissue overlying the extensor mechanism. The sagittal band rupture is most often seen on the radial side. In acute injuries, this is readily apparent. Each edge of the sagittal band is gently freed of surrounding soft tissue by blunt dissection to allow accurate reapproximation. This is accomplished using fine absorbable sutures (5-0 Vicryl) in a horizontal mattress fashion, with care taken to prevent overlap of the edges. The extensor tendon should be accurately centered over the MP joint and gentle motion should be performed to insure that it remains in place. If there is a tendency for the extensor tendon to sublux ulnarly, release of the ulnar sagittal fibers should be performed to help balance the repair. In more chronic cases, ulnar sagittal release is almost always necessary and the attenuated radial band is incised and overlapped to restore balance.[7] If the radial sagittal fibers are too attenuated to allow adequate repair or reefing, other adjacent tissues must be used. The junctura on the ulnar side of the affected tendon may be detached with as much length as possible, brought volar to the extensor tendon, and sutured to the radial aspect of the MP joint capsule with a stout absorbable suture (3-0 Vicryl).[13] If this is not possible, a distally based retrograde slip of extensor tendon may be fashioned on the radial side of the affected tendon and anchored to the deep intermetacarpal ligament[4] or passed around the lumbrical and sutured to itself.[8]

For all injuries and surgical procedures in zones 5 and 6, a large bulky compressive bandage is applied over a nonadherent dressing. The wrist is held in moderate extension and the MP joints are held in 0° of extension. The PIP and distal interphalangeal (DIP) joints should remain free.

For extensor tendon lacerations, the initial postoperative dressing is changed in 3 to 4 days and the patient is placed in a dynamic extension splint. The patient then begins a monitored rehabilitation program. The sutures are routinely removed about 2 weeks after surgery. When the MP joint capsule has been damaged, the drain is removed in 24 to 48 hours and dynamic splinting is begun when the wound is stable.

For patients with sagittal band rupture and repair, the postoperative dressing is changed in 2 weeks, the sutures removed, and a short arm cast applied with the fingers in the same position. PIP and DIP joint motion is encouraged to prevent the formation of extensor adhesions.

■ TECHNICAL
ALTERNATIVES

The most significant pitfall involved in zone 5 or 6 extensor tendon injury is failure to recognize the extent of the injury. Zone 6 lacerations are generally obvious, with drooping of the finger. Partial lacerations can be missed if careful evaluation of full extension of the MP joints, with and without resistance, is not performed. Lacerations proximal to the juncturae may be missed if weak extension through adjacent juncturae occurs. Missed complete lacerations almost always produce extensor lag. Missed partial lacerations may attenuate sufficiently to produce extension lag or they may rupture completely.

Technical difficulties in zone 6 are generally limited to the quality of repair. A frayed, badly damaged tendon may be difficult to repair neatly and without shortening. Careless repairs of tendons, which produce significant shortening, may introduce unnecessary iatrogenic diminution of finger range of motion. In addition, use of suture techniques that do not sufficiently grasp the tendon, such as the mattress and figure-of-eight techniques, may allow repair attenuation.

Missed lacerations of the MP joint capsule in zone 5 may lead to septic arthritis, with resultant destruction of the joint or severely decreased MP joint motion, neither of which are easily salvageable; both lead to markedly diminished hand function. Therefore, a high index of suspicion is necessary to fully investigate this injury.

Missed rupture of the sagittal bands in zone 5 can still be treated if recognized later but may require significant additional intervention to properly repair. A rupture treated early may require only repair of the sagittal fibers, whereas later repair may require ulnar sagittal band release and may also require use of adjunct tissues (e.g., juncturae or extensor slips) to adequately centralize and hold the central tendon. Surgical difficulties in repair usually involve inadequate repair or reefing of the injured radial fibers or inadequate release of the ulnar fibers, such that the central tendon redislocates into the ulnar metacarpal valley.

Postoperative management must consider the entire injury. Ideally, bony stability and skin coverage should be adequate to allow early dynamic extensor splinting. Dynamic splinting is probably more important in these complex injuries because of an increased likelihood of tendon adherence to soft tissue or bone. The dynamic splint should include all affected fingers in the outrigger and adjacent fingers to alleviate the pull of adjacent juncturae. It should be applied as soon as the wound is stable, generally 2 to 3 days after surgery in simple lacerations. This dynamic splint is formed of heat-sensitive plastic, holds the wrist in about 30° extension, passively pulls the MP joints into extension with rubber bands, and allows free active flexion (Fig. 15–3). The patient is instructed by the therapist to keep the splint on at all times and to perform finger flexion exercises several times per hour. A static splint with all joints in extension may be used at bedtime if the dynamic

■ REHABILITATION

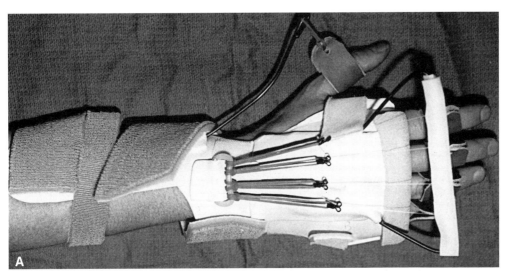

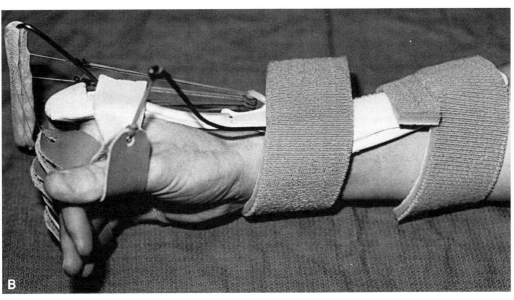

■ FIGURE 15–3
A and **B**, Dynamic extension splint for postoperative rehabilitation after extensor injury in zones 5 and 6.

splint is too unwieldy. A dynamic extensor splint with a dorsal block hood holding the MP joints in about 15° flexion is most efficacious in preventing extensor muscle activity during passive extension and active flexion.[10] This regimen is followed for 5 to 6 weeks, after which the splint is discontinued and gentle active flexion and extension begun.

For unreliable patients or for those who cannot fully cooperate, a static splint or cast holding the wrist in 30° extension and MP joints at 15° flexion, allowing and encouraging free PIP and DIP joint motion, may be used for 4 to 6 weeks.

■ OUTCOMES

Although studies have shown excellent results with dynamic splinting (98 to 100% good/excellent) in selected patients having simple lacerations,[2,5] no study has similarly documented results in multicomponent trauma. A recent study, however, has shown that 74% of patients without associated injury obtain good or excellent results in zones 5 and 6, whereas only 26% of those having associated injury (fracture, joint dislocation, skin loss) have good or excellent results.[9] These patients were all treated with static splinting and although not yet scientifically proved, it is inviting to think that the percentage of

■ FIGURE 15–4
A and **B**, Loss of motion (in degrees) at each joint after extensor injury in zones 5 and 6.

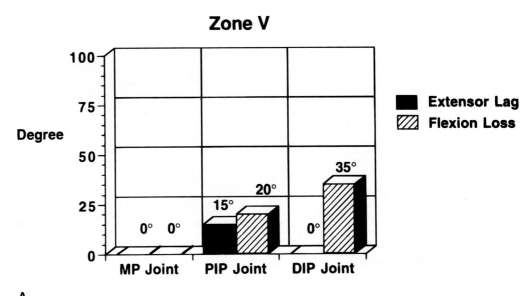

A

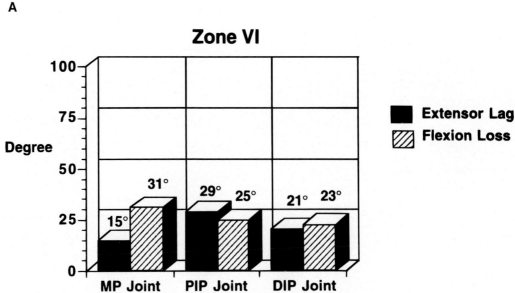

B

good and excellent results in extensor tendon lacerations with associated injury would improve with dynamic extensor splinting. In addition, the recognition that there can be an iatrogenic contribution to poorer results should also help to improve overall results. Lastly, it should be noted that when comparing the results of extensor injury in all zones, zone 5 had the best overall rate of good and excellent results (83%) and results in zone 6 were equivalent to those in zones 7 and 8 (63 to 68%).[9] Simple laceration of the joint capsule did not affect the quality of result in zone 5.

Quality of result after extensor tendon repair must include evaluation of both extensor lag and loss of flexion. Although extensor lag may be annoying to the patient, loss of flexion occurs more frequently and is a greater detriment to hand function. Zone 5 averaged no loss of flexion or extension at the MP joint but did lose motion at more distal joints.[9] Figure 15-4A and B show a comparison of motion loss at each joint after extensor tendon injury in zones 5 and 6. It is important to note that injury in one area can result in loss of motion at distant joints.

Injury to the extensor tendons in zones 5 and 6 is relatively common. Diagnosis of extensor damage is generally not difficult but obtaining a quality repair is. Gentle handling of these tendons is imperative because they easily fray and separate. The available literature shows that the quality of result is directly attributable to suture technique and postoperative rehabilitation; as a consequence, careful attention must be given to both.

References

1. Allieau Y, Asencio G, Rouzand JC: Protected Passive Mobilization After Suturing of the Extensor Tendons of the Hand. In: Tubiana R (ed): The Hand, Vol III, Philadelphia: WB Saunders, 1988:157–166.
2. Browne EZ Jr, Ribik CA: Early dynamic splinting for extensor tendon injuries. J Hand Surg, 1989; 14A:72–76.
3. Doyle JR: Extensor Tendons-Acute Injuries. In: Green DP (ed): Operative Hand Surgery, 3rd Ed, New York: Churchill Livingstone, 1993:1925–1954.
4. Elson RA: Dislocation of the extensor tendons of the hand. Report of a case. J Bone Joint Surg, 1967; 49B:324–326.
5. Evans RB, Burkhalter WE: A study of the dynamic anatomy of extensor tendons and implications for treatment. J Hand Surg, 1986; 11A:774–779.
6. Hung LK, Chan A, Chang J, Tsang A, Leung PC: Early controlled active mobilization with dynamic splintage for treatment of extensor tendon injuries. J Hand Surg, 1990; 15A:251–257.
7. Kettlekamp DB, Flatt AE, Moulds R: Traumatic dislocation of the long finger extensor tendon. A clinical, anatomical, and biomechanical study. J Bone Joint Surg, 1971; 53A:229–240.
8. McCoy FJ, Winsky AJ: Lumbrical loop operation for luxation of the extensor tendons of the hand. Plast Reconstr Surg, 1969; 44:142–146.
9. Newport ML, Blair WF, Steyers CM: Long term results of extensor tendon repair. J Hand Surg, 1990; 15A:961–966.
10. Newport ML, Shukla A: Electrophysiologic basis of dynamic extensor splinting. J Hand Surg, 1992; 17A:272–277.
11. Newport ML, Williams CD: Biomechanical characteristics of extensor tendon suture techniques. J Hand Surg, 1992; 17A:1117–1123.
12. Tubiana R: Surgical repair of the extensor apparatus of the fingers. Surg Clin North Am, 1968; 48(5):1015–1031.
13. Wheeldon FT: Recurrent dislocation of extensor tendons. J Bone Joint Surg, 1954; 36B:612–617.

LAWRENCE M.
LUBBERS,
PAUL A. COOK

16

Extensor Tendon Repairs in Zones 7–8

■ HISTORY OF THE
TECHNIQUE

Advances in zone 7 and 8 extensor tendon repairs have resulted from improved under-standing of suture technique, the biomechanics of the retinaculum, relative tendon excursion, and the importance of early motion in rehabilitation. The extensor tendons in zone 7 are unique. The extensor tendons in this zone are deep to the dorsal retinaculum. Reflections of the retinaculum onto bone create fibro-osseus tunnels, which act as pulleys to prevent bowstringing of the tendons with wrist extension. Lieber and co-authors,[16] Brand,[3] and Kaplan[14] found that each muscle-tendon unit is anatomically and biomechanically unique. There is significant tendon excursion at the distal forearm and wrist varying from 35 mm for the flexor carpi ulnaris to 55 mm for the extensor digitorum communis.[28] The large amount of excursion is important to each muscle tendon unit. For example, Newport and co-authors[22] reported that it is critical to repair these tendons at their proper lengths to avoid loss of flexion.

Zone 8 extensor tendon injuries pose two particular problems: proximal tendon retraction and inadequate suture purchase in the proximal tendon stump. Urbaniak and co-authors[25] tested different types of end-to-end tendon repair and found that the "grasping" suture techniques offer the greatest strength for flexor repairs. Newport and Williams[21] found that the modified Bunnell repair technique was only 50% as strong in extensor tendons as in flexor tendons, although it still provides the greatest strength for extensor tendon repairs. Advances in zone 8 have centered on the concepts of intramuscular tendon repair when the laceration occurs at the muscle tendon junction.[2] In these zones, an early mobilization program is increasingly important for good and excellent results.[20]

■ INDICATIONS AND
CONTRAINDICATIONS

One of the key principles of hand surgery is early accurate diagnosis and primary, if not immediate, surgical repair. Primary repair will almost always achieve superior results when compared with delayed primary repair. Secondary repair (after 10 days) is almost always impossible because of myostatic contracture of the muscle. Any questions of tendon continuity are best resolved by early exploration and definitive treatment.

Generally, any sharp laceration on the extensor surface of the forearm and wrist area that penetrates the subcutaneous tissue deserves careful consideration. McNicholl and colleagues[19] found that 33 patients had undetected tendon lacerations with 21 requiring repair in a group of 100 consecutive extensor surface lacerations. Chamay[5] noted that drooping of two fingers indicated transection of the extensor digitorum communis. Also, pain on resisted extension or difficulty moving a digit is usually a sign of a partial tendon transection. Occasionally, locally anesthetizing the injured area will permit a better examination.

Excessive contamination may warrant a delayed repair or repair concomitant with flap or other local tissue coverage. When tendon loss is encountered, an unacceptably tight end-to-end tendon repair must be avoided. In this situation, a primary transfer may be indicated. If the extensor digitorum communis is involved, a more distal side-to-side tendon repair can be used.

■ SURGICAL
TECHNIQUES

For tendon injuries distal to zone 7, local anesthesia often will suffice. Lacerations in zones 7 and 8 should be repaired in the operating room because the tendon stumps retract proximally, usually require a more extensive exploration for identification, are located in the deep layers, and may require intramuscular dissection. Therefore, local anesthesia will not suffice, and regional anesthesia is preferred.

For zone 7 injuries (the retinacular zone), the key anatomic landmarks are Lister's tubercle and the distal radioulnar joint. Dorsal compartments 1 and 2, which contains the extensor carpi radialis longus (ECRL) and extensor carpi radialis brevis (ECRB), are radial to Lister's tubercle. The extensor pollicis longus (EPL), in dorsal compartment 3, winds around Lister's tubercle at a very acute angle, creating inherent tension in this tunnel. Because of this inherent tension, the lacerated EPL tendon stumps tend to retract considerably. Compartment 4 is between Lister's tubercle and the distal radioulnar joint and contains the extensor digitorum communis (EDC) and the extensor indicis proprius (EIP). The extensor digiti minimi (EDM) is in the fifth dorsal compartment and is directly over the distal radioulnar joint and radial to the extensor carpi ulnaris (ECU) tendon sheath. The ECU can be isolated along the ulnar border of the wrist[24] and is more ulnar than dorsal. Extensor anatomy can be visualized in Figure 16–1.

When planning incisions, one should first inspect the wound and try to identify at least one of the two cut tendon ends. This will help determine if the tendon was cut in extension or flexion and helps decide the direction of incision extension. At this point, two separate approaches to designing incisions can be used. A proximal, limited incision will produce less scar than an extensile exposure, yet will provide visualization. This is best employed in single tendon injuries, in which proximal tendon retrieval is required. Extending the original laceration proximal offers the advantage of better visualization, but the incision may overlie the tendon repair (one must be careful to place the incision[s] away from the repair site and the site of excursion of the repaired tendon when possible). This technique is best for multiple tendon lacerations. Also, care should be taken to avoid incisions that extend toward the superficial branch of the radial nerve or the dorsal branch of the ulnar nerve. The skin and subcutaneous tissue can be elevated widely from a more dorsal central incision to expose nearly the entire width of zones 7 and 8 without violating neurovascular planes.

Intimate three-dimensional knowledge of the deeper anatomy is critical for accurate identification of the various tendon ends especially when multiple tendons are transected. It is usually easy to identify the wrist extensors by their size and anatomic position, as opposed to the digital extensors. In zone 7, the only structures at risk are the superficial branch of the radial nerve as it exits between the brachioradialis and extensor carpi radialis longus and the superficial sensory branch of the ulnar nerve as it pierces the dorsal fascia proximal to the ulnar styloid.

The retinaculum should be preserved. If this is not possible, it may be partially taken down.[6,26] If it is necessary to completely open the retinaculum, a Z-type retinacular incision will allow for adequate approximation of the edges at the time of repair. We reserve transplantation of the extensor retinaculum underneath the extensor tendons for arthritis

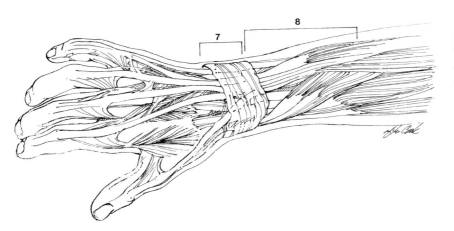

■ FIGURE 16–1
Zones 7 and 8 extensor tendon injury. Zone 7, dorsal retinaculum; zone 8, distal forearm.

surgery. The consequence of this maneuver is bowstringing of the extensor tendons. Most repairs should be performed with minimal bulk and without violation of the dorsal retinaculum. This will allow "potentially" normal tendon excursion underneath an undisturbed retinaculum.

The extensor indicis proprius has the most distal muscle belly of all of the finger extensors and the tendon can be found ulnar to the corresponding slip of the EDC. The abductor pollicis longus (APL) and extensor pollicis brevis (EPB) cross the radial wrist extensors in the distal forearm. When dissecting through the intermuscular planes near the midforearm, one needs to be mindful of the distally coursing branches of the posterior interosseous nerve. For the most part, these branches enter the muscles proximally.

Once all transected tendon ends are identified, each is aligned in preparation for repair. A combination of finger and wrist extension can be used to create end-to-end contact of the tendon stumps. The matching tendon ends are repaired with a braided nonabsorbable suture material in a modified Bunnell pattern. Suture of 0 or 2-0 caliber is used for wrist extensors and 4-0 or 3-0 caliber is used for digital extensors. This can be individualized based on tendon size. Next, a 5-0 nylon suture is used to approximate the tendon ends on the core suture, which prevent tendon separation and limits friction at the repair site.

The most common problems encountered in zone 8 injuries are retraction of the proximal tendon stump into the body of the muscle and a tapered proximal tendon stump (this is the zone where the tendon is in transition into the muscle). Placement of a grasping structure will usually require a wide exposure and more extensive dissection into the muscle belly to retrieve the proximal tendon stump (Fig. 16–2). It is especially important to use the modified Bunnell suture to grasp the proximal tendon stump, since there may not be substantial tendon substance. Suture placement in the proximal stump should avoid incorporating muscle, which results in muscle death and scar formation. Injuries involving only the proximal muscle belly (zone 9) do not hold suture well. Botte and co-workers[2] have advocated using a tendon graft to loop the muscle ends together.

If the retinaculum has been divided, it should be repaired. The repair of the retinaculum should not constrict the tunnel for the excursion of the repaired tendon. Generally, skin is repaired in two layers using an absorbable suture in the subcutaneous tissue and a nonabsorbable interrupted suture technique in the skin. Almost without exception, the wound should be drained to prevent a hematoma. A retained hematoma may result in scar adhesions and pain, which may prevent early mobilization of the repaired tendons.

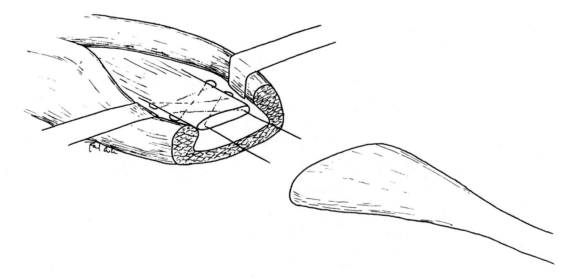

■ FIGURE 16–2

Technique of extensor tendon repair at the muscle tendon junction. The muscle belly must be split to identify the retracted extensor tendon stump to allow placement of a modified Bunnell stitch.

Initially, a bulky postoperative dressing is applied with the wrist extended 45°, the metacarpophalangeal (MP) joints flexed 20°, and the interphalangeal joints unsplinted. In most cases, a short-arm splint is applied for the immediate (i.e., up to 3 days) postoperative period. The elbow should be splinted at 90° when the repair is performed in muscles arising above the elbow. If there has been some delay and the repair is tight, the fingers may be extended farther and on a temporary basis. After the first few days, a decision must be made as to whether treatment will be static or dynamic.

One of the greatest problems in zones 7 and 8 injuries is failure to make an accurate and early diagnosis. Incomplete finger extension may represent a completely severed tendon at a proximal location because extension can be accomplished by the juncturae tendinae.[1] Proximal intramuscular tendinous lacerations can have some remaining muscle fibers crossing the laceration site, which also may produce incomplete extension. This gives a false idea that the tendon is intact because some extension is possible. Clinically missed diagnoses most often occur with injuries involving the extensor digiti minimi in zone 7. Surprisingly, the late complication is loss of finger flexion (rather than loss of extension) due to adhesions of the distal tendon end.

■ TECHNICAL ALTERNATIVES

Care must be taken not to confuse a laceration over zone 8 with a more proximal nerve injury. For example, the EIP, APL, and EPB are distally innervated.

The extensor tendon repair should not be excessively tight or a loss of function can occur.[22] When a loss of tendon substance precludes a direct repair, side-to-side transfer in the digital extensors usually works nicely.[1] In rare cases of mutilating injuries, a conjoined repair of all the finger extensors may be accomplished with relatively good success. Two-stage tendon reconstruction on the dorsal side of the hand is rarely indicated, but this technique may be useful when a coverage procedure is needed concomitantly. A transfer of a wrist motor to a digital extensor can be problematic. This technique provides inadequate excursion and can result in a loss of total active motion.

Both Lovett and McCalla[17] and Holm and Embrick[12] have addressed specific problems related to the EPL tendon. The EPL can occasionally pose special problems because of its unique angulation around Lister's tubercle. If tendon loss or if an attrition rupture is imminent from prior injury, then rerouting of the tendon dorsal to the retinaculum is appropriate (this results in a more direct line of pull). It is, in general, better to repair the EPL in its bed to avoid devascularization of the tendon.[17] If triggering of the EPL occurs around Lister's tubercle and is problematic, Wilson has found that rerouting is acceptable.[27] In cases in which the EPL tendon has ruptured in zone 7, it is usually not feasible to perform a direct end-to-end repair unless it is diagnosed almost immediately and rerouted. When an end-to-end repair cannot be achieved, an immediate transfer of the EIP to the distal stump of the EPL should be performed.

When tendon ruptures occur due to overzealous exercising, re-repair is indicated and can be achieved with a more extended Bunnell-type suture. Conversely, lack of early mobilization may allow excessive tendon adhesions, especially when associated with extensive overlying skin injury or with underlying bone injury near the site of tendon repair. In these situations, early motion is critical to prevent adhesions. If tendon adhesions develop despite early mobilization, it may be wise to wait up to 6 months before returning to the operative site for tenolysis. Usually, the results of tenolysis on the extensor surface of the forearm and wrist are good. To avoid the problems associated with rupture of the tendon repair and tendon adhesions, the protected postoperative splinting course must be individualized for each patient. For example, patients with evidence of early heavy scarring may have the splint removed as early as 3 weeks after surgery. In contrast, patients with early, full motion and an extensor injury to both the finger and wrist should remain splinted for up to 6 weeks to prevent attenuation of the repair sites.

The postoperative program, in our experience, is responsible for approximately 50% of the result. The key to a good result is individualized postoperative management and splinting. The initial dressing is changed on the second or third postoperative day and

■ REHABILITATION

rehabilitation is initiated. Although it is often safe to statically immobilize zone 7 and 8 injuries for up to 5 weeks, we prefer to start an early dynamic mobilization program (except for the most proximal zone 8 injuries).[27] We treat proximal zone 8 injuries statically. These injuries require additional healing time due to relatively weak muscle tissue and a small caliber of tendon for repair, which limits the strength of the grasping suture.

We use one of two dorsally based splints; a flat splint with a limited dynamic restraint or an outrigger with dynamic and static restraints. The flat splint places the wrist in 45° of extension and extends dorsally to the distal aspect of the proximal phalanges. An elastic strap is placed volarly, just distal to the MP flexion crease, which creates passive MP extension after finger flexion. Fifty to seventy percent of combined finger motion is permitted by the elastic loops (Fig. 16–3). The flat splint is used for patients with sharp tendon transections with high quality repairs and for patients who are highly motivated.[13]

For better control of the range of motion, an outrigger with both dynamic and static restraints is used. A finger loop is placed around the affected digit, just distal to the MP flexion crease, while the wrist is statically maintained in 45° of extension (Fig. 16–4). The static restraints are used to precisely limit the degree of MP flexion before the elastic component pulls the MP joint back to the extended position (Fig. 16–4). Usually, this type

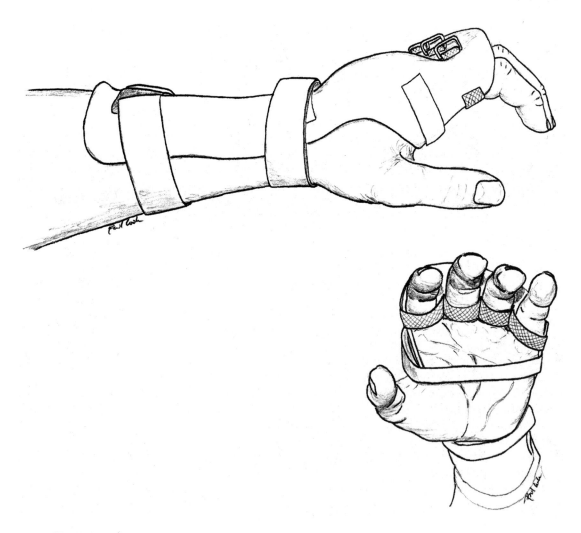

■ FIGURE 16–3

Dorsal forearm based splint for zones 7 and 8 extensor tendon injuries. The fingers are allowed moderate active flexion limited by elastic strapping.

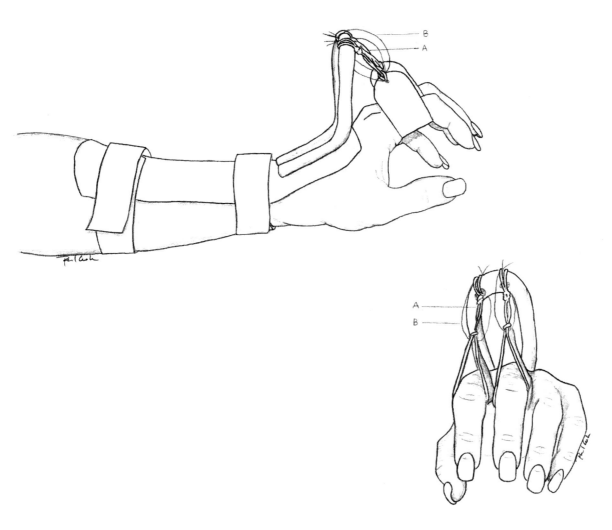

■ FIGURE 16–4

Dynamic dorsal forearm based splint for extensor tendon injuries in zones 7 and 8. The degree of flexion is adjusted by the static restraint, while the dynamic loop allows active flexion with passive extension. (**A,** dynamic loop; **B,** static restraint.)

of splinting is reserved for individual tendon injuries in which the tendon has been shredded and a less than optimal repair was performed.

Some authors, as exemplified by Blue and co-authors,[1] have advocated splinting extensor mechanism injuries for up to 8 weeks.[18] Others, such as Browne and Ribik,[4] Minamikawa and co-authors,[20] and Hung and co-authors,[13] have advocated early dynamic splinting for extensor tendon injuries. The physiologic bases for early passive motion of flexor tendons has been outlined by Duran and associates, who have shown that only 5 mm of tendon excursion will significantly aid in the prevention of tendon adhesions.[7] In a controlled study, Strickland and co-authors found a significant improvement in flexor tendon results with controlled passive motion compared with immobilization.[23] Gelberman and co-authors also have shown that intermittent passive mobilization has improved the strength at various time intervals following flexor tendon surgery when compared with lack of mobilization.[10,11] We extrapolate from the results and apply the principles of flexor tendon surgery to extensor tendon injuries in zones 7 and 8.

In all patients with zone 7 or 8 injuries, the wrist is held in 20° to 45° extension. The tendon excursion generated by finger flexion is used to prevent tendon adhesions in the initial stage of splinting. With single tendon injuries differential glide between tendons is stressed. Generally, the more massive the injury, the more crucial early immobilization.

With extensive injuries, combined finger motion is important. This technique avoids tension differentials among repair sites. As one approaches the fifth postoperative week, wrist motion is added to digital motion. The wrist portion of the splint can be changed from extension to neutral. Alternatively, exercise can be permitted without the splint. If static splinting was used, the extensor adhesions formed can usually be overcome because the flexor power is greater than the extensor power. Motion can be permitted as tolerated starting at the beginning of the fifth postoperative week. Thereafter, regular physical therapy should continue to help regain full motion and to restore differential glide.

Motion studies by Minimikawa and co-authors have found that less than 21° of wrist extension generates little or no glide of the extensor tendons in zones 5 or 6.[20] They also believe that end-to-end repair could be performed with up to 6.4 mm of tendon loss, without loss of flexor excursion, when the wrist was held in 45° of extension. These authors also found that in zone 7 injuries, 45° of wrist extension does not prevent adhesions but does protect the repair adequately. At this degree of wrist extension, there is little tension on the repaired extensor and little excursion of the extensor tendon with finger flexion. Furthermore, these authors believe that, in zone 8 injuries, the wrist should be held in only 10° to 20° of extension to achieve some glide at the repair site. Evans and Burkhalter stress the amount of excursion of the individual wrist and digital extensor tendons at the various levels of the forearm, wrist, and hand.[8,9] Their splinting program is quite elaborate and specific for each tendon group in each zone.[9]

If necessary, the splint should be checked and adjusted at least once a week. The splint is worn an average of 5 weeks (range, 4 to 7½ weeks). Usually in the last 2 weeks of treatment, the wrist splint is brought to a near 0° position of wrist extension (especially if the wrist extensors are involved) to prevent adhesions. Ideally by the eighth week, the wrist should be neutral and the fingers should come into full flexion without resistance.

Repairs performed at the proximal extent of zone 8 are relatively weak because of the lack of tendon substance. For this reason, prolonged extension splinting may be necessary to achieve a satisfactory result. Another unique situation, multiple tendon lacerations in the distal aspect of zone 8 requires individualized treatment. In this region, the individual tendons lack sheaths, as in zone 7, and are prone to intertendinous scarring and adhesions. Thus, we prescribe early individual tendon motion. With combined extensor and flexor tendon injuries and repairs, static splinting is combined with a mandatory passive motion program.

■ OUTCOMES

Most authors who have reported on extensor tendon repairs in zones 7 and 8 have described either good or excellent results.[26] Kelly found 97% excellent and 3% good results in 58 zone 7 injuries to the thumb extensor.[15] In contrast to 15 extensor tendon injuries in zone 7, only 33% were excellent and 57% good. His repairs were carried out with 4-0 monofilament wire, and rehabilitation consisted of 4 weeks of immobilization and 1 week of splinting.

More critical studies have yielded less spectacular results. Newport and co-authors[22] reported that 52% of patients with extensor mechanism injuries achieved either a good or excellent result. Results in zones 5 to 8 were better than in zones 1 to 4. Results of tendon repair in zone 7 combined with retinacular repair were no different from repairs in zones 6 and 8. The actual outcomes in zone 7 were 0 excellent, 6 good, and 3 poor. In zone 8, results were 1 excellent, 4 good, 2 fair, and 1 poor. In most cases, failure to achieve excellent results was due to overtightening the repair.[21,22] Poor results were associated with more complex injuries.

In summary, the results of tendon repairs in zones 7 and 8 are good. The final result is equally dependent on the quality of the surgical repair and the postoperative rehabilitation program. In general, we apply the following principles: (1) repairs are carried out using a core suture in a modified Bunnell pattern (avoid an excessively tight repair), (2) a simple stitch at the repair site keeps the tendon ends from sliding along the core suture, (3) early motion is important to prevent tendon adhesions, (4) the use of a dynamic splint for early range of motion helps prevent adhesions, especially in the retinacular area (zone 7—the only area in which the extensor tendons are in a synovial sheath).

References

1. Blue AI, Spira M, Hardy SB: Repair of extensor tendon injuries of the hand. Am J Surg, 1976; 132:128–132.
2. Botte MJ, Gelberman RH, Smith DG, Silver MA, Gellman H: Repair of severe muscle belly lacerations using a tendon graft. J Hand Surg, 1987; 12A:406–412.
3. Brand PW: Clinical Mechanics of the Hand, St. Louis: Mosby, 1985:192–309.
4. Browne EZ Jr, Ribik CA: Early dynamic splinting for extensor tendon injuries. J Hand Surg, 1989; 14A:72–76.
5. Chamay JCA: Extensor tendon lesions on the dorsum of the hand and wrist. In: Verdan C (ed): Tendon Surgery of the Hand, Edinburgh: Churchill Livingstone, 1979:129–134.
6. Doyle JR: Extensor tendons—acute injuries. In: Green DP (ed): Operative Hand Surgery, New York: Churchill Livingstone, 1988:2045–2072.
7. Duran RJ, Houser RG, Coleman CR, Stover MG: Management of flexor tendon lacerations in zone 2 using controlled passive motion postoperatively. In: Hunter JM, Schneider LH, Mackin EJ, Callahan MS (eds): Rehabilitation of the Hand, St. Louis: Mosby, 1994:273–276.
8. Evans RB, Burkhalter WE: A study of the dynamic anatomy of extensor tendons and implications for treatment. J Hand Surg, 1986: 11A:774–779.
9. Evans RB: Therapeutic management of extensor tendon injuries. Hand Clinics, 1986; 2: 157–169.
10. Gelberman RH, Woo SLY, Lothringer K, Akeson WH, Amiel D: Effects of early intermittent passive mobilization on healing canine flexor tendons. J Hand Surg, 1982; 7:170–175.
11. Gelberman RH, Amiel D, Gonsalves M, Woo S, Akeson WH: The influence of protected passive mobilization on the healing of flexor tendons: a biomechanical and microangiographic study. Hand, 1981; 13:120–128.
12. Holm CL, Erabrick RP: Anatomical consideration in the primary treatment of tendon injuries of the hand. J Bone Joint Surg, 1959; 41A:599–608.
13. Hung LK, Chan A, Chang J, Tsang A, Leung PC: Early controlled active mobilization with dynamic splintage for treatment of extensor tendon injuries. J Hand Surg, 1990; 15A:251–257.
14. Kaplan EB: Anatomy, injuries and treatment of the extensor apparatus of the hand and the digits. Clin Orthop, 1959; 13:24–41.
15. Kelly AP: Primary tendon repairs. A study of 789 consecutive tendon severances. J Bone Joint Surg, 1959; 41A:581–598.
16. Lieber RL, Fazeli BM, Botte MJ: Architecture of selected wrist flexor and extensor muscles. J Hand Surg, 1990; 15A:244–250.
17. Lovett WL, McCalla MA: Management and rehabilitation of extensor tendon injuries. Orthop Clin North Am, 1983; 14:811–826.
18. McFarlane RM, Hampole MK: Treatment of extensor tendon injuries of the hand. Can J Surg, 1973; 16:366–375.
19. McNicholl BP, Martin J, McAleese P: Subclinical injuries in lacerations to the forearm and hand. Br J Surg, 1992; 79:765–767.
20. Minamikawa Y, Peimer CA, Yamaguchi T, Banasiak NA, Kambe K, Sherwin FS: Wrist position and extensor tendon amplitude following repair. J Hand Surg, 1992; 17A:268–271.
21. Newport ML, Williams CD: Biomechanical characteristics of extensor tendon suture techniques. J Hand Surg, 1992; 17A:1117–1123.
22. Newport ML, Blair WF, Steyers Jr CM: Long-term results of extensor tendon repair. J Hand Surg, 1990; 15A:961–966.
23. Strickland JW, Glogovac SV: Digital function following flexor tendon repair in zone II: a comparison of immobilization and controlled passive motion techniques. J Hand Surg, 1980; 5:537–543.
24. Taleisnik J, Gelberman RH, Miller BW, Szabo RM: The extensor retinaculum at the wrist. J Hand Surg, 1984; 9A:495–501.
25. Urbaniak JR, Cahill Jr JD, Mortenson RA: Tendon suturing methods: analysis of tensile strengths. In: Hunter JM, Schneider LH (eds): American Academy of Orthopaedic Surgeons Symposium on Tendon Surgery in the Hand, St. Louis: Mosby, 1975:70–80.
26. Weckesser EC: Evalulation of results with tendon suture and tendon transplants. In: Jupiter JB (ed): Flynn's Hand Surgery, Baltimore: Williams & Wilkins, 1991:234–240.
27. Wilson RL: Management of acute extensor tendon injuries. In: Hunter JM, Schneider LH, Mackin EJ (eds): Tendon Surgery in the Hand, St. Louis: Mosby, 1987:336–343.

JOSEPH P. LEDDY
JEFFREY BECHLER

17

Flexor Tendon Avulsion from the Distal Phalanx

■ HISTORY OF THE TECHNIQUE

Avulsion of the profundus tendon insertion occurs most commonly in the ring finger[1–3,6,7] of young adult males participating in football, flag football, or rugby. However, the injury may occur in any finger or the thumb at any age in either sex. Von Zander[14] published the first case report in 1891. McMaster,[8] in 1933, showed that the tendon was the strongest link in the musculotendinous chain, and that a normal tendon usually ruptured either at its bony insertion or at the musculotendinous junction.

Before the report by Leddy in 1977,[6] the different types of injury were not classified, and a detailed treatment program had not been outlined. The authors classified this injury into three distinct types and treated them using well-established principles in flexor tendon surgery. If there was a large intra-articular fragment of bone attached to the flexor tendon, this was repaired by open reduction and internal fixation. If the tendon itself had avulsed from the distal phalanx, it was threaded back beneath the annular pulleys and reinserted into the base of the distal phalanx. These techniques were certainly not original with the authors, but this was the first report to classify this injury and to describe a technique for repair of each of the three types.

■ INDICATIONS AND CONTRAINDICATIONS

The injury often occurs when, in an attempt to make a tackle, the fingers grasp the pants or jersey of the opposing player. If the little finger misses and continues to flex and the opposing player pulls away, the ring finger, caught in the pants or jersey, is extended forcibly while the profundus tendon is maximally contracting. The tendon can be avulsed from the distal phalanx with or without a fragment of bone. The diagnosis is often missed initially because the radiographs are normal, and the patient can still flex his finger at the proximal interphalangeal (PIP) and metacarpophalangeal (MP) joints (Fig. 17–1). Unless the physician is aware of the entity, takes an accurate history, and tests specifically for active flexion of the distal interphalangeal (DIP) joint, the injury may not be recognized. Unfortunately, delay in diagnosis and treatment can severely compromise the final outcome.

When an avulsion of the flexor tendon insertion is recognized early, it should be reinserted into the distal phalanx to restore stability and active flexion to the DIP joint and to restore normal grip strength. Unless there is a medical contraindication to the procedure, in our opinion, consideration should be given to early reinsertion. If the injury is old and the tendon cannot be brought back out to the distal phalanx and reinserted, then obviously this technique would be contraindicated. Those old untreated cases that are relatively asymptomatic are best left alone in our opinion. If there is no instability at the DIP joint and no special requirement for active flexion at this joint, no surgical treatment is indicated. If there is instability of the DIP joint with weakness of pinch or recurrent dorsal dislocations, then fusion or tenodesis of the joint or flexor tendon grafting through the intact superficialis in one or two stages should be considered.[4,5,9,13,15]

It is well known that the flexor tendons in zone 2 have a dual source of nutritional supply (i.e., blood and synovial fluid). A thorough understanding of the vincular system bringing blood supply to the flexor tendons in zone 2 is important in the treatment of this injury. The profundus tendon receives blood supply from the short vinculum at the level of the distal end of the middle phalanx. It also receives blood supply from the long vincu-

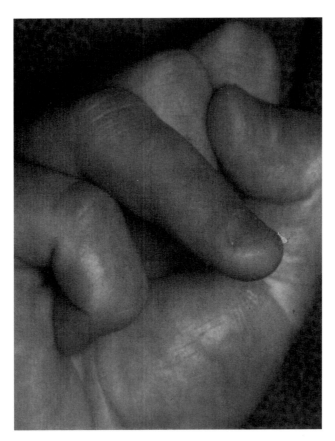

When the flexor digitorum profundus is avulsed, active flexion is absent at the DIP joint.

lum near the level of the PIP joint. The factors influencing the prognosis and treatment of this injury include (1) the level to which the tendon retracts; (2) the remaining nutritional supply of the avulsed tendon; (3) the length of time between injury and treatment; and (4) the presence and size of a bony fragment seen on radiographs.

Leddy and Packer[6,7] described three main types of avulsion of the profundus tendon insertion.

In type I, the tendon retracts into the palm after avulsion. Both vinculae rupture and therefore the blood supply is lost. The diffusion of nutrients from the synovial fluid is interrupted. There is no active flexion at the DIP joint, and there is a tender, swollen mass in the palm. This tendon should be reinserted within 7 to 10 days before it becomes contracted (Fig. 17–2).

Type II is by far the most common type. The tendon retracts to the level of the PIP joint, leaving the long vinculum at this level intact, thereby retaining some of the blood supply. Because the tendon remains in the sheath, presumably diffusion of nutrients from the synovial fluid continues. Rarely, a small fleck of bone is avulsed with the tendon and can be seen on lateral radiographs at the PIP joint level (Fig. 17–3). There is no active flexion at the DIP joint and there is pain, swelling, tenderness, and some loss of motion at the PIP joint level. This type is best treated by early reinsertion of the tendon into the distal phalanx. However, in contrast to type I injuries, the tendon can be reinserted at a later date because it has retained a better nutritional supply and does not become too contracted. It is possible to repair these up to 2 or more months after injury with a satisfactory result. In a type II injury, the tendon may first retract to the level of the PIP joint, but, at a later date, the long vinculum may rupture and the tendon may then slip into the palm, becoming a type I injury.

In a type III injury, a large bony fragment is avulsed by the profundus tendon. The A4 pulley prevents proximal retraction of this fragment. Both vinculae remain intact and tendon length and nutrition are preserved. There is swelling, ecchymoses, and tenderness

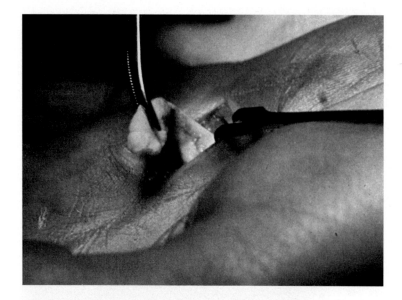

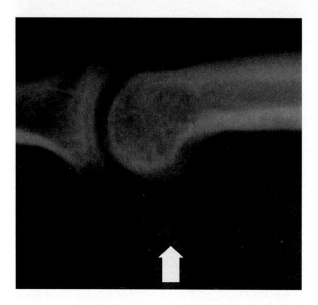

over the middle phalanx and inability to flex the DIP joint. The large bony fragment can be seen just proximal to the DIP joint on the lateral radiograph (Fig. 17–4). Early reinsertion of the fragment with internal fixation will give a satisfactory result (Fig. 17–5). Some authors have described a type III injury with a simultaneous avulsion of the profundus tendon from the fracture fragment. In this case, bony continuity should be restored by open reduction and internal fixation if possible. The avulsed flexor profundus tendon should then be treated as a type I or type II injury depending on the level of tendon retraction.

■ SURGICAL TECHNIQUES

General, axillary block, or intravenous regional anesthesia may be utilized depending on the preference of the surgeon. Our current preference is to use intravenous regional anesthesia (Bier block) supplemented with intravenous sedation. For type I and type II injuries, we use a palmar zigzag incision, exposing the flexor sheath (Fig. 17–6) from just proximal to the PIP joint to the area of the insertion of the profundus tendon on the distal phalanx. A transverse incision is made in the sheath just distal to the A2 pulley (Fig. 17–7). If the tendon is not found at this level, it has retracted into the palm and an incision is made in the palm at the base of the finger paralleling the distal palmar crease. There is

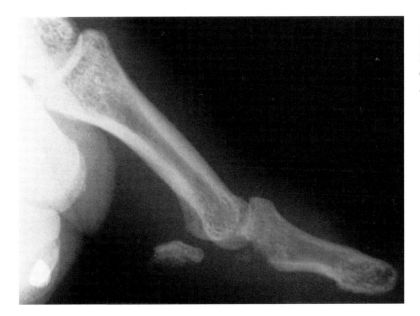

In a type III injury, a large bony fragment is caught just distal to the A4 pulley.

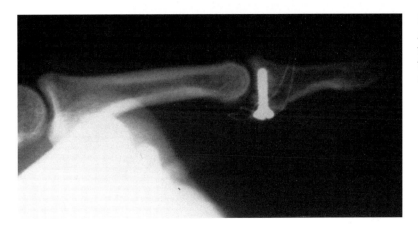

A type III injury was treated with open reduction and internal fixation using a screw and wire.

usually some hemorrhage within the sheath and an incision is made here just proximal to the A1 pulley exposing the flexor tendons. A small pliable catheter, such as an infant feeding gastrostomy tube, is then passed retrograde starting just distal to the A2 pulley and proceeding beneath the sheath and pulleys and through the superficialis decussation to exit proximal to the A1 pulley through the incision previously made in the sheath. The distal end of the flexor profundus tendon is then attached to the catheter with a nonabsorbable monofilament suture such as 4-0 Prolene. When the catheter is pulled distally, the profundus tendon is threaded back beneath the pulleys and through the superficialis chiasm to the level of the previously made incision in the sheath distal to the A2 pulley. The distal phalanx is then exposed by extending the zigzag incision distally and the area of avulsion of the tendon is visualized. We open the sheath distal to the A4 pulley and generally do not repair this section. The tube is passed distally through the remainder of the sheath under the A4 pulley into the distal window. Here it is brought out delivering the flexor tendon to the level of the DIP joint. The A4 pulley must be preserved, but it can be difficult to pass the distal end of the tendon beneath this structure (Fig. 17–8). It may be necessary to suture the fan-shaped portion of the distal tendon to itself to narrow its diameter. Once the tendon reaches the distal window, a Keith needle is used to hold it in place. A modified Bunnell 4-0 Prolene core suture is put into the tendon. It is not necessary to trim or otherwise prepare the tendon end. A cortical flap is then raised by hand with a sharp osteotome in the distal phalanx just distal to the palmar

■ FIGURE 17–6
Through a palmar zig-
zag incision, the annular
and cruciform pulleys are
visualized; there is blood
in the flexor sheath.

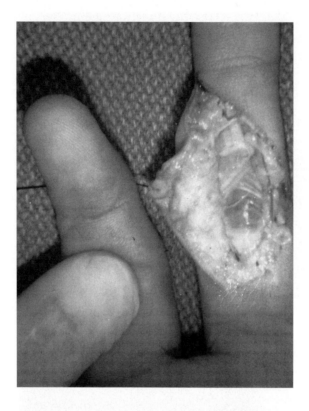

■ FIGURE 17–7
A transverse incision in
the sheath distal to A2
pulley exposes the distal
end of the avulsed ten-
don in a type II injury.

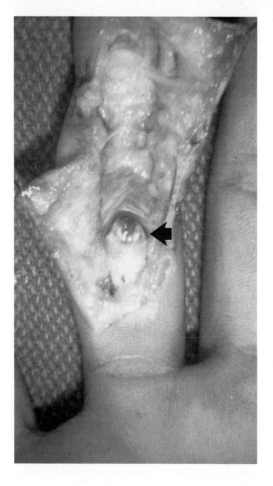

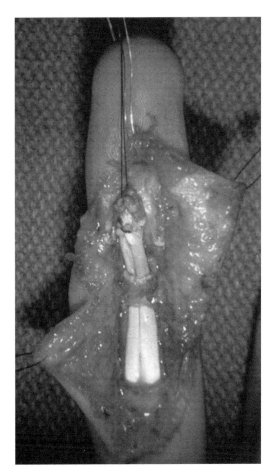

■ FIGURE 17–8
The avulsed tendon was passed beneath the A4 pulley and is ready for re-insertion under a cortical flap raised on the distal phalanx.

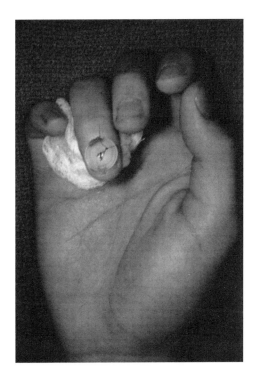

■ FIGURE 17–9
Normal tension has been restored after the tendon is reinserted into the distal phalanx; the suture is tied dorsally over a button.

plate. A bony trough is made by elevating the cortical flap exposing a bed of cancellous bone. A K-wire is then driven in the midline through the trough to exit on the dorsum of the finger through the base of the nail. The ends of the 4-0 Prolene suture are placed through the eye of a Keith needle, which is then placed in the hole made by the K-wire and pulled out through the base of the nail. The sheath between the A2 and A4 pulley is repaired with 6-0 Mersilene. The tourniquet should be deflated here, and good hemostasis should be obtained. Once this is accomplished, the tourniquet can be inflated again. When using a Bier block and intravenous sedation, it is usually not necessary to use more local anesthetic to complete the procedure. The finger is held in the flexed position and the Prolene suture is tied over a button on the dorsum of the finger after the distal end of the tendon has been pulled up into the bony trough (Fig. 17–9). No additional sutures in the tendon are used. The wounds are closed with 5-0 nylon, and a dorsal plaster splint is applied, holding the wrist in slight flexion, the MP joints in 60° to 70° of flexion, and the PIP and DIP joints in relative extension. All fingers are included in the splint.

If the tendon is found just distal to the A2 pulley (type II), a modified Bunnell 4-0 Prolene core suture is placed in the distal end. The suture ends are left long and passed under the sheath distally to exit distal to the A4 pulley. (This can be accomplished by attaching the suture ends to the infant feeding gastrostomy tube, which has been passed proximally underneath the A4 pulley and the sheath. Pulling the tube distally will deliver the suture ends into the distal window.) The tendon is passed in the sheath under the A4 pulley and is then reinserted into the distal phalanx as described above. If possible, the sheath just distal to the A2 pulley is repaired with interrupted sutures of 6-0 Mersilene. Skin closure and splinting are the same as in type I injuries.

In type III injuries, there is usually a large bony fragment held in place at the level of the A4 pulley. There may be some comminution of the fragment, a comminuted intra-articular fracture of the DIP joint, or both. Open reduction and internal fixation of the fragment usually will give a satisfactory result. However, the tendon may pull away from the bony[10,11] fragment. If this happens, reinsertion of the tendon after open reduction and internal fixation of the fragment is necessary. Postoperative care is the same. Active motion is instituted when bony healing permits.

■ TECHNICAL
ALTERNATIVES

Some surgeons prefer general or axillary block anesthesia. The procedure may even be accomplished with local nerve block. A mid-lateral incision may be used rather than the palmar zigzag approach. In a type I injury, the tendon in the palm can be retrieved by the method of Sourmelis and McGrouther.[12] In this case, the profundus tendon is attached side-to-side to the tube without exposing the distal tendon end if it is not present proximal to the A1 pulley. When the tube is pulled distally, the tendon is threaded back beneath the pulleys and through the superficialis chiasm to the level of the previously made incision in the sheath distal to the A2 pulley. There are different methods of attaching the FDP tendon to the distal phalanx. In our opinion, suturing the tendon to the surrounding soft tissues at the distal phalanx is not satisfactory. There is no periosteum left at the site of insertion and the remaining soft tissues are not strong enough to hold the tendon in place. Some surgeons create a bony trough as previously described and then pass the sutures around rather than through the distal phalanx. The sutures are then tied over a button. This is an acceptable alternative.

There are several pitfalls in the management of this injury. The largest one may be missing the diagnosis. One must test for active flexion at the DIP joint after the finger is injured. If the diagnosis and treatment are delayed, the outcome may be adversely affected. It is important to make the incision at the PIP level first to see if the tendon is held in place there by the long vinculum. If the palm is opened first and traction is put on the tendon, the intact vinculum may rupture converting a type II injury into a type I injury. A transverse incision should be made in the sheath at the distal edge of the A2 pulley. It can be extended distally if necessary along the side. One should preserve as much sheath intact as possible proximal to A4 because this makes it much easier to pass the tendon beneath this pulley. If the sheath is excised proximal to the A4 pulley, it can be difficult to pass the tendon beneath the sharp leading edge of this structure. Different types of core sutures can be used in the distal end of the tendon, such as a Kessler grasping suture. We prefer a 4-0 Prolene suture in a modified Bunnell fashion because it is easier to remove the suture by cutting one end beneath the button and then pulling the entire suture out in one piece. We prefer to close the sheath between the A2 and A4 pulley just before reinsertion of this tendon, but this is not necessary. All annular pulleys should be preserved. Loss of the A4 pulley will result in bowstringing and loss of motion. Care should be taken to avoid damage to the palmar plate when reinserting the tendon because this can cause a flexion contracture. The tendon should be reinserted in the proper place near the base of the phalanx. If it is put back too far distally, a flexion contracture may be produced. If the tourniquet is not deflated and hemostasis not achieved, a hematoma may develop and compromise the end result. Infection is rare.

We prefer to begin passive exercises in the splint as soon as the patient is comfortable enough to do so. We have not used early active motion in our postoperative program for this injury. After 3 weeks, the splint can be removed several times a day for gentle active exercises. It is reapplied to protect the repair until week 4, when it can be discontinued. The tendon suture and button can be removed at 3 to 4 weeks after surgery. At 4 weeks, range of motion exercises, particularly those isolating the profundus tendon, are performed several times a day. Gentle extension exercises are begun at 5 weeks, and splinting may be necessary to regain the last few degrees of extension at the DIP joint. The finger is protected for all sports activities for a minimum of 3 months. In a type III injury, postoperative care is the same. Active motion is instituted when bony healing permits.

■ REHABILITATION

There in no precise objective data in the literature detailing range of motion, pinch, and grip strength after treatment of this injury. In our experience, in those patients whose injuries are recognized immediately and who are treated with early reinsertion of the tendon, a satisfactory result can generally be anticipated. There may be a 10° to 15° loss of extension at the DIP joint, but flexion is full, and pinch and grip strength should approach normal.

Complications are rare but can include infection, skin slough, and loss of motion. These problems are treated in the standard fashion. Failure of the reinsertion can occur and, if recognized in time, can be treated by prompt re-exploration and repair.

■ OUTCOMES

References

1. Blazina ME, Lane C: Rupture of the insertion of the flexor digitorum profundus tendon in student athletes. J Am Coll Health Assoc, 1966; 14:248.
2. Carroll RE, Match RM: Avulsion of the profundus tendon insertion. J Trauma, 1970; 10:1109.
3. Chang WH, Thoms OJ, White WL: Avulsion injury of the long flexor tendons. Plast Reconst Surg, 1972; 50:260.
4. Goldner JL, Coonrad RW: Tendon grafting of the flexor profundus in the presence of a completely or partially intact flexor sublimis. J Bone Joint Surg, 1969; 51A:527–532.
5. Honner R: The late management of the isolated lesion of the flexor digitorum profundus tendon. Hand, 1975; 7:171–174.
6. Leddy JP: Avulsions of the flexor digitorum profundus. Hand Clinics, 1985; 1:77–83.
7. Leddy JP, Packer JW: Avulsion of the profundus tendon insertion in athletes. J Hand Surg, 1977; 2:66–69.
8. McMaster PE: Tendon and muscle ruptures. Clinical and experimental studies on the causes and location of subcutaneous ruptures. J Bone Joint Surg, 1933; 15:705–722.
9. Pulvertaft RG: The treatment of profundus division by free tendon graft. J Bone Joint Surg, 1960; 42A:1363–1371.
10. Robins PR, Dobyns JH: Avulsion of the insertion of the flexor digitorum profundus tendon associated with fracture of the distal phalanx. In: AAOS Symposium on Tendon Surgery in the Hand. St. Louis, C. V. Mosby, 1975:151–156.
11. Smith JH: Avulsion of the profundus tendon with simultaneous intraarticular fracture of the distal phalanx. Case report. J Hand Surg, 1981; 6:600–601.

12. Sourmelis SG, McGrouther DA: Retrieval of the retracted flexor tendon. J Hand Surg, 1987; 12B:109–111.
13. Stark HH, Zemel NP, Boyes JH, Ashworth CR: Flexor tendon graft through intact superficialis tendon. J Hand Surg, 1977; 2:456–461.
14. Von Zander: Trommlerlahmung Inaug. Dissertation. Berlin, 1891.
15. Wilson RL, Carter MS, Holdeman VA, Lovett WL: Flexor profundus injuries treated with delayed two-staged tendon grafting. J Hand Surg, 1980; 5:74–78.

THOMAS R.
KIEFHABER

18

Flexor Tendon Repairs in Zone 1

Until relatively recently, repair of the flexor digitorum profundus tendon in zone 1 or at any level within the flexor tendon sheath was considered foolhardy because the results were usually unsatisfactory. As an alternative to tenorrhaphy, Bunnell[2] recommended that the profundus tendon be advanced into bone if the laceration occurred near the dostal phalanx. Lacerations in the proximal aspect of zone 1 were treated by stabilizing the distal interphalangeal (DIP) joint by tenodesis or arthrodesis and converting the finger to a sublimis-only digit.

In the early 1960s, Verdan[21,22] and Kleinert[10,11] introduced new surgical techniques and rehabilitation programs that revitalized the interest in direct tendon repair. Other surgical pioneers offered technical improvements, and primary end-to-end suture of the profundus tendon in the proximal half of zone 1 is now the procedure of choice. Profundus advancement is still preferred for lacerations occurring in the distal aspect of zone 1.

■ HISTORY OF THE
TECHNIQUE

An attempt should be made to repair the profundus tendon when it is disrupted by laceration or avulsion. The profundus tendons of the ulnar digits provide a significant contribution to power grasp and the profundus to the index finger allows precision pinch. Certain manual tasks such as playing a stringed instrument require precise DIP joint control that can only be attained with an intact and mobile profundus tendon. The functional improvement provided by a successful profundus tendon repair usually justifies the time and expense of the surgery and rehabilitation.

Sharp disruption of the profundus tendon must be suspected with any laceration to the volar half of the digit. Observation of the finger's resting posture often suggests the diagnosis of a complete profundus division. The DIP joint of the involved digit assumes an extended posture, throwing the finger out of the hand's normal flexion cascade. Profundus disruption should also be suspected when the tenodesis that occurs with passive wrist extension does not cause DIP flexion. Complete profundus laceration is confirmed when the patient fails to generate any active DIP flexion while the proximal interphalangeal (PIP) joint is blocked in full extension.

A high index of suspicion must be maintained if closed avulsions of the profundus tendon are to be accurately and rapidly diagnosed. The involved digit is often swollen and tender over the flexor tendon sheath. Any closed injury to the digit should prompt the examiner to use the tests mentioned above to confirm the continuity of the profundus tendon.

Partial profundus lacerations are more difficult to diagnose. Active DIP flexion is retained but usually is painful, especially when tested against resistance. Tenderness along the flexor tendon sheath at a site distant from the laceration suggests bleeding within the sheath, and the examiner should suspect a partial tendon laceration. Triggering can be caused by a flap of tendon catching on the edge of the fibro-osseous tunnel and should prompt a thorough surgical inspection. The tendon must be visualized proximal and distal to the skin laceration because extending the digit for surgical inspection may pull the injured tendon segment into the fibro-osseous tunnel and out of view.

Repair of incomplete profundus tendon lacerations is controversial.[17] Some authors believe that an unrepaired incomplete laceration increases the chances of entrapment, rupture, or triggering.[15] Other studies have demonstrated that suturing decreases the strength of the tendon.[4] Lacerations that involve more than 60% of the diameter of the tendon

■ INDICATIONS AND
CONTRAINDICATIONS

should be repaired with a core suture and epitenon stitch. Small beveled lacerations are treated with excision of the flap or repair with an epitenon suture.

The most frequently encountered contraindication to zone 1 flexor tendon repair is a lengthy delay between injury and diagnosis. After 4 weeks, a myostatic contracture develops and the tendon ends become swollen. Passage of the contracted, bulbous tendon stump through the annular pulleys is difficult and the creation of a smooth repair that glides through the flexor tendon sheath is nearly impossible.[9] Other contraindications to primary tendon repair include segmental tendon loss,[17] wounds so heavily contaminated that they can not be rendered clean by surgical debridement, or severe soft-tissue injury with loss of skin over the flexor tendon sheath.[9,18,19] Fractures and nerve injuries are not contraindications to tendon repair.[18,19] Primary tenorrhaphy can also be performed in injuries that render the A4 pulley incompetent but the pulley must be securely repaired or reconstructed at the same surgical sitting. Reconstruction of a poorly performed tenorrhaphy is difficult or impossible. Primary tenorrhaphy should only be attempted by surgeons who are familiar with the anatomy, practiced in modern repair techniques, and supported by trained rehabilitation specialists.[9,13,18,19]

■ SURGICAL TECHNIQUES

Zone 1 of the flexor tendon sheath extends from the middle phalanx insertion of the superficialis tendon to the distal phalangeal attachment of the flexor digitorum profundus. The fibro-osseous tunnel in zone 1 is composed of the thin C3 and A5 retinacular thickenings and the tough, broad, mechanically important A4 pulley. Even though the profundus tendon is the sole occupant of zone 1, creating a repair that glides through the tight and constricting A4 pulley presents all of the same challenges encountered in producing a successful zone 2 repair. Meticulous attention must be given to the details of tendon handling, suture technique, management of the fibro-osseous canal, and rehabilitation.

Complete relaxation of the profundus muscle provided by general or regional anesthesia and tourniquet hemostasis is necessary for a successful zone 1 flexor tendon repair. Exposure of the flexor tendon sheath is obtained through a Bruner zigzag or mid-lateral approach. Even though it is difficult to develop, I prefer the mid-lateral incision because it has the theoretic advantage of separating the healing skin and subcutaneous tissue from the tendon and sheath repair. To prevent any scar contracture from causing a postoperative flexion contracture, the mid-lateral incision should be kept dorsal to the axis of rotation of the PIP and DIP joints. The axis can be found by flexing the PIP and DIP joints and identifying the most dorsal extent of the flexor creases. The incision is designed by connecting these points and extended distally by proceeding obliquely from the lateral side of the DIP joint to the pulp of the digit. Proximal exposure is obtained by extending the incision from the lateral extent of the metacarpophalangeal (MP) flexion crease obliquely to the distal palmar crease. The neurovascular bundle is found midline and palmar to the skin incision.[13] The flap is carefully separated from the nerve and artery, which are left with the dorsal skin and subcutaneous tissue.

Before openings are made in the flexor tendon sheath, the injury should be studied to determine whether the repair must be performed proximal or distal to the A4 pulley. The repair can be completed proximal to the A4 pulley if flexion of the DIP joint delivers the distal profundus stump at least 5 mm past the proximal edge of the A4 pulley. In this situation, an opening should be created proximal to the A4 pulley. Lister[12] has recommended an L-shaped incision that has a transverse component at the pulley edge and a proximally directed longitudinal component along the lateral border of the tendon sheath. This technique creates a funnel-shaped opening that facilitates passage of the repair under the A4 pulley. When the repair must be performed distal to the A4 pulley, open the flexor tendon sheath at the distal edge of A4 and avoid making the proximal window.

The proximal end of the profundus can be located by observing the contour of the flexor tendon sheath or identified by palpation. The long vincula usually prevents retraction of the profundus tendon past the A2 pulley.[17,19] At this level, it should be retrieved through either a small transverse incision between the A1 and A2 pulleys or between pulleys A2 and C1. If the tendon retracts into the palm, the incision should be extended proximally until the tendon can be located by direct observation. Attempts to blindly retrieve a proximally retracted tendon with a tendon retriever are injurious and should be avoided. The tendon retriever may damage the tendon sheath or if introduced into the palm, may inadvertently grasp a neurovascular bundle.[19,20]

The tendon ends may be trimmed sparingly to remove loose edges and to improve end-to-end apposition[9] but extensive debridement or shortening should be avoided.[19] The core sutures should be placed in the proximal and distal ends of the profundus as soon as they are identified and debrided. This avoids further damage to the epitenon and aids in the passage of the tendon through the flexor tendon sheath. For end-to-end repair, I prefer a 4-0 braided nonabsorbable suture using the combined Kessler-Tajima technique described by Strickland.[19] The tendon stump is stabilized by grasping the central core of the cut end with a small Bishop-Harmon forceps. The tendon surface should not be touched with the forceps because the epitenon may be broken, creating a focus for adhesion development. The suture needle is passed into the lateral aspect of the core and exits along one side of the tendon about 4 mm from the cut edge. Half of the suture is pulled through the tendon. A small locking stitch is placed proximal to the point of suture exit. The needle is then passed transversely across the tendon, keeping the suture in the palmar half of the tendon to avoid damage to the blood supply. Another locking stitch is placed in the opposite tendon wall, distal to the transverse component of the suture. Finally, the suture is passed into the lateral wall and out the cut end.

Rarely is the distal profundus stump long enough to allow completion of the repair proximal to the A4 pulley; for this reason, the proximal end of the profundus must be passed all the way to the distal flexor tendon sheath window in preparation for repair. The suture is first led through the sheath with a pediatric feeding tube that has been inserted into the distal window and threaded proximally. Both limbs of the core suture are passed through a hole in the feeding tube and then drawn through the flexor tendon sheath as the tube is pulled distally and removed[17] (Fig. 18–1). Gentle traction is then applied to the core suture, pulling the tendon distally through the pulley system. It is often difficult to pass the tendon under the A4 pulley but it can usually be coaxed into the proximal opening with a Freer elevator.[12] In stubborn cases, the opening can be slightly enlarged using pediatric urethral dilators. After the proximal tendon stump is delivered into the distal window, a 25-gauge needle is passed through the tendon to prevent proximal retraction and to allow the repair to be performed without tension.

The tenorrhaphy now proceeds much as it would in zone 2; however, rolling the profun-

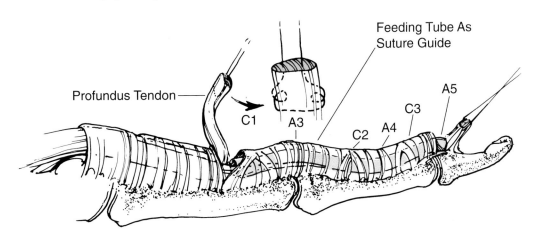

■ FIGURE 18–1
Retrieval of the profundus tendon. Rethreading the flexor tendon through the fibro-osseous tunnel begins by making a transverse opening between the annular pulleys, extracting the tendon stump. A core suture is placed and the suture ends are guided through the pulley system by a pediatric feeding tube or tendon retriever. Traction on the core suture guides the stump back under the pulleys.

■   FIGURE 18–2
Flexor tendon repair in
zone 1. The profundus
tendon is held distal to
the A4 pulley with a
transversely placed 25-
gauge needle. A running
epitenon suture is placed
in the back wall of the
tendon repair, the core
sutures are tied, and the
epitenon stitch is com-
pleted around the palmar
surface.

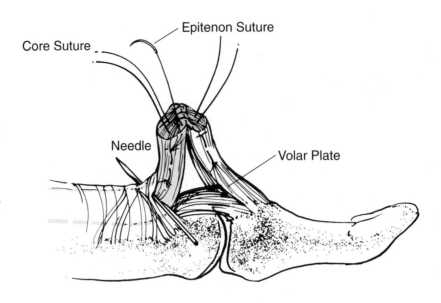

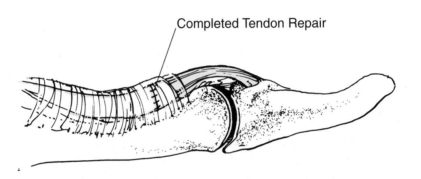

■   FIGURE 18–3
Flexor tendon repair zone 1. Uninhibited gliding of the flexor tendon under the A4 pulley is essential to the success of a zone 1 repair. Some of the A4 pulley may be excised but at least
half must be maintained. A bulky or bulbous tendon repair should not be accepted.

dus tendon to expose its dorsal surface is frequently impossible. This difficulty can be
overcome by placing the 6-0 running epitenon suture into the back wall before tying the
core sutures (Fig. 18–2). The stitch enters the epitenon about 3 mm from the repair site
and exits 1 mm from the cut surface. By reversing this sequence in the opposing tendon
end, the edges are inverted and a smooth repair surface is created. An attempt should be
made to bury the knot that begins and ends this running stitch. The core sutures are then
secured, burying the knots within the repair surface. The core sutures must not be overly
tightened or the tendon ends will collapse together in an accordion-like fashion. The final
step is to complete the epitenon suture around the palmar surface of the tendon. The 25-
gauge needle is removed and the excursion of the repair tested by a combination of passive
flexion of the DIP joint and gentle traction on the profundus tendon through one of the
proximal windows. The repair must glide through the A4 pulley without binding (Fig.
18–3). If the repair binds at the distal end of the A4 pulley, a small part of the pulley may
be opened[19] or excised[17] but at least 50% of the pulley must be left intact. The tenorrhaphy
should be taken down and redone instead of rendering the A4 pulley incompetent. It is
rarely possible to close the A5 pulley, and it may be excised. The proximal openings of
the flexor tendon sheath should be closed with a running 6-0 nylon suture.

The wound is copiously irrigated and the skin closed with 5-0 nylon horizontal mattress
sutures. A nonadherent bandage is applied from the fingertips to the elbow, incorporating

a dorsal blocking splint that allows complete extension of the PIP and DIP joints but flexes the wrist to 30° and the MP joints to 70°. The common profundus muscle belly of the ulnar digits necessitates immobilization of all three fingers when any member of the group is injured. All four digits should be immobilized when the index finger profundus is damaged. The surgical dressing is removed and the rehabilitation program is started 3 to 5 days postoperatively. The sutures are removed 10 to 14 days after surgery.

The primary decision facing the surgeon treating a zone 1 flexor tendon injury is whether to attempt a primary repair or commit the patient to a reconstructive procedure. Barring the excessive passage of time, unfavorable wound conditions, or extensive soft-tissue loss, a primary or delayed primary repair should be performed. The results of repair are usually superior to tendon grafts or two-staged reconstructions. Beyond the initial decision to repair the profundus tendon, the surgeon is challenged with a host of technical decisions, including the choice of direct repair or advancement, which suture material and technique to employ, and how to best rehabilitate the patient.

Lacerations of the profundus tendon in the distal portion of zone 1 are better suited to advancement into bone than to end-to-end tenorrhaphy. Creating a tendon-to-bone juncture is technically simpler than a mid-substance repair but overly aggressive advancement produces a flexion deformity of the injured digit and loss of active flexion in the adjacent digits, secondary to the quadriga effect.[14] The relatively independent index finger profundus can be advanced up to 1.5 cm[14] but profundus advancement in the ulnar three digits should be limited to 1 cm.[9,17] Profundus advancement begins by exposure of the proximal and distal tendon ends. My preference for the proximal core suture is a double-needle 4-0 stainless steel suture coupled with a pull-out loop. The suture is placed using a nonlocking Bunnell technique. The core suture is then threaded through the tendon sheath and used to pull the tendon distal to the A4 pulley. The attachment site should be planned in the proper anatomic location to decrease the risk of a DIP flexion contracture—a complication that frequently occurs after an excessively distal insertion. Using a No. 15 blade, the distal tendon stump is subperiosteally elevated from the proximal 3 to 4 mm of the distal phalanx. Care should be taken to avoid damaging the palmar plate or completely releasing the attachment to the distal phalanx.[17] A rongeur is used to create a trough 3 mm wide and parallel to the joint line; the cortical bone must be penetrated and cancellous bone exposed. Drill holes are placed at the radial and ulnar edges of the trough to accept the pull-out sutures. Some surgeons prefer to create a suture exit site through the nail plate.[17] As an alternative, the nail can be avoided completely by directing the drill holes parallel

■ TECHNICAL ALTERNATIVES

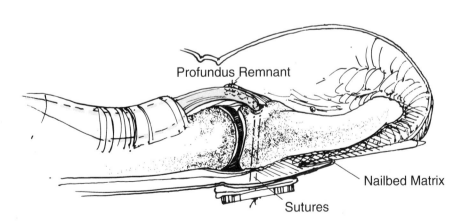

■ FIGURE 18–4
Flexor tendon advancement into the distal phalanx. The flexor tendon is advanced into a cancellous trough in the distal phalanx and secured with a pull-out wire. The palmar plate should not be disturbed and any remaining stump of the profundus tendon can be used to reinforce the repair. The pull-out suture should exit proximal to the germinal matrix to avoid a nail-plate deformity.

to the joint surface, exiting proximal to the germinal matrix (Fig. 18–4). After making the drill holes, the DIP joint is flexed, the core sutures are passed through the bone, and the profundus tendon is advanced into the cancellous trough. A folded piece of adaptic is used to pad the button and the suture is tied. The 25-gauge needle is removed and the repair inspected. The remaining flap of the distal tendon stump is sutured on top of the repair, using 4-0 braided nonabsorbable suture. Full DIP flexion is passively tested to assure that the repair does not bind on the distal edge of the A4 pulley. If necessary, a small portion of the A4 pulley may be resected. Dressing care and rehabilitation proceed, using the same protocol as a tenorrhaphy. The pull-out wire is removed 6 weeks after the repair.

The choice of skin incision must be made by giving consideration to the shape and extent of the laceration that caused the profundus disruption. The mid-lateral approach can be used in most circumstances, including profundus avulsion and transverse or short oblique lacerations. Necrosis of the skin flaps does not result unless the intersection angle of the two incisions is excessively oblique. Long oblique lacerations should be extended in a Bruner zigzag approach. The surgical exposure starts at the pulp of the digit and proceeds proximally, alternating between the ulnar and radial extent of the joint flexion creases, and ends at the distal palmar crease.

Creating a profundus repair that glides freely beneath the constricting A4 pulley presents formidable technical challenges but it is generally agreed that the pulley must be preserved.[13,17–19] Loss of the pulley allows bowstringing of the flexor tendon, which can lead to flexion contractures, loss of DIP flexion, tendon adhesions, and rupture of additional pulleys. If rendered incompetent by the original injury or surgical mishap, the A4 pulley should be reconstructed by one of the many techniques that are available.

■ REHABILITATION

Postoperative mobilization can be managed by one of the three techniques described for rehabilitation of zone 2 flexor tendon repairs. The Duran-Houser[5,18] technique uses static splinting combined with controlled passive motion. The modified Kleinert program[23] employs a rubber band that provides dynamic flexion while the patient actively extends the digit to the limits of a dorsal blocking splint. The use of a continuous passive motion machine[17] is the third and least frequently used rehabilitation option. Each method has its advantages and possible complications. Excellent results can be obtained with the Kleinert program but flexion contractures of the PIP joint are a frequent complication.[3,8,16,17] The Duran program is simple, well tolerated by patients, and easy to monitor. It is my rehabilitation program of choice.

Three to 5 days after surgery, the original dressing is removed and a forearm-based dorsal blocking splint is fabricated. A laceration of the index finger necessitates inclusion of all four digits but a disruption of one of the ulnar three profundus tendons allows the index finger to be left out of the splint. The therapist instructs the patient to passively flex each joint independently and the digit compositely into the palm. The exercise is repeated six times a day. Four weeks postoperatively, active flexion exercises are begun. Recent studies suggest that superior results can be obtained by modifying the program to allow passive flexion/active maintenance (place and hold) exercises before the traditional starting time of 4 weeks.[3,7] This change has been tried with promising early results but is yet unproved and therefore should be used cautiously. The splint is discontinued 6 weeks postoperatively and gentle resistance strengthening is begun. Full unrestricted activity is allowed 3 months after the repair.

■ OUTCOMES

The outcomes and expected complications of zone 1 flexor tendon repairs are difficult to learn from the literature because most authors combine zone 1 and zone 2 repairs into a single group. The few available reports that isolate zone 1 injuries suggest that good to excellent results can be achieved in 60 to 75% of individuals.[6] One study[7] reports an active DIP flexion arc of about 42°. Tenolysis may be successfully employed to improve results but ultimately, the final DIP motion is directly related to the quality of the initial repair. If the repair binds on the A4 pulley, no amount of postoperative therapy or reconstructive surgery will restore active flexion.

Adhesions are the most frequently encountered complication after zone 1 flexor tendon repairs.[17,18] Other complications include wound sepsis, cold intolerance, and triggering.[9,17] Rupture of the repair can occur any time in the first 3 months and has been reported to occur with a frequency of 3 to 6%.[20] Ruptures that are immediately recognized should be re-repaired.[1] Some complications are specific to repairs in zone 1, such as DIP flexion contracture from excessive profundus advancement, a distal insertion site onto the distal phalanx, or loss of the A4 pulley. Advancing the profundus more than 1 cm or flexor tendon adhesions can lead to flexion loss in adjacent digits secondary to the quadriga effect.

Other complications appear to be related to the rehabilitation method chosen. Dynamic flexion devices can lead to PIP flexion contractures.[3,8,16,17] Close supervision by the surgeon and therapist is essential to avoid this complication. It is tempting to overcome a developing flexion contracture with passive extension but one author[8] reports an unacceptably high rate of tendon dehiscence with this maneuver.

The techniques of flexor tendon repair and rehabilitation are constantly changing. Basic science research is increasing our understanding of tendon healing and adhesion formation. Surgeons are refining suture techniques and therapists are striving to improve the rehabilitation protocols. As our knowledge and experience increase, it is hoped that we will see an improvement in the functional results obtained after zone 1 flexor tendon repair.

References

1. Allen BN, Frykman GK, Unsell RS, Wood VE: Ruptured flexor tendon tenorraphies in zone II: repair and rehabilitation. J Hand Surg Am, 1987; 12:18–21.
2. Bunnell S: Surgery of the Hand, 3rd ed. Philadelphia, JB Lippincott, 1956, pp. 520.
3. Cannon N, Strickland JW: Therapy following flexor tendon surgery. Hand Clin, 1985; 1: 147–165.
4. Cooney WP, Weidman K, Malo D, Wood MB: Management of acute flexor tendon injury in the hand. Instr Course Lect, 1985; 34:373–381.
5. Duran RJ, Houser RG: Controlled Passive Motion Following Flexor Tendon Repair in Zones 2 and 3. In: AAOS: Symposium on Tendon Surgery in the hand. 1975:105–114.
6. Edinburg M, Widgerow AD, Biddulph SL: Early postoperative mobilization of flexor tendon injuries using a modification of the Kleinert technique. J Hand Surg Am, 1987; 12:34–38.
7. Evans RB: A study of the zone I flexor tendon injury and implications for treatment. J Hand Ther, 1990; :133–148.
8. Gerbino PG, Saldana MJ, Westerbeck P, Schacherer TG: Complications experienced in the rehabilitation of zone I flexor tendon injuries with dynamic traction splinting. J Hand Surg Am, 1991; 16:680–686.
9. Kleinert HE, Cash SL: Management of acute flexor tendon injuries in the hand. Instr Course Lect, 1985; 34:361–372.
10. Kleinert HE, Kutz JE, Ashbell TS, et al: Primary repair of lacerated flexor tendons in ''No Man's Land.'' J Bone Joint Surg, 49A:577, 1967.
11. Kleinert HE, Kutz JE, Cohen M: Primary repair of zone 2 flexor tendon lacerations. *In* AAOS Symposium on Tendon Surgery in the Hand. St. Louis, C.V. Mosby Co., 1975, pp. 91–104.
12. Lister G: Incisions and closure of flexor tendon sheath during primary repair. Hand, 1983; 15(2):123–135.
13. Lister G: Pitfalls and complications of flexor tendon surgery. Hand Clin, 1985; 1:133–146.
14. Malerich M, Baird R: Permissable limits of flexor digitorum profundus tendon advancement—an anatomic study. J Hand Surg, 1987; 12A:30–33.
15. Schlenker J, Lister G, Kleinert HE: Three complications of untreated partial tendon lacerations of flexor tendons: entrapment, rupture, and triggering. J Hand Surg, 1981; 6: 392–396.
16. Schneider LH, McEntee P: Flexor tendon injuries. Treatment of the acute problem. Hand Clin, 1986; 2:119–131.
17. Steinberg DR: Acute flexor tendon injuries. Orthop Clin North Am, 1992; 23:125–140.
18. Strickland JW: Management of acute flexor tendon injuries. Orthop Clin North Am, 1983; 14: 827–849.
19. Strickland JW: Flexor tendon injuries part 2: flexor tendon repair. Orthop Rev, 1986; 15:49–69.

20. Tonkin M, Lister G: Flexor tendon surgery—today and looking ahead. Clin Plast Surg, 1986; 13:221–242.
21. Verdan C: Primary repair of flexor tendons. J Bone Joint Surg, 42A:647–657, 1960.
22. Verdan C: Practical considerations for primary and secondary repair in flexor tendon injuries. Surg Clin North Am, 44:951–970, 1964.
23. Werntz JR, Chesher SP, Breidenbach WC, Kleinert HE, Bissonnette MA: A new dynamic splint for postoperative treatment of flexor tendon injury. J Hand Surg Am, 1989; 14:559–566.

19

Flexor Tendon Repairs in Zone 2

A restoration of gliding function after injury in the tendon sheath area of flexor tendons is a major issue in hand surgery.[27,38] The main problem is the formation of restrictive adhesions between the tendon and the tendon sheath or other tissues. Despite increased knowledge about tendon healing, the introduction of refined surgical techniques, and the use of sophisticated postoperative rehabilitation programs, individual results after tendon repair in zone 2 remain highly unpredictable.

Two different methods can be used for reconstruction of lacerated flexor tendons within the tendon sheath: free tendon grafting and direct tendon repair. Free flexor tendon grafts were first described by Lexer in 1912.[16] Bunnell[2] advocated this method in 1922 and favored secondary grafting (i.e., performing the free tendon transplantation after the primary injury had healed). He formulated a moratorium on suturing lacerated flexor tendons within the flexor tendon sheath, an area he called "no man's land." It was assumed that flexor tendons lacerated within the flexor tendon sheath had a limited intrinsic capacity to heal and that adhesions that invaded the repair site from the periphery brought reparative cells and nutrition to the healing tendon (extrinsic healing). These adhesions also limited tendon excursion, however, and led to poor outcomes from primary repair. Peacock[30] recognized the importance of migrating peripheral cells and did not consider the tendon cells capable of collagen production. Potenza[33] found that mechanical separation of the tendon from the sheath delayed tendon healing, as it delayed the invasion of peripheral cells. A cellular response of the tendon was reported by Lindsay and coworkers in 1959.[19] They described adhesions as not being essential to the healing process but being a result of inflammatory reaction. The concept of an intrinsic healing capacity of flexor tendons was established by Matthews and coworkers,[29] Eiken and coworkers,[8] and Lundborg in 1974–1976.[24] It has not been possible to determine the relative contribution of the intrinsic and extrinsic healing to the total repair process. Along with the fact that diffusion has been recognized as a major nutrient pathway to the tendons, as shown by Lundborg and coworkers[23] and Manske and coworkers,[26] there seems to be a rationale for trying to totally avoid postoperative adhesions.[9]

The concept of "no man's land" was redefined by Posch,[32] Verdan,[41] Kleinert,[14] and Kessler and Nissim,[11] who established that primary flexor tendon repair is the preferred method of treatment in the appropriate clinical setting.[27,38] They refined the surgical technique and published clinical results from primary repair that were equal to the results achieved by tendon grafting. Posch[32] and Verdan[41] performed partial resections of the tendon sheath and resected the sublimis tendon. Verdan used blocking pins in the sutured tendons. Kleinert[13] improved the results by introducing controlled passive motion, using rubber band traction and preserving the tendon sheath and sublimis tendon.

Direct repair of isolated tidy lacerations of flexor tendons in zone 2 is indicated as an emergency or delayed primary procedure in most cases when a trained hand surgeon and rehabilitation resources are available. Appropriate instruments and loupe magnification should be available. Additional injuries to the digit are relative contraindications to direct repair. The more scar tissue likely to be formed and the more immobilization required, the greater the contraindication for direct repair. Digital nerve injury is usually no contraindication if, despite simultaneous nerve repair, early controlled mobilization can be allowed. Phalangeal fractures induce such severe adhesions that tendon repair is indicated

■ HISTORY OF THE TECHNIQUE

■ INDICATIONS AND CONTRAINDICATIONS

only when the osteosyntheses are so strong that they allow early mobilization. Severe damage to critical pulleys requires pulley repair or reconstruction. During healing, the pulleys should be unloaded; therefore, staged tendon grafting is indicated rather than primary tendon repair. A major skin defect requiring some kind of flap is usually a contraindication to direct tendon repair. In digits requiring revascularization or replantation, however, primary tendon repair should be performed when possible because of the difficulties involved in performing re-explorations in these digits. Debridement of the tendon ends is usually not necessary but when debridement results in shortening of more than 1 cm of the profundus tendon, direct repair is probably contraindicated and grafting should be performed instead to avoid flexion contracture.[25]

■ SURGICAL TECHNIQUES

Axillary block or general anesthesia should be used for flexor tendon repair. According to the modification of Verdan's zone system,[15] zone 2 extends from the distal palmar crease to a point between the middle and the distal digital crease (Fig. 19–1A). In my opinion, the principles of zone 2 tendon surgery are valid all the way to the distal digital crease (i.e., the distal interphalangeal [DIP] joint and the A5 pulley [zone 1]) (Fig. 19–2).

Tourniquet control is mandatory during this operation but it should be deflated before closure of the wound. Adequate access to the injured tendon is an absolute necessity for atraumatic and correct tendon surgery. The original laceration usually has to be extended for better exposure. A skin marker is used to plan the incision line. Bruner zigzag incisions should be attempted but often have to be modified because of the direction of the primary wound (Fig. 19–1B). The incision should be carried far enough distally and proximally

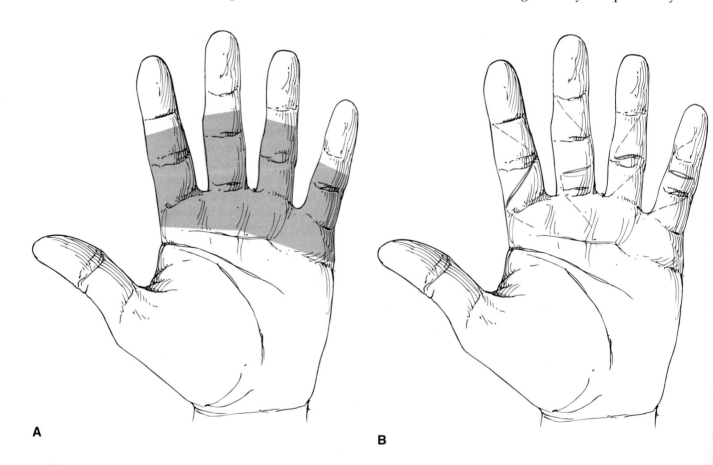

A   B

■ FIGURE 19–1

A, Hand with the shaded area indicating zone II for the flexor tendons. **B**, Alternative skin incisions that are basically variations of the standard Bruner incision. The preferred variation in each case is determined by the location and orientation of the original laceration.

so that the retracted tendon ends can be found in the exposed tendon sheath, usually the distance of one phalanx in both directions. The surgeon should avoid narrow skinflap tips because insufficient circulation to a narrow tip may cause partial flap necrosis, a severe complication. The tips of the flaps can be made wider by curving the incisions instead of producing narrow sharp angles. The tip angle should not be less than 90°. Longitudinal incisions should be placed only in the mid-lateral line and may be used alternating with a Bruner incision (Fig. 19–1B).

The volar digital neurovascular bundles are parallel and located on either side of the tendon sheath. The digital nerves are volar to the arteries. When the artery has been injured by a volar laceration, it is likely that the nerve is also injured. The flexor tendon sheath consists of a continuous synovial sheath and an interrupted fibrous retinacular sheath.[5] The latter starts proximally at the level of the metacarpal head, which corresponds to the distal palmar crease. The fibrous parts are called annular (A) and cruciform (C) pulleys. The A2 and A4 pulleys are attached to the phalanges and are biomechanically the most important (Fig. 19–2). They should never be incised.

The hand is positioned with the dorsum against the operating table and stabilized (e.g., with a lead hand). The skin is incised and fine skin hooks are used to elevate the skin flaps. The lateral tips of the skin flaps are dissected superficial to Grayson's ligaments, so that the neurovascular bundles are not injured. Note that the flaps have to carry some subcutaneous tissue to ensure perfusion. The neurovascular bundles are situated deep to Grayson's ligaments. These ligaments are transected and released from the flexor tendon sheath as the elevation of the skin flap approaches the base of the flap. Grayson's ligament is carried in the flap, protecting the neurovascular bundle.

The goal of the tendon repair is to restore exact anatomy and function by performing atraumatic surgery. Numerous modifications have been tried to achieve less traumatic techniques and thereby less inflammatory response and adhesion formation. Suture materials, needles, and suture techniques have been refined to lessen inflammatory response, gaping, negative effects on the circulation, and to increase the strength of the repair. The Kessler grasping technique or one of its modifications is now the most favored method of direct tendon repair. It is combined with a running coaptation suture.[11,28,38,40] The tendon repair should be performed in the cruciate pulley areas between the annular pulleys. If further incisions in the tendon sheath are needed to reach the tendon, L-shaped incisions in the synovial sheath should be used with the transverse part of the incision, always away from the annular pulley.[22] By this technique, a cornet-shaped entrance to

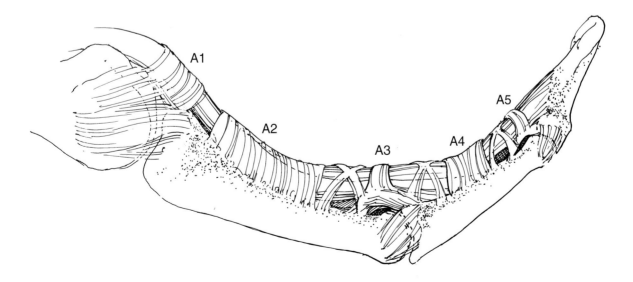

■ FIGURE 19–2
The flexor tendon sheath with the annular pulleys A1–A5, with cruciate pulleys in between.

the pulley is developed that facilitates the passage of the tendon end. Incisions of the annular pulleys should be avoided. A complete cut of the A2 or A4 pulleys should never be performed. You should rather abandon the attempt to do a direct tendon repair and instead choose tendon grafting. If the proximal tendon end is retracted try to flex the wrist and massage the palm in a distal direction. Try just a couple of times to grip the tendon with a tendon retriever or a fine hemostat; if this is not successful, extend the incision proximally as necessary or to the base of the digit. A separate proximal incision can be placed in the palm at the level of the distal palmar crease. A skin incision continuing across the proximal digital crease is not useful because this is at the level of the A2 pulley, which should not be incised anyway. The tendons are exposed proximal to the A1 pulley. A Silastic tube or a silicone rod can be used to find the right channel for the profundus tendon through the decussation of the superficialis tendon or through another long segment of the sheath. It can also be used to deliver the tendon from the proximal exposure into the distal exposure. The tendon probe, silicon tube, or rod is most often inserted into the tendon sheath distally and delivered through the incision into the palm, sutured to the proximal tendon end, and then pulled out through the distal exposure. If both the flexor digitorum profundus (FDP) and flexor digitorum superficialis (FDS) tendons are retracted and cannot be retrieved together, the FDS tendon is first repaired. The proximal end may be sutured to a probe or rod and pulled distally and a primary repair performed. The FDP is then brought through the repaired FDS tendon, as described above. The position of the FDP tendon is then secured with a 1-inch straight needle put transversely through both the tendon sheath and tendon.

Touching the tendon surface is avoided as much as possible. When the tendon must be grasped, it is done with a jeweler's forceps in the cut transverse surface. This grip is used while placing the core suture in the tendon, trying to keep the same grip without change through the whole procedure. At least 1 cm of each tendon end must be available for surgery outside the annular pulley. The suture should be passed 1 cm through the tendon to create a safe grasping stitch. If 1 cm of the tendon end is not available, the tendon has to be retracted to the opposite side of the annular pulley and the tendon core suture placed at this level. It is practical to first bring the needle through the sheath under the pulley in a retrograde direction before performing the core suture. The needle, suture material and tendon are then returned under the annular pulley, and the core suture is continued in the other tendon end.

Core suture materials should be 4-0 or 3-0 braided polyester or multi- or monofilament stainless steel.[12] The latter should be avoided in cases having a level of injury at the proximal interphalangeal (PIP) or metacarpophalangeal (MP) joints because fatigue develops in the suture material from the postoperative flexion exercises. Special cutting needles of good quality must also be used.

If possible, both FDP and FDS tendons should be repaired. The vincular system may be better preserved, as is independent joint flexion. There is less tendency for hyperextension in the PIP joint. When the FDS injury is at the level of the two slips, the tendon repair begins with these. If the tendon slip is large enough, a traditional core suture is used. Otherwise, a figure-of-eight suture is sufficient. The knot is placed on the dorsal side, away from the FDP tendon. There is usually room for only one suture in each slip.

For the FDP repair, I prefer to use a modified Kessler suture, with one suture buried in the tendon gap, although I am not comfortable with the deposition of suture material in the tendon gap, where it may disturb healing. To apply the Kessler suture take a firm grip with the jeweler's forceps in the transected surface of the profundus tendon and bring the needle through this surface in the center of the tendon and parallel to the collagen fibers at least 1 cm along the tendon. Then bring the needle through the surface, just volar to the midline. The needle is then brought laterally and a couple of millimeters back toward the tendon end and reentered into the tendon in a transverse direction, positioned volar to the longitudinal part of the suture. By this arrangement, a half-hitch is formed, grasping about 25% of the cross-sectional tendon area. The needle is taken out of the tendon, brought toward the midline of the volar surface a couple of millimeters from the

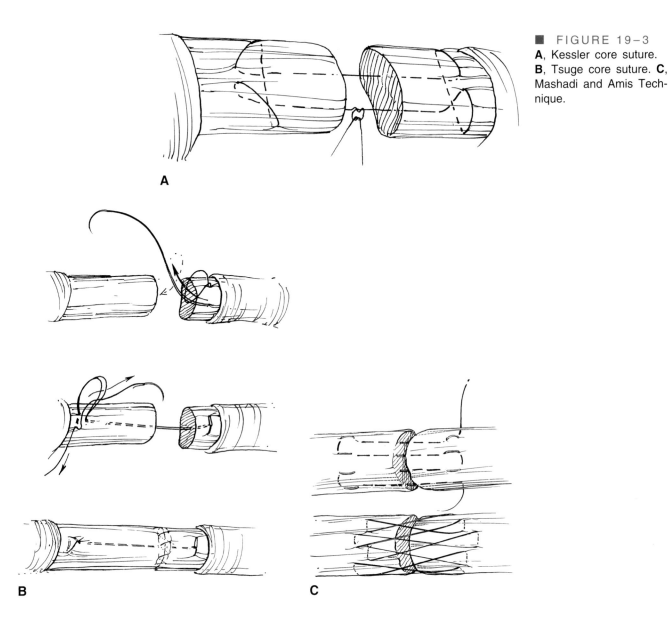

■ FIGURE 19–3
A, Kessler core suture.
B, Tsuge core suture. **C**,
Mashadi and Amis Technique.

transverse stitch, re-entered into the tendon, and taken longitudinally, passing dorsal to the transverse stitch. This procedure is repeated in the other tendon end. Finally, the tendon ends are brought together and the tension of the suture is adjusted to eliminate gaps or bulkiness. The visible part of the core suture should then be four diagonally oriented sutures on the volar surface, one in each corner (Fig. 19–3A). The tendon repair is completed by a running epitendinous (peripheral) suture, using a 6-0 or 5-0 monofilament suture. This suture is not just a tidying-up suture; attention recently has been drawn to the considerable contribution of this suture to repair strength and resistance to gap formation. Different modifications have been suggested.[18,28] My preferred technique is described by Mashadi and Amis[28] (Fig. 19–3C). It achieves superior anchorage by making the transverse passes across the tendon fiber direction within the fibers. The grasps should be made 5 mm from the tendon ends. The longitudinal passes are also placed in the tendon to minimize suture material on the tendon surface, reducing foreign body reaction. Eversion of the edges is avoided by bringing the suture to the epitenon at the cut tendon ends. When the needle is introduced into the transected surface from outside, it is helpful to first place the backside of the needle tip on the longitudinal outside surface of the tendon and to then withdraw the needle until the tip suddenly falls down into the cut surface. This maneuver corrects eversion and the needle tip usually ends up in the epitenon. Multiple passes in a running configuration multiply the strength of the suture material. The dorsal surface is reached by rotating the tendon 180°. The rotation may be impossible and should be avoided if a vinculum is still intact close to one of the cut tendon ends. In such a case, either the dorsal peripheral suture can be relinquished or the dorsal part of the peripheral suture can be from inside before tying the core suture, as described by Sanders.[38]

The stabilizing straight needle is removed after the tendon repair has been finished, and the excursion of the tendon repair is inspected during passive flexion/extension to determine whether it is likely to catch or bind on the pulley system. Necessary corrections are performed. If redoing the tendon repair is considered, additional trauma to the tendon ends has to be anticipated. Sometimes a better alternative is a partial release of the pulley to gain more space in the sheath. This can be accomplished by performing an oblique incision across the pulley, then lengthening and suturing it.

Partial lacerations to more than 50% of the tendon cross-section should always be repaired because of the risk of a secondary rupture. A regular core stitch with a 4-0 polyester suture is used. If the injury involves less than 50% of the cross-section, it often should be repaired to avoid the risk of having the tendon edge trapped in the sheath or the injured profundus trapped at the entrance of the decussation of the superficialis tendon. A peripheral running suture with 6-0 or 5-0 monofilament is used.

Although the procedure is technically demanding, it should be remembered that a direct correlation exists between the time spent in the wound and the amount of trauma inflicted to the tissues by the surgeon. It is also important to keep the tissues moist throughout the procedure to reduce the trauma of desiccation to the tendon surface.

From personal clinical and experimental experience, I believe that closure of the tendon sheath is important. From a mechanical perspective, it prevents the repaired tendon from catching the sheath edges, especially the pulleys. It does not seem to be important in preventing adhesions. The sheath is closed by a running suture, using 6-0 monofilament. Before closing the skin, the tourniquet should be deflated and hemostasis obtained to decrease the tendency of fibrosis. It is important to thoroughly close the skin if early mobilization is planned, and I recommend a running suture with small grasps, using 5-0 monofilament nylon. The running suture is tied at each tip of the skin flaps and also once in between to prevent partial separation of the skin edges.

The whole hand (including all digits) is put into a bulky dressing and a dorsal splint applied to keep the wrist in 20 to 30° of flexion, the MP joints of the fingers in maximum flexion, and the interphalangeal joints in neutral position. This dressing is kept for about 2 days and then replaced, depending on the method chosen for early controlled mobilization.

■ TECHNICAL
ALTERNATIVES

The anatomy of the superficialis tendon along the proximal phalanx requires special attention because the two slips spiral around the profundus tendon. After sectioning of the slips, the proximal and distal ends rotate in different directions and present to the surgeon in a 180° rotated position relative to the other. The slips must be derotated to restore correct anatomy.

The Kessler suture may be modified by a second locking grasp at each corner to improve stability; the drawback is increased difficulty when the final suture tension is set because the suture will not glide. Another alternative to the described modified Kessler suture is to place the knot on the surface of the tendon, as originally suggested by Kessler, but this may induce irritation of the sheath and the possibility of a trigger phenomenon. Some authors[38] advocate the use of a separate suture in each tendon end, thereby ending with two knots. This sometimes facilitates the procedure, especially the advancement of the tendon ends in the sheath, but doubles the problem with the knots.

Improper core suture placement can easily occur when performing a Kessler suture. The difficulty is the positioning of the transverse limb volar to the longitudinal limb. If the transverse limb is instead placed dorsal to the longitudinal limb, the suture loop does not lock around the tendon fibers, and a Nicoladoni suture is performed instead, with less strength. Inadequate tension when tying the core suture may result in gaping, which increases the risk of adhesions and rupture. Tension that is too high results in a bulky repair, with increased risk of catching the tendon sheath and impairment of tendon gliding.

The core suture technique of Tsuge[39] is a good alternative to the modified Kessler suture. Defino and coworkers[4] compared Kessler and Tsuge (see Fig. 19–3) sutures and found no significant differences. Both techniques use a grasping stitch that is applied in the relatively avascular volar half of the profundus tendon, have equal strength, and cause limited deprivation of the blood supply to the tendon ends. Great interest has recently been focused on the development of stronger suture techniques. The reason for this is a trend in postoperative rehabilitation toward controlled active mobilization at an earlier stage to protect against the development of adhesions. There are several alternate epitendinous sutures in common use. The most common is probably the running over-and-over peripheral stitch, which is simple to perform. Running sutures are stronger than those that are interrupted. Traditional horizontal mattress sutures use longitudinal grasps in the tendon tissue and are not as strong as the Mashadi-Amis technique,[28] which uses transverse passes across the tendon fiber direction. If considerable eversion problems exist at the cut tendon ends, the suture may pass over the laceration site completely superficial to the tendon surface, as described by Halsted and Silfverskiold,[35] but this increases the risk of foreign body reaction and the development of adhesions.

Treatment of the tendon sheath has gained considerable interest. The concept of intrinsic tendon healing drew attention to the synovial environment and its influence on the development of adhesions between a repaired tendon and its parietal tendon sheath.[7] Closure of the tendon sheath was thought to help the synovial environment and thereby decrease adhesion formation. Free transplantation of tendon sheath from toe flexors has been described by Eiken and coworkers[7] as a treatment of tissue defects in the tendon sheath to prevent adhesions. The method was used in combination with secondary reconstruction using two-stage tendon grafting. Slightly improved flexion was achieved but a simultaneous tendency for flexion contracture was seen, resulting in no improvement of overall total active motion.

Peterson and coworkers[31] reported that closure of the flexor tendon sheath after primary tendon repair in chickens did not improve tendon gliding, as measured biomechanically. Despite repair, it was reported that the flexor tendon sheath did not maintain its synovial characteristics histologically and it was concluded that an entirely new sheath was formed. Furthermore, there are also reports[1,21,34] claiming that closure of the tendon sheath in man is not superior to leaving it open. It should always be remembered that if the attempted tendon repair turns out to be too complicated and the operative result is not technically satisfying, an alternative treatment is tendon grafting. When indicated, grafting should be performed immediately, either as a one- or two-stage procedure, depending on the presence of associated injuries.

Rupture of the primary tendon repair should usually be treated with re-exploration and a second direct repair within a couple of days.

Pulley injury may cause bowstringing of the flexor tendon, an increase in the moment arm, and a flexion contracture in the interphalangeal joint. Injury to a single pulley usually passes without notable effects. Two or more consecutive injured pulleys, however, are likely to impair function and should be repaired. The most important pulleys are A2 and A4. If pulley tissue is lost, a reconstruction of these pulleys is performed, usually using a tendon graft.[17] The more extensive the additional injuries, the greater the indication is for converting the attempted direct tendon repair into a two-stage tendon grafting procedure.

■ REHABILITATION

The dressing is changed and the exercise splint applied 2 days after tendon repair. The splint has wrist flexion of 10 to 20° and MP joint flexion of 70 to 80°. Rubber band flexion traction is combined with active finger extension in the splint every hour.[10,20] Passive flexion exercises are also performed after temporary removal of the rubber band. Isolated DIP and PIP joint exercises are performed to maximize differential tendon gliding between

■ FIGURE 19–4
A thermoplastic splint used for rubber band passive flexion–active extension exercises. Monofilament line attached to the bands passes through metal eyes in the palm to pull the fingers into flexion. Active extension is used to straighten the fingers against the resistance of the rubber bands.

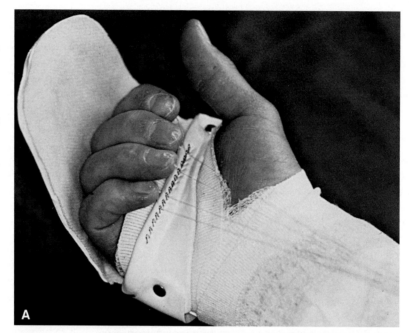

A

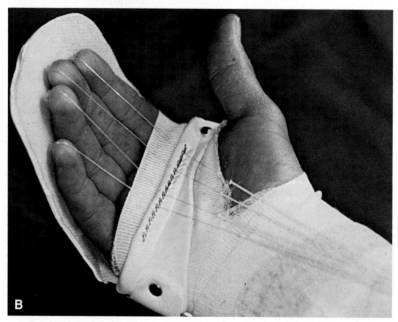

B

the FDP and FDS tendons.[6,37] These exercises are also started at 2 days and performed every hour during the daytime. To avoid the quadriga phenomenon, all four digits are included in rubber band traction. The splint should have an important bar or external pulley system in the palm to bring the rubber bands down to the distal palmar crease (Fig. 19–4). When using this method, it is important to be aware of the significant risk of developing flexion contractures in the PIP joints. I therefore tell the patients to remove the rubber bands at night and immobilize the digits with an elastic bandage, with interphalangeal joints in a straight (safe) position in the same dorsal splint.

The patients are seen twice a week during the first 2 weeks. There is usually no urgency to remove the skin sutures. The early mobilization program stresses the wound, and a wound dehiscence may be a serious complication, with development of an inflammatory reaction and the risk of infection. The skin sutures are removed after 2 to 3 weeks, when the skin is well healed. Rubber band traction is continued for a total of 3 weeks and replaced by active flexion and extension exercises while remaining in the dorsal splint during the fourth week. The splint is then removed, wrist range-of-motion exercises started, and free active motion allowed without resistance during the fifth week, with slight resistance during the sixth week. After 6 weeks, limited resistance is permitted, defined as easy daily activities. Moderate resistance should be avoided until 8 weeks and unrestricted resistance until 12 weeks postoperatively. It is important to note that the patient who improves rapidly during rehabilitation is especially at risk to rupture the repair, just because he or she "is doing so well." If flexion contracture is developing, a dynamic interphalangeal extension splint is introduced about 6 weeks after the operation.

The importance of continuity in the rehabilitation program and cooperation with dedicated hand therapists can not be overemphasized; it is an important requirement if flexor tendon surgery is to be successful.

Different controlled mobilization programs indicate that 70 to 75% of the patients have excellent or good results and 10 to 20% have poor results. This also includes the published results from controlled active mobilization.[3,36] The reported frequencies of rupture of the tendon repair is in the range of 3 to 20%. The definition of excellent and good is not uniform in the literature. The American Society for Surgery of the Hand[14] has recommended defining "excellent" as having 100% (of corresponding contralateral digit) active range of motion (MP + PIP + DIP) and "good" as having 75 to 99%. Strickland[38] suggests that "excellent" be defined as total active motion (PIP + DIP) in the range of 75 to 100% of normal and "good" in the range of 50 to 74%. Kleinert's criteria[14] are based on residual flexion contracture and extension deficit. "Excellent" is defined as a pulp-to-distal palmar crease distance of less than 1 cm and an extension deficit of 1 to 15°. "Good" is defined as a pulp-to-distal palmar crease distance of 1 to 1.5 cm and an extension deficit of 16 to 30°.

■ OUTCOMES

References

1. Amadio PC, Hunter JM, Jaeger SH, Wehbe MA, Schneider LH: The effect of vincular injury on the results of flexor tendon surgery in zone 2. J Hand Surg 1985; 10A:5:626–632.
2. Bunnell S: Repair of tendons in the fingers. Surgery, Gynecology and Obstetrics 1922; 35: 88–97.
3. Cullen KW, Tolhurst P, Lang D, Page RE: Flexor tendon repair in zone 2 followed by controlled active mobilization. J Hand Surg, 1989; 14B:392–395.
4. Defino HLA, Barbieri CH, Goncalves RP, Paulin JBP: Studies on tendon healing. A comparison between suturing techniques. J Hand Surg, 1986; 11B:444–450.
5. Doyle JR: Anatomy of the finger tendon sheath and pulley system. J Hand Surg, 1988; 13A: 473–484.
6. Duran RH, Houser RG: Controlled passive motion following flexor tendon repair in zones 2 and 3. In: American Academy of Orthopaedic Surgeons symposium on flexor tendon surgery in the hand. St Louis: C.V. Mosby, 1975:105–114.
7. Eiken O, Hagberg L, Lundborg G: Evolving biological concepts as applied to tendon surgery. Clin Plast Surg, 1981; 8:1–12.
8. Eiken O, Lundborg G, Rank F: The role of the digital synovial sheath in tendon grafting. An experimental and clinical study on autologous tendon grafting in the digit. Scand J Plast Reconstr Surg 1975; 9:182–189.
9. Gelberman RH, Woo SL, Lothringer K, Akeson WH, Amiel D: Effects of early intermittent passive mobilization on healing canine flexor tendons. J Hand Surg, 1982; 7:170–175.
10. Hagberg L, Selvik G: Tendon excursion and dehiscence during early controlled mobilization after flexor tendon repair in zone II: An x-ray stereophotogrammetric analysis. J Hand Surg, 1991; 16A:669–680.
11. Kessler I, Nissim F: Primary repair without immobilization of flexor tendon division within the digital sheath. An experimental and clinical study. Acta Orthop Scandinav, 1969; 40: 587–601.
12. Ketchum LD: Suture materials and suture techniques used in tendon repair. Hand Clin, 1985; 1:43–53.

13. Kleinert HE, Kutz JE, Ashbell TS, Martinez E: Primary repair of flexor tendons in "no man's land." J Bone Joint Surg 1967; 49A:3:577.
14. Kleinert HE, Kutz JE, Atasoy E, Stormo A: Primary repair of flexor tendons. Orthop Clin North Am 1973; 4:865–876.
15. Kleinert HE, Verdan C: Report of the Committee on Tendon Injuries. J Hand Surg 1983; 8: 794–798.
16. Lexer E: Die Verwehtung der freien Sehnentransplantation. Arch Klinic Chir 1912; 98:918.
17. Lin GT, Amadio PC, An KN, Cooney WP, Chao EYS: Biomechanical analysis of finger flexor pulley reconstruction. J Hand Surg 1989; 14B:278–282.
18. Lin GT, An KN, Amadio PC, Cooney WP: Biomechanical studies of running suture for flexor tendon repair in dogs. J Hand Surg, 1988; 13A:553–558.
19. Lindsay WK, Thomson HG: Digital flexor tendons. An experimental study (Part I). The significance of each compartment of the flexor mechanism in tendon healing. Br J Plast Surg 1959; 12:289–316.
20. Lister GD, Kleinert HE, Kutz JE, et al: Primary flexor tendon repair followed by immediate controlled mobilization. J Hand Surg, 1977; 2:441–451.
21. Lister GD, Tonkin M: The results of primary flexor tendon repair with closure of the tendon sheath. J Hand Surg, 1986; 11A:5:767.
22. Lister GD: Indications and techniques for repair of the flexor tendon sheath. Hand Clin, 1985; 1:85–95.
23. Lundborg G, Holm S, Myrhage R: The role of the synovial fluid and tendon sheath for flexor tendon nutrition. An experimental tracer study on diffusional pathways in dogs. Scand J Plast Reconstr Surg, 1980; 14:99–107.
24. Lundborg G: Experimental flexor tendon healing without adhesion formation. A new concept of tendon nutrition and intrinsic healing mechanisms. A prelininary report. Hand 1976; 8: 235–238.
25. Malerich MM, Baird RA, McMaster W, Erickson JM: Permissable limits of flexor digitorum profundus tendon advancement—An anatomic study. J Hand Surg, 1987; 12A30–33.
26. Manske PR, Lesker PA: Comparative nutrient pathways to the flexor profundus tendons in zone II of various experimental animals. J Surg Res 1983; 34:83–93.
27. Manske PR: Flexor tendon healing. J Hand Surg, 1988; 13B:237–245.
28. Mashadi ZB, Amis AA: Strength of the suture in the epitenon and within the tendon fibres: Development of stronger peripheral suture technique. J Hand Surg, 1992; 17B:172–175.
29. Matthews P, Richards H: The repair potential of digital flexor tendons. J Bone Joint Surg 1974; 56B618–625.
30. Peacock EE: Fundamental aspects of wound healing relating to the restoration of gliding function after tendon repair. Surgery, Gynecology and Obstetrics, 1964; 119:241–250.
31. Peterson WW, Manske PR, Kain CC, Lesker PA: Effect of flexor sheath integrity on tendon gliding: A biomechanical and histologic study. J Orthop Res, 1986; 4:458–465.
32. Posch JL: Primary tenorrhaphies and tendon grafting procedures in hand surgery. Archives of Surgery, 1956; 73:609–624.
33. Potenza AD: Critical evaluation of flexor tendon healing and adhesion formation within artificial digital sheaths. J Bone Joint Surg, 1963; 45A:1217–1233.
34. Saldana MJ, Ho PK, Lichtman DM, Chow JA, Dovelle S, Thomes LJ: Flexor tendon repair and rehabilitation in zone II open sheath technique versus closed sheath technique. J Hand Surg, 1987; 12A6:1110–1113.
35. Silfverskiold KL, May EJ: Flexor tendon repair in zone II with a new suture technique and an early mobilization program combining passive and active flexion. J Hand Surg, 1994; 19A: 53–60.
36. Small JO, Brennen MD, Colville J: Early active mobilization following flexor tendon repair in Zone 2. J Hand Surg, 1989; 14B:383–391.
37. Strickland JW, Glogovac SV: Digital function following flexor tendon repair in Zone II: A comparison of immobilization and controlled passive motion techniques. J Hand Surg, 1980; 5:537–543.
38. Strickland JW: Flexor tendon surgery. Part 1: Primary flexor tendon repair. J Hand Surg, 1989; 14B:3:261–272.
39. Tsuge K, Ikuta Y, Matsuishi Y: Intratendinous tendon suture in the hand: A new technique. The Hand 1975; 7:250–255.
40. Urbaniak JR, Cahill JD, Mortenson RA: Tendon suturing methods: analysis of tensile strengths. In: American Academy of Orthopaedic Surgeons: Symposium on tendon surgery in the hand. St. Louis: Mosby Co., 1975:70–80.
41. Verdan C. Primary repair of flexor tendons: J Bone Joint Surg 1960; 42A:4:647–656.

ROBERT FALENDER
DANIEL P. MASS

20

Flexor Tendon Repairs in Zones 3–5

Much has been written regarding the treatment of injuries to the flexor tendon of the hand. Most research has focused on clinical follow-up studies and basic research of tendon injuries in zones 1 and 2. The literature has shown that obtaining a good result after a repair in these zones is difficult. Bunnell[2] coined the term "no man's land" to emphasize the difficulties associated with injuries in this area. Since the work of Verdan[15,16] Kleinert[6–8] and others[3,4,11,12] most surgeons now agree that primary repair in these zones should be attempted when possible. Many of these studies reported empirically that tendon injures in zones 3, 4, and 5 can do well if basic surgical principles are followed. Although injuries in zones 3, 4, and 5 are not uncommon[13,14] the reported functional and subjective results are not well-documented. Our philosophy is to repair injured structures acutely when possible. If the repair is performed within 3 weeks, there is little difference in the total active motion follow up, especially in zone 5. Early reports noted that repair of all structures in zone 5 was responsible for dense adhesions, limiting digital motion.[16] With the advent of early mobilization techniques in flexor tendon surgery, results have improved.[5]

■ HISTORY OF THE TECHNIQUE

The primary repair of flexor tendon injures is indicated in tidy wounds (Figure 20–1A and B). Because these injuries are usually associated with nerve and vascular injuries, they require prompt attention. Relative contraindications to repair of injuries in zones 3, 4, and 5 include those associated with vascular damage or those associated with severe contamination or mutilation, as caused by snowblowers, chainsaws, lawnmowers, and farm machinery. After assessment and thorough debridement of the wounds, repair of injured structures is performed in a stepwise manner. The skeleton is stabilized first with internal fixation (e.g., wires, screws, and plates). Fractures, both displaced and nondisplaced, require internal fixation prior to tendon repair to allow postoperative rehabilitation. This is followed by repair of the vascular and nerve structures by microsurgical techniques. Finally, the flexor tendons are repaired. In our opinion, an absolute contraindication to primary tendon repair is extensive skin loss or segmental tendon defects. Soft-tissue coverage, either by free tissue transfer or local flap coverage, should be done first. Segmental tendon defects can be repaired with interposition tendon grafts. After 3 to 4 days, a delayed primary repair of the tendons can be considered if the wound is clean and closed.

■ INDICATIONS AND CONTRAINDICATIONS

Preoperatively, the patient should receive a first generation cephalosporin antibiotic such as cephalexin or its equivalent. A general anesthetic or axillary block (our preference) should be performed by the anesthesiologist. After a sterile prep and drape, the arm is exsanguinated, either by elevation or with a stretch elastic wrap, and the tourniquet is then inflated.

Basic principles are important to all repairs. Flexor tendon repair should be performed in an operating room with loupe magnification. Electrocautery should be used for meticulous hemostasis. An attempt should be made to repair all injured structures. The injured structures are exposed by proximal and distal extension of the traumatic wound. In wounds with injuries to multiple structures, the skeleton is stabilized first, the tendons are repaired,

■ SURGICAL TECHNIQUES

■ FIGURE 20–1
A and **B**, Posteroanterior and lateral views of a zone 5 volar wrist laceration. The normal flexion cascade of the index finger is lost. The flexor digitorum profundus and flexor digitorum suoperficiallis tendons to the index finger were completely cut, while those to the long and ring were partially cut.

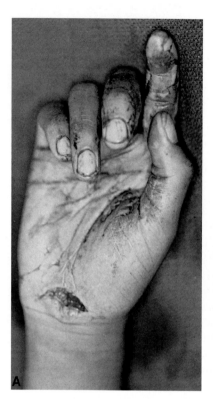

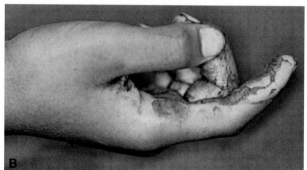

and finally, the injured arteries and nerves are repaired. However, if there has been a long period of ischemia, the bone is temporarily stabilized and one or more arteries repaired to reestablish distal perfusion. Even though single-vessel injuries may be ligated if the hand shows no evidence of preoperative hypo-vascularity,[5] our preference is to repair a single vessel laceration.[12] All nerve injuries are repaired at the time of initial operation, with the use of microepineural technique and group fascicular suture. All wound edges should be debrided, and all nonviable tissue is removed. All hemorrhagic synovium is explored and removed carefully, examining for injured tendons that may be retracted into the synovium or muscle. The tourniquet is deflated prior to skin closure or prior to microsurgical repair of the arteries. The skin is closed with 4-0 nylon interrupted sutures. Small rubber drains are placed to allow post-op drainage.

In Zone 5 injuries, the wound is also extended proximally and distally. The incisions must provide the exposure necessary for the repair. Transverse lacerations may be extended proximal and distal at right angles to the original wound. Angled lacerations may be extended in a zig-zag manner. Skin flaps are retracted with 4-0 nylon sutures. The volar antebrachial fascia is incised to expose the muscle fascia. The muscle fascia is preserved by dissecting along longitudinal planes between the muscle. This is important because muscle tissue does not hold a suture, whereas the fascia does. Necrotic tissue is resected, the hematoma evacuated, and all injured structures identified. The neurovascular structures are repaired first and the preserved muscle fascia is then approximated with 0 or 2-0 absorbable Vicryl sutures using a horizontal mattress stitch. If muscle substance has been lost and there is tension on the repair, the palmaris longus or long toe extensor tendon can be harvested and used as an interweaving tendon graft suture to relieve tension.[11]

In the distal forearm, injuries often occur at the musculotendinous junction, where identification of the proximal ends can be very difficult. There is usually a confluence of muscle into tendon over a long distance in the forearm, and the cut end of the tendon often retracts into the substance of the muscle and is surrounded by hematoma. Careful exploration of the muscle ends reveals tendinous material for adequate suturing.

Within the distal 5 cm of the forearm, the distal ends of the lacerated tendons are easily identified by grasping the center of the tendon with a mosquito hemostat, avoiding epitenon damage and gently pulling to flex the associated digits. Other fingers may flex along with the correct finger, because of interconnections between tendons or their synovial sheaths. In this case, one should apply light resistance on the pulp of the suspected finger and feel for resistance. The proximal tendon ends are more difficult to identify. The distal ends should be examined and noted for the angle of the laceration and the cross-sectional area. The profundus tendons are flat and multi-stranded, whereas the superficialis tendon, flexor pollicis longus, and the index finger profundus are more oval. Each tendon is identified, tagged, and approximated. The tendons are then repaired with a 4-0 Ethibond[2] core suture, using modified Kessler suture technique (Fig. 20–2A). The center of the tendon is grasped and the needle is driven through the cut end, exiting distally. The suture is then placed transversely and placed back into the tendon substance to exit through the cut end. This suture placement allows the knots to be buried in the substance of the tendon. The proximal ends are identified and then matched with their respective distal ends by matching the cross-sectional area and angle of laceration. The profundus tendons are repaired first, followed by the superficialis tendons. A 4-0 Ethibond core suture is placed into the proximal end, using a modified Kessler technique, as described earlier. The tendon ends are approximated and the sutures tied, burying the knots within the tendon substance.

Zone 4 tendon injuries are rare because of the depth of the structures and the protection provided by the transverse carpal ligament and carpal bones. The median nerve is most often injured. The traumatic wound is extended in the palm, in line with the long axis of the ring finger and in a zig-zag manner, both proximally and distally. Skin flaps are retracted with a 4-0 nylon retaining stitch. The median nerve and recurrent motor branch are identified, as are the proximal and distal ends of the transverse carpal ligament. Attempts are made to repair the tendons either proximal or distal to the transverse carpal ligament in a manner similar to that recommended for repair of zone 2 injuries around the A2 and A4 pulleys. However, if the median nerve is lacerated, the transverse carpal ligament must be opened. If the transverse carpal ligament must be opened, it is incised in a step cut manner, beginning radially through the proximal half of the ligament, then progressing transversely before finishing the division along the distal ulnar side (Fig. 20–3A and B). The swollen, hemorrhagic tenosynovium is removed.[6] The tendons are repaired with 4-0 Ethibond, using a Kessler stitch as the core suture and a 6-0 nylon as the epitendinous suture. Following tendon repair, the step-cut transverse carpal ligament ends are sutured with 3-0 absorbable suture (Fig 3C) in a lengthened position. Postoperative tendon bowstringing at the wrist is prevented by repair of this ligament.

Zone 3 is located between the distal end of the transverse carpal ligament and the A1 pulley. Zone 3 injuries are usually associated with the most collateral structural damage, including injuries to the common digital nerves, the superficial arch, motor branch of the median nerve, and the lumbrical muscle. At this level, proximal retraction of the proximal tendon end is prevented by the lumbrical muscle. The wounds are extended in Z-fashion proximally and distally. If the proximal tendon end cannot be easily retrieved, a second longitudinal incision in the distal forearm should allow identification. A core suture of 4-0 Ethibond is placed as described earlier (Fig 2A). The proximal tendon is then passed through the carpal tunnel if necessary. The two core sutures are tied and a 6-0 epitendinous nylon stitch is also performed (Fig 2B). If the lumbrical muscle is minimally injured, it can be sutured at the tendon repair site to provide a blood supply to aid in healing. The lumbrical muscle should not be advanced proximally, however, or a lumbrical plus[10] imbalance (attempted profundus flexion tightens the lumbrical) and proximal interphalangeal (PIP) joint extension could occur. Finally, the common digital nerves, arteries, and superficial arch are repaired using microsurgical techniques.

After tendon repair, in either of Zones 3, 4, or 5, the tension in the flexor tendons should be similar and the cascade of the resting fingers returned to normal. This relationship is best assessed by inspecting the hand from different perspectives, prior to wound closure (Fig. 20–4).

■ FIGURE 20–2
A, The tendons are repaired with a 4-0 Ethibond suture, using a modified Kessler technique. **B,** After tying the core suture, a running epitendinous stitch is placed using a 6-0 nylon suture.

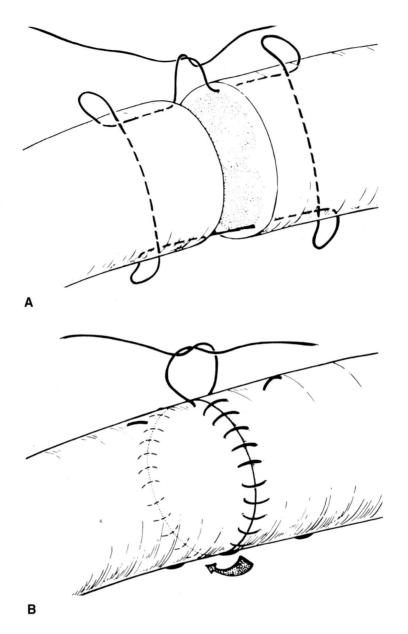

A

B

At the end of the surgery in zones 3 and 4, before the splint is applied, a 2-0 nylon suture is placed through each nail for postoperative dynamic motion. Alternatively, the hand therapist can "crazy glue" a bra hook to the fingernail at the time dynamic splinting is initiated.

The postoperative dressing is applied in a manner that allows early therapy to commence. For proximal zone 5 muscle belly repairs, however, a long arm cast with the elbow flexed at 90 degrees, the wrist at 30 degrees, the metacarpophalangeal (MP) joints at 60 degrees, and interphalangeal (IP) joints straight is applied and maintained for 4 weeks before active motion is started. Distal zone 5 injuries are immobilized in a dorsal plaster splint, with the wrist in 40 degrees of flexion, the MP joints in 30–60 degrees of flexion, and the IP joints straight. Zone 4 injuries, in which the transverse carpal ligament is repaired, are splinted with the wrist in neutral to 10 degrees of flexion, the MP joints in 80 degrees of flexion, and the IP joints straight. Zone 3 injuries are placed in a dorsal blocking splint.

Fortunately, complications are few in the three proximal zones. Most complications can be avoided by good surgical techniques and postoperative management.

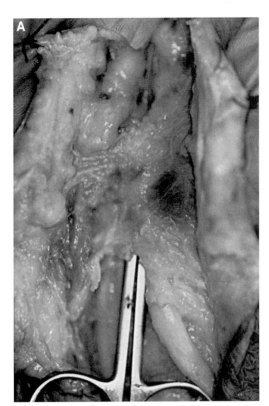

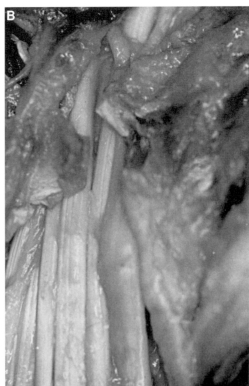

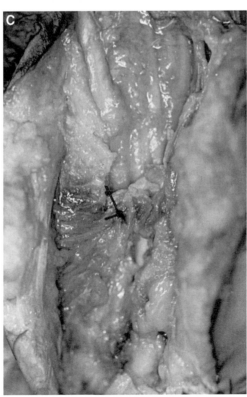

■ FIGURE 20–3
A, The transverse carpal ligament, overlying the scissors in this cadaver dissection, must at times be opened to achieve Zone 4 flexor tendon repairs. **B,** The transverse carpal ligament is step-cut from proximal radial to distal ulnar. **C,** The ligament is closed in a lengthened position.

■ FIGURE 20–4
After tendon repair, the
resting cascade of the fingers is returned to
normal.

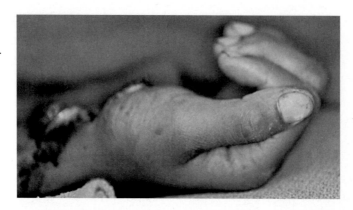

■ TECHNICAL
ALTERNATIVES

If end to end repair of a profundus tendon is not possible, the distal end is sutured to an adjacent profundus tendon. If end to end repair of the sublimis tendon is not possible, it is not repaired and the patient is left with a profundus finger. Interposition tendon grafts can also be performed in areas in which there is tendon substance loss. If the transverse retinacular ligament is irreparable from the injury, the palmaris longus or long toe extensor is used to loosely reconstruct the ligament. The tendon is weaved through the available tissue and sutured to itself. The postoperative regimen is the same as for repair of the transverse carpal ligament.

Adhesions are the most common problem because of the trauma of the injury and the surgical intervention. The lacerated tendon should be handled by the cut end only, avoiding more trauma to the epitenon, which leads to increased areas for adhesions to form. Gap formation at the repair site leads to adhesions and weakening of the musculotendinous unit. The core stitch must be strong, nonabsorbable, and approximate the tendon. The repair site may be "tidied" with a 6-0 nylon epitendinous suture.

Probably most important, is strict adherence to a well-planned, well-regimented postoperative rehabilitation protocol, managed on a daily basis by a trained hand therapist. It is very important that the therapist educate the patient about the post-operative protocol and motivate the patient to follow the exercise program. Failure to obtain stable skeletal fixation hinders early motion and leads to stiffness.

Zone 5 complications are fortunately few because of the excellent blood supply in the area. The major problem is muscle weakness due to the denervation of the muscle belly distal to the laceration. Other major complications are due to delay in diagnosis, misdiagnosis, inability to perform primary repairs, wound infection, segmental muscle and tendon injury, and insufficient skin coverage. Secondary repairs can be performed within 3 weeks of injury, but results may be compromised. Beyond 3 weeks, permanent musculotendinous unit shortening occurs. This requires reconstruction or tendon transfers to correct.

Tendon transfers may become necessary to correct loss of intrinsic muscle innervation from median and ulnar nerve injuries.

■ REHABILITATION

Following flexor tendon repair, therapy plays a major role in functional recovery. Although there is less excursion of the tendons in zones 3 through 5 than in zones 1 and 2, we recommend a combination of modified Kleinert[6,7] rubber-band range of motion, with the Duran[4] passive range of motion protocols. The modification of the Kleinert method includes placing the rubber band through a palmar pulley to obtain full distal interphalangeal joint flexion and therefore more profundus excursion. Another modification of the protocol is to remove the rubber bands at night and splint the IP joints in extension to avoid PIP joint flexion contractures. Finally, each finger must be exercised separately, by both protocols of tendon gliding to prevent the adhesions between adjoining tendons and loss of independent finger motion. The initial therapy is conducted for 4 weeks. The splint is then changed to place the wrist in neutral position and the rubber bands are removed.

MP joint extension blocks are continued as active flexion of the individual digits is done gently for the next 4 weeks. After the second 4 weeks, resisted flexion and extension exercises are begun. Tenolysis is rarely needed[8,14] and should not be considered until the wounds are soft and full passive motion is obtained in the fingers. Timing for tenolysis is from 3–9 months.

In children, who are unable to cooperate with the postoperative therapy protocol, a long arm cast is applied for 3 weeks. At the end of this time, the cast is removed and the patient allowed to start active motion.

Although there is little follow-up information or basic research on injuries in zones 3,4, and 5, good results from tendon repairs can be expected if good surgical technique is followed and a good postoperative therapy protocol is maintained. We believe all injured structures should be repaired. The major factors influencing a good result are recovery from the nerve injury or the loss of tissue from an untidy injury that causes a delay in treatment.

■ OUTCOME

References
1. Botte M, Gelberman R, Smith DG, Silver MA, Gellman H: Repair of severe muscle belly lacerations. J Hand Surg, 1987; 12A:406–412.
2. Bunnell S: Surgery of the Hand. Philadelphia: Lippincott, 1944.
3. Carroll RE, Match RM: Common errors in the management of wrist lacerations. J Trauma, 1974; 14:553–562.
4. Duran RJ, Houser RG: Controlled passive motion following flexor tendon repair in zones 2 and 3. In American Academy of Orthopedic Surgeons: Symposium on tendon surgery in the hand. St. Louis, C.V. Mosby, 1975:105–114.
5. Gelberman RH, Blasingame JP, Fronek A, Dimick MP: Forearm arterial injuries. J Hand Surg, 1979; 4:401–408.
6. Kleinert H, Kutz JE, Atasoy E, Stormo A: Primary Repair of Flexor Tendons. Orthop Clin North Am, 1973; 4:865–876.
7. Kleinert HE, Kutz JE, Cohen MJ: Primary repair of Zone 3 Flexor Tendon Lacerations. In American Academy of Orthopedic Surgeons: In Symposium on tendon surgery in the hand. St. Louis, C.V. Mosby, 1975:91–104.
8. Kleinert HE, Schepel S, Gill T: Flexor tendon injuries. Surg Clin North Am, 1981; 61:267–286.
9. Lister G: The Hand: Diagnosis and Indications. Chapter 1. London: Churchill Livingston, 2nd ed., 1987:1–106.
10. Parker A: The "lumbrical plus" finger. J Bone Joint Surg, 1971: 53B:236–239.
11. Potenza AD: Current concepts of tendon healing and repair. In American Academy of Orthopedic Surgeons: Symposium on tendon surgery in the hand. St. Louis, C.V., Mosby 1975:18–47.
12. Potenza AD: Flexor tendon injuries. Orthop Clin North Am, 1970; 1:355–373.
13. Puckett C, Meyer VH: Results of treatment of extensive volar wrist lacerations: The spaghetti wrist. Plast and Reconstru Surg, 1985; 75:714–721.
14. Stefanich RJ, Putnam MD, Peimer CA, Sherwin FS: Flexor Tendon Lacerations in Zone 5. J Hand Surg, 1992; 17A:284–291.
15. Verdan C: Tendon Surgery of the Hand. London, Churchill Livingston, 1979.
16. Verdan C: Half A Century of Flexor Tendon Repair. Current Status and Changing Philosophies. J Bone Joint Surg, 1972; 54A:472–491.

PART
III

Irreducible Dislocations

21

Irreducible Volar Dislocations of the Proximal Interphalangeal Joint

The anatomy of the proximal interphalangeal (PIP) joint has been elegantly described.[1,3-5] The key to PIP joint stability is the strong conjoined attachment of the paired collateral ligaments and the volar plate into the volar third of the middle phalanx. This ligament box has a three-dimensional configuration that strongly resists PIP joint displacement (Fig. 21–1). For displacement of the middle phalanx to occur, the ligament box must be disrupted in at least two planes.[4] Furthermore, for volar displacement to occur, a significant injury must occur to the extensor mechanism.[3-6,9-14,16,17]

Volar dislocation of the PIP joint is an uncommon injury, reputed to be difficult to treat and having an uncertain outcome.[14,15] These clinical difficulties are frequently attributed to the relative inexperience of the initial treating physician. Problems can also occur because of the failure to make the distinction between a purely volar dislocation and a volar rotatory dislocation.[6] A straight volar dislocation is easily reduced and is always associated with a rupture of the central slip. After reduction, it must be treated as an acute closed boutonniere deformity. Volar rotatory dislocations of the PIP joint are difficult and sometimes impossible to reduce. The volar plate and the collateral ligament on the convex side of the angular finger deformity are ruptured[14] and the extensor mechanism is disrupted longitudinally between the central slip and one of the lateral bands.[7,9,13] The injury to the extensor mechanism may be between the central slip and the lateral band on the same[3,4,6,9,10,12,17,19] or opposite[2,9,11,13,16] side of the collateral ligament injury. In either case, the head of the proximal phalanx buttonholes through the extensor mechanism. If the rent in the extensor mechanism is on the same side of the central slip as the collateral ligament injury, the involved condyle will become trapped between the central slip dorsally and the volarly displaced lateral band (Fig. 21–2A). If the injury to the extensor mechanism is on the opposite side of the central slip, both the central slip and ipsilateral lateral band will be trapped volarly beneath the involved condyle (Fig. 21–2B).

The principles of surgically treating this injury are directly related to the anatomy of the injury and have been well described by Dray and Eaton,[3] Thompson and Eaton,[18] and Peimer and coworkers.[14]

A volar rotatory dislocation of the PIP joint is not considered to be irreducible until an adequate attempt at closed reduction has failed. Because of the interposition of part of the extensor mechanism in the joint, the usual reduction maneuver of traction and middle phalangeal extension tends to tighten the soft tissue encircling the condyle and to block reduction. Many of these dislocations can be reduced, however, by applying gentle traction and rotation while holding both the metacarpophalangeal (MP) and PIP joints flexed. This maneuver relaxes the volarly displaced lateral band or lateral band and central slip so that with rotation, the obstructing portion of the extensor mechanism is disengaged from behind the condyle. When necessary, further relaxation of the extensor mechanism can be accomplished by modest wrist extension.[18] If the joint reduces, active range of motion is assessed. If the PIP joint resubluxes or does not demonstrate full active extension, an injury to the central slip of the extensor mechanism is assumed. Treatment in this case is

■ HISTORY OF THE TECHNIQUE

■ INDICATIONS AND CONTRAINDICATIONS

■ FIGURE 21–1
A, The quadrangular collateral ligament, by its insertion on the phalanx and volar plate, overlaps and reinforces the volar plate insertion into the middle phalanx. **B**, The accessory ligament represents a proximal thinning of the collateral ligament. The central volar plate also becomes membranous proximally, permitting this portion of the capsule to fold on itself in full flexion.

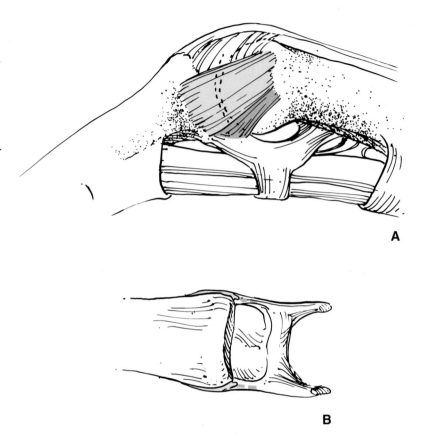

A

B

identical to that of an acute closed boutonniere deformity. If there is full strong extension of the PIP joint, the injured anatomy consists of a unilateral rupture of a collateral ligament (which is now presumably restored to its anatomic alignment), a partial volar plate injury, and a longitudinal injury to the extensor mechanism between the central slip and one of the lateral bands. Therefore, guarded active range of motion exercises may be started immediately, with dynamic extension splinting, but must be monitored closely (Fig. 21–3).

■ SURGICAL
TECHNIQUES

The irreducible volar dislocation of the PIP joint must be treated surgically. The ideal anesthetic for either closed or open reduction of a volarly dislocated PIP joint is a digital block at the lumbrical canal level. This may be supplemented by including the dorsal sensory branches of the radial or ulnar nerves or both. This block has the advantage of sparing the intrinsic musculature, affording the opportunity to assess the full strength of active PIP joint extension. Thus, extensor mechanism competence may be documented once the reduction is accomplished. One-half percent bupivacaine without epinephrine is used because it provides excellent postoperative pain relief.

A brachial pneumatic tourniquet is employed. The extensor apparatus of the finger is exposed with a straight dorsal midline incision. It should be about 4 cm in length, centered over the PIP joint. This affords excellent access to both sides of the extensor mechanism, which is important because the tear may be on either side of the central slip. This incision also minimizes the risk of injury to the dorsal branch of either digital nerve and generally heals well without hypertrophy.

Dissection proceeds to the level of the peritenon. Full-thickness flaps are raised from the peritenon and are retracted with stay sutures. The flap on the convex side of the finger deformity may need a little more development because of the location of the injury to the extensor mechanism. At this junction, the head of the proximal phalanx is seen buttonholing through the extensor mechanism. On the side of the collateral ligament injury, either the ipsilateral lateral band or the central slip with the lateral band is seen coursing

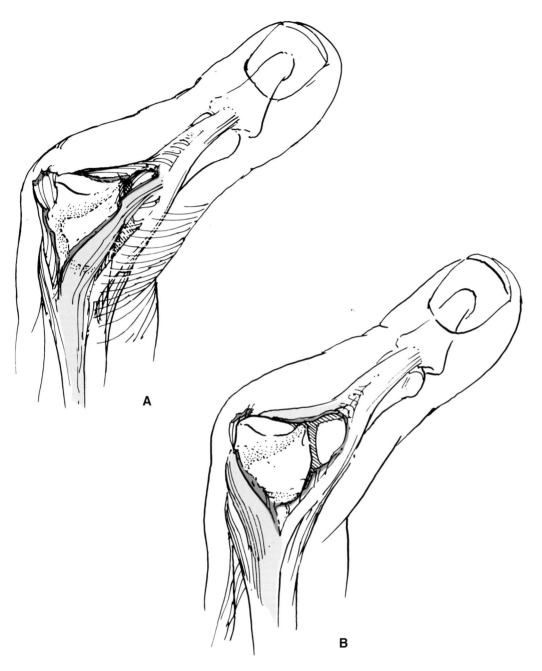

■ FIGURE 21–2

A, The collateral ligament injury and the longitudinal tear in the dorsal apparatus are on the same side of the PIP joint. The lateral band is interposed volar to the condyle. **B**, The collateral ligament injury and the longitudinal tear in the dorsal apparatus are on opposite sides of the PIP joint. The lateral band and central slip are both interposed volar to the condyle.

through the PIP joint. These tendons engage the volar flare of the condyle of the proximal phalanx and prevent reduction (Fig. 21–2A and B). Using a dental probe, the displaced central slip or lateral band is teased from underneath the involved condyle and the joint is reduced.

The tourniquet is now deflated and hemostasis is obtained. When the effect of the tourniquet on intrinsic and extrinsic extensor function has reversed, active extension of the PIP joint is evaluated and should be excellent, barring an injury to the central slip. Likewise, active congruous finger flexion is evaluated. After reexsanguination, the tourniquet is again inflated. Repair of the ruptured collateral ligament is generally unnecessary. The extensor mechanism is then examined. The rent between the central slip and the involved lateral band is repaired using 4-0 nylon simple sutures, tied with absolute square knots. Care is taken to cut the tails of the suture flush on the knot to prevent sensitivity over the knots in the extended postoperative period. If the involved lateral band is too tattered,

■ FIGURE 21–3
A and **B**, Radiographs of a volar rotatory dislocation of the PIP joint of a long finger.

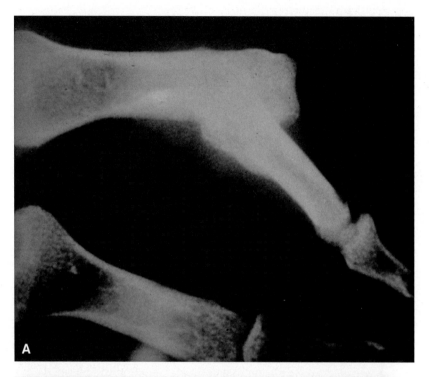

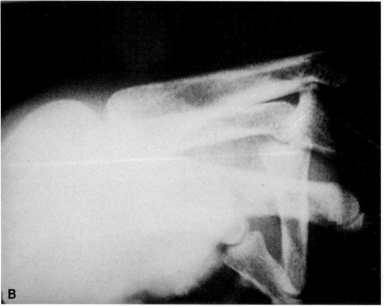

however, it may be resected, allowing PIP joint extension by the opposite lateral band and central slip. If hemostasis is excellent, no drains are necessary. Otherwise, a small silicone feeding tube is used through the distal end of the incision. The wound is then closed with interrupted 5-0 nylon horizontal mattress sutures. A bulky compression dressing is applied, using large gauze fluffs between the fingers and 3-inch rolled gauze for the circumferential portion. Appropriate cast padding is applied. The tourniquet is deflated and removed from the arm with the underlying cast padding to prevent a continued venous tourniquet. Local pressure for 10 minutes is applied to the involved finger to enhance hemostasis. Anterior and posterior splints are then applied from the forearm to the tips of the fingers. The fingers are held with the MP joints in comfortable flexion

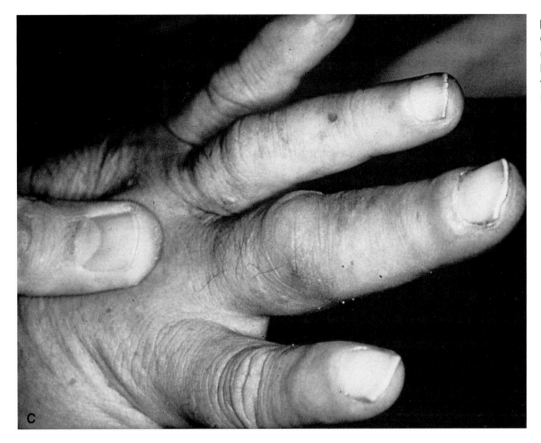

■ FIGURE 21–3
C, After closed reduction using the technique outlined in the text. Note the full active extension at PIP joint.

(around 30 to 40°) and the interphalangeal joints in extension. The hand is kept elevated above the heart in the early postoperative period to minimize swelling.

Some surgeons believe that volar rotatory dislocations are always irreducible and thus require surgical intervention.[2,8–11,13,16,17,19] Others believe that open reduction is mandatory, not only to reduce the interposed extensor mechanism but also to repair it. Still others believe that it is appropriate to repair the torn collateral ligaments and sometimes the volar plate.[2,7,9,11,12,16,17]

The primary technical alternative for this operation is the surgical approach. I have described a midline dorsal approach, which is my present preference. A similar curved dorsal incision has also been recommended by Inoue and Noboru,[7] Meyn,[10] and Peimer and coworkers.[14] An alternative approach is the mid-lateral approach, described by Dray and Eaton.[3] The advantage of the midline dorsal approach is that it allows the surgeon to more easily address the range of injuries to the dorsal apparatus.

The most important thing to verify, after the reduction has taken place by either closed or open means, is the integrity of the central slip of the extensor mechanism. In open cases, this may be documented by both visual inspection and testing the strength of full active extension. If a closed reduction is obtained, this is done by the latter. If an injury to the central slip is suspected, static extension splinting is necessary to prevent the development of a chronic boutonniere deformity or chronic volar subluxation of the joint.

The patient is seen the first postoperative day for examination and drain removal as necessary. The hand is kept in the bulky dressing, with the finger in extension and elevation is continued until 5 to 7 days postoperatively. At this time the dressing is removed; wound sensitivity should be diminished. If there has been no injury to the central slip of the extensor mechanism, active range of motion is begun using a forearm-based dynamic extension splint. This may be alternated with a static extension splint for rest and nighttime

■ TECHNICAL ALTERNATIVES

■ REHABILITATION

use. At 3 weeks postoperatively, the dynamic splint may be discarded. The night splinting is continued for another 3 weeks. If the central slip has been injured, a static splint is used to hold the PIP joint in extension for 3 weeks. Active motion and splinting, as described above, is then begun.

As with any severe ligamentous injury to the PIP joint, the patient should be advised the day of the injury that rehabilitation is required and that it will be a tedious and prolonged process. This should be reinforced at each subsequent examination. Maximum recovery may be expected to take up to 1 year postinjury.

If the central slip of the extensor mechanism is not injured and the early rehabilitation process is properly monitored, one can expect to regain at least 90° of flexion at the PIP joint with perhaps a slight flexion contracture.[7,9-11,13,16] If the central slip is injured, a less favorable result can be expected, although the results are not as extensively documented.

References

 1. Bowers WH, Wolf JW Jr, Nehil J, Bittinger S: The proximal interphalangeal joint volar plate. I. An anatomic and biomechanical study. J Hand Surg, 1980; 5:79–88.
 2. De Smet L, Vercauteren M: Palmer dislocation of the proximal interphalangeal joint requiring open reduction: a case report. J Hand Surg, 1984; 9A:717–718.
 3. Dray GJ, Eaton RG: Dislocations and Ligament Injuries in the Digits. In: Green DP (ed): Operative Hand Surgery, 3rd Ed, Vol I, New York: Churchill Livingston, 1993:767–776.
 4. Eaton RG: Joint Injuries of the Hand, Springfield, IL: Charles C. Thomas, 1971:3–34.
 5. Eaton RG, Littler JW: Joint injuries and their sequelae. Clin Plast Surg, 1976; 3:85–98.
 6. Green DP: Dislocations and Ligamentous Injuries of the Hand. In: Evarts CM (ed): Surgery of the Musculoskeletal System, 2nd Ed, Vol 1, New York: Churchill Livingston, 1989:384–448.
 7. Inoue G, Noboru M: Irreducible palmar dislocation of the proximal interphalangeal joint of the finger. J Hand Surg, 1990; 15A:301–304.
 8. Johnson FG, Greene MH: Another cause of the irreducible dislocation of the proximal interphalangeal joint of a finger: a case report. J Bone Joint Surg, 1966; 48A:542–544.
 9. Kilgore ES, Newmeyer WL, Brown LG: Post-traumatic trapped dislocation of the proximal interphalangeal joint. J Trauma, 1976; 16:481–487.
10. Meyn MA Jr: Irreducible volar dislocation of the proximal interphalangeal joint. Clin Orthop, 1981; 158:215–218.
11. Murakami Y: Irreducible volar dislocation of the proximal interphalangeal joint of the finger. Hand, 1974; 6:87–90.
12. Neviaser FJ, Wilson JN: Interposition of the extensor tendon resulting in persistent subluxation of the proximal interphalangeal joint of the finger. Clin Orthop, 1972; 83:118–120.
13. Ostrowski DM, Neimkin RJ: Irreducible palmar dislocation of the proximal interphalangeal joint. A case report. Orthopedics, 1985; 8:84–86.
14. Peimer CA, Sullivan DJ, Wild DR: Palmar dislocation of the proximal interphalangeal joint. J Hand Surg, 1984; 9A:39–48.
15. Posner MA, Kapila D: Chronic palmar dislocation of proximal interphalangeal joints. J Hand Surg, 1986; 11A:253–258.
16. Posner MA, Wilenski M: Irreducible volar dislocation of the proximal interphalangeal joint of a finger caused by interposition of an intact central slip: a case report. J Bone Joint Surg, 1978; 60A:133–134.
17. Spinner M, Choi BY: Anterior dislocations of the proximal interphalangeal joint: a cause of rupture of the central slip of the extensor mechanism. J Bone Joint Surg, 1970; 52A:1329–1336.
18. Thompson JS, Eaton RG: Volar dislocation of the proximal interphalangeal joint. J Hand Surg, 1977; 2:232.
19. Wong JTM: Extensor mechanism preventing reduction of finger. Med J Aust, 1978; 1(2):101.

22

Irreducible Dorsal Dislocations of the Metacarpophalangeal Joint

The first description of an irreducible dorsal metacarpophalangeal (MP) joint dislocation is attributed to Malgaigne in 1855.[14] In 1876, Farabeuf described in detail the difference between reducible and irreducible dorsal dislocations of the MP joint of the thumb.[9] Farabeuf first used the term "complex dislocation" in reference to irreducible dorsal dislocations of the MP joint of the fingers. Based on his cadaver studies and operative experience, he recommended a dorsal approach for surgical reduction of the entrapped palmar plate.

In 1957, Kaplan[13] reported in what has become a landmark article a single case of an irreducible dorsal dislocation of the MP joint of the index finger. In this article, he describes in great detail the pathologic anatomy of the injury. In addition to entrapment of the palmar plate between the base of proximal phalanx and the head of the metacarpal, Kaplan believed that the head of the metacarpal was locked in a grid of soft tissue, consisting of the natatory ligament and palmar plate, flexor tendons and pretendinous band, lumbrical muscle, and the superficial and deep transverse metacarpal ligament (Fig. 22–1). Based on this pathologic anatomy, Kaplan recommended a palmar approach for surgical reduction of this injury. After publication of Kaplan's article, the palmar surgical approach became the favored technique for surgical reduction of the complex MP dislocation.[1-3,11]

A detailed description of the pathologic anatomy of the irreducible dorsal MP dislocation of the small finger was provided by Baldwin and coworkers in 1967.[2] In the case of the small finger, the entrapping grid about the head of the metacarpal was found to be the abductor digiti minimi, the flexor tendons, the natatory ligament, and the superficial and deep transverse metacarpal ligaments. Baldwin also advocated a palmar approach to the surgical reduction of this injury.

In 1973, Green and Terry[11] reported on their series of operative management for complex dislocations of the MP joint. They employed a palmar exposure and warned about the vulnerability of the radial digital nerve to the index finger and of the ulnar digital nerve to the small finger. They emphasized that the interlocking grid about the metacarpal head was not nearly as important as the entrapped palmar plate in rendering the joint irreducible. Operative experience indicated that the entrapped palmar plate was incompletely detached from the deep transverse metacarpal ligament. Tension through these retained connections maintained the position of the entrapped palmar plate despite attempts at open reduction. Extrication of the palmar plate could not be achieved until the residual connections between the palmar plate and deep transverse metacarpal ligament were released. They also emphasized the importance of early motion after surgical reduction in achieving an acceptable functional result.

In 1975, Becton and coworkers reintroduced the dorsal approach proposed by Farabeuf. It was their contention that the dorsal approach provided access to associated osteochondral fractures, prevented possible injury to the vulnerable digital nerves, and allowed full exposure of the entrapped palmar plate, which was the primary pathology preventing reduction.[6] The dorsal approach was also favored by Bohart and coworkers in their series reported in 1982.[7] The literature has yet to support the superiority of one approach over another. Depending on the situation, dorsal,[7,10] palmar,[1-3,11] or combined[4,16] approaches have been used in the reduction of this dislocation.

■ HISTORY OF THE
TECHNIQUE

■ FIGURE 22–1
An anatomic drawing demonstrating the entrapping grid of soft tissue surrounding the metacarpal head. The soft-tissue structures are the lumbrical muscle, flexor tendons, natatory ligament, palmar plate, and superficial transverse metacarpal ligament.

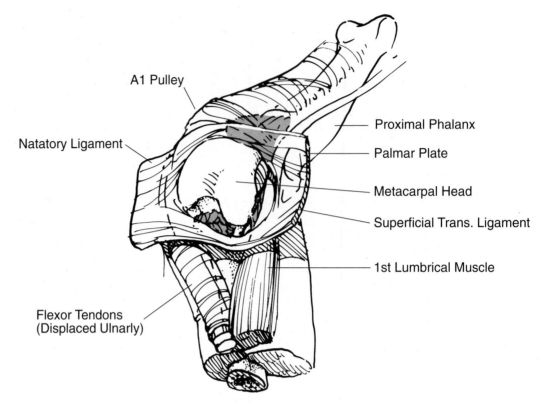

A1 Pulley

Natatory Ligament

Proximal Phalanx

Palmar Plate

Metacarpal Head

Superficial Trans. Ligament

1st Lumbrical Muscle

Flexor Tendons
(Displaced Ulnarly)

■ INDICATIONS

Simple dorsal dislocations present clinically with the proximal phalanx hyperextended 90° on the head of the metacarpal. The interphalangeal joint rests in compensatory flexion. Although there is palmar prominence of the metacarpal head, no puckering or dimpling of the palmar skin is detected. Radiographic visualization of the MP joint space is difficult on the anteroposterior (AP) projection. Lateral views clearly demonstrate the dislocation and the relatively perpendicular positioning of the proximal phalanx relative to the dorsal head of the metacarpal (Fig. 22–2).

In complex dislocations of the MP joint, the proximal phalanx is only slightly hyperextended on the head of the metacarpal, and the MP joint appears less deformed than it does in simple dorsal dislocations. In addition to palmar prominence of the metacarpal head, dimpling of the palmar skin is sometimes present, produced by traction along fibrous bands bridging the skin to deeper fascial structures. Radiographs may demonstrate a widened joint space on the AP projection (Fig. 22–3). The presence of a sesamoid bone within the joint space is pathognomonic of a complex dorsal MP dislocation. On a lateral view, the palmar base of the proximal phalanx lies on the dorsal aspect of the metacarpal head, and the longitudinal axes of the proximal phalanx and metacarpal are relatively parallel (Fig. 22–4).

The protruding metacarpal head may place adjacent digital neurovascular bundles on tension. These structures are at risk of injury on a palmar approach for open reduction. This is particularly true in the index finger for the radial digital neurovascular bundle and in the small finger for the ulnar digital neurovascular bundle.

Although complex dislocations are considered irreducible, in most situations at least one attempt at closed reduction is worthwhile. When attempting closed reduction of either the simple or complex MP dislocation, the reduction maneuver is the same. The MP joint should first be hyperextended; with force applied to the dorsal base of the proximal phalanx, reduction then should be attempted by translation along the contour of the metacarpal head. To achieve the comfort and relaxation required for reduction, a regional block or field block anesthetic is advised. Instillation of sterile fluid or anesthetic into the joint space before reduction may help dislodge the entrapped palmar plate. Application of pure

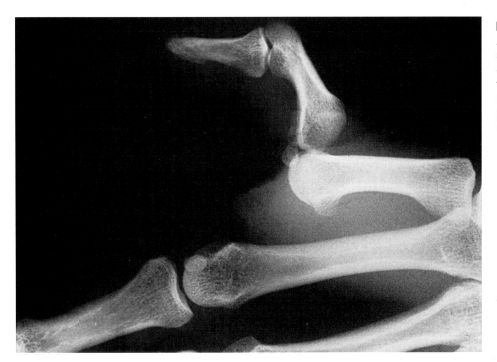

■ FIGURE 22–2
A lateral radiograph of a simple dorsal dislocation of the MP joint of the thumb. The proximal phalanx rests in a nearly perpendicular relation to its metacarpal.

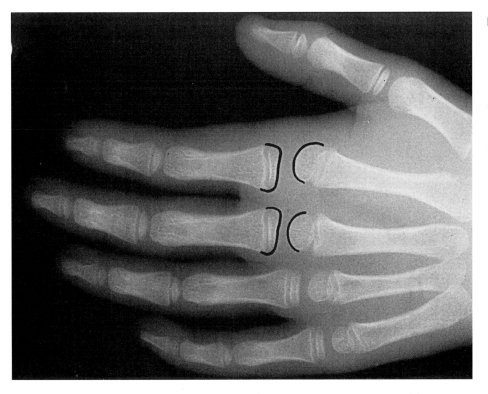

■ FIGURE 22–3
Posteroanterior radiograph of an adolescent's hand, with a complex dislocation of the MP joint of the index finger. Note the widened joint space of the MP joint of the index finger, compared with the MP joint of the adjacent middle finger.

longitudinal traction only tightens the noose of entrapping soft tissues about the neck of the metacarpal and changes the position of the proximal phalanx to the metacarpal from perpendicular to parallel. This maneuver may convert a simple dislocation to one that is complex.[9,15] Use of a low-energy fluoroscopic unit may be helpful in aiding the reduction maneuver.

Failure to achieve a complete concentric reduction of a dorsal MP joint dislocation is

■ FIGURE 22–4
Lateral radiograph of a
complex dorsal disloca-
tion of the MP joint of
the thumb in an adoles-
cent. The joint space is
widened and the proximal
phalanx rests in a dor-
sally translated but relatively parallel position to
its metacarpal.

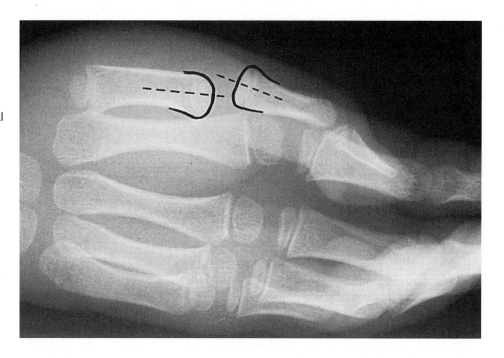

■ FIGURE 22–4
Lateral radiograph of a
complex dorsal disloca-
tion of the MP joint of
the thumb in an adoles-
cent. The joint space is
widened and the proximal
phalanx rests in a dor-
sally translated but relatively parallel position to
its metacarpal.

the primary indication for surgical intervention. Open dislocations are also an indication for operative intervention. They should be treated as open fractures, with thorough soft-tissue debridement and joint irrigation in an operating theater and with adequate anesthesia.

■ SURGICAL
TECHNIQUES

Open reduction of irreducible dorsal MP dislocations is best performed under either general or regional block anesthesia. A well-padded pneumatic tourniquet should be applied to the upper extremity for hemostasis. In the unreduced state, the proximal base of the proximal phalanx rests on the dorsal head of the metacarpal. The metacarpal head projects as a prominence into the distal palm. Palpation of these landmarks helps to localize the joint in the presence of posttraumatic swelling and hemorrhage. The pathologic anatomy varies somewhat with the digit involved and has been previously described.

A linear or gentle curvilinear incision placed dorsally over the affected MP joint is used to approach the dislocation. A linear incision is made through the midline of the extensor hood, splitting this structure. Next, the dorsal capsule is incised longitudinally. At this point, the articular base of the proximal phalanx and entrapped palmar plate should be in view. The palmar plate is split longitudinally through its midline and a Penfield elevator or similar instrument is used to tease the palmar plate over the head of the metacarpal (Fig. 22–5). Once this has been accomplished, a reduction maneuver similar to that described for a closed reduction is used to translate the base of the proximal phalanx around the metacarpal head into a reduced position. At this point, the articular surfaces of both joints can be visualized for evidence of cartilage damage and fixation of any osteochondral fractures that may be present. Small periarticular defects may best be managed by excision when unstable and too small for fixation. For fracture stabilization, fine K-wires may be used; for larger fragments, screw fixation may be acceptable. Under fluoroscopic control, a complete reduction through a full range of motion should be ensured. The point of recurrent dorsal instability should be noted and used as a guide for postoperative protection. Displaced complete tears of the collateral ligament can be repositioned and repaired by intrasubstance suture, suture anchor, or pull-out suture technique.

Capsular closure is accomplished by a running or interrupted absorbable suture. The extensor hood is closed with interrupted sutures of 4-0 braided synthetic nonabsorbable suture. Skin closure is with 5-0 nylon or polypropylene.

A well-padded bulky hand dressing with a dorsal splint is applied, holding the MP

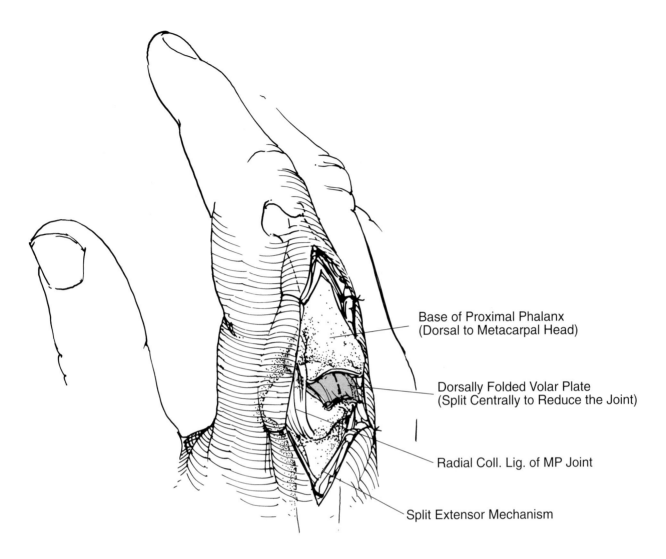

Base of Proximal Phalanx
(Dorsal to Metacarpal Head)

Dorsally Folded Volar Plate
(Split Centrally to Reduce the Joint)

Radial Coll. Lig. of MP Joint

Split Extensor Mechanism

■ FIGURE 22–5
A dorsal surgical approach to the MP joint of the index finger, with a complex dorsal dislocation. Note the longitudinal skin incision, longitudinal splitting of the extensor mechanism, the
proximal phalangeal base resting on the metacarpal head with the interposed palmar plate, and
the dotted surgical line, showing a longitudinal splitting of the plate.

joints in 40 to 60° of flexion and the interphalangeal joints in extension. This dressing is
kept in place for the next 2 or 3 days, during which time the patient is instructed to keep
the extremity elevated and dry. The procedure is typically performed as an outpatient
basis and the patient released with appropriate oral pain medication.

An alternative palmar approach to reduction has been advocated by Kaplan and others.[1-3,8,11] A palmar approach may also be considered in an open dislocation that involves
a palmar wound. By palpation or fluoroscopy, the palmar prominence of the metacarpal
head is identified. In the case of an open dislocation, the wound is usually transverse and
may be extended proximally and distally by oblique incisions. For closed dislocations, a
Bruner or transverse incision, with proximal and distal extensions as necessary, may be
used. Division of the soft tissues immediately deep to the palmar skin should proceed
with caution because a digital neurovascular bundle may be prominently draped over
the metacarpal head and easily injured. Once the neurovascular structures have been
identified, they can be protected. Next, the superficial transverse metacarpal ligament or

■ TECHNICAL
ALTERNATIVES

palmar aponeurotic pulley and frequently the A1 pulley of the flexor sheath must be divided to relax the soft-tissue noose about the metacarpal head and to expose the entrapped palmar plate. To extract the palmar plate, it is necessary to completely release the incomplete tear of the palmar plate from the deep transverse metacarpal ligament. With the joint hyperextended, the proximal edge of the palmar plate is teased or pulled over the dorsal head of the metacarpal. If this cannot be accomplished, it may be necessary to longitudinally split the palmar plate to free it. Once the palmar plate is extricated, the reduction maneuver is as described for the dorsal approach. With the joint reduced, the palmar plate (if previously split) is repaired using nonabsorbable 4-0 suture. It can be reanchored to bone if desired by pull-out suture or suture anchor. This is required only in cases in which the joint is unstable to extension. Because the articular surfaces and joint space are not easily visualized from the palmar approach, fluoroscopic examination or intraoperative radiographs of the joint after reduction are appropriate to rule out associated fractures. As with the dorsal approach, a full range of motion should be confirmed and the postreduction stability determined. Advocates of the palmar approach emphasize the importance of visualizing the pathologic anatomy and the potential to diminish the risk of late instability by repair or reattachment of the palmar plate. For the unwary surgeon, there is significant potential for injury to the digital neurovascular bundle. The literature has failed to show improved results or less frequent redislocation with the palmar approach over the dorsal approach. There is no question that the dorsal approach is easier and less risky. The dorsal approach is also best for management of most fracture dislocations and for chronic dorsal dislocations, which require release of the contracted dorsal capsule and collateral ligaments in addition to extrication of the entrapped palmar plate.

■ REHABILITATION

Results are inversely related to the length of immobilization.[11,15] After 2 to 3 days of elevation and immobilization, pain and swelling should be improved. After removal of the surgical dressing, a hand-based dorsal block splint is applied across the MP joint, limiting extension within the range of stability determined at surgery. Radiographs are taken to confirm that the reduction has been maintained. Range of motion exercises should be started immediately. The patient is instructed in hourly active and passive range of motion exercises within the splint. Dynamic splinting and taping may be required if difficulties are encountered regaining flexion. Measures for edema control and elevation are taken as necessary. A forearm-based safe-position splint holding the MP joints in maximum flexion and interphalangeal joints fully extended is provided for night wear in patients with problems of swelling and slow return of motion. Sutures are removed and a follow-up radiograph is obtained 10 to 14 days after surgery. Additional radiographs beyond this time are needed only when there is an associated fracture or problems arise with recovery. Prolonged discomfort and poor return of motion suggest redislocation. When redislocation occurs, reduction by closed or open technique is necessary. Normally, the joint is inherently stable after reduction unless there is an associated fracture or other concomitant ligament injury.

By 3 weeks postoperatively, the extension block should be brought to a neutral position and worn protectively. Active extension exercises with the splint removed are initiated. By 5 weeks postoperatively, the dorsal block splint may be discontinued and the joint protected by buddy taping between adjacent proximal phalanges. Passive extension to a neutral position may be performed in the absence of full extension. Rarely is dynamic or static extension splinting necessary if motion has been started early.

■ OUTCOMES

Results after early open reduction of complex dorsal MP dislocations are good, with return of painless functional motion at the MP joint if there is no articular damage, fracture, nerve or tendon injury and after an appropriate therapy program. McLaughlin noted that return of motion was inversely proportional to the length of immobilization.[15] In his series, patients mobilized more than 2 weeks rarely regained more than 20° of flexion. The patients immobilized for shorter periods of time gained more motion, although improvement was gradual, improving up to 1 year after injury. In Green and Terry's series, the only patient not regaining normal motion was immobilized for 10 days.[11] This is in contrast to Murphy and Stark, who reported three patients with complex dorsal dislocations immobilized for 2 weeks after open reduction and who subsequently regained normal motion.[16] Excellent results, with full restoration of motion after open reduction of acute complex MP dislocations, have been obtained when motion was initiated within days of surgery.[6,7,12] Results of open dorsal MP dislocations have not been as good as those of surgically managed closed complex dorsal dislocations.[12]

Results after reduction of chronic dislocations are influenced by the length of time since injury, prior nonsurgical and surgical management, the condition of the articular cartilage at the time of successful reduction, and the extent of soft-tissue release required for reduction. Mclaughlin reported that complex dislocations treated more than 10 days postinjury had poor results.[15] It was his recommendation that these patients were best managed by arthrodesis. Murphy and Stark's series of closed dislocations of the MP joint of the index finger included six patients with untreated dislocations ranging from 3 weeks to 5 months after injury.[16] Both palmar and dorsal incisions were required for reduction of these injuries and a K-wire was used to transfix the joint for 3 weeks. These authors reported return of functional motion in all patients but none achieved full restoration of motion.[16] Barenfeld and Wesley reported on a single case of late management of a complex dorsal dislocation of the index finger, in which they were able to achieve normal range of motion.[4] Joints that develop posttraumatic arthritis may be treated by arthroplasty or arthrodesis.

References

 1. Andersen JA, Gjerloff GC: Complex dislocation of the metacarpophalangeal joint of the little finger. J Hand Surg, 1987; 12B:264–266.
 2. Baldwin LW, Miller DL, Lockhart LD, Evans EB: Metacarpophalangeal-joint dislocations of the fingers. J Bone Joint Surg, 1967; 49A(8):1587–1590.
 3. Barash HL: An unusual case of dorsal dislocation of the metacarpophalangeal joint of the index finger. Clin Orthop, 1972; 83:121–122.
 4. Barenfeld PA, Weseley MS: Dorsal dislocation of the metacarpophalangeal joint of the index finger treated by late open reduction. J Bone Joint Surg, 1972; 54A:1311–1313.
 5. Barry K, McGee H, Curtin J: Complex dislocation of the metacarpophalangeal joint of the index finger: a comparison of surgical approaches. J Hand Surg, 1988; 13B(4):466–468.
 6. Becton JL, Christian JD Jr, Goodwin HN, Jackson JG III: A simplified technique for treating the complex dislocation of the index metacarpophalangeal joint. J Bone Joint Surg, 1975; 57A(5):698–700.
 7. Bohart PG, Gelberman RH, Vandell RF, Salamon PB: Complex dislocations of the metacarpophalangeal joint: open reduction by Farabeuf's dorsal incision. Clin Orthop, 1982; 164(4):208–210.
 8. Eaton RG: The Digital Metacarpophalangeal Joint. In: Joint Injuries of the Hand, Springfield, Ill: Charles C. Thomas, 1971:35–47.
 9. Farabeuf LM: De la luxation du pouce en arriere. Bull Mem Soc Chir Paris, 1876; 11:21–62.
10. Fultz CW, Buchanan JR: Complex fracture dislocation of the metacarpophalangeal joint. Clin Orthop, 1988; 227:255–260.
11. Green DP, Terry GC: Complex dislocation of the metacarpophalangeal joint. J Bone Joint Surg, 1973; 55A(8):1480–1486.
12. Hunt JC, Watts HB, Glasco JD: Dorsal dislocation of the metacarpophalangeal joint of the index finger with particular reference to open dislocation. J Bone Joint Surg, 1967; 49A(8): 1572–1578.
13. Kaplan EB: Dorsal dislocation of the metacarpophalangeal joint of the index finger. J Bone Joint Surg, 1957; 39A(5):1081–1086.
14. Malgaigne JF: Treatise on Fractures, translated from the French by John H. Packard, MD [Traite Des Fractures et Des Luxations], Philadelphia: JB Lippincott, 1859:500–507.
15. McLaughlin HL: Complex "locked" dislocation of the metacarpophalangeal joints. J Trauma, 1965; 5:(6):683–688.
16. Murphy AF, Stark HH: Closed dislocations of the metacarpophalangeal of the index finger. J Bone Joint Surg, 1967; 49A(8):1579–1586.

23

Irreducible Perilunate Dislocations

■ HISTORY OF THE TECHNIQUE

Perilunate dislocations comprise about 3% of all injuries to the carpus.[11] The pathomechanics resulting in a perilunate dislocation were first described by Mouchet and Tavernier in 1919.[9] The mechanism they described was one of hyperextension. In 1980, Mayfield and coworkers studied the pathomechanics and specific pattern of ligament disruption in progressive perilunar instability that led to first a dorsal perilunate dislocation and subsequently a volar lunate dislocation. They described not only hyperextension but forced intracarpal supination as being involved in the pathomechanics of these injuries.[17] Because these injuries are part of a continuum, we discuss both perilunate and lunate dislocations but limit the discussion in this section to the treatment of irreducible dislocations that are unstable to such a degree or present a sufficient time after the initial injury to make closed reduction impossible.

One of the earliest described treatments of lunate dislocations which present late was by McBride in 1933.[18] Although follow-up was limited, based on a series of six patients that were treated by open reduction of the lunate he concluded that reduction rather than excision was the preferred treatment method. In 1944, MacAusland stated that he preferred excision of the lunate in cases that presented more than 6 weeks after injury.[15] Alternatively, Campbell and coworkers suggested proximal row carpectomy as the preferred treatment for chronic perilunate dislocations.[5] Siegert and coworkers, in 1988, advocated open reduction of the perilunate or dorsal perilunate dislocations, suggesting that the results of open reduction were superior to the results of excision of the lunate. Furthermore, they stated that late open reduction, even as long as 35 weeks after the injury, could provide good results.[20] Weir, in 1992, also recommended open reduction of lunate or perilunate dislocations as late as 6 months after the initial injury.[23]

The specific approach for open reduction has varied. Initially, most authors preferred a dorsal approach.[1,6-8,14,16,18,22] Alternatively, several authors have described and preferred the volar approach.[2,3,5,13,16,21] Eggers[12] devised an ulnar approach because of his concern that a direct volar approach would result in flexor tendon adhesions. Campbell and colleagues[4] reported on a series in which they used a dorsal approach in some patients; in others, they used a volar approach. They noted no avascular necrosis in any of the patients in whom they used a volar approach, which is a concern previously presented by other authors. Later, Campbell, and coworkers[5] stated that they favored the dorsal approach, both to better reduce the scaphoid and to appropriately debride the capitolunate space. They proposed using a combined volar and dorsal approach when the lunate was significantly displaced or decompression of the median nerve was necessary. Dobyns and Swanson[10] also advocated combined dorsal and volar approaches.

Minami and coworkers[19] compared open scapholunate interosseous ligament (SLIL) repair and reconstruction in patients having lunate and perilunate dislocations with patients having lunate and perilunate dislocations that did not have the SLIL ligament repaired or reconstructed. They recently reported that clinical and radiographic results suggest that repair or reconstruction of the SLIL during open reduction can prevent or reduce the occurrence of carpal instability and improve clinical results.

■ INDICATIONS AND CONTRAINDICATIONS

If the patient has a dorsal perilunate or volar lunate dislocation that cannot be anatomically reduced by closed means, reduction should be accomplished by open reduction. If

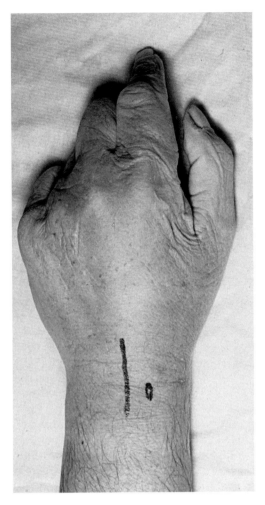

■ FIGURE 23–1
The planned longitudinal incision for the dorsal approach, located ulnar to the mark over Lister's tubercle.

the wrist has remained dislocated for a sufficient time, typically several weeks or more, the likelihood of a successful closed reduction is decreased. If degenerative changes have occurred within the carpal articulations, the likelihood of having reasonable motion without significant pain is low. Furthermore, although in the acute and subacute dorsal perilunate and lunate dislocations closed reduction may be possible, it is my preference to also address these injuries with an open reduction, pin fixation, and ligamentous repair.

The forces acting on the individual carpal bones of the proximal row are significant, and I believe that they cannot be adequately managed by closed treatment and cast immobilization alone. Neither do I believe that closed reduction and percutaneous pin fixation is an adequate treatment, even when a reduction can be obtained.

The patient is placed in the supine position, with the hand on an arm table. A tourniquet is placed on the upper arm. Either regional or general anesthesia is used. The surgical approach begins with a dorsal longitudinal incision on the dorsum of the wrist, just ulnar to Lister's tubercle (Fig. 23–1). The skin incision is carried down to the extensor retinaculum. The dorsal venous complex of the wrist should be saved whenever possible, and a dissection plane is extended radially and ulnarly over the extensor retinaculum. A stepcut incision is made in the extensor retinaculum over the fourth dorsal compartment, leaving a radial- and an ulnar-based flap (Fig. 23–2). The terminal branch of the posterior interosseous nerve is identified on the floor of the fourth dorsal compartment, lying immediately to the ulnar side of the septum separating the third and fourth compartments. A segment of this nerve is resected, making sure to cut the nerve proximal to the distal end

■ SURGICAL
TECHNIQUES

■ FIGURE 23–2
The step-cut incision in
the extensor retinaculum
is highlighted by dots in
this photograph.

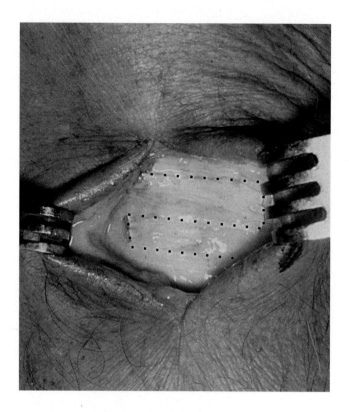

■ FIGURE 23–2
The step-cut incision in the extensor retinaculum is highlighted by dots in this photograph.

of the radius. The extensor tendons are retracted. The proximal pole of the capitate is often evident in the wound at this point. In some cases, the dorsal ligamentous and capsular disruption is significant and identification of individual ligament remnants is difficult. The substance of the dorsal portion of the SLIL, lunotriquetral interosseous ligament, dorsal transcarpal ligament, and dorsal radiocarpal ligaments are generally identifiable. The capsular incision is extended distally, and any adhesions are incised from the scaphoid, lunate, and triquetrum to assist in relocating the perilunar carpus or the lunate, depending on whether the injury is a dorsal perilunate dislocation or a volar lunate dislocation. An initial period of longitudinal traction of 10 lb may be helpful before attempting the reduction. Reduction is attempted by exerting axial traction of the carpus with the wrist in neutral. With counterforce against the palmar aspect of the lunate, the wrist is brought into flexion, with continued axial traction of the carpus. When the reduction is accomplished, axial compression is applied while the wrist is brought back into neutral or slight extension. When the reduction cannot be accomplished adequately and atraumatically, a volar incision is made. The volar incision is similar to the classic open carpal tunnel approach. It is about 1 cm ulnar and parallel to the thenar crease and begins at the level of the fully abducted thumb distally and extends to the proximal wrist crease. When necessary, the incision can be extended obliquely in an ulnar direction 1 to 2 cm proximal to the proximal wrist crease. Volarly, the incision is extended through subcutaneous tissue to the level of the transverse carpal ligament, which is incised in line with the skin incision. The flexor tendons and median nerve are reflected radially. At the base of the carpal tunnel, a perilunar rent can often be identified, coinciding with the space of Poirier in dorsal perilunate dislocations. In volar lunate dislocations, the lunate is often flexed in a palmar direction, and the distal concavity of the lunate faces proximal and lies just volar to the distal volar aspect of the radius. After completion of the dorsal and volar approaches, the lunate is reduced under direct vision from the volar approach by manually derotating and pushing it back in between the capitate and radius, while gentle axial traction is applied to the hand. The volar rent, which runs through the space of Poirier, is repaired with simple interrupted nonabsorbable sutures. The proximal wrist and mid-carpal joints are then examined through the dorsal capsule incisions for any osteochondral or chondral lesions. Free fragments are excised. The reduction of the scapholunate and triquetrolunate joints is assessed; if there is any difficulty in obtaining and maintaining anatomic reduction, additional measures should be used. The carpal alignment may be enhanced by positioning the wrist in more or less radioulnar deviation, with radioulnar compression of the proximal carpal row. Additionally, dorsally placed K-wires can be used as joysticks to assist carpal reduction. A Richards scaphoid staple reduction clamp can also be used to assist in the reduction. A single hole, using a 0.062-inch diameter K-wire, is made at the dorsal aspect of the proximal pole of the scaphoid and a second hole is made in the dorsal aspect of the radial side of the lunate, considering the palmar flexed position of the scaphoid and the extended position of the lunate. The arms of the scaphoid fracture reduction clamp are placed into the holes once the scaphoid and lunate have been properly derotated, and the reduction clamp is used to anatomically reduce the scapholunate joint (Fig. 23–3A and B). While maintaining the scapholunate reduction, at least two and preferably three or more nonparallel 0.045-inch–diameter K-wires are used to percutaneously pin the scapholunate joint, and an additional pin may be placed across the scaphocapitate joint to maintain the reduction (Fig. 23–4). Once the scapholunate joint has been pinned, the reduction clamp is removed and the lunotriquetral joint is reduced manually or in a similar manner with the aid of the scaphoid reduction clamp. The radioscaphoid and radiolunate joints should not be pinned. Once the reduction and pinning has been accom-

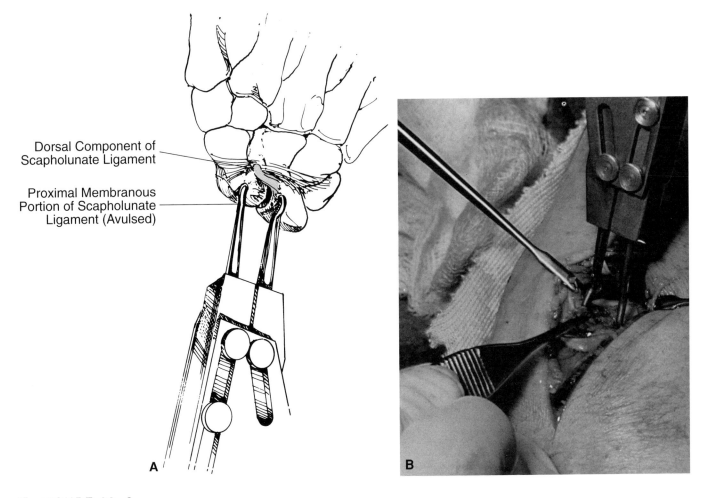

Dorsal Component of
Scapholunate Ligament

Proximal Membranous
Portion of Scapholunate
Ligament (Avulsed)

A   B

■ FIGURE 23–3
A, A diagram of a scaphoid reduction clamp used to reduce the scapholunate joint. One prong of the clamp is inserted into the scaphoid and one into the lunate. **B**, A photograph of the reduction clamp applied intraoperatively.

■ FIGURE 23–4
Percutaneous pinning of
the scapholunate joint is
done while the reduction
of the scaphoid and the
lunate is maintained by
the reduction clamp.

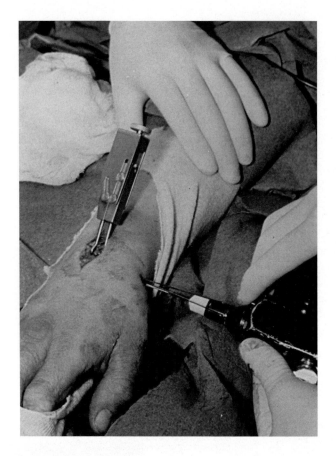

plished, radiographs are obtained to confirm the reduction in both anteroposterior and lateral projections. Although generally it is stated that the radius-lunate-capitate axes should be colinear, considering anatomic variability, radiolunate and capitolunate angles of less than 15° are usually acceptable. Direct visualization from the mid-carpal joint of the anatomic reduction of the proximal carpal row is the best way to determine whether the reduction is anatomic. Once the reduction has been confirmed radiographically, the dorsal transverse carpal ligament is repaired. If needed, additional holes are placed in the dorsal rim of the proximal half of the scaphoid and the dorsal rim of the lunate and triquetrum to assist in the repair of the dorsal segment of the scapholunate and lunotrique-tral interosseous ligaments and the dorsal transverse carpal ligament. In the case of a volar lunate dislocation, the dorsal radiocarpal sling ligament and capsule are reattached to the dorsal lip of the lunate. Repairs are performed with 4-0 nonabsorbable sutures. Finally, the capsular incision is repaired, followed by the extensor retinaculum, and the skin is closed with simple interrupted sutures on both the dorsal and volar approaches.

■ TECHNICAL
ALTERNATIVES

Arthroscopically assisted reduction has been proposed as an alternative to closed or open reduction. This technique involves reduction and multiple pin placement under direct arthroscopic visualization. Chronic dislocation is a contraindication to this technique; even in acute cases, the reliability and long-term results of this technique remain unknown. In the open reduction technique, an alternative to suturing ligaments to the bones through drill holes is the use of suture-anchoring devices to facilitate the reattachment of the ligaments and capsule. Pitfalls such as the use of too few pins for fixation or the parallel placement of the pins may result in loss of reduction of the carpus. Pin-tract infections may result in the compromise of fixation and also cause a loss of reduction. Pin-tract infections should be treated with supression antibiotic techniques. Patients who lose reduction should be offered an opportunity to have another open reduction and internal fixation procedure.

The wrist and forearm are immobilized in a long arm splint with the forearm in pronation for 4 weeks. The wrist is then immobilized in a short arm splint for an additional 6 weeks. Radiographs are obtained postoperatively at 1, 2, and 4 weeks to assess carpal alignment and pin position. The sutures are removed at 2 weeks postoperatively. Any sign of pin-tract inflammation or drainage should be treated with suppressant antibiotics until pin removal. The pins are removed at 8 to 10 weeks postoperatively. The wrist is placed in a removable short arm volar splint, and gentle active range of motion exercises are begun.

■ REHABILITATION

Carpal instabilities, particularly dorsal intercalated segment instabilities, are reported to occur frequently after reduction of perilunate dislocation without ligamentous repair. Results of open reduction and repair for late dorsal perilunate and volar lunate dislocations are not well documented in the literature. Generally, it is believed that satisfactory results can be obtained. Excellent results are rarely listed, however. Virtually all of these patients have some stiffness and permanent limitation of motion. Rehabilitation is often slow, and it takes several months for a patient to regain the motion, which is often only 50% of their preinjury normal wrist range of motion.

■ OUTCOMES

References

1. Adkison JW, Chapman MW: Treatment of acute luntae and perilunate dislocations. Clin Orthop, 1982; 164:199–207.
2. Bohler L: The Treatment of Fractures, 4th English Ed, Baltimore: William Wood, 1935: 235–247.
3. Bohler L: The Treatment of Fractures, 5th English Ed, New York: Grune & Stratton, 1956: 826–854.
4. Campbell RD Jr, Lance EM, Yeoh CB: Lunte and perilunar dislocations. J Bone Joint Surg, 1964; 46B:55–72.
5. Campbell RD Jr, Thompson TC, Lance EM, Adler JB: Indications for open reduction of lunate and perilunate dislocations of the carpal bones. J Bone Joint Surg, 1965; 47A:915–937.
6. Cave EF: Retroulnar dislocation of the capitate with fracture or subluxation of the navicular bone. J Bone Joint Surg, 1941; 3:830–840.
7. Cave EF: Injuries to the Wrist Joint. Instr Course Lect, 1953; 10:9–24.
8. Davis GG: Treatment of dislocated semilunar carpal bones. Surg Gynecol Obstet, 1923; 37: 225–229.
9. Destot E: Traumatismes Du Poignet Et Rx. Paris: Masson Et Cie, 1923.
10. Dobyns JH, Swanson GE: Fracture conference: a 19-year-old with multiple fractures. Minn Med, 1973; 56:143–149.
11. Dobyns JH, Linscheid RL: Fractures and Dislocations of the Wrist. In: Rockwood CA Jr, Green DP (eds): Fractures in Adults, 2nd Ed, Vol 1, Philadelphia: JB Lippincott 1984:411–509.
12. Eggers GWN: Anterior dislocation of os lunatum. J Bone Joint Surg, 1933; 15:394–400.
13. Hill NA: Fractures and dislocations of the carpus. Orthop Clin North Am, 1970; 1:275–284.
14. Keenan CB, Wilkie AL: Dislocation of the semilunar bone of the wrist. Can Med Assoc J, 1929; 20:639–641.
15. MacAusland WR: Perilunar dislocation of the carpal bones and dislocation of the lunate bone. Surg Gynecol Obstet, 1944; 79:256–266.
16. Mahorner HR, Meade WH: Operation for dislocated semilunar bone of the wrist. Surgery, 1939; 5:249–259.
17. Mayfield JK, Johnson RP, Kilcoyne RK: Carpal dislocations: pathomechanics and progressive perilunar instability. J Hand Surg, 1980; 5:226–241.
18. McBride ED: An operation for late reduction of the semi-lunar bone. South Med J, 1933; 26: 672–676.
19. Minami A, Kaneda K: Repair and/or reconstruction of scapholunate interosseous ligament in lunate and perilunate dislocations. J Hand Surg, 1993; 18A:1099–1106.
20. Siegert JJ, Frassica FJ, Amadio PC: Treatment of chronic perilunate dislocations. J Hand Surg, 1988; 13A:206–212.
21. Taleisnik J: Wrist: anatomy, function, and injury. American Academy of Orthopaedic Surgeons Instr Course Lect 1978; 27:61–87.
22. Watson-Jones R: Carpal semilunar dislocations and other wrist dislocations with associated nerve lesions. Proc R Soc Med, 1929; 22:1071–1086.
23. Weir IGC: The late reduction of carpal dislocations. J Hand Surg, 1992; 17B:137–139.

PART

IV

Fracture Fixation of the Phalanges

24

Percutaneous Pin Fixation of the Diaphysis of the Phalanges

Percutaneous pin fixation of small bone fractures was first advocated by Tennant in 1924.[13] He pushed a steel phonograph needle through metacarpal fracture fragments to act as a "retaining pin." After Kirschner described in 1927 the use of small traction wires made from chrome-plated steel piano wire measuring 0.7 mm (0.028 inch) to 1.5 mm (0.062 inch) in diameter,[10] Bosworth reported successfully treating a fifth metacarpal neck fracture by closed reduction and percutaneous pinning with two Kirschner wires (K-wires) under fluoroscopic control.[2] This technique did not become popular until the 1940s, when power drills became available.[10] When Vom Saal reported his results after closed reduction and percutaneous intramedullary fixation of a variety of metacarpal and phalangeal fractures in 1953, Littler commented that "[o]ne is encouraged in the use of such radical fixation because of the grave necessity of maintaining the architecture of the hand in its perfect form ."[14] Twenty years later, in 1973, Green and Anderson described their technique of closed pinning of phalangeal fractures using crossed K-wires.[4] Although instrumentation has improved significantly, the techniques and principles described by Vom Saal and refined by Green and Anderson are used routinely today to treat small bone fractures in the hand.

■ HISTORY OF THE TECHNIQUE

Phalangeal shaft fractures may be spiral, oblique, transverse, or comminuted. Generally, proximal phalangeal fractures shorten and angulate apex volarly because of the strong pull of the interosseous muscles. Middle phalangeal fracture angulation depends on the location of the fracture with respect to the flexor digitorum sublimis tendon insertion. Fractures proximal to the sublimis insertion angulate apex dorsally because of the strong pull of the tendon on the distal fragment; those distal to the sublimis insertion angulate apex volarly.[9]

■ INDICATIONS AND CONTRAINDICATIONS

Percutaneous pin fixation is indicated for those unstable phalangeal shaft fractures in which an adequate reduction can be obtained but not maintained by closed methods. Long oblique and spiral oblique fractures that are initially in good position present a relative indication for percutaneous pin fixation because they frequently displace despite cast or splint immobilization (Fig. 24–1). This technique prevents fracture displacement, allows tendon gliding and early motion of adjacent joints, and avoids the soft-tissue disruption associated with open reduction and internal fixation. Minimally comminuted transverse fractures should be indicated for this operation with caution (Fig. 24–2).

Inadequate closed reduction of a fracture (angulation greater than 10° in any plane, more than 2 mm of shortening, less than 50% bony apposition, or any malrotation)[11,12] constitutes a contraindication to percutaneous pin fixation. Thus, simple fractures with soft-tissue interposition and comminuted fractures with markedly displaced or rotated fragments require open reduction. In addition, comminuted fractures wherein key fragments may be displaced or rotated by the fixation pin should be treated by open methods.

This procedure should be performed in an operating room or minor surgical suite, using aseptic technique. An experienced surgical assistant is essential because the fracture must be reduced and held by one individual while K-wires are driven across the fracture site by a second. Digital block anesthesia is performed (except in small children, in whom

■ SURGICAL TECHNIQUES

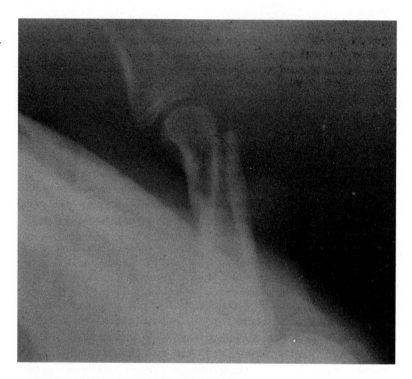

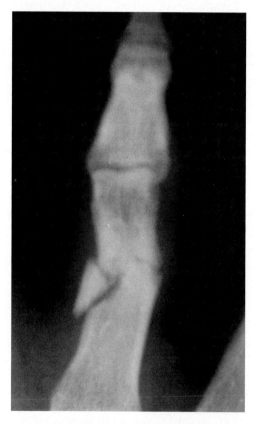

general anesthesia may be required) using 1% lidocaine and 0.25% bupivacaine (both without epinephrine) mixed in equal parts to provide rapid onset of local anesthesia and postoperative pain relief, respectively. Local infiltration in the digit is avoided because it obscures cutaneous landmarks.

Closed reduction is performed before the surgical prep and checked fluoroscopically. I prefer to use a mini–C-arm such as the FlouroScan (FluoroScan Imaging Systems, Inc., Northbrook, IL); it provides excellent visualization of small bones while minimizing irradiation scatter.[3] The hand is held as closely as possible to the image-detection device to provide the largest field of vision and minimize magnification. If closed reduction is deemed inadequate, this procedure is aborted, a tourniquet is applied, and preparations are made for open reduction of the fracture. If the reduction is adequate, the upper extremity is prepped and sterilely draped while instrumentation for percutaneous pin fixation (a minor hand tray and an air-powered pencil or pistol-grip microwire-driver with a rapid release chuck) is opened and the mini–C-arm is sterilely draped. The method of closed reduction and K-wire fixation employed depends on fracture pattern, location, and displacement.

Spiral and long oblique fractures are best reduced by longitudinal traction applied manually or with finger traps. A large towel clip or fracture clamp is then applied perpendicular to the longitudinal axis of the bone to stabilize the reduction and apply compression across the fracture site. Rotational alignment is evaluated by inspecting the plane of the fingernails and by checking for abnormal crossing of the fingers as the metacarpophalangeal (MP) and interphalangeal (IP) joints are flexed. Two or three 0.028-inch K-wires are introduced near the mid-lateral line, avoiding the lateral bands and extensor aponeurosis, and drilled transversely across the fracture site (Fig. 24–3). The clamp is then removed. The reduction and pin placement are checked fluoroscopically and the finger is moved through a full range of motion to verify tendon gliding. If tendon gliding is limited, the pin most likely to have transfixed the extensor mechanism is removed and repositioned and range of motion is reassessed.

Transverse and short oblique fractures of the proximal phalanx are reduced by flexing the MP joint 90°, so that the collateral ligaments stabilize the proximal fragment. The distal fragment is then reduced onto the proximal fragment by applying longitudinal traction with the proximal interphalangeal (PIP) joint flexed. The reduction is verified clinically and fluoroscopically. A 0.035- or 0.045-inch K-wire is introduced laterally at the retrocondylar fossa of the proximal phalangeal head and drilled longitudinally across the fracture site to lodge in the opposite cortex proximally (Fig. 24–4). Compression is applied across the fracture site as the pin is advanced to prevent distraction of the fracture fragments. The pin should be angled slightly dorsal in the anteroposterior plane to accommodate the slight dorsal curve of the phalanx. Pin placement is made easier by first placing a free pin over the finger as a fluoroscopic guide to correct pin alignment. A second K-wire is then introduced at the opposite retrocondylar fossa and drilled longitudinally, so that the two wires cross in the phalangeal medullary canal. This technique may be used in transverse and short oblique fractures of the middle phalanx as well as selected comminuted phalangeal shaft fractures if the comminution is limited.

K-wires may be cut off just beneath the skin or left protruding 5 to 6 mm and bent 90° to prevent pin migration. A sterile dressing and plaster splint, immobilizing the involved and adjacent fingers in the functional or "safe"[5] position, is applied.

Selection of K-wires is determined by the size of the phalanx. Generally, 0.045- and 0.035-inch K-wires are used in the proximal phalanges of large and average-sized adults; 0.035- and 0.028-inch K-wires are used in small adults and children. These techniques are applicable to middle phalangeal fractures, using 0.035-inch K-wires in larger adults and 0.028-inch K-wires in small adults and children.

■ TECHNICAL ALTERNATIVES

Percutaneous pin fixation may be difficult to perform, even when aided by fluoroscopy. The surgeon should be familiar with alternative methods of percutaneous fixation, so that a different technique can be employed if difficulties are encountered intraoperatively.

For transverse, short oblique, and short spiral fractures located in the proximal half of the phalanx, it may be easier to advance the pins from proximal to distal, introducing them at the proximal phalangeal base adjacent to the MP joint articular surface (Fig. 24–5). The pin is lodged in the small bony shelf, lateral to the articular surface, aligned with a guide pin, and drilled into the opposite cortex distally.

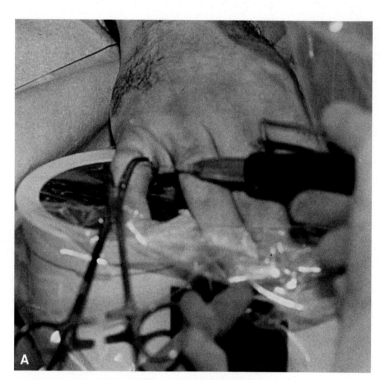

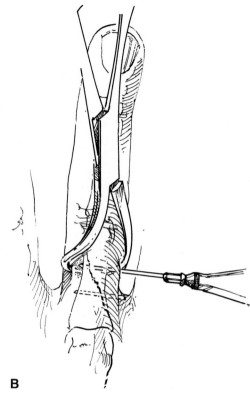

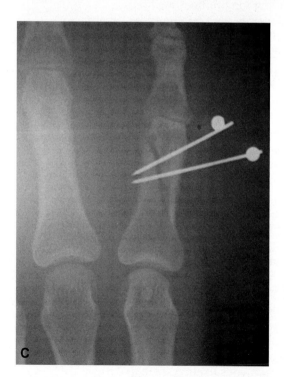

■ FIGURE 24–3

A, An unstable long oblique fracture of the proximal phalanx is reduced under fluoroscopic control; the hand rests on the sterilely draped image detection unit of the mini–C-arm. A large towel clip maintains the reduction as an 0.028-inch K-wire is driven across the fracture. **B**, Diagram of fracture reduction and pin placement. Note the position of the towel clip points, maintaining the reduction. **C**, Postoperative PA radiograph. Two 0.028-inch K-wires stabilize the fracture.

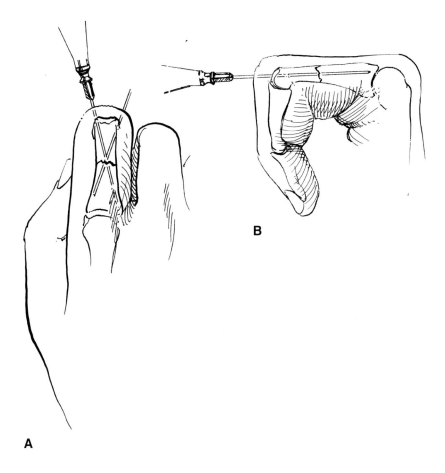

■ FIGURE 24–4

Crossed intramedullary K-wire fixation of a transverse proximal phalangeal fracture. **A**, With the PIP joint flexed, a 0.035-inch K-wire is introduced in the retrocondylar fossa of the proximal phalanx and drilled across the fracture site to lodge in the opposite cortex proximally. A second 0.035-inch K-wire is introduced in the opposite retrocondylar fossa, such that the two wires cross within the medullary canal just proximal to the fracture site. **B**, Lateral view demonstrating pin placement. Note the slight dorsal direction of the pin with respect to the long axis of the bone.

Transverse and short oblique proximal phalangeal fractures may be stabilized with a single 0.045-inch K-wire introduced through the metacarpal head. The K-wire is introduced just lateral to the extensor tendon with the MP joint in 80° to 90° of flexion and advanced longitudinally across the fracture into but not through the PIP subchondral cortex (Fig. 24–6). Because this single pin does not provide rotational stability, plaster or thermoplastic splints applied postoperatively are removed only for pin care. Range of motion exercises are not performed until the pin is removed at 3 weeks. Although this method simplifies pin placement, it precludes early range of motion exercises, violates an otherwise normal joint, and may damage the extensor hood over the MP joint. It is a useful technique in fractures associated with burn or crush injuries, in which MP joint immobilization in flexion is desired to prevent extension contractures.

Placement of crossed K-wires is difficult, especially when there is significant soft-tissue swelling around the PIP joint. The most common errors are to traverse the medullary canal without crossing the fracture site and to lever the fracture site open as the pin is advanced. Penetration of the soft tissue distal to the PIP joint, lodging the pin on the small shelf of bone in the retrocondylar fossa, and use of a guide pin to determine the correct drilling angle are helpful in obtaining accurate pin placement. Application of compression across the fracture site while pins are advanced prevents fracture distraction.

■ FIGURE 24–5
A PA radiograph of an unstable short oblique fracture of the ring finger proximal phalanx stabilized with two 0.045-inch crossed K-wires introduced in the proximal fragment and advanced distally.

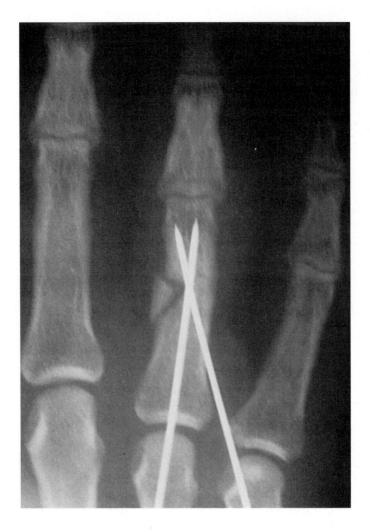

■ REHABILITATION

The postoperative dressing and splint are removed at 3 to 5 days postoperatively and a light dressing is applied. The patient is placed in a well-molded plaster or thermoplastic hand-based splint, which maintains the MP joints of the involved and adjacent digit at 80 to 90° of flexion and the IP joints in full extension. The splint is removed 3 to 5 times per day for active and passive range of motion exercises under the supervision of a trained hand therapist. When pins are left protruding from the skin, pin care with peroxide is performed twice daily.

Pins are removed at 3 to 4 weeks postoperatively when the fracture site demonstrates minimal tenderness to palpation and no pain with stress; they may be left an additional 1 to 2 weeks if the fracture remains tender or joint range of motion is limited. Buried pins are removed in the office, using local anesthetic and sterile technique. Radiographs obtained after pin removal should show no change in the position or alignment of the fracture fragments. Radiographic evidence of fracture healing may not be evident for 2 to 3 weeks after clinical healing has occurred; thus, rehabilitation initially should be based on the clinical exam. After pin removal, if the fracture site is not tender and there is no pain or motion with stress testing, active assisted and passive range of motion exercises are continued. For an additional 2 to 3 weeks, the patient's removable splint is applied for heavy activities such as lifting, carrying, and sports activities and the finger is buddy taped for light activities. Resisted exercises and unrestricted activities are initiated at 6 to 8 weeks postoperatively or when radiographs demonstrate bony union. Patients may return to light duty employment after pin removal and to full duty employment when union is apparent radiographically, usually by 6 to 8 weeks postoperatively.

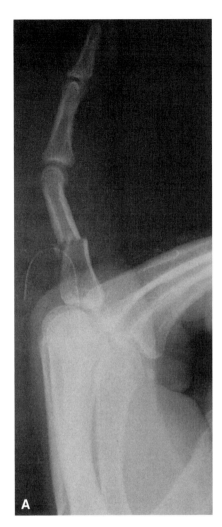
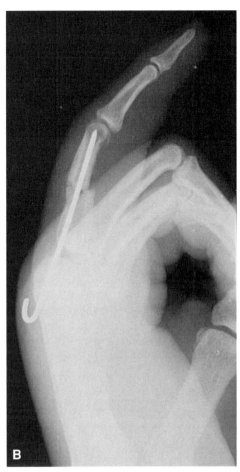

■ FIGURE 24–6

A, Preoperative lateral radiograph of an unstable transverse proximal phalangeal fracture of the index finger. **B**, The fracture is stabilized with a single longitudinal 0.045-inch K-wire. Note the point of entry of the pin in the small juxtarticular cortical ridge of bone in the proximal phalanx. Lodging the pin here provides leverage for longitudinal placement. The pin was introduced with the MP joint in flexion; it does not traverse the index metacarpal head.

Several studies have demonstrated good to excellent results in about 90% of patients having phalangeal fractures treated with percutaneous fixation,[1,4,6] a finding that prompted Jupiter and Belsky to comment that many surgeons consider K-wire fixation to be the "gold standard" for skeletal fixation in the hand.[7] The reported incidence of superficial pin-tract infections ranges from 0 to 10%.[1,4,6,14] Early pin-tract infections usually respond to oral antibiotics and improved pin care but may necessitate early pin removal. Nonunion, delayed union, and malunion may result when K-wire fixation is improper.[1,8] Most of the poor outcomes reported are a result of loss of motion in the IP joints. Range of motion can be maximized by obtaining an accurate reduction, demonstrating intraoperatively that the extensor expansion and lateral bands move freely, and encouraging early active range of motion combined with extension splinting of the IP joints during rest periods.[1,5]

■ OUTCOMES

References

1. Belsky MR, Eaton RG, Lane LB: Closed reduction and internal fixation of proximal phalangeal fractures. J Hand Surg, 1984; 9A:725–729.

2. Bosworth DM: Internal splinting of fractures of the fifth metacarpal. J Bone Joint Surg, 1937; 19:826–827.
3. Gehrke JC, Mellenberg DE Jr, Connelly RE, Johnson KA: Technique tips: the fluoroscan imaging system in foot and ankle surgery. Foot Ankle, 1993; 14:545–549.
4. Green DP, Anderson JR: Closed reduction and percutaneous pin fixation of fractured phalanges. J Bone Joint Surg, 1973; 55A:1651–1654.
5. James JIP: The assessment and management of the injured hand. Hand, 1970; 2:97–105.
6. Joshi BB: Percutaneous internal fixation of fractures of the proximal phalanges. Hand, 1976; 8:86–92.
7. Jupiter JB, Belsky MR: Fractures and Dislocations of the Hand. In: Browner BD, Jupiter JB, Levine AM, Trafton PG (eds): Skeletal Trauma; Fractures, Dislocations, Ligamentous Injuries, Philadelphia: WB Saunders, 1992:923–1024.
8. Jupiter JB, Koniuch M, Smith RJ: The management of delayed unions and nonunions of the tubular bones of the hand. J Hand Surg, 1985; 4:457–466.
9. McNealy RW, Lichtenstein ME: Fractures of the metacarpals and phalanges. West J Surg Obstet Gynecol, 1935; 43:156–161.
10. Meals RA, Meuli HC: Carpenter's nails, phonograph needles, piano wires, and safety pins: the history of operative fixation of metacarpal and phalangeal fractures. J Hand Surg, 1985; 10A:144–150.
11. Pun WK, Chow SP, So YC, et al: A prospective study on 284 digital fractures of the hand. J Hand Surg, 1989; 14A:474–480.
12. Stern PJ: Fractures of the Metacarpals and Phalanges. In: Green DP (eds): Operative Hand Surgery, New York: Churchill Livingstone, 1993:695–758.
13. Tennant CE: Use of steel phonograph needle as a retaining pin in certain irreducible fractures of the small bones. JAMA, 1924; 83:193.
14. Vom Saal FH: Intramedullary fixation in fractures of the hand and fingers. J Bone Joint Surg, 1953; 35A:5–16.

THOMAS L. GREENE

25

Open Pin Fixation of the Diaphysis for Phalangeal Fractures

Small pins and wires were among the earliest devices used for the internal fixation of phalangeal fractures.[6] As the principles of stable fixation and early motion evolve, these devices have less frequent use as the sole means of fixation. Biomechanical studies have demonstrated the inferiority of K-wire fixation alone, compared with plates, screws, or composite wiring techniques.[2,5,7] The tension-band principle of fracture fixation was introduced by Pauwels[8] and applied to fracture surgery by Weber.[9] The incorporation of wire loops about Kirschner pins (composite wiring) for fixation of the long bones of the hand has developed from these earlier techniques of fracture surgery.[1,3,4]

Stability of fracture fixation is enhanced by interfragmentary compression. A composite of bone, pin, and wire can achieve this compression to promote primary bone healing and permit early motion of the finger.

■ HISTORY OF THE TECHNIQUE

Closed fractures that are displaced, angulated, or rotated that cannot be treated by closed means, including percutaneous pinning, are the prime indications for the use of open pin techniques. Oblique and spiral fractures are considerably easier to treat than transverse fractures (Fig. 25–1). The small diameter of the diaphysis may make proper placement of two pins across but close enough to a transverse fracture a difficult maneuver. Open fractures without bone loss are amenable to composite wiring. When there is bone loss or extensive comminution at the fracture site, pin placement in firm cortical bone may not be possible, or the fracture may displace when compression is applied as the wire loops are tightened.

■ INDICATIONS AND CONTRAINDICATIONS

Anesthesia is with either a digital block, using a longer-acting agent such as bupivicaine, or a brachial plexus block. The time required for the procedure dictates this choice, based on patient tolerance of a brachial pneumatic tourniquet. For middle phalanx fractures, an alternative is the use of a digital tourniquet. Some degree of visual magnification is necessary to properly manipulate the delicate soft tissues and small bone fragments encountered in these procedures.

The surgical approach created to expose the fracture probably has as much of an effect on the ultimate functional result as any other factor. The close proximity of the skin, the extensor and flexor tendon mechanisms, and the periosteum to each other and the fracture predisposes to adhesions between soft tissues and bone, induced by the injury itself and the surgical insult. The approach to a closed fracture should be through a dorsolateral incision of sufficient length to allow skin retraction without excessive tension or struggle. The adventitial layers between the extensor mechanism and the subcutaneous tissue and periosteum should be left as undisturbed as possible. The phalanx is approached through periosteum volar to the edge of the extensor mechanism. When proximal exposure of the phalanx is required, the lateral band and oblique fibers of the extensor hood should be excised on the exposed side.

The use of composite wiring techniques requires minimal periosteal stripping. Only the bone immediately adjacent to the fracture needs to be exposed to prepare the fracture

■ SURGICAL TECHNIQUES

■ FIGURE 25–1
Preoperative radiograph
of an oblique proximal
phalanx fracture.

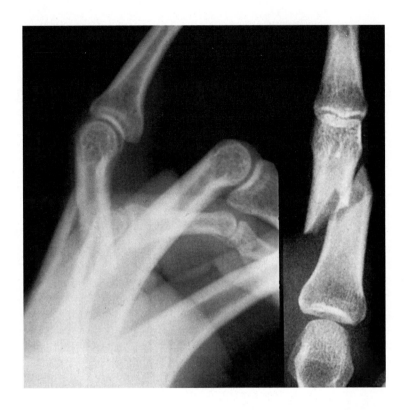

■ FIGURE 25–2
Examples of pin-and-wire
fixation techniques for
transverse and short
oblique phalangeal frac-
tures. (Reproduced with
permission from Greene
TL, Noellert RC, Belsole
RJ, Simpson LA: Com-
posite wiring of metacar-
pal and phalangeal frac-
tures. J Hand Surg,
1989; 14a: 665–669.)

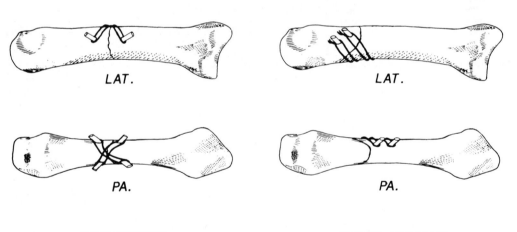

LAT.   LAT.

PA.   PA.

TRANSVERSE   SHORT OBLIQUE

surfaces for reduction. One should avoid placing any retractors along the volar surfaces because this may promote adherence of the flexor tendons in the sheath or to the fracture. Anatomic fracture reduction is obtained and temporarily held by a fine bone–holding clamp. Failure to obtain accurate interdigitation of the fracture surfaces at this stage results in translation or rotation of the fragments when compression is applied.

Once the fracture is reduced, an assessment of the fracture geometry is required. Nearly all fractures involving two fragments can be stabilized with two Kirschner pins. For an oblique or spiral fracture, two pins are placed perpendicularly to the plane of the fracture and are equally spaced along the length of the fracture (Figs. 25–2 and 25–3). The pins should be as centrally located within each fragment as possible and should not be too close to the spiked ends of fragments, which would risk fracturing. Transverse fracture patterns require crossed pinning in most cases. Retrograde placement of two pins in one of the fragments first is usually easier than fixation after reduction. A small intramedullary

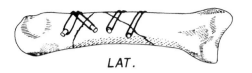
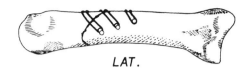

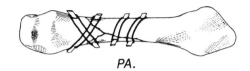
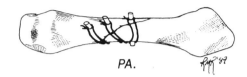

COMMINUTED   LONG OBLIQUE/SPIRAL

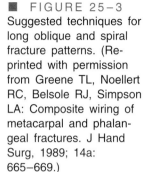

■ FIGURE 25–3
Suggested techniques for long oblique and spiral fracture patterns. (Reprinted with permission from Greene TL, Noellert RC, Belsole RJ, Simpson LA: Composite wiring of metacarpal and phalangeal fractures. J Hand Surg, 1989; 14a: 665–669.)

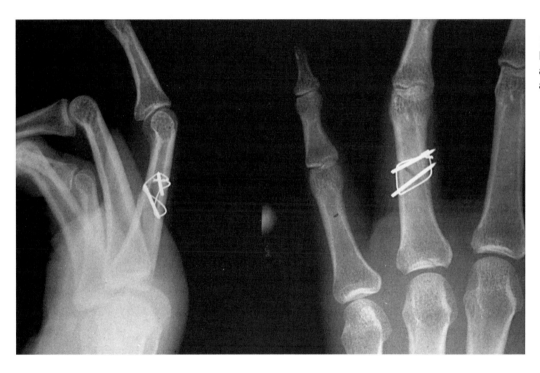

■ FIGURE 25–4
Postoperative radiograph after composite wiring fixation.

canal and thick cortices in the mid-diaphysis may make composite wiring the less favored technique for transverse fractures. Modifications in the placement rules occasionally need to be made to avoid pin impingement in tendons and to allow clear visualization of the end of each pin placed. Kirschner pins of 0.035-inch diameter are inserted with a power driver in the predetermined positions. An 18-gauge hypodermic needle may be used as a guide. The pin point should only protrude from the opposite cortex by 1 or 2 mm; this should be just enough to allow the wire loop to engage it. The bone-holding clamp is then removed. Alignment and rotation of the finger are checked visually and may be done radiographically at this time (Fig. 25–4).

Stainless steel wire suture (26-gauge) is used to create the wire loops. One strand may be folded in half, making a narrow loop, and the looped end gently curved to facilitate placement. The looped wire is passed beneath the soft tissues dorsal to the phalanx, over the end of the pin in the far cortex (opposite the side of insertion), pulled snugly to cinch it against the bone, and the free ends are pulled tightly as they are wrapped around the other end of the pin close to bone. While maintaining tension, the two ends are twisted together several times. The wire ends are trimmed, leaving about 2-cm tails. A large needle holder is used to complete the tightening of the braid. As the loop is tightened, compression of the fracture can be observed. Deformation of the twisted wire is noted by a loss of its surface shine at the braid. Breaking the wire occasionally during the early learning curve for this technique serves to enhance the surgeon's feel for the yield point of the metal. The wire braid is trimmed to a length of 2 or 3 mm and bent against the bone, away from the extensor mechanism. The remaining length of Kirschner pin in the near cortex is trimmed as close to the bone as possible. The finger is then moved through a full range of motion to be sure of proper alignment and free excursion of the extensor mechanism.

The periosteum is closed as much as possible with 4-0 polyglycolic acid sutures. The postoperative dressing should consist of fluffed gauze that provides gentle compression to the digit and also allows some freedom of movement of the finger joints. The wrist may be splinted in extension to facilitate digital motion and promote a safe position for the finger joints. Splinting of the digit is not required because the stability of fixation achieved permits early active motion and rehabilitation.

■ TECHNICAL ALTERNATIVES

Oblique and spiral fractures may be fixed with interfragmentary screws 2.0 or 1.5 mm in diameter. As opposed to insertion of Kirschner pins, the drilling and tapping of the small holes required for these screws is more difficult and unforgiving of the slightest technical error. Composite wiring would be the suitable technique to salvage a failure of screw fixation. Tranverse fractures may be more suitably stabilized with a lateral miniplate and screws or proximally inserted intramedullary pins.

The major problems inherent to the open treatment of phalangeal fractures are related to the soft tissues enveloping the fracture site. Pin and wire impingement in the extensor mechanism contributes to these inherent problems and should be avoided.

Adherence of the extensor mechanism to the overlying skin—but more importantly to the fracture—is responsible for the greatest difficulties in restoring mobility. The use of miniplates and interfragmentary screw fixation requires considerably more soft tissue dissection and stripping, which increases the potential for adhesions and stiffness and is a major disadvantage to their use for phalangeal fractures.

■ REHABILITATION

The goals of rehabilitation after open repair of a phalanx fracture should be to decrease edema and restore full active motion to the digit in the shortest time. A delay of even a few days before beginning active and gentle passive range of motion exercises may promote adherence of gliding soft tissues and early periarticular fibrosis.

Active motion of the digits is encouraged immediately after surgery within the confines of the dressing. An advantage of using a long-acting local anesthetic with a digital block technique is the freedom of movement without pain that it affords, thus increasing patient compliance and confidence in their rehabilitation.

An aggressive active exercise program is begun on the second or third postoperative day. The dressing is minimized to permit freedom of movement. Edema is controlled by active motion, elevation, and elastic taping. A supervised hand-therapy program is instituted after surgery if the patient has difficulty regaining active motion in the first 7 to 10 days. Occasionally, a digital block anesthetic administered in the postoperative period can greatly enhance active motion and break early adhesions. The sutures are removed at about 10 days postoperatively. Passive motion, with or without dynamic splinting, is begun at 3 weeks if motion has not returned to a nearly normal range. A hand-based extension splint for the interphalangeal joints typically suffices for most early contractures. A spring extension splint can be used for more resistant and persistent flexion contractures after the fourth week. Resistance exercises begin when fracture union is assured radiographically, usually 4 to 6 weeks postoperatively. Static splinting of the interphalangeal joints in extension is done during periods of sleep when an extensor lag is noted. This may need to be continued for 6 to 8 weeks or longer.

One should continue a rehabilitation program as long as there is soft-tissue swelling in response to stretching or exercise or there is a soft end point to passive motion of the digit that is associated with pain. Expectations for normal motion after phalangeal fractures treated by open means are not often realistic. The minimum goal should be a digit that flexes to touch the palm and extends enough to avoid being an interference to overall hand function.

The fractures treated by open pinning techniques represent a highly selected group from all phalangeal fractures and consist of the most comminuted, displaced, or unstable fractures that would by definition do poorly with closed treatment. The addition of a surgical insult to the soft-tissue envelope about the phalanx is an unfortunate necessity. These factors would be expected to contribute to less than full motion in many cases.

■ OUTCOMES

Twenty-one phalangeal fractures treated by composite wiring achieved a mean total active motion (TAM) of 215° (standard deviation [SD], 40°).[3] There was no statistical difference between the TAM of open (mean 192°, SD 41°) and closed fractures (mean 232°, SD 42°). The presence of a nerve, tendon, or arterial injury was the only factor that had a negative influence on the final result (mean TAM, 182°; SD 39°; $p<.05$). No instances of malunion, nonunion, loss of reduction, or tendon rupture were noted. These results indicate that open pin fixation can be a valuable technique for the treatment of selected phalangeal fractures.

References

1. Belsole R: Stabilizing hand fractures with tension bands. In: Spiegel PG (ed): Topics in Orthopaedic Trauma. Baltimore: University Park Press, 1984: 57–67.
2. Gould WL, Belsole RJ, Shelton WH: Tension band stabilization of transverse fractures: An experimental analysis. Plast Reconst Surg, 1984: 73: 111–115.
3. Greene TL, Noellert RC, Belsole RJ, Simpson LA: Composite wiring of metacarpal and phalangeal fractures. J Hand Surg, 1989: 14A: 665–669.
4. Greene TL, Noellert RC, Belsole RJ: Treatment of unstable metacarpal and phalangeal fractures with tension band wiring techniques. CORR, 1987: 214: 78–84.
5. Mann RJ, Black D, Constine R, Daniels AN: A quantitative comparison of metacarpal fracture stability with five different methods of internal fixation. J Hand Surg, 1985: 10A: 1024–1028.
6. Meals RA, Meuli HC: Carpenter's nails, phonograph needles, piano wires, and safety pins: the history of operative fixation of metacarpal and phalangeal fractures. J Hand Surg, 1985: 10A: 144–150.
7. Rayhack JM, Belsole RJ, Shelton WH: A strain rescording model: Analysis of transverse osteotomy fixation in small bones. J Hand Surg, 1984: 9A: 383–387.
8. Segmuller A: Surgical stabilization of the skeleton of the hand. Baltimore: Williams & Wilkins, 1977.
9. Weber BK: Grundlagen und Moglichkeiten der Zuggurtungs-osteosynthese. Chirurg, 1963: 35: 81–86.

ALAN E. FREELAND,
MICHAEL E. JABALEY

26

Screw Fixation of the Diaphysis for Phalangeal Fractures

■ HISTORY OF THE TECHNIQUE

The first recorded use of screws for bone fixation was by Berenges-Ferand in 1870. Lane used buried screws to fix an oblique fracture of the tibia and fibula while simultaneously introducing his "no touch" surgical technique in 1894. Lambotte introduced operative treatment for phalangeal fractures in 1904 and wrote further about it in his *Chirurgie: Operatoire des Fractures* in 1914. Screw fixations were among the techniques described and recommended.[10]

In 1952, Peterson introduced the use of drill guides and emphasized the importance of proper drill size in relation to the core and thread diameters of the screw. He also recommended countersinking the cortical bone to more evenly distribute the force of the screw head over a larger area, thereby decreasing the risk of fragmentation. In the hand, this provides the additional advantage of decreasing the prominence of the screw head in relation to both the bone and adjacent soft tissues.[10]

Progressive refinements in metallurgy, design, and biomechanics led to the development of mini-fragment screws by Heim and Mathys in 1970.[12] These screws are proportionate in size to the small bones of the hand. Specific instruments of similar metal were designed for their insertion. Recently, even smaller self-tapping titanium screws have been applied to simple (single fracture line) low-demand phalangeal fractures.

■ INDICATIONS AND CONTRAINDICATIONS

Mini-screw fixation can be selected for stabilization of displaced or otherwise unstable oblique or spiral proximal or middle phalangeal diaphyseal fractures in which the fracture length approximates twice or more of the diameter of the fractured diaphyseal bone. Although there may be exceptions to this guideline with slightly shorter fractures, the importance of this parameter is that the fracture must be of sufficient length to allow firm placement of two or more screws. Additionally, the fracture fragments must be of sufficient size that the largest drill bit diameter is a third or less than the diaphyseal diameter where it is used—again, as a precaution to prevent fragmentation.

A mini-screw may be thought of as a K-wire with threads and a head. It has an advantage over a K-wire because it applies greater stability through compression.[7] This biomechanical advantage must be balanced against the potential fracture devascularization and scar formation that result from the incision and dissection necessary for implant application. When mini-screws can be applied transcutaneously, in closed fractures that must be opened to achieve reduction, and in open fractures wherein little or no additional dissection is necessary for mini-screw application, these implants provide an advantage in stability. This is important in maintaining anatomic reduction, reducing pain, and allowing earlier and more intensive rehabilitation. This is especially true when there is adjacent tendon injury and in the polyfractured or polytraumatized digit or hand. Screws are preferable to less rigid implants when patient noncompliance is anticipated. Screw fixation is generally reserved for mature adult bone but exceptions may occur, particularly in adolescents with more severe fractures. Smaller screws of about 2.0 mm diameter or less are usually selected for phalangeal fractures but larger diameter screws may be chosen for a more secure fixation, for osteopenic bone, or to replace an unstable smaller screw.

Intravenous regional, axillary, or even local block anesthesia is sufficient for phalangeal fracture fixation in most cases. General anesthesia is indicated for more complex injuries or at the preference of the patient or the anesthesiologist.

The proximal phalanx is surrounded by collagenous structures, including a sophisticated dorsal extensor mechanism, a dual extrinsic flexor system, and periarticular capsular and ligamentous structures. When injured, either by trauma or surgery, these tissues tend to undergo a proliferative fibroblastic response.[6-8] Additionally, the one-wound-one-scar principle of tissue healing directs the healing of all involved tissues toward consolidation into a single cicatrix.[14] This translates into loss of motion in many cases. To minimize this tendency in fractures of the proximal phalanx, a surgical approach that achieves stable fracture fixation and allows motion of adjacent soft tissues is important.[10,12,16]

The classic and most commonly performed surgical exposure of the proximal phalanx uses a dorsal tendon-splitting approach[15] (Fig. 26–1). This incision can result in the inclusion of the extensor apparatus in the scar formed between the overlying skin and fractured bone and consequently may diminish tendon excursion.

Conversely, the mid-axial incision (Figs. 26–2 and 26–3) allows adequate phalangeal access, avoids the extensor apparatus to a large degree, and minimizes the risk of flexion contracture or scar hypertrophy because of its neutral position in relation to digital motion. It undergoes no change in length on flexion or extension of the digit.[8,13] It can be extended as far proximally and distally as necessary for phalangeal exposure by curving dorsally. Incisions on the ulnar side of the index, middle, and ring fingers and on the radial side of the small finger are preferable to avoid damage to the lumbrical tendons and working surfaces. In the small finger, the surgeon must choose between a radial incision that jeopardizes the lumbrical tendon and an ulnar incision that imperils the resting surface and occasionally, the abductor insertion.

■ SURGICAL TECHNIQUES

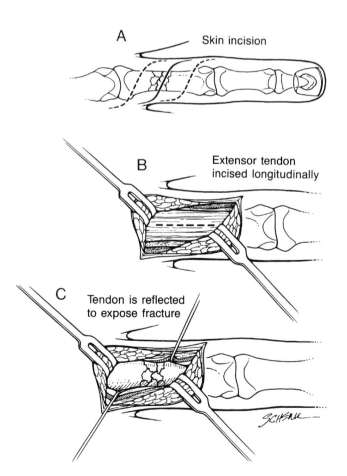

A Skin incision

B Extensor tendon incised longitudinally

C Tendon is reflected to expose fracture

■ FIGURE 26–1
A, The dorsal skin incision is obliquely angled over the extensor tendon to minimize postoperative adhesions between these two tissues. The incision can be positioned proximally or distally to enhance exposure. **B**, The extensor tendon is split longitudinally, **C** providing excellent phalangeal exposure.[8,15] (Adapted from Pratt DR: Exposing fractures of the proximal phalanx of the finger longitudinally through the dorsal extensor apparatus. Clin Orthop, 1959; 15:22–26.)

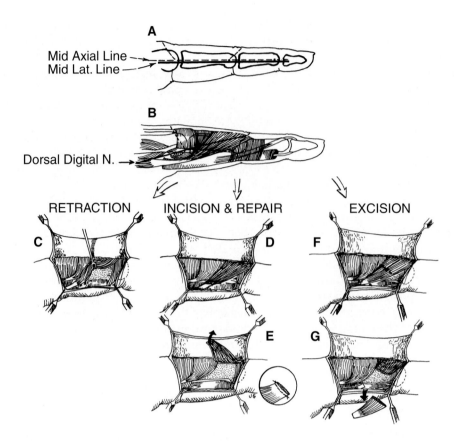

A

Mid Axial Line
Mid Lat. Line

B

Dorsal Digital N.

RETRACTION   INCISION & REPAIR   EXCISION

C   **D**   **F**

E   **G**

■ FIGURE 26–2

A, A mid-axial incision connecting the centers of joint rotation is placed 1 to 2 mm dorsally to the anatomic mid-lateral position. The mid-axial line connects the points made at the dorsal extremes of the flexion creases of the MP and interphalangeal joints when the finger is fully flexed.[13] **B**, The incision can be extended as a flap along the skin creases over the dorsal proximal, distal, or both aspects of the finger. The dorsal digital nerve should be sought and spared when possible or mobilized with the dorsal portion of the incision or flap. The neurovascular bundle is left undisturbed volarly. **C**, For more distal phalangeal fractures, the lateral band can be mobilized and retracted. **D** and **E**, Mid-phalangeal, proximal, or both phalangeal fractures may require more extensive exposure by lateral band incision, mobilization, and repair,[4,5,9] **F** and **G**, or by excision of a triangle of the oblique dorsal fibers and the adjacent lateral band.[8] The periosteum may then be incised and reflected sufficiently to expose the fracture site. (Re-

The configuration or plane of the fracture, location of an accompanying wound, or the preference of the surgeon dictate the location and orientation of the operative incision. The fracture should be reduced and provisionally stabilized by fracture-reduction clamps, K-wires, or both. If the surgical exposure is awkward, the hand can be positioned away from the hand table by bending the elbow and allowing the hand to rest on the patient's chest or abdomen and operating on it in this position. It may be returned to the hand table as necessary for fluoroscopic and standard radiographic evaluation.

In closed fractures, a manipulative closed reduction can sometimes be performed with or without the assistance of sharply pointed tenacular clamps, K-wires, or both using a radiolucent hand table and fluoroscopic radiographic or standard radiographic monitoring. Screws then may be inserted either transcutaneously or through a limited incision, using the precepts detailed above.[11]

Should implant removal be necessary or should tendon adhesions occur, the mid-axial approach to the proximal phalanx may again be used and the implant or implants removed. Tenolysis of both extensor and flexor tendons often may be completed simultane-

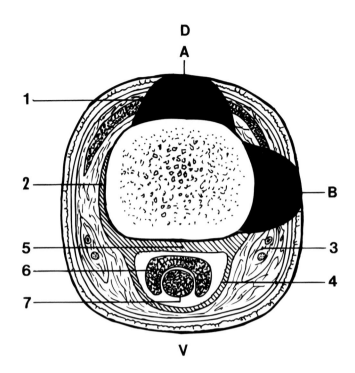

■ FIGURE 26–3
Finger phalanges (**D**=**dorsal; V**=**volar**) are surrounded by collagenous structures: (**1**) dorsal extensor apparatus, (**2**) collateral ligaments, (**3**) transverse and oblique retinacular ligaments, Cleland's and Grayson's ligaments, (**4**) flexor tendon sheath, (**5**) volar plate, and (**6** and **7**) flexor tendons. When injured, as by incisions, these structures form scar and fields of collagen, either dorsally (**A**) or laterally (**B**).[8,16]

ously. Excision of the scarred portions of the extensor apparatus may be more likely to result in functional improvement than tenolysis if the remaining uninvolved tendon is sufficient in structure and strength to operate and extend the interphalangeal joints.[10,12,16]

Screw design is based on that of a simple tool—the inclined plane. Diagonal placement of threads wrapped around a central core allows the torsional force applied through the head of a screw to compress fracture fragments, thereby stabilizing them. The lag-screw principle is used whenever a screw crosses a fracture. To apply the principle, the diameter of the hole in the proximal fragment should be slightly greater than the thread diameter of the selected screw. This allows the screw to slip through this hole without contact and produces a gliding hole. A concentric hole of screw core diameter is drilled in the distal fragment. A countersink is used next to enlarge the proximal portion of the near cortex to accommodate the screw head adjacent to the gliding hole. A depth gauge is used to determine screw length. The distal hole is then threaded with a tap, the diameter of which is the same as the thread diameter of the screw. This hole is then known as the threaded hole (screws with self-tapping tips can eliminate this step). A screw of appropriate diameter and length is selected.

As the screw is introduced, it slides through the proximal gliding hole (Fig. 26–4), the head engages the countersunk area of the proximal cortex, the distal portion purchases the threaded hole, and compression is achieved. The screw should fasten the entire width of the distal cortex but should not exceed one full turn of the screw thread through it. This avoids attritional injury to adjacent soft-tissue structures. Tightening should be achieved by using a three-jaw chuck grip with the thumb, index, and middle fingers on the screw driver, using firm but not excessive force to achieve stable purchase without causing fracture. This sensory feedback technique of touch can be acquired as a part of a surgeon's training. Laboratory testing has shown that the torque generated is about 6 lbs.

■ FIGURE 26–4
A gliding hole is drilled in the proximal cortex and a threaded hole in the distal cortex. Note the seating of the screw head in the countersunk proximal cortex.[10]

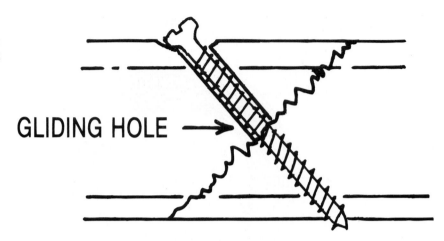

GLIDING HOLE ⟶

When space permits, more than two screws may be inserted to increase fracture stability. The maximum number of screws that may be inserted can be estimated by dividing the fracture length by the bone diameter at the fracture site. Fewer large-diameter screws can be used than small-diameter screws. The increased stability of an extra screw may be especially significant on a border digit (such as the index finger), which must sustain greater force due to both repetitive and forceful pinching and grasping. Screws should not be placed any closer to each other or to the fracture borders than three screw diameters. This avoids stress risers and consequent bone shattering.

In addition to the number of screws, the configuration of their placement is important to fracture stability. First, the fracture must be reduced anatomically. Some "preload" may be applied by reduction forceps. This force is transferred to or assumed by the lag screws.

A screw placed perpendicular to the long axis of bone provides the greatest resistance to shear fracture displacement.[1] Such a screw is called a neutralization screw. Although interlocking bony interstices at the fracture site may prevent shear and even rotational displacement, it is usually prudent to have at least one neutral screw to counteract these potential forces.

A screw applied perpendicular to the fracture has the greatest compressive force.[1] This screw is called a compression screw. After placing one neutralization screw, additional screws may be placed in compression. Two or more screws act to dissipate the rotational forces on the other.

Oblique, extraarticular proximal phalangeal fractures are the result of pure shearing forces and require one neutralization screw. Additional screws may be applied in the compression mode for maximum stability or as the fracture configuration permits (Fig. 26–5A and B).

In spiral fractures (due to a combination of shear and torsional forces), one or more points may be found along the fracture that allow the placement of a screw that is perpendicular to both the fracture and the long axis of the bone. A single screw satisfying both these requirements is an optimal screw. Additional screws may be placed in the compression mode for maximum fracture stability or as fracture and incisional circumstances allow (Fig. 26–6A and B).

Skin closure is accomplished with 4-0 or 5-0 nylon sutures. A soft, sterile, bulky conforming hand dressing is applied, with the hand and wrist in the position of function. If desired, a continuous passive motion machine is applied after surgery to decrease edema and pain. Alternatively, the hand and wrist may be functionally positioned and supported by one or more plaster splints. A sling is provided and the hand is initially kept elevated above the heart level. Gentle, active digital motion is allowed in the hand dressing when splints are used and appropriate therapy instituted when they are removed.

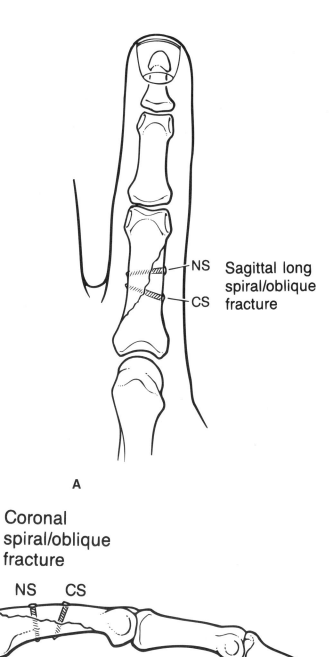

A

Coronal
spiral/oblique
fracture

B

■ FIGURE 26–5

A, A sagittal spiral oblique phalangeal fracture. The plane of the fracture requires dorsal screw insertion. **B**, A coronal oblique phalangeal fracture. The plane of this fracture allows screw insertion through a mid-axial incision. In both **A** and **B**, **CS** is the compression screw and **NS** is the neutral screw. Interdigitating fracture interstices complement fixation. Incision and screw placement may be adjusted to variations in the fracture between the coronal and the sagittal planes.

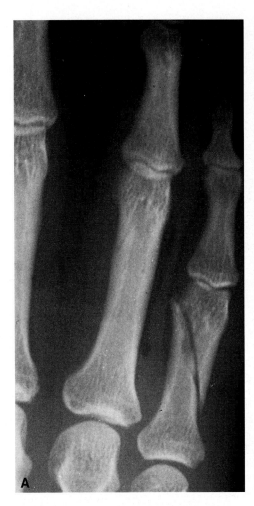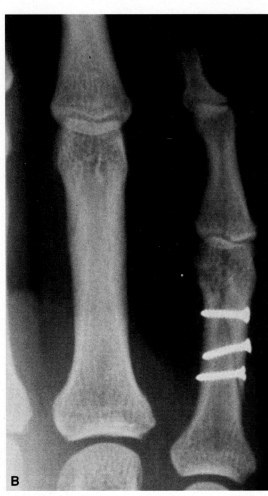

■ FIGURE 26–6
A, A radiograph of a displaced sagittal spiral oblique proximal phalangeal fracture demonstrates overriding of the fragments and shortening. **B**, The distal screw is an optimal screw. The two proximal screws are placed in the compression mode. A long fracture and smaller screws allows the placement of three screws on this border digit. Three screws, each inserted in the compression mode, allow maximum stability of the configuration and at least 50% more stability than two screws.

■ TECHNICAL
ALTERNATIVES

K-wire fixation is the standard against which other methods of internal fixation of displaced, unstable, spiral oblique phalangeal shaft fractures are measured. K-wires may be introduced through the skin and drilled directly into the bone after closed or indirect manipulative reduction. Although adjacent fracture reduction and sufficient stabilization are paramount, final functional outcome after proximal phalangeal fractures is perhaps even more directly correlated to adjacent soft-tissue damage and subsequent scarring. When applied transcutaneously, K-wires minimize soft-tissue trauma and this is their major advantage. In contrast, K-wires have no compressive force and little resistance to loosening. Loosening is related to motion and time and can be minimized by controlling motion during rehabilitation. Fortunately, the splinting effect of the wires is only required for 3 to 4 weeks. It should be kept in mind that K-wires must penetrate deep structures and may migrate, causing tendon irritation or rupture, skin irritation, and pin-tract infection.

Screw fixation also has potential pitfalls. First, it depends on sufficient bone mineralization. For patients with osteopenia, a larger screw size with wider threads and greater pitch may be necessary to obtain sufficient purchase. Furthermore, a screw may strip during application. When redirecting, redrilling, or the application of a larger screw does not provide sufficient fixation, adjunctive K-wire stabilization may be necessary or K-wires may be needed as a contingent or alternative method of internal fixation. Sometimes, traction, external fixation, or other methods of fracture immobilization may be necessary. Finally, a potential disadvantage of screw fixation may be the need for later removal but most implants may be left in place permanently with no adverse consequences.

The recovery of motion and prevention of contracture of the injured finger (especially the proximal interphalangeal [PIP] joint) are the principle goals of rehabilitation. When screws can be inserted without creating excessive scar, they offer a decided advantage over K-wires because they are more stable, allowing better pain control and more intensive rehabilitation. Firm fracture fixation with screws can also assure timely primary fracture healing and avoid the incorporation of adjacent soft tissues into external bony callus.

Rehabilitation is divided into artificial and overlapping stages. These include tissue healing, recovery of motion, and flexibility; increase in strength, power, and endurance; and finally, regained ability of the patient to perform activities of daily living, work, and recreation. While these steps are occurring, every effort must be made to prevent, control, and eliminate edema. Steps are also taken to minimize, soften, mobilize, and desensitize scar tissue.

We have found the early application of a dorsal wrist support splint with a metacarpophalangeal (MP) joint block, dorsal outrigger, rubber band, and sling distal to the PIP joint to be an important adjunct in the rehabilitation of proximal phalangeal fractures (Fig. 26–7A and B). The PIP joint extensors are weak and have a poor moment arm. The fracture brace described above assists the patient in recovering full finger extension, whereas the powerful finger flexors may work against it in the simultaneous recovery of finger flexion. This brace is usually applied 3 to 10 days after surgery. A light dressing secured by burn net allows finger flexibility while protecting the incision. The fracture brace is usually removed 3 ½ to 4 weeks after fracture fixation if full PIP joint extension has been achieved. If not, the brace is continued until this objective is accomplished or motion plateaus. At 6 weeks postoperatively, more intensive dynamic extension splinting of the PIP joint may be necessary to overcome residual flexion contracture.

In most cases, at 4 weeks, a wrist support splint is applied to properly position the wrist for optimal digital flexion and extension power. The injured finger can be buddy splinted to an adjacent finger to prevent snagging and to supplement motion. Splinting usually can be discontinued 6 to 8 weeks after injury and surgery. Efforts at progressively regaining

■ REHABILITATION

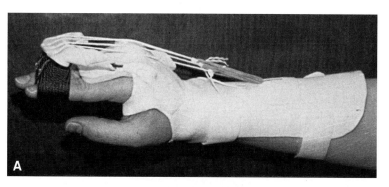

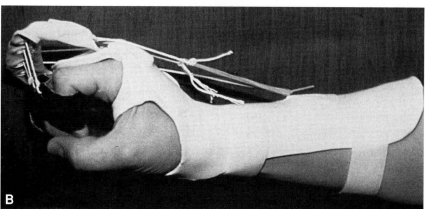

■ FIGURE 26–7
A, A standard dynamic fracture brace is used for rehabilitation after proximal phalangeal fracture fixation. The MP extension block allows the brace to give a dynamic extension assist to the PIP joint. **B**, Flexion exercises are initiated by the strong finger flexors.

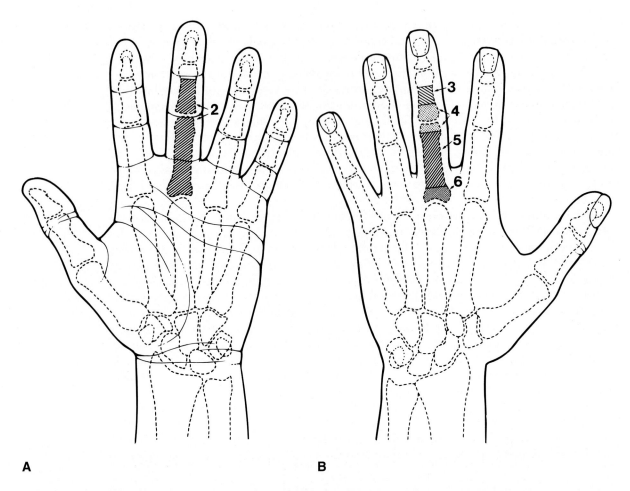

A   **B**

■ FIGURE 26–8

A, "No person's land" for hand fractures encompasses flexor tendon zone 2 and **B**, extensor zones 3 through 6.[6] (Reproduced with permission from Duncan RW, Freeland AE, Jabaley ME, Meydrech EF: Open hand fractures: an analysis of the recovery of active motion and of complications. J Hand Surg, 1993; 18A:387–95.)

strength, power, and endurance are then undertaken within the patient's pain and functional tolerance. An important guiding principle during rehabilitation is that the patient's condition not be aggravated by excessive effort. Returning to activities of daily living, work, and recreation are the final stages of rehabilitation and may be phased in—once again, according to the patient's tolerance and functional capabilities.

■ OUTCOMES

The tendency of the soft tissues about the proximal and middle phalanges to form scar has led some authors to refer to this as the "no person's land" of hand fractures (Fig. 26–8A and B).[2,4-6] Stiffness due to tendon adhesions, joint contracture, or a combination are the most frequent and serious complications of finger fractures. In 1976, Crawford reported encouraging results with the operative treatment of four spiral oblique proximal phalangeal fractures using screw fixation. Each of these four patients achieved a painless complete range of digital flexion and extension.[3] Subsequent authors[4,5,9] have reported that about 90% or more of their patients have recovered 70% or more of their digital motion after screw fixation. These included excellent results (recovery of 85% or more of total active digital range of motion) in 55 to 95% of patients. When loss of motion occurred, it most frequently was that of extension at the PIP joint. The functional mid-range of motion was preserved in these patients.

Up to 10% of patients had poor results (loss of 50% or more of total active digital range of motion). Usually this occurred in association with loosening of fixation and minor malunion (less than 10° angulation) during the rehabilitation and recovery period. Increasing soft-tissue injury (especially in the case of open fractures) and comminution (when present) were felt to have an adverse affect on final outcome as measured by total active digital motion. No nonunions or infections were reported. Aching and cold intolerance, when present, generally resolved after 1 year.

References

1. Arzimanoglon A, Skiadaresis SM: Study of internal fixation by screws of oblique fractures in long bones. J Bone Joint Surg, 1952; 34A:219–223.
2. Burkhalter WE: Closed treatment of hand fractures. J Hand Surg, 1989; 14A:390–393.
3. Crawford GP: Screw fixation for certain fractures of the phalanges and metacarpals. J Bone Joint Surg, 1976; 58A:487–492.
4. Dabezies EJ, Schutte JP: Fixation of metacarpal and phalangeal fractures with miniature plates and screws. J Hand Surg, 1986; 11A:283–8.
5. Diwaker HN, Stothard J: The role of internal fixation in closed fractures of the proximal phalanges and metacarpals in adults. J Hand Surg, 1986; 11B:103–108.
6. Duncan RW, Freeland AE, Jabaley ME, et al: Open hand fractures: an analysis of the recovery of active motion and of complications. J Hand Surg, 1993; 18A:387–95.
7. Eaton R, Hastings Hill II: Point/counterpoint: closed reduction and internal fixation versus open reduction and internal fixation for displaced oblique proximal phalangeal fracture. Orthopedics, 1989; 12:911–916.
8. Field LD, Freeland AE, Jabaley ME: Midaxial approach to the proximal phalanx for fracture fixation. Contemp Orthop, 1992; 25:133–137.
9. Ford DJ, El-Hadidi S, Lunn PG, Burke FD: Fractures of the phalanges: results of internal fixation using 1.5 mm and 2.0 mm AO screws. J Hand Surg, 1987; 12B:28–33.
10. Freeland AE, Jabaley ME, Hughes JL: Stable Fixation of the Hand and Wrist, New York: Springer-Verlag, 1986.
11. Freeland AE, Roberts TS: Percutaneous screw treatment of spiral oblique finger proximal phalangeal fractures. Orthopedics, 1991; 14:384–388.
12. Heim U, Pfeiffer KM: In collaboration with Meuli HC (eds): Small Fragment Set Manual. Technique recommended by the ASIF Group (Swiss Assoc for Study of Internal Fixation), New York: Springer-Verlag, 1974.
13. Littler JW: Hand, Wrist and Forearm Incisions. In: Littler JW, et al (eds): Symposium on Reconstructive Hand Surgery, St Louis: CV Mosby Co, 1974.
14. Peacock EE, Van Winkle W: Surgery and biology of wound repair, Philadelphia: WB Saunders, 1970:333.
15. Pratt DR: Exposing fractures of the proximal phalanx of the finger longitudinally through the dorsal extensor apparatus. Clin Orthop, 1959; 15:22–6.
16. Segmuller G: Surgical Stabilization of the Skeleton of the Hand, Baltimore: Williams and Wilkins, 1977.

27

Plate Fixation of the Diaphysis for Phalangeal Fractures

■ HISTORY OF THE TECHNIQUE

The earliest plates developed for fracture fixation were designed for the larger bones of the skeleton. It was not until the early 1970s that small plates suitable for phalangeal fracture fixation were introduced. Heim and co-authors described the proper technical application of many plates in the phalanges in their monograph entitled *The Small Fragment Set Manual*.[7] Subsequently, several clinical investigators described successful miniplate applications to the phalanges.[2,8] As the applications expanded, an awareness of limitations and complications also developed. As a result of this process, which has continued well into the 1980s, hand surgeons have gradually developed a clearer sense of the indications for plate fixation of the phalanges.[4]

■ INDICATIONS AND CONTRAINDICATIONS

The indications for plate fixation of middle and proximal phalangeal fractures should be approached conservatively. The application of miniplates usually requires additional dissection for adequate exposure and plate application. This has the potential to be significantly disadvantageous in the fingers, where both extensor and flexor tendons closely approximate bone, increasing the possibility that postoperative adhesions will limit long-term motion. In addition, most available plates are large relative to the bones to which they are affixed, making sizing and contouring of the plates a challenge. The relatively large size of the plates also implies that it is nearly impossible to access the bone for plate placement without mobilizing either flexor or extensor tendons, and the prominence of the plates after application has a tendency to deform the overlying tendons and disturb their excursion.

With these considerations in mind, it can be stated that the primary indication for plate fixation of a phalanx begins with the concept of fracture instability. Instability is defined as a fracture that cannot be reduced to a satisfactory position by closed means alone or when satisfactorily reduced, predictably will not remain in that position. Although most unstable phalangeal fractures can be fixed by alternative methods (such as percutaneous pinning, open reduction and pin fixation, or open reduction and screw fixation),[5] those phalangeal fractures with extensive diaphyseal comminution or a segmental loss of bone are difficult to stabilize with nonplating techniques. Comminuted phalangeal fractures, especially in the presence of bone loss, are therefore best suited to plate fixation. It is worth mentioning that because of the nature of the injury, these are often open fractures. Another unusual circumstance, in which instability may be an issue, is pathologic fractures. Plate fixation, however, would be appropriate only in a histologically proved benign lesion associated with a fracture.

Another circumstance in which plate fixation of a fracture may be indicated, even in the presence of less severe instability, is in association with flexor tendon lacerations (Fig. 27–1).[3] In this situation, early passive or even active metacarpophalangeal (MP) and proximal interphalangeal (PIP) joint motion is required for optimal outcome after the tendon repair. Plate fixation of the phalanges often provides the stability necessary for the appropriate rehabilitation program. When a hand surgeon also pursues a relatively vigorous motion program after extensor tendon injuries, specifically those in extensor zones 3 through 5, plate fixation of the phalanges can again be performed to facilitate rehabilitation.

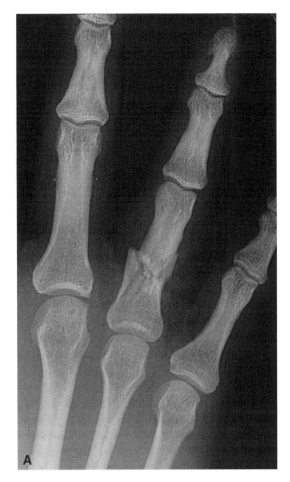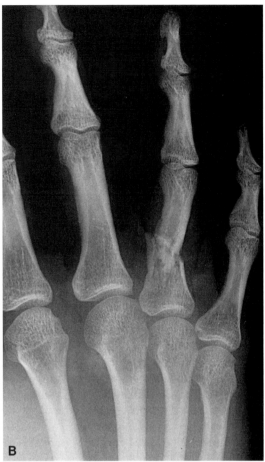

■ FIGURE 27–1

A, Posteroanterior and **B**, lateral radiographs of an open comminuted fracture of the diaphysis of the proximal phalange in a 42-year-old man. The fracture was open volarly and associated with laceration of the two flexor tendons.

Dorsal or dorsal lateral plating of the middle and proximal phalanges should be approached with different expectations. Dorsal plating of the proximal phalanx offers some interference with the extensor mechanism and can limit finger joint motion. Dorsal plating of the middle phalanx, however, inevitably interferes with the extensor mechanism. Plating of the middle phalanx should only be used in salvage procedures, wherein little distal interphalangeal joint motion is anticipated.[5]

The use of miniplates for phalangeal fixation is contraindicated for a variety of reasons. First, the appropriateness of less complex methods of fixation to stabilize the fracture should be excluded. Second, plates are indicated in the presence of more advanced, complex injuries; it must be determined, given all associated factors, that finger salvage rather than amputation is the most appropriate treatment for the patient. Third, the magnitude of comminution must not exclude the technical feasibility of building a stable construct; too much comminution excludes plate fixation. Finally, when the fracture is open and contaminated, it must be convertible to a clean wound before plate application. When this is not possible, an alternative approach to treatment is required.

The time required for this operation usually precludes the use of regional intravenous anesthesia; axillary blocks or general anesthesia are usually recommended. A pneumatic tourniquet is applied about the upper arm, the arm is exsanguinated, and the tourniquet

■ SURGICAL
TECHNIQUES

is inflated. The surgical approach is a longitudinal midline incision on the dorsum of the finger. It usually extends from the PIP joint distally to the MP joint proximally. It would be positioned more distally for fixation of the middle phalanx. The incision may have to be relatively long to allow mobilization of the skin and subcutaneous tissues volarward on both sides of the finger. In the case of open fractures, the laceration is incorporated into the longitudinal incision. The skin flaps are sewn volarly, using 4-0 nylon sutures.

This exposes the underlying dorsal apparatus. The interval between the contribution from the extensor digitorum communis and the "wing tendon" is identified. The dorsal apparatus is divided longitudinally along this interval. Adequate exposure often involves dividing the distal portion of the sagittal bands proximally and mobilization of the lateral band distally. The lateral band is retracted volarly during the bone fixation. Usually, the approach can be through either the medial or lateral aspect of the dorsal apparatus; seldom is an approach through both sides required. The choice of one side or the other depends on the anatomy of the fracture and should be planned preoperatively, based on radiographic features and the nature of the associated injuries.

The underlying periosteum is divided longitudinally and elevated from the bone to the minimal extent possible to allow plate application. The fracture hematoma is irrigated away and the fracture ends cleaned with small curettes. Small fragments of comminuted bone are set aside in saline. The fracture is then reduced, using interdigitations to judge the quality of the reduction. When the fracture fragments are reduced and well-aligned, the plate is applied. When possible, the plate is clamped in place, using small plate- or bone-holding clamps or a hemostat. Screws are then inserted, using the appropriate 1.5-mm drill, 2-mm tap, and 2-mm screws.

Whenever possible when applying plates, it is best to minimize the amount of soft-tissue release and mobilization required for plate and clamp application. If the application of plate-holding clamps is difficult secondary to limited soft-tissue exposure, the technique can be modified. After initially manually reducing and applying the plate, the location of the holes required for the screws can be marked through the plate holes. The reduction can then be displaced and the plate applied to one end of the bone alone. The bone-and-plate construct is then reduced to the other fragment, compression is applied, and the other end of the plate is applied. Although this method can require less soft-tissue dissection, it should be done only by surgeons with considerable experience in miniplate application.

After plate fixation, intraoperative fluoroscopy with spot films or plain posterolateral and lateral radiographs for confirmation of reduction and quality of hardware fixation are recommended.

After confirmation of reduction and fixation, the wounds are thoroughly irrigated. The periosteum is closed, to the extent possible, with 4-0 absorbable sutures. Similarly, the dorsal apparatus is closed using 4-0 absorbable sutures. The skin is closed using interrupted 5-0 or 6-0 nylon sutures. A dressing of Xeroform, fluffs, volar and dorsal apposition splints (to include the forearm, wrist, and to project over the fingers) is applied. The wrist should be immobilized in 30° of extension, the MP joints flexed 45°, and the interphalangeal joints positioned near 0°. If the long, ring, or small fingers are operated, they are all included in the postoperative dressing. If the index finger is operated, it is included with only the long finger in the postoperative dressings.

■ TECHNICAL
ALTERNATIVES

One of the pitfalls in miniplate application to the phalanges is the use of screws that are too long. Given dorsal or dorsal lateral plate application, the screws have the potential to project through the volar aspect of the bone. Because the flexor tendon closely approximates the volar surface of the bone, abrasion of the flexor tendon over time is possible, setting the stage for flexor tendon rupture. Prevention of volar screw projection can be minimized by careful measurement of screw hole depths, palpation of the volar surface of the bone with instruments after plate fixation, and careful review of intraoperative radiographs.

In the presence of a volar laceration and an open phalangeal fracture, especially when tendon or nerve repairs are planned, a volar approach to plate application may seem inviting. This strategy should be avoided because of the sheath disruption required for adequate exposure, plate bulk that interferes with flexor tendon gliding, and difficulties with surgical access if the plate later requires removal.

Very distal or proximal phalangeal fractures may not be amenable to standard miniplate applications because these plates may interfere with the joint capsule or ligaments. In these specific periarticular fractures, an alternative method of fixation using minicondylar plates may be appropriate.[1] They have the advantage of being placed laterally, minimizing interference with tendons, and can be used to fixate intraarticular components of the fracture. In fractures with slightly larger proximal or distal fragments, L-shaped or T-shaped plates may also be used.

In fractures with segmental loss or in comminuted fractures in which fragments are devitalized or irreducible, bone grafting may be of value. The decision to graft is made intraoperatively, after reduction and plate application. There are no specific guidelines for use in making the decision but I am more inclined to add bone graft than not. The dorsal aspect of the ipsilateral distal radius, between the second and third compartments just proximal to Lister's tubercle, is easily accessed as a donor site. The volume and quality of bone obtained from this site are appropriate for these phalangeal fractures.

The dressings are removed at 3 to 7 days postoperatively. When there is minimal swelling and the wounds are healing well, a forearm-based thermoplastic splint is fitted. The patient is started on active range of motion exercises, to be performed vigorously in nonoperated fingers and gently in the operated finger. This approach is continued until 4 weeks postoperatively. At that time, the forearm-based splint is exchanged for a hand-based thermoplastic splint and the patient started on more aggressive active motion exercises for the operated finger also. The splint is discontinued at 6 weeks postoperatively, and modified activities of daily living are allowed. The splint is continued for protection during more strenuous activities. Radiographs should be completed at about this time to confirm

■ REHABILITATION

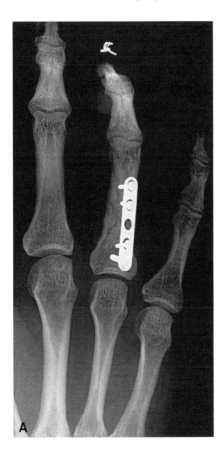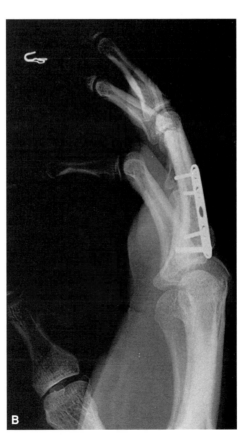

■ FIGURE 27–2
A, Posteroanterior and **B**, lateral radiographs after application of a four-hole AO miniplate. Primary bone grafting from the distal radius contributed to successful healing of the fracture.

bone healing (Fig. 27–2). At 8 weeks postoperatively, passive range of motion exercises into flexion and extension are added to the program. At 12 weeks postoperatively, the patient is returned to unrestricted activities. Additional modified therapy programs may be required, depending on residual impairments.

In the presence of associated soft-tissue injuries, such as flexor tenorrhaphies or digital neurorrhaphies, the therapy program must be modified. Generally, if the fracture fixation was stable, the rehabilitation required for the associated injury takes precedence over that for the fracture. For example, a patient who had an open reduction and internal fixation of a proximal phalanx along with a flexor digitorum profundus or flexor digitorum superficialis tenorrhaphy would be entered into a routine flexor tendon rehabilitation program, without regard for the phalangeal fracture.

■ OUTCOMES

The results of plate fixation of the phalanges are best judged in terms of union rates and the resulting active range of motion. The reported union rates for plated phalangeal fractures range from 83 to 100%.[6,9] Hastings[6] reported that all 11 plated phalanges in a larger series of internally fixed metacarpals and phalanges healed. When open fractures of comparable severity require additional soft-tissue exposure to achieve internal fixation, the range of motion is less than if the exposure is not required. There does not appear to be a difference among types of fixation, however, if stable fixation is achieved.[3]

The associated rates of nonunion, malunion, and infections are also important. Nonunion and malunion rates are about 15%.[9] The infection rates may be low because none are reported by Hastings[6] or by Stern and co-authors.[9] Plate removal from the phalanges is common, however. Plate removal may be required for either discomfort because of plate prominence or in association with other secondary procedures such as a tenolysis.

Although these analyses help to define expected results from the technique of plate fixation, there are other intangible features that are difficult to quantitate. It is not possible to quantitate the advantages that the stability of plate fixation brings to the care and rehabilitation of associated injuries, especially of the tendons and nerves. It is also difficult to compare the advantages of plate fixation with less stable methods of fixation in similar clinical circumstances. Although plate fixation of phalangeal fractures is rarely indicated and the successful use of the technique depends on considerable experience and careful preoperative planning, the technique can be valuable in treating selected phalangeal fractures.

References

1. Buchler U, Fischer T: Use of a minicondylar plate for metacarpal and phalangeal periarticular injuries. Clin Orthop, 1987; 214:53–58.
2. Dabezies EJ, Schulte JP: Fixation of metacarpal and phalangeal fractures with minimal plates and screws. J Hand Surg, 1986; 11A:283–288.
3. Duncan RW, Freeland AE, Jabaley ME, Meydrech EF: Open hand fractures: an analysis of the recovery of active motion and of complications. J Hand Surg, 1993; 18A:387–394.
4. Freeland AE, Jabaley ME, Hughes JL: Indications for Stable Fixation. In: Freeland AE, Jabaley ME, Hughes JL (eds): Stable Fixation of the Hand and Wrist. New York: Springer-Verlag, 1986:28–30.
5. Freeland AE, Jabaley ME, Hughes JL: Transverse and Short Oblique Phalangeal Fractures. In: Freeland AE, Jabaley ME, Hughes JL: Stable Fixation of the Hand and Wrist. New York: Springer-Verlag, 1986:84–89.
6. Hastings H II: Unstable metacarpal and phalangeal fracture treatment with screws and plates. Clin Orthop, 1987; 214:37–42.
7. Heim U, Pfeiffer KM, Meuli HC: Small Fragment Set Manual. New York: Springer-Verlag, 1974.
8. Melone CP: Rigid fixation of phalangeal and metacarpal fractures. Orthop Clin North Am, 1986; 421–435.
9. Stern PJ, Wieser MJ, Reilly DG: Complications of plate fixation in the hand skeleton. Clin Orthop, 1987; 214:59–65.

28

Pin Fixation of a Mallet Fracture

An understanding of the mechanisms and anatomy of a mallet finger with an intraarticular fracture injury helps to ensure success of surgical treatment. The generally accepted etiology of mallet finger or "baseball" finger is axial compression of the distal joint associated with sudden flexion of the distal phalanx against an actively functioning extensor tendon. This causes avulsion of a portion of the distal phalanx. Small fragments, as well as larger fragments, may show significant displacement (Fig. 28–1). Although the injury often occurs from a baseball striking the tip of the finger, it may also result from activities as innocuous as tucking in a bed sheet or retrieving an article from beneath a seat cushion. The extensor tendon pull is almost one and a third times the applied load in static equilibrium.

The mechanism of injury of intraarticular fracture of the interphalangeal joint of the thumb is similar to that of the distal interphalangeal (DIP) joint of the finger. Actually, the function of this joint in the thumb may be more important than that of the DIP joint and anatomic restoration more crucial. As in the finger, the deforming forces are the extensor pollicis longus on the fracture fragment and the flexor pollicis longus on the remaining distal phalanx. Literature on mallet thumb is limited and deals primarily with injuries of tendon origin.[2,7,10]

Mallet finger deformity with an intraarticular fracture of the distal phalangeal joint can be treated either operatively[6,12] or nonoperatively.[8,15] Since the earliest descriptions, operative treatments of this injury have been controversial. Watson-Jones wrote "preserve us from the proposals recently made of intramedullary fixation by pins driven through the pulp across the phalanges and interphalangeal joints."[14] Bunnell used this quotation while discussing a paper presented by Cassells at the Annual Meeting of the American Academy of Orthopaedic Surgeons in Chicago, Illinois, January 30, 1956. Subsequently, Cassells and coworkers[1] and Pratt and coworkers[11] published similar techniques within 3 months of each other in 1957.

The development of small, sharp K-wires (0.028-inch) and high-torque pneumatic drills have made operative treatment of these small fracture fragments more feasible. I have found that an open approach to the fracture through a dorsal H-shaped incision, with anatomic realignment of the dorsal cortex of the distal phalanx and pin fixation with two 0.028-inch K-wires, is a reliable approach for anatomic restoration of this intraarticular fracture.

In fractures of articular surfaces, anatomic reduction by surgery is usually required when displacement occurs to the extent that joint congruity is lost. The end joint in the finger, however, may be different because satisfactory finger function may be regained despite mild arthrosis or even fusion of the DIP joint. Although deformity of the joint may develop when joint congruity is not restored, reasonable fracture healing and joint alignment are still possible.

Indications for operative treatment presume that the surgeon is skilled in treating fractures of small bones. He or she must have loupe magnification available, access to a fully equipped surgical facility, and the technical expertise to successfully complete the procedure. Too often, mallet fractures and other injuries of the extensor mechanism are relegated to the most junior member of the surgical team, with suboptimal results.

The aforementioned problems aside, indications still include fracture involving more than 30% of the articular surface of the distal phalanx and some degree of joint subluxation.

■ HISTORY OF THE TECHNIQUE

■ INDICATIONS AND CONTRAINDICATIONS

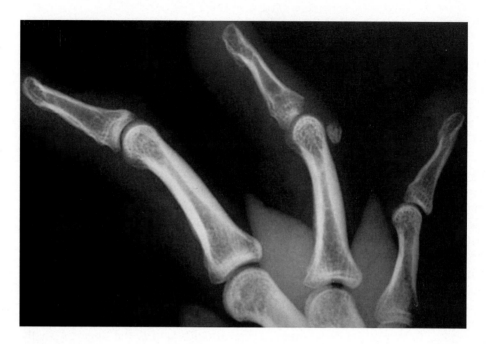

■ FIGURE 28–1
Displaced mallet fracture. The fragment, although relatively small, lies over the distal metaphysis of the middle phalanx.

The patients selected for operative treatment should demonstrate a need or desire for gaining full range of motion of the distal phalanx. They must fully understand that anatomic restoration of the joint will avoid the dorsal deformity that develops with mallet finger; however, a dorsal scar may remain. Although full extension is more likely with operative treatment, some degree of limitation in flexion of the DIP joint may occur.[6] The patient must be reliable and have a clear understanding of the goal of treatment: to restore anatomic position of the fracture. The patient must protect the delicate fixation for 4 to 6 weeks. Patients planning to return sooner than this to contact sports, strenuous activities, or manual labor should be treated nonoperatively.

■ SURGICAL
TECHNIQUES

Success in the operative treatment of displaced intraarticular fractures of the distal phalanx depends on several factors. First and foremost, the surgeon must have a clear understanding of the goal of the procedure and in-depth knowledge of the anatomy of the extensor mechanism and DIP joint. The procedure should be either performed or closely supervised by an experienced hand surgeon.

Digital block anesthesia using 2% lidocaine is most effective. The anesthetic is introduced either dorsally, between the metacarpal heads, or through a palmar approach with a 25-gauge needle (or smaller). The needle is introduced on the radial and ulnar sides of each digit directly over the neurovascular bundle, so that the proper digital nerves (or more proximally, common digital nerves) are fully anesthetized. Most importantly, the injection should also anesthetize the dorsal cutaneous branch as it supplies sensation to the area of the incision of the dorsal aspect of the DIP joint. Plain radiographs or image intensification must be available intraoperatively to evaluate the reduction and K-wire placement.

My preferred exposure[6] is through a dorsal H-shaped incision (Fig. 28–2). Dissection is carried through the dorsal subcutaneous tissue. Most of the dorsal veins must be sacrificed, although the more radial or ulnar veins may be saved. To avoid partial skin sloughing, flaps are mobilized deep to the epitenon of the extensor mechanism. These flaps should be held by stay sutures and the wound kept moist with saline or lactated Ringer's solution throughout the procedure. The dorsal 30% of the radial and ulnar collateral ligaments of the DIP joint are taken down to adequately mobilize the distal phalanx. At this point, loupe magnification of at least 2.5× power becomes valuable.

The secret to successful anatomic restoration of the fracture and subsequent restoration of function lies in leaving the extensor mechanism intact and attached to the fracture fragment of the distal phalanx. The joint is copiously irrigated, fracture fragments and

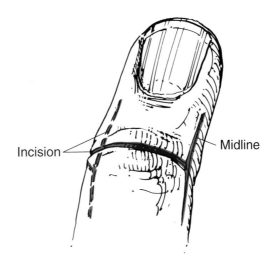

A dorsal H-shaped incision for adequate exposure of a mallet fracture. Note that the longitudinal extensions proximally and distally are at the axis of rotation of the DIP joint.

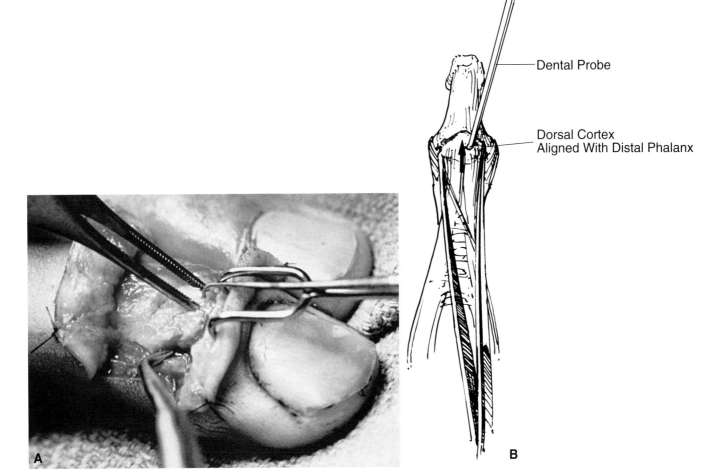

■ FIGURE 28-3

A, The surgical exposure showing the flaps mobilized deep to the epitenon of the extensor mechanism. The DIP joint is reduced and the fragment held in place while visualizing the dorsal cortex of the distal phalanx. The dorsal third of the collateral ligaments have been excised to facilitate exposure and reduction. **B**, A diagram indicates how the reduction is maintained by aligning the dorsal cortex of the distal phalanx.

hematoma evacuated, and reduction obtained by anatomic alignment of the dorsal cortex of the distal phalanx (Fig. 28–3A and B). Small instruments such as a dental probe, Freer elevator, and fine-tooth forceps are important in holding the reduction. Regardless of the size of the fracture fragment, a 0.028-inch K-wire is passed retrograde through the dorsal third of the fracture surface in the distal phalanx. This is done such that the wire passes through the distal phalanx just below the sterile matrix of the nailbed, avoiding the undersurface of the nail. The dorsal fragment is then held anatomically reduced, with the DIP joint in neutral position and the pin driven back across the fracture site, securing the fragment and the DIP joint. The second pin is then passed through the fragment into the distal phalanx, further stabilizing the fracture fragment (Fig. 28–4A and B). The surgeon usually has only one opportunity because multiple attempts at fixation result in comminution of the fragment, which further compromises any hope of stabilization.

In certain large fragments, the "kabob" technique, as described by Lister,[5] may be sufficient stabilization, without the need for the second K-wire. If the fracture fragment seems large for a 0.028-inch K-wire, a second wire should be added rather than using a larger wire. The second wire adds torsional stability and is less likely to "fracture" the fragment. Anatomic reduction of the fragments is verified by posteroanterior and lateral radiographs

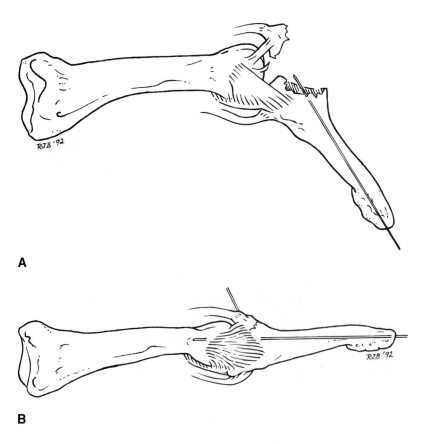

A

B

■ FIGURE 28–4

A and **B**, With the fracture site exposed on the articular surface of the distal phalanx, a 0.028-inch K-wire is passed retrograde through the dorsal third of the fracture surface of the distal phalanx. This is done carefully, such that the wire passes through the distal phalanx below the sterile matrix of the nailbed, avoiding the undersurface of the nail. The dorsal fragment is then held reduced anatomically with the DIP joint in neutral position. The pin is driven back across the fracture site, securing the fragment and the DIP joint, if possible. A second pin is then passed through the fragment into the distal phalanx, which further stabilizes the fracture fragment. If the fragment is not fixed by the first K-wire (Kabob technique), it is imperative that the second K-wire do so to maintain fracture stability.

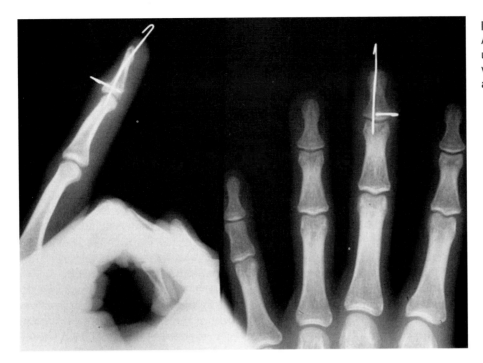

■ FIGURE 28–5
An anatomic reduction using 0.028-inch K-wires, verified by posteroanterior and lateral radiographs.

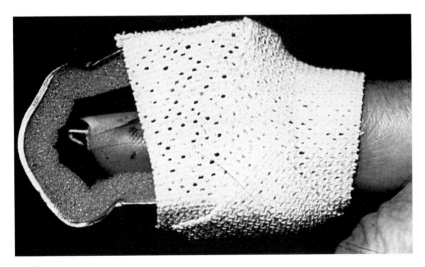

■ FIGURE 28–6
An alumafoam splint in which the foam is cut out over the dorsally placed 0.028-inch K-wire. Once the transarticular pin is removed, the splint may be removed intermittently to allow DIP joint flexion.

(Fig. 28–5); the skin is closed with nylon, and a bulky dressing with plaster splint is applied.

The splint immobilizes not only the DIP joint but extends across the wrist onto the forearm to neutralize the flexor musculature. The first dressing change should be made between 24 and 48 hours. At that time, a smaller alumafoam splint is applied to stabilize the DIP joint (Fig. 28–6).

Jupiter and Sheppard[10] have described the use of a tension band wire for fixation, Nunley and Urbaniak[9] the use of a small interfragmentary screw, and numerous authors the technique of a pull-out or intraosseous wire.[4] Although these procedures are technically possible, reproducibility may be difficult, the required exposure somewhat greater, and the risk of further fracture and comminution of the distal fragment significant. Stark and coauthors[12] report excellent results with internal fixation. Conversely, Wehbé and Schneider[15] strongly recommend closed treatment, with the only exception being a dorsal bump.

■ TECHNICAL
ALTERNATIVES

This nonoperative approach avoids the potential complications of infection, pin breakage, fragmentation of the fracture, and loss of reduction.

My experience is that open reduction and internal fixation with anatomic reduction results in full extension of the finger but often, between 10 and 20° of flexion at the DIP joint is lost.[6] Nevertheless, this technique allows maximum fracture stabilization, anatomic reduction, and less risk of fracture comminution.

Hamas and coworkers[3] described a technique in which the fracture fragment remains attached to the collateral ligaments and the extensor mechanism is divided transversely. This complicates fracture healing by introducing the undesirable problem of tendon healing. Stark recommends a dorsal lazy-S–shaped skin incision. A wider exposure is possible, however, through a dorsal H-shaped incision. This allows better visualization of the dorsal cortex and extends volar to the mid-axial line of the finger to permit the collateral ligaments to be mobilized. The dorsal skin flaps must be deep to the epitenon. If these flaps are too thin, skin sloughing of the corners is possible. An alternative is to make the dorsal flap triangular; however, a similar risk of sloughing exists at the tip or apex of the triangle.

■ REHABILITATION

Rehabilitation of operative treatment of mallet finger fracture begins with removal of the forearm-based splint. Active motion of the metacarpophalangeal and the proximal interphalangeal joints to the finger is crucial in preserving good finger and hand function and must be started early despite discomfort at the site of the surgical wound. At 4 to 6 weeks, once fracture healing has begun (as evidenced by minimal local tenderness at the site of the fracture), the transarticular K-wire may be removed, leaving the remaining K-wire to hold the fracture in place. Active DIP joint flexion may then be started with blocking of the joint. When 2 to 3 more weeks have elapsed, the remaining K-wire may be removed and more active motion begun with resistance. Should any degree of displacement or discomfort develop at this point, splinting should be immediately reinstituted. To avoid refracture, splinting should be continued for an additional 6 weeks at night and during strenuous activities to avoid refracture. Depending on the patient's progress, this program may or may not require the supervision of a hand therapist.

■ OUTCOMES

Multiple incisions and techniques have been described for fixation of intraarticular fractures of the distal phalanx. The basic principles of fracture management, as applied to intraarticular fractures, also apply to the DIP joint fracture.

Before proceeding with operative treatment of fractures of the DIP joint of the finger or interphalangeal joint of the thumb, the surgeon should carefully consider the goals of treatment. Is the patient compliant? Is the return of nearly normal function of the DIP joint or interphalangeal joint likely? Is it in the best interest of the patient? For example, a self-employed uninsured farmer who will be required to pay for his procedure may prefer conservative nonoperative treatment. Surgery would delay his return to gainful employment and the postoperative regimen may delay his return to work even longer. He may feel that being treated surgically is not in his best interest, particularly when reasonable results are possible with nonoperative treatment.[15]

Finally, is the surgeon comfortable with the technical expertise required, including being facile with loupe magnification and use of small surgical instruments similar to those required for a microsurgical procedure?

Stern and Kastrup[13] reviewed a large series of mallet fractures treated at several institutions near Cincinnati, Ohio. They found a relatively high incidence of osteomyelitis, loss of fracture fixation, and pin breakage. Their concerns are borne out by the concerns in this chapter. When the basic principles of fixation of intraarticular fractures are followed (i.e., anatomic restoration of joint congruity combined with early range of motion), normal or nearly normal joint range of motion is possible.[6,12]

References

1. Cassells SW, Strange TB: Intramedullary wire fixation of mallet finger. J Bone Joint Surg 1957; 39A(3):521–526.
2. Din KM, Meggitt BF: Mallet thumb. J Bone Joint Surg 1983; 65B(5): 606–607.

3. Hamas RS, Horrell ED, Pierret GP: Treatment of mallet finger due to intra-articular fracture of the distal phalanx. J Hand Surg 1978; 3(4):361–363.
4. Jupiter JB, Sheppard JE: Tension wire fixation of avulsion fractures in the hand. Clin Orthop 1987; 214:113–120.
5. Lister GD: The Hand Diagnosis and Indication, Edinburgh: Churchill Livingstone, 1984:48.
6. Lubahn JD: Mallet finger fractures: a comparison of open and closed technique. J Hand Surg 1989; 14A(2):394–396.
7. Miura T, Nakamura R, Torii S: Conservative treatment for a ruptured extensor tendon on the dorsum of the proximal phalanges of the thumb (mallet thumb). J Hand Surg 1986; 11A(2): 229–233.
8. Niechajev IA: Conservative and operative treatment of mallet finger. Plast Reconstr Surg 1985; 76(4):580–585.
9. Nunley J, Urbaniak J: Treatment of Extensor Tendon Injuries of the Hand. In: Orthopaedic Surgery Updates Series, Vol 2/Lesson 12, Princeton, NJ: Continuing Professional Education Center, Inc, 1982:2–7.
10. Patel MR, Lipson L-B, Desai SS: Conservative treatment of mallet thumb. J Hand Surg 1986; 11A(1):45–47.
11. Pratt DR, Bunnell S, Howard LD: Mallet finger. Classification and methods of treatment. Am J Surg 1957; 93:573–579.
12. Stark HH, Gainor BJ, Ashworth CR, Zemel NP, Rickard TA: Operative treatment of intra-articular fractures of the dorsal aspect of the distal phalanx of digits. J Bone Joint Surg 1987; 69A(6):892–896.
13. Stern PJ, Kastrup JJ: Complications and prognosis of treatment of mallet finger. J Hand Surg 1988; 13A(3):329–334.
14. Watson-Jones R: Fractures and Joint Injuries. Vol. II. 4th ed. Baltimore, Williams & Wilkins, 1955.
15. Wehbé MA, Schneider LH: Mallet fractures. J Bone Joint Surg 1984; 66A(5):658–669.

29

Screw Fixation for Unicondylar Fracture of the Phalanges

■ HISTORY OF THE TECHNIQUE

Intraarticular unicondylar fractures of the distal aspect of the proximal phalanx are common injuries in young, athletic patients.[7,8] This fracture pattern can also be seen in the distal portion of the middle phalanx, although far less frequently. Historically, these injuries have been treated by a variety of protocols, including conservative splint management, closed reduction and percutaneous pin fixation, and open reduction with pin or screw fixation.[8] Several studies have highlighted the propensity of unicondylar fractures to displace with closed treatment.[2,8] Combined with the heightened awareness of secondary degenerative joint changes in nonanatomically reduced fractures, this has led to a more aggressive treatment protocol over the last several decades.[1-8] The introduction of miniscrews to the armamentarium of the hand surgeon has provided the opportunity for stable and rigid internal fixation of these inherently unstable fractures for appropriate joint surface reduction and early range of motion. Despite these advantages, screw fixation of unicondylar fractures is demanding, having little room for error because of the small size of the fracture fragments.

■ INDICATIONS AND CONTRAINDICATIONS

Nondisplaced unicondylar fractures (as documented by anteroposterior, lateral, and oblique radiographs) represent a relative indication for open reduction and internal fixation using miniscrews because of the high propensity for these fractures to displace. Alternatively, nondisplaced fractures may be treated with splinting if careful follow-up is performed. Any displacement at the fracture site (1 mm or more) or any open fracture represent absolute indications for open reduction with stable internal fixation (Fig. 29–1). The use of a miniscrew for fracture fixation is appropriate if the fragment is large enough to accept the screw without danger of fragment comminution. Any fracture fragment having a length of more than 1 cm is generally amenable to screw fixation. Four classes of fracture pattern have been described, of which classes I and II are appropriate for screw fixation. Class III and IV fractures are more appropriately treated by K-wire fixation or intraosseous wire techniques (Fig. 29–2).

■ SURGICAL TECHNIQUES

A bloodless field is essential for screw fixation of unicondylar fractures and is best accomplished by axillary block or general anesthesia with exsanguination and the use of a pneumatic tourniquet on the involved extremity. Either of two different surgical approaches, lateral or dorsal, can be appropriate, depending on the anatomy of the fracture. If the fracture fragment is large, having little or no comminution at the articular surface, a mid-axial or lateral incision provides excellent exposure and minimal disruption of the extensor and flexor tendons.[1] The incision should be at least 3 cm in length, with two thirds proximal to the proximal interphalangeal flexion crease and a third distal. This incision should be on the side of the finger that contains the fracture fragment. Dissection is done using a knife through the subcutaneous tissues over Cleland's ligament, which is released, and the extensor hood mechanism is retracted dorsally (Fig. 29–3A). This approach provides excellent exposure of the proximal phalanx, fracture fragment, and collateral ligaments. Injury to the digital neurovascular bundle volarly and the extensor hood mechanism dorsally should be avoided on exposure.

If any comminution exists at the joint surface, a dorsal approach provides a more effective means of joint reduction. A straight longitudinal incision in the midline of the finger

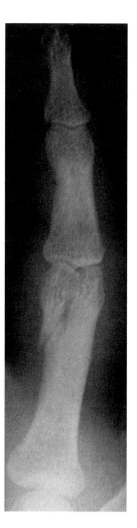

■ FIGURE 29–1
Posteroanterior radiograph, showing a displaced unicondylar fracture of the proximal phalanx.

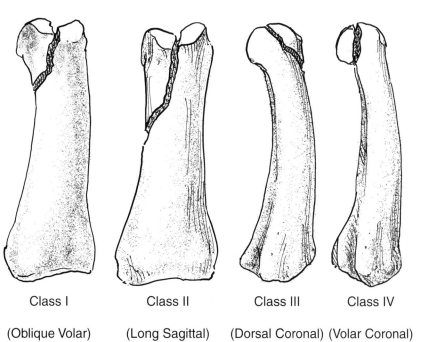

■ FIGURE 29–2
The four patterns of distal unicondylar fractures, demonstrating that class I and II fractures are particularly amenable to operative screw fixation.

Class I	Class II	Class III	Class IV
(Oblique Volar)	(Long Sagittal)	(Dorsal Coronal)	(Volar Coronal)

■ FIGURE 29–3
A, Optimal distal screw placement at the area just proximal to the collateral ligament origin. Screw orientation should be from perpendicular to the shaft axis to a line slightly proximal in alignment. **B**, The screw head should be counter-sunk and a second screw (or K-wire) placed proximally, space permitting, to aid in rotational control.

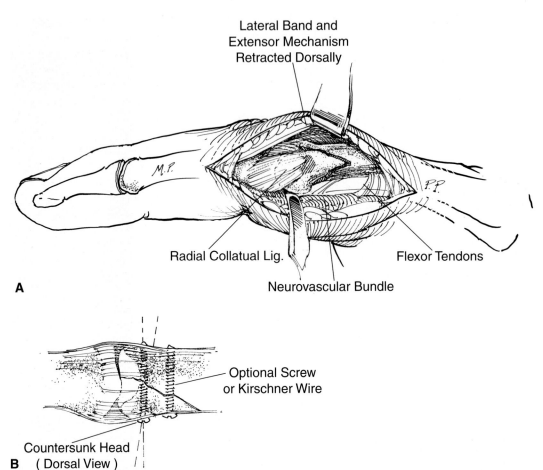

Lateral Band and
Extensor Mechanism
Retracted Dorsally

M.P.

P.P.

Radial Collatual Lig.

Neurovascular Bundle

Flexor Tendons

A

Optional Screw
or Kirschner Wire

Countersunk Head
B   (Dorsal View)

is performed and should be at least 3 cm in length. Most of the incision should be proximal to the dorsal proximal interphalangeal (PIP) joint crease because distal exposure is limited by the central slip insertion in the deep plane. Using a knife, the extensor tendon is split in the midline. Excellent exposure to the fracture is obtained by this technique and it allows adequate reduction under direct visualization. Placement of screws using this exposure is more difficult because of impingement from the retracted extensor tendon mechanism. This disadvantage is outweighed in patients who have a comminuted intercondylar articular surface because reconstruction can be done under direct vision.

The next step in this operation is fracture reduction and the placement of screws. The use of a low-radiation minifluoroscopy unit can greatly aid in this technique. With large fracture fragments, using the lateral approach, at least two 1.5-mm diameter miniscrews can generally be placed from the fracture fragment into the proximal phalangeal shaft using a standard lag technique with overdrilling of the near cortex. The fracture surfaces should be cleared of clot or callus. An indirect reduction technique of the joint can usually be accomplished through this approach without great difficulty. Reduction may be maintained by a tenaculum clip or by a small K-wire (always less than 1 mm in diameter in case a screw must be placed through the same tract). Intraoperative radiographic confirmation of reduction should be undertaken before placement of any screws. Because of the overlying extensor hood, efforts should be made to avoid any prominence of the screw head. For this reason, slight countersinking of the screw heads is appropriate and angulation of the screw should not be excessive. Because of the normal fracture plane orientation, slight proximal angulation of the screw is appropriate because it provides better interfragmentary compression. When the fracture fragment is too small to safely place two screws, one screw should be centrally placed just proximal to the origin of the collateral ligament and augmentation of fixation should be undertaken, if possible, with a supplementary K-wire to aid in rotational stability. The K-wire should be cut flush with the bony surfaces. This central screw is crucial for rigid fixation and should be placed with extreme care. When the size of the fracture fragment permits, a second screw is then placed proximally, taking care to not comminute the fragment further, providing additional rotational control (Fig. 29–3B). The minifluoroscopy unit can then be used intraoperatively to confirm reduction and fixation (Fig. 29–4).

In fractures having intercondylar comminution, appropriate joint debridement should be performed before fragment reduction. If any significant gap (more than 1 mm) exists, bone graft augmentation should be performed to provide resistance to compression during the screw fixation for appropriate joint reconstitution. A reduction clamp or temporary K-wire is placed to maintain the reduction. With careful retraction of the extensor tendon hood, a transverse screw is placed in the same manner as was previously described. A second screw or K-wire should then be placed proximally to aid in rotational control. If the bone graft placed in the intercondylar notch does not support compression, the screw should be placed in a nonlag fashion to avoid inappropriate excessive joint compression and narrowing.

Wounds in either exposure are copiously irrigated with normal saline and closed. The advantage of the lateral technique is that no repair of the extensor tendon mechanism is required. The skin is closed using a 5-0 interrupted nylon suture and a horizontal mattress technique. With the dorsal approach, a tight tendon closure using interrupted figure-of-eight 4-0 nonabsorbable sutures should be employed. Because early range of motion is always initiated, it is important that the tendon repair have closely spaced sutures, so that postoperative dehiscence of the tendon does not occur. With the longitudinal incision and an appropriate repair, early motion does not lead to tendon problems and most likely

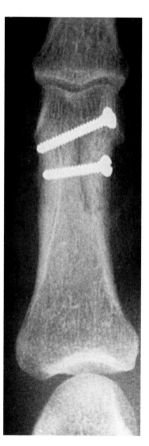

■ FIGURE 29–4
Posteroanterior radiograph, demonstrating placement of a 1.5-mm screw just proximal to the collateral ligament origin and with slight proximal angulation, aiding in interfragmentary compression.

reduces secondary adhesions. A sterile bulky dressing with fluffs placed between the fingers is generally applied in the immediate postoperative period, and early range of motion exercises (both active and passive) are begun as soon as postoperative soft-tissue swelling is reduced (generally 5 to 7 days). Careful elevation of the hand is important in the immediate postoperative period because of the propensity of swelling around the PIP joint.

■ TECHNICAL
ALTERNATIVES

An excellent alternative technique during the dorsal approach is to use an incision in the extensor mechanism between the central extensor tendon and the lateral band. This approach, used on the side of the central extensor tendon that contains the fracture fragment, allows easier placement of the transverse screw during fracture fixation. It also provides the advantage of not disrupting the central extensor tendon itself. Its disadvantage lies in not providing the same amount of exposure to the intercondylar notch that can be accomplished using a tendon-splitting approach.

Some surgeons favor transfixing the fracture fragment by placing the screw from the intact cortex into the fracture fragment itself. This technique does not allow indirect reduction of the joint surface by cortical alignment and requires a significant degree of preoperative reduction to avoid significant screw protrusion through the fragment. The exposure using this technique is somewhat easier because of the relative lack of trauma from the fracture but is generally outweighed by the difficulty in obtaining fracture alignment.

An alternative technique for fracture fixation is the use of multiple K-wires. This technique imparts less rigidity to fracture fixation, which can be improved by using three or more wires, and provides fixation with frequently less soft-tissue dissection and trauma. Excellent functional results, with little risk of loss of reduction, can be obtained using this method and may frequently be superior to those using screw fixation.

The major pitfalls in screw fixation of unicondylar fractures can be avoided with careful technique. Placement of the distal screw should always be just proximal to the origin of the collateral ligament. If a screw is placed in the collateral ligament itself, the collateral ligament may lose some of its normal excursion, inhibiting postoperative range of motion. Any toggle of the drill bit should be avoided because fixation of the fracture fragment relies on one cortex per screw. If excessive toggle occurs during drilling, little bony "thread" is cut by the tap, resulting in poor interfragmentary compression and in the worst cases, loss of fixation of the screw. The proximal screw should be tightened gently because its placement at the sharp apex of the fracture fragment can impart secondary splitting if the screw is overly tightened. Screws should be placed close to a perpendicular line from the axis of the phalanx. Slight angulation of the screw in a proximal direction aids in interfragmentary compression, although overangulation results in a prominent screw head and inhibition of extensor tendon mechanism glide.

■ REHABILITATION

With appropriate stable fixation of unicondylar fractures, active and passive range of motion under the supervision of a hand therapist may be initiated as soon as soft-tissue swelling has resolved (generally 5 to 7 days). Passive motion should be gentle and not overly aggressive for the first 3 weeks. A protective molded plastic splint should be made by a hand therapist, immobilizing the metacarpophalangeal (MP), PIP, and distal interphalangeal (DIP) joints (hand-based). The splint should be worn at all times, except during range of motion exercises. This type of splint allows wound care and edema control measures to be performed concurrently. Edema control using techniques such as Coban (3M, St. Paul, MN) wrapping aids in improving range of motion by reducing soft-tissue motion impingement. Sequential radiographs should be taken on a weekly basis for 3 weeks in the postoperative period to ensure that rehabilitation is not causing any fracture fragment displacement. Protective splinting should be full time for 4 weeks and then used during sleep or with manual activities thereafter until the fracture is completely healed.

■ OUTCOMES

Intraarticular unicondylar fractures of the proximal phalanx have a high propensity for PIP joint stiffness despite appropriate screw fixation and anatomic reduction. A total active arc of motion at the PIP joint of about 80° is the average in patients undergoing this type of fixation.[8] The patient should be warned that some loss of motion should be expected; it is only the rare patient who attains a normal range of motion after sustaining this type of fracture pattern. Patients rarely lose any significant degree of MP joint motion but an occasional patient has DIP joint stiffness. Generally, this DIP joint loss of motion is not functionally significant, with most of the impairment in the digit coming from secondary PIP joint motion loss.

The infection rate from this procedure is low, regardless of the fixation method used. The propensity for developing an infection late in treatment, however, would be greater in those patients who undergo fracture fixation using percutaneous K-wires. Nevertheless, with appropriate pin care in a vigilant patient, this risk is relatively minimal. Fixation failure of the fracture fragment is frequently noted when only one K-wire is used for the definitive reduction.[8] In all cases, an attempt should be made to obtain multi–K-wire fixation when this treatment method is used. The use of a single screw for fracture fixation does not appear to have an increased incidence of fracture fixation failure.[8] Despite this observation, augmentation of single screw fixation with a second K-wire adds to fracture stability.

Few data are available on the incidence of secondary posttraumatic arthritis occurring at the PIP joint. Generally, when appropriate reduction is obtained, significant problems with secondary arthritis do not appear to occur in the first few years after fracture fixation.[8] This observation may be consistent with future long-term results because the fracture line courses through the intercondylar notch, a relatively protected area relative to joint forces. Further long-term follow-up studies are needed to determine the exact incidence of late posttraumatic arthritis is in this injury.

References

1. Barton NJ: Fractures of the hand. J Bone Joint Surg, 1984; 66B:159–167.
2. Bloem JJAM: The treatment and prognosis of uncomplicated dislocated fractures of the metacarpals and phalanges. Arch Chir Neerl, 1971; 23:55–65.
3. Brown PW: The management of phalangeal and metacarpal fractures. Surg Clin North Am, 1973; 53:1393–1437.
4. Hastings HH II, Carrol C IV: Treatment of closed articular fractures of the metacarpophalangeal and proximal interphalangeal joints. Hand Clin, 1988; 4:503–527.
5. Kilbourne BC: Management of complicated hand fractures. Surg Clin North Am, 1968; 48: 201–213.
6. London PS: Sprain and fractures involving the interphalangeal joints. Hand, 1971; 3:155–158.
7. McCue FC, Honner R, Johnson MC Jr, Gieck JH: Athletic injuries of the proximal interphalangeal joint requiring surgical treatment. J Bone Joint Surg, 1970; 52-A:937–955.
8. Weiss APC, Hastings HH II: Distal unicondylar fractures of the proximal phalanx, J Hand Surg, 1993; 18A:594–599.

RICHARD L. UHL
WILLIAM F. BLAIR

30

Open Reduction and Internal Fixation of Proximal Interphalangeal Joint Fracture Dislocations

■ HISTORY OF THE TECHNIQUE

Fracture dislocations of the proximal interphalangeal (PIP) joint are difficult to treat, and the outcome following such an injury can be somewhat unpredictable.[15] The injury is usually caused by hyperextension at the PIP joint, often during sports.[6] In mild hyperextension injuries, the volar plate starts to tear from the base of the middle phalanx, sometimes taking a small fleck of bone with it. In the more significant fracture dislocation, a large fragment is avulsed from the base of the middle phalanx. Attached to this fragment is the volar plate and most of the collateral ligament structure. The central extensor tendon remains attached to the middle phalanx, pulling it into the dorsal, dislocated position.[4]

Early attempts at open reduction were considered unsatisfactory because of difficulty with joint exposure and fracture stabilization, and closed treatment was advocated.[8,10,11] Wilson and Rowland[15] later presented a series of 15 PIP fracture dislocations treated by open reduction and internal fixation (ORIF). Their method consisted of a midlateral approach, detachment of the collateral ligaments, volar plate, and, occasionally, the dorsal capsule, and even the central slip of the extensor. The fracture fragments were pinned using a small Kirschner wire, with an additional wire inserted across the PIP joint, if needed. In delayed cases, they advocated an intraarticular osteotomy to restore the joint surface. The fingers were immobilized 4 to 8 weeks after surgery to allow the fractures and repaired tissues to heal.

Dray and Eaton[4] advocated a volar approach, with careful handling of the flexor tendons. This approach has the advantage of allowing access to both sides of the joint, and leaves the extensor mechanism undisturbed. With the development of the miniscrew, fractures without comminution could be secured with a single screw, inserted using the volar approach.[5]

Properly performed, the volar approach provides excellent visualization of the fracture and adequate space for insertion of wires or a miniscrew for fracture fixation. Preservation of the important flexor sheath allows early postoperative motion.

■ INDICATIONS AND CONTRAINDICATIONS

Following a hyperextension injury to the PIP joint, radiographs in two planes are essential for diagnosis and treatment planning. The injury is commonly best seen on the lateral radiograph (Fig. 30–1).

If the PIP joint is stable after closed reduction, then usually at least a portion of the collateral ligament remains attached to the base of the middle phalanx. These injuries are ordinarily best treated by closed means.[4,6,15] If the joint is unstable only in full extension, then prevention of extension by the use of a dorsal block splint or wire will allow early flexion while keeping the joint reduced.[1,9,14] None of these closed methods directly align the articular surface.

Open reduction and internal fixation is indicated when the joint remains subluxed after closed reduction or when the volar fragment represents a major portion (40%) of the articular surface and does not reduce by closed means.[4–6,15] Open injuries should be treated

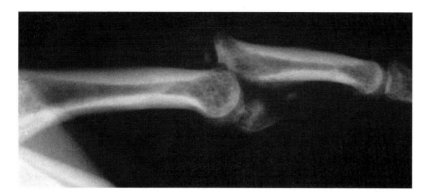

■ FIGURE 30-1
Lateral radiograph of a 26-year-old man who injured his finger while catching a basketball. There is a dorsal dislocation of the PIP joint with a large volar lip fracture.

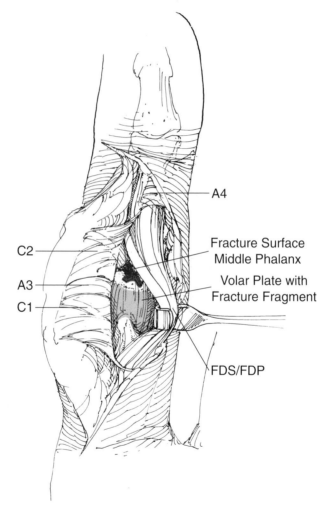

■ FIGURE 30-2
The flexor tendon sheath is mobilized, and the flexor tendons are retracted. This exposes the volar plate, which is attached to the fracture fragment.

with irrigation and debridement, but do not necessarily require ORIF if stable after reduction.[4]

This procedure is best performed under regional or general anesthesia. A tourniquet is used to provide a bloodless surgical field.

■ SURGICAL
TECHNIQUES

We recommend the volar approach. This provides access to both sides of the joint and allows fixation (whether screw or pin) to safely be inserted perpendicular to the fracture plane.[4,5,15] The flexor sheath is approached using a volar zigzag (Brunner) incision. The skin flaps are carefully elevated from the underlying flexor sheath and sewn back. The PIP joint lies beneath the A3 pulley and the volar lip fragment is just distal to this. The sheath is opened by making a transverse incision at the distal edge of the A2 pulley, and a second transverse incision is made just proximal to the A4 pulley. The portion of the sheath containing the C1, A3, and C2 pulleys is then elevated from its ulnar border and hinged on the radial border. This exposes the flexor tendons.

The flexor tendons are retracted with a small retractor or small rubber drain to expose the volar plate (with the lip fragment attached) and the fracture site (Fig. 30–2). Releasing the distal corners of the volar plate from the fracture fragment allows the fracture site to be better exposed. The fracture site is then cleared of small fragments and hematoma.

The joint is then reduced by gentle flexion and longitudinal traction. A soft "clunk" is often felt as the joint is reduced. Traction is then released, and the joint is allowed to redislocate. The reduction maneuver is repeated, and the soft "clunk" is again appreciated. This sequence accomplishes one of the most important steps in this operation—the confirmation of joint reduction.

With the joint reduced, a 0.035- or 0.045-inch wire is inserted dorsally from distal to proximal, across the dorsal aspect of the PIP joint. The wire can either transfix the joint or function as a dorsal block. At this stage in the procedure, radiographic confirmation of joint reduction is mandatory. This is most easily done with a quality image intensifier. Reduction of the joint, and not the fracture, should be confirmed by the concentric appearance of the joint surfaces.

If the volar fragment is large and not comminuted, a single 2.0-mm screw can be used to fix the fragment.[5] More commonly, the fragment is small or comminuted, and fixation with a single screw would not be sufficient. We prefer the use of small, smooth wires (0.028 inches), inserted from volar to dorsal. The flexor tendons are first pulled to one side, allowing access to one corner of the fracture fragment. The fragment is manipulated into place using the tip of a tissue forceps. Once the fragment is reduced, the first wire is inserted. The flexor tendons are then pulled in the other direction, the reduction checked, and the second wire inserted. Although the pins can be inserted parallel, the geometry of the exposure makes it easier to direct the pins slightly toward the midline (Figs. 30-3A

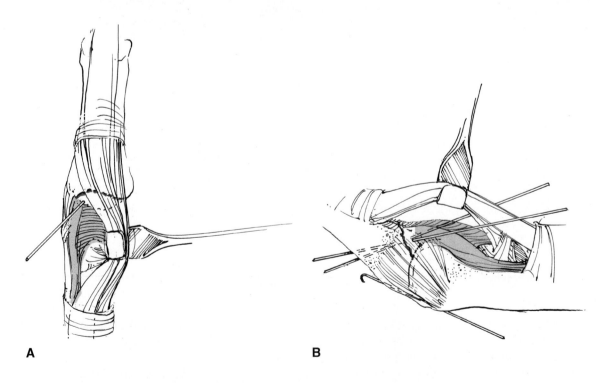

A   B

■ FIGURE 30–3
A and B, After inserting a pin dorsally to prevent the PIP joint from subluxing dorsally, the fracture is reduced. It is pinned with two small K-wires.

and 30-3B). The crossing of the pins also helps keep the volar fragment from pulling away.

Once inserted, the wires are then pulled from dorsally, until the tips are flush with the surface of the fragment. Cutting the tip of the wire, before it is brought flush with the volar fragment, will widen the end slightly and increase the holding power within the small fragment.

Intraoperative confirmation of joint and fragment reduction as well as pin placement is again checked using an image intensifier (Figs. 30-4A and 30-4B). All pins are then bent,

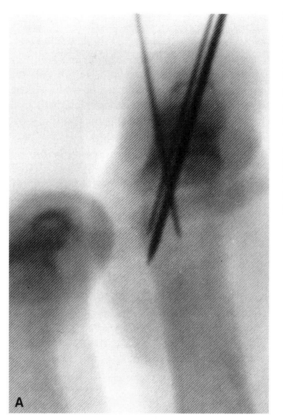

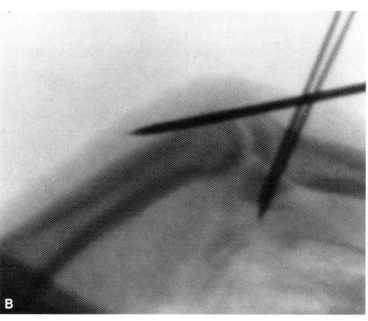

■ FIGURE 30–4
A, Intraoperative PA fluoroscopic image shows the wires crossing to hold the fragment. **B,** An intraoperative lateral fluoroscopic image shows reduction of the PIP joint (held with a dorsal pin) and reduction of the volar lip fracture (held with 2 smaller crossed pins, inserted volarly, and brought out dorsally).

cut, and left out through the skin. The window made in the flexor sheath is closed using interrupted 5-0 absorbable sutures. The skin is closed, and a bulky dressing and protective splint is applied.

■ TECHNICAL
ALTERNATIVES

Early attempts to treat PIP fracture dislocations by splinting in extension resulted in several associated complications, including finger joint stiffness, continued subluxation, joint disruption, and skin necrosis from the splint application.[10] Treatment in extreme flexion will reduce the joint and fracture fragment[11] but may result in a fixed flexion contracture.[7,8,13] The fracture fragments and joint subluxation can be controlled by skeletal traction, but the techniques are cumbersome, and the articular surface is not precisely aligned with these closed methods.[1,10] Other procedures designed to facilitate motion, such as extension block splinting and the use of a dorsal extension block wire, can produce a good end result, in the right type of injury.[9,14]

Often, the degree of comminution can only be appreciated once the fracture site is exposed. The fracture should be approached volarly as described and evaluated. If the fragment is comminuted, volar plate arthroplasty (VPA) may be a better treatment choice then ORIF.[4] Similarly, if the lip fragment becomes comminuted after attempting ORIF, the procedure can be converted to VPA since the volar plate has been preserved with this approach. Other surgical approaches do not provide this alternative.[5,15]

A comminuted volar lip also can be replaced with a homograft, but the long-term results of this technically difficult method are unknown.[3] Injuries in which the entire base of the middle phalanx is crushed (pilon fractures) are occasionally treated by ORIF, but often may do better with traction or external fixation.[12]

Late cases in which the fracture has healed are probably best treated with excision of the fragments and volar plate arthroplasty,[4] although osteotomy of the volar lip has been described.[15]

■ REHABILITATION

Early motion, with the proper precautions, is essential in the rehabilitation of this injury. Instituting motion depends on the fixation technique. If screw fixation alone was possible, supervised motion can be started on the first postoperative day.[5] When the dorsal pin is used as an extension block, flexion is started at 10 days. If the dorsal pin transfixes the joint, the start of active flexion must be delayed until the dorsal pin is removed at 4 weeks.

At the first postoperative visit, the protective splint is removed, and a hand-based thermoplastic splint is applied. The splint is removed regularly for gentle, active range of motion exercises at 10 days or 4 weeks depending on the dorsal pin technique. The crossed pins holding the volar lip fragment are usually removed at 6 weeks. After removal, the splint is discontinued and the joint protected by buddy taping. More aggressive range of motion exercises, using both joint isolation and composite motion techniques, are encouraged. Active assisted and passive flexion exercises are started at 8 weeks after surgery. If the recovery of motion is progressing slowly, the use of dynamic orthoses may begin at 10 weeks after surgery. It may take up to 12 months to regain full motion at the PIP joint following this injury.

■ OUTCOMES

Fracture dislocations of the PIP joint are serious injuries. The final outcome depends on reduction of the dislocation, restoration of the articular surface, rehabilitation,[15] but most importantly on the initial injury itself.[2] Fractures that are not comminuted, which can be more readily restored, will do better than those in which the articular surface is comminuted.

The outcome for ORIF of the PIP fracture dislocation is not well described in the literature. The final motion in the 15 patients in Wilson and Rowland's series[15] averaged 12° to 86°, with 6 patients having postoperative pain. The two patients reported by Green and co-authors[5] averaged 3° to 98°. Similar final motion has been obtained in our experience. In the ideal case, where the articular surface can be restored, motion started early, and the patient cooperative, a near full range of motion, with some residual discomfort can be anticipated (Figs. 30-5A and 30-5B).

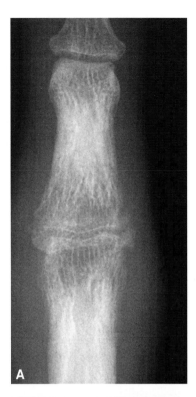

■ FIGURE 30–5
A and B, PA and lateral radiographs taken 3 months after surgery. The joint is reduced and the fracture healed.

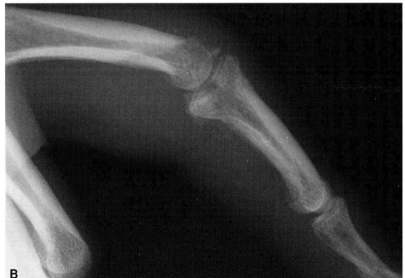

The eventual outcome of a PIP fracture dislocation can be improved with accurate diagnosis, precise surgical reconstruction of the articular surface when possible (volar plate arthroplasty when not), and attentive rehabilitation to regain motion.

References

1. Agee JM: Unstable fracture dislocations of the proximal interphalangeal joint. Treatment with a force couple splint. Clin Orthop, 1987; 4:101–112.
2. Belsole R: Physiological fixation of displaced and unstable fractures of the hand. Orthop Clin North Am, 1980; 11:393–404.
3. Bury TF Stassen LPS, van der Werken C: Repair of the proximal interphalangeal joint with a homograft. J Hand Surg, 1989; 14A:657–658.

4. Dray GJ, Eaton RG: Dislocation and ligament injuries in the digits. In: Green DP (ed): Operative Hand Surgery, 3rd Ed, New York: Churchill Livingstone, 1992:767–797.

5. Green A, Smith J, Redding M, Akelman E: Acute open reduction and rigid internal fixation of proximal interphalangeal joint fracture dislocation. J Hand Surg, 1992; 17A:512–517.

6. Hart DP, Blair WF: Acute dorsal fracture dislocation of the proximal interphalangeal joint of the finger. J Iowa Med Soc, 1983; 73:359–363.

7. Incavo SJ, Morgan JV, Hilfrank BC: Extension splinting of palmar plate avulsion injuries of the proximal interphalangeal joint. J Hand Surg, 1989; 14A:659–661.

8. Lee MLH: Intra-articular and peri-articular fractures of the phalanges. J Bone Joint Surg, 1963; 45B:103–109.

9. McElfresh EC, Dobyns JH, O'Brien ET: Management of fracture-dislocation of the proximal interphalangeal joints by extension-block splinting. J Bone Joint Surg, 1972; 54A:1705–1711.

10. Robertson RC, Cawley JJ, Faris AM: Treatment of fracture-dislocation of the interphalangeal joints of the hand. J Bone Joint Surg, 1946; 28:68–70.

11. Schulze HA: Treatment of fracture dislocations of the proximal interphalangeal joints of the fingers. Milit Surg, 1946; 99:190–191.

12. Stern PJ: Fractures of the metacarpals and phalanges. In: Green DP (ed): Operative Hand Surgery, 3rd Ed, New York: Churchill Livingstone, 1992:719–758.

13. Sprague BL: Proximal interphalangeal joint injuries and their initial treatment. J Trauma, 1975; 15:380–385.

14. Viegas SF: Extension block pinning for proximal interphalangeal joint fracture dislocations: Preliminary report of a new technique. J Hand Surg, 1992; 17A:896–901.

15. Wilson JN, Rowland SA: Fracture-dislocation of the proximal interphalangeal joint of the finger. Treatment by open reduction and internal fixation. J Bone Joint Surg, 1966; 46A: 493–502.

PART
V

*Fracture Fixation
of the Metacarpals*

31

Percutaneous Pin Fixation of the Diaphysis of the Metacarpals

Percutaneous pin fixation of small bone fractures was first advocated by Tennant, who in 1924 used a steel phonograph needle as a "retaining pin" for a metacarpal fracture.[19] In 1927, Kirschner described the use of small traction wires made from chrome-plated steel piano wire measuring 0.7 mm (0.028 inch) to 1.5 mm (0.062 inch) in diameter. Ten years later, Bosworth reported successfully treating a fifth metacarpal neck fracture by closed reduction and percutaneous pinning with two of these K-wires under fluoroscopic control.[2] This technique did not become popular until the 1940s, when power drills with rapid release chucks became available.[15] Vom Saal reported his results after closed reduction and percutaneous intramedullary fixation of a variety of metacarpal and phalangeal fractures in 1953, prompting Littler to comment that, "[o]ne is encouraged in the use of such radical fixation because of the grave necessity of maintaining the architecture of the hand in its perfect form."[20] Although instrumentation has improved significantly, the techniques and principles described by Vom Saal are routinely used today and this "radical fixation" is still considered by many to be the "gold standard" for fracture fixation in the hand.[10]

HISTORY OF THE TECHNIQUE

Metacarpal shaft fractures may be transverse, spiral, oblique, or comminuted. Transverse fractures tend to shorten and angulate volarly (fracture apex dorsal) as the strong pull of the interosseous muscles on the proximal phalanx flexes the distal fragment (Fig. 31–1).[14] Shortening rarely exceeds 3 to 4 mm; it is limited by the deep transverse metacarpal ligaments. Shortening of the central rays may produce a noticeable cosmetic defect because these knuckles are normally more prominent than those of the border rays. Angulation results in palmar prominence of the metacarpal head, which may cause pain with gripping; psuedoclawing with digital extension due to metacarpophalangeal (MP) joint compensatory hyperextension; and a dorsal bump, which may be cosmetically unacceptable to the patient. Spiral and oblique fractures tend to malrotate as they shorten (Fig. 31–2). Malrotation produces abnormal crossing of the fingers as they are flexed.

INDICATIONS AND CONTRAINDICATIONS

Most metacarpal shaft fractures may be treated by closed reduction and splinting. Percutaneous pin fixation is indicated when an adequate reduction can be obtained but not maintained by closed methods. In addition, long oblique and long spiral fractures that are initially in good position represent a relative indication for the use of this technique because of their propensity to displace despite splinting.

Inadequate closed reduction of a metacarpal shaft fracture (as evidenced by less than 50% bony aposition, more than 10° angulation in the index and long fingers or more than 20° in the ring and small fingers,[7,17,18] or more than 3 to 4 mm shortening[3,7] or any malrotation)[7] constitutes an absolute contraindication to percutaneous pin fixation. Thus, simple fractures with soft-tissue interposition and comminuted fractures with marked displacement or rotation of fragments require open reduction. In addition, comminuted fractures with key fragments that may be displaced during pin placement (e.g., a large butterfly fragment) are best treated by open methods.

This procedure should be performed in an operating room or minor surgical suite, using aseptic technique. An experienced surgical assistant is essential because the fracture must

SURGICAL TECHNIQUES

■ FIGURE 31–1
A and **B**, Preoperative posteroanterior and lateral radiographs of a displaced transverse fifth metacarpal shaft fracture. Note prominence of the metacarpal head in the palm from 60° of volar angulation of the distal fragment.

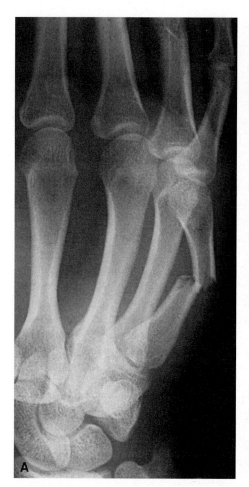
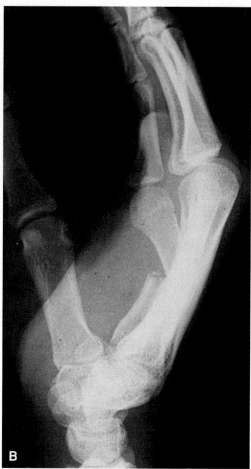

be reduced and held by one individual while K-wires are driven across the fracture site by another. Wrist block anesthesia is performed (except in small children, in whom general anesthesia may be required) using 1% lidocaine and 0.25% bupivacaine, both without epinephrine, mixed in equal parts to provide rapid onset of local anesthesia and postoperative pain relief, respectively. A tourniquet is not necessary.

Closed reduction is performed after induction of regional anesthesia but before the surgical prep and verified fluoroscopically. I prefer to use a mini–C-arm such as the FluoroScan (FluoroScan Imaging Systems, Inc., Northbrook, IL); it provides excellent visualization of small bones while minimizing irradiation scatter.[8] When an adequate closed reduction cannot be obtained, this procedure is aborted, a tourniquet is applied, and preparations are made for open reduction of the fracture. When an adequate reduction is obtained, the upper extremity is sterilely prepped and draped while instrumentation for percutaneous pin fixation (a minor hand tray and an air-powered pencil- or pistol-grip microwire-driver with a rapid release chuck) is opened and the mini–C-arm is sterilely draped.

Metacarpal shaft fractures are best reduced by flexing the MP joint 90° to tighten the collateral ligaments. The flexed digit can then be used as a lever arm to derotate the distal fragment. If rotational control cannot be obtained in this fashion, the distal metacarpal can be grasped percutaneously with a large towel clip or fracture clamp and rotated (Fig. 31–3A). Longitudinal traction and upward pressure on the metacarpal head applied through the flexed proximal phalanx correct distal fragment shortening and palmar angulation, respectively. The reduction is verified fluoroscopically before pin placement.

There is no "best" technique for percutaneous pin fixation of metacarpal shaft fractures.

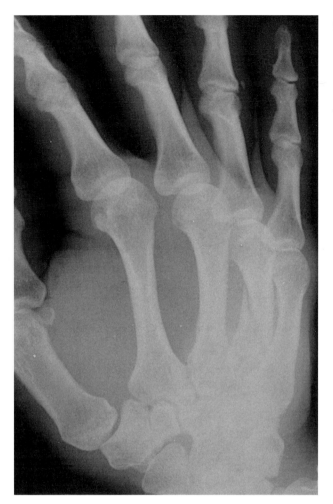

■ FIGURE 31–2
A preoperative radiograph in an oblique projection, showing a displaced long spiral fourth metacarpal shaft fracture. The fracture has rotated and shortened about 3 to 4 mm.

The method employed depends on the fracture pattern, the fracture location, and the experience of the surgeon.

Transverse and short oblique metacarpal shaft fractures may be stabilized with crossed intramedullary pins. A 0.045-inch K-wire is introduced laterally at the retrocondylar fossa of the metacarpal head and drilled longitudinally across the fracture site to lodge in the opposite cortex proximally (Fig. 31–3B and C). Pin placement is simplified by first placing a free pin over the hand as a fluoroscopic guide to determine the optimum location for soft-tissue penetration and pin angle, with respect to the metacarpal shaft. Longitudinal placement is facilitated by lodging the pin in the small shelf of bone in the retrocondylar fossa proximal to the collateral ligament origin. A second 0.045-inch K-wire is introduced in the opposite retrocondylar fossa and drilled longitudinally, so that the two wires cross in the metacarpal medullary canal. After pin placement, the adequacy of reduction is verified by checking the plane of the fingernails and by flexing the fingers fully to document that the fingers do not cross abnormally and that tendons glide freely. If tendon excursion is limited, K-wires may be removed one at a time (to avoid loss of reduction) and repositioned.

Long spiral fractures may be fixed by introducing two or three 0.035-inch K-wires through the dorsum of the hand adjacent to the extensor tendons (Fig. 31–4). The pins are advanced transversely across the fracture site, perpendicular to the long axis of the metacarpal. The pins should just traverse the far cortex of the metacarpal; if advanced too far, damage to the neurovascular structures in the palm may occur. Care should be taken not to skewer the extensor tendons with the pins. Although this technique can be employed

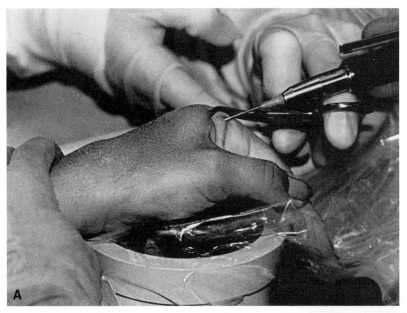

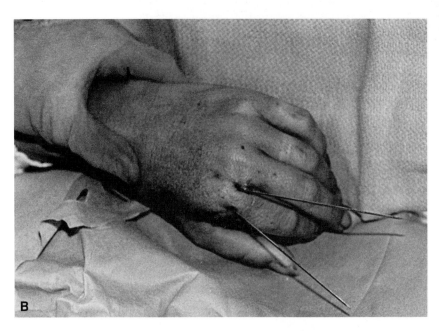

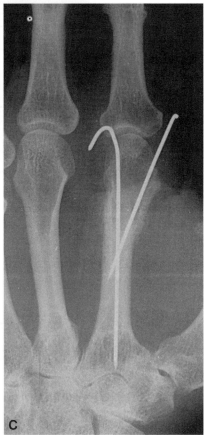

■ FIGURE 31–3

Crossed K-wire fixation of a transverse or short oblique metacarpal shaft fracture. **A**, Intraoperative photograph demonstrates the use of the sterilely draped mini–C-arm detection device as
the hand table. The metacarpal head is grasped percutaneously with a large towel clip and
held by the assistant to control rotation and alignment of the distal fragment. Note that the K-
wire penetrates the skin distal to the metacarpal head. **B**, Intraoperative photograph demonstrates the position of two intramedullary crossed K-wires. **C**, A postoperative radiograph illustrates pin placement.

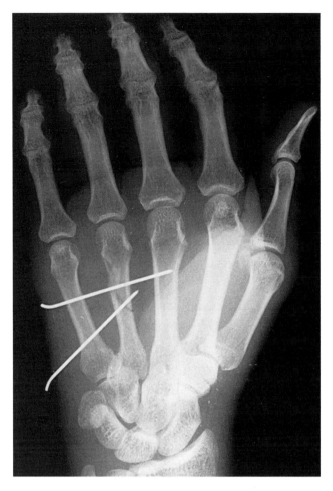

■ FIGURE 31-4
Postoperative posteroanterior radiograph of a long spiral fracture of the ring metacarpal stablized with two transverse 0.045-inch K-wires. The distal pin was advanced transversely into the long metacarpal shaft to enhance stability. The proximal pin just penetrates the cortex.

in the long and ring metacarpals, it is much easier in the border rays (i.e., thumb, index, and small).

Pins are cut, leaving 5 to 6 mm protruding from the skin and bent 90° to prevent migration. A sterile dressing and a short arm plaster splint, immobilizing the involved and adjacent fingers in the functional or "safe" position,[9] are applied in the operating room.

The percutaneous pin fixation methods discussed above can be technically difficult. The surgeon should be familiar with several alternative methods, so that if difficulties are encountered intraoperatively, a different technique can be employed.

■ TECHNICAL ALTERNATIVES

Any type of metacarpal shaft fracture may be stabilized with transverse K-wires passed through an adjacent intact metacarpal (Fig. 31–5). The intact metacarpal functions like an external fixator frame. A 0.045-inch K-wire is introduced transversely through the dorsum of the hand into the distal metacarpal fragment, passes through both cortices of the fractured metacarpal, then into the neighboring normal metacarpal shaft. A second 0.045-inch K-wire is introduced into the distal fragment, parallel to the first. These wires should be as far apart as possible, while remaining within the shaft of the distal fragment to maximize control of angulation. In the mobile ring and small metacarpals, a third 0.045-inch K-wire is placed through the proximal fragment to prevent displacement from carpometacarpal (CMC) joint motion. Pin placement in the long and ring metacarpals is facilitated by flexing the small CMC joint and cupping the hand.

Transverse and short oblique metacarpal shaft fractures may be stabilized with a single intramedullary 0.045- or 0.062-inch K-wire introduced through the articular surface of the metacarpal head adjacent to the extensor tendon (Fig. 31–6). The pin is directed slightly dorsally and may be lodged in the cortex of the proximal fragment or drilled out the

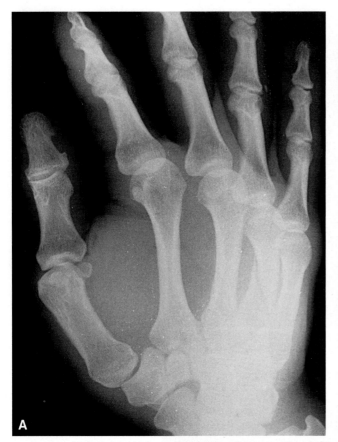

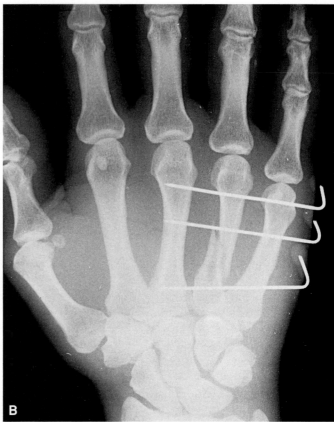

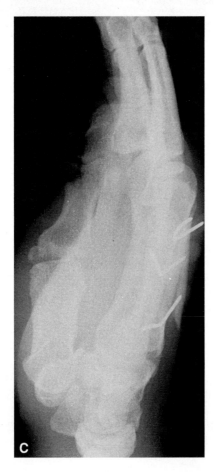

■ FIGURE 31–5
Percutaneous transverse
pin fixation of a long spiral ring metacarpal frac-
ture to an adjacent intact
metacarpal. **A**, Preoperative oblique radiograph
demonstrates mild short-
ening and malrotation. **B**
and **C**, Postoperative
posteroanterior and lat-
eral radiographs demon-
strate restoration of
length and correction of
malrotation after place-
ment of three transverse
0.045-inch K-wires. Note
use of pin proximal to
the fracture site to stabilize the mobile ring and
small CMC joints.

dorsal metacarpal cortex proximal to the fracture site and withdrawn in a retrograde fashion until it no longer enters the MP joint. It is left protruding from the skin and bent 90° to prevent migration. This single pin does not control rotation at the fracture site; supplemental splinting is required. A sterile dressing and volar-dorsal short arm plaster splints are applied in the operating room and left in place for 3 to 4 weeks postoperatively. Splints are changed only if they become loose or examination of the pin site is indicated clinically. Range of motion exercises are delayed until 3 to 4 weeks postoperatively, when the pin is removed in the office. This technique simplifies pin placement but violates the articular cartilage of an otherwise normal joint and risks damage to the extensor tendons as the pin is advanced out the dorsum of the metacarpal. It is most useful in treating young children, in whom early range of motion exercises are not indicated, or for distal shaft fractures in adults.

■ REHABILITATION

The postoperative dressing is replaced at 3 to 5 days with a removable plaster or thermoplastic short arm splint, which maintains the involved and adjacent digits and the wrist in the functional position. The splint is removed for pin care twice daily with peroxide and for range of motion exercises. Gentle active and passive range of motion exercises are performed three to five times daily under the supervision of a trained hand therapist. Patients may resume light activities of daily living and light-duty employment with their splint on.

Pins are removed in the office 3 to 4 weeks postoperatively when the fracture site is not tender to palpation and radiographs demonstrate early callus formation. Pin removal may be delayed 1 to 2 weeks if clinical or radiographic examination suggests slow healing. After pin removal, pain and motion with stress of the fracture site are assessed. When

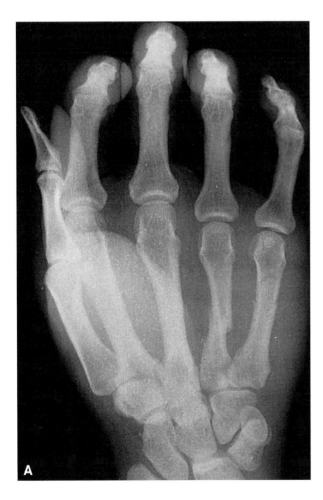

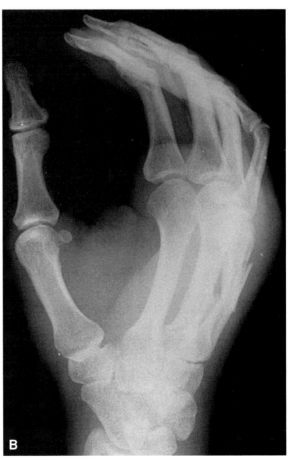

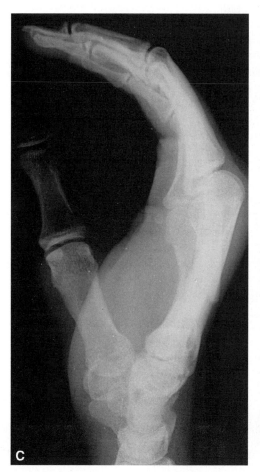

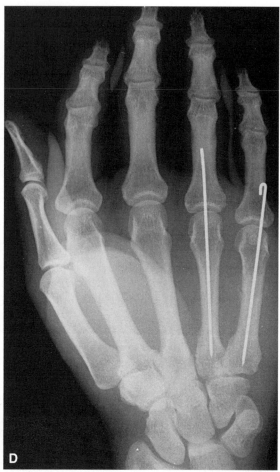

present, external splinting and gentle active range of motion exercises are continued until clinical and radiographic evidence of union is present. When absent, strengthening exercises are initiated and the patient may resume unrestricted activities of daily living. Sports activities and work requiring heavy lifting or carrying may be resumed 1 to 2 weeks later when the pin sites have healed and strength is adequate.

■ OUTCOMES

Although many authors recommend the use of percutaneous K-wire fixation to treat unstable metacarpal shaft fractures when a satisfactory reduction can be obtained but not maintained by closed methods,[1,4,6,10,12,13,16,18,20] much of the evidence supporting the use of this technique is anecdotal. For example, Vom Saal[20] reported a "satisfactory" outcome in 40 patients treated with intramedullary fixation of unstable fractures of the metacarpals and phalanges followed by early mobilization. Most patients returned to work within 3 days of treatment without the use of external splints. The incidence of malunion, delayed union, and nonunion are not mentioned. Three patients developed "weeping" at their pin sites; two were treated with dressings, and one with antibiotics. No other complications were noted.

Treatment of metacarpal fractures by transverse K-wire fixation to the intact adjacent metacarpals was reviewed by Berkman and Miles.[1] They reported that 20 patients in a military population returned to light-duty activities 1 day postoperatively without the use of external splints and regained full function rapidly. No incidents of pin-tract infection, loss of reduction, or residual stiffness were reported by the authors. The "gratifying results"[1] reported by Berkman and Miles were substantiated in an excellent retrospective review by Lamb and coworkers.[12] They reviewed 66 fractures in 50 patients. There were no instances of delayed or nonunion and about half of the patients regained full active

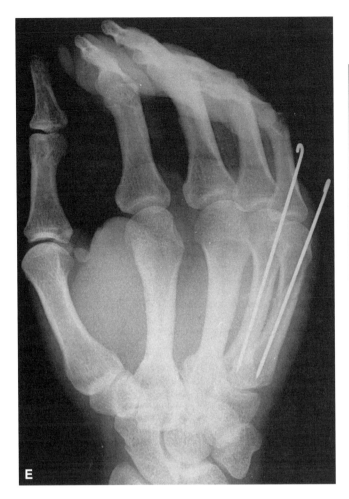
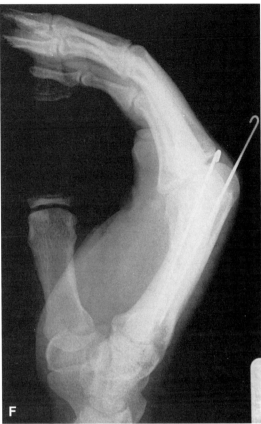

■ FIGURE 31–6

A through **C**, Preoperative posteroanterior, lateral, and oblique radiographs of the right hand. The transverse fracture of the ring metacarpal is shortened, flexed, and malrotated. The short obliqe fracture of the small metacarpal is minimally displaced. **D** through **F**, Postoperative posteroanterior, lateral, and oblique radiographs. Note the dorsal position of the pins in the metacarpal heads. These K-wires have not been advanced out the dorsal cortex proximally.

use of their hand within 6 weeks postoperatively. Complications included subjective complaints of weakness or pain in 44% patients, a finding that was closely correlated with residual deformity, a 13% incidence of extensor lag of less than 20° at the MP joint, and a 9% incidence of PIP joint flexion contracture, which the authors ascribed to external splinting postoperatively. Grip strength was normal or nearly normal in 75% of their patients at the time of follow-up.

More recently, Diwaker and Stothard[5] have reported their results in 90 closed fractures of the proximal phalanges and metacarpals. Forty-five stable fractures were treated conservatively with immobilization for an average of 3.1 weeks. Of the unstable fractures, 16 (eight metacarpal and eight proximal phalangeal) were treated with percutaneous K-wire fixation and immobilization for an average of 4.1 weeks; 29 (20 proximal phalangeal and nine metacarpal) were treated with AO miniscrew fixation and immobilization for an average of 2 weeks. The authors evaluated patient satisfaction, residual deformity, total active range of motion, grip strength, length of immobilization, and time to return to work. Although their data suggest that AO fixation is superior to both cast immobilization and K-wire fixation, the only statistically significant difference (p<.05) noted between their treatment groups was in the average time to return to work; the AO-treatment group averaged 6.2 weeks, compared with 10.1 weeks for the K-wire treatment group. These results do not reflect the time lost from work or the morbidity associated with hardware removal, which the authors recommend routinely. The authors do not mention the type or incidence of complications encountered in the different treatment groups.

Complications of percutaneous K-wire fixation of metacarpal shaft fractures include pin-tract infections, loss of motion, and delayed union, malunion, and nonunion. The reported incidence of superficial pin tract infections varies from 0 to 10%.[1,9,20,18,20] Pin-tract infections usually respond to oral antibiotics and improved pin care but may necessitate early pin removal. Delayed union, malunion, and nonunion may result if improper K-wire fixation is employed.[11] Range of motion can be maximized by obtaining an accurate reduction, demonstrating intraoperatively that the extensor tendons move freely, and encouraging early active range of motion exercises combined with splinting in the functional or "safe" position during rest periods.[1,6,9,11,12]

References

1. Berkman EF, Miles GH: Internal fixation of metacarpal fractures exclusive of the thumb. J Bone Joint Surg, 1943; 25:816–820.
2. Bosworth DM: Internal splinting of fractures of the fifth metacarpal. J Bone Joint Surg, 1937; 19:826–827.
3. Brown PW: The management of phalangeal and metacarpal fractures. Surg Clin North Am, 1973; 53:1393–1437.
4. Clifford RH: Intramedullary wire fixation of hand fractures. Plast Reconstr Surg, 1953; 11:366–371.
5. Diwaker HN, Stothard J: The role of internal fixation in closed fractures of the proximal phalanges and metacarpals in adults. J Hand Surg, 1986; 11B:103–108.
6. Flatt AE: Fractures. In: The Care of Minor Hand Injuries, 3rd Ed, St. Louis: CV Mosby Co, 1972:196–216.
7. Freeland AE, Jabaley ME, Hughes JL: Oblique and Spiral Metacarpal Shaft Fractures. In: Stable Fixation of the Hand and Wrist, New York: Springer Verlag, 1987:55–57.
8. Gehrke JC, Mellenberg DE Jr, Connelly RE, Johnson KA: Technique tips: the fluoroscan imaging system in foot and ankle surgery. Foot Ankle, 1993; 14:545–549.
9. James JIP: The assessment and management of the injured hand. Hand, 1970; 2:97–105.
10. Jupiter JB, Belsky MR: Fractures and Dislocations of the Hand. In: Browner BD, Jupiter JB, Levine AM, Trafton PG (eds): Skeletal Trauma: Fractures, Dislocations, Ligamentous Injuries, Philadelphia: WB Saunders Co, 1992:923–1024.
11. Jupiter JB, Koniuch M, Smith RJ: The management of delayed unions and nonunions of the tubular bones of the hand. J Hand Surg, 1985; 4:457–466.
12. Lamb DW, Abernethy PA, Raine PAM: Unstable fractures of the metacarpals: a method of treatment by transverse wire fixation to intact metacarpals. Hand, 1973; 5:43–48.
13. Lipscomb PR: Management of fractures of the hand. Am Surg, 1963; 29:277–282.
14. McNealy RW, Lichtenstein ME: Fractures of the metacarpals and phalanges. West J Surg Obstet Gynecol, 1935; 43:156–161.
15. Meals RA, Meuli HC: Carpenter's nails, phonograph needles, piano wires, and safety pins: the history of operative fixation of metacarpal and phalangeal fractures. J Hand Surg, 1985; 10A:144–150.
16. Opgrande JD, Westphal SA: Fractures of the hand. Orthop Clin North Am, 1983; 14:779–810.
17. Smith RJ, Peimer CA: Injuries to the metacarpal bone and joints. Adv Surg, 1977; 2:341–374.
18. Stern PJ: Fractures of the metacarpals and phalanges In: Green DP (ed): Operative Hand Surgery, 3rd Ed, New York: Churchill Livingstone Inc, 1993:695–758.
19. Tennant CE: Use of steel phonograph needle as a retaining pin in certain irreducible fractures of the small bones. JAMA, 1924; 83:193.
20. Vom Saal FH: Intramedullary fixation in fractures of the hand and fingers. J Bone Joint Surg, 1953; 35A:5–16.

32

CHARLES D.
JENNINGS

Open Pin Fixation of the Diaphysis of the Metacarpals

Kirschner, a renowned German surgeon of the early nineteenth century, used a thin steel wire stretched taut by a tension bow for skeletal traction. Kirschner developed this method of traction out of concern for the high infection rate caused by the use of larger diameter pins, now known as Steinmann pins.[2] Interestingly, Kirschner never used these small wires for internal fixation of the hand. Tennant in 1924 was the first to report pin fixation of a hand fracture in the American literature. He used a steel phonograph needle for the fixation of a metacarpal fracture. Later, in 1937, Bosworth reported the fixation of a displaced fracture of the fifth metacarpal neck using K-wires.[11] Sixty-eight years later, K-wire fixation is still an important part of our armamentarium for skeletal fixation of the hand. For the past 20 years, the ease and accuracy of K-wire insertion has been greatly enhanced by the use of powered drivers with automatic chucks.

■ HISTORY OF THE
TECHNIQUE

Generally, open K-wire fixation is still widely used for metacarpal fractures despite several authors showing that AO plate and screw fixation is superior.[1,10,14,16] The remaining question is: how strong does the fixation have to be? The answer to this comes from the surgeon's proper analysis of the strength of fixation versus the estimated activity of the patient. There are four indications for open reduction of metacarpal shaft fractures: 1) failure to achieve or maintain satisfactory alignment of an isolated transverse fracture by closed means, 2) multiple displaced metacarpal fractures, 3) an isolated oblique or comminuted fracture with unacceptable shortening or rotation, and 4) open metacarpal shaft fractures.[13]

■ INDICATIONS AND
CONTRAINDICATIONS

In the case of closed transverse fractures of the metacarpal shaft, an attempt should be made to treat by closed means. If acceptable alignment can be maintained by splint or cast, open reduction is contraindicated. If acceptable reduction is not well-maintained by closed technique, percutaneous fixation as previously described can be used. Residual angulation of more than 10° in the index and long metacarpal shafts and more than 20° in the ring and little metacarpal shafts is an indication for open reduction.[6,18] Percutaneous techniques often require more protection than open fixation and little or no active exercise may be allowed after their insertion.[5,15,20]

In the case of oblique or comminuted fractures, open reduction and internal fixation is often required to correct rotation or excessive shortening. Five degrees of metacarpal rotation can cause 1.5 cm of digital overlap at the fingertip.[14] The patient must be able to fully flex the fingers to assess rotational alignment. If necessary, an anesthetic must be used to assess rotation. In the literature, the minimum allowable metacarpal shortening varies from 2 to 4 mm.[3,6,9] Rigid fixation may be obtained by multiple K-wires inserted at right angles to the fracture line. This can be done quickly, compared with insertion of compression screws.

In the case of multiple metacarpal fractures, open techniques are more suitable for several reasons. Soft-tissue interconnections (transverse metacarpal ligaments and interosseous muscles) between fractured metacarpals are no longer stabilizing structures as they are for isolated fractures, making it more difficult to hold by external means. Early motion is important to counteract the effects of the more extensive soft-tissue damage.

In the case of open metacarpal fractures, the opportunity for stable fixation is immediately available because of the necessity for thorough wound debridement. The stability afforded by internal fixation allows early rehabilitation of soft-tissue structures and carries no additional risk of infection, assuming that the wound has been adequately cleaned. K-wire fixation, although weaker than plate and screws, theoretically carries less risk of infection because there is less metal and less requirement for soft-tissue stripping. A contra-indication to the use of internal fixation might be the presence of soft-tissue loss, bone loss, or both, with or without gross contamination. In this setting, external fixation may be appropriate primary care.

■ SURGICAL TECHNIQUES

Anesthesia for open reduction of metacarpal fractures may be either regional or general. Local infiltration is not adequate for this type of work. A regional anesthetic (axillary, supraclavicular, or Bier block) that blocks muscle contraction is preferable to a more distal anesthetic such as a wrist block. Open reduction of the metacarpals is best accomplished by a straight longitudinal incision directly overlying the fractured metacarpal. When multiple metacarpals are involved, three may be exposed through one incision, and all four metacar-pals may be exposed through two longitudinal incisions. One incision may be placed between the index and long metacarpals and the other incision placed between the long and ring metacarpals. By gentle retraction of soft-tissue structures to one side, exposure of more than one bone is easily obtained. If needed, oblique extension can be made on either or both ends to facilitate exposure.

After the skin incision, careful blunt dissection of the subcutaneous tissues is required to protect small dorsal sensory nerves. The extensor tendons may be retracted to one side for exposure of the underlying periosteum. If necessary, the junctura tendinae may be divided to facilitate exposure but should be repaired at the completion of the procedure. Periosteum is incised longitudinally and an attempt should be made to preserve this for closure over the fixation devices. An attempt should also be made to minimize further damage to interosseous muscles because this can predispose to fibrosis and contracture.

A few technical points need to be mentioned regarding insertion of K-wires. The most commonly used K-wire in my experience is 0.045 inch. This has the right balance of rigidity and flexibility. To prevent adjacent soft-tissue damage, the K-wire is easily bent, using a fine needle-nosed plier or heavy needle holder. There are two types of K-wire points, spatula and trocar. The trocar point is favored because it has cutting power equal to that of the spatula and is easier to control when inserting into cortical bone at an oblique angle. The spatula point has a greater tendency to ride out of the hole initially than does the trocar point.[12] In addition, more solid bony fixation is possible if lower speeds are used for K-wire insertion. Lower speed lessens the bone necrosis, which occurs as the result of the heat of friction around the pin. Whenever there is significant soft-tissue movement next to the fracture, such as overlying tendon gliding or immediately adjacent joint motion, the protruding end of the pin must be bent to a right angle and turned so that the tip rests against bone or away from the moving soft-tissue structure. It is important to firmly hold the K-wire next to the bony cortex with a large needle holder to provide a fulcrum for bending the K-wire. Otherwise, the bone acts as the fulcrum, which causes loosening. A small metal neurosuction tube can be used as a bending lever if the protruding part of the pin is short. Cross-pinning can be executed retrogradely or from the outside of the cortex.[4,13] A 14-gauge hypodermic needle tip pushed firmly against the cortex will stabilize the K-wire tip acting as a pin guide.[13]

Transverse fractures of the metacarpal shaft tend to angulate dorsally because of the predominance of flexion forces from intrinsic muscles and extrinsic flexor tendons. This tendency is enhanced because of the greater flexion moment arm, resulting from the meta-carpal anatomy. This angulation must be resisted by a tension-band wire. Tension-band wires must often be used to enhance the rigidity afforded by K-wires.[8] The most commonly used size for tension band wires are either 26-gauge or 28-gauge monofilament stainless steel wire. Hypodermic needles may be used for passage of wires through bone. A 0.035-inch K-wire is used to drill the hole and a 20-gauge needle is passed through the hole to act as a guide for a 26- or 28-gauge wire.[7,19] Tension bands can be in a figure-of-eight configuration, with the crossing of wires in the region of the fracture, either looping around

K-wires or through transverse holes in the cortex. Because the metacarpal fracture tends to angulate apex dorsally, the crossed portion of the tension band should be placed over the dorsal cortex and the transverse hole should be dorsal to the mid-frontal plane of the metacarpal. The wire should be twisted four to five times and the end bent, so that it is facing the bone surface rather than the soft tissue. The tightness of the wires should be such that maximum tension is obtained short of the wire breaking. The point of wire breaking can be determined by the appearance of dullness at the base of the wire twist.

Fixation of transverse fractures can be accomplished in one of several ways. In the border metacarpals of the thumb, index, or little fingers, I prefer crossed K-wires inserted in the frontal plane supplemented by a figure-of-eight tension band looping around the ends of the K-wires and crossing over on the dorsal side of the fracture site (Fig. 32–1). The tension-band wire resists the predominant tendency for the metacarpal to angulate apex dorsally.

Another technique that can be used in any of the metacarpals is the longitudinal insertion of two parallel K-wires. They are introduced distally at an acute angle to the dorsal cortex and are passed down the medullary canal and into the medullary canal of the proximal fragment adjacent to the volar cortex of the proximal fragment. Two K-wires afford rotational stability but they must be supplemented with a dorsal figure-of-eight tension-band wire, which is looped through the cortex of the proximal fragment and around the protruding pins in the distal fragment. Because the ends of the wires are close to the joint, soft-tissue irritation should be prevented by bending the wires at 90°, cutting them off, and turning them such that the tips face the cortical bone (Fig. 32–2).

When attempting to fix the long and ring metacarpals, it is difficult to insert crossed K-wires in the frontal plane but adequate fixation and resistance to dorsal angulation can be achieved by inserting K-wires in crossed configuration in the sagittal plane. This must be supplemented by a wire-loop tension-band between the two wires protruding dorsally (Fig. 32–3). I recommend that the two dorsally protruding ends be bent at 90° and turned, so that the ends do not protrude dorsally into the extensor tendon. In the long and ring metacarpals, a figure-eight tension band may be used alone when there is good interlocking of fragments to prevent rotation.[17] On the index and little metacarpals, rotatory stability is more critical and at least one oblique or two crossed K-wires should be used.[17]

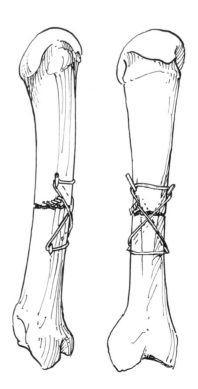

■ FIGURE 32–1
Crossed K-wires, with dorsal figure-of-eight tension-band wires.

■ FIGURE 32–2
Parallel K-wires for rotational fixation, with figure-of-eight tension-band wires.

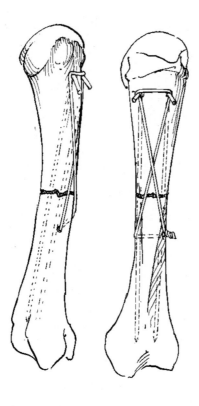

■ FIGURE 32–3
Fixation of long and ring metacarpal fractures, using crossed K-wires in the sagittal plane with a tension-band loop.

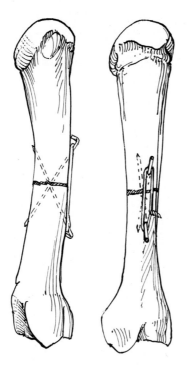

In the case of oblique fractures, exposure of the fracture site must be adequate to achieve anatomic alignment of the fracture. Once the reduction is obtained, the fragments are held with a clamp. The fracture can then be fixed by two or three K-wires inserted as far apart as possible at 90° to the plane of the fracture and to the longitudinal axis of the metacarpal. The 0.045-inch diameter K-wires are the most commonly used. One must be certain that each pin engages both cortices and that the pin is no less than 3 mm away from the fracture

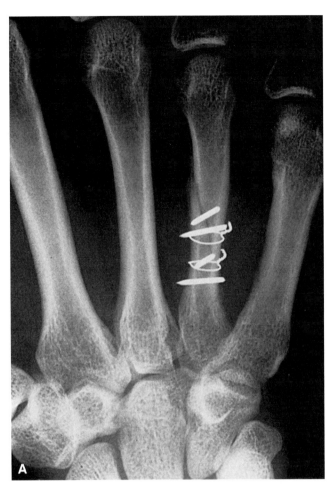

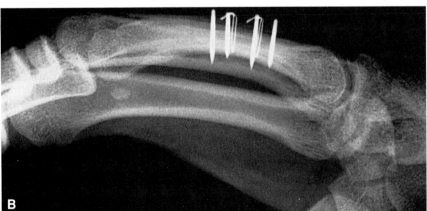

■   FIGURE 32–4
A, Posteroanterior radiograph and **B**, lateral radiograph of a long oblique fracture fixed, using four transverse K-wires with cerclage wiring.

line. Supplemental cerclage wires may be inserted to counteract any significant angulatory forces (Fig. 32–4). Comminuted or short oblique fractures are fixed with a longitudinal K-wire for alignment, supplemented by transverse or oblique K-wires to secure individual fragments (Fig. 32–5). Cerclage wires are occasionally necessary to prevent longitudinal collapse.[9] These fractures often require more protection postoperatively than long oblique or transverse fractures.

Attempts should be made to close periosteum over the hardware. It should be assured that the sharp edges of the pin do not impinge on the overlying gliding extensor tendon structures. Subcutaneous closure layer is not necessary. The skin can be closed using the suture of choice. A bulky dressing should be applied using a dorsal splint to immobilize

■ FIGURE 32–5
K-wire fixation for short
oblique or comminuted
fractures.

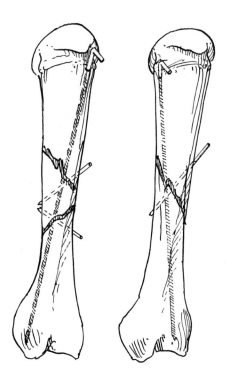

the wrist in 30 to 40° of extension and the metacarpophalangeal (MP) joint in 60° or more of flexion. Even with isolated metacarpal fractures, it is preferable to immoblize all meta-carpals and proximal phalanges initially. The interphalangeal joints may be left free to begin early motion. After 3 to 5 days, dressings may be changed, wounds inspected, and splints reapplied.

■ TECHNICAL
ALTERNATIVES

Plate and screw fixation using tension band principles espoused by AO is the preferred technique for open fixation of transverse fractures.[1,10,14,16] When properly executed, this technique allows more aggressive rehabilitation of soft-tissue structures than does the K-wire technique. Plate and screw fixation is exacting, however, with little room for error, and requires more soft-tissue stripping and additional time to complete the procedure. With oblique fractures, screws may be used instead of or in combination with K-wires. Lag technique must be used. This provides more rigid fixation than K-wires alone.

■ REHABILITATION

The goal of rehabilitation is to achieve fracture healing in good alignment, with restora-tion of strength and motion in 12 to 16 weeks. Generally, it has been my practice to keep the patient in a removable splint for 6 to 8 weeks, depending on the rate of fracture healing. The splint should extend above the wrist, holding the wrist in 30 to 40° of extension, and extend distally to the proximal interphalangeal joints, holding the MP joints in 60° of flexion. The splint needs to protect only the injured rays. Radiographs should be taken at l, 3, and 8 weeks. The splint may be periodically removed to perform active exercise. K-wire fixation requires more restrained activity than plate and screw fixation. Unrestricted activity with any kind of internal fixation is risking disaster, however. Careful follow-up at weekly or every other week intervals by surgeons or therapists is necessary to assure a properly graded exercise program according to the patient's range of motion and reliabil-ity. Metacarpophalangeal joint extension contracture is a risk. This can be prevented by careful attention to splinting the MP joint in flexion and proper intermittent exercise, emphasizing full active MP flexion. Extensor tendon adherence is also a risk and must be prevented by intermittent active extension exercises.

The typical duration of closely supervised therapy for these injuries should be about 8 to 12 weeks. Additional improvement may be expected beyond this period. Often, the patient and surgeon are too impatient. Slow improvement in strength and range of motion can be seen up to 1 year after open reduction.

The results of open reduction and K-wire fixation of metacarpal shaft fractures are generally good if enough stability is achieved to allow early active motion to the extent required to prevent adhesions. Accurately measuring the strength of fixation against the activity of the patient demands the utmost in judgment from the surgeon and is a major factor in determining the outcome. The literature is generally lacking any sizable series that show outcomes of open pin fixation of the metacarpal shaft.

■ OUTCOMES

References

1. Black DM, Mann RJ, Constine RM, Daniels AU: Comparison of internal fixation techniques in metacarpal fractures. J Hand Surg, 1985; 10A:466–472.
2. Boyes JH: On the Shoulders of Giants, Philadelphia: JB Lippincott 1976:181–184.
3. Brown PW: The management of phalangeal and metacarpal fractures. Surg Clin North Am, 1973; 53:1393–1437.
4. Edwards GS, O'Brien ET, Heckman MM: Retrograde cross-pinning of transverse fractures. Hand 1982; 14:141–148.
5. Flatt AF: Fractures. In: Care of Minor Hand Injuries, 3rd Ed, St. Louis: CV Mosby, 1972.
6. Freeland AE, Jabaley ME, Hughes JL: Stable Fixation of the Hand and Wrist, New York: Springer-Verlag, 1986.
7. Gingrass RP, Fehring B, Matloub H: Intraosseous wiring of complex hand fractures. Plast Reconstr Surg, 1980; 66:383–391.
8. Greene TL, Noellert RC, Belsole RJ: Treatment of unstable metacarpal and phalangeal fractures with tension band wiring techniques. Clin Orthop, 1987; 214:78–84.
9. Gropper PT, Bowen V: Cerclage wiring of metacarpal fractures. Clin Orthop, 1984; 188: 203–207.
10. Lister G: Intraosseous wiring of the digital skeleton. J Hand Surg, 1978; 3:427–435.
11. Meals RA, Meuli HC: Carpenter's nails, phonograph needles, piano wires, and safety pins: the history of operative fixation of metacarpal and phalangeal fractures. J Hand Surg, 1985; 10A:144–150.
12. Namba RS, Kabo JM, Meals RA: Biomechanical effects of point configuration in Kirschner-wire fixation. Clin Orthop, 1987; 214:19–22.
13. O'Brien ET: Fractures of the Metacarpals and Phalanges. In: Green DP (ed): Operative Hand Surgery, 2nd Ed, New York: Churchill Livingstone, 1988:709–775.
14. Opgrande JD, Westphal SA: Fractures of the hand. Orthop Clin North Am, 1983; 14:779–792.
15. Pulvertaft RG: Operative Treatment of Injuries of the Phalangeal and Metacarpal Bones and Their Joints. In: Furlong R (ed): Operative Surgery, 2nd Ed, Philadelphia: JB Lippincott, 1969.
16. Ruedi TP, Burri C, Pfeiffer KM: Stable internal fixation of fractures of the hand. J Trauma, 1971; 11:381–389.
17. Segmueller G: Principles of Stable Internal Fixation in the Hand. In: Chapman JM (ed): Operative Orthopaedics, Philadelphia: JB Lippincott, 1988:1213–1218.
18. Smith RS, Peimer CA: Injuries to the metacarpal bones and joints. Adv Surg, 1977; 2:341–374.
19. Scheker LR: Department of technique: a technique to facilitate drilling and passing intraosseous wiring in the hand. J Hand Surg, 1982; 5:629–630.
20. Vom Saal FH: Intramedullary fixation in fractures of the hand and fingers. J Bone Joint Surg, 1953; 35A:5–16.

HILL HASTINGS, II
MARK S. COHEN

33

Screw Fixation of the Diaphysis of the Metacarpals

■ HISTORY OF THE
TECHNIQUE

The application of miniscrew fixation to metacarpal shaft fractures represents a natural evolution from the techniques used in the larger tubular bones. In 1958, Kilbourne and Paul first reported on the use of screw fixation alone in metacarpal shaft fractures and actually recommended against its use.[5] In that same year, Muller, Allgower, and Willenegger founded the Swiss Association for the Study of Internal Fixation dedicated to the science and practice of skeletal fixation. In 1964, Heim and Mathys developed the small fragment set and in 1970 the minifragment set. Today, miniscrew fixation alone is widely accepted as a viable and successful alternative in the treatment of appropriate metacarpal diaphyseal fractures. Unique anatomic considerations in the hand regarding soft-tissue coverage, closely approximated gliding tendons, and the precision of the minidrills and screws in relation to the thinner cortices of the metacarpal shaft require special knowledge and experience when applying these implants to the hand.

■ INDICATIONS AND
CONTRAINDICATIONS

The indications for internal screw fixation of metacarpal fractures include displaced spiral and long oblique patterns that cannot be reduced and maintained by closed techniques of immobilization. These fractures have a tendency for malrotation (evidenced by a gap on radiographs), shortening, and apex dorsal angulation. Additional indications for stable internal fixation include significant soft-tissue injury, compromising cast treatment, and associated skeletal or tendon injuries that require stable skeletal fixation for rehabilitation.

The goal of osteosynthesis is to use the minimum hardware necessary to hold the fracture in stable anatomic alignment to prevent displacement during rehabilitation. The advantage of using screws alone, when indicated, is to minimize dissection and periosteal stripping, which lead to bone devascularization and scar formation. Screws are also low profile, with little tendency to compromise tendon gliding or protrude beneath the thin dorsal skin of the hand.

Preoperatively, good quality anteroposterior, lateral, and oblique radiographs out of plaster are needed to properly evaluate the fracture pattern. We routinely use the image intensifier intraoperatively to further evaluate the fracture before making the skin incision. It is most important to ensure that the fracture does not involve a butterfly fragment, which in most cases contraindicates screw fixation alone. A general rule of thumb is that the fracture length must be at least two times the metacarpal diameter at the level of the fracture for screw fixation to be used alone. If the fracture is less oblique, a single compression screw must be protected from torsional and bending forces by the addition of a neutralization plate. Screw fixation alone is also inadequate in cases of significant bone loss or comminution. Although some authors believe that a plate should be used on the border digits to help neutralize torsional forces, we treat all metacarpal fractures similarly, based on the aforementioned principles.

■ SURGICAL
TECHNIQUES

Open reduction of metacarpal fractures requires longitudinal incisions. These are usually offset from the underlying metacarpals to decrease adhesions between the extensor tendons and the skin. For isolated injuries, the incisions are usually made on the radial border of the index metacarpal and the ulnar border of the small finger metacarpal. The middle and ring metacarpals are approached through a longitudinal incision between these bones. These incisions may be extended proximally or distally with a V or Y extension. When adjacent metacarpal fractures exist, a single incision placed in the common interosseous space provides adequate exposure for both injuries. Careful dissection is undertaken to preserve the dorsal venous drainage of the hand. Sensory branches of the ulnar and radial nerves must also be protected and retracted out of the way.

Most extensor tendons do not run coaxially with the metacarpals and can be safely retracted with preservation of their peritenon. Occasionally, a junctural tendinum must be sacrificed to gain distal exposure. The periosteum is sharply elevated 2 to 3 mm away from the fracture margin on both the proximal and distal fragments to expose the fracture. Once exposed, Homan or small Bennett retractors are often helpful to aid in retraction. Soft tissue, hematoma, and periosteum are gently removed from the cortical fracture margins with a small curette or elevator. An important and often neglected aspect of metacarpal fixation is the need to open the fracture to define its "personality." This ensures the identification of nondisplaced butterfly fragments or hidden comminution, which may make screw fixation alone inadequate. In addition, the three-dimensional anatomy of the fracture is better appreciated to plan for optimal intrafragmentary screw placement and anticipate the direction for subsequent drilling.

The fracture is next anatomically reduced. Care must be taken to achieve interlocking of all fracture margins to maximize stability and allow compression. The fragments can then be gently held in a reduced position with a bone forceps, taking care to not fracture the thin spikes proximally and distally. Proper rotation is now confirmed by passively flexing the involved digit and comparing it with the adjacent fingers. Most metacarpal fractures are best fixed with 2-mm minicompression screws. A minimum of two and

■ FIGURE 33–1
The closest safe position for a screw relative to a bone edge (shaded hole). Screws should not be placed less than three screw diameters from the nearest cortical margin. Less than this risks fragmentation of the screw hole and nearby cortex.

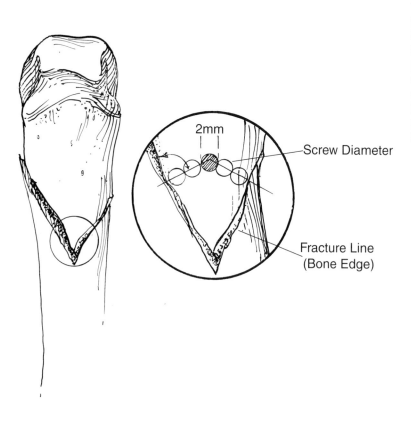

sometimes three screws can be used for intrafragmentary compression. Occasionally, the third screw can be a 1.5-mm diameter screw when it is deemed necessary.

The position and direction of the screws are critical to success. A screw placed too close to a fracture margin or fracture apex risks fragmentation near the hole on countersinking and screw tightening. Depending on bone quality and fracture configuration, a safe guideline is that a screw should not be placed less than three thread diameters away from the nearest bone edge (Fig. 33–1). Screws positioned perpendicular to the fracture line provide the greatest intrafragmentary compression. These are best in resisting torsional load but are less able to resist axial forces. Screws positioned perpendicular to the longitudinal axis of the shaft best resist axial loading. In the past, it was recommended that one screw be placed perpendicular to the fracture and one perpendicular to the shaft. Alternatively, both screws could be directed in a plane that bisected two perpendiculars—one to the fracture and the other to the long axis of the bone (Fig. 33–2). We now advise placing all screws perpendicular to the fracture line to maximize intrafragmentary compression.

The sequence of osteosynthesis begins with the 1.5-mm drill to perforate both near and far cortices (Fig. 33–3). Although some advise drilling the glide hole first with the 2-mm drill, we believe it is important to drill first with the finer 1.5-mm drill to maximize the accuracy of screw placement. Care must be taken to plan for the position of the additional screws when placing this first drill hole. Marking the entry point of subsequent screws (especially the screw nearest the fracture spike) with a marking pen is often helpful in this regard.

Drill guides and tap sleeves must be used with the minifragment screws. These avoid soft-tissue injury and decrease toggle, which can compromise fixation. Precise and gentle handling of the instruments is crucial to success because there is generally only one chance for optimal screw placement in the thin metacarpal diaphysis. The new AO minicompressed air system is helpful in performing this delicate work (Fig. 33–4).

■ FIGURE 33–2
The optimal directions of screw placement in metacarpal shaft fractures. **A**, Screws placed perpendicular to the long axis of the bone provide the greatest resistance to axial loads. **B**, Screws placed perpendicular to the plane of the fracture provide the best intrafragmentary compression and greatest stability to torsional forces. **C**, Screws placed in a plane that bisects these perpendiculars was previously recommended as a compromise.

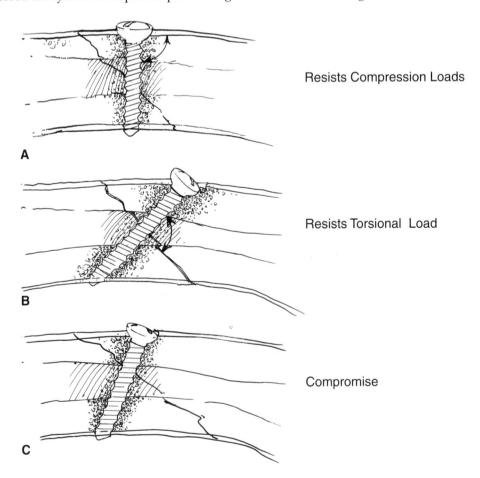

Resists Compression Loads

A

Resists Torsional Load

B

Compromise

C

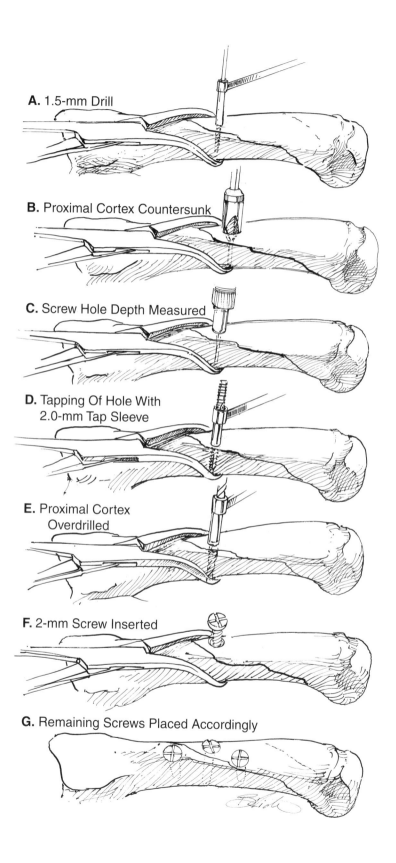

A. 1.5-mm Drill

B. Proximal Cortex Countersunk

C. Screw Hole Depth Measured

D. Tapping Of Hole With 2.0-mm Tap Sleeve

E. Proximal Cortex Overdrilled

F. 2-mm Screw Inserted

G. Remaining Screws Placed Accordingly

■ FIGURE 33–3
The sequence of steps in placing 2-mm intrafragmentary compression screws in a metacarpal diaphysis. **A,** Both cortices are initially drilled using the 1.5-mm drill bit and drill guide. **B,** The proximal cortical hole is enlarged with the countersink. **C,** The depth of the screw is measured. **D,** The hole is tapped with the 2-mm tap and tap sleeve. **E,** The proximal cortex is overdrilled. Care is taken to avoid drilling beyond the first cortex. **F,** The 2-mm screw is inserted in a lag fashion. **G,** Additional screws are similarly inserted, adjusting to the rotational nature of the fracture.

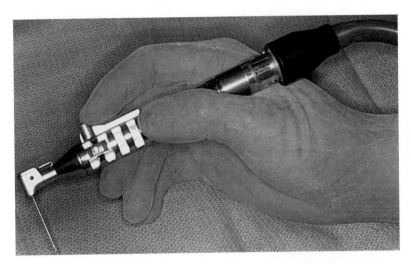

■ FIGURE 33–4
The new AO mini-compressed air system (Synthes, Paoli, PA) is designed to be held like a pencil. Power is controlled by a slide switch adjusted with the index finger. This device aids in performing the delicate work of metacarpal screw fixation.

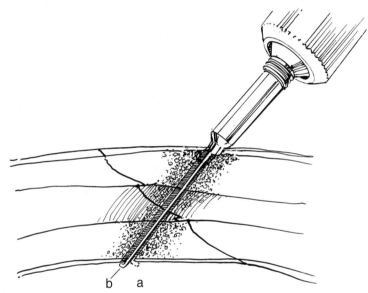

■ FIGURE 33–5
Placement of the depth gauge away from the fracture in obliquely placed lag screws. **A**, Placing the depth-gauge tip on the near cortex may underestimate the optimum screw length. **B**, By placing the tip of the gauge away from the fracture, the correct screw length is achieved.

b   a

a. Incorrect Placement of Depth Gauge May
   Underestimate Screw Length Needed
b. Correct Screw Length Determined

After drilling, the proximal cortical hole is deepened with the countersink. This device improves compression by enlarging the surface contacted by the screw head, thus distributing the force of the head over a greater surface area. Near a fracture apex, care must be taken not to overcountersink. This can weaken the cortical surface of the spike and increase the likelihood of fragmentation. Without diverting vision from the fracture, the countersink is exchanged for the depth gauge. Ideally, the compression lag screw should have one full thread showing through the distal cortex. When the measured length falls between two lengths, the longer is chosen. Optimal screw length is ensured in these obliquely placed screws by placing the depth-gauge hook away from the fracture. This avoids undersizing the screw length, which can compromise fixation (Fig. 33–5).

A 2-mm tap is next used with a tap sleeve to tap both cortices. The proximal cortex is then overdrilled with the 2-mm drill, taking care to not drill beyond the first cortex. The 2-mm lag screw can then be inserted and gently tightened. The second and possibly third screws are inserted in a similar manner, adjusting their positions for the rotational changes of the fracture (Fig. 33–6).

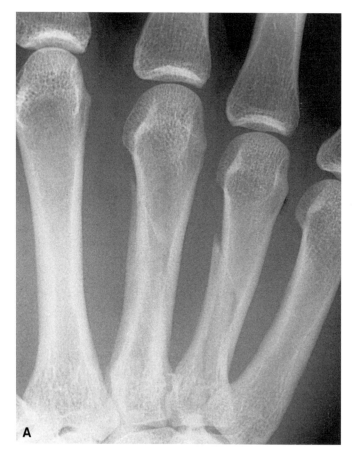
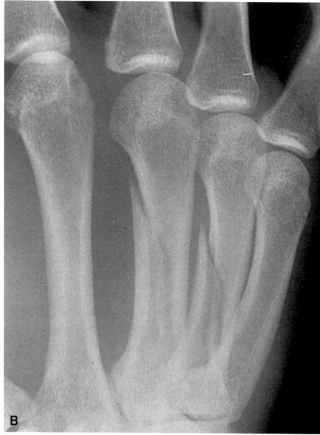

■ FIGURE 33–6

A and **B**, Radiograph of spiral diaphyseal fractures of middle and ring finger metacarpals.

Most complications of metacarpal screw fixation relate to improper technique and lack of experience. As previously stated, these tubular bones are quite fragile, and successful screw fixation requires meticulous attention to detail. The first error of fixation involves inadequate exposure. Although excessive dissection and periosteal stripping are not required, one must be able to visualize the entire fracture out to the proximal and distal apices to determine its configuration and rule out hidden comminution and nondisplaced fracture lines. These may make fixation by screws alone inadequate.

■ TECHNICAL ALTERNATIVES

A fully anatomic reduction must be obtained before initiating screw placement. The miniscrews will not aid in reducing cortices that are not aligned. Placing screws in this manner may lead to stripping of the cortex or fragmentation of the fracture spikes. Clamps and forceps will also damage the thin bony apices if they are applied too vigorously.

The configuration of screw placement must be determined and understood before placing the first screw. All too often, the inexperienced surgeon attempts to place the first screw directly in the center of the fracture, making fixation by additional screws alone impossible. One must always remember to avoid placing screws less than three screw diameters from the nearest fracture margin. During the actual sequence of drilling and tapping, it is crucial for the surgeon to use the drill and tap sleeves and to keep his "eye on the ball." Tapping or placing a screw in an incorrect plane can distract the fragments, thereby fragmenting a spike or stripping a well-placed initial lag screw. Occasionally, a stripped screw can be salvaged by placing a 2.7-mm screw or redrilling the distal cortex in a new plane. Both of these are clearly suboptimal.

Lastly, bone grafting should be considered for any significant cortical defects. If any questions remain regarding the rigidity of fixation, one should not hesitate to add a neutralization plate to protect the intrafragmentary fixation.

■ FIGURE 33-6
(continued) **C,** Radiograph of spiral diaphyseal
fractures of middle and
ring finger metacarpals.
D, Intrafragmentary screw
fixation has been per-
formed using multiple 2-
mm screws. Note the ro-
tation of the screws with
the spiral fracture pat-
terns.

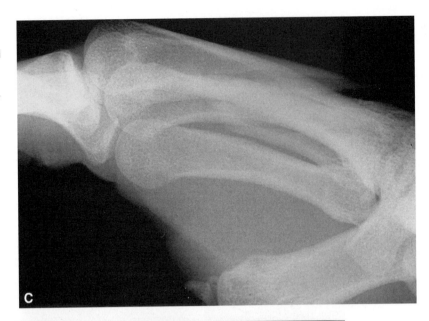

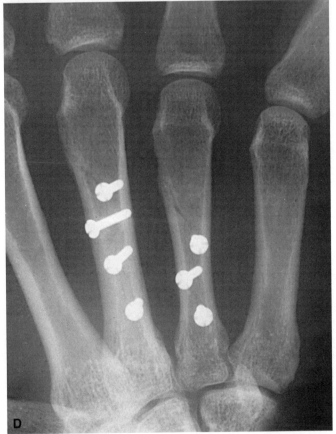

■ REHABILITATION   Rehabilitation after fixation requires close communication between the therapist and
the surgeon. Only the surgeon knows the quality of the fixation, regardless of the appearance on roentgenograms. Barring associated nerve or tendon injuries requiring special
protection, most range of motion programs are begun 1 to 2 days postoperatively. At this
point, edema control is initiated and active and passive motion are begun. Edema is a
proteinaceous fluid that evolves into scar tissue, ultimately limiting motion and function.

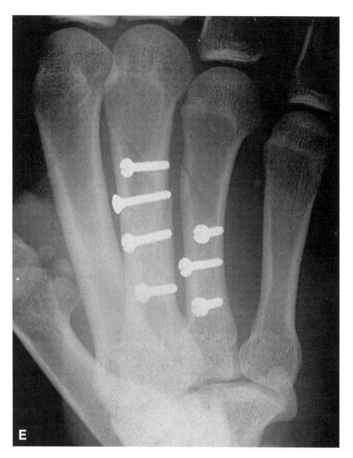

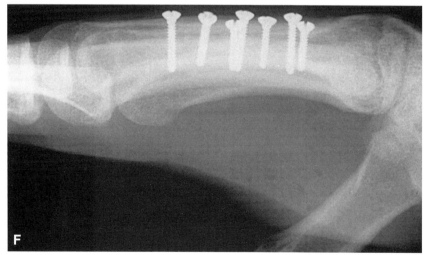

■ FIGURE 33–6 *(continued)* **E** and **F,** Intrafragmentary screw fixation has been performed using multiple 2-mm screws. Note the rotation of the screws with the spiral fracture patterns.

Postsurgical swelling must be controlled with the appropriate elevation and compressive dressings. Motion programs also help reduce edema by the pumping action of the digits, which promotes resorption of this transudate.

If fixation is deemed "rigid," as in a long spiral fracture in a young patient with good bone stock and excellent screw purchase, little postoperative immobilization is necessary. We simply "buddy tape" the digit to the adjacent finger for support when initiating an active and passive motion program. Exercises should emphasize isolated metacarpophalangeal flexion, composite flexion to form a fist, and long extensor tendon excursion by combined metacarpalphalangeal extension and interphalangeal flexion. A night splint in the position of function is often helpful to further aid in edema control. Once the wound is stable, we often incorporate a silicone elastomer putty under the splint at night to help prevent scar thickening on the dorsum of the hand.

At 3 to 4 weeks postoperatively, assuming the fracture site is not painful and alignment has been maintained, progressive strengthening may be initiated with a soft foam ball or putty. By 6 to 8 weeks postoperatively, protection is no longer needed but we advise avoiding contact sports for an additional 2 to 3 weeks unless protected by "buddy tape."

If fixation is deemed semirigid (but stable), such as in a short oblique fracture with marginal bone quality, the rehabilitation program is modified appropriately. Active range of motion exercises are initiated at about 7 to 14 days postoperatively and the fixation is protected between exercise periods with a custom splint in the position of function. Passive range of motion is delayed until 4 to 6 weeks postoperatively in these cases.

■ OUTCOMES

With the proper internal fixation techniques and postoperative rehabilitation, one can expect excellent results with internal fixation of diaphyseal metacarpal fractures. Although no clinical reports specifically address metacarpal screw fixation alone, several support the efficacy of internal fixation for unstable metacarpal diaphyseal fractures.[1-4,6] In these series, there have been no reports of loss of fixation, nonunion, or infection in appropriately treated metacarpal shaft fractures with screws. Total active motion is recorded to be about 97% of normal when screws, plates, or both are applied to the metacarpal.[2] Screw fixation provides stable anatomic reduction with the minimum of soft-tissue dissection and allows early functional rehabilitation of the traumatized hand. Once mastered, the techniques outlined above will provide the surgeon with gratifying results and satisfied patients.

References

1. Crawford GP: Screw fixation for certain fractures of the phalanges and metacarpals. J Bone Joint Surg, 1976; 58A:487–492.
2. Dabezies EJ, Schutte JP: Fixation of metacarpal and phalangeal fractures with miniature plates and screws. J Hand Surg, 1986; 11A:283–288.
3. Hastings H: Unstable metacarpal and phalangeal fracture treatment with screws and plates. Clin Orthop, 1987; 214:37–52.
4. Jabaley ME, Freeland AE: Rigid internal fixation in the hand: 104 cases. Plastic Reconstr Surg, 1986; 77:288–297.
5. Kilbourne BC, Paul EG: The use of small bone screws in the treatment of metacarpal, metatarsal and phalangeal fractures. J Bone Joint Surg, 1958; 40A:375–383.
6. Ruedi TP, Burri C, Pfeiffer KM: Stable internal fixation of the hand. J Trauma, 1971; 11: 381–389.

ALAN E. FREELAND,
WILLIAM B. GEISSLER

34

Plate Fixation of Metacarpal Shaft Fractures

In 1885, Halsted visited Hansmann, who was developing his nickel, copper, and tin plate in Hamburg, Germany. Halsted acquired several of these plates from Hansmann. This plate had a small right angle on one end that protruded from the skin, as did the screws. As a result of this protrusion, the wounds were frequently contaminated or infected. The plate was used to stabilize diaphyseal fractures in long bones; it was left in place for 4 to 8 weeks and then removed. Halsted plated a fracture of the humerus at Roosevelt Hospital in New York about the time that Hansmann first presented his plate to the Deutsche Gesellschaft fur Chirurgie in 1886. In 1890, Halsted used Hansmann plates at the Johns Hopkins Hospital at about the same time that he introduced the use of rubber gloves. In 1893, in a major departure from standard operating technique, Halsted began to use buried screws for plate fixation rather than screws that penetrated the skin.

In 1902, Lambotte introduced the term "osteosynthesis." Soon after, he developed the first modern plate, a plate that was completely buried and was intended to be permanent or to be removed in a later independent operation. He fixed a metacarpal fracture with an aluminum plate and two cerclage wires in 1904. In 1913, Lambotte discussed the use of plates to stabilize metacarpal and phalangeal fractures in his book, *Chirurgie: Operatoire des Fractures*.

In 1909, Lane developed a system of plates and screws. In 1914, he postulated that fractured bone ends held in firm apposition by plates healed primarily.

From 1900 to 1950, many progressive refinements were made in the design, metallurgy, and biomechanics of plates. Between 1956 and 1958, Bagby and Janes developed the first self-compressing bone plate. They used the principle of offset screws to produce compression at the fracture site. Significantly, they noted that compression did not speed the rate of healing but did help to assure it by improving stability. In a separate study, they described the histology of primary contact and gap healing that resulted from their compression plate fixations.

In 1958, Muller, Allgower, and Willenegger led a group of European surgeons in the foundation of the Swiss Arbeitsgemeinschaft fur Osteosynthesefragen or Association for the Study of Internal Fixation. This group combined the talents of physicians, biologists, engineers, and metallurgists to develop principles for design, metallurgic composition, instrumentation, and technique of application of implants for internal fixation. They emphasized from the beginning the importance of research, education, training and technique, and documentation so that continuing progress could be made in this field. Heim and Mathys developed a minifragment set, with plates and screws for bones in the hand and foot in 1970. Heim, Pfeiffer, and Meuli wrote the *Small Fragment Set Manual* in 1974, which was revised and updated in 1982 and 1988.[11] This manual describes the proper technical application of miniplates in the metacarpals. Subsequently, several clinical investigators have described both successful miniplate applications to the metacarpals and some of the techniques used and problems and complications encountered.[4,6,9,10,15,20-22]

■ **HISTORY OF THE TECHNIQUE**

The stability of metacarpal fractures is dually determined by fracture configuration and periosteal (and surrounding soft tissue) disruption. Fracture displacement is an indicator of periosteal disruption and consequently, fracture stability. Fracture configuration and displacement are also treatment and outcome determinants. Outcome is influenced addi-

■ **INDICATIONS AND CONTRAINDICATIONS**

tionally by the extent and severity of adjacent soft-tissue injury. Vascular disruption at the fracture site and consequent adjacent scar formation closely parallel the increasing gravity of soft-tissue injury. Thus, crush and open injuries are more serious than those that are low-energy derived and closed.

Metacarpal shaft fractures may be affected by angular, rotational, shortening, or combined deformities. Angulation is usually dorsal, resulting from unbalanced intrinsic muscle forces. Generally, the hand can accommodate up to 10 to 15° more dorsal angulation than afforded by the carpometacarpal joint motion at the base of the fractured metacarpal. As a guideline, this means that about up to 10 to 15° of dorsal angulation may be accepted in the second and third metacarpals, 30 to 35° in the fourth metacarpal, and 50 to 55° in the fifth metacarpal. Projection of the metacarpal head into the palm, clawing on extension of the fractured digit, loss of knuckle contour, severe unsightly angulation, and frank fracture instability may justify closed or open reduction and internal fixation, whether or not fracture angulation exceeds the above guidelines.[7] Patient age, the presence or absence of systemic disease, occupational considerations, bone mineralization, and the wishes of the patient or the patient's family are additional considerations.

Rotational deformity generally is unacceptable. In oblique or spiral fracture configurations, separation of the fracture fragments by a radiolucent line on plain radiograph may be the earliest indication of a rotational deformity. With the fingers extended, rotational malalignment is masked by divergence of the fingers. A small rotational deformity may result in a substantial overlap of the fingers when they are closed to form a fist.[16]

Metacarpal shortening of up to 4 mm is fairly well tolerated without much functional loss.[1,3] The deep transverse metacarpal ligaments of intact metacarpals constrain shortening in adjacent fractured metacarpals. The correction of excessive shortening is achieved in concert with that of angulation and rotation by closed manipulation or open reduction.

Closed simple (single fracture line) fractures that can be reduced by closed manipulation and maintained by functional casting or bracing or by transcutaneous K-wire techniques need not be opened or plated. Fractures that cannot be adequately reduced or maintained within the confines of the above guidelines are candidates for open reduction and plate fixation. Open, comminuted, and multiple metacarpal fractures, especially those with bone loss, often require plate fixation for sufficient or optimal stability.

■ SURGICAL
TECHNIQUES

Regional intravenous or axillary block anesthesia is usually adequate for the operative treatment of metacarpal fractures. General anesthesia may be indicated for multiple or difficult fractures or at the discretion of the patient or anesthesiologist.

Although sharp, designed, low-energy incisions are less destructive than blunt, random, high-energy, traumatic soft-tissue laceration or disruption,[5] their impact on outcome must be considered by the surgeon. The concept of one-wound-one scar[17] (unit scar) is useful in evaluation, treatment selection, prognostication, and rehabilitation. Incisional contour and placement are shaped and positioned to avoid mobile deep structure incorporation with the fracture and skin as much as possible without seriously compromising exposure and structural fixation of the bone (Fig. 34–1A and B). The hand—with its adjacent intrinsic muscles, a thicker and more mobile covering, and the absence of extensive and sophisticated ligamentous and tendinous force couples—is more tolerant to injury and forgiving to function after surgery than the fingers.

Plate Application   Plates have anatomic names for their form, such as straight, "T," or "L" tubular or dynamic compression plates. There are also long straight and minicondylar reconstruction plates used to bridge defects with comminution or loss and to incorporate bone grafts. Reconstruction plates can be custom cut to the desired length at the time of surgery. They also can be contoured by bending in all three planes, whereas conventional tubular plates only can be contoured in two planes. Bending should only be carried out in one direction in any one or more planes, even if incrementally. Bending a plate back for correction of a previously applied contour decreases plate fatigue strength and life.

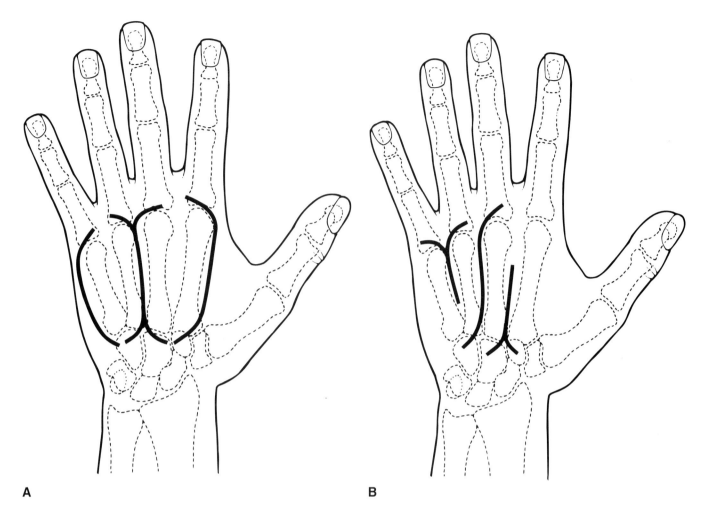

A   B

■ FIGURE 34–1

A, Longitudinal incisions are offset from the fractured metacarpal to spare the extensor tendon or tendons from excessive scarring to contiguous skin and bone. Two adjacent diaphyseal fractures can be approached through a single incision. **B,** These are additional incisional modifications for two adjacent metacarpal fractures proximally, distally, and at different levels.

Plates also have functional names for the physiologic way in which they are applied. This includes neutralization, compression (tension banding), and buttress plating. Bridging or strutting plates are a subtype of neutralization plate. A plate may perform one or even two of these functions. When performing two functions, a plate may neutralize and compress or it may neutralize and buttress. It can never buttress and compress because these are diametrically opposed functions.[19]

Several factors affect bone-plate construct stability and strength. The bending strength of a plate is proportionate to the cube of its thickness. Tubular and reconstruction plates are of adequate thickness to provide sufficient stability for most metacarpal fractures. Thicker mini-dynamic compression plates are occasionally necessary.

The bending strength of a plate is inversely proportionate to the cube of its length. Plates must provide sufficient length for screws to purchase three or preferably four cortices on either side of a diaphyseal fracture. Despite the decreased bending strength of a longer plate, this disadvantage is often more than compensated by the increased stability provided by the purchase of bone and cortex by additional screws. The number of screws applied, screw core diameter, screw thread diameter, the pitch of the screw, the area of bone and especially cortex purchased between the threads, the mineralization of the bone, cortical thickness, and the physiologic application of the plate are additional factors affect-

■ FIGURE 34–2
Minicondylar plate design allows application dorsally or laterally for periarticular metacarpal diaphyseal fractures, with or without bone loss.

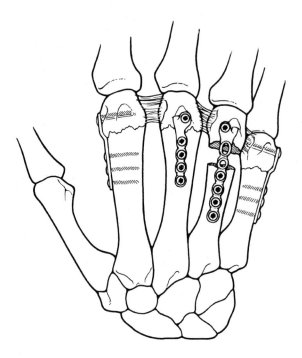

ing bone-plate construct stability. Occasionally, we have used screws one size larger than the plate size (e.g., 2.7-mm screws in a 2-mm plate) for additional stability.

For mid-diaphyseal fractures, plates conventionally are applied dorsally on the tension side of the fractured bone, where dorsal angulation tends to occur. Exceptions may occur because of fracture configuration, wounding, or at the discretion of the surgeon.

When a fracture is near the diaphyseal metaphyseal junction, "T," "L," or minicondylar plates are used because their design allows the placement of more screws and better fixation in the metaphysis than a straight plate. "T" and "L" plates must be applied dorsally but minicondylar plates are more versatile because they are smaller and have a lower profile. This allows lateral as well as dorsal application (Fig. 34–2).[2]

Intraoperatively, the surgeon often can manipulate metacarpal fractures into a reduced or nearly reduced position by making a fist with the patient's hand, with or without the Jahss' maneuver.[13] The rotational deformity is largely corrected, and further fine adjustment can be affected by using the proximal phalanx as a lever to rotate the distal fragment indirectly or by open anatomic reduction. The position of the fingernails and the relation to the scaphoid tubercle are further indicators of rotational alignment.

Transverse Fractures   For transverse diaphyseal fractures, straight plates are used in the compression mode. Four- to six-hole plates with at least four cortices secured by screws on either side of the fracture are usually sufficient (Fig. 34–3A through C). Screws adjacent to the fracture may be placed so that they diverge slightly away from it to assure firm purchase in the far cortex without bone fragmentation (Fig. 34–4A through F).

Transverse fractures at the metaphyseal diaphyseal junction are secured by "T," "L," or minicondylar plates. The plate chosen, fracture configuration, accessibility, wounding, and the preference of the surgeon influence whether the plate is placed dorsally or laterally.

Short Oblique and Spiral Fractures   Short oblique or spiral fractures (fracture line less than two times the diameter of adjacent bone) ordinarily have only the capacity for one lag screw across the fracture. A single lag screw can seldom support a diaphyseal fracture alone (Fig. 34–5A through B). Consequently, a plate is applied to neutralize bending and rotational forces (Fig. 34–6).

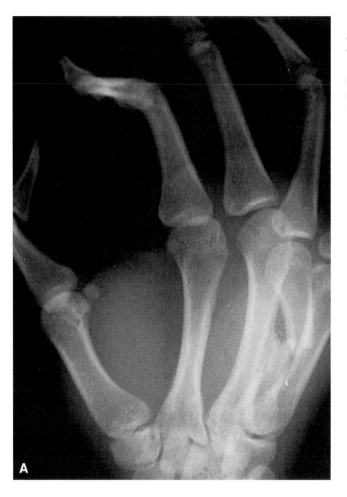

■ FIGURE 34-3

A, A transverse displaced closed diaphyseal fourth metacarpal fracture is shortened, angulated, and slightly supinated. Swelling prevents reduction.

Open Fractures   Open fractures generally have or require sufficient fracture exposure for adequate wound care that plate fixation can be applied with little additional dissection. The additional stability provided by plate fixation is an adjunct against infection and protects the repairs of other deep structures (tendons, nerves, blood vessels). Plate fixation also controls pain and allows earlier and more intensive functional rehabilitation. Transverse and short oblique or spiral fractures are treated by the techniques described above. With comminuted fractures having major fragments, the fragments can be reduced and fixed by compression lag screws and then incorporated into the proximal and distal metacarpal fragments by a neutralizing bridging or strut plate. Fractures with irreparable comminution or bone loss present special problems with fixation and bone grafting.[8,14]

Multiple Metacarpal Fractures   When two or more metacarpals are fractured and displaced, the intrinsic stability of the hand is substantially compromised. Although not imperative, this is often a strong indication for internal fracture fixation. Severe extraarticular fracture angulation should alert the physician to look at adjacent metacarpal bases for fracture, dislocation, or combined injury.

Reducible closed simple (single fracture line) extraarticular metacarpal fractures frequently can be treated by closed manipulation and functional cast bracing. When additional stabilization is required, percutaneous transfixation wires are an excellent method.[18] Reducible closed oblique or spiral fractures usually require fixation because of their unstable configuration. The transfixation wires are left in place for 4 weeks. The hand is further protected in a position of function by splinting. Although there may be temporary tethering of the interosseous muscles, this is usually of little consequence to final functional

■ TECHNICAL
ALTERNATIVES

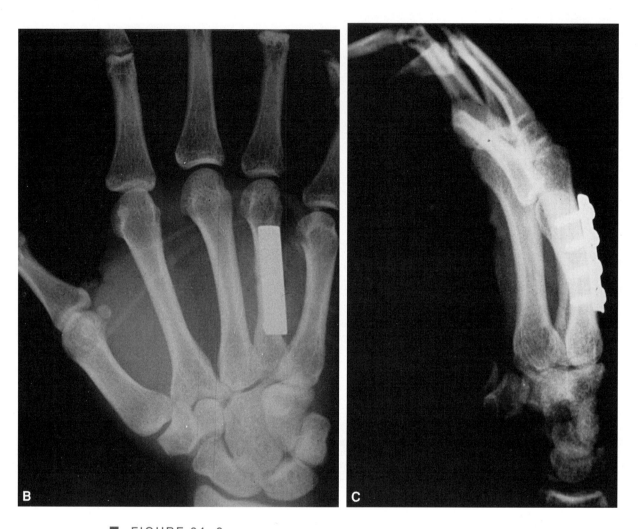

■ FIGURE 34–3
(continued) **B** and **C**, A dorsal 4-hole tubular plate is applied, using the principles outlined in Fig. 34–4.

outcome. This minimally invasive method of closed reduction and internal fixation has the combined advantages of high reliability in achieving fracture union and little additional scar formation to impair functional recovery.

Completely displaced transverse fractures are frequently accompanied by swelling that prevents a closed reduction. When these fractures require open reduction, wiring techniques may be chosen in preference to plate fixation when the reduction can be performed with a less extensive incision.

Fractures of oblique, spiral, or combined configuration longer than twice the diameter of the bone are called long oblique or spiral oblique fractures. These fractures can accept and be stabilized by two or more miniscrews.

■ REHABILITATION

Stable anatomic fracture position is paramount for pain control and rehabilitation. Once this is achieved in the finger metacarpals, the hand should be placed in the position of function and splinted. Gentle progressive active range of motion exercises are instituted within the patient's pain and functional tolerance. Buddy splinting to an adjacent intact digit is an excellent method of preventing painful or disruptive snagging of an injured finger. Although most hand functions are performed in the mid-range of digital motion,[12] extremes of motion are important. Full flexion is important for grasping and pinching activities and for strength, power, and endurance. If the patient lacks full extension of the

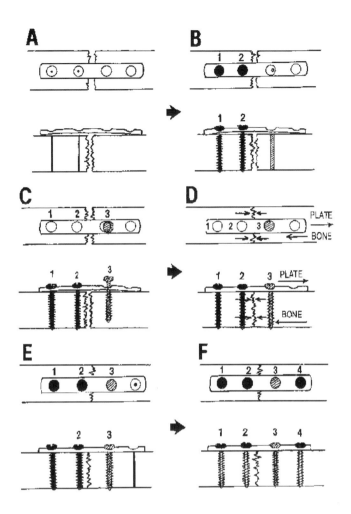

■ FIGURE 34-4

This diagram demonstrates a reduced transverse metacarpal diaphyseal fracture with a gap of less than 1 mm. **A,** Two neutral (centered) holes are drilled on the left side of the fracture. The plate has a graduated bend of about 5° centered at the middle of the plate with no acute bend or buckling, especially at the level of the screw holes. **B,** Two neutral (centered) screws are placed on the left side of the fracture site. A drill hole is placed eccentrically, away from the fracture site in the screw hole adjacent to the fracture on the right side of the plate. **C,** A screw is inserted in the eccentric drill hole. **D,** As the screw is tightened and the screw head engages the plate, translation of the plate and bone in opposite directions cause compression at the fracture site. **E,** After compression is obtained, a neutral drill hole is centered in the remaining plate hole or holes. **F,** A neutral screw is then inserted completing fixation. (Reprinted with permission from Freeland AE, Jabaley ME: Management of Hand Fractures by Stable Fixation. In: Habal MB, et al (eds): Advances in Plastic and Reconstructive Surgery, Vol 2, Chicago: Year Book Medical Publishers, Inc., 1986:106–107)

digit, he or she will have trouble placing it in a pocket, glove, or other confined areas. Splinting the proximal interphalangeal joint of a finger in full extension may be useful, especially during therapy sessions, to achieve a full arc of digital flexion and extension through the metacarpophalangeal joint and to avoid extensor tendon adhesions to the injured metacarpal.

It is additionally important to maintain the metacarpophalangeal joint in at least 50° of flexion during rehabilitation, so that the collateral ligaments at the metacarpophalangeal joint can be maintained at their longest diameter. Positioning and rehabilitation of the hand with the metacarpophalangeal joint in this position minimize the risk of ligament

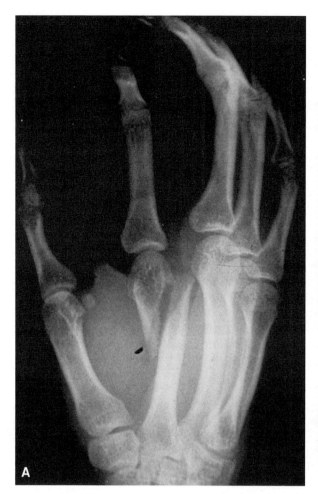

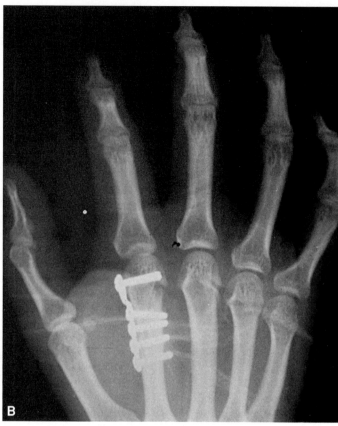

■ FIGURE 34–5

A, A closed displaced oblique index metacarpal fracture at the diaphyseal metaphyseal junction is unstable. **B**, Open reduction is secured, using a lateral minicondylar plate in the buttress mode. This plate also neutralizes the bending and rotational forces on the lag screws applied through the plate in accordance with the principles outlined in Fig. 34–6 II B.

and capsular contracture. Should this occur, capsulectomy or sufficient collateral ligament origin release, particularly of the band portion of the ligament, may be necessary if intensive hand therapy alone cannot overcome this deficit.

Extensor tendon adhesions to a fractured metacarpal can occur independently or frequently coexist with nonunion and malunion. In the hand, these respond well to tenolysis. When a fracture is clinically and radiographically healed, any retained metallic implant can be removed at the time of tenolysis. When tendon adhesions occur in concert with nonunion or malunion, firm stable fixation, usually by a miniplate, is preferable so that vigorous rehabilitation can be instituted immediately after surgery to maintain any operative functional gain achieved by tenolysis.

■ OUTCOMES

Plate fixation of finger metacarpal diaphyseal fractures is reliable in terms of biomechanical stability. Outcome is more closely related to the extent and severity of soft-tissue damage. Although sharp, designed, low-energy incisions are less destructive than blunt, random, high-energy, traumatic soft-tissue disruption, their impact on outcome must be considered by the surgeon. Consequently, we prefer closed reduction and transcutaneous transfixation wiring techniques for single, simple, low-demand metacarpal fractures and in

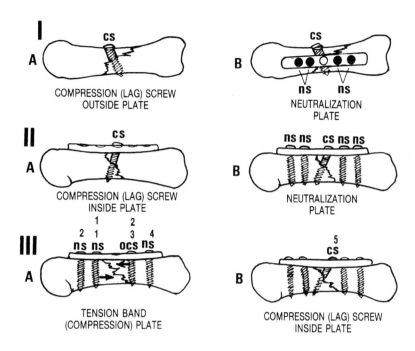

■ FIGURE 34-6

Whenever a screw crosses a fracture, the lag screw principle should be applied. By using the lag screw principle and drilling a gliding hole the same size or just slightly larger than the screw thread diameter across the proximal cortex of the fracture, compression can be achieved when the screw threads purchase the far cortex. This is accomplished by inserting a drill guide into the gliding hole and drilling the same diameter as the screw core. The core hole is then threaded with a tap. When self-tapping screws are used, this step is eliminated. When the screw is inserted, it glides through the proximal fragment and purchases the distal threaded fragment, compressing the fracture. Whenever a screw crosses the fracture site, the lag-screw principle should be applied. Straight plates are used for diaphyseal fractures. "T," "L," or mini-condylar plates are used at the metaphyseal or diaphyseal junction. A lag screw may be applied either outside (I) or inside (II and III) of a neutralization plate. If applied inside the plate, the lag screw may be applied first with the remaining screws placed in neutral position in the plate (II). This is a pure neutralization plate. For stronger plate-bone construct when circumstances allow, the lag screw may be applied after fracture compression (III). Such a plate compresses the fracture, as does the lag screw. The plate also neutralizes the bending and rotational forces on the lag screw.

osteopenic bone. Tendon adhesions and joint stiffness are rare sequelae with transfixation pinning.[18]

Plating is reserved for those single simple fractures requiring open reduction or for multiple metacarpal or hand fractures and for fracture configurations where pinning is inapplicable, less reliable, or biomechanically insufficient. It is also used for open fractures to enhance biomechanical stability when exposure of the fracture is partially or completely made by the initial injury. Increased fracture stability is a real advantage when adjacent skin, tendons, nerves, and blood vessels require repair or reconstruction. Plate fixation of simple (single fracture line) closed finger diaphyseal fractures achieve good (70 to 85%) to excellent (86 to 100%) total active digital range of motion in 90% or more of injured fingers.[4,6,20,22] Of the fingers having good or excellent motion, 75% are excellent and more than 50% have a full range.[6]

Results with plating of grades I and II open fractures closely approximate those of closed fractures in terms of recovery of digital motion. More severe fractures have fewer results in the good or excellent categories and 25% or more fingers have poor (less than 50%)

recovery of digital motion.[5] This is probably due more to injury severity than to implant selection or application. Although exact data are not available, tendon injury probably potentially compromises functional outcome.

Infection, nonunion, and amputations are rare, ranging from 0[4,6,22] to 2%.[20] Malunion is also unusual and was not reported in three series,[4,6,22] whereas it occurred in 6% of fractures in another.[20] Plate removal was performed for cause, usually discomfort due to prominence, as a secondary procedure in 8 to 25% of fractures.

References

1. Bloem JJAM: The treatment and prognosis of uncomplicated dislocated fractures of the metacarpals and phalanges. Arch Chir Neerl, 1971; 23:55–65.
2. Buchler U, Fischer T: Use of a minicondylar plate for metacarpal and phalangeal periarticular injuries. Clin Orthop, 1987; 214:53–58.
3. Butt WD: Fractures of the hand III. Treatment and results. Can Med Assoc J, 1962; 86: 815–822.
4. Dabezies EJ, Schulte JP: Fixation of metacarpal and phalangeal fractures with minimal plates and screws. J Hand Surg, 1986; 11A:283–288.
5. Duncan RW, Freeland AE, Jabaley ME, Meydrech EF: Open hand fractures: an analysis of the recovery of active motion and of complications. J Hand Surg, 1993; 18A:387–394.
6. Ford DJ, El-Hadidi S, Lunn PG, Burke FD: Fractures of the metacarpals: treatment by AO screws and plate fixation. J Hand Surg, 1987; 12B:34–37.
7. Freeland AE, Geissler WB: Malunions and Nonunions of the Hand. In: Kellam J, Johnson K (eds): Malunions and Nonunions, New York: Raven Press. In press.
8. Freeland AE, Jabaley ME, Burkhalter WE, Chaves AMV: Delayed primary bone grafting in the hand and wrist after traumatic bone loss. J Hand Surg, 1984; 9:22–28.
9. Freeland AE, Jabaley ME, Hughes JL: Stable Fixation of the Hand and Wrist. New York: Springer-Verlag, 1986.
10. Hastings H II: Unstable metacarpal and phalangeal fracture treatment with screws and plates. Clin Orthop, 1987; 214:37–42.
11. Heim U, Pfeiffer KM: In collaboration with Meuli HC: Small fragment set manual. Technique recommended by the ASIF Group (Swiss Association for Study of Internal Fixation), New York, Springer-Verlag, 1974.
12. Hume MC, Gellman H, McKellop H, Brumfield RH Jr: Functional range of motion of the joints of the hand. J Hand Surg, 1990; 15A:240–243.
13. Jahss SA: Fractures of the metacarpals: a new method of reduction and immobilization. J Bone Joint Surg, 1938; 20:178–186.
14. Littler JW: Metacarpal reconstruction. J Bone Joint Surg, 1947; 29A:723–737.
15. Melone CP: Rigid fixation of phalangeal and metacarpal fractures. Orthop Clin North Am, 1986; 17:421–435.
16. Opgrande JD, Westphal SA: Fractures of the hand. Orthop Clin North Am, 1983; 14:779–792.
17. Peacock EE, Van Winkle W: Surgery and biology of wound repair. Philadelphia: WB Saunders, 1970:333.
18. Raskin KB, Melone CP Jr, Prazier JI, Segalsnan K: Closed pinning of unstable metacarpal fractures. Paper presented at the 46th ASSH Annual Meeting, October 5, 1991, Orlando, FL.
19. Rosen H: Plate fixation, AO Basic and advanced fracture couses, 1987, Davos, Switzerland.
20. Segmuller G: Surgical Stabilization of the Skeleton of the Hand. Baltimore: Williams & Wilkins, 1977.
21. Simonetta C: The use of "AO" plates in the hand. Hand, 1970; 2:43–45.
22. Stern PJ, Wieser MJ, Reilly DG: Complications of plate fixation in the hand skeleton. Clin Orthop, 1987; 214:59–65.

35

THOMAS F.
DeBARTOLO

Screw Fixation of Bennett's Fracture

Edward H. Bennett (1837–1907), Professor of Surgery at Trinity College (Dublin, Ireland) reported his observations concerning an oblique intraarticular fracture involving the base of the thumb metacarpal in 1882.[17] The particular fracture pattern to which the pseudonym Bennett's fracture applies occurs as a result of an axially directed force on a partially flexed thumb metacarpal, resulting in a two-part intraarticular fracture. One fracture fragment of variable size is composed of the medial volar base of the first metacarpal. This segment is never displaced and is held in its anatomic position by the deep palmar "beak" ligament. The second fracture fragment, which may or may not be displaced, is the remaining portion of the first metacarpal. When the applied force is sufficient to cause displacement, it is this larger metacarpal fragment that is displaced radially and dorsally (Fig. 35–1). It is also supinated by the unchecked pull of the abductor pollicis longus (APL), whereas the adductor pollicis pulls the first metacarpal head in a palmar direction.

■ HISTORY OF THE TECHNIQUE

The Bennett's fracture has been the focus of much clinical study, which reflects the following: 1) it occurs commonly, the ratio being ten males to one female; 2) two thirds involve the dominant hand; 3) about 50% occur in patients younger than 30 years of age;[8] and 4) different fracture displacement patterns exist with associated injury to the metacarpophalangeal joint.[12]

Bennett's original recommended treatment consisted of closed reduction by thumb extension and immobilization. Previous clinical studies of patients with Bennett's fracture have suggested that less than anatomic reduction does not lead to significant symptomatic first carpometacarpal (CMC) joint arthritis.[4,5]

Consequently, more aggressive surgical treatment has remained controversial. More recent clinical studies are changing our concepts about treating Bennett's fracture. A study by Livesley, with an average 26-year follow-up of patients having conservatively managed Bennett's fractures, found that patients had decreased thumb range of motion (especially extension), diminished pinch strength, and radiographic evidence of degenerative arthritis in 88% of the CMC joints.[14]

Recent advances in understanding of the pathomechanics of injuries to articular cartilage generally and of the development of articular cartilage degeneration at the trapeziometacarpal joint particularly, combined with the continuing clarification of the natural history of Bennett's fracture, are beginning to define optimum treatment. Experimentally induced intraarticular fractures with fragments that allow anatomic reduction and internal fixation with compression heal with virtually normal articular cartilage.[3] Osteoarthritis of the trapeziometacarpal joint develops primarily on the palmar compartment of the first metacarpal, the contact area between the thumb metacarpal and the trapezium in lateral pinch. Articular cartilage injury occurs in the aging joint in proportion to the attrition of the anterior oblique ligament, an aging process that allows shear forces to be generated as the first metacarpal translates on the trapezium with lateral pinch.[16] A Bennett's fracture that heals with intraarticular displacement (Fig. 35–2) permanently translocates a significant proportion of the articular surface of the first metacarpal, thereby predisposing the patient to posttraumatic arthrosis. Therefore, when fracture fragment size is sufficient, I recommend open reduction and internal fixation with a screw.

■ FIGURE 35–1
In an acute Bennett's
fracture, the small medial
volar base of the first
metacarpal is undis-
placed, and the remain-
ing portion of the first
metacarpal is displaced
radially and dorsally.

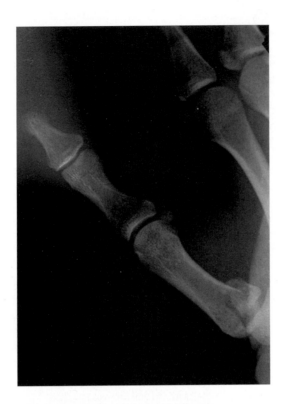

■ FIGURE 35–2
In a Bennett's fracture
that heals in a displaced
position, a significant portion of the articular surface of the first metacarpal is translocated,
predisposing to posttrau-
matic arthrosis.

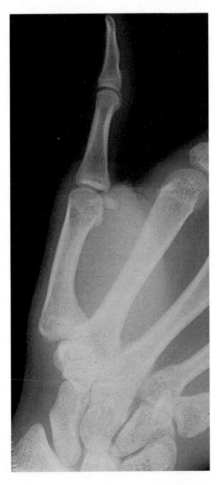

In a Bennett's fracture, the fragment sizes and the amount of displacement can be difficult to interpret using routine radiographs. A true lateral radiograph of the first CMC joint can be especially helpful. This projection is obtained by placing the palm of the injured hand on a radiographic cassette, pronating the hand 20°, and directing the beam 15° proximally from the vertical.[1]

If the fracture is nondisplaced, reduction can be maintained by closed percutaneous pinning of the first metacarpal to adjacent bony structures.[19] If the radiographic assessment of the fractured first metacarpal base demonstrates 1) displacement of the articular surface equal to or greater than 1 mm in any plane, 2) a truly two-part fracture, and 3) that the smaller fracture fragment is at least a third of the articular surface, open reduction internal fixation with a screw is the patient's best treatment option. An open Bennett's fracture is also an indication for meticulous debridement in addition to immediate screw fixation.

When there are more than two fracture fragments, the pattern of fracture is a Y- or T-type intraarticular fracture of the first metacarpal base. This type of fracture pattern is termed a Rolando's fracture. Internal fixation of a Rolando's fracture with a single screw is not technically possible and a first metacarpal base fracture exhibiting intraarticular comminution is an absolute contraindication for the use of a single screw for internal fixation. When confronted with a patient who has an acute Rolando fracture, it is important to recognize that successful open reduction and internal fixation of this type of fracture pattern is difficult to achieve and it is my recommendation that internal fixation of this fracture should only be undertaken by a surgeon fully trained and experienced in the internal fixation of small fractures. When the fracture fragment size is small, the screw thread diameter must be less than 30% of the length of the fragment's cortical surface to avoid iatrogenic fracturing of the fragment, and the surgeon should be prepared to stabilize the fragment with multiple K-wires rather than a screw.

If the patient's fracture is closed but the surrounding soft tissue has been severely traumatized, closed reduction and percutaneous pinning, oblique traction,[2] or application of an external fixator[10] rather than open reduction and internal fixation should be considered.

Once the operation is indicated, the injured extremity should be splinted and elevated until operative treatment can be performed. In discussing the risks and expectations of treatment with the patient, I also discuss anesthesia alternatives and usually recommend a regional anesthetic. I likewise notify the anesthesia consultant of my preference for a regional anesthetic.

In the operating room, the anesthetized patient is placed in a supine position, a pneumatic tourniquet is applied, and the prepped and draped extremity is positioned on an extremity table. The patient is given a broad-spectrum antibiotic agent prophylactically.

A curved radiovolar approach to the first CMC joint is employed, using the demarcation between dorsal and palmar skin. The incision is drawn to extend distally along the radial border of the metacarpal shaft just volar to the extensor pollicis brevis tendon (EPB). Under tourniquet control, with low-power loop magnification, the incision is made and the flap is elevated and retracted distally and volarly. This exposes the fine branches of the radial sensory nerve, which are protected. The nerve branches may be carefully mobilized along their ulnar border and gently retracted in a dorsoradial direction. To avoid desiccation of the nerve branches and soft tissues, moist sponges or frequent irrigation of the tissue is necessary. The key anatomic landmark is the insertion of the APL on the displaced first metacarpal fragment. The fracture and capsule of the first CMC joint are visualized as the thenar musculature, the superficial abductor pollicis brevis, and the deep opponens are subperiosteally stripped from the volar and proximal aspect of the first metacarpal (Fig. 35–3A). The joint is opened transversely, allowing evacuation of the hematoma and visualization of both articular fragments. The capsule between the small, undisplaced metacarpal fragment and the trapezium is not released. After directly viewing the fracture fragment size, the specific internal fixation device (2-mm screw, 2.7-mm screw, or multiple K-wires) to be used should be confirmed.

With the articular fracture exposed, the surgical site is copiously irrigated and carefully debrided until anatomic reduction can be confirmed. The interval between the APL and

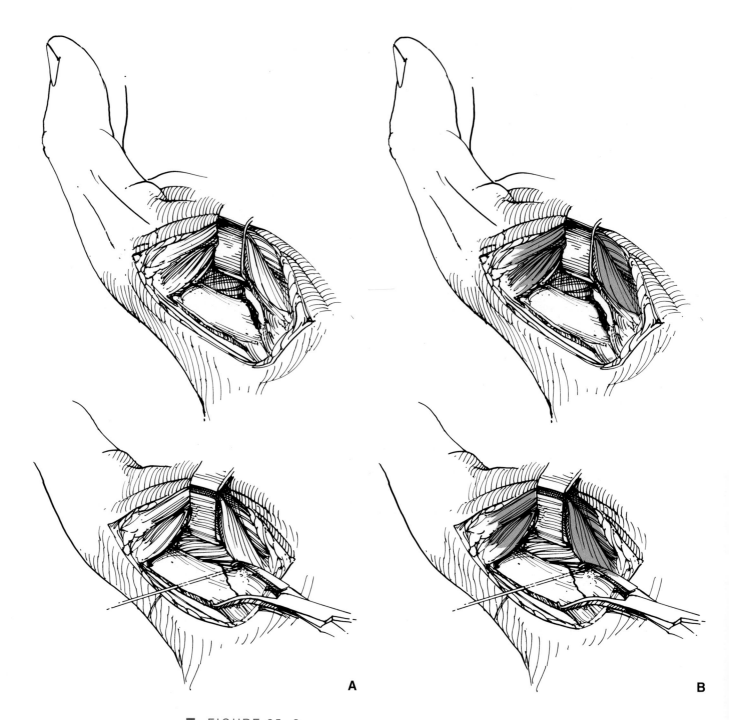

■ FIGURE 35–3
A, The surgical exposure is volar to the EPB tendon; the thenar muscles are elevated, using subperiosteal dissection. **B**, The reduction is temporarily stabilized with a distally placed 1-mm K-wire.

the EPB is exposed and prepared to serve as the portal of fixation. Reduction is obtained as the assistant applies longitudinal traction on the thumb and rotates the thumb as directed by the surgeon. The surgeon completes reduction with a small bone or nerve hook and secures the anatomic reduction with small reduction forceps. I then stabilize the reduction with an 0.8-mm or 1-mm K-wire placed through the fixation portal parallel but slightly distal to the desired final screw position (Fig. 35–3B). The provisional K-wire fixation allows removal of the reduction forceps and final inspection, confirming anatomic

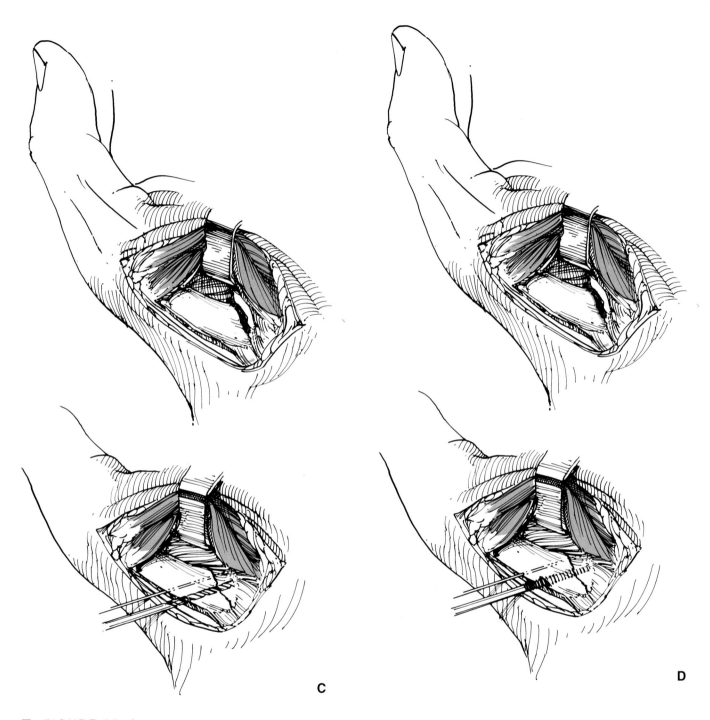

C

D

■ FIGURE 35–3
(continued) **C**, A 2-mm drill hole is made through both fracture fragments, perpendicular to the fracture plane. **D**, The hole is tapped with a 2.7-mm tap.

reduction of the articular fracture fragments. When reduction is not satisfactory, the exposure is extended by Z-division of the APL and further subperiosteal stripping of the thenar musculature. When reduction is satisfactory and the fracture fragment size is compatible with the use of a 2.7-mm cortical screw, the reduction forceps are reapplied and a 2-mm drill hole is made through both fracture fragments in the position of optimal screw alignment, perpendicular to the fracture plane in the cross-section (Fig. 35–3C). The hole is then measured and tapped using the 2.7-mm tap (Fig. 35–3D). A 2.7-mm drill is used

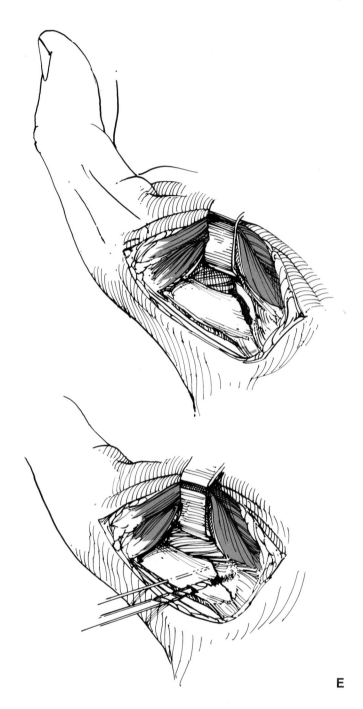

■ FIGURE 35–3

(continued) **E**, The outer hole is over-drilled with a 2.7-mm drill. The appropriately sized 2.7-mm cortical screw is inserted and tightened, producing a lag-screw effect.

to convert the tapped hole through the main (lateral) fragment into a gliding hole (Fig. 35–3E). The appropriately sized 2.7-mm cortical screw is then inserted and tightened.[7,9] The provisional K-wire fixation is removed, and the anatomic reduction is visually confirmed. If a Z-tenomyotomy of the APL was performed, it is repaired with interrupted braided synthetic sutures, such as 4-0 Ticron (Davis-Geck, Ontario, Canada). The thenar musculature is also loosely reapproximated to the periosteum of the thumb metacarpal using a similar suture. The skin is closed with interrupted sutures of the fine nylon. The wound is sterilely dressed, and a thumb spica splint is applied.

In the operative management of a patient having a Bennett's fracture, the surest way to avoid intraoperative pitfalls is with preoperative planning. Proper radiographic assessment of fracture patterns, fracture fragment size, and fragment displacement is critical. Attentive handling of the soft tissues intraoperatively is also important. Injury to the sensory branches of the superficial radial nerve can result in painful neuromas and prolonged disability.[13] Correct mobilization, gentle retraction, moistening the tissues, and protecting the nerve branches while drilling, tapping, and inserting the screw are the keys to avoiding neuroma formation. Proper soft-tissue handling is also critically important in fracture exposure. The capsulotomy of the first CMC joint should be limited. The capsule between the small undisplaced metacarpal fracture fragment and the trapezium is not opened and the attachment of the anterior oblique ligament must be maintained.

Once the fracture has been exposed and an anatomic reduction with provisional K-wire fixation has been obtained, it is important to maintain manual compression across the fracture site during the steps of internal fixation. Failure to maintain compression frequently results in a slight step off or rotational irregularity at the articular surface, which compromises the clinical outcome.

Comminution of the volar fragment, either unanticipated or as a result of attempted internal fixation, makes anatomic restoration of the articular surface impossible. This intra-articular situation can be salvaged with excision of the comminuted fragments and reconstruction of the volar anterior oblique ligament, using a portion of the flexor carpi radialis tendon.[6]

Therapy after screw fixation of a Bennett's fracture is usually not extensive and can be performed on a home program basis. Sutures are removed at 7 to 10 days and the plaster

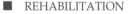

■ TECHNICAL ALTERNATIVES

■ REHABILITATION

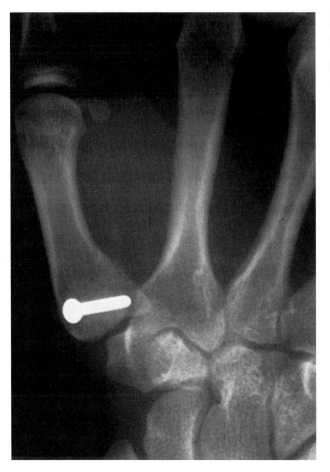

■ FIGURE 35–4
An anatomically reduced Bennet's fracture with 2.7-mm cortical screw fixation.

splint is replaced with a removable thermal plastic spica splint, fabricated by the hand therapist. The patient is instructed to use this splint at all times, except during exercise. Active range of motion exercises are initiated at this point. They include circumduction of the thumb, opposition of the thumb pulp to the pulps of digits II through V, and flexing the tip of the thumb to the fifth metacarpal head. The patient is instructed to perform these exercises three times a day, with ten repetitions of each exercise. The patient is advised against using the hand for resistive gripping or pinching during this time. One week after active exercise is initiated, the fit of the splint and the progress of thumb motion should be reevaluated by the hand therapist. At the 4- to 6-week point, the splint can be discontinued if the physician believes that the fracture is both clinically and radiographically healed (Fig. 35–4). Reincorporation of the hand into daily activity should be the focus at this time. Athletes are able to return to active competition without protection usually in 6 to 8 weeks.[18]

■ OUTCOMES

Complications after a Bennett's fracture can include limited thumb index web span, joint mobility, and pinch ability.[11] The therapist must recognize these sequelae and initiate edema-control measures, splinting, and exercise as needed. Because of the ability of the patient to begin early mobilization after screw fixation, however, these complications are usually avoided.

A patient with a Bennett's fracture that has been successfully treated, by anatomic reduction and stabilized by compression screw fixation which allows early protected range of motion, should anticipate normal painless motion, with minimal long-term risk of posttraumatic arthrosis. The above supposition is confirmed in a continuous series of 94 patients having Bennett's fractures, 44 of which were treated openly with single lag-screw fixation. There were no infections, no nonunions, and no mechanical failures of internal fixation. Ninety percent of patients were pain free, 93% of patients had full range of thumb and hand motion, and 89% had pinch strengths that were equal to the uninvolved side. Radiographic and clinical signs of posttraumatic arthrosis were present in only 2% of patients.[15]

References

1. Billing L, Gedda KO: Roentgen examination of Bennett's fracture. Acta Radiol, 1952; 38: 471–476.
2. Breen TF, Gelberman RH, Jupiter JB: Intra-articular fractures of the basilar joint of the thumb. Hand Clin, 1988; 4:491–501.
3. Buckwalter JA: Mechanical injuries of articular cartilage. Iowa Orthop J, 1992; 12:50–57.
4. Cannon SR, Dowd GSE, Williams DH, Scott JM: A long-term study following Bennett's fracture. J Hand Surg, 1986; 11B:426–431.
5. Charnley J: The Closed Treatment of Common Fractures, London: E & S Livingstone, 1968.
6. Eaton RG, Lane LB, Littler JW, Keyser JJ: Ligament reconstruction for the painful thumb carpometacarpal joint: a long-term assessment. J Hand Surg, 1984; 9A:692–699.
7. Foster RJ, Hastings H: Treatment of Bennett, Rolando, and vertical intra-articular trapezial fractures. Clin Orthop, 1987; 214:121–129.
8. Gedda KO: Studies on Bennett fractures: anatomy, roentgenology and therapy. Acta Chir Scand Suppl, 1954; 193–195.
9. Heim U, Pfeiffer KM: The Hand. In: Internal Fixation of Small Fractures, New York: Springer-Verlag, 1988:179–245.
10. Jakob RP: Frame fixation of the first metacarpal to the second metacarpal. In: The Small External Fixator: AO Bulletin, May 1983; 33–35.
11. Kasch M, Mullins P, Fullenwider L: Hand Therapy Review Course Study Guide. Hand Therapy Certification Commission, Garner, NC, 2nd Ed, 1991, Section 9-9.
12. Kjaer-Peterson K, Anderson K, Laughoff O, et al: Combined basal metacarpal fracture and ligament injury to the metacarpophalangeal joint of the thumb. J Bone Joint Surg, 1991; 73B: 176–177.
13. Linscheid RL: Injuries to the radial nerve and wrist. Arch Surg, 1965; 91:942–946.
14. Livesley PJ: The conservative management of Bennett's fractures/dislocation: a 26-year follow-up. J Hand Surg, 1990; 15B:291–294.

15. Moutet F, Tourne Y, Bettega G, Guinard D, Massart P, Lebrum CH: 44 cases of lag screw fixation out of 94 Bennett's fractures continuous series, value and limits of the procedure. Abstracts V International Congress of Hand Surgery, 1991, Paper 4-2-22.

16. Peltier LF: The classic—on fracture of the metacarpal bone of the thumb (E.H. Bennett). Clin Orthop, 1987; 220:3–6.

17. Rettig AC: Current concepts and management of football injuries of the hand and wrist. J Hand Ther, 1991; 4:42-9.

18. Wagner CJ: Method of treatment of Bennett's fracture—dislocation. Am J Surg, 1950; 80: 230–31.

19. Pellegrini VD Jr: Osteo arthritis of the trapeziometacarpal joint: the pathophysiology of articular cartilage degeneration. I, anatomy and pathology of the aging joint. J Hand Surg, 1991; 16A:967–74.

ALLEN T. BISHOP,
MICHAEL E. RETTIG

36

Pin Fixation of the Fifth Carpometacarpal Joint

Fracture-dislocations and dislocations of the small finger carpometacarpal (CMC) joints are relatively rare injuries. Isolated CMC dislocations were reported by Blandin (1844), Malgaigne (1855), and Bourguet (1853),[32] but none of these involved the small finger. An isolated dislocation of the fifth metacarpal base was first described in 1918 by McWhorter.[4,24] Palmar dislocation of multiple CMC joints (index through small) was reported by Vigouroux in 1856, and of all five metacarpal bases in 1873 by Rivington.[1,32] Since then, many cases of dislocations and fracture-dislocations involving the small finger ray have been reported.

Of all solitary CMC dislocations, 50% involve the fifth metacarpohamate joint.[7] Its greater susceptibility to injury is due in part to its peripheral position, as well as its greater laxity and mobility. Simultaneous dislocation of other CMC joints is more frequent than an isolated small finger CMC joint injury. A review of the recent literature by Mueller demonstrated simultaneous dislocation of 2, 3, 4, and 5 to be most common (42 cases) followed by 4 and 5 (17 cases), 1, 2, 3, 4, and 5 (6 cases), 5 alone (5 cases) and 3, 4, and 5 (2 cases).[25] Fracture-dislocations reported in the literature show a similar distribution. In a recent series from the Mayo Clinic, 9 of 13 cases involved the small finger. Only one of these was a solitary injury.[9]

Injuries of the CMC joints include sprains, carpe bossu, simple dislocations, and fracture-dislocations,.[17] Classification of the more severe fracture-dislocations and dislocations is useful in planning treatment. They may be described by direction of dislocation (palmar-ulnar, palmar-radial, or dorsal), by presence and type of carpal fracture(s), and as solitary or part of a multiple ray injury pattern. Cain and co-authors[4] divided fifth CMC dislocations into pure dislocations, dislocation with marginal hamate fractures, dislocation or subluxation with dorsal hamate comminution, and dislocation associated with a coronal hamate body fracture. This classification was later modified by Garcia-Elias and co-authors to include midcarpal injuries resulting in digital ray instability, and was applied to all CMC injuries (Table 36–1).[9] Each ray should be classified individually based on this method. Different patterns are often seen in adjacent digits.

Injuries to the ulnar side CMC joints occur from a variety of mechanisms, including direct blows to the palm,[9,15,31,32] dorsally applied forces to the hand with the wrist flexed,[9,29] and a direct axial force transmitted along the metacarpal shaft, generally applied when a clenched fist strikes an unyielding object (Fig. 36–1).[3,4,19,23] In rare circumstances, a crush or blast mechanism may produce a similar injury.[8,10] Depending on the precise vector of the force, rate of loading, and the intrinsic properties of the stabilizing ligaments and the bone, either a metacarpohamate dislocation or a fracture-dislocation will occur. The pattern of injury may be isolated to the fifth ray but more commonly involves multiple CMC joints. The fifth CMC joint is involved in approximately 80% of all multiple dislocations.[7,25] Most (approximately 80%) of all dislocations are dorsal, occurring from the mechanisms described previously. Most palmar dislocations are caused by direct blow and crush injuries.[15,20]

In the case of an isolated small finger CMC joint fracture-dislocation, the entire fifth ray is displaced, leaving the radial intra-articular fragment of the base of the metacarpal undisplaced on the hamate.[30] The metacarpal will usually dislocate ulnarward and dor-

TABLE 36–1 GARCIA ELIAS MODIFIED CAIN CLASSIFICATION:

Type		Description	Treatment
I		Dislocations	Closed reduction, percutaneous pin
	A	without fracture	
	B	with small dorsal chip fracture	
II		Major dorsal carpal fracture	Open reduction, internal fixation
III		Coronal carpal fracture (involving CMC and mid-carpal joints)	Same
IV		Mid carpal dislocation	Same, ligament reconstruction
	A	without palmar ligament avulsion fracture	
	B	with a palmar ligament avulsion fracture	

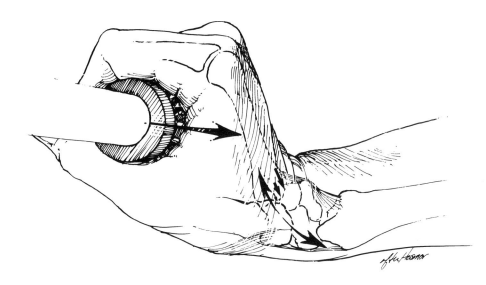

■ **FIGURE 36–1**
Many carpometacarpal dislocations occur with a combination of a lever-type force and an axial load. This results in dorsal compression fracture of one or more of the metacarpals.

sally in the direction of the force acting tangential to the articular surface.[21] The unopposed pull of the extensor carpi ulnaris, attached to the major fracture fragment, causes the displacement and contributes to the instability after closed reduction.[2,6,30] Less frequently, anterior or palmar fifth CMC dislocations may occur, with either simultaneous radial or ulnar translation.[2,7]

Injury of multiple rays may result in either dorsal or palmar subluxation of the involved metacarpals, depending on the direction of the applied force. Most result from a high velocity injury, such as a motor vehicle accident. Closed reduction may be difficult to obtain due to massive edema, interposed fracture fragments or ligaments, and overlapping of metacarpal bases.[13] Ligament injury and muscle forces crossing the joint tend to make closed treatment of these injuries difficult without stabilization. This fact was recognized by McWhorter, who in 1918 described open treatment of an isolated fifth CMC joint dislocation, maintaining reduction with a catgut suture through the torn ligaments.[24] Several years earlier (1905), Lop also had described open reduction of a chronic anterior fifth CMC dislocation.[22] Although some authors have since described satisfactory functional results with closed treatment, most advocate stabilization with pin fixation.[2,5,9,14,15,18,20,21,23,30] When significant intra-articular fractures are present, these are best performed in an open fashion. Simple dislocations may be treated percutaneously, provided an adequate closed reduction is obtained.

Carpometacarpal joint dislocations often occur with significant soft tissue laceration.[15,31,32] Soft tissues other than skin are frequently involved, including digital extensor tendons. The median nerve is not infrequently injured acutely, particularly in multiple palmar dislocations. Chronic compression in neglected dorsal or palmar dislocations will require release at the time of open reduction.[9,33] The deep motor branch of the ulnar nerve may be injured due to its proximity to the palmar aspect of the hamate and fifth CMC joint, particularly in coronal hamate body fractures. Metacarpal base fractures are commonly associated injuries, at times with significant compression and comminution of the articular surface.[13]

■ INDICATIONS AND CONTRAINDICATIONS

Pin fixation of the small finger CMC joint is indicated for most fracture-dislocations and dislocations of the joint, in conjunction with closed or open reduction. Fixation is generally necessary because of the inherent instability of these injuries.[5,12,13]

Percutaneous fixation of CMC joint injury is contraindicated in the presence of an inadequate reduction. Suspicion of ligamentous interposition (incomplete reduction), presence of displaced articular fragments, open injury with extensive soft tissue injury, and old and neglected dislocations require open reduction.[23] Chronic dislocation or incomplete reduction of the metacarpal bases will lead to a significant disruption in the hand mechanics, with resultant complaints of pain and weakness.[9] Carpal fracture nonunion is common with delayed treatment, as is painful arthritis.[9] Significant intra-articular fractures require open or possibly arthroscopic inspection to minimize the incidence of late posttraumatic arthritis.

Injury to the CMC joints is frequently overlooked on initial examination (40% of a recent large series of fracture-dislocations).[9] Missed diagnoses and delay in treatment result in poorer outcomes, frequently requiring carpal tunnel release for increasing digit hypesthesia and weakness as well as increased need for hamate-metacarpal arthrodesis.[9] A careful and systematic examination of the wrist would in all cases identify palpable deformity or tenderness in the area, prompting adequate evaluation of the injury by radiographic studies. Findings on examination include swelling, tenderness and ecchymosis on the dorsum of the hand, and pain to palpation of the CMC area. In dorsal dislocations, a prominence on the dorsum of the wrist may be noted, as well as malrotation of fingers. Wrist and digit motion will be diminished.

Subtle radiographic findings may be missed by a casual review. Standard PA and lateral projections will generally demonstrate the injury. PA projections will show the four finger CMC joints to approximate the letter "M" in configuration, and the opposing joint surfaces to be parallel and the joint space symmetric. No overlapping of joint surfaces should be seen, provided the hand is flat on the table (Figs. 36–2 and 36–3G).[7] A distinct cortical

■ FIGURE 36–2
The second through fifth CMC joints will normally demonstrate a "parallel M" configuration on a properly positioned PA radiograph, with a joint space of 1 to 2 mm.

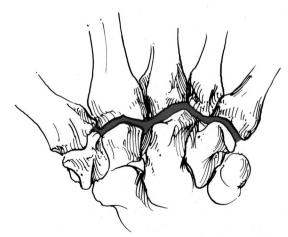

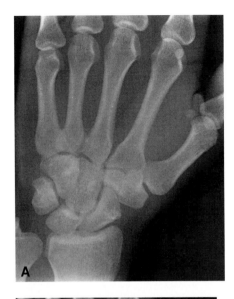

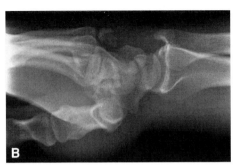

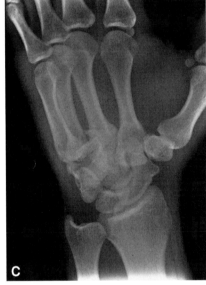

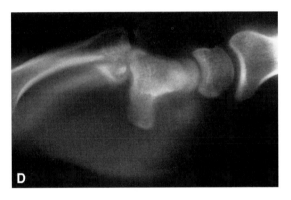

■ FIGURE 36–3
Fracture-subluxation of fifth CMC joint resulting from a motor cycle accident. **A,** PA view. Note abnormality of distal ulnar aspect of hamate, suggesting a dorsal rim fracture. **B,** Lateral view demonstrating abnormal widening of the CMC joint due to dorsal displacement of the fifth metacarpal base. Note the dorsal hamate fracture. **C,** A pronation-oblique view is often useful to visualize CMC injuries of the ulnar aspect of the hand. **D,** A lateral trispiral tomogram is the best method of accurately visualizing individual CMC joints. This individual demonstrates both a dorsal hamate fracture and a fifth metacarpal base fracture not visualized on standard projections.

rim is seen at apposing margins when the joint is viewed in profile. A standard lateral projection will demonstrate a lack of parallelism between opposing carpal and metacarpal bones. Comparison with the contralateral wrist will demonstrate widening of the anteroposterior diameter of the distal carpus due to the joint subluxation or dislocation (Figs. 36–3B and 36–3H).[9] A 30° pronation oblique view may be helpful for injuries of the fourth and fifth rays (Fig. 36–3C).[2] In our experience, lateral trispiral tomography with 1 to 2 mm increments was by far the most effective method of diagnosis, because the morphology, articular congruence, and amount of displacement can be assessed in detail for each CMC joint (Fig. 36–3D). Computed tomography scans also may be of some value.[4,23]

The anatomy of the CMC region provides a stable second and third metacarpal. They support the mobile metacarpals of the thumb, ring, and small fingers, which allows spatial adaptation of the hand through its distal transverse arch. The proximal transverse arch is made up of the distal carpal row and its associated ligamentous structures. It is fixed and provides needed stability for the mobile first, fourth, and fifth rays. The base of the second metacarpal has an inverted V-shape formed by both radial and ulnar styloids that match the distal aspect of the trapezoid. The third metacarpal keys into the distal capitate. Only minimal flexion-extension of these joints is allowed (1° to 3°).[12]

■ SURGICAL
TECHNIQUES

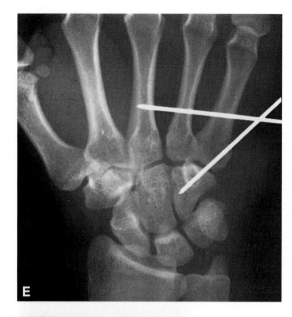

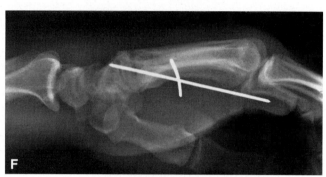

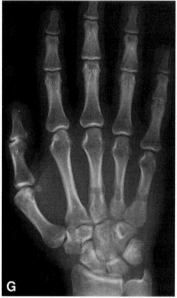

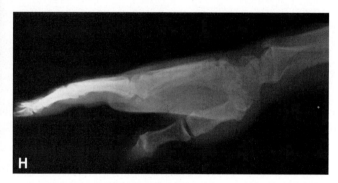

■ FIGURE 36–3*(continued)*
E and F, Stabilization with two 0.062-inch K-wires. Note restoration of joint congruency and normal CMC width on the lateral view. **G and H,** Postoperative radiographs demonstrating maintenance of anatomic reduction. Note normal width of CMC joint in lateral projection.

In contrast, the ulnar two CMC joints, formed by the hamate and fourth and fifth metacarpals, allow considerable motion. The distal articular surface of the hamate is relatively flat, separated into two surfaces by a shallow ridge.[21] The articular surface of the base of the fifth metacarpal is not horizontal, but somewhat oblique, oriented from ulnar proximal to radial distal.[21] The slope of this articular surface contributes to the instability after small finger CMC dislocation or fracture-dislocation. The ring finger CMC joint has a flexion-extension arc of 10° to 15°, and the small finger CMC joint approximately 15° to 30°.[28] Rotary motions also are present, which contribute to the normal cupping of the palm in grasp and in opposition of the small finger to the thumb.[2,18] This distal transverse arch motion is lost in ulnar-sided CMC dislocations.

The stability of the CMC joint of the small finger depends on the articular surfaces of the bones and on the ligaments and muscles attached to them.[2] Ligamentous support is provided by the dorsal and palmar CMC ligaments, of which the dorsal are more discrete and substantial.[13] The sturdy interosseous ligament between the two metacarpals also stabilizes this joint.

The extensor carpi ulnaris is the primary deforming force on the CMC joint of the small finger in isolated dislocations.[21] It inserts on the dorsoulnar aspect of the small finger metacarpal base. Through this insertion, the extensor carpi ulnaris causes ulnar and proximal displacement of the base of the metacarpal following an injury to the static stabilizers of the joint. The resultant displacement is similar to a Bennett's fracture of the first metacarpal.[2] The flexor carpi ulnaris, through the pisometacarpal ligament, also contributes to displacement of the small finger metacarpal base in dislocations and fracture-dislocations, as do the hypothenar muscles and the extrinsic digit flexors and extensors crossing the injured joints.

Adequate anesthesia and muscle relaxation are needed for appropriate closed reduction of CMC injuries. Regional anesthesia (axillary block) or general anesthesia is appropriate for percutaneous pin fixation. Longitudinal traction applied vertically or horizontally is appropriate, followed by gentle direct pressure over the bases of the dislocated metacarpals. The hand may be positioned vertically with the elbow flexed 90° and weights applied to the arm for distraction. We prefer use of a radiotransparent hand fracture table specially equipped for horizontal traction (Fig. 36–4). Approximately 5 pounds of traction will suffice. Standard radiographs or fluoroscopy in traction will allow assessment of the reduction, and fluoroscopy will greatly facilitate pin placement. This allows the surgeon to continue immediately with open reduction if needed without need for additional repreparing and draping of the extremity.

Following reduction by longitudinal traction and closed manipulation, pins are placed percutaneously while traction maintains the reduction. Most authors advocate percutaneous K-wire fixation for small finger CMC dislocations. For isolated fifth finger CMC injuries, the metacarpal may be reduced and transfixed to the ring metacarpal[13,21] or fixed to the hamate by a single percutaneous longitudinal Kirschner wire[26] or oblique pin driven from the dorsoulnar metaphyseal flare of the metacarpal into the hamate (Figs. 36–3E, 36–3F, and 36–5A).[28] Such obliquely driven pins must not penetrate palmarly, and thereby possibly impale the deep motor branch of the ulnar nerve.

Multiple dislocations require accurate relocation and fixation of each metacarpal base

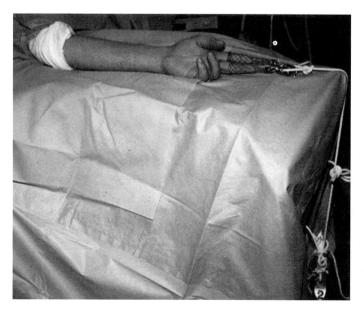

■ FIGURE 36–4
Longitudinal traction and gentle pressure applied to the metacarpal bases will reduce the dislocation unless soft tissue interposition is present. Failure to obtain adequate reduction of the dislocation or intraarticular fractures requires open reduction. A hand fracture table with a traction apparatus and radiolucent surface is ideal, allowing both closed reduction with fluoroscopic control and open reduction, if required.

to its carpal articulation or to a stable adjacent metacarpal. Either longitudinal (intramedullary) wires placed through the metacarpal head and advanced proximally across the CMC joint or oblique and transverse wires through the shaft or proximal metaphysis are useful.[4,14,20] Longitudinal intramedullary K-wires, as described by Kleinman, provide excellent stability with a minimum of hardware and are relatively easily placed, particularly when multiple CMC joints require fixation. The metacarpophalangeal (MP) joint is held in 60° of flexion. This draws the sagittal band distal to the metacarpal head and places the collateral ligaments under tension. The Kirschner wire (0.045 inch) is then introduced into the ulnar or radial collateral recess to avoid the extensor tendon, which lies more centrally and dorsally over the midaxis of the joint (Fig. 36–5B). If desired, the K-wire may be advanced proximally with the wrist flexed to exit through the skin of the dorsal wrist. It may then be withdrawn into the metacarpal head under image intensifier control. K-wire position is confirmed by biplanar fluoroscopy as the wire is advanced. Conventional radiographs with a 30° pronation oblique view will confirm appropriate K-wire placement and joint reduction. The digit is inspected for any sign of malrotation. The pins are then either bent with a Frazier suction tip 90° to the skin surface or covered with a pin cap. Kinking or tenting of the skin is corrected with judicious relaxing incisions to minimize pin tract infection problems, and a bulky compressive dressing with a plaster splint is applied. This is changed to a fiberglass cast at 10 to 14 days, followed by pin removal at 6 weeks.

The percutaneous wires should be left in place for at least 6 weeks in adults.[20] The wrist is immobilized during this period of time. Immobilization of the MP joints in flexion will improve stability at the site of injury.

■ FIGURE 36–5
K-wires are placed percutaneously for stabilization of CMC dislocations. **A,** Oblique placement of K-wires from the fifth metacarpal base into the hamate is easily accomplished under fluoroscopic control. **B,** Intramedullary placement in the shaft of the fifth metacarpal is accomplished by introduction of the wire into the collateral recess of the metacarpal head. The wire is then driven across the fifth metacarpal-hamate joint into the hamate body.

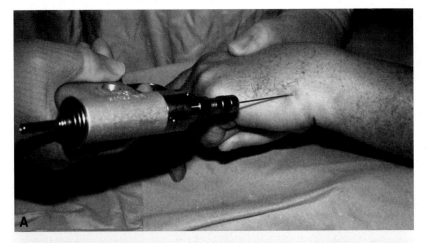
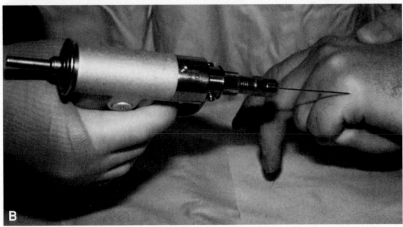

Closed reduction of the carpal-metacarpal joint is difficult to maintain and is not advised.[13,16,25,32] In Hartwig's series of closed treatment, one of four "successfully" treated cases had significant residual dorsal subluxation at 4 months. None of those treated with pinning had any subluxation.

Open reduction is necessary when an adequate closed reduction cannot be obtained due to interposed fracture fragments or ligament, marked swelling obscuring bony landmarks, delayed treatment, open fracture dislocation, and variants with depressed fractures of the fifth metacarpal or hamate.[11,13,16,28,31] An adequate reduction should have no residual subluxation or articular gap or step-off. Once reduction is obtained, it should be maintained with open K-wire placement or internal fixation. Should open reduction prove necessary, a longitudinal incision directly overlying the fifth CMC joint allows adequate visualization of an isolated dislocation. If multiple joints are involved, a modified longitudinal incision is safest, and extended as needed to visualize all four CMC joints.[11] This allows preservation of major dorsal veins as well as dorsal sensory branches of the radial and ulnar nerve.[28]

Advances in small joint arthroscopy currently allow placement of small arthroscopes into the CMC joints. It is likely that additional experience will allow arthroscopically guided reduction and pinning of some CMC joint fracture-dislocations in the future.

Use of rigid internal fixation (lag screws or miniplates) may allow earlier wrist and digit motion and thereby minimize morbidity. It is most applicable in type II fractures with a single large dorsal carpal margin fragment that, when reduced, restores joint stability.

Symptomatic CMC derangement after injury may require an arthrodesis, with distraction and grafting of the foreshortened metacarpal.[9,17] In the absence of significant subluxation, soft tissue interposition arthroplasty of the fifth CMC joint may be considered with dorsal capsule or tendon graft.

The critical problems to avoid are failure to recognize a CMC joint injury and failure to adequately treat a recognized problem. A high index of suspicion and a careful physical examination will lead to clinical suspicion of CMC injury. This must be confirmed with appropriate imaging studies, including lateral trispiral tomograms, to properly evaluate individual CMC joints. Percutaneous pin fixation is applicable for single or multiple dislocations with minimal articular injury (Garcia Elias et al's type I), after a satisfactory closed reduction is obtained. Large displaced fracture fragments, coronal fractures involving the hamate body or midcarpal joint, and midcarpal instability associated with CMC injury should be managed by open reduction and fixation.

■ TECHNICAL ALTERNATIVES

Cast immobilization is generally necessary for 4 to 6 weeks, at which time pin removal is performed. Earlier pin removal may lead to joint subluxation and symptoms. Digit range of motion can be allowed in limited fashion immediately, particularly at the proximal and distal interphalangeal joints. If longitudinal K-wires are used, the MP joints should be immobilized in the "safe" position until wire removal. At 6 weeks, rehabilitation efforts are begun at the wrist and MP joints. Extrinsic extensor tightness may require stretching, ultrasound, and other modalities. Supervised hand therapy is important throughout the postoperative recovery period.

■ REHABILITATION

Unrecognized sprains and impaction injuries to the CMC joints may lead to carpal bossing, pain, and ganglion formation. Conservative management is usually appropriate, with occasional surgical treatment for relief of symptoms.[17,27,28] Untreated or inadequately treated dislocations or fracture-dislocations may result in pain, loss of grip strength, limited wrist and finger motion, and symptoms of median or ulnar compressive neuropathy due to proximal migration and displacement of the metacarpal bases.[13] Fracture nonunion is common in undiagnosed fracture-dislocations.[9] Degenerative arthritis may occur late, occasionally despite appropriate management. Provided alignment is adequate, joint space narrowing may be minimally symptomatic.[13]

Garcia-Elias and co-authors found final functional outcome was most dependent on timely recognition and treatment. The method of reduction and stabilization used were less

■ OUTCOMES

important.[9] Patients with delayed treatment had an increased incidence of mild residual symptoms including weakness of grasp and pinch.

References

1. Bergfield TG, DuPuy TE, Aulicino PL: Fracture-dislocations of all five carpometacarpal joints: A case report. J Hand Surg, 1985; 10A:76–78.
2. Bora FW Jr, Didizan NH: The treatment of injuries to the carpometacrpal joint of the little finger. J Bone Joint Surg, 1974; 56A:1459–1463.
3. Bowen TL: Injuries of the hamate bone. Hand, 1973; 5:235–238.
4. Cain JE, Shepler TR, Wilson MR: Hamatometacarpal fracture-dislocation: classification and treatment. J Hand Surg, 1987; 12A:762–767.
5. Clement BL: Fracture-dislocation of the base of the fifth metacarpal. A case report. J Bone Joint Surg, 1945; 27:498–499.
6. Dommisse IG, Lloyd GJ: Injuries to the fifth carpometacarpal region. Can J Surg, 1979; 22: 240–244.
7. Fisher MR, Rogers LF, Hendrix RW: Systematic approach to identifying fourth and fifth carpometacarpal joint dislocations. A J Radiol, 1983; 140:319–324.
8. Garcia-Elias M, Abancó J, Salvador E, Sánchez R: Crash injury of the carpus. J Bone Joint Surg, 1985; 67B:286–289.
9. Garcia-Elias M, Bishop AT, Dobyns JH, Cooney WP, Linscheid RL: Transcarpal carpometacarpal dislocations, excluding the thumb. J Hand Surg, 1990; 15A:531–540.
10. Garcia-Elias M, Dobyns JH, Cooney WP, Linscheid RL: Traumatic axial dislocations of the carpus. J Hand Surg, 1985; 14A:446–457.
11. Green DP, Anderson JR: Closed reduction and percutaneous pin fixation of fractured phalanges. J Bone Joint Surg, 1973; 55A:1654–1663.
12. Gunther SF: The carpometacarpal joints. Orthop Clin North Am, 1984; 15:259–277.
13. Hartwig RH, Louis DS: Multiple carpometacarpal dislocations. J Bone Joint Surg, 1979; 61A: 906–908.
14. Harwin S, et al: Volar dislocation of the bases of the second and third metacarpals. J Bone Joint Surg, 1975; 57A:849–851.
15. Hazlett JW: Carpometacarpal dislocations other than the thumb. A report of 11 cases. Can J Surg, 1968; 11:315–323.
16. Hsu JD, Curtis RM: Carpometacarpal dislocations on the ulnar side of the hand. J Bone Joint Surg, 1970; 52A:927–930.
17. Joseph RB, Linscheid RL, Dobyns JH, Bryan RS: Chronic sprains of the carpometacarpal joints. J Hand Surg, 1981; 6:172–180.
18. Ker HR: Dislocation of the fifth carpo-metacarpal joint. J Bone Joint Surg, 1955; 37B:254–256.
19. Kimura H, Kamura S, Akai M: An unusual fracture of the body of the hamate bone. J Hand Surg, 1988; 13A:743–745.
20. Kleinman WB, Grantham S: Multiple volar carpo-metacarpal joint dislocation. A case report. J Hand Surg, 1978; 3:377–382.
21. Lilling M, Weinberg H: The mechanism of dorsal fracture dislocation of the fifth carpometacarpal joint. J Hand Surg, 1979; 4:340–342.
22. Lop: Luxation irreductible du cinquieme droit; reduction sanglant. Guerison operatoire et fonctionelle. Gaz des Hopitaux, Paris 1905;78:1455.
23. Marck KW, Klasen HJ: Fracture-dislocation of the hamatometacarpal joint: A case report. J Hand Surg, 1986; 11A:128–129.
24. McWhorter GL: Isolated and complete dislocation of the fifth carpometacarpal joint: Open operation. Surg Clin Chicago, 1918; 2:793–796.
25. Mueller JJ: Carpometacarpal dislocations: Report of five cases and review of the literature. J Hand Surg, 1986; 11A:184–188.
26. North ER, Eaton RG: Volar dislocation of the fifth metacarpal. J Bone Joint Surg, 1980; 62A: 657–659.
27. Petri PWR, Lamb DW: Fracture-subluxation of the base of the fifth metacarpal. Hand, 1974; 6:82–86.
28. Rawles JG Jr: Dislocations and fracture-dislocations at the carpometcarpal joints of the fingers. Hand Clinics North Am, 1988; 4:103–112.
29. Roth JH, de Lorenzi C: Displaced intra-articular coronal fracture of the hamate treated with a Herbert screw. J Hand Surg, 1988; 13A:619–621.

30. Sandzen SC: Fracture of the fifth metacarpal. Hand, 1973; 5:49–51.
31. Shephard E, Solomon DJ: Carpo-metacarpal dislocation. J Bone Joint Surg, 1960; 42B:772–777.
32. Waugh RL, Yancey AG: Carpometacarpal dislocations with particular reference to simultaneous dislocations of the bases of the fourth and fifth metacarpals. J Bone Joint Surg, 1948; 30A:397–404.
33. Weiland AJ, Lister GD, Villareal-Rios A: Volar fracture-dislocations of the second and third carpometacarpal joints associated with acute carpal tunnel syndrome. J Trauma, 1976; 16: 672–675.

37

External Fixation of the Metacarpals

■ HISTORY OF THE TECHNIQUE

External fixation for fractures of the hand has not been as widespread as the use of external fixation in major long bone fractures or wrist fractures. Miniaturization of external fixation devices was necessary to fit the small bones of the hand. Using readily available materials, Crockett[3] reported rigid fixation of metacarpals and phalanges using K-wires bonded with acrylic resin. Jaquet designed a mini-fixator in 1976 for use in the hand, which required minimal dissection of soft tissue and provided rigid bony stability, yet allowed active range of motion of adjacent joints and tendon excursion.[6] More recently, other designs have become available, using the same concepts mentioned above.[9,13]

■ INDICATIONS AND CONTRAINDICATIONS

External fixation should be considered in the following metacarpal injuries:

1. Open fractures, especially those with heavily contaminated wounds[2,6]
2. Fractures that are too comminuted for internal fixation[4,7]
3. Extensive loss of bone substance, in which case maintaining proper length of the metacarpal is difficult[2,9]
4. Fractures associated with complex wounds with extensive soft-tissue loss[6] (e.g., gunshot wounds,[1] shotgun wounds,[11] farm machinery injuries,[12] or complex industrial injuries)[1,11,13-15]
5. Infected fractures or nonunions, especially those having failed internal fixation devices such as K-wires, screws, or plates[12]
6. Arthrodesis of infected joints[12]

External fixation can be used as the definitive method of fracture fixation, especially when frequent dressing changes for wound care are necessary, for comminuted fractures and infected fractures. In the complex hand injuries, external fixation is often used as a temporary device to maintain metacarpal length at the time of initial debridement. It may then be removed a few days later at the time of definitive bone reconstruction if rigid internal fixation can be obtained.[9,11] Internal fixation and external fixation should not be considered as being mutually exclusive because it may be necessary to combine internal and external fixation to provide the necessary rigidity for fracture healing. The principles guiding the use of external fixation for the metacarpals are also applicable to proximal and middle phalangeal fractures.

External fixation is contraindicated when firm fixation with the pins in the bone is not possible (e.g, osteoporosis). It should not be used when simpler methods of fracture management, such as closed techniques or open pinning, will provide equally satisfactory results. Intraarticular fractures of the head or base of metacarpals or phalanges are usually more amenable to open reduction and internal fixation but external fixation may be used for comminuted fractures or combined with internal fixation as a load-sharing device when rigid internal fixation is not achievable.

■ SURGICAL TECHNIQUES

The procedure is begun under regional or general anesthesia in the operating room under the usual orthopaedic skin and wound preparation. In open fractures, extensive debridement of the wound may be necessary before fracture stabilization. Fixation of the fracture should be done before repair of tendons, nerves, muscles, or vessels. Because firm fixation by two pins and four cortices on each side of the fracture is recommended for rigid fixation,[16] the fracture pattern and location is critically evaluated by review of radiographs and direct inspection of the fractured bone. It is preferable to insert the pins through a separate incision placed to avoid skin tension postoperatively rather than to insert the pins percutaneously.[8] Once the incision is made for the pins, the bone is exposed by blunt or sharp dissection to avoid sensory nerves. If possible, it is important to avoid tendons that, if impaled by the pins, will limit tendon excursion and adjacent joint motion.[15] The plane of insertion of the pins in metacarpals with a free border (i.e., first, second, and fifth) should be the straight mid-lateral plane, thus easily avoiding extensor tendons. Pin insertion in the third and fourth metacarpals is usually at a 45° angle to this plane. For phalanges, a straight lateral approach avoiding the tendons is preferred.

I prefer to use the Mini Hoffmann External Fixation System (Howmedica, 359 Veterans Blvd, Rutherford, NJ 07070) because it is specifically designed for small bone fixation. Because of their rigidity, the preferred fixation pins are the 2-mm half pins for metacarpals and either 2-mm or 1.5-mm half pins for the phalanges. Two-millimeter pins require predrilling with a 1.5-mm drill. The following technique is recommended for the Mini Hoffman External Fixation.

Use the minidrill guide to align the drill holes in the desired plane. Drill through both cortices with the 1.5-mm drill bit. Leave the drill in place to act as an anchor to position the guide for the second hole. Drill the second hole. Select the proper length 2-mm half-pin and insert it by hand with the pin driver into a predrilled hole until the blunt end of the pin protrudes through the distant cortex, determined by visual inspection, palpation, radiographs, or all three methods. Insert the second pin through the predrilled hole. Insert the second set of pins into the intact bone on the other side of the fracture, generally parallel to the first set. This point is not critical because the Mini Hoffmann device has universal joints to adjust nonparallel pin placement. Apply the pin holder to each set of pins. Apply a swivel clamp to each pin holder. Connect the clamps to a 3-mm connecting rod of appropriate length (Fig. 37–1).

Reduce the fracture by manual manipulation and traction to restore the length of the bone. Although the image intensifier may be helpful it is usually not necessary. Tighten the clamps and check the fracture alignment and position visually in all three planes, including axially, and by intraoperative radiographs. Repair other structures as indicated. Give routine antibiotics for 24 to 48 hours in open fractures. Employ routine postoperative pin-care techniques.

■ TECHNICAL ALTERNATIVES

Before actually attempting external fixation in the operating room, familiarization with the equipment and the technical details for using the Mini Hoffmann or any external fixator (including practice in the laboratory) is strongly recommended.

The above description is for straightforward single metacarpal or phalangeal fractures. Multiple fractures and more complex fracture patterns may need more complex frames, including double frames and pins applied in multiple planes.[6] The Mini Hoffmann External Fixation System has a versatile design, allowing complex frames designed by the surgeon to fit a particular need. Ensuring that there is no skin tension on the pins is critical to preventing pin-tract infection.[8] An inexpensive yet quick method of making an external fixation frame uses methylmethacrylate resin (Figs. 37-2 and 37-3).[3,4,11,13] A distinct disadvantage in using this method is an inability to easily complete intra- or postoperative adjustments.

Transmetacarpal K-wire fixation to an adjacent intact metacarpal is a simple alternative technique to maintain metacarpal length and alignment in comminuted metacarpal fractures or with bone loss, particularly as a temporary fixation method before definitive bone grafting.[10]

■ REHABILITATION

Rigid external fixation allows easy dressing changes and wound cleansing techniques as necessary. Early range of motion is begun as soon as wound conditions permit (Fig. 37–4A and B).[5] Ideally, for an isolated single metacarpal fracture that has been rigidly fixed with an external fixator, range of motion exercises begin the first postoperative day and progress to patient tolerance. When the patient cannot perform active range of motion exercises because of pain, gentle passive range of motion exercises by an experienced hand

■ FIGURE 37–1
Unilateral Mini Hoffmann
External Fixation System,
used for a comminuted
metacarpal shaft fracture.
Note that two 2-mm half-
pins are inserted parallel
to each other and into intact cortices on either
side of the fracture site.
Bone grafting is neces-
sary to heal this fracture.

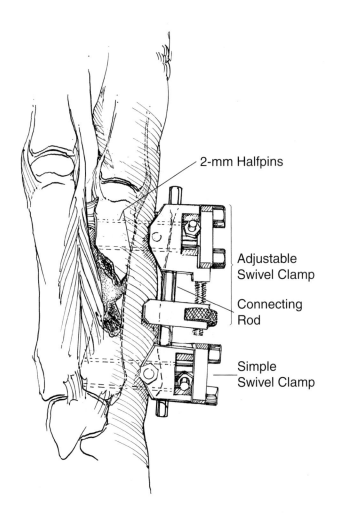

2-mm Halfpins

Adjustable
Swivel Clamp

Connecting
Rod

Simple
Swivel Clamp

■ FIGURE 37–2
Posteroanterior and lat-
eral radiographs of K-
wires and methylmethac-
rylate cement used as an
external fixator to treat a
nonunion of the distal
phalanx with bone loss.
In this case, cement was
applied to both ends of
the pins and the fixator
was left on for 8 weeks
after bone graft.

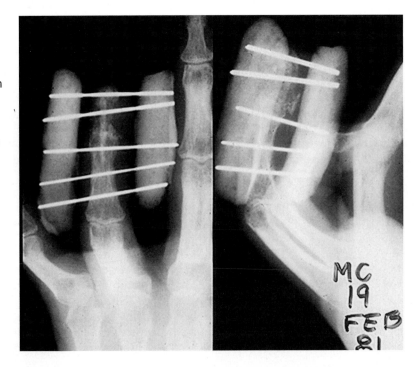

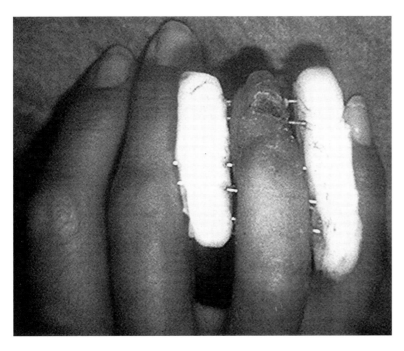

■ FIGURE 37–3
The clinical appearance of a K-wire and methylmethacrylate cement construct in place on the distal finger.

therapist allow maximum gain in motion. Edema control measures will be necessary. The postoperative rehabilitation program must be individualized to each patient, depending on fracture stability, the wound requirements, and the need to protect tendon, nerve, or vascular repairs. It is important to emphasize to the patient not to overload the fixator, causing fracture or loosening of the pins. Daily peroxide cleansing of the pins minimizes pin-tract infection. Pin fracture or loosening, or pin-tract infection may require premature removal of the external fixator.

The external fixator is left on until sufficient fracture healing and rigidity has occurred, usually about 6 to 8 weeks after injury. Once fracture healing seems adequate by radiographs, loosening of the external fixator and gently manually stressing the fracture for motion will reveal whether the fracture has healed clinically. When there is no motion, the external fixator may be removed in the office and generally no further casting or splinting is necessary.

Freeland[6] reported that 14 of 20 severe open fractures of the hand that were treated with external fixation healed with good anatomic alignment, whereas two healed with mild deformity. Parsons and coworkers[10] reported on external fixation of 37 unstable fractures of the hand (23 metacarpals), with an average healing time of 4.8 weeks and 94% excellent or good results in a mean of 6.3 weeks. There were no nonunions and two delayed unions. Bilos and Ekestrand[1] and Smith and coworkers[15] have reported good fracture healing with external fixation in proximal phalangeal fractures, especially difficult gunshot wounds, resulting in good metacarpalphalangeal motion but some stiffness of the interphalangeal joints.

■ OUTCOMES

It is apparent from these studies that external fixation in the hand can give both an excellent rate of fracture healing and functional results by allowing early range of motion. Complications can be minimized by following the principles outlined above. Attention to details, as outlined by Green,[8] are also helpful for someone who is not familiar with external fixators. The surgeon treating hand fractures should consider external fixation for the uncommon metacarpal and phalangeal fracture problems, as outlined in the Indications section of this chapter.

■ FIGURE 37–4
A, The Mini Hoffmann External Fixation System used for rigid fixation to obtain arthrodesis of an infected distal interphalangeal joint. **B**, In a lateral view, the Hoffmann fixator holds the arthrodesed distal interphalangeal joint in mild flexion, while the proximal interphalangeal joint is actively flexed to 90°, which speeds rehabilitation of the hand.

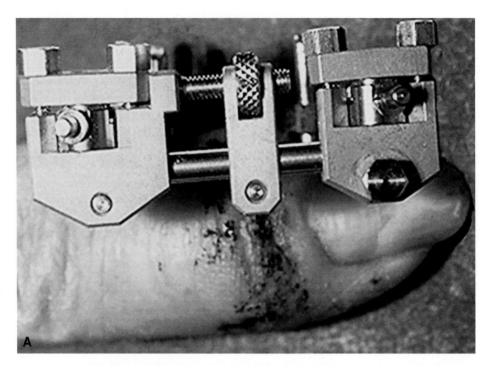

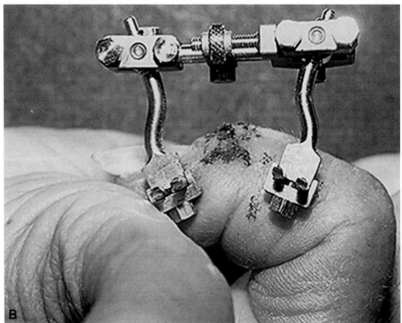

References

1. Bilos ZJ, Eskestrand T: External fixator use in comminuted gunshot fractures of the proximal phalanx. J Hand Surg, 1979; 4:357–359.
2. Chait LA, Cort A, Braun S: Metacarpal reconstruction in compound contaminated injuries of the hand. Hand, 1981; 13:152–157.
3. Crockett DJ: Rigid fixation of bones of the hand using K wires bonded with acrylic resin. Hand, 1974; 6:106–107.
4. Dickson RA: Rigid fixation of unstable metacarpal fractures using transverse K-wires bonded with acrylic resin. Hand, 1975; 7:284–286.
5. Dobyns JH, Linscheid RL, Cooney WP: Fractures and dislocations of the wrist and hand, then and now. J Hand Surg, 1983; 8:687–690.

6. Freeland AE: External fixation for skeletal stabilization of severe open fractures of the hand. Clin Orthop, 1987; 214: 93–100.

7. Green DP, Rowland SA: Fractures and Dislocations of the Hand. In: Rockwood CA, Green DP, Bucholz RW (eds): Fractures in Adults, 3rd Ed, Philadelphia: JB Lippincott, 1991:464–488.

8. Green SA: Complications of External Fixation; Causes, Prevention and Treatment, Springfield: Charles C. Thomas, 1981:12–34.

9. Jupiter JB, Belsky MR: Fractures and Dislocations of the Hand. In: Browner BD, Jupiter JB, Levine AM, Trafton PG (eds): Skeletal Trauma, Philadelphia: WB Saunders, 1992:958–959.

10. Parsons SW, Fitzgerald JAW, Shearer JR: External fixation of unstable metacarpal and phalangeal fractures. J Hand Surg, 1992; 17B:151–155.

11. Peimer CA, Smith RJ, Leffert RD: Distraction-fixation in the primary treatment of metacarpal bone loss. J Hand Surg, 1981; 6:111–124.

12. Pritsch M, Engel J, Farin I: Manipulation and external fixation of metacarpal fractures. J Bone Joint Surg, 1981; 63A:1289–1291.

13. Riggs SA, Cooney WP: External fixation of complex hand and wrist fractures. J Trauma, 1983; 23:332–336.

14. Scott MM, Mulligan PJ: Stabilizing severe phalangeal fractures. Hand, 1980; 12:44–50.

15. Smith RS, Alonso J, Horowitz M: External fixation of open comminuted fractures of the proximal phalanx. Orthop Rev, 1987; 16:937–941.

16. Stuchen SA, Kummer FJ: Stiffness of small-bone external fixation methods: An experimental study. J Hand Surg, 1984; 9A:718–724.

PART VI

Fracture Fixation of the Wrist

ANTON J. FAKHOURI,
ROY A. MEALS

38

Pin Fixation of Scaphoid Fractures

MacLennan first proposed the use of wires for scaphoid fractures in 1911;[12] internal fixation of scaphoid fractures at that time was considered impractical, however.[21] Three decades later, Geissendorfer recommended fixation of scaphoid fractures with K-wires.[8] During this period, scaphoid fractures were uniformly treated with little or no external immobilization, and only a few advocated the use of wire or other internal fixation devices. Dehne and coworkers described percutaneous pinning of displaced scaphoid nonunions in 1964.[5] They used only one pin, which crossed both the trapezioscaphoid and radiocarpal joints; however, half the pins broke. During the past two decades, it became more evident that poor treatment of scaphoid fractures enhances the risk of nonunion and malunion and the subsequent risk of long-term pain and functional disability.[1,2,11,14,19] Thus, fixation of displaced fractures has become accepted as the standard of care. Although the use of screw fixation has gained popularity, many hand surgeons continue to rely on pin fixation for the treatment of scaphoid fractures.[1-4,15,18,20,21]

■ HISTORY OF THE TECHNIQUE

Most hand surgeons agree that fractures displaced more than 1 mm or angulated more than 20° should be reduced and internally fixed.[1] Inherently unstable fractures are considered to be an indication for surgical intervention. These include proximal pole fractures that compromise less than 25% of the scaphoid, comminuted fractures, and scaphoid fractures that are associated with a perilunate dislocation.

■ INDICATIONS AND CONTRAINDICATIONS

Several approaches and techniques are useful. Closed reduction and percutaneous pinning of acute fractures may be indicated before an open reduction, unless the fracture is comminuted or is in the vertical oblique orientation (Fig. 38–1). These fractures are unstable and difficult to reduce. In addition, comminuted fractures may need bone grafting. Closed reduction and percutaneous pinning has the advantage of minimizing further damage to the scaphoid's blood supply, but an acceptable reduction and satisfactory K-wire placement may be difficult to achieve.

There are several approaches and techniques that are useful. Open reduction can be performed through an anterior, posterior, or lateral approach. The lateral approach is technically difficult and requires osteotomy of the radial styloid. The anterior approach gives good visualization of the fracture site and allows easy access for bone grafting of comminuted acute fractures and nonunions.

Although the anterior approach is more versatile, there are instances when the dorsal approach is more appropriate. Concomitant distal radius and scaphoid fractures can both be approached dorsally to avoid an extra incision. A Herbert screw for proximal third fracture is placed through a dorsal incision.[6] The scaphoid can be pinned from the same dorsal approach if an attempt at Herbert screw fixation fails. Also, an anterior approach may in certain circumstances disturb the carpal alignment by dividing important radiocarpal-stabilizing ligaments.[7] The union rate, however, has been similar for both approaches.[7]

Closed Reduction Percutaneous Pinning An axillary block or general anesthesia is preferred because Bier block anesthesia may result in severe pain and further displacement of the fracture during limb exsanguination. Facilities for open reduction and internal fixation should be immediately available in the event that closed reduction is unsuccessful.

■ SURGICAL TECHNIQUES

■ FIGURE 38−1
Scaphoid fracture types
(Russe's classification).
A, Transverse. **B**, Horizontal oblique. **C**, Vertical
oblique. The vertical
oblique type is an un-
stable fracture.

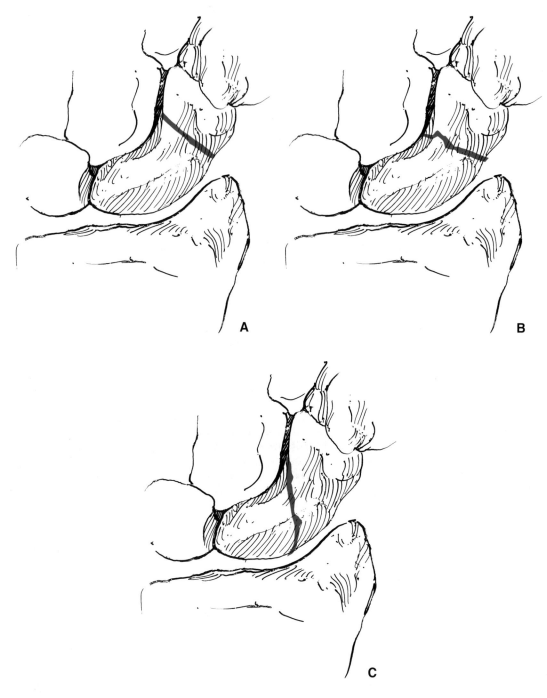

After induction of anesthesia, the hand is suspended in Chinese finger traps, with the
elbow flexed 90° and about 7 lbs of traction applied to the arm. Under the guidance of
image intensification, closed reduction is attempted by manipulating the wrist alternately
into radial and ulnar deviation until the fragments are properly aligned. Often, the distal
fragment is flexed with respect to the proximal fragment. Radial deviation and flexion of
the wrist flexes the proximal fragment and aligns it with the already flexed distal fragment.
When the reduction remains inadequate, dorsally directed pressure on the scaphoid tubercle helps to extend the distal fragment. Anteriorly directed counter-pressure is applied
on the dorsum of the capitate and lunate. This maneuver rotates the lunate and the attached
proximal scaphoid fragment into flexion.[3] The alignment of the fracture fragments can be
confirmed on lateral fluoroscopy.

When both lateral and posteroanterior views show adequate reduction, prepare to percutaneously pin the fracture because cast immobilization alone will not hold the reduction. The tubercle of the scaphoid is at the distal wrist flexion crease, and this surface landmark should be used for initiating the pinning, which should be performed under fluoroscopy guidance. Two parallel 0.045-inch K-wires are inserted from the scaphoid tubercle across the fracture. The wires are directed proximally, dorsally, and ulnarly, parallel to the longitudinal axis of the scaphoid. Proximally, the pins must not protrude from the scaphoid. Posteroanterior and lateral radiographs are obtained to make final and precise assessment of the reduction and fixation. Reduction is acceptable when the fracture is displaced less than 1 mm and angulated less than 20°. Because the pins may be required for 4 months, the ends are best cut short and left subcutaneously. A short arm thumb spica splint, changed to a cast of similar configuration when the swelling has subsided, protects the fracture and the internal fixation. The cast should be well molded and incorporate the thumb up to the level of the interphalangeal joint. The wrist is placed in neutral position with respect to both flexion–extension and radial–ulnar deviation. The cast should be changed frequently as the swelling gradually subsides. We routinely change the cast and obtain radiographs every 4 weeks.

Open Reduction and Pinning: Anterior Approach   A regional block is satisfactory unless iliac crest bone graft is needed, in which case general anesthesia is recommended. Occasionally, however, we have harvested iliac bone graft under local anesthesia with intravenous sedation.

A longitudinal incision is made over the flexor carpi radialis tendon (Fig. 38–2A). The incision begins 3 cm proximal to the distal wrist flexion creases and extends distally to the scaphoid tubercle. A slight radial oblique extension onto the thenar eminence helps to expose the distal pole. The sheath of the flexor carpi radialis tendon is incised and the tendon retracted ulnarly. The dorsal portion of the flexor carpi radialis tendon sheath is incised in line with the direction of the tendon. This obviates the need to identify the radial artery. When present, the superficial branch of the radial artery is identified and

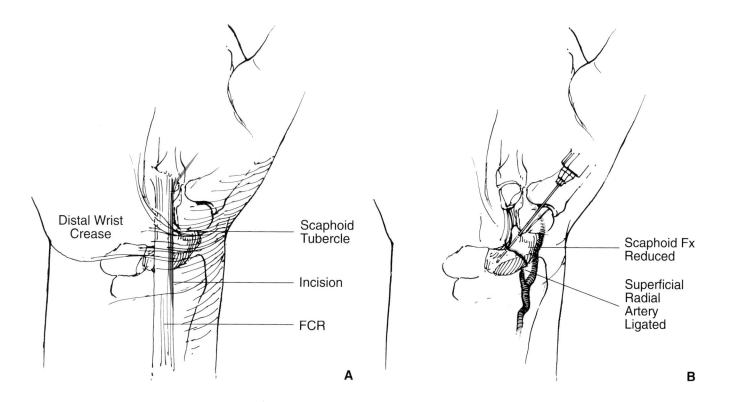

Distal Wrist Crease

Scaphoid Tubercle

Incision

FCR

Scaphoid Fx Reduced

Superficial Radial Artery Ligated

A

B

■ FIGURE 38–2
Anterior approach. **A**, An
incision is made over the
flexor carpi radialis tendon. The superficial
branch of the radial ar-
tery is ligated, the cap-
sule incised, and the fracture reduced. **B**, A 0.045-
inch K-wire is inserted
from the scaphoid tuber-
cle coaxial with the axis
longitudinal of the scaphoid. **C**, A second K-wire
is inserted parallel to the
first.

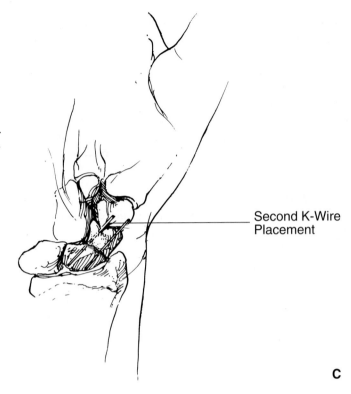

Second K-Wire
Placement

C

ligated. A self-retaining retractor is used to separate the capsule medially and laterally.
No special attempt is made to specifically identify and retract the flexor digitorum superficialis, flexor digitorum profundus, or flexor pollicis longus tendons. The wrist joint capsule
is then exposed and incised longitudinally, parallel to the axis of the radius. It is unnecessary to open the trapezioscaphoid joint capsule, as described for the Herbert screw technique. Generally, the dissection is less extensive than that described for the Herbert screw
insertion and nonunion fixation techniques. The capsule is reflected from the scaphoid
medially and laterally for short distances to expose the fracture site and the scaphocapitate
and radioscaphoid joints. The capsule is not routinely elevated from the distal radius
unless bone graft is harvested from the distal radius.

A thin periosteal elevator is used to manipulate the fragments into reduction while
applying longitudinal traction to the thumb and holding the wrist in ulnar deviation and
extension. When the fracture is difficult to reduce, a perpendicular 0.035-inch K-wire is
inserted into one or both fragments to be used as a joystick.

For comminuted acute fractures, bone graft from iliac crest or distal radius is used. To
obtain bone graft from the distal radius, the skin incision is extended slightly more proximally. The pronator quadratus is stripped subperiostially ulnarly to expose the metaphyseal area of the radius. An osteotome is used to remove a 1 × 1 cm window before
curetting the cancellous bone.

The fracture is reduced and percutaneously pinned, using a 0.045-inch K-wire from the
scaphoid tubercle in a proximal, dorsal, and ulnar direction across the fracture and toward
the proximal pole (i.e., in the longitudinal axis of the scaphoid; Fig. 38–2B). The wire must
not violate the radiocarpal joint. Another wire is inserted parallel to the first (Fig. 38–2C).

When the fracture is comminuted or there is any concern regarding the stability of the
fracture after the insertion of the two K-wires, an extra 0.045-inch K-wire is inserted. To
check on the stability of the fixation, the wrist is moved in radial and ulnar deviation to
demonstrate any possible motion at the fracture site.

For comminuted fractures, the bony and cartilaginous fragments are debrided and the
fracture reduced by aligning the noncommunited portion of the fracture edges, and insert-

ing the K-wires in the same manner as described above. When the fracture appears adequately reduced, the wires are pulled back flush with the fracture. Cancellous bone graft is packed in the defect. The K-wires are then advanced across the fracture toward the proximal pole of the scaphoid. For more extensive comminution, corticocancellous bone is used in a manner similar to that for nonunion fixation techniques.

Obtain posteroanterior, lateral, and scaphoid oblique radiographs to confirm adequate reduction and K-wire placement. The joysticks are removed and the K-wires cut, so that they can be palpated under the skin for easy removal at a later time. The capsule is closed tightly with nonabsorbable suture. A short arm thumb spica splint is converted to a cast after the skin sutures are removed.

Open Reduction and Pinning: Dorsal Approach   A longitudinal incision is centered over Lister's tubercle (Fig. 38–3). This allows access to the wrist through the third compartment and leaves the fourth compartment undisturbed. The extensor pollicis longus is identified

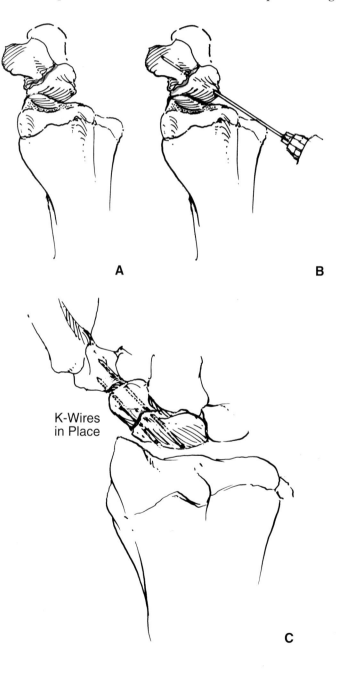

A   **B**

C

K-Wires
in Place

■ FIGURE 38–3
Dorsal approach. The wrist is flexed, the fracture reduced, and two to four 0.045-inch K-wires are inserted from the proximal aspect of the scaphoid to the scaphoid tubercle coaxial with the longitudinal axis of the scaphoid. The K-wires should exit through the scaphoid tubercle. **A**, Lateral view. **B**, Wrist flexed with a K-wire being inserted. **C**, Posteroanterior view, with two parallel wires in place.

in the third compartment, and the overlying extensor retinaculum is opened. Distally, the radial wrist extensors are retracted ulnarly and the extensor pollicis longus radially. The dorsal wrist capsule is exposed and incised parallel to the axis of the scaphoid. The capsule is reflected from the distal radius to facilitate exposure. The dissection near the area of the dorsal ridge of the scaphoid is minimized to preserve its blood supply. The scaphoid is gently freed from the overlying capsule. The fracture is identified and hematoma and debris are removed from the fracture site with a curette. The wrist is maximally flexed to expose the proximal fragment. K-wires are inserted perpendicularly to be used as joysticks to facilitate control of the fracture fragments, as previously described for the anterior approach. The distal fragment has a tendency to flex, with respect to the proximal fragment. The distal fragment is extended until it becomes well-aligned with the proximal fragment. The reduction is maintained with dorsally directed pressure on the scaphoid tubercle to keep the distal scaphoid fragment in extension. With the wrist acutely flexed and radially deviated, a 0.045-inch K-wire is inserted, starting in the most proximal aspect of the proximal pole. (Flexing and radially deviating the wrist brings the proximal fragment into flexion, which becomes aligned with the already flexed distal fragment.) The K-wire is directed anteriorly and radially toward the scaphoid tubercle. Another K-wire is inserted parallel to the first. Both wires should exit anteriorly in the region of the scaphoid tubercle. If the fracture is unstable, a third K-wire is inserted. The K-wires should be withdrawn distally, so that the proximal tips are not protruding into the radiocarpal joint. Multiple radiographic views are obtained to confirm fracture reduction and satisfactory placement of the K-wires. The wires are cut distally, so that they are easily palpated under the skin. The capsule is repaired with nonabsorbable suture and a short arm thumb spica splint is applied.

■ TECHNICAL
ALTERNATIVES

Many other fixation techniques have been described for acute scaphoid fractures, including open reduction and internal fixation with Herbert screws, noncannulated conventionally shaped screws, blade plates, staples; even an external fixation method has been described.[1,9,10,13,15-17,19] K-wire fixation and Herbert screw stabilization are the most accepted techniques. The Herbert screw has gained much attention during the past few years. Its appeal comes from the potential for early mobilization of the wrist. Its insertion, however, is technically difficult and fraught with intraoperative complications. It also requires more extensive exposure, compared with that required for K-wires. K-wire fixation is technically easier and offers an alternative after an unsuccessful attempt at Herbert screw fixation.

The radial artery, as it courses from the anterior forearm, is in close proximity to the scaphoid, and this important vessel is at risk from poorly directed K-wires. Also, extensive dorsal exposure of the scaphoid strips the bone of its nutrient vessels, further jeopardizing prompt fracture healing.[1] Be wary of approaching distal pole fractures through the dorsal approach because it gives a limited view of the distal part of scaphoid. The anterior approach requires division of some of the radiocarpal ligaments, which can disturb the carpal alignment.[7] This risk can be minimized by limiting capsular and ligament dissection and by tightly repairing the capsule.

■ REHABILITATION

At 10 to 14 days postoperatively, when the swelling has subsided, the sutures are removed and a short arm thumb spica cast is applied. The cast incorporates the proximal segment of the thumb but leaves the interphalangeal joint free. The wrist is placed in neutral flexion–extension and radial–ulnar position. We do not routinely use long arm casts postoperatively for scaphoid fractures. The K-wires are left in place until there are radiographic signs of fracture healing. Radiographs are obtained every 4 weeks out of plaster, followed by recasting as necessary.

During the casting period, the patient should exercise the fingers to avoid stiffness. There may be considerable stiffness of the wrist after the cast is removed. Hand therapy with passive and active motion and strengthening of the wrist is beneficial.

■ OUTCOMES

Fractures that are displaced more than 1 mm have a 55% nonunion rate and 50% avascular necrosis rate.[19] Unless treated properly, displaced fractures are associated with many problems, including radioscaphoid and intercarpal arthritis.[1,19] Although K-wire fixation is probably the most commonly used technique, most papers discuss compression screw technique.[9,19] It has been our observation that the union rate by K-wire fixation, whether by open or closed technique, is comparable with the Herbert screw technique.

References

1. Amadio PC, Berquist TH, Smith DK, Ilstrup MS, Cooney WP III, Linscheid RL: Scaphoid malunion, J Hand Surg, 1989; 14A:679–687.
2. Cooney WP, Dobyns JH, Linscheid RL: Fractures of the scaphoid: a rational approach to management. Clin Orthop, 1980; 149:90–97.
3. Cooney WP, Linscheid RL, Dobyns, JH: Fractures and Dislocations of the Wrist. In: Rockwood CA, Green DP, Bucholz PW: Fractures in Adults, 3rd Ed, Philadelphia: JP Lippincott, 1991: 638–647.
4. Cosio MQ, Camp RA: Percutaneous pinning of symptomatic scaphoid nonunions, J Hand Surg, 1986; 11A:350–355.
5. Dehne E, Deffer PA, Feighney RE: Pathomechanics of the fracture of the carpal navicular. J Trauma, 1964; 4:96–113.
6. Demaagd RL, Engber WD: Retrograde Herbert screw fixation for treatment of proximal pole scaphoid nonunions. J Hand Surg, 1988; 13A:604–612.
7. Garcia-Elias M, Vall A, Salo, JM, Lluch AL: Carpal alignment after different surgical approaches to the scaphoid: a comparative study. J Hand Surg, 1988; 13A:604–612.
8. Geissendorfer H: Welche Veralteten Kahnbeinbruche der Hand Eignen Sich zue Nagelung. Zentralbl Chir, 1942; 69:421.
9. Herbert TJ, Fisher WE: Management of the fractured scaphoid using a new bone screw. J Bone Joint Surg, 1984; 66B:114–123.
10. Huene DR, Huene DS: Treatment of nonunions of the scaphoid with Ender compression blade plate system. J Hand Surg, 1991; 16A:913–922.
11. Mack GR, Bosse MJ, Gelberman RH, Yu E: The natural history of scaphoid nonunion. J Bone Joint Surg, 1984; 66A:504–509.
12. MacLennan A: The treatment of fracture of the carpal scaphoid and the indications for operation. Br Med J, 1911; 2:1089.
13. Matti H: Ueber die Behandlung der Navicularefrakture und der Refracture patellae durch Plombierung mit Spongiosa. Zentrabl Chir, 1937: 64:2353–2359.
14. Ruby LK, Stinson J, Belskey MR: The natural history of scaphoid nonunion: a review of fifty-five cases. J Bone Joint Surg, 1985; 67A:428–432.
15. Russe O: Fracture of the carpal navicular: diagnosis, nonoperative treatment and operative treatment. J Bone Joint Surg, 1960: 42A:759–768.
16. Shapiro JS: Power staple fixation in hand and wrist surgery: new application of an old fixation device. J Hand Surg, 1987; 12A:218–227.
17. Shaw JA: Biomechanical comparison of cannulated small bone screws: a brief follow up study. J Hand Surg, 1991; 16A:998–1001.
18. Stark HH, Rickard TA, Zemel NP, Ashworth CR: Treatment of ununited fractures of the scaphoid iliac bone grafts and Kirschner wire fixation. J Bone Joint Surg, 1988; 70A:982–991.
19. Szabo RM, Manske D: Displaced fractures of the scaphoid. Clin Orthop, 1988; 230:30–38.
20. Taleisnik J: Fractures of the Carpal Bones. In: Green DP (ed): Operative Hand Surgery, 2nd Ed, New York: Churchill Livingstone, 1988:813–840.
21. Taleisnik J: The Wrist, New York: Churchill Livingstone, 1985:105–142.

39

Surgical Technique Using the Herbert Compression Screw for Scaphoid Fractures

■ HISTORY OF THE TECHNIQUE

After fractures of the distal radius, the scaphoid fracture statistically dominates skeletal injuries about the wrist.[11] Fortunately, an increase in our clinical index of suspicion, combined with sophisticated imaging techniques, has decreased the incidence of the missed scaphoid fracture. Concurrently, we now better understand the implications of scaphoid displacement and malunion, making assessment of scaphoid fractures all the more important. With this cumulative knowledge, there is justified emphasis on a more aggressive approach in the treatment of scaphoid fractures.

McLaughlin in 1954 is credited with first recommending open reduction and screw fixation of the fractured scaphoid.[9] Credit should also be given to Fisk for his work on scaphoid fractures and associated carpal instability.[2] This chapter discusses the indications and technique of the Herbert compression bone screw in the care of acute scaphoid fractures. The basis for this material was first published in the American literature by Herbert and Fisher in the *Journal of Bone and Joint Surgery* in 1984,[6] and I attended the first workshop held in this country by Dr. Herbert in Dallas, Texas, in 1986, which was hosted by Dr. Peter Carter and Zimmer, Inc.

The Herbert double-threaded bone screw engages both fracture fragments and has no screw head, permitting it to be countersunk beneath cartilage without protrusion into adjacent joints. It does not require removal. Special instrumentation facilitates proper placement of the screw (Fig. 39–1), which has threads of a greater pitch on the leading edge, allowing compression across the fracture line during insertion.

■ INDICATIONS AND CONTRAINDICATIONS

The debate regarding closed or open treatment with internal fixation of scaphoid fractures is ongoing. The scaphoid fracture is most often an injury in young and active patients. Although this population may tolerate a period of cast immobilization, the mean time for fracture healing in a cast is probably close to 3 months. Successful nonoperative treatment may require some patients to wear a cast considerably longer. With Herbert bone screw fixation, 2 to 6 weeks of cast or splint immobilization suffices. One can also anticipate greater primary healing rates with this system.[1,3,6]

The Herbert system is indicated in all cases of trans-scaphoid perilunate fracture dislocations; in addition, in patients with bilateral wrist injuries or multitrauma, earlier mobilization achieved with internal fixation of the fractured scaphoid greatly benefits rehabilitation. It should also be considered with radiographic evidence of intercarpal instability because the scaphoid is the stabilizing intercalated link between the proximal and distal carpal rows. Because of this, the integrity of scaphoid architecture must be respected.

There are few contraindications to Herbert screw fixation of the scaphoid. Anesthetic risks are minimized by an axillary regional block. In the presence of an open contaminated wound, the basic principles of staged surgical care are applicable. When the scaphoid fracture is nondisplaced, a philosophic decision of open or closed treatment is made based on pragmatic patient needs. When nonoperative care is elected, there are no substantive data favoring a long or short arm plaster but including the thumb and modestly flexing and radially deviating the wrist in the plaster applies some compressive and stabilizing forces across the fracture line.

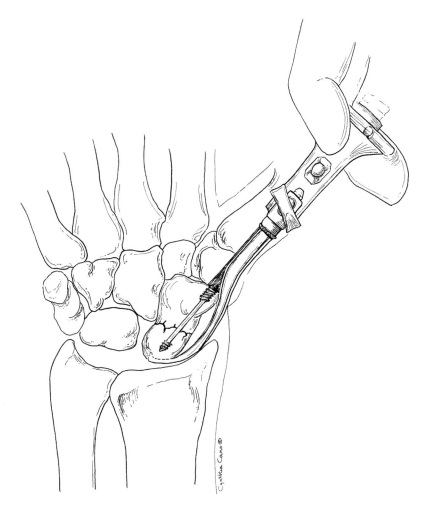

The Herbert jig, the screwdriver within the cannula, and the screw in the scaphoid. The screw head is buried beneath the articular cartilage and the screw is perpendicular to the fracture line.

The scaphoid articulates with the radius and four additional carpal bones (lunate, capitate, trapezoid, trapezium). Hence, fractures of this bone are always intraarticular, making principles of anatomic reduction, rigid fixation, and early motion relevant. As is the femoral neck, the scaphoid bone is "at risk" because of its blood supply.[5] Intercarpal instability is also associated with scaphoid fractures that are displaced or malunited. Indeed, retrospective reviews of scaphoid injuries suggest that with nonunion or malunion, degenerative arthritis ultimately develops in all cases.[8,10] Therefore, aggressive treatment of this fracture seems reasonable and appropriate.

It is my opinion that any displaced fracture (more than 1 to 2 mm) needs open reduction and internal fixation. Even patients having no demonstrated fracture displacement may be candidates for this technique because few individuals can afford months of cast immobilization and its socioeconomic impact. Similarly, with a small proximal pole fracture (proximal one third or less) in which the risk of avascular necrosis is greater, screw fixation through a dorsal approach is recommended. Finally, with an inclination angle of the fracture line of more than 45° to the horizontal plane, this fracture is unstable and in need of fixation with compression (Fig. 39–2).

The traditional and justified question, "What would you do if it were your wrist?" finds this author, should he break his scaphoid, electing surgery and anticipating return to work in 2 to 3 weeks.

Critical radiographic assessment of the scaphoid fracture is best made by an anteroposterior radiograph of the wrist in ulnar deviation and a true lateral view. Ulnar deviation of the wrist extends the scaphoid and therefore elongates its appearance, making the

■ FIGURE 39-2
An unstable fracture with
an inclination angle
greater than 45°.

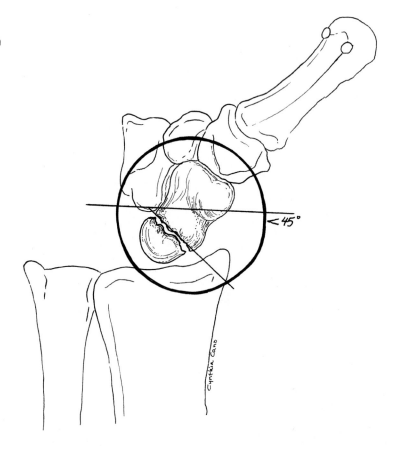

fracture line more apparent. The lateral view demonstrates the flexion angle of the scaphoid, and a comparison lateral of the opposite normal wrist can facilitate the diagnosis if a displaced and hyperflexed distal scaphoid fragment is suspected. In problematic cases, lateral tomograms or magnetic resonance imaging provide the most secure analysis of scaphoid position within the carpus.

■ SURGICAL
TECHNIQUES

Surgery of the closed scaphoid fracture is not a medical emergency unless associated with an irreducible perilunate dislocation. Indeed, if surgery is elected after a period of cast immobilization, surgery should be delayed and casting discontinued for perhaps 2 weeks to better mobilize the wrist for easier surgical exposure. Even a modestly stiff wrist, which can be present after a fracture and brief cast immobilization, makes surgery more difficult. General or axillary block anesthesia is required for surgery because proper wrist positioning requires complete muscle relaxation.

A palmar radial zigzag incision is outlined from the proximal third of the thumb thenar muscles to two fingerbreadths proximal to the wrist flexion crease (Fig. 39-3). This incision is radial to the major landmark, the flexor carpi radialis (FCR) tendon. Using the tendon sheath as a guide to the volar wrist capsule ensures protection of the palmar cutaneous branch of the median nerve to the ulnar side and the radial artery to the radial side of the capsular incision. The superficial palmar branch of the radial artery must be sacrificed with this exposure. It normally passes into the palm just proximal to the tuberosity of the scaphoid, a landmark that can be easily palpated. The proximal third of the thenar muscles are split in line with the incision, well proximal and radial to their innervation.

The floor of the FCR tendon sheath is opened longitudinally, safely exposing the palmar aspect of the distal radius and the scaphoid. The distal transverse fibers of the pronator quadratus muscle define the proximal extent of the incision, the carpometacarpal (CMC) joint, the distal extent.

As the radioscaphoid joint is entered, the important radioscaphocapitate (RSC) ligament

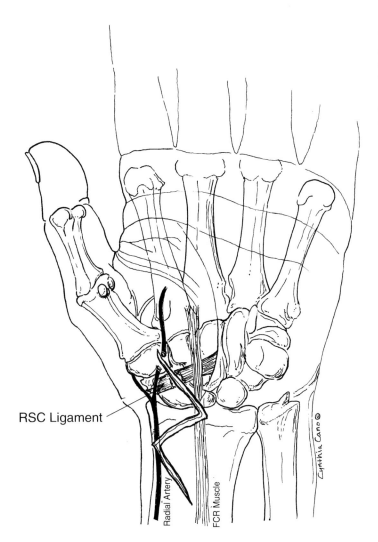

A zigzag incision for adequate exposure of a fractured scaphoid. The RSC ligament is marked. It can be a cause of scaphoid fracture fragment displacement.

RSC Ligament

Radial Artery

FCR Muscle

is identified and cut, anticipating its repair during closure (Fig. 39–3). Recognition of the ligament is facilitated by wrist extension and radial deviation because ligament tension defines its location. Sharply elevating the capsule ulnarward from the volar lip of the radius exposes the proximal scaphoid. The FCR tendon, as it dives radially and dorsally behind the scaphoid tuberosity toward its insertion into the trapezium or second metacarpal, is in jeopardy. Flexion of the wrist at this juncture relaxes and protects the tendon. The exposure must be complete enough to see clearly the distal end of the radius and its elliptical scaphoid fossa and the scaphotrapezial (ST) joint.

With completion of the distal extension of this incision, it is an opportune time to open the ST joint, sharply releasing the capsule from the scaphoid tuberosity, so that it may be repaired later. Ligament release is performed circumferentially—again anticipating the proximity of the FCR tendon on the ulnar side. The purpose of this capsulotomy is to permit elevation of the distal pole of the scaphoid for proper placement of the compression screw in the long axis of the bone. Placement of temporary K-wires in the scaphoid can be helpful at this phase of the operation in a nondisplaced fracture; they can be used later as a cantilever to elevate the distal pole for proper screw placement. Throughout this dissection, the scaphoid fracture can easily be visualized, enhanced by wrist extension and ulnar deviation. The more proximal the fracture is in the scaphoid, the more wrist extension and deviation is needed for exposure. Longitudinal traction in conjunction with a firm dorsal bolster proximal to the wrist further facilitates good scaphoid exposure.

With a displaced fracture, the next step is to anatomically reduce the fracture fragments.

In transverse fractures, the deformity is usually one of distal pole flexion; in oblique fractures, there is often a medial or lateral shift. Depending on the fracture angle of inclination from the horizontal plane of the forearm, the distal fragment can be displaced radially or ulnarly. In conjunction with this shift, the distal pole also has a tendency to pronate as it falls into flexion. Anatomic reduction is aided by once again extending and ulnarly deviating the wrist and applying longitudinal traction to the radial side of the hand, thereby opening the scaphoid compartment and eliminating compressive displacing forces. The Herbert screw set contains the instruments necessary for the reduction and fixation of the scaphoid fragments. A Freer elevator, present in the set, aids in achieving the anatomic reduction and then palpating the smooth contour of the reduced scaphoid. Again, temporary K-wire fixation can hold this reduction before the application of the jig.

The hook of the jig is placed on the large proximal pole of the scaphoid, well dorsal to ensure proper alignment and placement of the screw. Traction is maintained while the barrel of the device is placed on the articular surface of the scaphoid within the scaphotrapezial joint; hence the need to elevate the distal pole palmarly. The small, specially designed hook elevator facilitates this maneuver, and this elevator must be placed ulnarly and dorsally on the distal pole before inserting the barrel into the compression jig (Fig. 39–4). One or two K-wires across the fracture line can make this technically demanding part of the procedure easier because the wires can also be used to assist in gently elevating the reduced distal scaphoid. Position of the scaphoid and the jig should be verified by radiographs at this juncture. The barrel-hook assembly should ideally rest about 50° radial to the longitudinal axis of the scaphoid. Any error should favor an increased angle, which would place the screw more dorsal in the scaphoid, protecting against possible violation

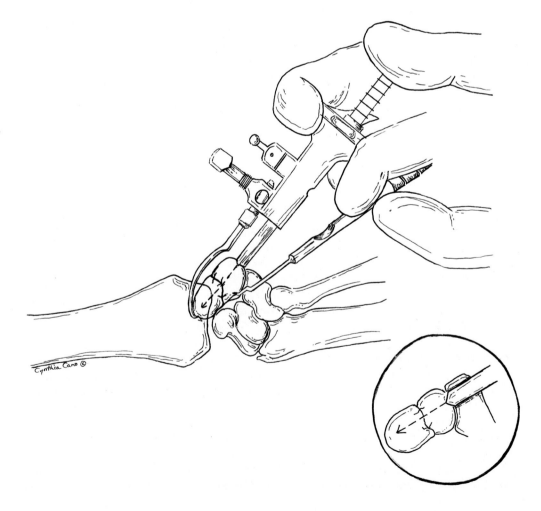

■ FIGURE 39–4
The Herbert instrumentation, demonstrating the hook of the jig placed well dorsal on the proximal pole of the scaphoid. The elevator lifts the dorsal pole. A trough can be made in the trapezium for easier positioning of the jig, cannula, and screw.

of the anterior cortex during screw placement. The jig and cannula should be applied as tightly as possible because the maximum compressive forces across the fracture line actually occur at this time.

Once the compression device is properly and securely placed, the most difficult part of the procedure is completed. Care must be taken, however, to not dislodge the jig during the drilling procedure because realigning the drill holes is difficult. The two drills and the tap are hand-held and prepare the path for the screw. The length of the screw is read directly from the cannula. When inordinate pressure is required to start the first drill through the distal cortex of the scaphoid, a K-wire can be used to facilitate the drilling. The Herbert screws are sized in even millimeter lengths. One can err on the side of the shorter screw because an additional 360° turn is made to bury the screw beneath the articular surface of the scaphoid to protect cartilage integrity. The jig is removed before the final turn of the screw.

Closure is conducted with the wrist in a neutral or modestly flexed posture, thereby facilitating reapproximation of the RSC ligament. A snug capsular closure is important but no specific repair of the scaphotrapezial ligaments needs to be performed. The muscle-splitting incision at the base of the thenar muscles often falls together without sutures before skin closure. A well-padded short arm splint is applied to include the thumb, and the CMC and metacarpophalangeal (MP) joints. This splint is changed to a cast in 7 to 10 days. Immobilization is continued for 2 to 6 weeks. The variable time of protection is clearly based on assessment of fracture stability, patient compliance, and lifestyle.

When a fracture of the proximal pole occurs representing 25% or less of the scaphoid, a dorsal approach is favored. Fortunately, these small proximal pole fractures, although more prone to delayed or nonunion, do not as often demonstrate the flexed posture seen with wrist fractures. They are unstable, however. The dorsal approach is recommended for this type of fracture.

The dorsal incision is longitudinal and just ulnar to Lister's tubercle between the third and fourth compartments (Fig. 39–5). With wrist flexion and ulnar deviation, the broad, convex proximal pole of the scaphoid is well visualized. In a fresh fracture, curettage and bone grafting at the fracture site are not recommended because it damages cartilage and can increase the chance of avascular necrosis. K-wires can be used to hold position while the Herbert screw is inserted free-hand, using manual compression. Without the jig, there is less compression applied to the fracture site. The Herbert miniscrew is recommended for these small proximal fractures because there is only a modest cross-sectional area of bone at best, and the smaller screw diameter allows a greater area for bone healing around the screw. The longitudinal axis of the scaphoid is directed toward the base of the abducted thumb, which is used for directional alignment during screw placement. There is no cannula to read screw length, and a short screw is all that is required. The screw is advanced beneath cartilage. Closure and mobilization schedules are similar to the palmar approach. These proximal pole fractures are slower to heal, yet there is less tendency toward loss of wrist motion.

■ TECHNICAL ALTERNATIVES

The Herbert bone-screw system is technically demanding. Clearly, a wide exposure facilitates comfort with the procedure. The pronator quadratus proximally and the CMC joint distally define the extent of the incision but one can extend beyond these landmarks if necessary. Elevating the capsular structures radially and ulnarly is also important but the need to preserve the integrity of the FCR tendon often finds wrist flexion helpful during this phase. Once the scaphoid is exposed, wrist extension and ulnar deviation provide the best exposure; therefore, it is important to mobilize the wrist for a time before surgery when stiffness exists. Sterile traction has also been helpful for scaphoid visualization, reduction, and fixation.[*]

When mobilizing the scaphoid to obtain reduction and jig placement, it is necessary to cut circumferentially the ST ligaments to elevate the scaphoid palmarly. Without sufficient

[*] The Carter Sterile Traction Hand Surgery Table. Innovation Sports, 7 Chrysler, Irvine, CA 92718

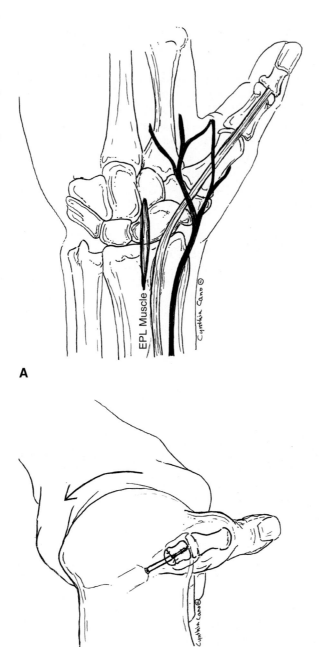

EPL Muscle

A

B

elevation, the barrel and cannula and, resultantly, the screw may be too palmar for the natural concave surface of the scaphoid. The proximal pole of the scaphoid, which articulates with the elliptical fossa of the radius, is the largest articulating surface of the scaphoid. Its size and convexity may lead to a common error of placing the compression device too palmar, thereby potentiating anterior placement of the screw and causing a flexion force with compression. As a result, screw placement can actually create the flexion deformity one is trying to correct.

Such a flexion posture shortens the scaphoid and leads to a dorsal intercalated segmental instability pattern of the wrist. Ideally, screw placement should be in the mid-coronal plane of the scaphoid and perpendicular to the fracture line.

If proper screw placement in the longitudinal axis of the scaphoid is particularly difficult to achieve, a small trough can be made on the palmar aspect of the trapezium with bone rongeurs to ensure better positioning of the jig and cannula (Fig. 39–4). The placement of temporary K-wires remains a useful support mechanism throughout the reduction, manipulation, and screw fixation of the scaphoid.

In the event of comminution, a bone graft must be considered to achieve stability and restoration and maintenance of scaphoid length during compression. When comminution occurs, compression forces across the fracture site without grafting can cause shortening and a flexion posture of the scaphoid, the so-called "humpback" deformity. This deformity is almost predictable without a graft or when the screw is placed palmar to the mid-coronal plane of the scaphoid. It is worth emphasizing that the compression jig hook should be well dorsal on the proximal pole because of the concave palmer surface of the scaphoid to restore the normal flexion posture of the scaphoid as the intercalated link between the proximal and distal carpal rows.

The bone graft should be harvested from the superior crest, taking with sharp osteotomes a small wafer of bone that includes the superior cortical crest and the inner and outer cortical tables (Fig. 39–6). The cancellous surfaces are placed between the proximal and distal fracture fragments, and either the inner or outer cortical table will be architecturally congruent against the capitate. Bone rongeurs are used to remove excessive bone. Ideally, the superior iliac cortical surface of the graft fits just below the palmar surface of the scaphoid, giving the graft stability and eliminating the tendency for graft extrusion as compression is applied across the fracture line and the graft. Use of bupivacaine with epinephrine minimizes bleeding during harvesting of the graft and postoperative pain.

Closure is best achieved with absorbable sutures because there is little soft-tissue coverage of this constant contact area of the wrist. Nonabsorbable sutures may lead to an uncomfortable foreign body granuloma, especially over the tuberosity of the scaphoid.

■ REHABILITATION

Immobilization is variable, depending on the needs and lifestyle of the patient, but a splint should precede a circumferential cast because of the rich vascularity in the surgical exposure and the potential for postoperative swelling. When changing to a short arm

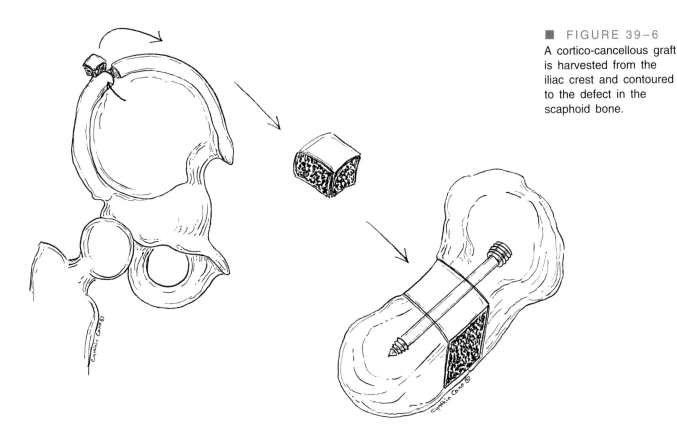

■ FIGURE 39–6
A cortico-cancellous graft is harvested from the iliac crest and contoured to the defect in the scaphoid bone.

thumb spica cast, gradual wrist extension is desired because most patients lose some extension range when the operated wrist is compared with the contralateral normal side. Six weeks postoperatively, most patients are back to normal activities. If, however, the fracture is a small proximal pole or if comminution requires a bone graft, further immobilization, depending on radiographic evidence of healing, may be necessary.

Occupational therapy to achieve better wrist motion can be valuable for these patients. The patient should be forewarned, however, that there may be a modest loss of wrist motion. Improvement in motion, strength, and comfort can be expected for 6 months or more after this operation.

■ OUTCOMES

Studies of nonoperative scaphoid fracture treatment suggest that primary healing rates are 90 to 95%.[4,7] Yet many acute fractures are missed and untreated and in those series addressing nonsurgical care, many patients are lost to follow-up. In essence, I believe that nonunion has a greater incidence than published reports indicate, especially in cases in which the scaphoid fracture is displaced or involves a small proximal pole.

Those caring for scaphoid fractures have embraced the Herbert compression bone-screw system with enthusiasm. The technique represents a step forward in the care of the problematic scaphoid fracture. Based on my experience and that of Dr. Peter Carter (personal communication), healing rates of 95% or greater in fractures treated primarily with this method, and healing rates of 100% in nondisplaced scaphoid fractures can be expected.[6] It must be emphasized that the operation is technically demanding. Many scaphoid fractures heal using cast immobilization, K-wire fixation, or both. Therefore, a surgeon should not be rigidly committed to this technique as the only way of achieving union in a fractured scaphoid. Presently, however, the Herbert compression screw achieves as closely as possible the goals of anatomic reduction, rigid fixation, and early motion.

References

1. Bunker TD, McNamee PB, Scott TD: The Herbert screw for scaphoid fractures. J Bone Joint Surg, 1987; 69B:631–634.
2. Fisk GR: Carpal instability and the fractured scaphoid. Ann R Coll Surg, 1970; 46:63–76.
3. Ford DJ, Khoury G, El-Hadidi S, Lunn PG, Burke RD: The Herbert screw for fractures of the scaphoid. A review of results and technical difficulties. J Bone Joint Surg, 1987; 69B:124–127.
4. Gelberman RH, Wolock BS, Siegel BR: Current concepts reviews. Fractures and non-unions of the carpal scaphoid. J Bone Joint Surg, 1989; 71A:1560–1565.
5. Gelberman RH, Menon J: The vascularity of the scaphoid bone. J Hand Surg, 1980; 5:508–513.
6. Herbery TJ, Fisher WE: Management of the fractured scaphoid using a new bone screw. J Bone Joint Surg, 1984; 66B:114–123.
7. Herndon JH: Scaphoid fractures and complications. American Academy of Orthopaedic Surgeons. Monograph Series, 1993.
8. Mack GR, Bosse MJ, Gelberman RH, et al: The natural history of scaphoid non-union. J Bone Joint Surg, 1984; 66A:504–509.
9. McLaughlin HL: Fractures of the carpal navicular (scaphoid) bone: some observations based on treatment by open reduction and internal fixation. J Bone Joint Surg, 1954; 36A:765–774.
10. Ruby LK, Stinson J, Belsky MR: The natural history of scaphoid non-union. J Bone Joint Surg, 1985; 67A:428–432.
11. Taliesnik J: Fractures of the Carpal Bones. In: Green DP (ed): Operative Hand Surgery, New York: Churchill Livingstone, 1988:813–873.

40

External Fixation for Fractures of the Distal Radius

Fractures of the distal radius are common. Most are well treated by closed means but unfortunately, because of a long-standing belief that any fracture about the distal radius is benign, more complex fractures have historically been undertreated and as a result have resulted in significant problems and complications. Recognition of the complexity of certain fractures involving the distal radius has prompted investigation into developing methods for surgical stabilization and articular reconstruction. External fixation has become a mainstay in the hands of the surgeon managing complex fractures about the distal radius.[1,2,4,5,7-9,11-13,20,23]

Several classification systems have been described for fractures of the distal radius. Combining some of the principles of other classification schemes, Cooney and coworkers and Rayhack and associates have developed a universal classification system that is quite helpful in the diagnosis and treatment of distal radius fractures.[3,16] This classification system divides these fractures into four groups (Fig. 40–1): type I: nonarticular, nondisplaced; type II: nonarticular, displaced (this type can further be broken down into those that are reducible and stable, those that are reducible and unstable, and irreducible); type III: intrarticular fractures, nondisplaced; and type IV: intraarticular fractures that are displaced (again with three subgroups: reducible and stable, reducible and unstable, and irreducible). The components of the fracture pattern indicating an unstable condition include significant volar or dorsal comminution; widely spread or depressed articular fragments; angulation of the major fragments in any plane greater than 10°; significant displacement (more than 5 mm) of the major distal fragments away from the shaft; significant extension of the comminution into the radiocarpal articulation or radioulnar articulation; and significant fracture of the neck or head of the ulna (not simply the ulnar styloid).

Methods of external fixation have been widely used to manage fractures of the distal radius throughout this century. They have undergone periods of popularity and disfavor, with some authors[26] reporting dismal failures, whereas others[5,7,11,20] have reported marked success in its use. It must be remembered that a method of fixation is only as good as the technique of the surgeon applying it. It should be applied for the proper reasons, safely, with an understanding of the physiology and biomechanics of the anatomic region and the fracture itself, with great attention paid to limiting sources of potential complication.[18,19,21-24]

Indications for use of external fixation include unstable intraarticular fractures of the distal radius, unstable extraarticular fractures of the distal radius unmanageable by noninvasive closed means, open fractures, fractures with nerve injuries, bilateral injuries, and a fracture in a patient with impaired contralateral function. The external fixation device obviates the need for cast immobilization and allows early finger mobility, pronation, and supination in addition to elbow and shoulder motion. It requires compliance for pin-site care, with the patient taking an active role in the performance of postoperative rehabilitation.

Contraindications include noncompliant patients. This may be somewhat difficult to assess in the emergency setting. When there is evidence that the patient may be noncompliant (e.g., intoxication, drug abuse, combative nature), it may be beneficial to initially

■ HISTORY OF THE
TECHNIQUE

■ INDICATIONS AND
CONTRAINDICATIONS

309

■ FIGURE 40–1
The "universal" classification system for distal radius fractures.[19,20]

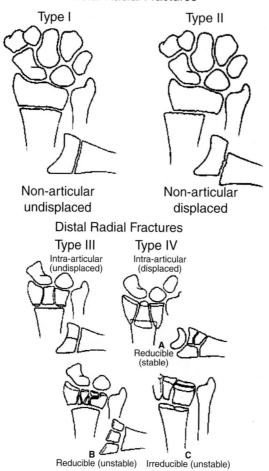

FIGURE 40–1
The "universal" classification system for distal radius fractures.[19,20]

Classification of
Fractures
by Treatment

Distal Radial Fractures

Type I   Type II

Non-articular   Non-articular
undisplaced   displaced

Distal Radial Fractures

Type III   Type IV
Intra-articular   Intra-articular
(undisplaced)   (displaced)

A
Reducible
(stable)

B   C
Reducible (unstable)   Irreducible (unstable)

splint the patient and get to know the patient over the first few days after injury to assess his or her ability to comply with the rigorous demands of postoperative rehabilitation and pin care. Other contraindications include stable, minimally displaced fractures; fractures of the distal radius with concomitant metacarpal or radial fractures at or near the site of proposed pin insertion; and unstable but extraarticular irreducible distal radius fractures that will require open reduction and may be better treated with internal plate fixation.

■ SURGICAL
TECHNIQUES

Principles of Application   The first step in the use of external fixation in unstable distal radius fractures is the choice of an external fixation device. A diverse spectrum of devices exists, ranging from pins and plaster through a variety of half-frame designs; to fixators with articulated joints, which allow early motion; to complex circular frames, such as the Ilizarov device.[6] The type, size, shape, and configuration of the fixator is not critical as long as it is one that works well in the hands of the treating surgeon. It is not my intention to recommend any one fixation device but to provide a "generic" approach to fixator selection and application to aid the reader in choosing a reliable fixator. Generally, ideal fixator design should provide satisfactory fracture visualization. That is, it should not block key radiographic views. Radio-opaque external fixators that are in direct lateral line with the hand and wrist can, for example, block a true lateral view of the reconstructed distal radius. This problem can be circumvented by using offset pin terminals, which elevate the bar more dorsally and provide adequate visualization of the lateral aspect of the wrist or by using a radiolucent device.

The fixation device should also be easy to apply. Preferably, the pins can be inserted, the device applied to the implanted half-pins, and after assembly has been performed, a reduction maneuver can be performed and the device locked in place. The device should be forgiving enough so that when initial reduction is not adequate, the device may be loosened and a gentle repeat reduction may be performed.

Principles of Ligamentotaxis Biomechanically, the external fixation device uses the principle of "ligamentotaxis": the technique by which physiologic tension is developed through the soft tissues traversing the joint. This physiologic soft-tissue tension helps mold the fracture fragments back into alignment and holds the fracture out to length while providing angular alignment and rotational control. Through ligamentotaxis, the external fixator provides stability, maintains soft-tissue tension to help prevent capsular contractures, and controls length, as well as angular and rotational alignment. It does not, however, ensure precise small fragment control nor does it prevent late collapse.

Limited Open Surgical Approach This procedure should be performed in the operating room, using either a regional anesthetic block or general anesthesia. The patient's arm is prepped and draped and laid out on a radiolucent hand table, and a small image-intensifier is draped and positioned for easy entry and withdrawal.

After exsanguination with an elastic wrap, a pneumatic tourniquet around the upper arm is inflated to 100 mm Hg above the patient's systolic pressure. The hand and arm are positioned with the radial aspect facing upward, and a point about 10 cm proximal to the radial styloid directly overlying the radial border of the distal forearm is demarcated. This is the central point of the proximal incision, which measures 2.5 cm (Fig. 40–2). The skin and subcutaneous tissue are divided and retracted. In the subcutaneous tissues, one must be careful to look for overlapping branches of the lateral antebrachial cutaneous nerve. These should be carefully bluntly dissected and retracted and protected. The fascia overlying the forearm musculature is then noted. The interval between the brachioradialis volarly and the extensor carpi radialis longus dorsally is easily seen. The point of separation of these two tendons marks their myotendinous junction and the emergence of the radial sensory nerve from beneath the brachioradialis. It is important to fully free the fascia overlying these muscles, gently mobilize them, and ensure that the radial sensory nerve is fully mobilized and not tethered. It may then be carefully retracted out of the way; in this interval, the periosteum of the radius is scored and elevated, using small Carroll elevators, which are then sequentially replaced with small Bennett retractors. These retractors fully expose the radius throughout the 2.5-cm span of the incision, protect the periosteum, and carefully retract and protect the radial sensory nerve and branches of the lateral antebrachial cutaneous nerve. Drill guides are then used for central placement of the drill bit. These are inserted with power under direct vision, using sharp new drill bits, with constant irrigation to prevent thermal injury.[22]

The size of the drill bit should be equal to the core diameter of the threaded half-pin to be used. When two drill bits have been inserted, the second is removed and replaced with a threaded half-pin by hand until both cortices are engaged. The initial drill bit is then removed and again replaced, using the drill guide with a second threaded half-pin. When this has been completed, any bone fragments are removed from around the drill holes, appropriate placement is documented with the image intensifier, the soft tissues are allowed to relax back into place, and the skin is approximated, using simple sutures of monofilament nylon.

The distal incision is then made over the dorsoradial border of the index metacarpal, measuring 2.5 cm from just proximal to the tubercular flare at the base of the index metacarpal distally along its shaft (Fig. 40–3). Careful blunt subcutaneous dissection is performed

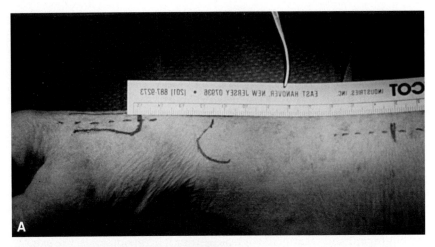

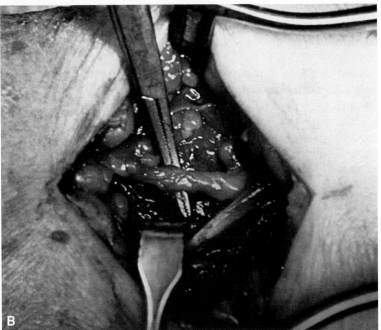

■ FIGURE 40–2

A, Incisions for the limited open approach for pin placement in the radial aspect of the forearm and hand. The forearm incision is centered about 10 cm above the radial styloid, whereas the hand incision is placed over the dorsoradial aspect of the base of the index metacarpal. **B,** The proximal incision overlying the radial aspect of the forearm at the distal third provides access to the radial sensory nerve (being demonstrated by the hemostat).

to identify, retract, and protect the terminal branches of the radial sensory nerve in this area. The deeper interosseous fascia is divided, demonstrating the dorsal "clear space" along the dorsoradial aspect of the index metacarpal between the first and second dorsal interosseous muscles. Along this plane, a No. 15 scalpel blade is used to elevate the first dorsal interosseous from the shaft of the index metacarpal as far proximal as its attachment along the tubercle at the base of the metacarpal. In this area, the capsular attachment and insertion of the extensor carpi radialis longus tendon is also elevated in a continuous sheet with the first dorsal interosseous downward along the radial border of the base of the metacarpal. This maintains integrity of the first dorsal interosseous without any mid-substance rents or tears. A drill guide is then placed at the base of the index metacarpal and directed transversely, toward the base of the middle finger metacarpal. The trajectory

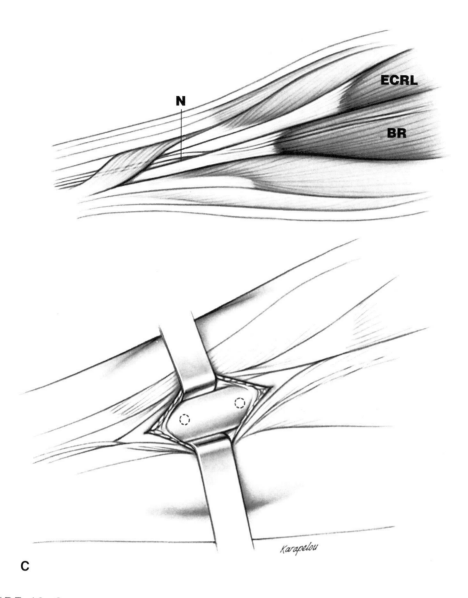

C

■ FIGURE 40–2

(continued) **C**, The myotendinous junction of the brachioradialis and extensor carpi radialis lon-gus demarcates the emergence of the radial sensory nerve from under the brachioradialis. At this point, it is quite safe to retract the nerve, incise the periosteum, and retract it with Bennett retractors for complete visualization of the radius for central predrilling and fixator pin insertion. (From Seitz W, Putnam MD, Dick HM: Limited open surgical approach for external fixation of distal radius fractures. J Hand Surg, 1990; 15A:2:288–293.)

of the planned drill insertion is then confirmed on the image intensifier to prevent violation of the carpometacarpal joints. The power drill is used to insert a drill bit across the bases of the index and middle metacarpals through their four cortices. Using the drill guide again, a second drill bit is inserted centrally through only the shaft of the index metacarpal distally. This is removed and replaced with a self-tapping threaded half-pin, after which the first drill bit is removed from the bases of the index and middle metacarpal and replaced with a threaded self-tapping half-pin. This provides total distal purchase of six cortices and avoids violation of the intermetacarpal space and its interosseous muscle (Fig. 40–4). Once radiographic confirmation of appropriate pin position has been made, the first dorsal interosseous muscle is allowed to fall back into its anatomic position, and the skin is approximated around the fixator pins, using simple sutures of monofilament nylon.

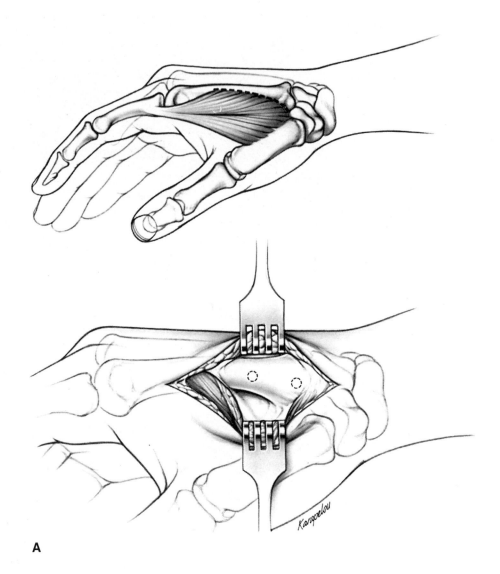

A

■ FIGURE 40-3

A, The distal pin site incision for the limited open approach is made over the dorsoradial aspect of the index metacarpal base. This exposes the adjacent shaft of the metacarpal for direct access for central predrilling and insertion of the fixator pins. (From Seitz W, Putnam MD, Dick HM: Limited open surgical approach for external fixation of distal radius fractures. J Hand Surg, 1990; 15A:2:288–293.)

At this point, the fixation device is applied to the pins in its loosened mode. The hand is then held by the surgeon as though to shake hands, and gentle traction is applied in the longitudinal direction. The assistant applies gentle countertraction in the other direction at the level of the distal humerus while stabilizing the applied but unfastened fixator. With his other hand, the surgeon gently applies compression and molds the fracture fragments back into alignment while maintaining tension across the wrist. When the surgeon feels that the fragments are back in alignment, the assistant uses the wrench to secure all fasteners and lock the fixation device in place. Assessment of reduction is then performed initially under the image intensifier and then with plain radiographs. When adjustments need to be made in the reduction, they can be performed with adjustment of the fixator, adding or subtracting tension, changing rotational or angular settings, or reloosening the device and performing a complete re-reduction.

Plain radiographs must be assessed at this point to ensure that overdistraction has not

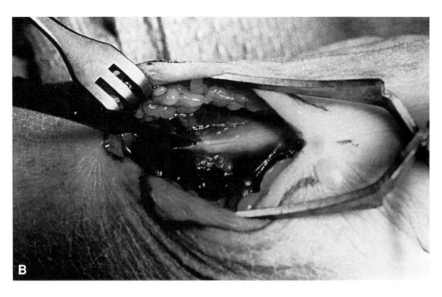

■ FIGURE 40–3
(continued) **B**, The first dorsal interosseous muscle is sharply elevated from the tubercular flair at the base of the index metacarpal along its shaft, using a No. 15 scalpel blade. This maintains the integrity of the first dorsal interosseous, preventing any tears or rents in the substance of the muscle.

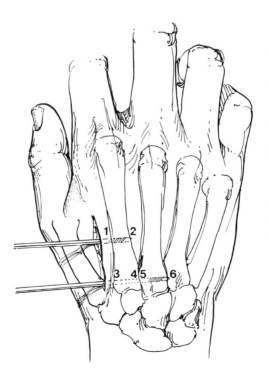

■ FIGURE 40–4
Distal pins are inserted through the bases of the index and middle metacarpals, avoiding violation of the carpometacarpal joints, and a second pin is inserted through the shaft of the index metacarpal only, avoiding violation of the second interosseous muscle compartment, giving purchase in a total of six cortices.

occurred, that there is no evidence of intercarpal ligamentous injury or carpal bone fracture, and that an adequate articular restoration has been achieved. Critical assessment of these radiographs should reveal 1 mm of increased space in the radiocarpal articulation, compared with the mid-carpal articulation. This demonstrates development of enough ligamentotaxis to provide physiologic tension through the radiocarpal ligaments, preventing contracture, while avoiding overdistraction. There should be normal scapholunate and lunotriquetral orientations in all planes, and anatomic restoration of the scaphoid and lunate fossae must be achieved to less than 1 mm of step-off. There should not be a large subarticular void in the metaphyseal bone of the radius, the radioulnar joint should be congruous, and the ulna should be reduced in the sigmoid notch on both the posteroanterior and lateral views. The wrist should not be hyperflexed but should be essentially in a neutral position (Fig. 40–5). When these parameters have not been met, augmentation is necessary, with some degree of internal fixation and in some cases, bone grafting.[20]

Augmentation of external fixation for management of complex distal radius fractures uses limited internal fixation in the form of K-wires as internal sutures to elevate and secure articular fragments in place and to provide additional subchondral support. After

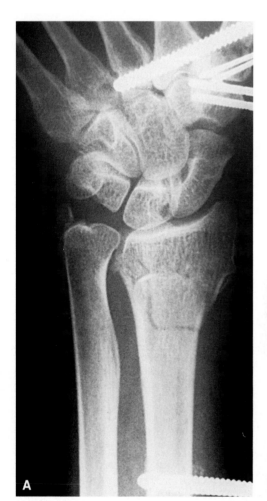
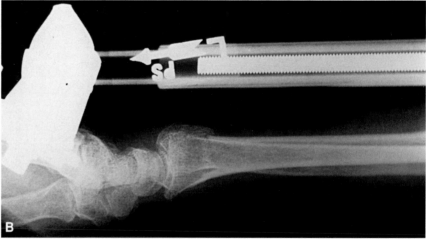

■ FIGURE 40–5
A, Anteroposterior, and **B**, lateral radiographs demonstrate restoration of normal alignment in a comminuted intraarticular fracture of the distal radius that has been managed with external fixation. There is enough ligamentotaxis to provide tension on the radiocarpal ligamentous structures, which hold the fracture fragments in anatomic alignment while the wrist remains in a relatively neutral position, as seen on the lateral view.

overall length and alignment have been achieved with the external fixation device, should articular step-off, depression, impaction, or comminution prevent restoration of a congruent joint surface, a 0.062-inch K-wire is inserted percutaneously, obliquely into the tip of the radial styloid fragment. This fragment, which tends to be laterally displaced and rotated, is then manipulated into position by holding the K-wire freehand until it is properly aligned with the shaft of the radius. It is then driven obliquely across the contralateral cortex of the more proximal radial shaft, fixing it in place as a "buttress" against which the lunate facet fragments may be elevated and wedged into place. This is performed by inserting another 0.062-inch K-wire held freehand into the fracture site from a dorsal approach and "teasing" or levering the lunate fossa fragments back up into proper alignment with the scaphoid fossa of the radial styloid. Once these are returned to their proper level, transverse subchondral K-wires are inserted from the radial side, creating a subartic-

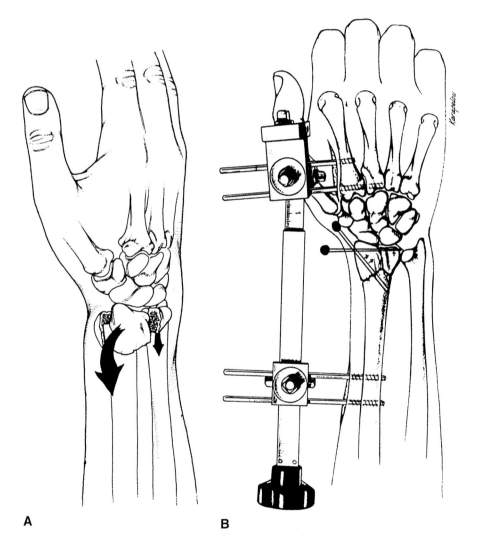

A   **B**

■ FIGURE 40–6

A, The major radial styloid fragment tends to be rotated laterally and proximally, whereas the lunate fossa fragments tend to be impacted and shortened in unstable intraarticular fractures of the distal radius. **B**, After restoration of length and alignment by the external fixation device, return of articular congruity is achieved by means of percutaneously placed K-wires. An initial K-wire inserted into the tip of the radial styloid restores normal orientation and is then transfixed to the more proximal intact ulnar side of the shaft of the radius. This acts as a buttress, against which the lunate fossa fragments can be percutaneously "teased" back into alignment and held by transverse subarticular K-wires.

ular support and resistance to recollapse (Fig. 40–6). In this way, the articular surface can usually be realigned without actually opening the fracture site. If, however, some of the fracture fragments are severely rotated and displaced and cannot be realigned, it may be necessary to open the dorsum of the joint for reduction under direct vision.

■ TECHNICAL
ALTERNATIVES

Alternative means of managing irreducible and extraarticular fractures or intraarticular fractures with minimal fragmentation include open reduction and internal fixation using a buttress plate and screws, providing the ability to restore anatomy, remove soft tissue (frequently the pronator quadratus) from an interposed position between the fracture fragments, and achieve a solid fixation without need in most cases for additional external support. It is important to remember that plates used on the distal radius function biomechanically as "buttresses." Therefore, they should be placed along the volar surface when there has been significant volar displacement of the distal fragment and conversely along the dorsal surface when there has been significant dorsal displacement of the distal fragments.[15]

In younger patients having such fractures, in which there is dorsal displacement and good bone stock, intrafocal pinning as described by Kapandji has been of value, although when this technique has been used in older patients, significant resorption around the intrafocally placed K-wires has resulted in displacement and less than satisfactory outcomes.[10,24]

Although transulnar pinning has been recommended by Rayhack and coworkers, this technique "locks up" the distal radioulnar joint by the passage of K-wires across the intact ulna into the fractured radius. Proximal rotational forces of pronation and supination applied to the radius also generate torsional forces that could exceed the holding capacity of smooth K-wires. Nonetheless, Rayhack and colleagues have reported some good short-term results with this technique.[16]

Relatively high rates of complication have been reported in some series when external fixation has been used to manage unstable fractures of the distal radius.[8,17,26] Critical assessment of where and how complications occur, however, usually indicates a breakdown in strict adherence to principles. In most cases, failure begins at the pin–bone interface. This is the site of linkage between the fixator and the patient. Failure to maintain a healthy pin–bone interface can result in pin breakage or loosening, loss of fixation, loss of reduction, infection, fracture through the bone at the site of pin insertion, and damage to the surrounding soft-tissue structures.[21]

Those factors influencing the pin–bone interface include the actual insertion of the pin by the surgeon, the mechanism by which the pin is inserted, the choice of size and thread of the pin, and the aftercare.[21-23] Central placement of the pin provides a round hole, whereas eccentric drilling provides a more ovoid hole, removing more cortical bone. When the drilling is eccentric, an open section defect can be generated, which severely weakens the torsional strength of the bone and may predispose to fracture.[22] Central placement can more reliably be performed when the bone is directly visualized through a limited open approach rather than inserted percutaneously by "feel."[18]

Osteopenic bone has been blamed for poor fixation and therefore poor results of external fixation of distal radius fractures in the older patient.[17] Yet these patients are in particular need of optimal treatment to maintain independence and can be successfully treated with few complications using 4-mm pins, with strict adherence to principles.

The method of drilling also has a direct impact on the pin–bone interface. When a power drill is used with sterile irrigant for cooling, a smooth round cortical hole is developed. This is more difficult to achieve through hand-drilling techniques. Slow-motion video has demonstrated a considerable "wobble factor" that occurs when hand drilling is performed, resulting in significant microfractures and an "out-of-round" pilot hole, with cortical fragmentation.[22]

Attempts to save small amounts of time by using a "self-drilling self-tapping" fixation pin can also cause cortical fragmentation because the pin tips have minimal thread. Also, the pins must be inserted almost a full centimeter beyond the tips until adequate bicortical thread purchase can be achieved. This runs the risk of damaging deeper soft-tissue structures and tethering muscles and tendons. The small savings in time really does not warrant replacement of the simple two-step process of predrilling and inserting of fully threaded self-tapping pins.[22]

Recently, some articulated fixators have emerged that are intended to allow wrist motion during fracture healing. No evidence exists, however, that motion does not also take place through the fracture. Ultimately, results have not demonstrated improved motion over well-performed static external fixation.

■ REHABILITATION

Immediately after surgery, the patient is started on active and active assisted range of motion of the fingers, elbow, and shoulder, including forearm pronation and supination. The patient is usually kept overnight and on the second postoperative day instructed in activities of daily living while active mobilization of all joints continues. On the fourth postoperative day, the bulky soft dressing is removed and the patient is educated about pin-site care. For the next week, the patient cleans the pin sites with a sterile cotton-tipped swab and hydrogen peroxide twice daily: once in the morning and once in the evening. On about the tenth postoperative day, the few sutures around the pin sites and bone graft portal are removed, the patient begins to cleanse the pin sites twice daily with isopropyl alcohol on a cotton-tipped swab and is allowed to shower, permitting clean, running tap water over the fixation device and pin sites. Immediately on completing the shower, the pin sites are carefully dried with a clean towel and then cleansed with an alcohol-soaked cotton-tipped swab.

Activities of daily living training continues and as soon as the patient is adequately in control of the hand and arm, he or she is allowed to drive an automobile. Many patients return to work within the first week, performing sedentary activities with the fixator in place. Gentle resistive exercises are begun at about the tenth day and progressive resistive exercises are begun with the fixation device in place over the next 3 weeks. The patient is seen in the physician's office for follow-up radiographs and clinical evaluation at 1, 3, and 6 weeks after surgery. Based on clinical stability and radiographic evidence of healing, the fixation device is removed in the office or the ambulatory suite, requiring at most mild intravenous sedation between the sixth and eighth weeks after surgery. In most cases, patients have already regained most of their pronation and supination by this time and at the time of fixator removal there is usually between 35° and 45° of dorsiflexion and palmar flexion of the wrist noted immediately. The therapist fabricates a thermoplastic resting splint for the patient for comfort and protection for the next 4 weeks but this is removed daily for bathing and exercises, which are done both at home and periodically in the rehabilitation department. Strengthening exercises continue and at about the tenth week, work and sports-hardening exercises commence and continue over the next 3 months.

■ OUTCOMES

Clinical experience in the application of external fixation for the management of distal radius fractures using the techniques described here has afforded rewarding clinical results. In a large general population of patients among all ages, using a detailed objective and subjective rating score system, we have reported good and excellent results, ranging from 89 to 97%, with a low rate of complications. Younger patients tend to develop these fractures as the result of high-energy trauma, with more localized soft-tissue injury and in our hands have tended to run an acceptable (good or excellent) result of about 89%. In a recently reported series of older patients (greater than 65 years) good or excellent results were obtained in 95% of patients.[25]

Although the use of external fixation has been associated with poor results in the management of unstable fractures of the distal radius, these poor results frequently are the result of breakdown in technique and lack of adherence to the principles in this chapter. Successful outcomes can be achieved with careful evaluation by the surgeon to determine the pattern of the fracture, recognize associated soft-tissue injury, and avoid needless fracture manipulation. Careful well-visualized pin insertion and the use of a fixator frame that is stable, that provides adequate visualization, and that is forgiving enough to allow re-reduction also minimize complications. The physician must also recognize the need for augmentation with internal fixation and bone grafting, provide early functional rehabilitation, and educate the patient about the importance of his or her role in the rehabilitation program, pin-site care, and regular follow-up. In this way, "pattern recognition" leads to appropriate immediate management, whereas the surgical technique and rehabilitation program satisfy the early goals of stable fixation, with minimal immobilization of adjacent joints providing early motion of these joints and allowing tendon excursion about the fracture site. Ultimately, adherence to these principles should lead to fulfillment of the long-term goals of restoration of normal anatomy and articular congruity with return of normal (or nearly normal) motion, strength, function, and comfort.[23,24]

References

1. Andrianne Y, Donkerwolcke M, Kinsenkamp M, et al: Hoffman external fixation of fractures of the radius and ulna. A prospective study of 53 patients. Orthopedics, 1984; 7:845.
2. Cooney WP, Linscheid RL, Dobyns JH: External pin fixation for unstable Colles' fractures. J Bone Joint Surg, 1979; 61A:840–845.
3. Cooney WP, Dobyns JH, Linscheid RL: Complications of Colles' fractures. J Bone Joint Surg, 1980; 62A:613–619.
4. Cooney WP: External fixation of distal radius fractures. Clin Orthop, 1983; 180:44–49.
5. Cronier P, Talha A, Toulemonde JL, Jaeger F, Guntz M: Results of distraction by external metacarporadial fixation in fractures of the distal end of the radius: a presentation of 97 cases. J Chir, 1991; 128:8–12.
6. Frykman GK, Tooma GS, Boyko K, Henderson R: Comparison of eleven external fixators for treatment of unstable wrist fractures. J Hand Surg, 1989; 14A:247–254.
7. Horesh Z, Volpin G, Hoerer D, Stein H: The surgical treatment of severe comminuted intraarticular fractures of the distal radius with the small AO external fixation device: a prospective three-and-one-half-year follow-up study. Clin Orthop, 1991; 263:147–153.
8. Jakim I, Pieterse HS, Sweet MBE: External fixation for intraarticular fractures of the distal radius. J Bone Joint Surg, 1991; 73B:302–306.
9. Jupiter JB, Knirk JL: Intraarticular fractures of the distal end of the radius in young athletes. J Bone Joint Surg, 1986; 68:647–659.
10. Kapandji A: Intrafocal pinning of fractures of the distal end of the radius 10 years later. Ann Chir Main Memb Super, 1987; 6:57–63.
11. Kongsholm J, Olerud C: Comminuted Colles' fractures treated with external fixation. Arch Orthop Trauma Surg, 1987; 106:220.
12. Kongsholm J, Olerud C: Plaster cast versus external fixation for unstable intraarticular Colles' fractures. Clin Orthop, 1989; 241:57–65.
13. Leung KS, Shen WY, Leung PC, Kinninmonth AWG, Chang JCW, Chan GPY: Ligamentotaxis and bone grafting for comminuted fractures of the distal radius. J Bone Joint Surg, 1989; 71B: 838–842.
14. Melone CP: Articular fractures of the distal radius. Orthop Clin North Am, 1984; 15:217.
15. Putnam MD, Seitz WH Jr: Advances in fracture management in the hand and distal radius. Hand Clin, 1989; 5:455–470.
16. Rayhack JM, Langworthy JN, Belsole RJ: Transulnar percutaneous pinning of displaced distal radius fractures: a preliminary report. J Orthop Trauma, 1989; 3:107–114.
17. Roumen RMH, Hesp WLEM, Bruggink EDM: Unstable Colles' fractures in elderly patients: a randomized trial of external fixation for redisplacement. J Bone Joint Surg, 1991; 73B:307–311.
18. Seitz WH Jr, Putnam MD, Dick HM: Limited open surgical approach for external fixation of distal radius fractures. J Hand Surg, 1990; 15A:288–293.
19. Seitz WH Jr, Froimson AI, Brooks DB, et al: Biomechanical analysis of pin placement and pin size for external fixation of distal radius fractures. Clin Orthop, 1990; 251:207–212.
20. Seitz WH Jr, Froimson AI, Leb R, Shapiro JD: Augmented external fixation of unstable distal radius fractures. J Hand Surg, 1991; 16A:1010–1016.
21. Seitz WH Jr, Froimson AI: Reduction of treatment related complications in the external fixation of complex distal radius fractures. Orthop Rev, 1991; 20:169–177.
22. Seitz WH Jr, Froimson AI, Brooks DB, et al: External fixator pin insertion techniques: biomechanical analysis and clinical relevance. J Hand Surg, 1991; 16:560–563.

23. Seitz WH Jr: External fixation of distal radius fractures. Indications and technical principles. Orthop Clin North Am, 1993; 24:255–264.
24. Seitz WH Jr: Complications and problems in the management of distal radius fractures. Hand Clin, 1994; 10:117–123.
25. Seitz WH Jr, Froimson AI: External fixation of unstable distal radius fractures in the senior population: "How old is too old?" Orthop Trans, 1994; 17:579.
26. Weber SC, Szabo RM: Severely comminuted distal radius fractures as an unsolved problem. Complications associated with external fixation and pins and plaster techniques. J Hand Surg, 1986; 11A:157–165.

MATTHEW D.
PUTNAM

41

Radial Styloid Fractures

■ HISTORY OF THE
TECHNIQUE

Fractures of the radial styloid are uncommon, particularly when compared with the more common Colles fracture. Original descriptions of the fracture were rendered at a time when the important function of the radial styloid as a point of ligament origin was less understood.[5,8,9,11,18] Perhaps this incomplete understanding of the anatomy accounts for the historic lack of emphasis on accurate reduction of the radial styloid.

Regardless, the report of Bacorn and Kurtze began a clearer understanding of disabilities associated with distal radius fractures.[6] Reasons postulated for impairment after fracture include incongruity of the joint surface, radial shortening, a decreased angle of radial inclination, and cartilage pressure abnormalities. With specific note to the radial styloid, recent improvements in our knowledge of radial carpal ligament origin dramatize the importance of radial styloid fracture reduction.[4–6,14,20,22,26]

The probable location of critical ligament supports in relation to a radial styloid fracture are shown in Figure 41–1. From this figure, it is clear that progressively larger fractures destabilize the volar radiocarpal ligaments. Worse, a large fracture can be associated with a tear of the scapholunate (SL) interosseous ligament complex.[1,7,12–14,16,24,25,27] Thus, for reasons of joint congruity, joint alignment, and ligament integrity, displaced fractures of the radial styloid should be accurately reduced.

Ellis is perhaps the first to have advocated open fixation of large fracture fragments about the distal radius.[10] And, although Ellis' technique was directed at Barton's fracture, others have reported successful outcomes and few complications when performing open reduction and internal fixation (ORIF) of radial styloid fractures.[12,17,29]

Radial styloid fracture patterns almost always contain at least one repairable fracture fragment. This differs substantially from some distal radius fractures wherein the number and size of fracture fragments preclude direct uncomplicated ORIF. Furthermore, it is essential to visualize the joint surface directly in complex AO class C-type fractures, whereas extensive joint surface visualization may not be as critical or necessary for some radial styloid fractures.[23] However, the joint surface congruity must be restored and stabilized.

■ INDICATIONS AND
CONTRAINDICATIONS

Radial styloid fractures may alter load transfer across the radioscaphoid fossa. Depending on the degree of displacement, degenerative change could ensue if the displacement is not corrected. Displacement of 2 mm has been defined as acceptable in the literature; this is the maximum displacement that we allow before reducing the fracture (Fig. 41–1).[15] The location of the fracture will directly affect carpal ligament stability as the fracture will variably involve ligaments originating from the region of the radial styloid. As the fracture fragment enlarges, a greater number of ligaments are potentially compromised (Fig. 41–2).

Figure 41–3 and Table 41–1 outline our strategy for management of radial styloid fractures.[17,19,21,23,26,28,30] Essentially, anatomic reduction is required for all fractures. The treating physician should always remember to assess the integrity of intercarpal ligaments after initial reduction of the styloid fracture.

■ SURGICAL
TECHNIQUES

A small number of patients will have a nondisplaced radial styloid fracture. However, all of these fractures should be regarded as unstable. In addition to application of a long arm thumb spica (LATS) cast for nondisplaced fractures we obtain at least one comparative

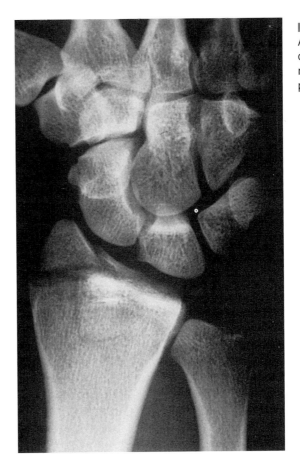

■ FIGURE 41–1
A PA radiograph of a radial styloid fracture with more than 2 mm of displacement.

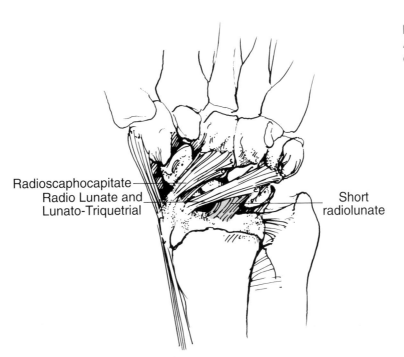

■ FIGURE 41–2
Anatomy of the volar radiocarpal ligaments.

Radioscaphocapitate
Radio Lunate and
Lunato-Triquetrial

Short
radiolunate

■ FIGURE 41–3
Anatomic zones through which the radial styloid fractures. Location-based Treatment Strategy: I, closed management if carpus stable (LATS); II, reduction accomplished through lateral or arthroscopic approach (evaluate carpal ligaments); III, reduction accomplished using dorsal approach (evaluate carpal ligaments).

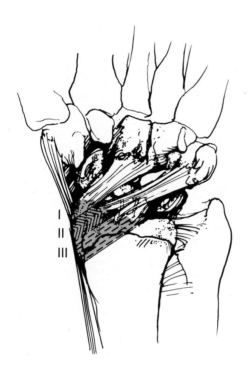

TABLE 41–1 A STRATEGY FOR TREATING RADIAL STYLOID FRACTURES BASED ON AMOUNT OF DISPLACEMENT

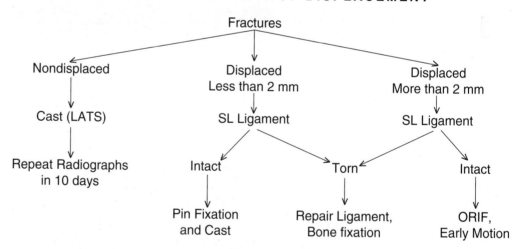

radiograph in the first 10 to 14 days to determine if progressive displacement exists. The purpose of the LATS cast is to reduce forces exerted by the brachioradialis, which is a potential destabilizer because of its attachment to the radial styloid. If the fracture is displaced initially or at follow-up, it should be treated as below.

Fractures that are displaced should be reduced and stabilized internally. Generally, we use an axillary block, a C-arm fluoroscope with freeze-frame capability, powered drills and wire drivers, and a complete selection of hand instruments. The C-arm is used to help place the surgical incision. Most often we use a transverse skin incision (Fig. 41–4). However, if the scapholunate ligament is damaged or substantial comminution is present, we use a dorsal incision between the third and fourth compartments.

The transverse incision has been developed to minimize risk to the superficial radial nerve and vascular structures and to improve the appearance of the scar. Once deep to the skin, the orientation of the dissection is longitudinal. Neurovascular structures are

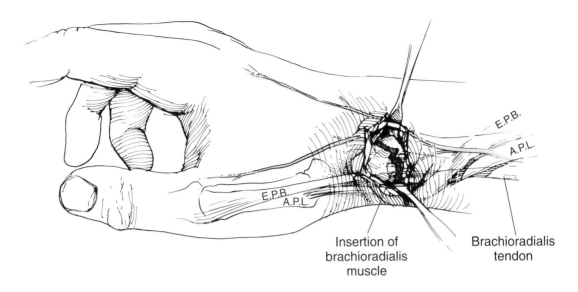

E.P.B.

A.P.L.

E.P.B.
A.P.L.

Insertion of
brachioradialis
muscle

Brachioradialis
tendon

■ FIGURE 41–4
A transverse lateral approach for internal fixation of the radial styloid.

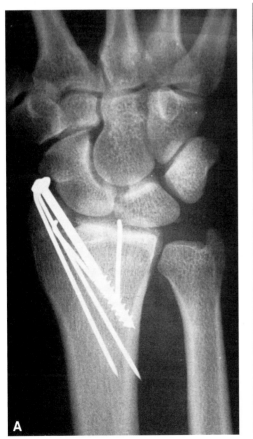

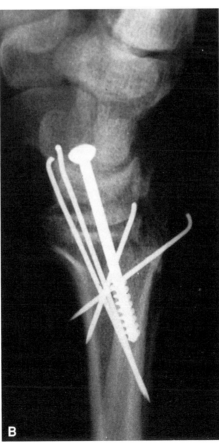

A

B

■ FIGURE 41–5
A and B, PA and lateral radiographs after internal fixation of a radial styloid fracture through a transverse approach. Ligamentous integrity was assessed using C-Arm fluoroscopy.

mobilized and carefully retracted. Tendons of the first dorsal compartment may be mobilized by partially or completely releasing the tendon sheath, and possibly by releasing the brachioradialis. However, care must be taken not to detach ligament origins from the styloid pieces; therefore, joint inspection and irrigation is completed through the fracture site. While using a traction apparatus, the quality of reduction is ascertained using the C-arm fluoroscope in addition to direct visualization of the fracture site. We use a combination of cancellous lag screw fixation and smooth wire placement to stabilize the fracture. We believe the addition of a second fixation device is important to assist in controlling rotation of the fracture fragments (Fig. 41–5). The fracture fragment is frequently not large enough to support more than one screw. However, there is no specific contraindication to more than one screw if the fracture fragment is of sufficient size. The surgeon should avoid placing the fixation screw(s) into the distal radioulnar joint or into the interosseous space in a fashion that limits pronation or supination. Also, when comminution exists, the surgeon must be careful not to narrow the radius by exerting too much compression across the fracture. This point deserves emphasis because a reduction that changes the shape of the articular surface is potentially as damaging as an intra-articular step-off. Also, there should be no restriction of radiocarpal motion. The final construct is evaluated with fluoroscopy to assess the quality of fixation.

Closure is completed in a standard fashion using a bulky soft tissue dressing with splint support for the first 24 to 48 hours after surgery. Figure 41–6 shows postoperative radiographs of a patient treated by this method.

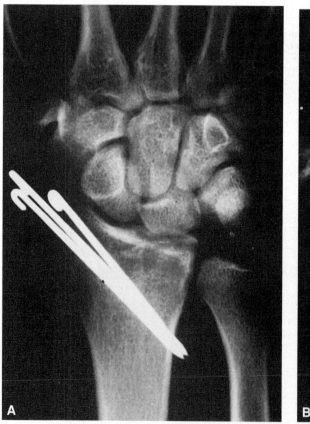
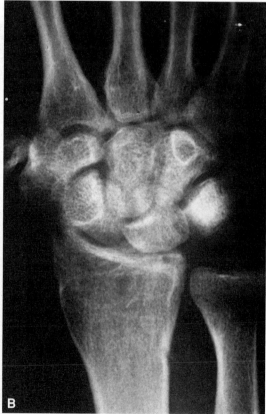

■ FIGURE 41–6

A, A postoperative radiograph of an internally fixed radial styloid. An SL ligament injury was not appreciated. **B,** Six months later, a carpal instability pattern is more apparent, and the cartilage space is narrowed in the lunate fossa.

The standard dorsal approach is used when there is comminution of a large radial styloid fragment or when the SL ligament is disrupted. The basic goals of this approach are to obtain a clear view of the joint surface, the proximal intercarpal ligaments, and the region of metaphyseal comminution. The longitudinal incision is placed in the internervous plane between the radial and ulnar sensory nerves. The extensor retinaculum is incised obliquely over the fourth dorsal compartment, facilitating later closure. A longitudinal dorsal capsular incision and radial periosteal elevation techniques are used. This facilitates visualization of the fracture fragments, the SL ligaments, and the joint surfaces. Using this approach, it is possible to elevate the periosteum radially to the volar tip of the radial styloid. This approach can be used in combination with a laterally placed external fixator. This is important to note, because many fractures that require this approach also may benefit from external fixation neutralization.

After visualization of the fracture and carpal ligaments, reduction should be accomplished using indirect methods to the degree possible. Fragment stabilization, in the presence of substantial comminution, is improved by placement of a bone graft. We use copious cancellous graft obtained from between the inner and outer tables of the iliac crest. Fixation, using this approach, is done with interfragmentary screws, neutralization screws, neutralization plates, K-wires, or interosseous wires. External neutralization should be considered for fractures that cannot be completely stabilized solely using internal fixation methods.

This incision is closed in layers. The soft tissue can be approximated over an accurately contoured plate and the extensor retinaculum can be loosely closed. We place a temporary hemovac in the subcutaneous tissues for up to 24 hours. A bulky compression dressing with the forearm placed in supination and the fingers free to extend is used for 24 to 48 hours. The splint is appropriately modified if an external fixator is in place.

The largest fracture fragments potentially exit at the interval between the scaphoid and lunate fossa and in this region may extend into the SL ligament, thereby destabilizing the scapholunate articulation. Figure 41–6 depicts a progressive, originally unrecognized, scapholunate instability occurring subsequent to a radial styloid fracture. It should be noted that the initial surgical treatment reduced the styloid fragment but did not restore the relationship between the scaphoid and lunate. Figure 41–6A demonstrates original pin fixation of the fracture. Figure 41–6B shows the carpal position 3 months after injury.

If the SL ligament is damaged, the scaphoid should be stabilized to the lunate using fixation pins as minimum treatment. A more formal open ligament repair or augmentation might be appropriate in younger patients whereas conversion to a proximal row carpectomy or other salvage procedure could be considered for an older patient, particularly if arthritis is already present.

A final note of caution concerns the comminuted radial styloid fracture. In this situation, it is possible with compression to change the shape of the scaphoid fossa and thereby induce post-traumatic degenerative joint disease. To prevent this situation, the surgeon should consider placement of bone graft and noncompressive, neutralization fixation.

The role of arthroscopy for treating this fracture is expanding. Ligament and fracture line visualization can be accomplished and reduction facilitated in less comminuted radial styloid fractures. However, the goal of anatomic reduction and perhaps early postoperative mobilization should remain the standard, and the means by which this goal is achieved (open versus arthroscopic technique) is less important.

■ TECHNICAL ALTERNATIVES

The early focus of rehabilitation efforts should be prevention of stiffness and pain in the areas of the upper extremity not directly involved in the injury. Mobilization of the wrist itself will depend on the stability of fixation. Less comminuted fractures should be sufficiently stable after ORIF to allow early, protected active assisted range of motion of the wrist. We continue splint protection for 6 weeks after surgery in all patients. Control of edema, mobilization of the fingers and forearm, and utilization of the shoulder have proven to be the keys to success.

■ REHABILITATION

Altissimi and co-authors[1] note that radial styloid fractures associated with intercarpal injuries resulted in early onset of arthrosis in more than 50% of their patients. Le-Nen and co-authors,[16] Bassett,[3] Bilos and co-authors,[7] and Mayfield and co-authors[20] found similar difficulties in treating this often complex fracture. These authors conclude that the accuracy of joint surface reduction and the identification and stabilization of any ligamentous injuries are the two most important variables in determining whether a successful outcome will be achieved.

Radial styloid fractures require careful assessment. Their original benign appearance can hide significant ligamentous injury and scaphoid fossa irregularity. At a minimum, a well-molded LATS cast is required with radiographs checked at intervals. Displaced and comminuted fractures require reduction and internal stabilization with attention to possible need for ligament stabilization. If open reduction and internal fixation is completed, fixation should be stable enough to allow early mobilization. To reiterate, the surgeon must remain attentive to prevent the development of ligamentous instability.

References

1. Altissimi M, Mancini GB, Azzara A: Perilunate dislocations of the carpus. A long term review. Ital J Orthop Traumatol, 1987; 13:491–500.
2. Bacorn RW, Kurtzke JF: Colles' fracture. A study of two thousand cases from the New York State Workman's Compensation Board. J Bone Joint Surg, 1953; 35A:643–658.
3. Bassett RL: Displaced intraarticular fractures of the distal radius. Clin Orthop Rel Res, 1987; 214:148–152.
4. Berger RA, Blair WF: The radioscapholunate ligament: A gross and histologic description. Anat Rec, 1984; 210:393–405.
5. Berger RA, Kauer JMG, Landsmeer JMF: Radioscapholunate ligament: A gross anatomic and histologic study of fetal and adult wrists. J Hand Surg, 1991; 16A:350–355.
6. Berger RA, Landsmeer JMF: The palmar radiocarpal ligaments: A study of adult and fetal human wrist joints. J Hand Surg, 1990; 15A:847–854.
7. Bilos ZJ, Pankovich AM, Yelda S: Fracture dislocations of the radiocarpal joint. J Bone Joint Surg, 1977; 59:198–203.
8. Edwards HC: Mechanism and treatment of backfire fractures. J Bone Joint Surg, 1926; 8: 701–717.
9. Eliason EL: Fractures of the Humerus, Radius and Ulna. New York, D. Appleton & Co., 1925.
10. Ellis J: Smith's and Barton's fractures: A method of treatment. J Bone Joint Surg, 1965; 47B: 724–727.
11. Fitzsimmons RA: Colles' fractures and chauffeur's fracture. Br Med J, 1938; 2:357–360.
12. Helm RH, Tonkin MA: The chauffeur's fracture: Simple or complex? J Hand Surg, 1992; 17B: 156–159.
13. Higgens TF, Weiss AC: Scaphocapitate syndrome: Case report and literature review. Contemporary Orthopaedics, July, 1993; :33–36.
14. Hixon ML, Stewart C: Microvascular anatomy of the radioscapholunate ligament of the wrist. J Hand Surg, 1990; 16A:279–282.
15. Knirk JL, Jupiter JB: Intraarticular fractures of the distal end of the radius in young adults. J Bone Joint Surg, 1986; 68A:647–659.
16. Le-Nen D, Riot O, Caro P, Le-Fevere C, Courtois B: Luxation fractures of the radiocarpal joint. Clinical study of six cases and general review. Annales de Chirurgie de la Main et du Membre Superieur, 1991; 10:5–12.
17. Letsch R, Schmit-Neuerburg KP, Towfigh H: Indications and results of plate osteosynthesis of the distal radius. Langenbecks Arch Chir, 1984; 364:363–368.
18. Pilcher LS: Fractures of the Lower Extremity or Base of the Radius. London, JB Lippincott, 1917.
19. Mah ET, Atkinson RN: Percutaneous Kirschner wire stabilization following closed reduction of Colles' fractures. J Hand Surg, 1991; 17:55–62.
20. Mayfield JK, Johnson RP, Kilcoyne RK: Carpal dislocations: pathomechanics and progressive perilunar instability. J Hand Surg, 1980; 5:226–241.
21. Munson GO, Galnor BJ: Percutaneous pinning of distal radius fractures. J Trauma, 1981; 21: 1032–1035.
22. Ogden JA, Beall JK, Conlogue GJ, Light TR: Radiology of postnatal skeletal development, IV, distal radius and ulna. Skeletal Radiol, 1981; 6:255–266.

23. Putnam MD: Fractures and dislocations of the carpus including the distal radius. In: Gustilo RB (ed): Fractures and Dislocations, St. Louis: Mosby, 1992:553–593.

24. Rosenthal DI, Schwartz M, Phillips WC, Jupiter J: Fractures of the radius with instability of the wrist. AJR, 1983; 141:113–116.

25. Schmit-Neuerburg KP, Letsch R, Sturmer KM, Kosser K: Special forms of distal radius fractures. Langenbecks Arch Chir Suppl Verh Dtsch Ges Forsch Chir, 1990 (suppl. II); 667–674.

26. Siegel DB, Gelberman RH: Radial styloidectomy: An anatomical study with special reference to radiocarpal intracapsular ligamentous morphology. J Hand Surg, 1991; 16A:40–44.

27. Skelly WJ, Nahlglan SH, Hidvegi EB: Palmar lunate transtriquetral fracture dislocation. J Hand Surg, 1991; 16A:536–539.

28. Solgaard S: Angle of inclination of the articular surface of the distal radius. Radiologe, 1984; 24:346–348.

29. Tajima T, Salto H: A new classification of distal radius fractures and corresponding treatment methods. Handchir Mikrochir Plat Chir, 1991; 23:227–35.

30. Terry DW, Jr, Ramin JE: The navicular fat stripe: A useful roentgen feature for evaluating wrist trauma. Am J Roentgenol Radium Ther Nucl Med, 1975; 24:25–28.

CHARLES P. MELONE,
JR.
JOEL L. FRAZIER

42

Internal Fixation of Distal Radius Fractures: Volar Approach

■ HISTORY OF THE
TECHNIQUE

Unstable intra- and extraarticular distal radius fractures with volar displacement have historically been categorized by multiple eponyms and classification schemes. In 1838, Barton[1] described intraarticular distal radius fractures–dislocations that traditionally bear his name occurring in both dorsal and volar directions. The more frequently occurring pattern is characterized by volar displacement of an "anterior" marginal fracture of the distal radius, along with the adjacent carpus. Shortly thereafter, Smith[25] in 1847 described an extraarticular distal radius fracture with volar displacement of the hand and wrist with respect to the forearm. Subsequently, in 1957, Thomas[26] further categorized Smith's injuries into three fracture types. Briefly, the type II fracture, analogous to the volar Barton's fracture, is characterized by a marginal intraarticular fracture of the radius, with volar and proximal dislocation of the carpus.

Ellis[5] in 1965 advocated buttress-plating of the volar marginal fracture. His volar approach was through a longitudinal radiovolar incision of the distal forearm. This approach develops an interval between the flexor carpi radialis (FCR) and flexor pollicis longus radially and the pronator quadratus, sublimis tendons (FDS), palmaris longus and median nerve ulnarly. The pronator quadratus is divided at its origin on the radius to expose the anterior surface of the distal radius. The Ellis technique of buttress-plate fixation, noted even in recent references, does not insert screws in the distal fragment.[2-6,15,19,20,22,23] Although the buttress plate controls volar subluxation, it does not provide rigid stabilization of intraarticular comminuted fragments or prevent occasional delayed radial displacement. De Oliveira, in 1973,[4] recommended all volar Barton fracture–dislocations be openly reduced and internally fixed because of their frequent loss of closed reduction. He placed an alternative buttress plate with supplemental percutaneous K-wires through the radial styloid, using the volar longitudinal incision. His incision, also recommended by others,[20] was between the FCR medially and the radial vessels laterally. Also in 1973, Fuller[9] reviewed the patients of Ellis and recommended the Ellis plate fixation through his volar approach for the Smith's type II fractures. Simultaneously, in 1974 the Swiss Association for the Study of Internal Fixation (AO/ASIF) Group recommended in the technique manual a special T-plate or oblique T-plate placed on the palmar side of the radius for fixation of comminuted articular radial fractures with palmar displacement of fragments. The T-plate is secured with 3.5-mm fixation screws in the radial shaft and distal fragments. The unstable radial styloid is fixed either with a separate screw, as DePalma[2] preferred, or a K-wire. The AO/ASIF plate was placed through a long S-shaped incision on the distal forearm ulnar to the FCR and continued to the thenar crease. The median nerve and finger flexor tendons are retracted ulnarly and the FCR radially with the radial artery. The pronator is reflected on the distal radial surface. An alternative approach to expose the distal radioulnar joint is made by retracting the flexor tendons laterally, together with the median nerve and radial artery. The AO/ASIF[21] modified the wide exposure of the volar radius to provide additional access to decompress the median nerve and protect the soft tissues from intraoperative injury. This longitudinal volar forearm skin incision is made radial to the palmaris longus tendon and over the median nerve. At the distal forearm, the incision is slightly angled to cross the flexor crease and extend onto the palm. The median nerve is retracted radially with the FCR tendon. The palmaris longus, flexor

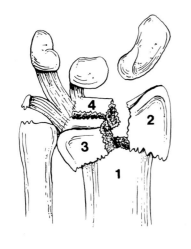

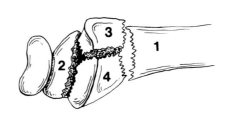

4-PART ARTICULAR FRACTURE
1. **SHAFT**
2. **RADIAL STYLOID**
3. **DORSAL MEDIAL**
4. **VOLAR MEDIAL**

■ FIGURE 42–1
Articular fractures comprise four basic components: 1) metaphyseal or shaft, 2) radial styloid, 3) dorsal medial, and 4) volar medial. (From Melone CP Jr: Distal radius fractures: pattern of articular fragmentation. Orthop Clin North Am, 1993; 24:239–253.)

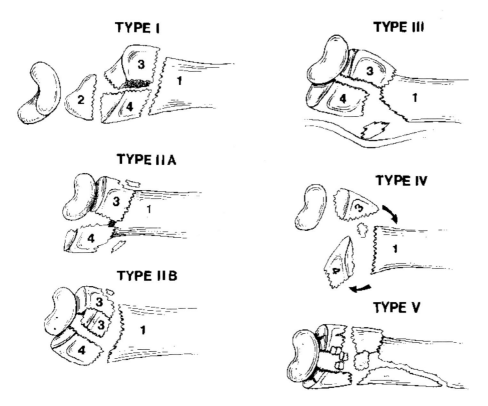

■ FIGURE 42–2
Displacement of the key medial fragments disrupts both the radiocarpal and distal radioulnar joints and is the basis for an increasingly comprehensive system of categorizing distal radius articular fractures. Compared with the type IIA injury, the type IIB fracture is characterized by greater comminution and displacement of the medial fragments, with articular disruption. The type V fractures are extensively comminuted and often extend from the articular surface into the diaphysis.

pollicis longus, and flexor mass are retracted ulnarly. The pronator is incised at its radial border.

In an effort to enhance the rational selection of treatment for intraarticular distal radius fracture, the Melone[16] classification places emphasis on displacement of the "medial complex" (Fig. 42–1). The medial complex consists of the medial fragments and their strong ligamentous attachments with the carpal bones and ulnar styloid. Its displacement is the basis for a useful scheme of incorporating six fracture types (Fig. 42–2). The type II fractures, characterized by displacement of the medial complex, are unstable because of excessive comminution. With posterior displacement, the dorsal medial fragment, traditionally termed the "die-punch" fragment,[24] is severely compressed by the lunate and lies in a position that is proximal to the palmar medial fragment. With anterior displacement, the palmar medial fragment and the carpus are in a proximal position relative to the dorsal medial fragment, a fracture configuration similar to the volar Barton's fracture or Smith's type II pattern. The type IIA fracture, in which the medial fragments are neither widely separated nor rotated, is generally reducible and amenable to closed methods of treatment. In general agreement with Green's[11] contention, the type IIA fracture with volar displacement is best treated by ligamentotaxis with an external fixation device. In contrast, the irreducible type IIB fractures are refractory to ligamentotaxis alone because of excessive medial complex displacement and thus require open reduction, internal fixation, and bone grafting. The type IIB fracture with volar displacement is predominantly encountered among younger males[2,4,6,10,13,14,20,25] sustaining high-energy injuries from falls or motor vehicle accidents, who often have a concomitant distal radius fracture, neuropathies, and flexor tendon injuries. In contrast to other distal radius fractures, this pattern is often well-suited to plate and screw fixation through a volar approach. In a similar fashion, the spike fragment in the type III fracture and the irreducible widely separated palmar medial fragment in the type IV fracture require a volar approach for restoration of the articular congruity in addition to repair of associated skeletal and soft-tissue injuries. The volar approach through the extended carpal tunnel incision for open treatment of these more complex displaced articular fractures of the distal radius was presented in 1986[19] and recently supported by others.[7,12]

■ INDICATIONS AND CONTRAINDICATIONS

In most cases employing high-quality radiographic films of injuries, readily identifiable radiographic signs of instability and reducibility can be promptly recognized and serve as a sound basis for optimal management. In uncertain cases, distraction views, tomography, or computed tomography can facilitate an accurate diagnosis.[16]

Radiographic signs of the irreducible die-punch fracture with volar displacement are greater comminution and displacement of the palmar medial fragment. The irreducible type II volar fracture requiring open reduction consistently has a radiocarpal step-off exceeding 5 mm, as viewed in the sagittal plane. Additional radiographic signs in the irreducible die-punch fracture include the double die-punch mechanism, whereby both the scaphoid and lunate impact the distal radius, causing greater fragmentation of the scaphoid articular facet and further displacement; extensive medial comminution, often resulting in five fracture components and profound instability; an off-set of the radiocarpal joint exceeding 2 mm; radial shortening exceeding 5 mm; and dorsal tilting of the radiocarpal joint in excess of 10°.

The type III spike fracture has a substantial volar fragment that projects from the metaphysis, in addition to the articular disruption similar to the type II fractures. This fragment can be clearly visualized on lateral radiographs as projecting vertically into the flexor compartment of the wrist. The restoration of this fragment through the volar approach is essential for the stability of the volar articular buttress supplied by this segmental portion of the metaphyseal cortex. Displacement of the spike fragment is indicative of injury to adjacent nerves and tendons, which require repair through a volar approach to the wrist.

The type IV fracture is characterized by wide separation or rotation of the medial fragments. Not infrequently, the palmar medial fragment is rotated 180°, causing its articular surface to face proximally, toward the radial shaft. The preoperative injury radiographs always reveal major biarticular disruption. The injury pattern always has extensive concomitant soft-tissue and skeletal damage, requiring open volar repair simultaneous with the open reduction and internal fixation for restoration of articular congruity.

Radiographic features of fracture instability include articular fragment separation of 2 mm or more that is prone to persistent and progressive joint incongruity; radial shortening in excess of 3 to 5 mm that is predisposed to further collapse; angulation or tilting of the radial articular surface exceeding 20° in the sagittal plane that disturbs the collinear radiocarpal alignment and congruity of the distal radioulnar joint; and metaphyseal comminution that involves both volar and dorsal radial cortices. The compressive forces can produce central articular fragmentation without soft-tissue attachments. These impacted and depressed fragments are irreducible not only by traction but also after open reduction and leave significant subarticular or metaphyseal voids, which require supplemental buttressing with iliac crest bone graft.

The AO/ASIF group classifies the volar articular margin fractures as a type B3 injury and emphasizes that this highly unstable fracture, because of extrinsic muscle forces, requires open reduction with internal fixation.[4,5,7,9,12,20,21]

Marked fracture impaction and cortical buckling, preventing closed reduction of distal radius fractures, are not limited to articular fractures. Although the extraarticular Smith's fracture is usually treated by closed means, occasionally, excessive cortical buckling with dorsal angulation and subluxation of the distal radioulnar joint can prevent full reduction by closed means. Restoration of radial alignment is achieved by a volar approach to the distal radius, direct fragment manipulation, and internal fixation with a volar buttress plate.[12]

Contraindications to the limited volar approach for distal radius fractures include successful, accurate, and stable restoration of the fracture by closed means through ligamentotaxis that is provided by external fixation, frequently supplemented with percutaneous internal fixation. Another contraindication is irreducible die-punch fractures or extraarticular fractures with dorsal displacement and comminution, requiring a dorsal approach for accurate reduction, placement of fixation, and adjunctive iliac crest bone grafting. Other types of fractures that are inappropriate for the volar approach are the Melone type V explosion fracture or the open AO-C3, with comminution extending from the articular surface to the diaphysis, requiring provisional stabilization by external fixation for revascularization or resurfacing procedures.

Because of the constant location of the irreducible palmar medial fragment at the volar aspect of the wrist and the frequent soft-tissue damage encountered in the flexor compartment, we preferentially approach the volar aspect of the distal radius through an extended carpal tunnel incision curved ulnarly across the wrist.

■ SURGICAL TECHNIQUES

The volar approach to the distal radius is performed under general anesthesia when preoperative planning predicts the necessity for adjunctive contralateral iliac crest bone graft. Axillary block regional anesthesia is acceptable if iliac bone graft is not anticipated. After placement of a well-padded proximal arm tourniquet and administration of prophylactic intravenous antibiotics, the injured upper extremity and contralateral hip are placed on an elevating pillow support and thoroughly prepped and draped into a sterile field. Under tourniquet control, the curvilinear incision centered over the wrist is extended distally across the mid-palm and proximally along the ulnar aspect of the forearm. After the transverse carpal ligament and antebrachial fascia are completely incised to expose and evacuate hematoma from the carpal tunnel, wrist, and forearm, a decompression of the median nerve is performed. Because of the characteristic medial fragment displacement, the dissection is extended between the ulnar neurovascular bundle and the flexor digitorum profundus (Fig. 42–3). The flexors, along with the median nerve, are retracted radially; the flexor carpi ulnaris and ulnar neurovascular bundle are retracted ulnarly. If the pronator quadratus has not been disrupted by the fracture, it can be excised along its radial insertion and reflected ulnarly (Fig. 42–4). This approach is beneficial in fractures wherein the medial complex is the focus of attention.

The critical step in the restoration of the distal radius articulations is precise reduction of the medial complex. With traction provided directly by an assistant or temporary use of an external fixator as a distraction device, the displaced palmar fragments are first reduced and provisionally stabilized to the dorsal medial fragment. The restored "medial complex" is then accurately fixed to the radial shaft.[19] Subsequent apposition of the medial fragments and the styloid preserves the radiocarpal joint, and replacement of the ulnar head in the sigmoid notch of the reduced medial fragments preserves the distal radioulnar joint.

The method of fracture fixation is contingent on the fracture fragment size and comminution. In the type II articular fractures, stabilization in many cases can be achieved with

■ FIGURE 42-3
The volar approach between the ulnar neurovascular bundle and flexor digitorum profundus/sublimis tendon mass with the medial complex exposed.

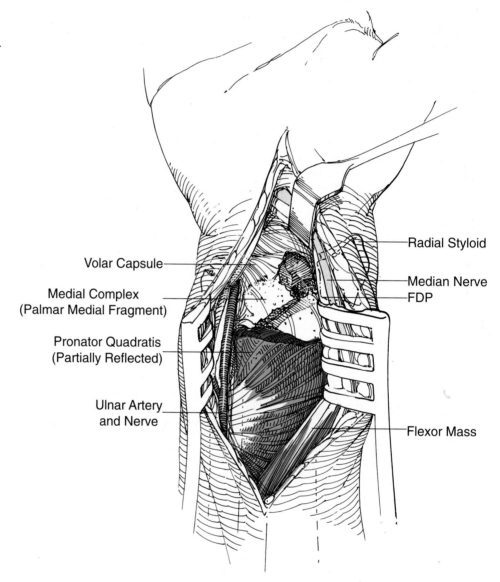

Volar Capsule

Medial Complex
(Palmar Medial Fragment)

Pronator Quadratis
(Partially Reflected)

Ulnar Artery
and Nerve

Radial Styloid

Median Nerve
FDP

Flexor Mass

plate fixation, as designed by the AO group, inserting screws in both the proximal and distal portion of the plate and therefore attaining secure fixation (Fig. 42–5A and B). Some cases require a combination of plates and K-wires. When there is an unstable radial styloid fracture fragment that is not secured by the distal fixation screws of the T-plate, supplemental fixation is provided by a percutaneous K-wire or separate oblique or transverse screw. In cases characterized by excessive comminution, resulting in bone defects between major fragments, and in cases with bone loss, primary iliac crest cancellous bone grafting and a corticocancellous strut graft provide additional stability and security against settling and collapse. In the extensively comminuted cases (Fig. 42–6A and B), stabilization with a minimum of three 0.045- or 0.063-inch K-wires has proved to be a successful method of internal fixation because multiple fragments, small fracture fragment size, extraarticular comminution, or bone loss generally precludes rigid fixation with compression screws or plates (Fig. 42–7A and B). After completion of stabilization with fixation and adjunctive bone grafting, the pronator quadratus muscle is repositioned and sutured radially.

After tourniquet deflation and hemostasis, the skin incision is closed over a 1/4-inch Penrose drain. A sterile fluff dressing is applied to protect all wounds. Further protection

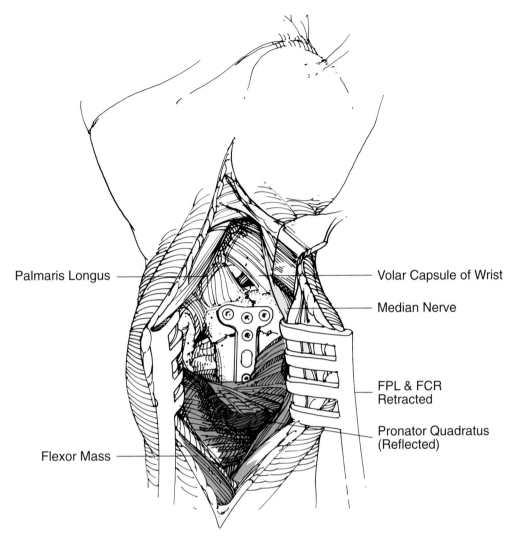

Palmaris Longus

Flexor Mass

Volar Capsule of Wrist

Median Nerve

FPL & FCR
Retracted

Pronator Quadratus
(Reflected)

■ FIGURE 42–4
The volar approach be-
tween the FCR and
flexor mass, with the
FCR, flexor pollicis lon-
gus, and median nerve
retracted radially. This approach gives access to
the radial styloid.

is provided by a volar plaster short arm thumb spica splint with external fixators. A long
arm thumb spica splint with the wrist in neutral pronation–supination and elbow in 90°
of flexion is applied when only internal fixation is used.

■ TECHNICAL
ALTERNATIVES

An alternative approach is between the FCR and palmaris longus, with radial retraction
of the median nerve, FCR, and radial artery, and ulnar retraction of the palmaris longus
with the flexor mass (Fig. 42–4). This approach is useful where access to the radial styloid
is necessary for placement of K-wires, compression screws, small T-plate, or oblique T-
plate. To assist in radiocarpal visualization, an accessory small longitudinal incision can
be made in the volar capsule at its ulnar aspect, thus avoiding the critical radiocarpal
ligaments arising from the radial styloid. Because of the deep concavity of the distal radius
articular facets, however, visualization is usually compromised. Restoration of radial alignment often is best assessed by two additional parameters: identification of the ulnar head
concentrically located in the sigmoid notch, as visualized through a small volar incision
in the radial ulnar joint capsule, and restoration of the volar metaphyseal cortical buttress.

Alternative rigid volar fixation can be provided by two one-quarter semitubular plates as
described by Freeland.[8] When the metaphyseal comminution prevents adequate proximal
fixation of the T-plate, two 2.7-mm reconstruction plates, which diverge distally, may be
substituted.[12] The external fixator is an adjunctive device that provides additional stability
and a sturdy method of immobilization with plate or K-wire fixation or both during the
process of fracture healing.

■ FIGURE 42–5
A, A lateral radiograph of a type IIB fracture with volar displacement. With volar and medial displacement exceeding 5 mm, this is an irreducible injury. **B,** Restoration of articular congruity is achieved by open reduction with plate and screw fixation. Secure fixation is attained by screws in both the proximal and distal portion of the plate.

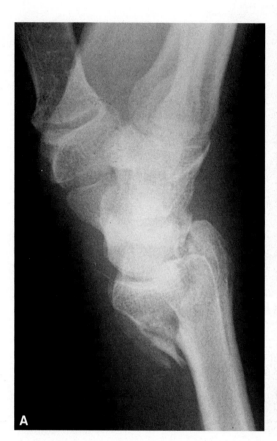

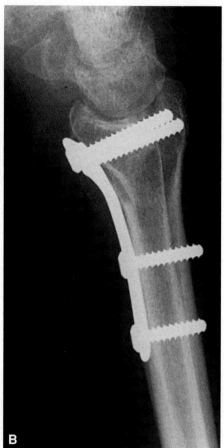

After confirmation of skeletal restoration by intraoperative radiographs, the soft-tissue injuries are repaired. One should perform a thorough decompression, neurolysis, epineurotomy, and evacuation of subepineural hematomas of the affected median or ulnar nerves. Nerve disruption from sharp laceration is addressed by a microscopic epineural suture repair. All tendon lacerations receive primary end-to-end suture repairs, despite the presence of frayed ends. Arterial lacerations, after resection of damaged ends, may be directly anastomosed or require an interposition vein graft for successful repair. When trauma and subsequent swelling extend into the intermetacarpal region, intrinsic releases may be necessary.[12] A fasciotomy of the flexor compartment may also be necessary for cases of prolonged ischemia.[17-19] Because of the frequent high-energy injury causing these fracture patterns, concomitant extrinsic or intrinsic wrist ligament injuries may occur, which may require reduction of the carpal bones and primary ligamentous repair.[12]

Avoiding the many pitfalls associated with unstable irreducible volar articular distal radius fractures requires extreme and meticulous attention to detail, from the initial assessment of the fracture pattern and associated soft-tissue injuries to the selection of appropriate fixation with adjunctive bone grafting and intraoperative handling of the soft tissue and bony structures.

To prevent postoperative loss of fracture reduction, the T-plate is contoured with a slight overbending to ensure that dorsal pressure is applied to the distal fragment with tightening of the proximal fixation screws. The plate should be provisionally secured at a distal hole to prevent proximal migration of the plate as the more proximal screws are sequentially placed. Exact screw length is necessary to prevent dorsal extensor tendon interference and potential rupture.[12]

Articular comminution, particularly central fragments with no soft-tissue attachments, should be indirectly reduced with a small elevator, buttressed with abundant packed

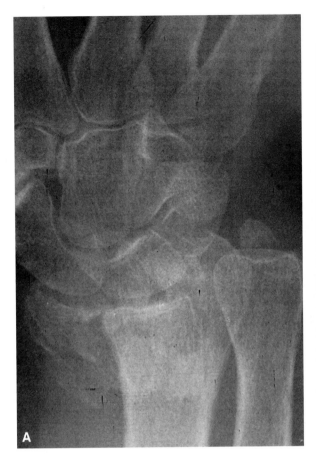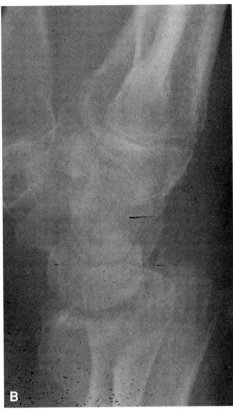

■ FIGURE 42–6
A and **B**, Posteroanterior and lateral radiographs of a type IIB fracture with volar displacement and considerable comminution.

cancellous bone graft, and secured with appropriately sized K-wires. Nonvascularized or free metaphyseal fragments should be removed and the void supplemented with cortico-cancellous bone graft.[12] The bone graft promotes faster healing and provides a bony buttress to prevent further collapse.[16]

Immediate postoperative elevation and encouragement of active digital motion is instituted. If concomitant tendon repair is performed, an appropriate tendon protocol for the level of injury is initiated with the hand therapist. Patient care of external fixation pins is not taught. The external fixation pins are exposed only during dressing changes in the office, about four times during the 8-week healing phase. Full active range of motion is expected within a week of surgery. If the patient fails to achieve this functional level, formal hand therapy with active and passive digital range of motion is initiated.

At 10 to 14 days postoperatively, sutures are removed and with internal fixation only, the long arm splint is converted to a cast that incorporates the thumb metacarpal and the humeral epicondyles. Except for those with tendon repairs, the digital joints are completely free for immediate active motion. With external fixator frames, the sutures are removed at the pin incisions and palmar incision. The volar plaster splint is replaced by a supplemental and protective volar short arm thumb spica thermoplastic splint. This splint provides supplemental comfort for the patient, additional support to the fracture, and protection for the exposed K-wires. Dry sterile gauze is reapplied at the skin/external fixator frame contact interface at each visit avoiding the need for daily pin care.

■ REHABILITATION

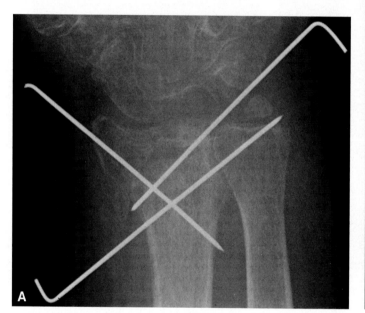
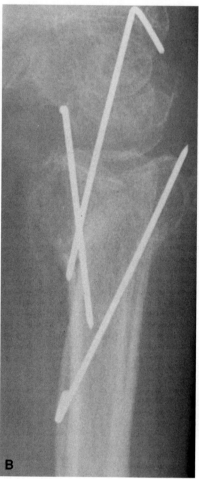

■ FIGURE 42–7

A and **B**, Posteroanterior and lateral radiographs after reduction and fixation through a volar approach. Because of the extensive comminution, stabilization of the small fragments was attained using multiple K-wires.

In most cases, after 6 to 8 weeks of total immobilization by an external fixator or cast, the immobilization is discontinued and fixation wires removed. An intensive therapy program supplemented with protective orthoplast splinting is initiated, consisting of gradual active and passive motion exercises, with progressive resistive strengthening of the wrist and forearm. Improvement is consistently observed for 6 months or more after the commencement of therapy. At 5 to 8 months postoperatively, depending on the severity of the fracture and concomitant soft-tissue injury, most patients return to their preinjury activity level.

■ OUTCOMES

Personal experience with unstable articular injuries involving the anterior margin of the distal radius has reinforced my conviction that an extensile volar approach facilitates an anatomic reduction of fracture components as well as meticulous repair of concomitant tissue damage. By restoring articular congruity of the type IIB articular fractures with volar displacement through a volar approach and stabilization, when suitable, by plate and screw fixation, a consistently high functional recovery is achieved. In patients with excessive comminution, K-wires with supplemental external fixation and adjunctive iliac bone grafting provide similar results. A preliminary review of these patients revealed a high level of satisfaction, with all returning to work, school, or sports activity by 8 months postoperatively. At follow-up, the overall range of wrist motion was 84% of the uninjured wrist, with an average loss (dorsopalmar flexion) of 20°. Grip strength averaged 90% of the uninjured side, and pinch strength averaged 81% of the uninjured side. All patients had excellent or good results using the Gartland-Werley rating system.

In a previous analysis of open treatment for type IV fractures with a characteristically displaced palmar medial fragment and soft-tissue damage within the flexor compartment, a volar approach yielded a successful result in most patients. No patient required a second operation.[19]

The rational management of distal radius articular fractures is contingent on recognition of the variable magnitude of articular disruption and skillful treatment based on specific fracture configurations. In more severe injuries, early detection and repair of frequent periarticular injuries are essential for a favorable recovery. The restoration of articular congruity with precise fixation and stabilization of the key medial fragments is the principal prerequisite for a successful outcome.

References

1. Barton JR: Views and treatments of an important injury of the wrist. Philadelphia Medical Examiner, 1838; 1:365–374.
2. Connolly JF: Smith's and Barton's Fractures. In: Depalma's The Management of Fractures and Dislocations, AF DePalma: 3rd Ed, Philadelphia: WB Saunders, 1981:1028–1032.
3. Crensaw AH: Intra-articular Fractures of the Distal Radius. In: Campbell's, Operative Orthopaedics, AH Crenshaw: 8th Ed, St. Louis: Mosby-Year Book Inc., 1992:1048–1053.
4. De Oliveira JC: Barton's fractures. J Bone Joint Surg, 1973; 55:586–594.
5. Ellis J: Smith's and Barton's fractures: a method of treatment. J Bone Joint Surg, 1965; 47B: 724–727.
6. Emmet JE, Breck LW: A review and analysis of 11,000 fractures seen in a private practice of orthopaedic surgery 1937–1957. J Bone Joint Surg, 1958; 40A:1169–1175.
7. Fernandez DC, Geissler WB: Treatment of displaced articular fractures of the radius. J Hand Surg, 1991; 16A:375–384.
8. Freeland AE, Jabaley ME, Hughes SL: Stable Fixation of the Hand and Wrist, New York: Springer-Verlag, 1986:117–122.
9. Fuller DJ: The Ellis plate operation for Smith's fractures. J Bone Joint Surg 1973; 55B:173–178.
10. Frykman GK: Fracture of the distal radius including sequelae-shoulder hand-finger syndrome, disturbance in the distal radio-ulnar joint, and impairment of nerve function: a clinical and experimental study. Acta Orthop Scand, 1967; 108:1–155.
11. Green DP: Pins and plaster treatment of comminuted fractures of the distal end of the radius. J Bone Joint Surg, 1975; 57:304–310.
12. Hasting H, Leibovic SJ: Indications and techniques of open reduction internal fixation of distal radius fractures. Orthop Clin North Am, 1993; 24:309–326.
13. Heim U, Pfeiffer KM: Small Fragment Set Manual: Technique Recommended by the ASIF Group. Berlin: Springer-Verlag, 1974:85–114.
14. King RE: Barton's fracture-dislocation of the wrist. In: Ahstrom JP Jr (ed): Current Practice in Orthopaedic Surgery, Vol 6, St. Louis: CV Mosby, 1975:133–144.
15. Mehara AK, Rastogi S, Bham S, Dave PK: Classification and treatment of volar Barton fractures. Injury, 1993; 24:55–59.
16. Melone CP Jr: Distal radius fractures: Pattern of articular fragmentation. Orthop Clin North Am, 1993; 24:239–253.
17. Melone CP Jr: Articular fractures of the distal radius. Orthop Clin North Am, 1984; 15: 217–239.
18. Melone CP Jr: Classification and management of intra-articular fractures of the distal radius. Hand Clin, 1988; 4:349–360.
19. Melone CP Jr: Open treatment for displaced articular fractures of the distal radius. Clin Orthop, 1986; 202:103–111.
20. Muller ME, Allgower M, Schneider R, Willenegger H: Manual of Internal Fixation Techniques Recommended by the AO Group, Berlin: Springer-Verlag, 1979:194–195.
21. Muller ME, Nazarian S, Koch P, Schatzker J: The Comprehensive Classification of Fractures of Long Bones, Berlin: Springer-Verlag, 1990:106–109.
22. Pattee GA, Thompson GH: Anterior and posterior marginal fracture dislocations of the distal radius. Clin Orthop, 1988; 231:183–195.

23. Rockwood CA Jr, Green DP: Fractures in Adults, 3rd Ed, Philadelphia: JB Lippincott, 1991: 585–600.

24. Scheck M: Long-term follow-up on treatment of comminuted fractures of the distal end of the radius by transfixation with Kirschner wires and cast. J Bone Joint Surg, 1962; 44:337–351.

25. Smith RW: A treatise of fractures in the vicinity of joints and on certain forms of accidental and congenital dislocations, Dublin: Hodges & Smith, 1847:129.

26. Thomas FB: Reduction of Smith's fracture. J Bone Joint Surg, 1957; 39B:463–470.

JESSE B. JUPITER

43

Internal Fixation of the Distal Radius: Dorsal Approach

Fractures of the distal radius remain among the most common of all skeletal injuries treated by extremity surgeons. Although many of these fractures are successfully treated by manipulation and immobilization with plaster support, it has become increasingly apparent, particularly with those individuals who place a high demand on their wrist, that the restoration of most extra- and intraarticular anatomy indeed correlates with function.[1,3,5] It has become evident also that articular fractures that unite with incongruity of 2 mm or more likely will result in symptoms of pain, weakness, and radiographic evidence of posttraumatic arthrosis.[4]

Several options have proved effective in maintaining a closed reduction of distal radius fractures. In addition to plaster immobilization, external skeletal fixation also has an important place in the management of these fractures.

Surgical exposure of the fracture becomes necessary when an acceptable reduction cannot be accomplished by manipulative means, when persistent loss of reduction precludes continued immobilization with plaster, or when high-energy injuries in which extensive soft-tissue trauma or associated skeletal injury require stable fixation of the distal radius. The initial experience with the operative approach may have been in association with the shearing fractures of the joint surface, which include reverse Barton's[6] and radial styloid fractures. These particular fracture patterns have proved to be unstable and representative of radiocarpal fracture–dislocations. These injuries are often seen in younger adults, and the use of open exposure and stabilization with plates and screws has become commonplace.

■ HISTORY OF THE TECHNIQUE

The indications for the operative approach to fractures of the distal radius through a dorsal incision are relatively well-defined. They are shearing fracture–dislocations with dorsal displacement (Fig. 43–1), impacted articular fractures that cannot be elevated by closed or percutaneous methods,[2] extraarticular fractures that have displaced in plaster and cannot be reduced by closed means, and combined skeletal and soft-tissue injuries involving complex fractures about the distal radius.

There are also absolute contraindications for an operative approach to fractures of the distal radius through a dorsal incision. These would include inadequate soft-tissue coverage or the inability to obtain adequate soft-tissue coverage, surgeon inexperience with the operative approaches to this complex skeletal region, and an unreliable patient.

■ INDICATIONS AND CONTRAINDICATIONS

Any surgical procedure in the skeletal system (but in particular in the area of the distal radius) should be preceded by adequate preoperative planning. This includes an understanding of the fracture anatomy, which may not be easily obtained by standard radiographs. Lateral and anteroposterior tomography may be helpful. If these techniques are not available, most centers today have the ability to perform computed tomography. Longitudinal traction and temporary plaster splint support may be recommended, not only as an initial procedure in the emergency ward but to allow a more accurate radiographic assessment of the fracture patterns. Actually, the most appropriate surgical approach frequently is selected only after careful and accurate radiographic assessment of the fracture. The preoperative planning should also consider the soft-tissue envelope. In the setting of

■ SURGICAL TECHNIQUES

A, Oblique and **B**, lateral radiographs of a shearing fracture–dislocation of the distal radius, with dorsal displacement.

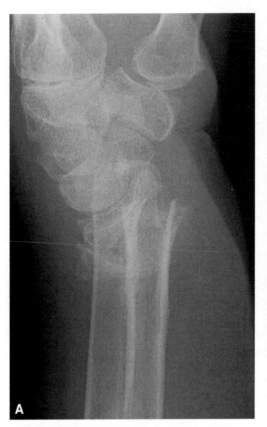

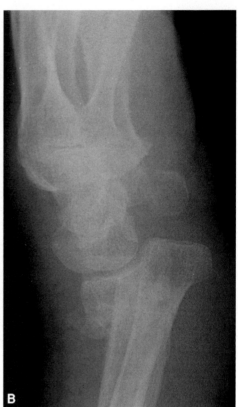

a compromised or swollen distal extremity, surgical intervention should be postponed until the soft-tissue trauma has improved.

With a clearer representation of the fracture pattern, classification of the fractures may be accomplished more accurately. Classification is important to understand the complexity of the fracture, the difficulty inherent in its treatment, and the prognosis of the injury. The most detailed classification is the AO system, which is organized in the order of increasing severity of the skeletal and articular lesions. This classification system divides the fractures into extraarticular (type A), partial articular (type B), and complete articular (type C).

Finally, when faced with the possibility of surgically treating a fracture with an impacted metaphysis or metaphyseal–diaphyseal comminution, the surgeon should prepare the patient for the possibility that autogenous cancellous bone graft may be required. Thus, preoperative discussion, appropriate surgical consent, and the necessary anesthesia (if iliac crest bone graft is to be used) should be planned in advance.

The choice of anesthesia depends on the complexity of the fracture, surgeon experience, and the requirements for autogenous bone grafting. In addition, it should go without saying that the level of confidence of the anesthesiologist toward regional anesthesia and the patient's overall medical condition play a major factor when selecting the anesthetic approach. Generally, axillary block or endotracheal anesthesia is preferable because the operative approach to these fractures may prove longer than anticipated. In cases of longer duration, the use of intravenous regional anesthesia may not adequately maintain an appropriate level of pain control.

When faced with a fracture that is relatively acute, provisional reduction can be obtained by manipulation and longitudinal traction, with or without the use of finger traps, which can be sterilized and hung over a pulley over the end of the hand table. Provisional reduction can also be obtained with the use of an external fixator to apply distraction before the surgical incision. This is particularly useful when dealing with those fractures that have extreme comminution both within the articular surface and extend into the diaphyseal–metaphyseal region. In addition, intraoperative fluoroscopy with the use of image intensification proves exceptionally helpful at this stage. Using surface anatomy, the location of the radiocarpal joint and the level of the fracture can be identified before making the skin incision. The use of intraoperative image intensification can greatly facilitate the placement of distractor pins in the second metacarpal and distal third of the radius.

After elevation and exsanguination of the limb, a pneumatic tourniquet is inflated. A straight longitudinal incision 7 to 10 cm in length is marked over the dorsal radius between the second and third extensor compartments. Once the skin incision is made, care must be taken to identify and preserve not only crossing sensory branches, in particular those off the radial nerve, but also large dorsal veins that are located in the area of the surgical incision. Preservation of these veins helps to minimize postoperative swelling.

At this point, the extensor retinaculum is opened between the second and third extensor compartments. The extensor pollicis longus tendon is identified and mobilized proximally and distally as it passes around Lister's tubercle. The fourth extensor compartment can now be elevated subperiosteally, which preserves the integrity of this compartment. This technique minimizes the commonly seen problem of extensor tenosynovitis, which can occur as the digital extensor tendons pass over the dorsally placed implants.

Exposure is facilitated by the placement of small Hohmann retractors along the radial and ulnar margins of the distal diaphyseal–metaphyseal junction of the radius. The fracture site can then be effectively exposed. With extraarticular shearing-type fracture–dislocations, the dorsal wrist capsule can be preserved because the accuracy of reduction is judged effectively by the resultant interdigitation of the fracture lines. When faced with intraarticular distortion, a longitudinal dorsal capsulotomy can provide direct exposure to the articular surface. Should this be required, the surgeon should not perform further stripping of the capsule off of the articular fragments but should open the fracture through the impacted fragments and under direct vision, elevate the articular fragments, maintaining as much soft-tissue attachment to these precarious fragments as possible.

At this point, particularly with impacted metaphyseal extraarticular fractures, fracture reduction is facilitated by the intraoperative placement of a small distractor. A 4-mm Schantz pin can be drilled into the distal metaphyseal fragment, parallel to the articular surface, and a second pin drilled perpendicular to the proximal fragment (Fig. 43–2).

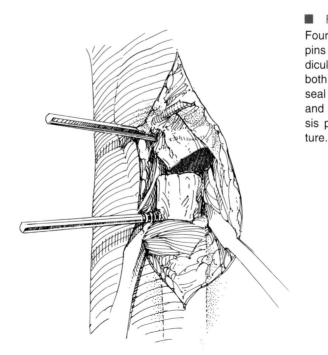

■ FIGURE 43–2
Four-millimeter Schantz pins are placed perpendicular to the radius in both the distal metaphyseal fracture fragment and in the distal diaphysis proximal to the fracture.

■ FIGURE 43–3
These pins are attached
to a small distractor,
which is used to carefully
and accurately control
fracture fragment position.

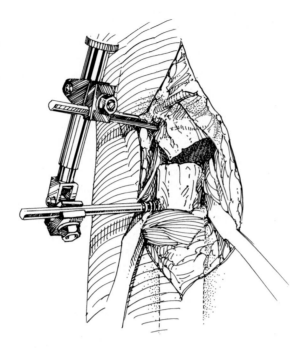

These pins are then assembled onto a small distractor, and fracture reduction can be performed under direct vision, with careful and gentle control over the fracture fragments (Fig. 43–3). In some cases, the indications for the surgical approach may have been a fracture that displaced while held in plaster. If the surgeon finds himself performing the dorsal approach in a fracture that has been immobilized for 2 weeks or longer, the surgeon should expect to see immature callous. This covers the fracture line and must be cautiously removed to allow exposure to the fracture lines. At this stage, the surgeon should recognize that the callous may be more prevalent than anticipated and certainly more than seen on the radiographs. The use of a small elevator facilitates disimpaction of the distal fragments while simultaneous distraction is performed.

Once accurate reduction is confirmed, both visually and on intraoperative radiographs, the stability of the fracture reduction is assessed. Impacted articular fragments require provisional Kirschner wire fixation, whereas the resultant defect that has occurred after disimpaction of the fragment is filled with cancellous bone graft. I prefer to use autogenous iliac crest bone graft, which can be obtained with the use of trephine biopsy needles. This minimizes exposure to the iliac crest and certainly diminishes the morbidity associated with bone grafting. Before any definitive fixation, the defects should be bone grafted to prevent the settling of the fracture during the course of healing. The bone graft is placed carefully in all of the defects and impacted with a small tamp to provide a compact cancellous support to the extra- and intraarticular reconstruction.

Definitive fixation is then performed. In most cases, when approaching the fracture through a dorsal incision, the use of a plate that is shaped in an angled "T" or straight "T" has been my preference. As with all fractures, plates should be contoured to meet the fracture rather than placing plates without direct contact in all of its arms. Caution should be exercised in this regard because these plates are relatively malleable, and tightening the screws can bring the bone to the plate, causing displacement of the fracture. Thus, in every instance, the surgeon should spend appropriate time to adequately contour the plate, using plate benders, pliers, or both, particularly curving the distal limbs of the angled "T" plate to fit the dorsal aspect of the distal radius.

Using a 2.5-mm drill bit and a 3.5-mm tap, the first screw should be placed in the distal radius, just proximal to the fracture line. The screw is measured and placed but not securely

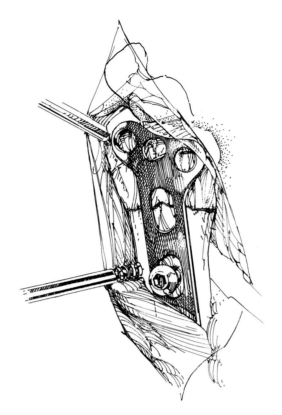

The first screw is placed in the distal radius, just proximal to the fracture line. It is not tightened completely to allow further correction of the position of the plate in relation to the fracture.

tightened to permit the plate to be shifted either proximally or distally and to some degree radially and ulnarly to sit appropriately over the fracture. Often, Lister's tubercle prevents the plate from seating adequately distally; it has been my preference to lower this tubercle, using a rongeur (Fig. 43–4). In many cases, the distal holes of the plate do not have to be filled with screws because the plate serves in most cases to "buttress" the restored articular and metaphyseal fracture fragments.

At this juncture, the fracture reduction is confirmed by obtaining true lateral and posteroanterior radiographs of the distal radius.

The remaining screws are placed—a second screw in the proximal fragment or if the surgeon believes it to be necessary, screws in the distal fragment. It is my preference in most cases not to place distal screws unless the bone is substantial; the fracture fragment is large, such as with a styloid fragment; or the fracture fragment tends to displace with application of the buttress plate alone.

The extensor retinaculum is reapproximated with nonabsorbable suture, leaving the extensor pollicis longus above the retinaculum. The tourniquet is released and hemostasis obtained. The skin is closed with interrupted sutures of 5-0 nylon suture. I prefer a bulky postoperative dressing and plaster splint, which is converted on the first postoperative day to an orthoplast splint. In most cases, active motion of the digits and wrist are initiated on the first postoperative day. The patient ordinarily has had a suction drain placed before wound closure, and the drain also is removed on the first postoperative day.

In some cases, when faced with more comminution than anticipated or displacement of the definitive plate and screws, the fracture can be treated by maintaining the intraoperative distractor, converting it to an external fixator with pins in the distal third of the radius and the second metacarpal, or combining either of these fixations with Kirschner wires. Kirschner wires with autogenous iliac crest bone graft may be more than adequate if axial loading on the wires is protected by the external fixator.

In some cases in which there is a single impacted fragment that can be manipulated by

■ TECHNICAL ALTERNATIVES

a percutaneously placed elevator, the use of an external fixator and Kirschner wires may suffice.

In the event that the surgery was performed in association with a high-energy lesion, the surgeon may be unable to close the wound without undue tension. Care should be taken when closing this type of wound. The use of temporary biologic dressing, split-thickness skin graft, or delayed primary closure is preferred.

■ REHABILITATION

Generally after internal fixation of fractures of the distal radius through a dorsal approach, I prefer to begin mobilization of the wrist, hand, and forearm on the first postoperative day. The use of a volar orthoplast splint for the first few weeks is recommended because it provides the patient with not only comfort but a sense of security. The functional loading of the fracture must be individualized, based on the type of fracture, the security achieved with the internal fixation, and the reliability of the patient. The use of autogenous bone graft helps to prevent settling of the articular fracture and enhance the rapidity of healing. The patient's fracture is monitored with radiographs; in the setting of ongoing union, functional loading can be increased. Activities of daily living, using the operated hand, are permitted 2 weeks after surgery. Loading is increased by permitting activities such as driving a car by 6 weeks postoperatively. Higher level performance activities, such as return to sports, are deferred until fracture union is assured, which is ordinarily not before 8 weeks postoperatively. If the patient is deemed unreliable and the surgery is undertaken to specifically restore widely displaced articular fragments, consideration should be given to the use of a Munster-type cast, which permits some elbow flexion and extension but immobilizes the wrist and forearm.

■ OUTCOMES

Generally, the shearing type two-part fracture dislocations of the carpus are well-treated with the operative approach through a dorsal incision (Fig. 43–5). Specifically, these are those shearing fractures in which the carpus and fracture fragment displace dorsally. Similar acceptable results have been seen with three- and four-part fractures in which the major displacement is dorsal.

■ FIGURE 43–5
A, Posteroanterior and **B**, lateral radiographs of the distal radius after plate and screw application and removal of the distractor and Schantz pins.

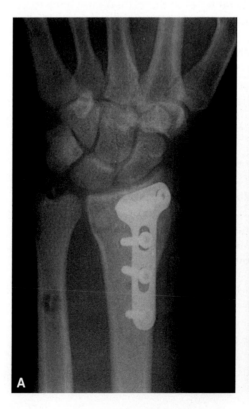
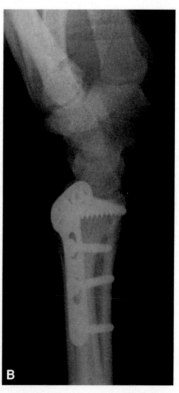

Conversely, with highly comminuted fractures, particularly in association with high-energy trauma, the results have not been as favorable. Although the extraarticular anatomy can be effectively restored, in some cases the extent of injury to the articular surface precludes anatomic restoration. The surgeon and patient should be prepared to accept a significant loss of wrist extension and flexion in addition to the possibility of posttraumatic arthrosis.

Prior reports of the operative treatment of fractures of the distal end of the radius have included a vast array of fracture patterns. Thus, it is difficult to glean the documented outcomes of the shearing fractures, as contrasted to the complex multifragmented articular fractures. My experience parallels that of Bradway and co-authors[3] and Melone,[5] who have reported that about two thirds of patients have good to excellent results without long-term sequelae such as posttraumatic arthritis.

The operative dorsal approach to fractures of the distal radius has proved its merit when articular fragments are not acceptably reducible by closed or percutaneous means.

References

1. Axelrod TS, McMurtry RT: Open reduction and internal fixation of comminuted intraarticular fractures of the distal radius. J Hand Surg, 1990; 15A:1–11.
2. Axelrod TS, Paley D, Green J, McMurtry RT: Limited open reduction of the lunate facet in comminuted intraarticular fractures of the distal radius. J Hand Surg, 1988: 12A:372–377.
3. Bradway J, Amadio PC, Cooney WP III: Open reduction and internal fixation of displaced, comminuted intraarticular fractures of the distal end of the radius. J Bone Joint Surg, 1989; 71A:839–847.
4. Knirk JL, Jupiter JB: Intra-articular fractures of the distal end of the radius in young adults. J Bone Joint Surg, 1986; 68A:647–659.
5. Melone CP Jr: Open treatment for displaced articular fractures of the distal radius. Clin Orthop, 1986; 202:103–111.
6. Thompson GH, Grant TT: Barton's fractures—reverse Barton's fractures. Confusing eponyms. Clin Orthop, 1977; 122:210–221.

44

Combined Internal and External Fixation for Fractures of the Distal Radius

Most distal radius fractures are relatively stable and can be successfully treated by closed methods. Unstable fractures with intraarticular extension require a different strategy.[5,7] This concept has been increasingly clear since Knirk and Jupiter demonstrated that accurate restoration of the articular surface of the distal radius was the most critical factor in achieving a successful clinical result.[8] The reduction and fixation can be achieved with either external fixation or internal fixation. Both techniques are suitable for specific fractures.

There is a subset of more complex fractures that are not well treated by either external fixation or internal fixation alone and appear to be best treated by a combination of the two techniques. This concept is appreciated when reviewing recent publications on internal fixation of distal radius fractures. These publications invariably include small subsets of patients who had both internal and external fixation, presumably because of increased magnitudes of comminution and displacement, and an inability to readily achieve a satisfactory reduction. Axelrod and McMurtry and Seitz and coworkers reported subsets of patients who underwent limited dorsal approaches along with external fixation for complex fractures.[1,13] Similarly, Bradway and coworkers treated four of 16 patients with a combination of external fixation and open reduction with K-wires.[3] Missakian and coworkers also treated ten of 32 patients with a combination of open reduction, internal fixation, and external fixation.[11] In none of these articles were the specific indications, techniques, or outcomes defined for patients who had combined internal and external fixation.

In recent years, presentations at national and international meetings have begun to define the specific role for the strategy of combined internal and external fixation for treating severe fractures of the distal radius. The strategy developed at the University of Iowa, beginning in 1989, has been used prospectively with minimal modification.[2] The strategy features volar and dorsal approaches, in addition to internal fixation and external fixation for the treatment of the more severe AO-C3 type fracture.

The primary indication for this operation is a severe intraarticular fracture of the distal radius, with volar and dorsal metaphyseal comminution (a fracture that would typically be classified as an AO-C3 type; Fig. 44–1). The classification of the fracture should be based on preoperative radiographic findings, usually taken after gross manipulation and protective splinting of the initial fracture (Fig. 44–2). Standard radiographs can be supplemented by plain tomography or computerized tomography to better define the fracture and assist with its classification. Associated carpal bone fractures, dislocations, or fracture dislocations are not reasons for rejecting this treatment strategy.

Contraindications to this operation include a successful attempt to achieve a closed reduction, despite the initial classification. This is most unusual, however, because ligamentotaxis is usually insufficient to correct the displacement or rotation of the fragments. Furthermore, the combined volar and dorsal approach should not be used to treat a fracture in which either a dorsal or a volar approach alone, with external fixation, could be successfully used. This latter technique is appropriate for AO-C2 fractures or for AO-C3

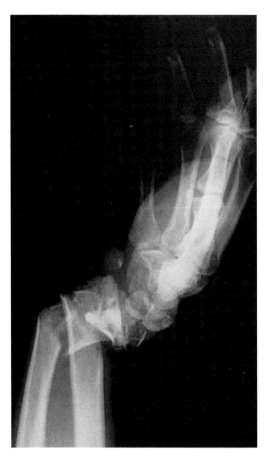

■ FIGURE 44–1
An oblique radiograph of the wrist of a 47-year-old male, with an AO-C3–type fracture of the distal radius.

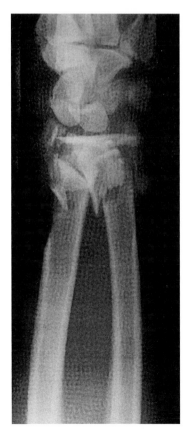

■ FIGURE 44–2
A posteroanterior radiograph of the distal forearm after an initial manipulation reveals extensive comminution, displacement, and rotation of the fragments.

fractures in which either the dorsal or the volar fragments are minimally displaced. This operation is contraindicated for open AO-C3–type fractures because these injuries probably require an alternative strategy.

■ SURGICAL
TECHNIQUES

The procedure is performed under general anesthesia. The injured upper extremity and the contralateral iliac crest are prepped and draped. The first step in the surgical procedure is a dorsal approach to the distal radius. Under tourniquet control, a longitudinal skin incision, centered over Lister's tubercle, is made. The third dorsal wrist compartment is entered, the extensor pollicis longus (EPL) tendon is mobilized and retracted radially. The fourth compartment is elevated from the dorsal aspect of the distal radius using subperiosteal dissection (Fig. 44–3). The capsular incision is then made transversely along the distal radial fracture fragments, although much of the dorsal capsular attachments to the radius fragments will be torn by the injury. A longitudinal capsular incision is then extended distally along the axis of the capitate. This allows visualization of the dorsal rim of the radius and the articular surfaces of the fragments. Next, a volar approach is performed through the flexor carpi radialis (FCR) sheath (Fig. 44–4). The distal radial corner of the pronator quadratus is sharply released; it is bluntly mobilized from the fracture fragments and retracted ulnarly. All fragments are mobilized and prepared for reduction but the volar radiocarpal ligaments are not released. An Orthofix (EBI Medical Systems, Parsippany, NJ) small-body fixator is then applied to the second metacarpal and distal

■ FIGURE 44–3
The dorsal approach is through the third compartment, with subperiosteal reflection of the fourth compartment.

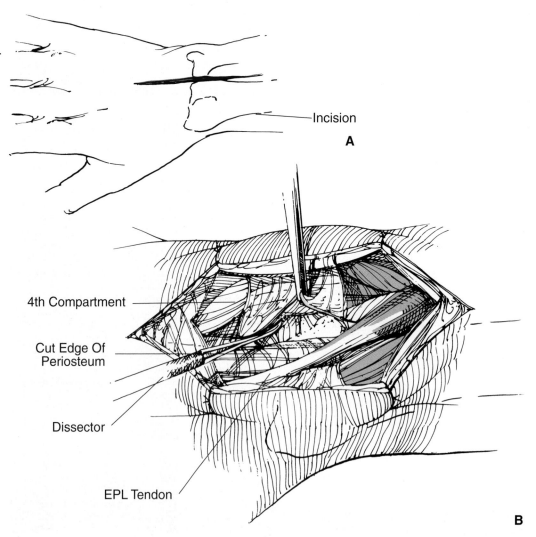

Incision

A

4th Compartment

Cut Edge Of
Periosteum

Dissector

EPL Tendon

B

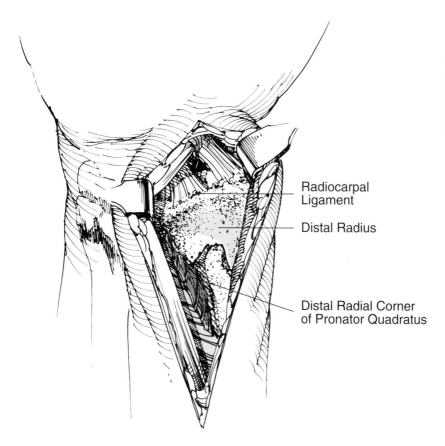

Radiocarpal
Ligament

Distal Radius

Distal Radial Corner
of Pronator Quadratus

■ FIGURE 44–4
The volar approach is through the FCR tendon sheath. After the tendon is retracted, the volar fragments are mobilized without releasing the volar carpal ligaments.

radius, using open techniques to expose the bone (Fig. 44–5). Firm longitudinal traction is applied along the forearm while firmly securing the elbow. Careful attention is given to the alignment and rotation of the hand relative to the forearm. The fixator is locked into place and the wrist is imaged with fluoroscopy. Confirmation of optimum alignment of the hand relative to the forearm in the posteroanterior and lateral projections is critical at this step. The axes of the capitate and radius should be collinear in all views. Reconstruction of the cortical shell and articular surface of the radius is then performed under direct visualization through both incisions. Anatomic reduction is usually accomplished by reducing and fixing fragments using a proximal-to-distal and volar-to-dorsal sequence. Fixation is accomplished primarily with smooth pins but neutralization plates or interfragmentary screws are appropriate for selected fractures patterns (Fig. 44–6). Extensive metaphyseal bone loss is invariable, and cancellous bone grafting from the iliac crest is usually required.

The dorsal capsular incision is closed with nonabsorbable sutures. The extensor retinaculum is closed beneath the EPL tendon and the pronator quadratus sutured to the lateral margin of the radius whenever possible. Skin closure is completed after tourniquet deflation.

On the first postoperative day, the patient is instructed on pin care, and supervised hand therapy is begun. Full-index active range of motion should be obtained within 2 weeks of surgery. The small pins are removed at 6 weeks. If radiographs confirm fracture repair, the external fixator is removed at 10 weeks. A thermoplastic wrist splint is provided, and progressive wrist motion exercises are begun.

The primary advantage of combined internal and external fixation is neutralization of the extremity (the hand relative to the forearm) and distraction across the radiocarpal joint. This allows fine manipulation and limited fixation of the multiple small fragments that occur in this fracture. Alternatives to this technique include either internal[3,10,11] or

■ TECHNICAL
ALTERNATIVES

■ FIGURE 44-5
The external fixator is then applied dorsoradially, using open approaches to centralize pin placement in the bone and to protect the superficial radial nerve.

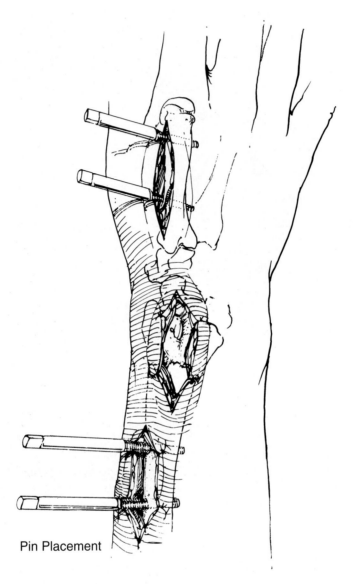

Pin Placement

external fixation[4,6,12] alone. Internal fixation is an alternative, although it must be performed without the advantages of the improved exposure afforded by the distraction. Also, it is difficult to obtain fixation that is rigid enough to resist collapse during postoperative immobilization. External fixation can also be used, but ligamentotaxis alone is usually not sufficient to derotate and then approximate the multiple fracture fragments.

Combinations of external fixation with percutaneous fixation[13] or limited fixation, with or without bone grafting,[9] have also been described for a less severe type of distal radius fracture.

The potential technical problems with this operation are many. Application of the external fixator must be done with single long incisions over both the metacarpal and the distal radius to avoid injury to the superficial branch of the radial nerve. Perhaps the most critical step in the operation is obtaining a truly neutral position of the hand and carpus relative to the forearm. This can only be confirmed using quality posteroanterior, lateral, and 30° supinated and pronated lateral intraoperative spot films. The opaque bodies of presently available external fixators can make this assessment difficult. The relation of the carpal bones to each other must also be carefully assessed, both pre- and intraoperatively, because distraction may reveal a previously unapparent carpal ligament injury. When present, the dorsal capsular incision must be extended, and anatomic reduction and pin fixation of subluxed carpal bones must be accomplished before distraction across the

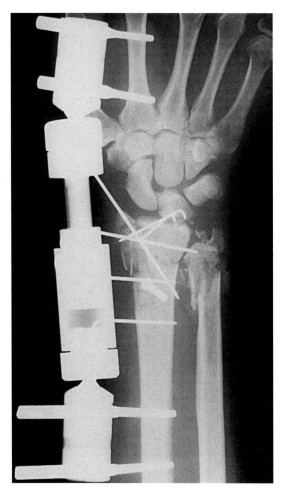

radiocarpal joint. The volar carpal ligaments should not be taken down during the volar approach to prevent devitalization of volar fragments and postoperative carpal instability. Centrally depressed, rotated, and impacted fragments are especially difficult to address and should be carefully assessed under direct visualization and with fluoroscopic views during the operation.

The approach to postoperative rehabilitation is critical to a quality long-term outcome. On the first postoperative day, the compression dressings are changed, and the patient or patient's family is instructed on daily pin-tract care. A hand therapist instructs the patient on active and passive range of motion exercises for the shoulder, elbow, and especially the fingers. The goal is the achievement of full active range of motion of the fingers within 14 days of the operation. The small K-wires are removed at 6 to 7 weeks. If posteroanterior and lateral radiographs confirm consolidation of the fracture and graft, the external fixator is removed at 10 weeks. A volar thermoplastic splint is applied. The patient begins active range of motion and progressive strengthening exercises for the wrist and forearm. During the next 3 months, motion and strength gradually improve, and most patients return to restricted employment 3 to 4 months postoperatively. At 6 months postoperatively, most patients can return to their preoperative activity level, including work-related activities. The motion and strength, however, continue to improve throughout a 2-year period.

■ REHABILITATION

Despite the relatively high potential for problems with surgery of this magnitude, the complication rates have been relatively low. Problematic pin-tract infections occur in about

■ OUTCOMES

■ FIGURE 44–7
A and **B**, At 2 years post-operatively, fragment and bone graft consolidation is complete. The articular surface is congruent and minimal osteoarthritis changes are present.

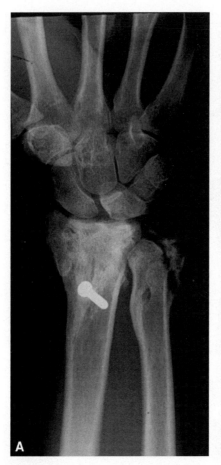
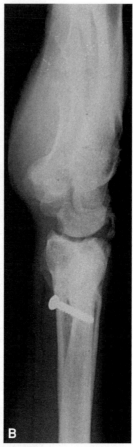

8% of patients. Overall patient satisfaction has been high, problems with activities of daily living have been minimal, and most patients have returned to regular work at about 5 months postoperatively. In my patients, at follow-up, the overall range of wrist motion was about 80% of the unaffected side. Mean grip strength was about 85% of the uninjured side. The restoration of radiographic variables was generally good, including 1° of dorsal tilt, 18° of radial inclination, radial length of 12 mm, and about a 0.5-mm increase in negative ulnar variance (Fig. 44–7). The severity of postoperative arthritis was absent to mild in 70%, moderate in 20%, and severe in 10%. Using the modified Green and O'Brien system, the following results were obtained: 57% excellent, 29% good, 14% fair, and 0% poor.[2]

This operation requires considerable expertise with both external fixator methods and internal fixation techniques for the radius. Each injury is complex and tends to be unique in some way, presenting a need for careful pre- and intraoperative planning and careful execution of each step in the procedure. Experience and mastery of this technique can provide good results after the treatment of this difficult clinical problem.

References

1. Axelrod TS, McMurtry RY: Open reduction and internal fixation of comminuted intra-articular fractures of the distal radius. J Hand Surg, 1990; 15A:1–11.
2. Bass RL, Blair WF, Hubbard PP: Combined internal and external fixation for treatment of AO-C3 fractures of the distal radius. J Hand Surg, 1995; 20A:373–381.
3. Bradway JK, Amadio PC, Cooney WP: Open reduction and internal fixation of displaced, comminuted intra-articular fractures of the distal end of the radius. J Bone Joint Surg, 1989, 71A:839–847.
4. Cooney WP, Linscheid RL, Dobyns JH: External pin fixation for unstable Colles' fractures. J Bone Joint Surg, 1979; 61A:840–845.

5. Fernandez DL, Geissler WB: Treatment of displaced articular fractures of the radius. J Hand Surg, 1991; 16A:375–384.
6. Jakim I, Pieterse HS: External fixation for intra-articular fractures of the distal radius. J Bone Joint Surg, 1991; 73B:302–306.
7. Jupiter JB: Current concepts review. Fractures of the distal end of the radius. J Bone Joint Surg, 1991; 73A:461–469.
8. Knirk JL, Jupiter JB: Intra-articular fractures of the distal end of the radius in young adults. J Bone Joint Surg, 1986; 68A:647–659.
9. Leung KS, Shen WY, Tsang HK, Chiu KH, Leung PC, Hung LK: An effective treatment of comminuted fractures of the distal radius. J Hand Surg, 1990; 15A:11–17.
10. Melone CP: Open treatment for displaced articular fractures of the distal radius. Clin Orthop, 1986; 103–111.
11. Missakian ML, Cooney WP, Amadio PC, Glidewell HL: Open reduction and internal fixation for distal radius fractures. J Hand Surg, 1992; 17A:745–755.
12. Sanders RA, Keppel FL, Waldrop JI: External fixation of the distal radial fractures: results and complications. J Hand Surg, 1991; 16A:385–391.
13. Sietz WH, Froimson AI, Leb R, Shapiro JD: Augmented external fixation of unstable distal radius fractures. J Hand Surg, 1991; 16A:1010–1016.

45

Trans-Scaphoid Perilunate Fracture Dislocation

■ HISTORY OF THE TECHNIQUE

Trans-scaphoid perilunate fracture dislocation is a relatively uncommon injury, although it is the most common form of complex carpal dislocation.[8,14,15] It is a high-energy injury, produced by wrist hyperextension. There is disruption of the palmar capsuloligamentous complex, starting radially and propagating through the carpus in an ulnar direction.[7,12,13] It has been termed a "greater arc" injury[13] and takes a transosseous route through the scaphoid and usually disrupts the lunotriquetral ligament (Fig. 45–1), resulting in a trans-scaphoid perilunate fracture dislocation. The distal scaphoid fragment usually dislocates dorsally, with the distal carpal row coming to rest on the dorsum of the lunate. The proximal scaphoid fragment and lunate usually remain coaxial with the distal radius (Fig. 45–2A and B). Rarely, the distal scaphoid and distal carpal row come to lie palmar to the proximal scaphoid and lunate.[2,7,8,21] Palmar dislocation of the proximal scaphoid and lunate as a unit has also been reported.[8,19]

Many variations of the trans-scaphoid perilunate fracture dislocation have been noted. The radial or ulnar styloids may be fractured, and osteochondral chip fractures of the capitate, hamate, or triquetrium can be present.[17] The scaphocapitate syndrome is an important variant to recognize and treat appropriately. In this case, the greater arc passes through the neck of the capitate and the proximal half rotates 90 to 180°, so that the articular surface of the head of the capitate is directed distally (Fig. 45–3).[7,20] Because initial radiographs can be confusing in these complex fracture dislocations, distraction films and comparison views of the contralateral wrist should be obtained.

Most authors agree that closed reduction is the initial treatment of choice, with surgical treatment reserved for failure to obtain or maintain adequate closed reduction. Cave, in 1941, was the first to advocate open surgical treatment.[4] He recommended a curved radial incision just volar to the first dorsal wrist compartment. The surgical approach to the scaphoid has since been modified by numerous authors but the standard incision is now centered just radial to the FCR tendon.

■ INDICATIONS AND CONTRAINDICATIONS

We initially attempt a closed reduction. Anesthesia of the wrist must be complete; this can be accomplished with intravenous regional (Bier), axillary block, or general anesthesia. Reduction is attempted after 10 minutes of longitudinal traction with finger traps. The patient's hand is then removed from traction while the surgeon manually maintains the longitudinal force on the extremity. One thumb stabilizes the lunate on the palmar aspect of the wrist, while the other hand extends the patient's wrist. A gradual palmarflexion force is applied to reduce the head of the capitate into the concavity of the lunate. If successful, a long arm thumb spica cast in neutral to slight wrist flexion is applied. Postreduction views are obtained to look critically at the reduction of the scaphoid and at the midcarpal joint. No amount of residual scaphoid fracture displacement nor any intercalated segment instability of the wrist can be accepted. When closed reduction successfully meets the above criteria, close follow-up is mandated. The stability of a closed reduction can be transient and radiographs should be checked twice during the first week, then on a weekly basis thereafter. Frequent cast changes may be necessary to maintain good three-point fixation as the swelling subsides beneath the cast.[5]

Although some authors believe that the inherent instability of this injury alone is enough

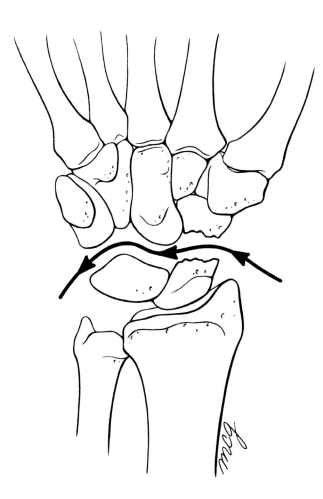

■ FIGURE 45–1
The path of injury in a trans-scaphoid perilunate fracture dislocation starts radially through the scaphoid and travels through the mid-carpal joint and out the lunotriquetral joint. This destabilizes the distal carpal row and with further wrist extension, usually leads to dorsal dislocation of the distal carpus. (Illustration by Margie Caldwell-Gill.)

to indicate open reduction and internal fixation,[1,14,15] we suggest that one closed reduction attempt always be made. When the perilunar carpal fracture dislocation cannot be reduced by closed methods, an open reduction should be performed unequivocally. Open reduction and fixation is also indicated when there is any subsequent displacement or fracture collapse or when static instability at the mid-carpal joint develops.[1,3,5,6,7,8,17] Open reduction and internal fixation is also indicated for those injuries that are open, irreducible,[11] associated with neurovascular injuries,[3,5,6,7,8,17] or in the presence of a scaphocapitate fracture complex.[5,7,8,20] For cases with scaphoid fracture comminution, we recommend open anatomic reduction, internal fixation, and bone grafting. When a closed reduction does not conform to the strict radiographic criteria mentioned above, early open reduction and alignment of the carpus as early as possible maximize the potential for bony healing and revascularization of the proximal pole of the scaphoid. Open reductions have been successful as long as 2[7,8] to 35[18] weeks after injury.

The following variables must be considered in operative management: timing; dorsal or palmar approach (or both); fracture fixation method; the need for bone grafting, median nerve decompression, or both,; and ligament repair or reconstruction.

■ SURGICAL TECHNIQUES

We recommend a palmar approach to expose, reduce, and stabilize the scaphoid fracture. A curvilinear 4-cm incision between flexor carpi radialis (FCR) and the radial artery is made, with the turn centered over the scaphoid tubercle (Fig. 45–4). After incising the antebrachial fascia, the FCR tendon is exposed and retracted ulnarly; the radial artery and its surrounding venae comitantes are carefully taken radially. The palmar wrist pericapsular fat and capsule are incised to expose the scaphoid. The fracture site is irrigated and cleaned of any interposed granulation tissue or clot.

■ FIGURE 45–2
A and **B**, Initial poster-oanterior and lateral radiographs of a trans-scaphoid perilunate fracture dislocation.

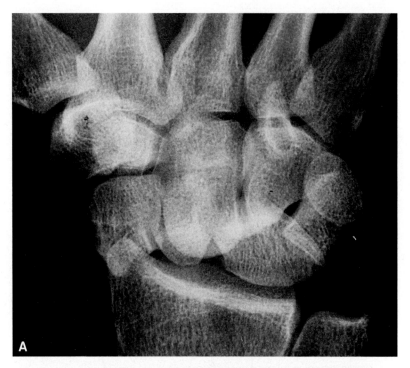

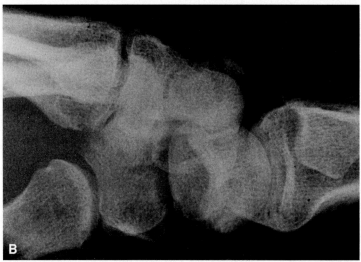

A reduction maneuver is effected. This step is facilitated by inserting two temporary 0.045-inch Kirschner pins, one into each fracture fragment, in a palmar-to-dorsal direction. These may then be used as "joysticks" to assist in fracture reduction. We prefer stabilization with a Herbert screw (Fig. 2C through E).[5,9,10] Proper positioning of the jig requires mobilization and distraction of the scaphotrapezial and radioscaphoid joints. Any "hump-back" deformity must be corrected. If there are any doubts regarding jig position, confirmatory radiographs should be obtained before screw placement. The Herbert screw must be inserted perpendicular to the fracture for maximum stability. When there is an oblique fracture line, a retrograde 0.045-inch Kirschner pin is placed first to prevent any shearing displacement that may occur with screw insertion. We have a low threshold for abandoning this means of fixation and using two retrograde 0.045-inch Kirschner pins when there is any difficulty in proper positioning of the jig or insertion of the Herbert screw. Pins give adequate stability and are easier to insert.

Significant palmar comminution or bone loss at the fracture site can be primarily bone

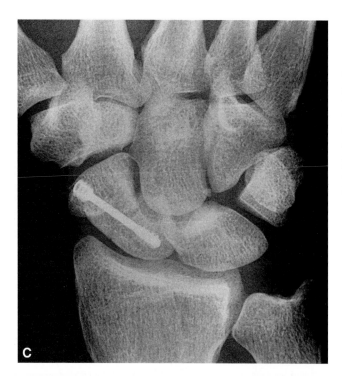

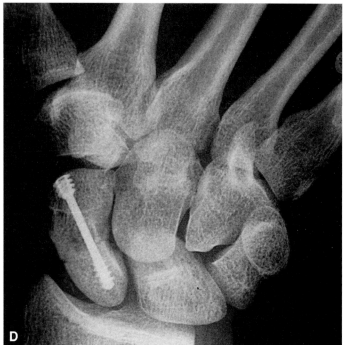

■ FIGURE 45–2 *(continued)* **C** through **E**, Posteroanterior, scaphoid, and lateral radiographs after open reduction and internal fixation with a Herbert screw performed through a palmar approach. The mid-carpal joint is reduced anatomically, and the carpal arcs have been restored.

grafted by extending the incision proximally. Distal radius bone graft is harvested after elevating the pronator quadratus. An associated radial styloid fracture (from which the radioscaphocapitate and radiolunate wrist ligaments originate)[11,13] should also be reduced and stabilized by this proximal extension. The radial artery and the dorsal sensory branch of the radial nerve must be protected.

Intraoperative fluoroscopy is useful. Permanent radiographs must also be obtained in the operating room after hardware placement to assure anatomic reduction; no fracture displacement or distraction is acceptable. To minimize iatrogenic articular injury, hardware should not protrude into the radioscaphoid or scapholunate joints. The mid-carpal

■ FIGURE 45–2
(continued)

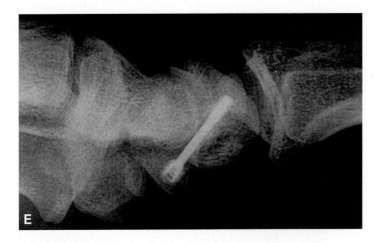

■ FIGURE 45–3
The scaphocapitate syndrome. The "greater arc" passes not only through the scaphoid but also through the neck of the capitate. Extensive ligamentous detachment allows the capitate head to rotate 180° on itself. Anatomic reduction requires derotation of the proximal fragment in the direction depicted by the arrow. (Illustration by Margie Caldwell-Gill.)

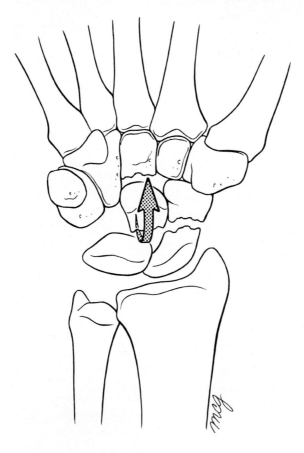

dislocation must be reduced and the carpal arcs restored. Critical review of the intraoperative radiographs for a static instability pattern of the lunate is essential; comparison contralateral wrist films are used to define normal intercarpal relations. Failure to line up the capitolunate articulation during reduction may lead to a late dorsal intercalated segment instability.[7,8] Residual volar intercalated segment instability after reduction of the scaphoid fracture mandates lunotriquetral joint reduction and pinning.[21] This is accomplished by manually reducing scaphoid flexion, using thumb pressure on the scaphoid tubercle, and then driving one or two 0.045-inch percutaneous Kirschner pins under fluoroscopy from the triquetrum into the lunate. An additional dorsal approach to the wrist may be required

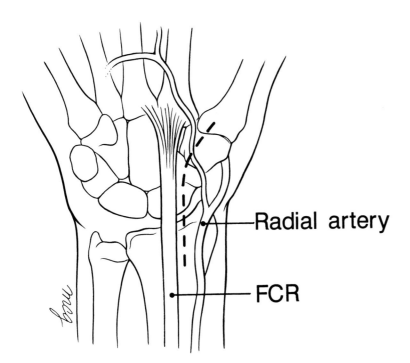

Radial artery

FCR

■ FIGURE 45–4
Recommended surgical
incision for the palmar approach to the scaphoid
fracture. It is parallel and
just radial to the FCR tendon and extends distally
and radially over the
scaphoid tuberosity. The
radial artery is retracted
to the radial aspect of
the wound. (Illustration by
Margie Caldwell-Gill.)

to accomplish this.[5,6] With anatomic restoration and internal stabilization of carpal bone alignment, primary interosseous ligament repair or reconstruction is not necessary.

The palmar wrist capsule and radiocarpal ligaments are closed with nonabsorbable suture. The FCR tendon and radial artery are allowed to fall back into position; skin closure is routine. A bulky, well-padded, long arm thumb spica splint is placed. Active and passive finger range of motion exercises are started immediately postoperatively.

With concomitant acute carpal tunnel syndrome, restoration of carpal alignment should adequately decompress the carpal canal.[1] Although return of median nerve function is anticipated, carpal tunnel release is indicated when there are progressive signs and symptoms of median nerve dysfunction after reduction.

Opinion in the literature varies regarding the optimal surgical exposure. Advocates of the palmar Russe-type approach[7,8,19,21] (Fig. 45–4) believe that it is easier to obtain an anatomic reduction and that this exposure is less injurious to the remaining dorsal blood supply of the scaphoid. Any cortical comminution of the scaphoid is more easily bone grafted. The palmar wrist capsuloligamentous complex is readily examined and repaired with this exposure.

■ TECHNICAL ALTERNATIVES

Proponents of a dorsal approach[1,11,14,15,17] believe that adequate visualization of the scaphoid fracture is attained while allowing direct exposure and manipulation of the mid-carpal and lunatotriquetral dislocations. Intrarticular or osteochondral fracture fragments and the capitolunate cartilaginous surfaces are readily observed from a dorsal approach. When the capitolunate joint cannot be reduced by closed manipulation or a palmar approach, a dorsal approach is useful to look for entrapped or impaled dorsal wrist capsule.[11]

A combined palmar and dorsal[5,6] surgical approach can be used for any combination of reasons mentioned above. Dorsal surgical exposure is obtained through a longitudinal incision centered over the carpus, just ulnar to Lister's tubercle. The third dorsal wrist compartment is entered, and the EPL tendon is reflected radially. The dorsal wrist capsule is incised between the second and fourth extensor compartments, exposing the capitolunate dislocation. A subperiosteal dissection of the distal radius beneath the second compartment exposes the scaphoid fracture site; a subperiosteal dissection beneath the fourth compartment allows access to the lunotriquetral joint.

The scaphocapitate syndrome[7,20] (Fig. 45–3), although uncommon, must be recognized. In addition to the scaphoid fracture, a capitate fracture occurs secondary to force directed against its neck by the distal radius in a hyperextended wrist. Six different patterns have been identified.[20] It is more readily diagnosed with the hand suspended in finger traps. The capitate is fractured transversely through its neck and with 180° rotation, the squared-off cancellous bed articulates proximally with the lunate concavity. The proximal capitate fragment is usually stripped free from the surrounding ligamentous attachments. It is preferable in this case to perform an open reduction through a longitudinal dorsal approach.[7,14] The proximal capitate fragment should first be derotated and the fracture fixed in anatomic position. Either Kirschner pins or a Herbert screw[9] may be employed. Reduction and stabilization of the capitate eliminates the space created at this fracture site, which allows easier reduction of the scaphoid fracture.[20] When the scaphoid cannot be anatomically reduced from this dorsal incision or there appears to be palmar comminution, it is helpful to add a palmar exposure to allow fixation and possible bone grafting, as described previously.

With the less commonly seen palmar trans-scaphoid perilunate dislocation, there is more extensive disruption of the lunotriquetral articulation and of the dorsal radiocarpal ligaments. A volar intercalated segment instability deformity may present itself immediately after reduction and fixation of the scaphoid fracture or gradually during follow-up. With this injury pattern, strong consideration should be given to a combined palmar and dorsal approach, combined with pinning of the capitolunate joint and the lunotriquetral joint.[21]

Trans-scaphoid perilunate dislocations are defined as chronic when they remain unreduced for more than 6 weeks. Surprisingly, some patients without a reduction can remain asymptomatic for many years. Median or ulnar nerve symptoms, pain and restricted mobility, and tendon rupture can eventually become disabling. Open reduction has been performed up to 35 weeks after injury but this should be done only if the cartilage is relatively well-preserved.[18] To assess the potential for late reduction of a chronic fracture dislocation, the surgeon should be able to distract the carpal bones with 25 or 30 lbs of finger trap traction.[6] Inability to do this suggests that a salvage procedure would be more appropriate. Salvage procedures in the presence of extensive cartilage loss and soft-tissue contracture include proximal row carpectomy or intercarpal, radiocarpal, or total wrist fusion.[6,14,16,18]

If delayed scaphoid union is apparent 4 to 6 months after reduction and no radiographic degenerative changes are seen, bone grafting and internal fixation of the scaphoid should be considered. A nonunion associated with periscaphoid arthrosis should be managed with a salvage procedure, as mentioned above.

■ REHABILITATION

We immobilize the extremity in a long arm thumb spica cast for a period of 6 weeks, followed by a short arm thumb spica cast for another 6 to 10 weeks.[14,15] When pins are used for scaphoid fixation, they are left in place for a minimum of 8 weeks[7,8] or until radiographic evidence of bone bridging is seen at the scaphoid fracture site.[1] Lunotriquetral or mid-carpal pins are left in place for 12 weeks. External immobilization should continue until there is radiographic union of the scaphoid. If there is any question, tomograms or a computed tomography scan of the scaphoid can be obtained.

Immediate postoperative finger mobilization is encouraged. After cast removal, exercises emphasizing active and passive wrist motion and grip strength are initiated. Referral to a hand therapist is essential.

Patients may return to limited work duties with the casted injured extremity. Unrestricted work is allowed only after scaphoid fracture healing and after 50% of normal wrist motion and 70% of normal grip strength have been regained. It may take up to 1 year for the patient to resume heavy work with the injured extremity.

■ OUTCOMES

Anatomic closed reduction was achieved in 67% in one series.[1] Of these patients, however, 59% lost reduction within the first 6 weeks. Closed treatment alone was successful in maintaining reduction in only 27%.

Scaphoid fracture union occurred in 73% of patients treated with closed reduction[8] and in 46%,[8] 88%,[15] and 100%[21] of patients treated operatively. Such figures are misleading because they represent small series. Additionally, irreducible and more complex fracture dislocations necessitate surgical intervention. Patients with anatomically healed scaphoids generally did well but worse results were seen in those who developed scaphoid malunions (humpback deformities).[8]

Functional outcomes were graded on a modified Green and O'Brien scale. With closed reduction alone, 33% good results were obtained, 44% fair, and 22% poor. In the same series, open reduction yielded 43% good, 38% fair, and 14% poor results.[5] In another study, those treated with closed methods had 55% good, 18% fair, and 27% poor results; surgical treatment led to 55% good, 9% fair, and 36% poor results.[8] Late scaphoid bone grafting was not as successful as primary bone grafting.[8] Two studies in which only open treatment was employed had 83%[15] and 80%[21] good results.

In one series, 60% of grip strength and 50% range of motion were recovered, regardless of whether open or closed treatment was rendered.[5] Seventy-five percent grip strength, 74% wrist extension, and 89% wrist flexion were obtained in another study with only open treatment.[21] Weak grip may persist for several years[15] but 82% of patients are able to return to either their original jobs or a modified job.[4] Those with volar dislocation of the lunate and proximal scaphoid pole had a worse prognosis.[8]

Median nerve symptoms were found in 16%,[1] 24%,[8] and 41%[15] of patients with this carpal fracture dislocation. In a series of seven patients having an associated median nerve injury, only one required a carpal tunnel release at 3 months after reduction.[15]

Avascular necrosis of the proximal pole of the scaphoid with this injury pattern ranges from 10% to 100%.[7] The reason for this disparity probably hinges on the definition of avascular necrosis: an increase in the radiographic density of the proximal pole is common, usually transient, and does not necessarily signify avascular necrosis.[7] Most proximal poles revascularize with fracture healing.

Appropriate treatment of a trans-scaphoid perilunate fracture dislocation includes attaining and maintaining an anatomic closed or open reduction. For those patients who require open treatment, we prefer a palmar approach to facilitate scaphoid reduction and bone grafting. A dorsal approach can be added to aid in reduction of the mid-carpal joint, if necessary.

References

1. Adkinson JW, Chapman MW: Treatment of acute lunate and perilunate dislocations. Clin Orthop, 1982; 164:199–207.
2. Aitken AP, Nalebuff EA: Palmar transnavicular perilunar dislocation of the carpus. J Bone Joint Surg, 1960; 42A:1051–1057.
3. Campbell RD, Thompson TC, Lance EM, Adler JB: Indications for open reduction of lunate and perilunate dislocations of the carpal bones. J Bone Joint Surg, 1965; 47A:915–937.
4. Cave EF: Retrolunate dislocation with fracture or subluxation of the mavicular. J Bone Joint Surg, 1941; 23:830–840.
5. Cooney WP, Bussey R, Dobyns JH, Linscheid RL: Difficult wrist fractures. Perilunate fracture-dislocations of the wrist. Clin Orthop, 1987; 214:136–147.
6. Cooney WP, Linscheid RL, Dobyns JH: Fractures and Dislocations of the Wrist. In: Rockwood CA, Green DP, Bucholz RW (eds): Fractures in Adults, 3rd Ed, Philadelphia: JB Lippincott, 1991:563–678.
7. Green DP, O'Brien ET: Classification and management of carpal dislocations. Clin Orthop, 1980; 149:55–72.
8. Green DP, O'Brien ET: Open reduction of carpal dislocations: indications and operative techniques. J Hand Surg, 1978; 3:250–265.
9. Herbert TJ: Use of the Herbert bone screw in surgery of the wrist. Clin Orthop, 1986; 202: 79–92.
10. Herbert TJ, Fisher WE: Management of the fractured scaphoid using a new bone screw. J Bone Joint Surg, 1984; 66B:114–123.
11. Jasmine MS, Packer JW, Edwards GS: Irreducible trans-scaphoid perilunate dislocation. J Hand Surg, 1988; 13A:212–215.

12. Johnson RP: The acutely injured wrist and its residuals. Clin Orthop, 1980; 149:33–44.

13. Mayfield JK, Johnson RP, Kilcoyne RK: Carpal dislocations: pathomechanics and progressive perilunar instability. J Hand Surg, 1980; 5:226–241.

14. Moneim MS: Management of greater arc carpal fractures. Hand Clin, 1988; 4:457–467.

15. Moneim MS, Hofammann KE, Omer GE: Transscaphoid perilunate fracture-dislocation. Result of open reduction and pin fixation. Clin Orthop, 1984; 190:227–235.

16. Neviaser RJ: Proximal row carpectomy for posttraumatic disorders of the carpus. J Hand Surg, 1983; 8:301–305.

17. Ruby LK: Fractures and Dislocations of the Carpus. In: Browner BD, Jupiter JB, Levine AM, Trafton PG (eds): Skeletal Trauma, Philadelphia: WB Saunders, 1992:1025–62.

18. Siegert JJ, Frassica FJ, Amadio PC: Treatment of chronic perilunate dislocations. J Hand Surg, 1988; 13A:206–212.

19. Stern PJ: Transscaphoid-lunate dislocation: a report of two cases. J Hand Surg, 1984; 9A: 370–373.

20. Vance RM, Gelberman RH, Evans EF: Scaphocapitate fractures. J Bone Joint Surg, 1980; 62A: 271–276.

21. Viegas SF, Bean JW, Schram RA: Transscaphoid fracture/dislocations treated with open reduction and Herbert screw internal fixation. J Hand Surg, 1987; 12A:992–999.

PART

VII

Distal Radioulnar Joint

WALTER H. SHORT
ANDREW K. PALMER

46

Dorsal Dislocation of the Ulna

Dorsal dislocation of the ulna is a complex clinical problem with a variety of causes. Under normal circumstances, the distal radioulnar joint performs several functions. It allows pronation and supination of the forearm to position the hand and wrist. Another function is to transfer load from the carpus to the radius and ulna. Interference with these two functions will cause pain, loss of motion, and decreased ability of the hand to be positioned for use.

Biomechanically, the distal radioulnar joint (DRUJ) is incongruous.[12] The radius of curvature of the sigmoid notch of the radius is greater than that of the corresponding articular surface of the ulna.[1] Besides the rotatory component of motion, there is a relative proximal-distal component to the motion. In pronation, the ulna becomes more ulnar positive. In grip, it also has been shown that the ulna becomes more ulnar positive.[6] Other studies have shown that, in pronation, the ulna contacts the sigmoid notch of the radius dorsally, while, in supination, the area of contact is in the volar aspect of the sigmoid notch.[3]

Several soft tissue structures seem to play a role in distal radioulnar joint stability. Johnson and Shrewsbury[9] in their study concluded that the pronator quadratus played an important stabilizing role. Kapandji[11] in his study suggested that the interosseous membrane helped in the stabilization of this joint. Spinner and Kaplan[5] stated that the sheath and tendon of the extensor carpi ulnaris (ECU) stabilized the joint in supination. Ekenstam[5] and Schuind[17] have suggested that the triangular fibrocartilage complex (TFCC) plays a role in stabilizing the distal radioulnar joint.

The known causes of dorsal dislocation of the DRUJ are many. They can be divided into bony abnormalities and loss of soft tissue constraints. Bony problems that lead to DRUJ instability will be discussed first followed by a discussion of soft tissue abnormalities.

Anatomically, the distance from the radius to the ulna stays fairly constant during pronation and supination. Fractures of the shaft of the radius or ulna with angulation may distort this relationship.[1] Galleazzi fractures are the best known example. If allowed to heal with an angular deformity, either rotation of the forearm will be limited or instability develops in the DRUJ. Rotational malalignments may also occur in shaft fractures of the radius and ulna. If allowed to heal in such a fashion, the relationship of the sigmoid notch of the radius and ulnar head will be altered. This may lead to instability problems of the DRUJ.

The problem arises if dorsal dislocation of the joint is recognized as a late sequelae after healing of the fracture. This may be due to several angular malalignments. A change in relative length of the radius and ulna may predispose to dorsal instability. Angular malalignments of the radius and ulna both in rotation or dorsal/volar angulation may cause incongruity of the joint. Treatment should first be directed to correcting the bony architecture to its normal geometry. One concern, however, is that soft tissue restraints to the distal radioulnar joint have become stretched or incompetent secondary to the bony deformity. Thus, it may be that even after correction of the bony deformity in chronic cases, soft tissue restraints may be too lax to insure stability of the joint. This would obviously decrease the chances of obtaining a good result.

Late treatment of dorsal instability of the DRUJ is a complex problem. In these cases, the dorsal dislocation of the ulna is longstanding, and it is not feasible to restore bony congruence to the joint and soft tissue restraints to the joint if they are nonfunctional.

■ HISTORY OF THE TECHNIQUE

The surgical treatment of dorsal subluxation described in this chapter is a combination of several procedures described by others. The procedure involves resection of the distal ulna which Watson and co-workers,[18] Bowers,[3] and Imbriglia and Mathews[7] have described. The use of either the pronator quadratus or other structures as an interposition arthroplasty has been described.[2,9,10] When the pronator quadratus is used, it is interposed into the space remaining between the radius and ulna.

The third portion of the operation requires stabilization of the DRUJ by the use of a portion of a tendon. Many authors have suggested that the ECU be used as a stabilizer, including Melone and Taras[13] and Webber and Maser.[19] Breen and Jupiter[4] suggested using both the ECU and FCU, while Hui[8] described using the FCU as a stabilizer of the distal radioulnar joint.

The operation described here is very similar to the procedure described by Melone and Taras[13] and Webber and Maser.[19] These authors recommended that it be used in rheumatoid surgery, but as described in this chapter it has been modified slightly for use in patients with post-traumatic instability.

■ INDICATIONS AND CONTRAINDICATIONS

Patients who have dorsal dislocation of the ulna are evaluated in several different ways. Physical examination should localize the pain to the DRUJ. The distal ulna is prominent dorsally. Usually there is restriction in pronation and supination movements and associated pain. Plain radiographs, including true lateral projections, show that the distal ulna is usually translocated dorsally. Computed tomography (CT) scans also are obtained and give important information about the advisability of surgery. The CT scan is done on both wrists in full pronation, neutral and full supination. The contralateral arm acts as the control. The CT scan allows assessment of the sigmoid notch of the radius and the forearm position of maximum subluxation and assists the surgeon in determining whether there is a position in which the joint reduces.

There are several criteria that should be met to indicate surgery. The pain should be localized to the DRUJ, and the CT or plain radiographs should show dorsal subluxation of the ulna. The CT scan also has the advantage of evaluating the contour of the sigmoid notch and ulnar head. In many cases of longstanding subluxation, the joint surfaces are irregular. Surgical treatment is only considered if splinting, anti-inflammatory agents, and activity modification have been unsuccessful in decreasing symptoms and improving function.

There also are several contraindications to the surgical procedure to stabilize dorsal subluxation of the DRUJ. Patients who have a malunion of a distal radius fracture or both bones forearm fracture may have concurrently dislocated the distal radioulnar joint. Treatment of this problem first requires corrective osteotomy of the malalignment. If persistent subluxation remains, then the patient can consider surgical stabilization of the ulna.

The surgical procedure can be performed on those patients who have had a Darrach procedure. Part of the surgical technique described may require partial resection of the distal ulna. Patients who have injuries to the wrist that would increase the likelihood of ulnar translocation of the carpus should not be candidates for this procedure. Other concerns that the surgeon should address before the surgery are co-existing arthritis or instability of the wrist that may mimic the subjective complaints of the person with DRUJ instability. The surgical procedure described requires the use of a portion of the ECU to stabilize the ulna. If this tendon is deficient or absent, then another approach to the problem would be advised.

■ SURGICAL TECHNIQUES

Stabilization of the chronically dislocated distal ulna is difficult to obtain, and clinical results can be, at times, disappointing. The surgical procedure described below involves three separate phases to the procedure. The first involves resection of the distal ulna while preserving the ulnar styloid. The second phase involves interposition of the pronator quadratus into the space previously occupied by the DRUJ. The third phase of the procedure stabilizes the distal ulna through use of the ECU tendon.

The surgical procedure is done under general anesthesia or axillary block anesthesia.

A tourniquet is used on the upper arm. After adequate anesthesia has been instituted, the arm is prepared and draped so that the entire forearm is in the surgical field. An 8 to 10 cm longitudinal skin incision is made over the dorsum of the wrist at the level of the prominent distal ulna. Using blunt dissection, the sensory branches of the ulnar nerve are protected. The ECU sheath is then exposed so that the entire length of the ECU tendon can be visualized. At this point in the dissection, the surgeon should be at the level of the antebrachial fascia, and the ECU tendon should be visualized below this fascia. Next, the skin flaps should be developed just superficial to the antebrachial fascia. Radial to the sixth dorsal compartment, the prominent distal ulna should be noticed. An incision is then made through the interval between the fifth and sixth dorsal compartments, and the distal ulna is exposed through this incision. Care should be taken not to incise any remnant of the TFCC. This incision into the distal radioulnar joint can then be analyzed so that the articular surface of the ulna and the sigmoid notch of the ulna can be visualized. One should see that the articular surfaces are irregular and incongruent.

The next step in the procedure is to remove the distal ulna. It is done in such a fashion so as to preserve the ulnar styloid as described by Bowers.[2] With the forearm in neutral position, an osteotomy is made in the distal ulna extending from the base of the ulnar styloid at the junction of the ulnar head and styloid and extending proximally and radially

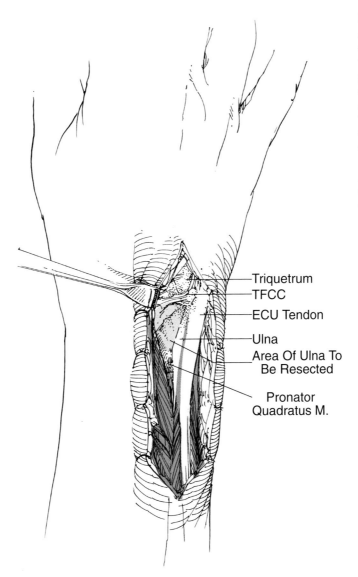

Triquetrum
TFCC
ECU Tendon
Ulna
Area Of Ulna To Be Resected
Pronator Quadratus M.

■ FIGURE 46–1
A 10-cm longitudinal incision is made just radial to the sixth dorsal compartment. Using blunt dissection, the distal aspect of the ulna is exposed. The dotted line shows the area of resection of the distal aspect of the ulna. To the ulnar aspect of the incision lies the extensor carpi ulnaris tendon.

exiting the radial aspect of the ulna just proximal to the distal radioulnar joint (Fig. 46–1). Care should be taken to keep the ulnar styloid in continuity with the remaining portion of the ulna. After completion of the osteotomy, the fragment of bone is removed. The remaining ulna is then contoured with a rongeur as the forearm is moved through pronation and supination. At this point in the operative procedure, the space created by the resection of the ulna should be palpated and visualized. There should be unrestricted pronation and supination without impingement of the radius and ulna.

At the depth of the wound lies the pronator quadratus. Using a periosteal elevator and blunt dissection, the origin of the muscle is reflected from the radius. The free edge of the pronator quadratus is then sutured to the periosteum along the dorsal edge of the sigmoid notch of the radius. This creates an interposition of muscle between the radius and ulna and would hopefully prevent bony contact during pronosupination (Fig. 46–2).

Upon completion of this portion of the surgery, attention is then turned to the ECU tendon. An incision is made in the sheath of the tendon although some portion of the extensor retinaculum should be preserved. After isolating the ECU tendon, a strip that is half the tendon in width and 10 cm long is mobilized proximally to distally, and it is left attached at its distal insertion.

After harvesting the ECU tendon, the distal aspect of the ulna is isolated. A curette is

■ FIGURE 46–2
After removal of the distal aspect of the ulna, the pronator quadratus is detached from the radius and transposed into the space created between the radius and ulna and attached to the dorsal aspect of the sigmoid notch of the radius.

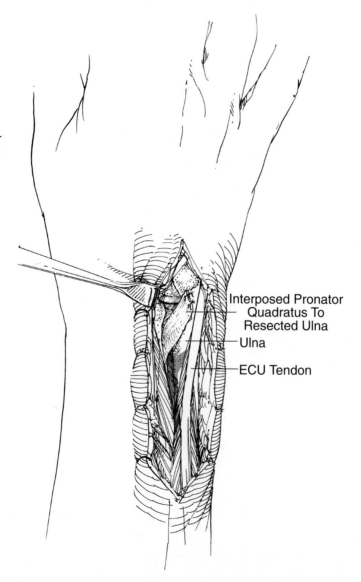

Interposed Pronator
Quadratus To
Resected Ulna

Ulna

ECU Tendon

then placed down the medullary canal of the ulna at the previously performed osteotomy site. The cancellous bone is then removed for a distance of 2 to 3 cm from the distal ulna. A drill hole is then made in the subcutaneous border of the ulna. This drill hole should be of the same diameter as the harvested ECU tendon, perpendicular to the long axis of the ulna and approximately 2 cm proximal to the end of the ulna (Fig. 46–3).

The end of the tendon graft is then passed through the end of the ulna and exited through the drill hole. Usually, this is accomplished by passing a suture through the tendon graft and then passing the suture through the medullary canal and drill hole. Once the graft is passed out of the bone, the free end of the tendon is woven through the distal end of the remaining, intact tendon three times. Tension is applied to the free end of the tendon graft. The amount of tension is considered appropriate when there is no subluxation of the ulna on pronation or supination of the forearm. The tendon graft is then sutured in multiple locations with nonabsorbable sutures (Fig. 46–4).

Before the incision is closed, the distal ulna is inspected, and the forearm is pronated and supinated. There should be no impingement of the ulna and radius. The ulna should not sublux dorsally relative to the radius. After the surgeon is assured that this does not happen, the general wound closure is begun. It is usually not possible to close the fascia

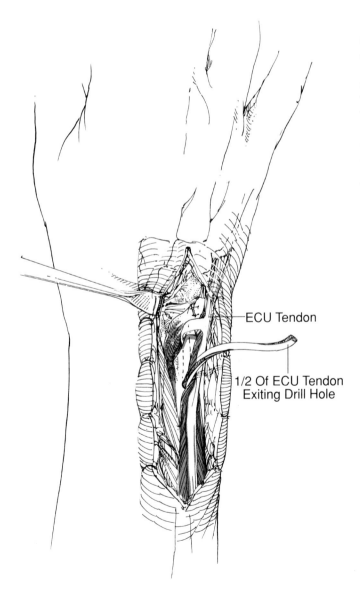

ECU Tendon

1/2 Of ECU Tendon
Exiting Drill Hole

■ FIGURE 46–3
One half of the extensor carpi ulnaris tendon is left attached distally and detached proximally. This tendon is woven through the medullary canal starting distally at the ulna and brought out through a drill hole approximately 2 cm proximal to the distal end of the ulna.

■ FIGURE 46–4
The tendon graft is then tightened and woven through the distal portion of the extensor carpi ulnaris tendon. It is then held in place with multiple sutures. Pronation and supination should reveal no subluxation of the distal ulna relative to the radius.

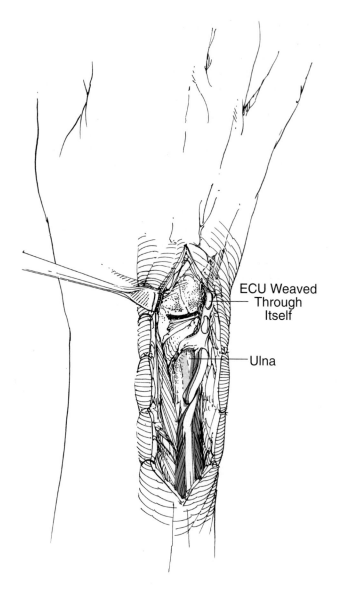

ECU Weaved
Through
Itself

Ulna

or retinaculum. The subcutaneous tissue is closed with absorbable sutures, and the skin is closed in a subcuticular fashion for better cosmesis.

■ REHABILITATION

Postoperatively, the arm is kept in neutral rotation either in a long arm or Munster cast for a period of 6 weeks. Physical therapy is then instituted by starting active range of motion exercises to increase mobility of the wrist. At this time, the patient may resume activity of daily living. Approximately 1 month later, passive motion and strengthening exercises are begun. At this point, the patient can resume work-related activities. It usually takes approximately 6 months to regain mobility and achieve the final clinical result.

■ OUTCOMES

Long-term follow-up results of any procedure for distal radioulnar subluxation are limited. The few studies that have been done have had a small sample size and a limited length of follow-up. Peterson and Adams[15] biomechanically studied several reconstructions and concluded that all fail to restore natural joint stability. In our experience, any procedure that attempts to stabilize the DRUJ can fail. The majority of our patients who undergo surgery for DRUJ have some relief of pain and increased mobility. Many continue to have symptoms, although to a less severe degree. In the future, the anatomic cause for this instability may be found. At that time, it is hoped that a surgical procedure can be designed that more accurately corrects the problem and diagnostic studies can be performed to ensure that the diagnosis is made earlier.

References

1. Aulicino PL, Siegel JL: Acute injuries of the distal radioulnar joint. Hand Clinics, 1991; 7: 283–293.
2. Bowers WH: Distal radioulnar joint arthroplasty: The hemiresection-interposition technique. J Hand Surg, 1985; 10A:169–178.
3. Bowers WH: Instability of the distal radioulnar articulation. Hand Clinics, 1991; 7: 311–327.
4. Breen TF, Jupiter J: Extensor carpi ulnaris and flexor carpi ulnaris tenodesis of the unstable ulna. J Hand Surg, 1989; 14A:612–617.
5. Ekenstam F, Hagert CG: Anatomical studies on the geometry and stability of the distal radioulnar joint. Scan J Plast Reconstr Surg, 1985; 19:17–25.
6. Friedman SL, Palmar AK: The ulnar impaction syndrome. Hand Clinics, 1991; 7:295–310.
7. Imbriglia JE, Mathews D: The treatment of chronic traumatic subluxation of the distal ulna by hemiresection interposition arthroplasty. J Hand Surg, 1993; 18A:899–907.
8. Hui FC, Linscheid RL: Ulnotriquetral augmentation tenodesis. A reconstructive procedure for distal subluxation of the distal radioulnar joint. J Hand Surg, 1982; 7:230–236.
9. Johnson RK, Shrewsbury MM: The pronator quadratus in motions and in stabilization of the radius and ulna at the distal radioulnar joint. J Hand Surg, 1976; 1:205–209.
10. Johnson RK: Stabilization of the distal ulna by transfer of the pronator quadratus origin. Clin Orthop Rel Res, 1992; 275:130–132.
11. Kapandji IA: The inferior radioulnar joint and pronosupination. In: Tubiana R (ed): The Hand, Philadelphia: W. B. Saunders, 1985:121–135.
12. Linscheid RL: Biomechanics of the distal radioulnar joint. Clin Orthop Rel Res, 1992; 275: 46–55.
13. Melone CP, Taras JS: Distal ulna resection, extensor carpi ulnaris tenodesis and dorsal synovectomy for the rheumatoid wrist. Hand Clinics, 1991; 7:335–343.
14. Mino DE, Palmer AK, Levinsohn EM: The role of radiography and computed tomography in the diagnosis of subluxation and dislocation of the distal radioulnar joint. J Hand Surg, 1981; 8:23–31.
15. Peterson MS, Adams BD: Biomechanical evaluation of distal radioulnar reconstructions. J Hand Surg, 1993; 18A:328–334.
16. Schuind F, An K-N, Berglund L, et al: The distal radioulnar ligaments: A biomechanical study. J Hand Surg, 1991; 16A:1106–1114.
17. Spinner M, Kaplan EB: The extensor carpi ulnaris: Its relationship to the stability of the distal radioulnar joint. Clin Orthop Rel Res, 1970; 68:124.
18. Watson HK, Ryu J, Burgess RC: Matched distal ulnar resection. J Hand Surg, 1986; 11A: 812–817.
19. Webber JB, Maser SA: Stabilization of the distal ulna. Hand Clinics, 1991; 7:345–353.

Volar Dislocation of the Ulna

■ HISTORY OF THE
TECHNIQUE

Forward subluxation, or, rarely, total luxation of the distal ulna, is a common concomitant of a considerably displaced Colles fracture. Isolated volar displacement of the ulna is an uncommon injury.

Uncomplicated anterior dislocation of the ulna was described for the first time by Desault[9] in 1791 as an incidental finding on a cadaver. He clearly pointed out that it is the distal radius that dislocates on the ulna and not vice versa. The next reference was 40 years later, by Dupuytren.

Volar dislocation of the ulna is frequently missed initially and therefore treated late. The history of treating this injury if discovered late is quite interesting. Although resection of the distal end of the ulna was reported by Moore in 1880, by van Lennep in 1897, by Angus in 1910, and by Tillmanns in 1911, the operation was popularized in an important article authored by Darrach in 1912.[7,8]

An alternative to resection of the head of the ulna was proposed in 1936 by Sauve and Kapandji.[22] They advised the production of a pseudarthrosis in the ulna at the level of the distal third with arthrodesis of the head of the ulna into its normal relation with the radius, so as to allow free pronation and supination, yet allow ulnar deviation of the hand at the wrist.

Many forms of treatment have been developed for long-term subluxation of the distal end of the ulna. Different types of external support, several methods of internal metallic support, and more than 20 types of internal soft tissue support have been recommended.[5,6,10–15,19]

■ INDICATIONS AND
CONTRAINDICATIONS

The volar dislocation of the ulna often is missed, and if the treatment is postponed more than 4 to 5 weeks, the condition is more difficult to treat.

A delay in diagnosis may be caused either by the patient's late presentation to the doctor or by failure to recognize key clinical features. There are some crucial clues that should give reason to suspect the diagnosis.

Dislocation of the distal radioulnar joint (DRUJ) is produced by displacement of the mobile radius and not the ulna. The term dislocation of the ulna is improper but has been accepted because of the clinical appearance of the distal ulna and because of common usage.

The clinical condition is usually caused by a major injury to the supinated and extended wrist. The ulna is dislocated not so often by a fall, which mostly results in a fracture, but more often by pulling of a heavy object or being struck by something heavy. If a major soft tissue injury is suspected, a thorough clinical investigation is important. A soft tissue injury of the DRUJ may result in dynamic or static instability. In a situation of static instability, the wrist is abnormally narrow, with loss of normal prominence of the distal ulna dorsally. Pronation is restricted and painful.

Radiographs may be misleading and even interpreted as normal, as it is difficult to get a true lateral view of the hand and wrist. Comparative radiographs of the contralateral normal wrist are always recommended. To get optimal information, a computed tomography (CT) scan of the DRUJ is the best procedure.[16] If the ulna is dislocated, this will easily be seen on the CT scan. With dynamic instability, the diagnosis is even more difficult. In this situation, the examiner can test the stability by stabilizing the hand and the radius with one hand and trying to dislocate the ulna in different forearm positions with the other. Often a click may be heard when the forearm is supinated and the ulna is dislocated, and another click when the ulna is reduced by pronating the forearm. Results of the examination should always be compared with the contralateral normal wrist.

The anatomic structures of importance in restoring stability in the DRUJ joint are now generally agreed upon, but their relative importance is not. I propose the following concept to explain a volar dislocation of the ulna without fractures. The ligaments of importance for a stable DRUJ are the triangular fibrocartilage (TFC), the ulnar carpal ligament (UCL), and the extensor carpi ulnaris (ECU) tendon sheath. An important prerequisite for stability is normal geometry of the joint.[1] The ulna also may dislocate in the volar direction in the following situations. If the dorsal radioulnar ligament is ruptured, the ulna may theoretically be dislocated volarly in supination with the help of the intact UCL. If the whole TFC is detached from the ulnar styloid, the ulna may dislocate volarly in supination with or without an intact UCL.

During the first 4 to 6 weeks after an isolated volar dislocation of the ulna, the condition may respond well to cast immobilization if an accurate closed reduction is obtained. A long arm cast with the forearm in full pronation should be used for 6 weeks to allow soft tissue healing.

If the volar dislocation is static and cannot be reduced, or if it is static because of a delayed diagnosis, the joint should be opened and reduced, the TFC and the UCL repaired, and the repair stabilized with K wires. If the joint has been dislocated for a long time, a CT scan of the joint should be obtained to exclude any degenerative joint changes. If such changes have occurred, a salvage procedure is recommended according to the surgeon's own experience. The most common procedures are those of Darrach, Bower, Sauve-Kapandi, and Milch.[5,7,8,15]

■ SURGICAL TECHNIQUES

The following text describes the procedure for treating a static volar dislocation of the ulna resistant to closed reduction.

The operation is preferably performed under axillary block using a tourniquet about the arm. The DRUJ is first approached by an angulated volar incision centered over the ulnar side of the flexor carpi ulnaris tendon. The ulnar nerve and artery are localized and protected as the antebrachial compartment is opened. The finger flexors are retracted while approaching the pronator quadratus muscle deeper in the wound. This muscle is incised and mobilized from the radius, as it is one of the main factors preventing reduction of the ulna. The volar capsule of the DRUJ can now be identified and incised. Usually this capsule is thickened because of early scarring. If the distal part of the interosseous membrane is involved in the scar tissue, which often is the case, it also has to be incised. The interosseous vessels and nerves must be protected during this release.

The arm is now rotated so that the dorsal side of the DRUJ can be approached. An angulated skin incision is centered over the ulnar head. Deeper dissection is performed with care to protect the dorsal branch of the ulnar nerve. The fifth and sixth extensor compartments are incised, and the extensor digiti minimi tendon to the small finger and the ECU tendon are retracted. The dorsal capsule of the DRUJ, which also may be scarred, is opened using a longitudinal incision. The DRUJ and the ulnar part of the radiocarpal joint are inspected. Any structure that interferes with the reduction, such as the position of the TFC complex, the ECU tendon, or the ECU sheath, must be released.[17,18] After this extensive soft tissue release, the ulnar head is reduced by manually distracting the radius and ulna and forcing the ulna posteriorly while the forearm is held in full pronation. Sometimes a more extensive division of the interosseous membrane is needed. The important anatomic structures contributing to DRUJ stability are evaluated. There are two main structures to consider. Either the TFC is avulsed from the base of the ulnar styloid, the so-called fovea region, or the styloid process is fractured at its base, and displaced along with the attached TFC and UCL ligaments. For the second option, the ulnar styloid process is reduced and stabilized with the "zuggurtung" technique. Two parallel 0.045 K-wires are inserted distally through the tip of the ulnar styloid and directed proximally. A transverse drill hole is made 2 cm proximally through the medial part of the ulna diaphysis.

A wire is brought through the drill hole and brought in a figure-of-eight fashion around the ends of the K-wires and tightened to get good compression over the fracture site.

If the TFC is avulsed from the ulnar styloid, it easily can be repaired. Drill holes are made from the foveal area of the ulnar styloid to the medial aspect of the ulna. Strong suture material is woven through the detached portion of the TFC and passed out through the drill holes. The suture is tightened over the medial aspect of the ulna with the forearm in neutral position (Figs. 47–1 and 47–2). This method previously has been well described by Hagert (personal communication). If the soft tissue release around the DRUJ has been successful, there should be no tendency for redislocation and, combined with a ligament repair, a K-wire is not needed to stabilize the DRUJ. To augment stability, the dorsal joint capsule is closed. Sometimes a fascial flap from surrounding tissue also can be used to augment stability. The pronator quadratus muscle is not reattached. Dorsally, the ECU tendon sheath is reconstructed to improve stability of the DRUJ and prevent dislocation of the tendon. One drain is placed volarly, and the skin is closed. After application of a

■ FIGURE 47–1
Avulsed TFC from the fovea area of the ulnar head.

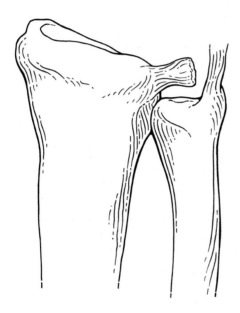

■ FIGURE 47–2
Reattachment of the TFC using drill holes through the ulna.

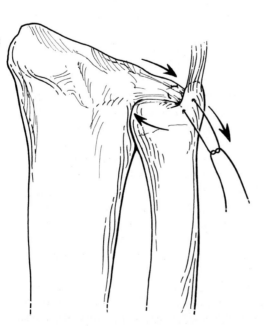

dressing, the radiocarpal joint, DRUJ, and the elbow are immobilized in an above elbow splint. The radiocarpal joint is placed in slight extension, the DRUJ in neutral position, and the elbow in 90° of flexion. Finger joints are left free for exercise. After 14 days, the sutures are removed, and the extremity is placed in a similar splint for another month.

At least 20 to 25 different procedures have been proposed for instabilities of the DRUJ. Some authors use local or grafted tissue to support the joint. Other authors use different tendons, preferably the ECU or the flexor carpi ulnaris tendon. The reports usually have been based on only one or two cases, and further experience is required. Many of the procedures include a tendon or fascial sling, which is passed through a drill hole in the distal radius, placed around the neck of the ulnar head, and attached to the radius.[14,19,] Over time, these operations do not prevent recurrent anteroposterior instability and they restrict rotation. I believe, as Bowers has observed,[5] that for a successful soft tissue reconstruction, the essential elements of the TFC-UCL should be reconstructed or substituted.[6]

■ TECHNICAL ALTERNATIVES

Before indicating an open reduction, an attempt at closed reduction should be made even as late as 7 to 8 weeks after injury. If the closed reduction is achieved, stabilization between the radius and ulna is important.[23]

Complications may occur with this procedure, especially in the volar exposure. Even in a healthy wrist, the volar capsule of the DRUJ is difficult to identify. In the dislocated condition, with abnormal anatomy, the scar tissue involving the pronator muscle, interosseous membrane, and the interosseous nerves and vessels, it is difficult to localize the ulnar head. As the incision is carried deep around the flexor tendons, care should be taken not to retract the ulnar nerve too vigorously.

In the dorsal exposure, careful identification and protection of the ulnar nerve is essential. The ECU tendon sheath should be reconstructed, as this structure is essential for stability of the ECU; luxation of this tendon can be very disabling.

I try to avoid pins through the DRUJ, as they also can cause complications. The pins can fatigue and break, as there always will be some motion of the forearm despite splinting above the elbow. Pin tract infection and pain may be associated clinical problems.

The assessment and achievement of an acceptable reduction is usually easy with the extensive soft tissue release I have described. If reduction is questionable, an image intensifier is used intraoperatively; plain radiographs also can be useful.

The splint is removed 6 weeks after surgery, and active motion of the immobilized joints is started. The patient's hand, forearm, and elbow are placed in a static splint. After another 2 weeks, resisted exercises are begun. Forearm rotation is the most difficult motion to achieve, and many months of rehabilitation may be needed. Sometimes a dynamic orthosis is used. Occasionally, a secondary procedure, such as capsulotomy of the DRUJ, is required to improve motion. This can only be performed after 6 months have passed.[2]

■ REHABILITATION

If the dislocation is recognized early, it can be reduced easily if the mechanism of injury is understood. After 6 weeks of above elbow immobilization, the expected result is excellent. Generally speaking, the earlier the recognition, the easier the reduction, and the better the result.

■ OUTCOMES

In static or recurrent volar dislocation, as mentioned previously, a wide range of solutions have been recommended in the literature. These include sling procedures, tendon procedures, and the Darrach procedure. Each author usually claims some success. According to Bowers, the reconstruction proposed by Boyes/Bunnel, which gives stability and capacity for rotation, provides the best results, although it does not attempt to directly reconstruct the UCL ligament.[5]

No prospective study of this clinical problem has been reported, likely because it is relatively rare.

My main experience has been gained through more than 100 corrective osteotomies, in which the often volarly displaced ulna had to be reduced and stabilized as well. In the cases with static or recurrent volar dislocation that I have treated, I have used reinsertion of the TFC as mentioned above, repair of the UCL if also injured, and raphing of the dorsal capsule of the DRUJ. By using this method, volar dislocation of the ulna has been resolved, although patients may have restricted forearm rotation, only about 60% of pronation, and 75% of supination. However, patients have been satisfied and function well in their activities of daily living and work. For these reasons, I consider this to be a valuable and effective operation in my practice.

References

1. af Ekenstam F, Hagart CG: Anatomical studies on the geometry and stability of the distal radioulnar joint. Scand J Plast Reconstru Surg, 1985; 19:17–25.
2. af Ekenstam FW: Capsulotomy of the distal radio ulnar joint. Scand J Plast Reconstr Surg, 1988; 22:169–171.
3. Axer A, Spann-Etzioni J: Dislocation of ulna at radio-ulnar joint without fracture of radius (report on 2 cases). Acta Med Orient, 1949; 8:54–57.
4. Burch-Jensen A: Luxation of the distal radio ulnar joint. Acta Chir Scand, 1951; 101:312–317.
5. Bowers: Distal radio ulnar joint. In: Green DP (ed), Operative Hand Surgery, 1st Ed, New York: Churchill Livingstone, 1982:756–761.
6. Boyes JH: Bunnel's Surgery of the Hand, 5th Ed, Philadelphia: J. B. Lippincott, 1970:299–302.
7. Darrach W: Anterior dislocation of the head of the ulna. Ann Surg, 1912; 56:802–803.
8. Darrach W: Habitual forward dislocation of the head of the ulna. Ann Surg, 1913; 57:1930.
9. Desault W: Extrait d'un memoire de M. Desault sur la luxation de l'extremite interieuse du radius. J Chir (Paris), 1791; 1:78.
10. Eliasson EL: An operation for recurrent inferior radio ulnar dislocation. Ann Surg, 1932; 96:27–35.
11. Fulkerson JP, Watson HK: Congenital anterior dislocation of the distal ulna. Clin Orthop, 1978; 131:179–182.
12. Kocks FJ: Anterior dislocation of the distal extremity of the ulna. Surgery, 1942; 12:41–45.
13. Liebolt FL: A new procedure for treatment of luxation of the distal end of the ulna. J Bone Joint Surg, 1953; 35A:261–262.
14. Lowman CL: The use of fascialata in the repair of disability at the wrist. J Bone Joint Surg, 1930; 12:400–402.
15. Milch H: Dislocation of the end of the ulna. Suggestion for a new operative procedure. Am J Surg, 19; 1:141–146.
16. Mino DE, Palmer AK, Levinson EM: The rule of radiography and computerized tomography in the diagnosis of subluxation and dislocation of the distal radio ulnar joint. J Hand Surg, 1983; 8:23–31.
17. Paley D, Rubinstein J, McMurty RY: Irreducible dislocation of the distal radio ulnar joint. Orthop Review, 1986; 15:(4)228–231.
18. Paley D, McMurty RY, Murray JF: Dorsal dislocation of the ulnar styloid and extensor carpi ulnaris tendon into the distal radioulnar joint: The empty sulcus sign. J Hand Surg, 1987; 12A:1029–1032.
19. Reagan JM, Bickel WH: Fascial sling operation for instability of the lower radio ulnar joint. Mayo Clinic Proc, 1945; 20:202–208.
20. Rose-Innes AP: Anterior dislocation of the ulna at the inferior radio ulnar joint. J Bone Joint Surg, 1960; 42B:515–521.
21. Sanders RA, Hawkins Bryan: Reconstruction of the distal radioulnar joint for chronic volar dislocation. A case report. Orthop, 1989; 12:1473–1476.
22. Suave, Kapandji: Nouvelle technique de traitement chirurgical des luxations recidivantes isolees de l'extremic inferieure du cubitus. J de Chir, 1936; 47:589–594
23. Schiller MG, af Ekenstam F, Kirsch PT: Volar dislocation of the distal radio-ulnar joint. J Bone Joint Surg, 1991; 73A:617–619.
24. Weseley MS, Barenfeld PA, Bruno John: Volar dislocation distal radioulnar joint, J Trauma, 1971; 12:1083–1088.

PART
VIII

Microsurgical Repairs

48

Neurorrhaphy at the Digital and Palmar Level

Digital nerve repair in the fingers and thumb appears to be a simple procedure and not very technically demanding. There are basic axioms regarding this treatment that are valuable, however. When they are applied appropriately, they provide reasonable surgical results. Pertinent historical milestones, regarding nerve repair, include Waller's physiologic description of degeneration and regeneration of peripheral nerves in the mid-1800s, Tinel's description of regenerating nerves published in the early 1900s, and Seddon's considerable research on peripheral nerve lesions and their repair.[1,3,7] Millesi contributed to Seddon's concepts regarding nerve grafting, and Moberg and others have done considerable work on sensibility testing after nerve repair.[5-7] Other authors have shown that surgical manipulation of peripheral nerves is associated with increased scar tissue formation and that this is detrimental to nerve regeneration.[4,5,7,10] The condensation of this tremendous amount of investigative work has led to current philosophies regarding nerve repair.[1-15]

I believe that at the level of the common and proper digital nerve, epineural suturing is satisfactory; whereas some may recommend interfascicular suturing, there is really little evidence to recommend that technique.[12,13] Probably the most important development in the last 20 years is the availability of excellent operating microscopes, and I believe that these should be used for all digital nerve repair.[9]

The indications for digital nerve repair are somewhat relative. The primary indication for digital nerve repair is anesthesia distal to a laceration or crush in a digit. The examination is performed for light touch and pin prick in the digital nerve distribution. I do not find two-point discrimination to be helpful; however, some surgeons disagree. In an injured hand, I believe that any sensory loss resulting from a laceration should be explored. Pseudomotor loss secondary to loss of sweat gland innervation is exhibited by dryness in the digital nerve distribution. An additional trick to help diagnose a digital nerve laceration is to place the injured part in water. Theoretically, because of the loss of pseudomotor activity, the affected skin will not wrinkle, compared with normally innervated skin.

Additionally, the decision to repair a digital nerve should be based on the anatomic location and subsequent deficit with a given injury. Certainly the repair of digital nerves beyond the level of the distal interphalangeal (DIP) joint is not only difficult but probably meddlesome. Simple suturing of the skin approximates these nerves near their point of arborization, and recruitment of collateral nerves is probably sufficient to provide a patient with reasonable protective sensibility on the tip of the finger. Repair of the digital nerve distal to the DIP joint is not indicated. Proximal to this level and up to the level of the mid-palm, digital nerve repair should be performed when sensibility is decreased on the radial borders of the index and long fingers and ulnar border of the small and ring fingers. Digital nerve lacerations to the thumb should always be repaired on both radial and ulnar sides. The functional loss from laceration of an ulnar digital nerve to a long finger and radial digital nerve to the ring and small fingers is minimal. Although repair of all digital nerves in the hand between the mid-palm and DIP joint is indicated, if the patient chose not to have an ulnar digital nerve to the long finger or radial digital nerve to the ring or small finger repaired, minimal deficit results. Patients and physicians should be aware

■ HISTORY OF THE TECHNIQUE

■ INDICATIONS AND CONTRAINDICATIONS

that digital nerve repair under no circumstance restores normal sensibility in the fingers.[1-15] Restoration of the sensibility to the palmar aspect of the thumb, however, is imperative because loss of protective sensation is a significant disability in that digit.

An additional major indication for digital nerve repair is the prevention of digital neuromas. It has been shown that these painful masses, although difficult to treat after formation, are reasonably well-prevented by digital nerve repair.[13]

■ SURGICAL TECHNIQUES

Anatomic considerations relative to digital nerve repair are somewhat simplistic. In the hand, these nerves are terminal branches of the median and ulnar nerves, with the median nerve supplying sensibility to the thumb, index, long, and radial half of the ring finger and the ulnar nerve supplying sensibility to the ulnar half of the ring finger and the small finger. These branches are common digital nerves, which then branch in the intermetacarpal space to form the terminal proper digital nerves, which join a digital artery and enter the finger. It should be noted that the digital nerves divide more proximally than the digital arteries. On entering the finger, the digital nerve is generally in a more midline and superficial position when compared with the digital artery. Both course on the palmar aspect of the finger, dorsal to Grayson's ligaments and palmar to Cleland's ligaments.

Once the decision for digital nerve repair is made, the technique of repair is important, and attention to detail is mandatory. I believe that all wounds in the hand and fingers should be surgically explored; in the presence of numbness in a digital nerve distribution, all structures in the finger should be visualized during the surgical procedure to make sure that they are in continuity passing through the laceration. This surgical procedure is generally performed with intravenous regional anesthesia or if the surgeon believes that multiple structures might need repair, general anesthesia. The flexor tendons and neurovascular bundles on either side of the finger must be identified. Bruner or zigzag incisions offer the best extensile exposure to the palm of the hand and finger. The laceration can generally be incorporated into modified Bruner incisions in some fashion and excellent exposure accomplished (Fig. 48–1). Frequently, in the finger the digital nerves can be

■ FIGURE 48–1
The fingers are approached through Bruner incisions, as marked on the small finger. With the laceration seen on the long finger, extensile exposure to identify the digital nerves can be accomplished through a modified Bruner incision, as marked on the ring finger. Once these skin flaps are retracted, exposure of digital structures is accomplished, as seen on the index finger.

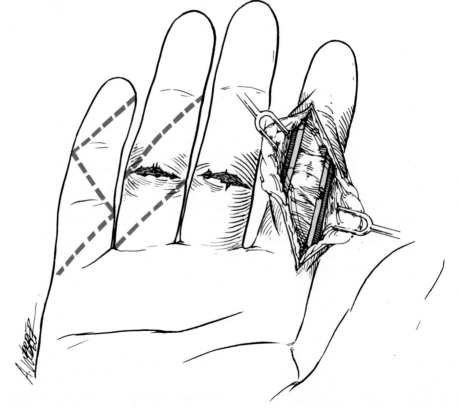

identified and repaired without extending the incisions, as can the various structures within the fingers. When possible, I try to use a limited exposure; however, if extension of the surgical exposure is necessary, this is always performed.

Timing of the repair is important, and although the literature states that nerve repair can be accomplished before 3 weeks after the laceration, I prefer to have the nerve repair completed by 7 to 10 days in tidy wounds. By this time, the contusions and injury directly to the nerves can be physically identified, and resection of damaged tissue can be performed.[4,12,13] In dirty or macerated wounds, soft-tissue concerns take precedence and secondary repairs or grafting may be necessary.

After prepping and draping the patient in the usual sterile fashion, the skin is marked to provide appropriate exposure of the palmar structures. When general anesthesia is used, the arm is exsanguinated and a tourniquet is inflated on the forearm or arm. Gross exploration is conducted under loupe magnification, using tenotomy or other scissors. After gross identification of the nerve, the microscope is brought into place. Under high-power magnification, the digital nerve is identified and trimmed of any necrotic or bruised tissue until normal fascicles are identified.[1,5,7,10,12-15] The fascicles, which can number between one and three, are then aligned and epineural suturing with the minimal number of sutures is performed to accomplish a tidy repair. Simple sutures are first placed on either side of the nerve anteriorly and then one in the midline posteriorly. The intervening epineurium is then sutured (Fig. 48–2). I believe that 10-0 nylon or Prolene sutures using BV 75 needle is the most appropriate suture to use, considering that when the nerve is under too much tension, these sutures do not hold. This is a reasonable test of the tension that the digital nerve can tolerate. According to Terzis[10] and others[5,6,12] work, tension cannot be accepted during a digital nerve repair. If there is any question about increased tension in the digital nerve repair, it should be grafted because holding a digit in flexion to oppose nerve ends can lead to contractures.

Closure of the wound is accomplished with simple sutures and postoperative care is standard for an open wound. The immediate postoperative bandage is a bulky bandage circumferentially around the finger to diminish swelling and a dorsal and palmar splint usually made of alumafoam.

■ REHABILITATION

Most sources state that splinting for a period of 3 weeks is useful after digital nerve repair; however, stiffness in the interphalangeal joints can occur during splinting. As long as there is no undue tension on the repair and full extension, range of motion can be initiated at about the time of suture removal.[1,13] Hand therapy after digital nerve repair is individualized, and many patients require no specific hand therapy. If stiffness develops in the metacarpophalangeal or interphalangeal joints, therapy and dynamic splinting are used. Generally, however, simple digital nerve lacerations are not associated with loss of motion in the fingers. Postoperatively, regeneration of the nerve is followed by Tinel's sign, which is paresthesia radiating distally from the level of nerve repair when the nerve is percussed. Because regeneration progresses at a rate of about 1 mm per day or an inch a month, the focus of percussion causing paresthesia migrates distally. As this migration occurs, sensibility is noted proximal to the Tinel's sign.[3]

■ OUTCOMES

Surgical results after the repair of digital nerves are somewhat inconstant. There are various factors that affect these results, including the amount of direct trauma to the nerve and the length of the nerve that has been traumatized. The greater the actual damage to the nerve, the larger the amount of scar tissue and the poorer the overall result. Age has a definite effect on the results after surgery, with children attaining better results than adults. Older patients attain the poorest results generally. Increased tension after repair leads to poor results. Nerve repair never results in normal sensibility; however, reasonable protective sensibility to light touch and pin prick can be attained, and two-point discrimination can approach normal in as many as a third of patients. More provocative tests, such as moving two-point discrimination, von Frey, and Semmes-Weinstein, generally show some deficit, however. That restoration of normal function is not possible should

■ FIGURE 48-2
A, The fascicles are trimmed, removing bruised or damaged tissue. **B** and **C**, Two anterior and one posterior sutures are placed to tack the nerve together. **D**, The intervening epineurium is sutured, completing the digital nerve repair.

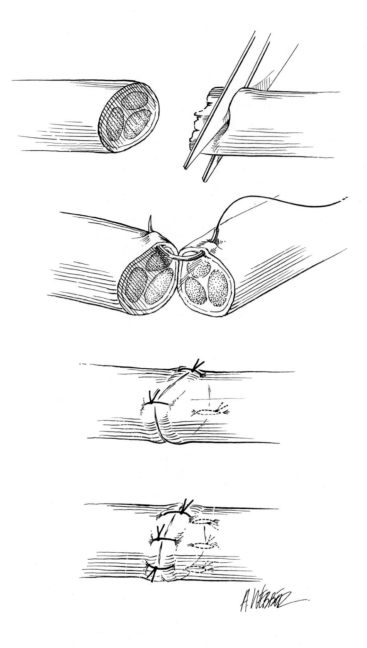

not be a deterrent to digital nerve repair because protective sensibility is nearly always accomplished and is a worthwhile goal.

References

1. Bunnell S: Surgery of nerves of the hand. Surg Gynecol Obstet, 1927; 44:145.
2. Gelberman R, Urbaniak J, Bright D, Leven L: Digital sensibility following replantation. J Hand Surg, 1978; 3:313–319.
3. Henderson WR: Clinical assessment of peripheral nerve injuries. Tinel's test. Lancet 1948; 2: 801–805.
4. Merle M, de Medinaceli L: Primary nerve repair in the upper arm. Hand Clin, 1992; 8: 575–585.
5. Millesi H, Meissl G, Berger A: The interfascicular nerve-grafting of the median and ulnar nerves. J Bone Joint Surg, 1972; 54A:727–749.
6. Moberg E: Nerve repair in hand surgery—an analysis. Surg Clin North Am, 1968; 48: 985–991.
7. Nicholson OR: Nerve repair in civil practice. Br Med J 1957; 2:1065–1071.

8. Poppen NK: Recovery of sensibility after suture of digital nerves. J Hand Surg, 1979; 4: 212–224.
9. Smith JW: Microsurgery of peripheral nerves. Plast Reconstr Surg 1964; 33:317–329.
10. Terzis J: The nerve hap: suture under tnsion vs. graft. Plast Reconstr Surg, 1975; 56:166–169.
11. Wilgis EFS, Maxwell GP: Distal digital nerve grafts: clinical and anatomical studies. J Hand Surg, 1979; 4:439–443.
12. Wilgis EFS: Nerve repair and grafting. Operative hand surgery 1988; 2:1373–1400.
13. Wray RC: Repair of sensory nerves distal to the wrist. Hand Clin, 1986; 2:767–772.
14. Young L, Wray RC, Weeks PM: A randomized prospective comparison of fascicular and epineural digital nerve repairs. Plast Reconstr Surg, 1981; 68:89–92.
15. Zachary RB, Holmes W: Primary suture of nerves. Surg Gynecol Obstet, 1946; 82:632–651.

PAUL A. COOK,
LAWRENCE M.
LUBBERS

49

Neurorrhaphy at the Forearm Level

■ HISTORY OF THE TECHNIQUE

From the 17th to the 19th century, nerve injury in the forearm was approached in one of two ways: passive neglect or amputation of the affected extremity. During this time, most surgeons believed the suture was a barrier to nerve regeneration. Lack of scientific knowledge led to many unusual methods of neurorrhaphy, including nerve flaps, tangential preparation, nerve-to-skin repairs, side-to-side repairs, transfixion sutures, and transplantation of the injured nerve to the side of an uninjured nerve. Advances in neuroanatomy and neurophysiology gradually improved the clinical care of nerve injuries. Baudens (1836) repaired nerves in the brachial plexus and reported his technique. In 1876, Bernard von Langenbeck reported success with Baudens' technique in median neurorrhaphy. As time progressed, optical magnification improved reapproximation and suture technique.

Observations by Tinel during World War I improved physical examination and clinical diagnosis. He described the symptoms of burning and tingling that helped the examining physician differentiate nerve irritation and regeneration. Sir Herbert Seddon's experiences during World War II provided insight into modern day neurorrhaphy: primary repair, secondary repair, and nerve grafting.[22] The next great advance in this era was identification of an individual nerve's internal topography. The internal neuroanatomy was studied extensively by Sir Sydney Sunderland in 1945,[23] and later by Jabaley and co-authors.[12] These studies led surgeons to improve previous neurorrhaphy techniques using a topographic map to assist in fascicular orientation. As magnification and science supported these improved techniques, the interpretation of results was improved by using 2-point discrimination—a new standard to judge the results of neurorrhaphy.[20]

Because each nerve has unique topography (fiber orientation), excursion, and ratio of motor-to-sensory fibers, the operative approach and results are individualized to each nerve. Significant determinants of clinical outcome are prompt neurorrhaphy and the quality of the first repair. Other significant determinants of outcome are patient-dependent and include compliance and participation in postoperative therapy. The surgeon can optimize certain variables: the time of neurorrhaphy, the tension of the neurorrhaphy, and the technique of neurorrhaphy. Other factors are beyond the surgeon's control: the mechanism and zone of injury, the condition of the nerve bed, the biochemistry of nerve repair as related to the trauma, identification of internal topography and realignment, the associated structural injuries, and the age of the patient.

Normal motion requires nerve excursion and each nerve is unique in regard to its inherent mobility (Table 49–1).[15,27] Peripheral nerves, with normal joint positioning and physiologic motion, undergo initial elongation and may experience 15% to 20% strain. Peripheral nerves are elastic in a safe zone and develop little tension. They have viscoelastic properties of creep (gradual elongation with time under a fixed tension) and stress-relaxation (relaxation of tension when stretched to a fixed point).[13] Certain amounts of strain create intraneural pressure and effectively limit perfusion. However, as the nerve lengthens, the nerve stiffens and the slope of the stress–strain curve acutely rises.[21] The increase in stiffness is from stretching of the connective tissue within the nerve. Retraction of the stumps occurs immediately due to elastic retraction, and an immediate repair easily corrects this retraction without consequence to local blood flow.

The injured nerve has altered biomechanical properties and exhibits increased stiffness.[1]

TABLE 49-1 EXCURSION OF PERIPHERAL NERVES IN THE FOREARM

Longitudinal Excursion of the Nerves at the Elbow

	proximal to elbow	distal to elbow
MEDIAN	7.3 mm (range 6–9)	4.8 mm (range 4–6)
ULNAR	9.8 mm (range 7–11)	3.0 mm (range 2–5)

Longitudinal Excursion of the Nerves at the Wrist

	proximal to carpal tunnel	distal to carpal tunnel
MEDIAN	14.5 mm (range 11–17)	6.8 mm (range 5–8)
ULNAR	13.8 mm (range 10–15)	6.8 mm (range 4–8)

Radial Sensory Nerve Excursion at the Wrist

full radial through ulnar deviation [15,27]	5.8 mm (range 5–8)

Therefore, reapproximation of a transected nerve should be slow (to avoid high peak tension within the nerve) and allow creep of the nerve tissue until the normal length relation is restored. Two key clinical considerations that arise when performing a delayed repair are: (1) significant increases in tension occur in the nerve with attempts at end-to-end repair, and (2) technical difficulty. If an end-to-end repair is achieved in this situation, significant tension is transmitted to the nerve and the repair site. Highet and co-authors[10,11] demonstrated that tension applied to nerve tissue, in humans and dogs, causes disseminated fibrosis along the segment exposed to tension, which causes a loss of elasticity and diminished potential excursion.

A primary repair can be classified into an immediate or delayed repair. This is based on the expired time between the injury and repair. An immediate primary repair is performed within 12 hours or less. A delayed primary repair occurs within the first 5 to 7 days after injury. Other authors have suggested that a primary repair can be performed within 4 weeks (this may be an acceptable timeline to categorize result; however, it is probably a delayed repair when assessing retraction, adhesions, and attempts at ease of end-to-end repair). When a repair is performed more than 7 days after injury, it is termed a secondary repair. The delayed technique has been used for many reasons: crush injuries, stretch injuries, contamination, and tissue loss. A greater potential for nerve regeneration was observed in the proximal stump after 7 days. At this time, the nerve is at peak metabolic activity and potentially would regenerate in less time.[9] This has biochemical advantages, yet the outcome of delayed repair has not clinically been shown to be advantageous. It seems that metabolic activity and optimal nerve sprouting do not parallel the quality of clinical results. Sprouting and alignment lead to connection, which is the most important factor contributing to a satisfactory result.[6,7] By performing an immediate repair, coaptation of equal caliber stumps theoretically provides optimal alignment and connections of axons. Primary neurorrhaphy has proven time and again to be the best technique for optimal suture neurorrhaphy. It permits identification of epineurial vessels for realignment, identification of fascicles in unaltered nerve stumps, correctable nerve retraction due to minimally altered nerve biomechanics, equal caliber stumps, and ability to compensate for nerve trimming and preparation. In fact, primary repair of the ulnar and median nerves has clinically demonstrated results superior to that of delayed repair in the forearm.[2,16]

The principles of neurorrhaphy that we use are similar to those outlined by Millesi and Terzis.[19] The first principle is preparation of the nerve bed, which is debridement of necrotic tissue followed by liberal irrigation of the nerve bed. This limits the inflammatory response and local scar formation. The second principle is sequential repair of other injured structures. Bone, tendon, muscle, and ligament should be repaired first and the neurorrhaphy performed as the last step before skin closure. The third principle is preparation of the nerve stumps before coaptation. The first step in preparation is a sharp transection by using "micro" trimming. In this step, the zone of nerve injury is defined and resected. This entails matching fascicles by creating clean transections and removing areas of unequal length. The fourth principle is coaptation without tension, while paying close attention to the "zone of attrition" or the gap between the stumps with normal joint motion. At the time of primary repair, direct end-to-end approximation can be achieved by joint positioning, transposition, and bone shortening in the presence of fractures and nerve deficits. We do not routinely use joint positioning for end-to-end repair. When performing secondary neurorrhaphy, these techniques will most likely be required due to nerve retraction, adhesions, and deficits. In addition, the bulb suture or stretch stitch can be used to achieve end-to-end anastomosis when retraction is limited. The fifth principle is adequate coverage of the neurorrhaphy site with muscle (or thick subcutaneous tissue) to protect the resultant neuroma. The final principle is adequate decompression of fascial structures or potential sites of compression proximal and distal to the neurorrhaphy site.

For the most part, anatomic landmarks are used as indicators of proper alignment. The nerve stumps are inspected to identify corresponding fascicles, groups of fascicles, and extraneural or intraneural branches. When groups are identified, the internal topography is drawn and mapped. The intraneural and extraneural branches are noted both proximally and distally and repaired first to assist in obtaining alignment. External landmarks, such as small surface blood vessels, also are useful for insight into the correct alignment. A gentle wipe of the proximal and distal stumps may squeeze the nerve into the correct rotation. Occasionally, mesoneural tissue tethers the nerve stumps and can assist in alignment.

It is helpful if the surgeon is knowledgeable about the internal topography of each nerve in the forearm before the regional suture techniques are applied.

■ SURGICAL TECHNIQUES

Peripheral nerve repair in the forearm level is best done under general anesthesia or with a proximal (axillary or supraclavicular) block. The patient is placed in the supine position. A pneumatic tourniquet is placed about the upper arm. The arm is exsanguinated and the tourniquet inflated. The specific technique for approximating the nerve can be either an external epineural repair, a group fascicular repair, or a fascicular repair. Although any technique can be used or used in combination, we most often repair forearm level nerve injuries using the external epineural technique.

The longitudinal vessels in the extrinsic epineurium are a helpful aid in alignment of the fascicles (Fig. 49–1). The first stitch should provide rotational realignment. This means the first stitch should align a known fascicle or intraneural branch such as the dorsal cutaneous fascicle of the ulnar nerve. The stitch perforates only the external epineurium. The neurorrhaphy is performed with 8–0 nonabsorbable suture (10–0 for smaller nerves) using 2 to 8 sutures in number. The epineurium is closed loosely. The nerve should be reapproximated with the minimum number of sutures to ensure apposition of the nerve ends. The suture should not violate the fascicles, and the nerve should not gap. If the nerve cannot be reapproximated with 8–0 suture, then too much tension exists in the repair. The repair must be performed without tension. It is important to remember this technique provides a physiologic splint for nerve repair because sutures do not penetrate any neural elements. Of the available techniques for repair, this technique seems to be the simplest and quickest. Optimum results are dependent on the realignment of fascicles and gentle coaptation of the epineurium by the suture line. Also, the external and internal epineurium can be gathered in one stitch for alignment and strength (Fig. 49–2).

The epineurial repair technique is most amenable to pure motor or sensory nerves, nerve repairs with indeterminate internal topography, and contusive or abrasive injuries. It can be used in the proximal forearm where the number of fascicles is higher and realignment is easier. In the distal forearm where the motor or sensory composition is more homoge-

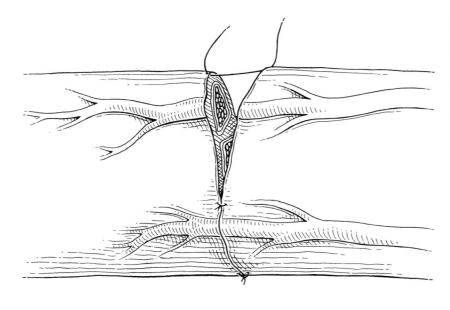

An epineural repair in which the stitch perforates only the external epineurium. The longitudinal vessels help with alignment. (After Cook).

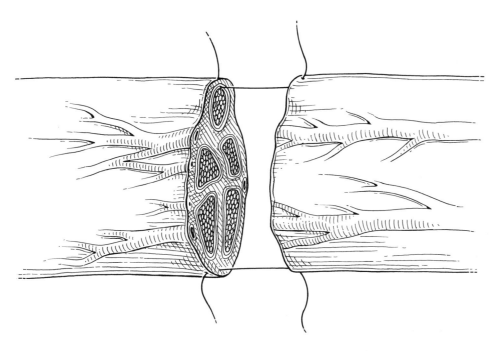

In an external and internal epineural alignment stitch, both layers are gathered in one stitch. (After Cook).

nous and fascicles are limited, such as the median nerve at the wrist, this technique can be used in combination with group fascicular repair. Magnification of 3.5× or better, retaining the epineurium, and limited tension are needed to optimize the result.

The group fascicular technique more accurately reapproximates fascicles by placing 2 to 3 sutures in the internal epineurium. The technique requires use of a microscope. The internal topography should be noted and mapped. The external epineurium is incised longitudinally, while protecting the internal epineurium, which covers a group of fascicles (Fig. 49–3). The margin of error is diminished by repairing the largest identifiable group first. Two to three sutures of 9–0 or 10–0 nonabsorbable suture are used for each group. This technique works best when repairing a nerve with a minimal number of groups and in cases in which the internal topography can be identified. However, one maligned group will result in complete malalignment. This technique requires considerable effort and

■ FIGURE 49–3
In a group fascicular repair the external epineurium is split longitudinally and sutures are placed in the internal epineurium. (After Cook).

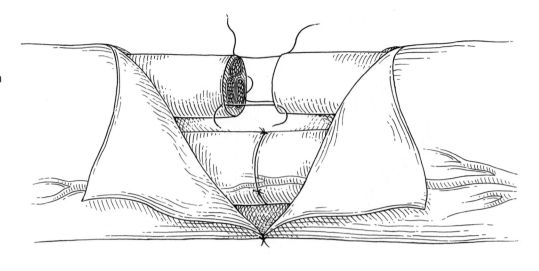

■ FIGURE 49–4
Fascicular repair may be used for partial nerve lacerations. The epineural layers are divided longitudinally and sutures are placed through the perineurium. (After Cook).

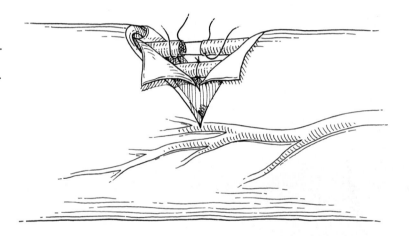

manipulation of the nerve. It should not be performed under tension in any circumstance, because tension at this level is transmitted to individual fascicles and will detrimentally affect their blood supply at the repair site. For this reason, supplemental sutures may be placed into the epineurium to transfer the tension away from the internal epineurium.

Further dissection of the nerve will expose individual fascicles—the fascicular technique. Longitudinally incising the external and internal epineurium is required for exposure. The perineurium must be preserved. The fascicular orientation must be understood to perform this technique. The suture material should consist of 10–0 or 11–0 material with only 2 sutures per fascicle. When performing this technique, the surgeon may use a large amount of suture material in a relatively small amount of tissue, so it is best performed in nerves with a maximum of five fascicles.[27] This stitch should not be used in a nerve that contains a large number of fascicles such as the median or ulnar nerves (30 to 40). A large number of fascicles can result in two problems: malalignment and scar secondary to excessive suture material. This type of repair is indicated in partially severed nerves (Fig. 49–4), either at one level or multiple levels, and in specialized branches where motor and sensory elements are identifiable yet are small in number. However, considerable manipulation, more dissection to identify individual fascicles, a large amount of suture material left in the nerve, and a lengthy operation are features of this repair. All these variables may result in increased scar formation and a less than optimal result.

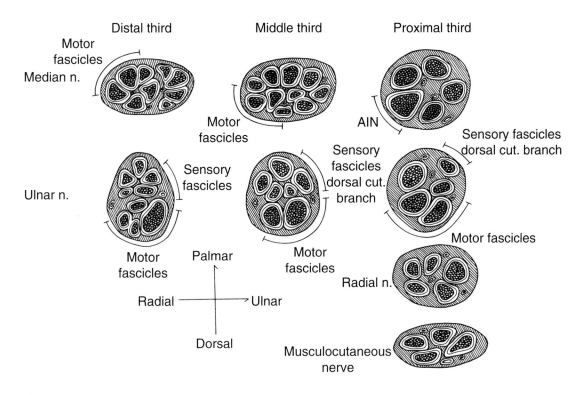

■ FIGURE 49–5
The regional internal topography of the nerves in the forearm is nerve and level specific.
Knowledge of these variations assist in planning repairs.

When visualizing and understanding nerve anatomy, it is easiest to think from distal to proximal as the nerve increases in caliber with addition of each branch (Fig. 49–5).

The Median Nerve—The Distal Third of the Forearm   The median nerve can be located at the distal third of the forearm between the palmaris longus and the flexor carpi radialis. The palmar cutaneous branch divides from the main body of the nerve 2 to 7 cm from the radial styloid and occasionally more than 8 cm proximally.[26] This branch travels within the epineurium of the median nerve another 15 to 25 cm proximally and can be dissected free over varying distances. This branch emerges from the radial, palmar sector of the median nerve, is radial to the flexor digitorum superficialis (FDS), and is adherent to the antebrachial fascia. At this level, the median nerve has approximately 30 fascicles with a sensory to motor ratio of 9:1. Before the identification of the leading edge of the distal aspect of the transverse carpal ligament, the recurrent motor branch is part of the main trunk. This branch is located radial and palmar and can be dissected free from the main trunk for varying distances that average 3 to 7 cm proximal to the radial styloid and occasionally more than 8 cm proximally. At 10 cm proximal to the radial styloid, the motor fascicles are located radially.[28] In this segment of the forearm, each terminal branch is represented by its own fascicular group. The most important consideration, at this level, is identifying the motor fascicles that are radial and palmar in the nerve. The technique we use when the fascicles can be identified is group fascicular often combined with an epineural repair for the sensory fascicles. Also, an inner and outer epineurial stitch can be used (Fig. 49–2).

The Median Nerve—The Middle Third of the Forearm   The median nerve can be located within the epimysium of the FDS on its dorsal surface. It can be approached between the flexor carpi radialis and radial side of the FDS or between the ulnar border of the FDS and the radial border of the flexor carpi ulnaris (FCU) (preferred approach). In this segment of the forearm, the median nerve is an isolated long segment of nerve without extraneural branches. In this region (20 to 30 cm), the nerve is circular and has a varying cross-sectional pattern with the motor fascicles located in a dorsal, radial position with 30 to 40 fascicles.[28] In this region of the forearm, the fascicles dispense and intermingle, which results in poor definition of fascicles or groups of fascicles. Because of the unpredictable internal anatomy of the fascicles, we perform an epineural repair unless intraneural branches can be identified. In this instance, we perform a group fascicular repair often combined with an epineural repair.

The Median Nerve—The Proximal Third of the Forearm   In the proximal forearm, the median nerve can be located between the brachialis and pronator teres. Further exposure will require ulnar retraction of the pronator teres and division of the lacertus fibrosis with potential elevation of the insertion of the pronator teres and radial origin of the FDS. This maneuver will expose the main body and the anterior interosseous nerve and branches to the finger flexors. The anterior interosseous nerve can be identified within the main body of the median nerve for approximately 6 cm proximally and is its largest motor branch. Isolated branches, such as the branch to the pronator teres, can be easily traced for 1.2 cm and then dissected another 10 cm proximally without evidence of interconnections.[12,18,23,28] Once the injury has occurred at this level, identification of groups of fascicles becomes much easier. This is due to intraneural localization of branch fiber systems. At this level, the surgeon is presented with two advantages; one is a branch that is pure motor and the second is the larger caliber branches in the main body of the nerve. We prefer to perform group fascicular repair at this level of injury, but an inner and outer epineurial repair can be used. When possible, the internal branching should be used for orientation of the repair.

One recommendation for suture technique is based on the internal topography at the level of the laceration. At the wrist, the motor branch is usually located palmar and can be repaired using the group fascicular technique combined with the epineural stitch for the surrounding sensory fascicles. At 3 to 8 cm proximal to the radial styloid, a group fascicular stitch will usually provide an optimal repair. From 8 cm to the anterior interosseous branch, the plexiform nature of the nerve lends to an epineural stitch. At and above the level of the anterior interosseous branch, we prefer to return to a group fascicular stitch.

The Ulnar Nerve—The Distal Third of the Forearm   The ulnar nerve can be located medial to the ulnar artery and radial to the FCU tendon beneath the antebrachial fascia. At the level of Guyon's canal (distal aspect of radial styloid), the ulnar nerve is made up of 15 to 25 fascicles, has a motor and sensory component, and has two distinct fascicular groupings.[28] The motor fascicles are dorsal to the abundant (12 to 14) sensory fascicles in the volar region. The fascicular orientation of the nerve can be identified for approximately 8 cm proximal to Guyon's canal. The sensory fibers to the small and ring fingers can be identified in the main sensory branch of the ulnar nerve 2 to 3 cm proximally to Guyon's canal. The dorsal cutaneous nerve is a separate nerve in the forearm. It can consistently be identified without interconnections for a range of 4.8 to 9.1 cm proximal to the radial styloid and up to 20 to 21 cm proximally.[12,23] In this region (10 cm proximal to the radial styloid), the motor fascicles maintain a dorsal position in the ulnar nerve with multiple sensory fascicles. The distinct internal topography of the dorsal cutaneous nerve can be used as a landmark to assist in achieving correct alignment. Because the motor and sensory fascicles can usually be easily distinguished, we recommend repairing this nerve at this level with a group fascicular technique. Occasionally, the motor fascicles can be repaired with a group fascicular technique and the surrounding sensory fascicles can be reapproximated with an epineural stitch.

The Ulnar Nerve—The Middle Third of the Forearm   At this level, the interval between the ulnar aspect of the FDS muscle and the radial aspect of the FCU muscle can be used to find the ulnar nerve. It lays adherent to the dorsal surface of the FDS muscle and medial to the ulnar artery. The dorsal cutaneous nerve can be isolated within the medial sector of the main body of the ulnar nerve. Similar to the median nerve in this region, the ulnar nerve's fascicles disperse and intermingle. However, adjacent to the fascicles containing the dorsal cutaneous fibers are the motor fascicles. If it is possible to identify these two separate fascicular groups, we prefer to perform group fascicular repair. If this is not possible, we perform a group fascicular repair of the internal branch of the dorsal cutaneous nerve. Again, this maneuver provides correct rotational alignment of the remaining fascicles so an epineural stitch can be used for the remaining repair.

The Ulnar Nerve—The Proximal Third of the Forearm   The ulnar nerve can be isolated as it exits the cubital tunnel and enters the forearm between the two heads of the FCU muscle. Division of the covering fascia and blunt dissection of the FCU muscle will allow access to the nerve. Access distal to this point can be gained between the FCU and the palmaris longus muscles. Twenty centimeters proximal to the radial styloid, the number of fascicles diminishes and the dorsal cutaneous nerve joins the main body of the nerve. Near the elbow a branch to the FCU muscle and a branch to the flexor digitorum profundus (FDP) of the ring and small finger are present. These two branches can be isolated for varying distances of 5 to 10 cm proximal to the elbow and can usually be identified in the radial, posterior sector of the nerve. Additionally at this level (30 cm), the ulnar nerve consists of 30 fascicles. Again, the internal branching system can be identified as we prefer to perform a group fascicular repair when possible.

Once again, the preferred type of repair is based on the internal anatomy at the level of laceration. At the level of the wrist or radial styloid, two distinct fascicular groups exist and, for this reason, group fascicular or epineural is recommended. When the laceration occurs in the mid to distal third of the forearm (10 cm from the radial styloid), motor fascicles can be identified dorsally with multiple sensory fascicles in the surrounding perineurium. In this region, we recommend a group fascicular stitch for the motor branch, which can be combined with an epineural stitch to repair the multiple sensory fascicles. The ulnar nerve, when lacerated in the proximal to mid forearm (20 cm proximal to the radial styloid), can be reapproximated with either a group fascicular or epineural stitch. Thirty centimeters proximal to the radial styloid motor branches to the FCU and flexor digitorum profundus muscles can usually be identified and a group fascicular stitch is recommended, which can be combined with an epineural stitch.

The Radial Nerve   As the radial nerve enters the forearm, it lies between the brachialis and the brachioradialis muscles. At this level, the nerve divides into the superficial radial nerve and the posterior interosseous nerve. The superficial radial nerve can be located within the epimysium of the deep surface of the brachioradialis and provides sensation to the thumb web space, the thumb, and a variable portion of the dorsum of the hand. The posterior interosseous nerve courses between the deep and superficial heads of the supinator and runs obliquely across the proximal radius to the wrist extensors. It comes to lie deep to the wrist extensors and superficial to the thumb abductors. This nerve provides motor fibers to the thumb and finger extensors and sensory afferents from the dorsal wrist capsule. Within the radial nerve, fascicles are large in size and small in number. This is beneficial in identification of the internal topography and fascicular realignment.[12,18,22,28] The internal topography of the radial nerve consists of two main fascicles. When the laceration occurs distal to the branch point of the posterior interosseous nerve and superficial radial nerve, the nerve is composed of two branches which are either pure sensory or pure motor with a limited number of fascicles. Therefore, an epineural or fascicular stitch technique can be used at the neurorrhaphy site. Proximal to this branching point in the radial nerve, two fascicles can be identified and a group fascicular or epineural stitch is optimal.

The Musculocutaneous Nerve   The musculocutaneous nerve exits the interval between the biceps brachii and the brachialis muscles and pierces the brachial fascia with the cephalic vein. This nerve has many branches that occur in a short segment and, thus, a complex fascicular arrangement with frequent branching. However, the internal topography becomes better defined in the forearm where the musculocutaneous nerve is sensory. Neurorrhaphy techniques that can be used are those used in pure motor or sensory nerves or nerves with a limited number of fascicles. The repair technique indicated in this situation includes both epineural and fascicular repairs.

After the neurorrhaphy has been completed, the operative site is inspected for hemostasis. Once hemostasis is achieved, the nerve repair site is inspected as the adjacent joints are ranged to determine limitations of motion. At this point, the surgeon must appropriately position the extremity to relieve tension at the site of repair. Once the position of the extremity is selected and the operative site is closed over a nonsuction drain, a splint is applied. This splint should be of substantial strength so it prevents joint motion of the operated extremity. The drain is removed on the second postoperative day.

■ TECHNICAL ALTERNATIVES

Neurohaphy has been advanced by an understanding of suture material, atraumatic needles, and improved technical skills. Despite the ease of stitch placement in difficult regions with marginal exposures, suture generates added trauma by altering fiber alignment and possibly increasing scar formation. For these reasons, new techniques of neurorrhaphy have been devised and tested. These techniques can be divided based on coaptation with and without suture.

Currently, two techniques that do not require suture coaptation are being tested: laser "welding" and fibrin adhesive without suture. These two techniques present several potential advantages such as no foreign material at the repair, a circumferential seal, and ease of application in difficult to expose areas.[14] A major deficiency is the strength of the repair, which is less than conventional suture techniques. However, an increased action potential[14] was observed in animal nerves repaired with laser neurorrhaphy versus standard neurorrhaphy techniques. Also, results in some animal models have demonstrated better neuromuscular function at 2 and 6 months than those repaired by an epineural suture technique.[3] When preparing the nerve for coaptation, the use of a laser may prove to be beneficial by eliminating the crush and twisting trauma of conventional preparation techniques. Perhaps the type of laser, the repair technique, and repair strength will be refined and improved sufficiently to justify its use for neurorrhaphy in the future.

Fibrin glue, an adhesive, has been studied in animals and in traumatic brachial plexus injuries.[8] The results of this technique were equivalent to conventional suture techniques. This technique is not approved by the Federal Drug Administration unless the fibrin is generated from the patient's own serum. We do not perform this technique because of the potential for nerve stump separation from diminished repair site strength. However, the lack of foreign material at the repair site is appealing.

Positive results of tubulization in peripheral nerve reconstruction have been established in animals. This technique is reliable for bridging nerve deficits. However, the nerve action potentials of vein-grafted nerves of rats were only 50% of those repaired by conventional suture techniques.[4] Recently, a prospective study was performed evaluating primary repair versus autogenous vein conduit for distal sensory nerve defects of 3 cm or less. Superior results were demonstrated in the primary repair group. However, patient satisfaction was high in the vein grafting group.[5] This is certainly a consideration when primary neurorrhaphy is unobtainable and the nerve graft material is limited.

Tubulation, as a method of sutureless nerve repair, can be performed using a variety of materials such as pseudosynovial sheaths, biodegradable polylactic acid tubes, biodegradable polyester tubes, polyglycolic acid tubes, silicone tubes nonperforated, silicone tubes perforated, and semipermeable and nonpermeable macropore. This technique has proven beneficial as a method of nerve repair across a gap. However, the best conduit material and the distance of potential regeneration vary in the literature.

In the office, the splint is changed to allow motion of the joints that minimizes tension at the site of repair. For instance, the wrist is flexed for a median nerve repair and flexion is permitted to limit adhesions, yet extension is limited by the splint. Because few injuries lacerate only nerve tissue, the rehabilitation program must incorporate other tissue mobilization programs specific to the individual injury. The tendon repairs are mobilized to maintain supple joints and to minimize tendon adhesions, yet protect the neurorrhaphy site.

Three weeks from the time of repair, the splint is adjusted to permit joint motion to the neural position. Gentle motion is initiated in the surrounding joints under direct supervision. This is an attempt to limit adhesions, which will limit nerve excursion and increase tension at the repair site. This restriction is maintained for another 3 weeks for a total splinting time of 6 weeks.

At 6 weeks postoperatively, the splint is removed. After this period of immobilization, a joint contracture is usually present and serves as an internal splint. This will protect the repair site until full motion is gradually regained. A few patients have ligamentous laxity and will require 2 to 3 weeks more immobilization. At the time of splint removal (6 weeks), the extremity is examined for sensory and motor function. At this point, the patient is started in therapy for strengthening, active assisted motion, sensory education, and other modalities.

After 6 weeks, Tinel's sign is used to assess and document the progression of nerve regeneration. If this sign fails to advance (at 2.5 cm per month), then consideration should be given to exploration and release of a constricting band, adhesions, or residual areas of potential compression. While the nerve is regenerating, it is of paramount importance to sustain the physiology of joints, musculotendinous units, and protect the anesthetic skin from pressure ulceration.

Results of major nerve repair in the forearm have generally been hard to analyze and compare due to the difficulty in measuring the sensory deficit and the lack of standardized tests to individually assess the results of motor recovery. However, several generalizations can be drawn from the literature. Many factors contribute to a poor result after neurorrhaphy. Birch, in a review of 2- and 7-year follow-ups of 108 median and ulnar nerve repairs after clean transection, identified six factors that he believed contribute to a poor result. These factors included poor surgical technique, failure to repair or ligate local arteries resulting in hematoma formation, lack of distal fascial release, a contaminated nerve bed that resulted in significant scar formation, age older than 21 years, and a delayed repair (more than 4 weeks after laceration).[2] In this review, excellent results were achieved only when neurorrhaphy was performed within 4 weeks of the injury and in almost all patients younger than 21 years of age (except one). However, a repair within 6 months of injury resulted in only 3 failures of 32. Two conclusions can be drawn from Birch's work: recovery is quicker after primary repair and the best outcome occurs in patients younger than 21 years old undergoing a primary neurorrhaphy at a distal site.

Merle and Amend reviewed 150 injuries to the median and ulnar nerves. This study suggested that age was the most significant factor for prognostication of neurorrhaphy. In patients older than 30 years, results of nerve repair began to decline, and repair in patients older than 60 years produced essentially a useless result. Also, patients involved in industrial accidents generally did poorly. The study demonstrated the utility of adequate blood supply to the nerve and repair site. Good and excellent results were obtained in 77% of patients without vascular injury. Another significant factor was the site of the laceration; a more distal laceration usually resulted in a better outcome. At the level of the wrist, 50% of nerves recovered to a good to excellent functional level, and 37% of patients with lacerations in the forearm demonstrated a good to excellent functional level.[16]

Generally speaking, when the neurorrhaphy is performed before significant nerve retraction (within 4 weeks), the nerve gap is eliminated as is the need for excessive dissection. The chance for an excellent result in the primary setting then depends on the age of the patient, fascial decompression, and application of basic principles of wound management. The limited literature provides evidence that a higher percentage of patients undergoing immediate repair have an excellent result.

References

1. Beel JA, Groswald DE, Luttges MW: Alterations in the mechanical properties of peripheral nerves following crush injury. J Biomech, 1984; 17:185–193.
2. Birch R, Raji ARM: Repair of median and ulnar nerves: Primary suture is best. J Bone Joint Surg, 1991; 73B:254–157.
3. Campion ER, Bynum DK, Powers SK: Repair of peripheral nerves with the argon laser. A functional and histological evaluation. J Bone Joint Surg, 1990; 72A:715–723.
4. Chiu DTW, Lovelace RE, Yu LT, et al: Comparative electrophysiologic evaluation of nerve grafts and autogenous vein grafts as nerve conduits: An experimental study. J Reconstr Microsurg, 1988; 4:303–312.
5. Chui DTW, Strauch B: A prospective clinical evaluation of autogenous vein grafts used as a nerve conduit for distal sensory nerve defects of 3 cm or less. Plast Reconstruct Surg, 1990; 86:928–934.
6. de Medinaceli L, Rawlings RR: Is it possible to predict the outcome of peripheral nerve injuries? A probability model based on prospects for regenerating neurites. Biosystems, 1987; 20–243.
7. de Medinaceli L: Functional consequences of experimental nerve lesions: Effects of reinnervation blend. Exp Neurol, 1988; 100:166–178.
8. Diao E, Peimer CA: Sutureless methods of nerve repair. In: Gelberman, Richard (ed): Operative Nerve Repair and Reconstruction. Philadelphia: J. B. Lippincott, 1991:307–308.
9. Ducker TB, Kempe LG, Hayes GH: The metabolic background for peripheral nerve surgery. J Neurosurg, 1969; 30:270–280.
10. Highet WB, Holmes W: Traction injuries to the lateral popliteal nerve and traction injuries to peripheral nerves after suture. Br J Surg, 1943; 30:212–233.
11. Highet WB, Sanders FK: The effect of stretching nerves after suture. Br J Surg, 1943; 30: 355–369.
12. Jabaley ME, Wallace WH, Heckler FR: Internal topography of major nerves of the forearm and hand: A current view. J Hand Surg, 1980; 5:1–18.
13. Kendall JP, Stokes IAF, O'Hara JP, Dickson RA: Tension and creep phenomena in a peripheral nerve. Acta Orthop Scand, 1979; 50:721–725.
14. Korff M, Bent SW, Havig MT, Schwaber MK, Ossoff RH, Zealer DL: An investigation of the potential for laser nerve welding. Otolaryngology—Head and Neck Surgery, 1992; 106: 345–350.
15. McClellan DL, Swash M: Longitudinal sliding of the median nerve during movements of the upper limb. J Neurol Neurosurg Psych, 1976; 39:566–570.
16. Merle M, Amend P, Cour C, Foucher G, Michon J: Microsurgical repair of peripheral nerve lesions. Peripheral Nerve Repair and Regeneration. 1986; 2:17–26.
17. Merle M, Medinaceli L: Primary nerve repair in the upper limb: Our preferred methods: Theory and practical applications. Hand Clinics, 1992; 8:575–586.
18. Millesi H, Terzis JK: Problems of terminology in peripheral nerve surgery. Microsurgery, 1983; 4:51–56.
19. Millesi H, Terzis JK: Nomenclature in peripheral nerve surgery. Clin Plast Surg, 1984; 11:1: 3–8.
20. Moberg E: Nerve repair in hand surgery: An analysis. Surg Clin North Am, 1968; 48:985–991.
21. Rydevik BL, Kwan MK, Meyers RR, et al: An in vitro mechanical and histologic study of acute stretching of rabbit tibial nerve. J Orthop Res, 1990; 8:694–701.
22. Seddon HJ: Nerve grafting. J Bone Joint Surg, 1963; 45B:447–461.
23. Sunderland S: The internal topography of the radial, median and ulnar nerves. Brain, 1945; 68:243–299.
24. Sunderland S, Bradley KC: The cross-sectional area of peripheral nerve trunks devoted to nerve fibres. Brain, 1949; 72:428–449.
25. Sunderland S: The anatomy and physiology of nerve injury. Muscle, 1990; 13:771–784.

26. Taleisnik J: The palmar cutaneous branch of the median nerve and the approach to the carpal tunnel. J Bone Joint Surg, 1973; 55A:1212–1217.
27. Wilgis EF, Murphy R: The significance of longitudinal excursion in peripheral nerves. Hand Clinics, 1986; 2:761–766.
28. Williams HB, Jabaley ME: The importance of internal anatomy of the peripheral nerves to nerve repair in the forearm and hand. Hand Clin, 1986; 2:689–707.

JOHN A. MCFADDEN
LEONARD GORDON

50

Arterial Repair at the Digital and Palmar Level

■ HISTORY OF THE TECHNIQUE

The surgical repair of small caliber blood vessels was first addressed in the literature in 1958 by Seidenberg and co-authors.[18] They demonstrated the technical feasiblity of repair of coronary, intracranial, and splanchnic vessels in dogs wieghing between 25 and 75 pounds. The fundamental principles of atraumatic technique and careful suture repair were established in this study even though these vessels seem rather large by today's standards. Interestingly, no mention of magnification was made. Numerous reports began to appear describing laboratory and clinical successes, new equipment and technology, and the successful repair of progressively smaller vessels.[3,4,10–13,15,18] In 1963, Jacobson noted that even very small technical errors resulted in thrombosis, and the use of an operating microscope was recommended. The relatively crude suture (7-0 silk) was noted to be limiting.[11] The same year, Holt described a sutureless arteriorrhaphy using coapting teflon rings with protruding pins, which is remarkably similar to the currently available 3M coupling device (Minneapolis, MN).[10] Chase and Schwartz challenged the need for expensive microscopy equipment by demonstrating the patency of 1.5-mm vessels repaired under $4\times$ loupe magnification.[3] Most surgeons, however, recognized the need for improved technology including high power magnification. Buncke and Schulz contributed the next major advance by emphasizing the need for appropriate suture material and microinstrumentation in addition to adequate magnification.[2] The silk suture used in previous studies suffered from three essential faults. The suture material was too tissue reactive, the needles were too large at the swage, and the suture diameter was simply much too large for the comparatively small vessel diameter. Buncke's group used a nonreactive nylon monofilament 10 μm in diameter. The needle was fashioned so that the swage was the same diameter as the suture. Although their overall patency rate in replanted rhesus monkey digits was poor, the equipment requirements and technical maneuvers for successful microanastomosis of vessels as small as 1 mm in external diameter was established.[2]

The application of microvascular techniques has made the successful repair of digital artery injuries commonplace. This was not the case before 1963. In that same year, Kleinert and Kasden reported the salvage of devascularized but attached fingers by repair of the digital arteries.[12] A similar report followed in 1965.[13] Then, in 1968, Komatsu and Tamai reported the successful replantation of a thumb and ushered in an era of widespread clinical application of microvascular surgery.[14] By the 1970s, large series of successful replantations were reported.[19]

Despite the wealth of interesting articles describing the evolution of microvascular surgery, little is written specifically on the repair of isolated palmar arch and digital arterial lacerations. This chapter will describe our approach to such injuries understanding that such wounds are often complex with injury of associated structures. A knowledge of the treatment of tendon, nerve, and osseous injury is assumed, and we will address the management of palmar arch and digital arterial trauma specifically. Arterial injuries to the thumb are unique and are described in the chapter on thumb replantation.

■ INDICATIONS AND CONTRAINDICATIONS

The most obvious indication for exploration and repair of palmar arch and digital artery lacerations is inadequate arterial inflow into a digit. If the finger is pale and lacking in capillary refill or if associated injuries demand immediate surgery, then the diagnosis is easy. A word of caution, however, is warranted. It is quite possible for both digital arteries to a finger to be transected and the finger may still have the appearance of adequate perfusion. This has fooled the emergency medicine physician or surgery resident on more than one occasion. The benign appearance of the injury may occur due to the influx or pooling of venous blood while the hand is dependent. The relatively low metabolic demand may not make the digit immediately cyanotic. Additionally, some arterial blood will find its way into the finger through the intact dorsal skin, although this is generally inadequate to sustain the injured part. Care must be taken to examine the hand in an elevated position. It is good practice to manually exanguinate the digit by gentle compression and then observe for the adequacy of refill. A finger with at least one intact artery should quickly refill and maintain good tissue turgor in the pulp space. This observation is made relative to the other uninjured fingers as peripheral vasoconstriction may affect all extremities. A good-quality, portable Doppler instrument should be able to detect the presence of absence of the digital arteries and is quite useful. In many institutions, it is common practice to repair cutaneous injuries and advise patients to return for elective flexor tendon or nerve repair. A thoughtful examination will help avoid the disastrous consequences of discharging a patient with an inadequately perfused finger. An assessment of all injured structures is made and an operative plan is formulated.

Regional or general anesthesia is used depending on the expected duration of the procedure. For procedures expected to last less than 2 hours, an axillary block is sufficient. For longer procedures, we most commonly use general anesthesia. The procedure is done under tourniquet control, and the contralateral lower extremity is also prepared if there is any suspicion that a vein graft may be required.

■ SURGICAL TECHNIQUES

The anatomy of the palmar arch and digital arteries is complex and warrants discussion to plan the operative procedure. Numerous variations exist, and there is no clear consensus as to the most common pattern. The clinically pertinent anatomic features are described herein.

The dominant source of blood supply to the fingers (thumb excluded) is derived from the superficial palmar arch. The superficial palmar arch is the termination of the ulnar artery and may have contributions from the radial artery or a persistent median artery. The ulnar artery courses through Guyon's canal bounded by the hook of the hamate radially, the pisiform ulnarly, the insertion of the transverse carpal ligament dorsally, and the volar carpal and piso-hamate ligaments volarly. The artery takes an abrupt turn at the hook of the hamate heading towards the radial side of the hand. The arch is convex toward the fingers and lies in a plane just deep to the palmar aponeurosis yet superficial to the branches of the median nerve. The arch is approximately at a level in line with a tangent drawn along the distal border of the radially adbucted thumb.

There are most commonly four major branches arising from the superficial palmar arch. The most ulnar is a proper digital artery supplying the ulnar side af the small finger. There are then three common digital arteries to the *small and ring, ring and long, and long and index* fingers before the vessel terminates in a radial direction. Each of these common digital arteries gives rise to two proper digital atreries to the sides of the two fingers of that web space[5–7,16,20–22] (Fig. 50–1). The origin of the digital artery to the radial side of the index finger is the source of some deliberation. Parks reported that in 50% of 50 cadaver hands, the proper radial digital artery to the index finger arose from the princeps pollicis artery, thus making it radial artery dominant.[17] Weathersby reported similar findings with 45% arising from the deep palmar arch.[21] Coleman and Anson, however, reported that in 77% of 265 hands examined, a fourth common digital artery arose from the superficial palmar arch, which then supplied the radial side of the index finger and ulnar side of the thumb.[5] For practical applications, it is best to remember that the radial digital artery to the index finger may be derived primarily from the ulnar artery or the radial artery, and one third of the time has a contribution from both the superficial and deep arches.

The superficial palmar arch may terminate as a small connecting branch to the first

■ FIGURE 50–1
The most common vascular pattern of the superficial palmar arch. The proper digital artery to the radial border of the index finger may arise from the deep arch. The thumb arterial supply is usually radial dominant.

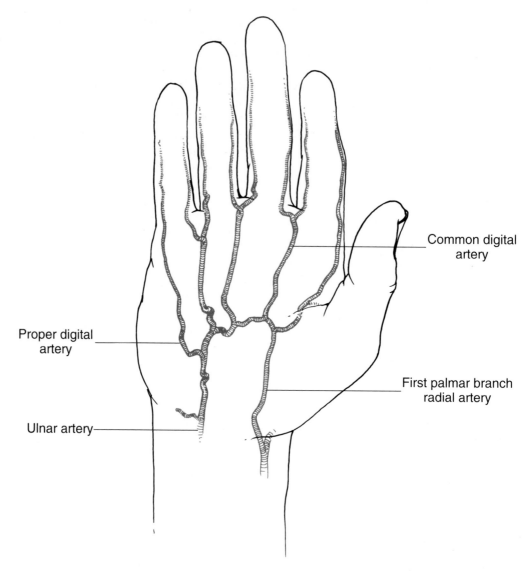

Common digital artery

Proper digital artery

First palmar branch radial artery

Ulnar artery

palmar branch of the radial artery or by direct communication to the princeps pollicis artery. Other connections between the superficial and deep systems include intermetacarpal perforating branches at the level of the web space that provide collateral circulation to the fingers when the common digital arteries are lacerated proximal to this level.[5,16,20]

The proper digital arteries course through the volar side of the finger along a line drawn just volar and parallel to the midlateral line of the finger. The vessels are deep to the digital nerves having made a transition, in the web space, from a more superficial location in the palm. Viewed in cross section, the digital arteries are subcutaneous to the glaborous palmar skin, superficial to Cleland's ligament, and deep to Grayson's ligament. The digital arteries are usually 1 to 1.5 mm in diameter in the adult patient, but both arteries to a given finger may not be the same diameter. A good rule to remember when referring to the digital arteries is that the index finger is usually ulnarly dominant, the small finger is radially dominant, and the arteries to the central two fingers are nondominant.[1]

The procedure is begun by using copious amounts of saline irrigation to remove all clot and foreign body from the wound. Under tourniquet control, the skin edges and any devitalized subcutaneous fat is debrided. All injured structures are identified.

Associated fractures and flexor tendon injuries are managed before repair of the arterial injury. In general, the repair sequence would include osseous stabilization first followed by flexor tendon repair, nerve repair, and then arterial repair. This prevents disruption of the delicate microvascular repair by doing "bigger" components of the operation, such as tendon repair, at a later time. This operative sequence also proceeds in a deep to superficial progression and facilitates exposure. Specific details for the repair of associated injuries appear elsewhere in the text.

The laceration is usually extended using the standard Brunner zigzag incision. These are fashioned so that the corners of the incisions are placed in flexion creases where appropriate. The flaps are elevated sharply taking care to avoid injury to the underlying neurovascular structures. The flaps are held open by tacking the skin edges to the adjacent palmar skin with interrupted 4–0 nylon sutures. A good quality hand retractor is essential for maintaining stability of the injured part during the repair process. We use the Tupper hand retractor.

There are essentially three approaches to repair of the injured digital artery (Fig. 50–2). The first and simplest approach to digital artery repair is direct repair of a clean laceration of the artery. This is often the case with lacerations from a sharp, clean object such as a knife or glass. In this setting, the artery can usually be mobilized enough to allow debridement of the damaged vessel end and completion of a primary arteriorraphy. The initial dissection is done under 3.5× loupe magnification. Once the vessel ends have been identified, the operating microscope is brought into the field and used for further dissection. Jewelers forceps and curved adventitial scissors are used to dissect the vessel ends. The vessel is

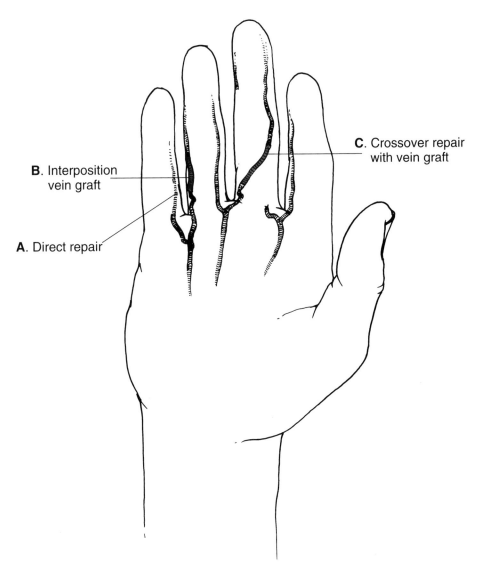

C. Crossover repair
with vein graft

B. Interposition
vein graft

A. Direct repair

■ FIGURE 50–2
Types of arterial repair at the digital level are: **A,** direct; **B,** reversed interposition vein graft; and **C,** crossover repair with vein graft.

carefully inspected for evidence of hemorrhage in the vessel wall that would indicate injury to the adventitia. The vessel end should be dissected back to the first uninjured branch and should have a normal appearance. A double approximating microvascular clamp is next applied with enough excess vessel length in the jaws of the clamp to allow debridement of the vessel ends. Straight microscissors are used to make a clean perpendicular cut at the vessel end. The adventitia is stripped from the vessel end with curved scissors. The vessel is gently dilated with vessel dilators, and any remaining thrombus is removed. The vessel is irrigated with heparinized saline solution at a concentration of 10 units of heparin per milliliter of solution.

The repair is then performed using 9–0 or 10–0 nylon suture as appropriate for the vessel size. Standard microsurgical technique is used.[8,9] The triangulation method of repair is the simplest and allows easiest visual access of the vessel lumen. Once the repair is completed, the microvascular clamps are removed and the finger reperfused. We usually allow a waiting period of about 10 minutes and then confirm patency of the repair.

In many cases, there may be tissue loss requiring repair of the injured artery by reversed interposition vein grafting. This is most commonly seen in power tool injuries. In these cases, the vessel ends are prepared under the operating microscope as was previously described. The resulting defect is measured, and a vein graft of appropriate length is harvested from the dorsum of the foot.

There are numerous small veins on the dorsum of the foot that serve well for vein grafting of the digital arteries. These can usually readily be seen through the skin and marked on the skin with a sterile marker. A tourniquet is next inflated, and the dissection is performed under tourniquet control. An Esmarch bandage is not used because having some blood in the venous side of the circulation facilitates visualization of the vein. An incision is made directly over the vein, and subcutaneous dissection is performed. We usually harvest more vein than is needed in case any technical difficulties require debridement of the end of the vein graft during the microanastomosis. Such may be the case if there is a valve right at the end of the cut vein. This would have to be removed before proceeding with arteriography. The side branches of the vein are doubly ligated with 8–0 nylon suture and divided. Both ends of the vessel are ligated with 6–0 silk. The distal end of the vessel is then marked with sterile ink for orientation as to direction of flow. The vein graft is then removed and the wound closed with 5–0 nylon suture. The vein graft is transferred to the hand for microscopic repair.

The vein graft is oriented so that the marked end of the graft is proximal and the unmarked end is distal. We usually perform the distal anastamosis first because this tends to be more difficult. The repair is made with the finger fully extended with a very slight amount of tension to the vein graft. It is important to avoid excess length of the vein graft to prevent tortuosity or kinking of the graft during flexion of the finger. Under the operating microscope, the distal anastamosis is performed using a standard microsurgical technique. The proximal end of the injured vessel and the vein graft are then placed in a double approximating clamp under very slight tension. The graft is trimmed to the appropriate length, and a microvascular repair is performed. Vascular clamps are removed, and the finger is reperfused.

The crossover method of digital artery repair can be performed with or without a vein graft and is used when the proximal and distal ends of the injured digital arteries cannot be matched on the same side of the finger. The proximal end of the injured vessel may only be usable on one side of the finger and a usable distal end on the contralateral side. If this is the case, the proximal vessel can be mobilized to allow it to cross over to meet the distal end of the contralateral digital artery. This may or may not require interposition vein graft, depending on the circumstances. The details of the microvascular repair are the same as described previously in this chapter. One must document this type of reconstruction by an appropriate drawing in the patient's chart so if future surgery, such as nerve or tendon reconstruction, is required, inadvertent injury to the repaired digital vessels can be avoided.

Injuries to the palm may occur at a level that is either distal to the palmar arch or through the palmar arch. Injuries that are distal to the palmar arch may or may not require vein graft for reconstruction. Injuries through the palmar arch often result in a loss of a portion of the arch requiring vein graft reconstruction. Each of these will be addressed separately.

The common digital arteries or proper digital arteries may be lacerated distal to the palmar arch. Brunner zigzag incisions are used for exposure, and microscopic dissection of the injured vessel ends is a prerequisite to the repair. After mobilization and debridement of the vessel ends, a standard microvascular arteriorrhaphy is performed.

Some injuries may result in a loss of a segment of the common digital or proper digital arteries or may cause a laceration through the bifurcation of two proper digital arteries from the common digital artery. An interposition vein graft is usually required. The vein graft is harvested as described previously. The only difference here is that, on occasion, it may be possible to harvest a Y-shaped vein graft from the foot to reperfuse two adjacent digital arteries simultaneously. Care must be taken with respect to direction of flow when configuring this graft. If a Y-shaped graft cannot be found, then one finger may be reperfused by a reverse interposition vein graft between the proximal common digital artery stump and the distal proper digital artery to the involved finger. The digital artery to the adjacent finger may then be repaired to this vein graft using an end-to-side anastomosis with or without additional vein graft (Fig. 50–3). It is important to note when using this

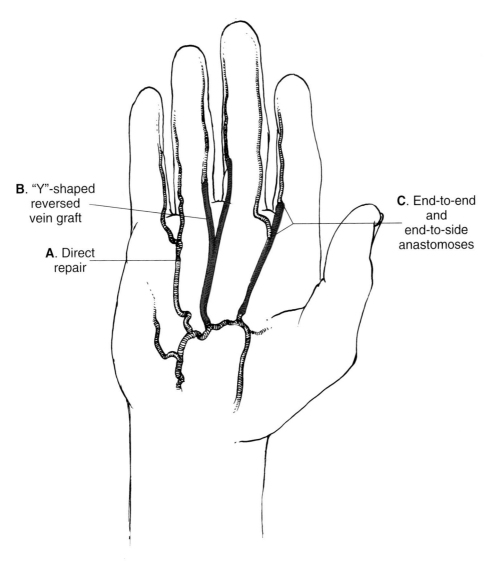

■ FIGURE 50–3
Types of arterial repair of the common digital arteries are: **A,** direct; **B,** a Y-shaped reversed vein graft; and **C,** a vein graft with an end-to-end and an end-to-side anastomosis.

B. "Y"-shaped reversed vein graft

A. Direct repair

C. End-to-end and end-to-side anastomoses

technique that two fingers may be dependent on one proximal anastomosis. Although theoretically one might object to this approach, we have had success in applying this technique.

Injuries to the palmar arch may cause the loss of vascular inflow to any or all of the fingers. This is a complex injury, which may require numerous microvascular anastmoses for reperfusion of all involved fingers. Simple lacerations of the palmar arch do not commonly cause a devascularizing injury to the finger. This is because of collateral circulation and contributions from the deep palmar arch. If a simple laceration to the palmar arch occurs, it is not unreasonable to treat it by simple ligation provided there is good vascular inflow into both sides of the injury. If there is no pulsatile backflow from the distal side of the injured palmar arch, then it is repaired using standard microsurgical technique. Most commonly, however, injuries to the palm are transverse and may cause destruction of a length of the palmar arch as it courses transversely across the palm. In these cases, vein graft reconstruction is required.

There are numerous ways to approach vein graft reconstruction of the palmar arch depending on the configuration of the injury. Obviously it would not be possible to describe the repair of every possible pattern of injury, but the basic principles remain the same. The arch is generally reconstructed with a reverse interposition vein graft, which is repaired to the ulnar artery or palmar arch proximally and the most radial devascular-

■ FIGURE 50–4
A typical configuration of a reconstructed superficial palmar arch; additional vein grafts can supplement the repair.

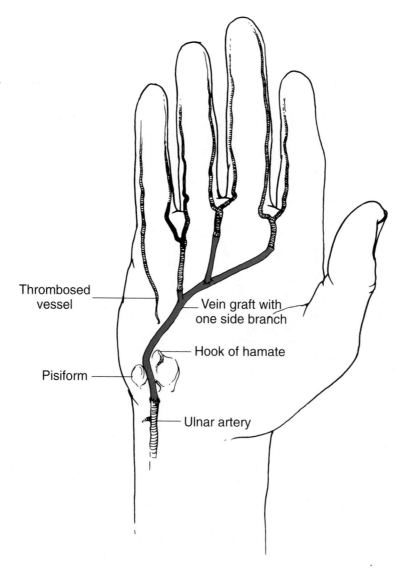

Thrombosed vessel

Vein graft with one side branch

Hook of hamate

Pisiform

Ulnar artery

ized finger distally (Fig. 50–4). In most patients, the thumb will be adequately perfused by inflow from the radial artery. If there is any evidence of an inadequate inflow into the thumb, however, it may be necessary to anastomose the reconstructed palmar arch to the princeps pollicis artery or ulnar digital artery to the thumb. Usually the outflow to the reconstructed arch will be repaired to the common digital branch to the long and index finger web space. This should provide adequate inflow into those two fingers. Next the common digital branch to the long and ring finger web space and the common digital branch to the ring and small web spaces are repaired to the vein graft. This could be done in an end-to-side fashion. A somewhat more elegant approach is to harvest a vein graft that has two or three appropriately sized side branches that can be used for repair to the common digital arteries. Obviously care has to be taken to preserve the direction of flow and avoid any venous valves.

Once repair of the injured arterial structures is completed, the wound is thoroughly irrigated and the skin flaps closed with interrupted 5–0 nylon sutures. Sterile dressings are applied with a large amount of gauze fluff dressings in the palm. A plaster splint is applied dorsally so as not to compress the repaired arterial structures.

After surgery, the patient is kept under close observation with the hand well elevated. We usually use at least 12 hours of recovery room or intensive care to allow "one on one" nursing. Any perceived failure of the microvascular repair would prompt re-exploration. Tobacco, caffeine, and other vasoconstriction substances are avoided. An anticoagulation protocol is initiated that consists of either low molecular weight dextran or systemic heparin. The dose of anticoagulant depends on the weight of the patient. For a 70-kg person, 30 ml/hr of intravenous dextran is administered after a loading dose of 500 ml. Heparin is generally given as a loading dose of 5000 units followed by continued infusion of 800 to 1000 units an hour while adjusting the partial thromboplastin time to 1.5 times the control. Systemic anticoagulation is discontinued on the seventh postoperative day, and 325 mg of aspirin is given daily for 1 month. Systemic anticoagulants have not conclusively improved the salvage rate for this type of injury; therefore, adverse side effects should be considered on an individual basis.

■ REHABILITATION

We begin early mobilization of the injured hand. A splint is fashioned from thermoplastic material about the fifth postoperative day. Obviously, the exact protocol for rehabilitation depends on associated injuries. For isolated arterial injuries, a palmar splint in the position of protection is applied. Full active range of motion is encouraged starting on the fifth day. The sutures are removed by 10 days postoperatively, and therapy is continued until the maximum range of motion has been achieved.

■ OUTCOMES

The outcome for repair of the digital arteries and palmar arch parallels the experience for replantation. An overall survival rate of 85% can be expected for the revascularized finger. The statistics, in fact, may be better because there is no venous component to the injury. Functional results depend on the associated injuries, and conclusions cannot be drawn from the discussion of the management of arterial injuries alone.

References

1. American Society of the Hand: Self-assessment examination, 1994. Englewood, CO: 1994:3.
2. Buncke HJ, Schulz WP: Experimental digital amputation and reimplantation. Plast Reconstr Surg, 1965; 36:62–70.
3. Chase MD, Schwartz SI: Consistent patency of 1.5 millimeter arterial anastomoses. Surg Forum, 1962; 13:220–222.
4. Cobbett JR: Microvascular surgery. Br J Surg, 1967; 54:842.
5. Coleman SS, Anson BJ: Arterial patterns in the hand based upon a study of 650 specimens. Surg Gynecol Obstet, 1961; 113:409–424.
6. Earley MJ: The arterial supply of the thumb, first web and index finger and its surgical application. J Hand Surg, 1986; 11B:163–174.
7. Edwards EA: Organization of the small arteries of the hand and digits. Am J Surg, 1960; 99:837–846.

8. Gordon L: Microsurgical reconstruction of the extremities: Indications, technique and post-operative care. New York: Springer-Verlag, 1988.

9. Green DP: Operative hand surgery, 3rd Ed, New York: Churchill Livingstone, 1993; 1039–1083.

10. Holt GP, Lewis J: A new technique for end-to-end anastomosis of small arteries. Surg Forum, 1960; 11:242–243.

11. Jacobson JH: Microsurgical technique in repair of the traumatized extremity. Clin Orthop, 1963; 29:132–145.

12. Kleinert HE, Kasden ML: Salvage of devascularized upper extremities including studies on small vessel anastomosis. Clin Orthop, 1963; 29:29–38.

13. Kleinert HE, Kasden ML: Anastomosis of digital vessels. J Kentucky Med Assoc, 1965; 63: 106–108.

14. Komatsu S, Tamai S: Successful replantation of a completely cut off thumb. Plast Reconstr Surg, 1968; 42:374–377.

15. Lendvay PG: Anastomosis of digital vessels. Med J Australia, 1968; 2:723–724.

16. Little JM, et al: Circulatory patterns in the normal hand. Br J Surg, 1973; 60:652–655.

17. Parks JP, Arbelaez J, Horner RL: Medical and surgical importance of the arterial blood supply of the thumb. J Hand Surg, 1978; 3:383–385.

18. Seidenberg B, et al: The technique of anastomosing small arteries. Surg Gynecol Obstet, 1958; 106:743–746.

19. Tamai S: Digit replantation. Clin Plast Surg, 1978; 5:195–209.

20. Warwick R, Williams PL: Gray's Anatomy, 35th British ed. Philadelphia: W. B. Saunders, 1973:656–657.

21. Weathersby HT: The artery of the index finger. Anatomical Record, 1955; 122:57–64.

22. Zbrodowski A: The anatomy of the digitopalmar arches. J Bone Joint Surg, 1981; 63B: 108–113.

LEIF T. ÖSTRUP
ANDERS BERGGREN

51

Mechanical Coupling of Vessels

Through almost a century, surgical innovators have presented various mechanical, nonsuture methods for quick and effective coupling of blood vessels. These techniques have ranged from simple cuff techniques using tubes made from absorbable or nonabsorbable materials; to the use of tissue adhesives, electrocoaptation, and laser energy; to rather complex stapling machines.[2,11,13,25] The concept of vascular anastomosis using rings incorporating small pins was revived by Holt and Lewis[10] in 1960, but the principal technique and instrumentation were described by Nakayama[15] and are used widely, both in the laboratory and in clinical surgery. The ring-pin technique necessitates only a 90° eversion of the vessel wall, in contrast to almost all other ''mechanical'' methods, in which a 180° eversion of the vessel is required. This difference is of vital importance in the anastomosis of either small vessels or rigid, arteriosclerotic human vessels.

With the evolution of microvascular surgery, it became obvious that each of these earlier coupling methods had serious disadvantages. Because the instruments and techniques were originally intended for larger vessels, they were awkward and inefficient when applied to small vessels.

Two mechanical anastomotic devices have been specifically designed for work under the operating microscope. Daniel and Olding[7] developed a three-part, absorbable cuff-and-collar device, which was used in 20 clinical microsurgical procedures, but their device, which required a 180° eversion of the vessel ends, was never marketed. In 1979, we began development and experimental trials of the UNILINK instrument system[17]—a ring-pin device that is now commercially available and in use worldwide as the 3M (St. Paul, MN) ''Precise'' Microvascular Anastomotic Device (PMAD).

■ HISTORY OF THE TECHNIQUE

The PMAD is currently applicable for the anastomosis of arteries and veins in the course of clinical revascularization, replantation, or vascularized tissue transfers in the hand, wrist, and distal forearm. It is applicable to the anastomosis of arteries and veins with an external diameter in the range of 0.8 to 2.8 mm. Different ring sizes with inner diameters of 1.0, 1.5, 2.0, and 2.5 mm are available, and larger ring sizes are under development. Although recommended mainly for fast and safe end-to-end anastomosis, it is possible to perform an end-to-side PMAD anastomosis, but this is technically more difficult and should normally not be attempted in thick-walled or mineralized human arteries.

In the hand, anastomosis is easy to perform in the fairly thin-walled radial and ulnar arteries at the wrist level, as well as in the large dorsal veins on the back of the hand. For arteries in the palm or wrist, the device is particularly useful and time-saving when vein grafts are being used to bridge arterial gaps. In finger replantations, the PMAD can be used for the dorsal veins of the finger but is often difficult to use on the digital arteries because of limited exposure and difficulties obtaining enough space to accommodate the ringholding wings.

Relative contraindications include the inability to obtain an optimal vessel/ring size match. The use of the device also can be problematic in very thick-walled, mineralized arteries, where intimal breakage during eversion or total obstruction of the ring by the thick walls can occur.

Vessel size discrepancy is not a major problem in venous anastomoses, because the vein wall is thin enough to be folded and plicated on the same pin if needed.[3] To date, we have not observed any disadvantages from leaving the anastomotic ring as a small piece

■ INDICATIONS AND CONTRAINDICATIONS

of "foreign body" in the wound. The rings have not been palpable, even in patients where the anastomosis was placed directly under a skin graft.

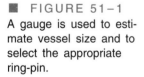

■ SURGICAL
TECHNIQUES

The PMAD consists of an autoclavable, multiple-use holding instrument, into which disposable wings, factory-loaded with a pair of ring-pins, are inserted. The tiny ring-pins each have 6 stainless steel pins that, during completion of the anastomosis, pass through corresponding holes on the opposite ring, securing the anastomosis by friction. Gauges for exact measurement of vessel diameter are included in the instrument system (Fig. 51–1).

Clamping, flushing, and preparation of the vessel ends before anastomosis are performed in the same manner as in standard microvascular procedures. The adventitia does not need to be stripped from the vessel, but can merely be pushed back to prevent it from being inverted into the lumen. However, in thick-walled vessels, it may facilitate eversion to strip or cut away adventitia from the immediate anastomotic area. The vessel ends in either arteries and veins should be carefully dilated, using a special, highly polished vessel dilator forceps. This procedure has not resulted in thrombus formation, either experimentally or clinically.

It is extremely important to choose the right ring-pin size for the vessel to be anastomosed. Using the measuring gauges, the inner diameter of the relaxed and fully dilated vessel should be roughly 10% larger than the chosen ring size. If a ring that is too large is chosen, the intima of the vessel wall will tear during eversion; or the use of a ring that is too small may result in luminal obstruction, especially in arteries.

The suitable, color-coded, disposable ring-holding wings are mounted in the instrument and introduced into the microscopic field. The vessel end is slipped through the ring, using a microhook or microforceps, and the everted vessel wall is mounted on the pins, distributing equal tension around the circumference. We prefer to do this in a triangular way, starting with the pin situated at the 12-o'clock position, then followed by pins at the 4- and 8-o'clock positions (Fig. 51–2), and finally by the three intermediate pins (Fig. 51–3). Other microsurgeons[12] prefer a "half-and-half" sharing technique, starting with the pins at the 12- and 6-o'clock positions. Great care must be taken that the intimal layer is impaled by each pin. If the pins perforate the vessel wall too far from the edge, incorrect apposition of the everted vessels results.

The other vessel end is mounted on the opposite ring-pin in the same way (Fig. 51–4), and the knob on the instrument handle is then simply turned clockwise (Fig. 51–5). This brings the two ring-pins together, and the anastomosis is completed. The joined ring pair

■ FIGURE 51–1
A gauge is used to estimate vessel size and to select the appropriate ring-pin.

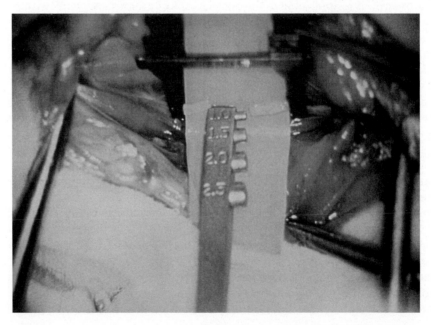

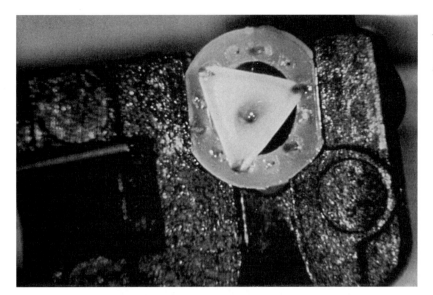

■ FIGURE 51–2
The triangulation technique for pinning the vessel onto the ring-pin.

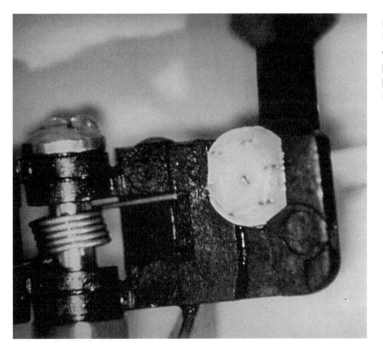

■ FIGURE 51–3
By passing the tissue over the intermediate pins, the vessel is completely mounted on the ring-pin.

is automatically ejected by the instrument and left free in the wound. Because the closing force in the disposable wings is often insufficient for complete ring closure one should always, just before ejection, slightly squeeze the wings with a small hemostat, to assure that the rings are closely locked together (Fig. 51–6). After release of the microvascular clamps, the anastomosis is checked, and there should normally be no leakage (Fig. 51–7).

To facilitate end-to-side anastomosis, we have used a specifically designed small balloon expander in the lumen of the recipient vessel, introduced through a transverse cut in the vessel wall.[19,21] After air inflation two to three times, to dilate the vessel wall and thus to ease the eversion procedure, the balloon is withdrawn and the ring-pin placed over the incision. The vessel wall is then everted over the pins and the donor vessel mounted on the opposite ring in the same manner as described above. Inherent in this mechanical technique of end-to-side anastomosis is the production of an incident angle between the two vessels of approximately 90°, which does not adversely affect blood flow.[14]

■ FIGURE 51–4
The same procedure is
completed on the other
ring-pin.

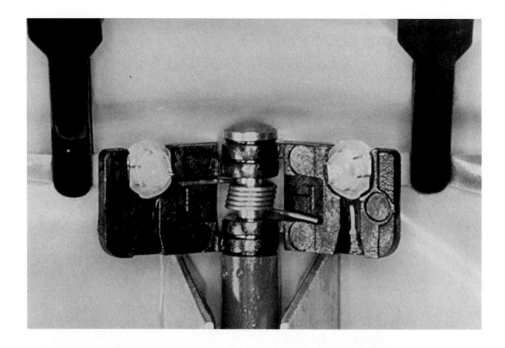

■ FIGURE 51–5
The jaws carrying the
ring-pins are approxi-
mated by turning the ap-
plicator knob.

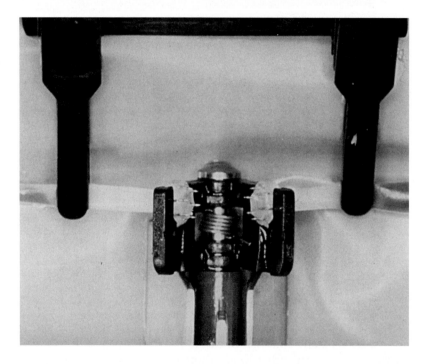

■ TECHNICAL
ALTERNATIVES

It is evident that the principal alternative to PMAD anastomosis is suture anastomosis. It must be stressed that conventional microvascular suture technique must be fully mastered in clinical replantation, revascularization, or free tissue transfer. The PMAD should not be regarded as a substitute for suture anastomosis—it should be considered an equally reliable complement to suture anastomosis.

The main advantage of the PMAD is that selected microvascular anastomoses can be accomplished more quickly and easier than suture techniques. With moderate training, a single operator can complete the whole anastomotic procedure in 2 to 5 minutes, and our experiences from microsurgical education and training show that it is much easier for the beginner in microsurgery to create a well-functioning vessel anastomosis with the PMAD

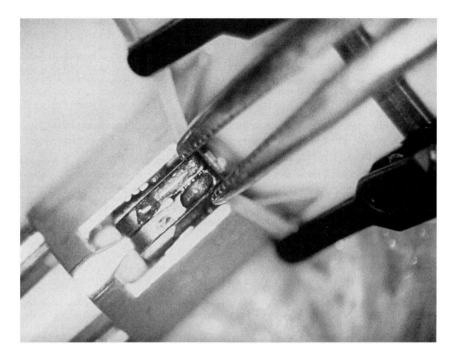

■ FIGURE 51–6
A fine hemostat is used to gently squeeze the opposed jaws, securing the ring-pins together.

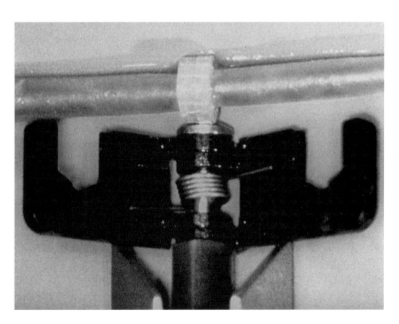

■ FIGURE 51–7
The completed anastomosis with the ring ejected from the jaws of the applicator.

than with suture technique. The experienced microvascular surgeon has a short learning curve using the PMAD.[1]

The speed of the method makes it particularly advantageous in interpositional vein grafting for venous or arterial defects, where regularly only one fourth of the length of time for suture anastomoses is needed.[8,20] This is even true when artificial polytetrafluoroethylene (PTFE) microvessel prostheses are inserted.[12]

With the PMAD method, as opposed to suture anastomosis, no foreign material is exposed in the vessel lumen, and the anastomosis can be readily inspected before closure, whereas suture anastomosis carries a risk of unrecognizable suture error. Conversely, a small amount of vessel length is "used up" by vessel eversion. If the anastomosis fails[24] everted vessel, together with the coupling rings, will have to be excised resulting in a difficult to address vessel deficit.[24]

■ REHABILITATION   The PMAD method and the incorporation of the ring-pin devices require no specific modifications in immediate or extended postoperative care. The rehabilitation in cases in which the devices are used should be guided by the care of associated structures such as bones and joints, tendons, nerves, and overlying skin or skin grafts.

■ OUTCOMES   Patency rates with the PMAD are fully comparable to patency rates generally accomplished by experienced microsurgeons with suture technique. In our clinical cases, the patency rate for critical PMAD-anastomoses was 98%,[4] and in clinical series presented by other investigators,[1,24] patency rates varied from 78% in acute trauma cases to 100% in elective free tissue transfers.

Apart from the numerous PMAD-anastomoses completed for technical, educational or training purposes, we have a total series of 379 controlled, experimental anastomoses (arteries and veins) with only two failures (thrombotic occlusions, both in arteries), which is a clear indication of the reliability and efficacy of the technique.

The hemodynamic consequences of anastomosing small blood vessels with the PMAD are minimal, and in principle similar to those observed after suture anastomosis.[5] Hemodynamic characteristics of the repaired vessel recover with the course of the normal healing process. Histological and SEM evaluation have shown a smooth, well healed and completely endothelialized anastomotic junction after 2 weeks.[3,6,18] Although the thickness of the vessel wall is usually reduced inside the anastomotic rings (due to atrophy of the media, most evident in arteries), there are no aneurysms, either in the short or long term.[23] The breaking strength of the anastomosis exceeds that of the normal, unoperated vessel.[19] In terms of patency, the PMAD is equal to suture anastomosis in vessels severely damaged by irradiation.[22] We consider the PMAD technique to be a dependable and efficient method if clinically anastomosing arteries and veins in the human hand and wrist.

■ ACKNOWLEDGMENT   We are deeply grateful to medical engineer Håkam Rohman, who with unique skills and imagination realized all our ideas (and quite a few of his own), and to engineer Wilhelm Ståhl for his never-failing, patient, and enthusiastic support.

References

1. Ahn CY, Shaw WW, Bern S, Markowitz B: Clinical experience with the 3M microvascular anastomotic-coupling device in free tissue transfer. J Reconstr Microsurg, 1992; 8:171–172.
2. Androsov PI: New method of surgical treatment of blood vessel lesions. Arch Surg, 1956; 73: 902–910.
3. Berggren A, Östrup LT, Lidman D: Mechanical anastomosis of small arteries and veins with the Unilink apparatus: a histologic and scanning electron microscopic study. Plast Reconstr Surg, 1987; 80:274–283.
4. Berggren A, Östrup LT, Ragnarsson R: Clinical experiences with the Unilink/3M Precise Microvascular Anastomotic Device in critical anastomoses. Scand J Plast Reconstr Hand Surg, 1992; in press.
5. Blair WF, Steyers CM, Brown TD, Gable RH: A microvascular anastomotic device: Part I. A hemodynamic evaluation in rabbit femoral arteries and veins. Microsurg, 1989; 10:21–28.
6. Blair WF, Morecraft RJ, Steyers CM, Maynard JA: A microvascular anastomotic device: Part II. A histologic study in arteries and veins. Microsurg, 1989; 10:29–39.
7. Daniel RK, Olding MD: An absorbable anastomotic device for microvascular surgery: clinical applications. Plast Reconstr Surg, 1984; 74:337–342.
8. Gilbert RW, Ragnarsson R, Berggren A, Ötrup LT: Microvenous grafts to arterial defects. The use of mechanical or suture anastomoses. Arch Otolaryngol Head Neck Surg, 1989; 115: 970–976.
9. Gilbert RW, Ragnarsson R, Berggren A, Östrup LT: Strength of microvascular anastomoses: comparison between the Unilink anastomotic system and sutures. Microsurg, 1988; 10:40–46.
10. Holt GP, Lewis FJ: A new technique for end-to-end anastomosis of small arteries. Surg Forum, 1960; 11:242.
11. Inokuchi K: A new type of vessel-suturing apparatus. Arch Surg, 1958; 77:954–957.
12. Lanzetta M, Owen E: Use of the 3M Microvascular Anastomotic system in grafting 1 mm

arteries with polytetrafluoroethylene prostheses: a long term study. Paper read at the 1st Meeting of the European Federation of Microsurgical Societies, Rome, 1992.

13. Mallina RF, Miller TR, Cooper P, Christie SG: Surgical stapling. Sci Am, 1962; 207:Vol 4: 48–56.

14. Nam DA, Roberts TL, Acland RD: An experimental study of end-to-side microvascular anastomosis. Surg Gynecol Obstet, 1978; 147:339–342.

15. Nakayama K, Tamiya T, Yamamoto K, Akimoto S: A simple new apparatus for small vessel anastomosis (free autograft of the sigmoid included). Surgery, 1962; 52:918–931.

16. Nylander G, Ragnarsson R, Berggren A, Östrup LT: The Unilink system for mechanical microvascular anastomosis in hand surgery. J Hand Surg, 1989; 14A:44–48.

17. Östrup LT, Berggren A: The Unilink instrument system for fast and safe microvascular anastomosis. Ann Plast Surg, 1986; 17:521–525.

18. Ragnarsson R: Mechanical microvascular anastomosis. Experimental and clinical evaluation of the Unilink system. Thesis. Linköping University Medical Dissertations, 1988; No. 279.

19. Ragnarsson R, Berggren A, Östrup LT, Gilbert RW: Arterial end-to-side anastomosis with the Unilink system. Ann Plast Surg, 1989; 22:405–415.

20. Ragnarsson R, Berggren A, Östrup LT, Franzén L: Microvascular anastomosis of interpositional vein grafts with the Unilink system. A comparative experimental study. Scand J Plast Reconstr Surg, 1989; 23:23–28.

21. Ragnarsson R, Berggren A, Östrup LT: Microvenous end-to-side anastomosis: an experimental study comparing the Unilink system and sutures. J Reconstr Microsurg, 1989; 5: 217–224.

22. Ragnarsson R, Berggren A, Klintenberg C, Östrup LT: Microvascular anastomoses in irradiated vessels: a comparison between the Unilink system and sutures. Plast Reconstr Surg, 1990; 85:412–418.

23. Ragnarsson R, Berggren A, Östrup LT: Long term evaluation of the Unilink anastomotic system. A study with light and scanning electron microscopy. Scand J Plast Reconstr Hand Surg, 1992; 26:167–171.

24. Steichen JB: Clinical results of vessel repair by the 3M Mechanical Anastomotic-Coupling Device. J Reconstr Microsurg, 1992; 8:173–174.

25. Vogelfanger IJ, Beattie WG: A concept of automation in vascular surgery: a preliminary report on a mechanical instrument for arterial anastomosis. Can J Surg, 1958; 1:262–265.

52

Replantation of Fingers

■ HISTORY OF THE
TECHNIQUE

In 1962, a surgical team led by Ronald Malt was the first to successfully reattach a completely amputated human limb.[32] Eventually, excellent experimental and clinical work supported the feasibility of reattaching amputated digits.[5,16] Subsequently, surgeons in Japan and China were among the first to report successful replantation of completely amputated digits. Major replantation centers in the United States, Japan, China, Australia, Germany, Switzerland, and Austria have participated in the successful replantation of several hundred digits, hands, feet, and limbs.[5,20,30,35]

The operating microscope, introduced in 1921 by Nylen for otologic surgery and mass-produced in 1953 by Zeiss, has been improved so that focus, magnification, and motion in multiple planes can be controlled with a foot-pedal switch. Originally modified jeweler's tools, today's microsurgical instruments have been improved to allow maximum control with minimum fatigue and strain for the surgeon. Microvascular approximators provide an atraumatic method for holding vessels much better than did the aneurysm clips originally used for replantation.

■ INDICATIONS AND
CONTRAINDICATIONS

Replantation of amputated upper extremity parts should be performed by surgeons who are trained in surgery of the hand and upper extremity and who have demonstrated competence in microvascular surgery. In most circumstances, especially those involving multiple digits, it is most desirable to use rotating teams of surgeons. Replantation surgeons generally should be available on a rotating basis 24 hours a day. Assistants should be familiar with the sequence of events, instruments, and other necessary equipment. It is essential to have institutional support, including surgical suites available 24 hours a day, intensive care units, and personnel to provide nursing and anesthesia care.

The final decision regarding replantation rests with the patient and the surgeon; consequently, there are no absolute indications for replantation of an amputated part. The most suitable candidate for digital replantation is a young, healthy person with multiple digital amputations (Fig. 52–1) or with an isolated thumb amputation. All factors should be carefully considered before a decision is made.

As noted previously, trained and interested personnel are integral to the success of any replantation effort. The absence of the essential preoperative, intraoperative, and postoperative personnel is a contraindication to replantation. Similarly, 24-hour availability of operating rooms with up-to-date and functional equipment and instruments is a requirement of successful replantation. If the facilities are not available, replantation is contraindicated.

Replantations have been reported in patients a few weeks old[2,3] and in those older than 70 years. The smaller digital vessels in young patients increase the technical difficulty of microvascular anastomoses. Postoperative anxiety may contribute to vasospasm, and rehabilitation of children may be less predictable than that of adults. Nevertheless, satisfactory functional results have been reported, and most authors consider replantation for amputations of almost any part in children, including some in the lower extremity.

Age alone is not a contraindication to replantation. While older patients may obtain satisfactory function after replantation of fingers, thumbs, and hands, they rarely obtain adequate sensibility, forearm and hand muscle strength, or coordination sufficient enough to warrant replantation of more proximal amputations. The patient's physiologic status and general activity level and the presence of other diseases should be carefully consid-

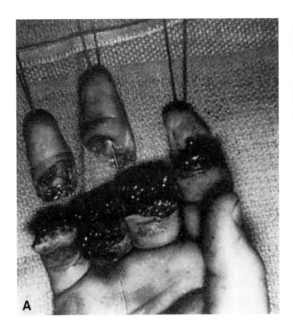

■ FIGURE 52–1
Multiple digital replantation: 20-year-old man with saw injury. **A,** Multiple digits amputated distal to flexor superficialis insertion.

ered. Because the potential for return of sensibility and motion is better after replantation at and beyond the tendinous portion of the forearm, replantation in older patients may be considered if their injury occurs more distally.

The following types of injuries may have the best outlook for survival and return of function following replantation: (1) clean, sharp amputations, (2) minimal local crush amputations, and (3) avulsion amputations with minimal proximal and distal vascular injury. Significant additional proximal and distal injury to the limb should not be present. Ring avulsion-degloving injuries may be revascularized and salvaged; however, the outlook for useful function is extremely uncertain after complete degloving or digital amputation.[40]

Despite dramatic results that have been obtained with the use of vein grafts and primary free tissue transfer for limb salvage, extensive crushing, avulsing, and segmental injuries at multiple levels damage the distal vascular tree sufficiently to frequently defeat replantation attempts. This is especially true with digital injuries. Ring avulsion amputations through the joint usually are best treated by closure of the amputation; however, satisfactory functional results can be obtained in patients with less severe ring avulsion injuries.[15,40]

Wounds with extensive soil contamination, especially from agricultural injuries, carry a high risk of infection and should be carefully evaluated before replantation.

Thumb amputations at almost any level should be considered for replantation,[32,43] even with nerve and tendon avulsion and joint involvement. If the thumb can be revascularized, sensibility can be restored with nerve grafts or a neurovascular island pedicle transfer, and motion can be obtained with tendon grafts or transfers. Replantation of single and multiple digits distal to the flexor digitorum superficialis insertion usually results in satisfactory function. Some patients do well without replantation of single digit amputations; such a replantation may be worthwhile for some musicians, patients with other special occupations, some children, and for other aesthetic or social reasons.[41] Replantation of a single digit also may be helpful if the remaining attached digits are severely damaged, especially with tendon and nerve injury over the proximal phalanx.

If multiple digits have been amputated, replantation of at least two digits in the long and ring positions should provide digits to use in combination with the thumb for pinch and for power grip.

In bilateral amputations, replantation on each side ideally should provide better function than bilateral prostheses. If replantation is not desirable because of extensive injuries on

■ FIGURE 52–1 *(continued)* **B and C,** Finger flexion and extension 7 months following replantation. Sensory return permits useful finger function. (From Wright PE II, Jobe MT: Microsurgery. In: Crenshaw AH, (ed): Campbell's Operative Orthopaedics, 8th ed, St. Louis: Mosby-Year Book, 1992.)

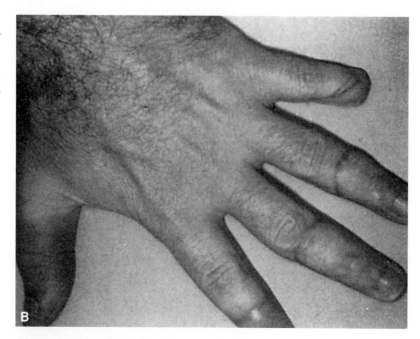

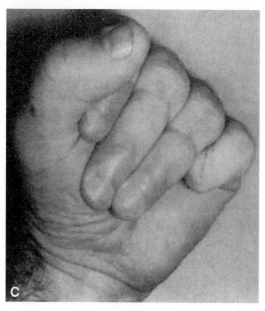

one side, the "best" side should be selected, and parts from one side may be attached to the opposite, more suitable stump.[2]

With some exceptions, replantation of single-digit amputations proximal to the flexor digitorum superficialis insertion and especially through the proximal interphalangeal joint usually results in poor function. The replanted digit usually is stiff and tends to impair the overall function of the remaining digits by getting in the way. The obvious exception to this generalization is an amputated thumb.

For parts with no muscle (digits), the allowable warm ischemia time may be 8 hours or more. Because the amount of skeletal muscle in digits is not significant, the risk to the patient is minimal if digits are replanted. Cooled digits have been replanted successfully at 30 to 94 hours and more after amputation.

If amputated parts have been frozen, placed in unphysiologic solutions such as formaldehyde or alcohol, or allowed to dry excessively, the chance for survival is so low that replantation attempts are futile.

After the amputated part has been retrieved, it may be rinsed with sterile saline, Ringer's lactate, or other physiologic solutions so that excess contamination is removed. The part should then be treated in one of two ways. It may either be wrapped with sterile gauze or other clean material, soaked in sterile Ringer's lactate or saline solution, and placed in a plastic bag, which is then sealed; or, it may be immersed in a plastic bag containing a physiologic solution such as Ringer's lactate or physiologic saline. The bag is then placed on ice in an insulated container so that the part is not touching the ice to avoid freezing of the part. Dry ice should not be used; neither should the part be warmed. No attempt should be made to clamp, dissect, ligate, or cannulate vessels on the amputated part because this may cause more vessel damage.

Amputated parts previously deformed or disabled because of some congenital or acquired disorder are not likely to function satisfactorily after replantation. Such conditions include scar deformity and contracture secondary to previous burns or mangling injury, residual deficits due to spinal cord or peripheral nerve injuries, and stroke-related deformities.

In polytraumatized patients, significant intracranial, thoracic, cardiovascular, or major intraabdominal visceral injuries may require lengthy lifesaving operations. Digits may be cooled to 4° C in a refrigerator and saved for later replantation if the patient's condition permits.

Patients with preexisting peripheral vascular disease may be poor replantation candidates if their vessels have an unsatisfactory appearance when inspected under the operating microscope. Digital replantation should be approached cautiously in patients with diabetes mellitus, rheumatoid arthritis, lupus erythematosus, other collagen-vascular diseases, or significant atherosclerosis. Chronic or uncontrolled medical illnesses such as coronary artery disease, myocardial infarction, peptic ulcer disease, malignant neoplasms, and chronic renal or pulmonary disease may increase the anesthetic risk enough to preclude replantation.

Replantation should be approached cautiously in patients with psychiatric illnesses. If the amputation is an act of self-inflicted mutilation or attempted suicide, replantation may have considerable risk of failure. If the amputated part is a focus in the patient's mental illness, it is likely that the part, if replanted, will be reinjured. If the amputation occurs as a true accident, especially in a patient whose mental illness is treatable, the outlook for replantation might be better. Valid psychiatric evaluation of patients with amputated parts in an emergency room is extremely difficult. The inability of patients with profound psychiatric illness to understand their fragile postoperative condition and to cooperate with the difficult rehabilitation process further complicates their care as replantation patients.

■ SURGICAL TECHNIQUES

While the patient is being evaluated and prepared, the replantation sequence is expedited if another surgeon of the replantation team takes the amputated part to the surgical suite to clean it and to evaluate the extent of injury.

While the amputated part is being dissected, the patient usually is given an axillary brachial plexus block with the long-acting local anesthetic bupivacaine. This, with monitored intravenous sedation, usually provides satisfactory anesthesia for digital or hand replantation in most adults and older children. For younger children, anxious patients, and patients with multiple digital or bilateral amputations, general anesthesia is preferable.

Pad the operating table well and apply a warming blanket to prevent excessive body cooling during prolonged surgery. Exsanguinate the limb and use a pneumatic tourniquet to provide a bloodless field for initial dissection of the stump and to control any subsequent significant bleeding. Deflate the tourniquet after the initial dissection, and reinflate it as needed during the procedure. Once the patient is comfortable, thoroughly cleanse the stump with an antiseptic solution and meticulously debride all debris and nonviable tissue.

Clean the part with povidone iodine and saline solution. Rinse with copious saline. Cool the part by placing ice in a pan, covering the ice with a sterile plastic drape, and then

■ FIGURE 52–2
Dissection of amputated digit. **A,** Incisions on radial and ulnar midline (broken lines) allow reflection of dorsal and palmar flaps. **B,** Carefully and gently dissect structures to be repaired using microsurgical instruments and meticulous technique.

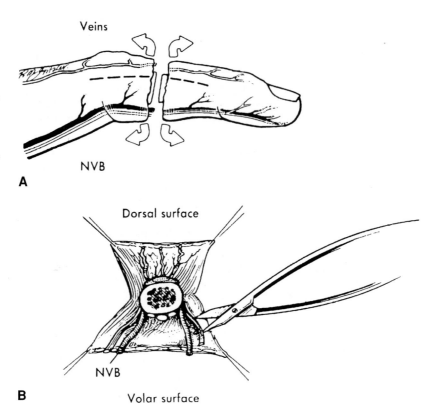

placing a sterile drape sheet over the plastic and ice. Place the part on the drape sheet for dissection under loupe or microscope magnification. Use a separate set of instruments to dissect the part on a field isolated from the amputation stump. If two teams are available, one team should work on the amputated part while the other works on the stump.

Expose the arteries, veins, nerves, tendons, joint capsule, periosteum, and other salvageable soft tissues in the amputated part. In digits, exposure is usually best achieved through radial and ulnar midlateral incisions. Dorsal and palmar flaps are reflected and the digital arteries and nerves are located in the palmar flap (Fig. 52–2). Careful, gentle, and meticulous dissection is required to locate satisfactory veins in the dorsal flap. After the arteries have been identified and marked with a small suture, dissect the veins from the dorsal skin flap. Three or four suitable veins usually are found on the dorsum of the digit between the metacarpophalangeal joint and the midportion of the middle phalanx. Distal to this point, there may be only one or two suitable veins. Although volar veins can be seen, they frequently are less than 1 mm in diameter and may not be suitable for anastomosis. Mark the veins with small sutures and proceed to prepare the vessels for anastomosis. Carefully preserve these small structures and use sutures of 8–0 or 9–0 nylon to mark them so that they can be easily located later. Final debridement of vessels is done using the operating microscope. Flexor and extensor tendons are identified and marked with sutures.

Although multiple vein grafts can be used to provide tension-free anastomoses, it is our practice to shorten bone so that vein grafts are unnecessary. Bone is shortened with a small oscillating saw if a cortical segment is to be removed (Fig. 52–3). Rongeurs are used to remove short spikes of bone. Protect soft tissues with small retractors or periosteal elevators if motorized instruments are used. The part of the digit having the most bone to spare usually is shortened. In digits this shortening rarely exceeds 1 cm.

The stump is then prepared. Use mid-lateral and ulnar incisions. Identify arteries, veins, and nerves with magnifying loupes or the operating microscope and tag them with sutures of 8–0 or 9–0 nylon. Dissect and debride flexor and extensor tendons and hold them with

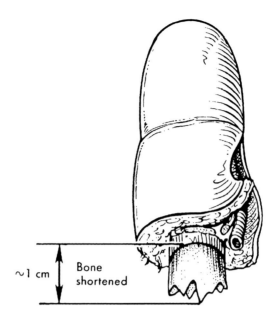

~1 cm | Bone shortened

4–0 nylon sutures for later repair. Tenorrhaphy may be expedited if 4-0 polyester suture is placed in the tendons as marking suture, using the surgeon's preferred intratendinous suture arrangement. Irrigate or debride clots from the proximal arterial stumps and open the stumps to allow free arterial flow. If no satisfactory flow can be achieved, additional dissection and vessel resection is needed. Prepare the bone in the amputation stump using a rongeur to form a transverse surface for bone reduction.

Internal fixation is done next in the digit. This is expedited by placing Kirschner wires in the amputated part before placing it on the amputation stump. A longitudinal Kirschner wire combined with an obliquely crossing Kirschner wire usually is sufficient (Fig. 52–4A). On occasion interosseous wires are used near joints (Fig. 52–4B). Plates and screws rarely are needed. If the amputation has occurred through a joint, or if the extensor mechanism is irreparable, arthrodesis usually is preferable (Fig. 52–4C).

If the amputation is clean and sharp, perfusing the digital arteries is unnecessary. If the part has been crushed or avulsed, ecchymoses along the vessels or abrasions and lacerations may signal distal vascular bed injury. In this situation gently perfuse the digital artery and vascular tree using a small Silastic catheter and heparinized Ringer's solution or saline. If there is no return of the perfusate or if it extravasates from vessels injured distally, blood flow is unlikely to be maintained after anastomosis. In such situations, unless in the surgeon's judgement there are other reasons to proceed, replantation should not be performed.

After all structures have been thoroughly cleansed, debrided, and identified, begin the repair. As indicated in the discussion that follows, certain conditions or circumstances will dictate a variation in the order of repair. The following is the usual order of repair: bone, extensor tendons, flexor tendons, arteries, veins, and nerves. If nerve repair will endanger repaired vessels, nerve repair should precede vessel anastomosis. The wounds are loosely closed and covered.

Bone fixation in digits usually is achieved by first shortening the bone and then using two parallel intramedullary axial Kirschner wires or a single axial Kirschner wire supplemented by an oblique Kirschner wire to control rotation (Fig. 52–4A). The technique chosen usually is the one that appears easiest at the time. Wires should be placed to allow joint motion, if possible. Occasionally when the amputation is near an undamaged joint, wire loops (3–0 or 4–0) may be inserted at right angles to each other through drill holes on either side of the fracture (Fig. 52–4B). Plates and screws rarely are indicated in digital replantation. Care must be taken to maintain axial and rotational alignment when more

A, Bone fixation is usually achieved with two parallel Kirschner wires, 1, or a single Kirschner wire supplemented with an oblique wire, 2. **B,** Wire loop fixation suitable for amputation near undamaged joint. **C,** Primary arthrodesis with crossed wires for amputation through irreparably damaged joint.

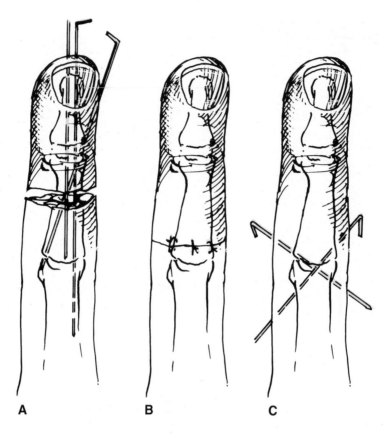

A   B   C

than one digit is replanted. Periosteal suture with 4–0 or 5–0 absorbable suture may be done after bone fixation.

Because of extensive damage to amputated parts or to the amputation stump, anatomic restoration of digits is at times impossible. In these situations a functioning part may be restored by moving digits from their original anatomic position to a more suitable position (Fig. 52–5). In bilateral digital amputations, parts from one hand may be better replanted to the opposite hand. Priority should be given to restoration of a thumb and replantation of a digit in the index or long position for pinch. Consideration also should be given to providing long, ring, and little digits for restoration of grip. When digital transposition is considered in bilateral amputations, the dominant hand usually is given priority.

Extensor tendons are repaired using nonabsorbable sutures. For injuries between the proximal and distal interphalangeal joints, individual mattress stitches or a roll stitch may be used. Tendons injured between the metacarpophalangeal and proximal interphalangeal joints are repaired with a roll stitch.

If the amputating injury involves crushing or avulsion of the part and if the amputation is through the digits proximal to the flexor digitorum superficialis insertion, or if tendon substance has been lost, flexor tendons are not repaired. Delayed tendon grafting is planned in these circumstances. Silicone rods may be inserted at the time of replantation if the condition of the wound is appropriate and if the extent of contamination and potential for infection are limited.

If the flexor tendons have been sharply severed, both tendons usually are repaired primarily for injuries proximal to the flexor digitorum superficialis insertion. Our usual tenorrhaphy involves a rectangular or abbreviated crisscross configuration of the suture using a single knot buried in the cut tendon end. Alternatively, separate sutures may be placed in each tendon end.[38] Nerve and vessel repairs are completed, and the tendon sutures are then tied to complete the tendon repair. This method makes vessel and nerve repair easier because the finger is not flexed until the tendon sutures are tied. Nonabsorb-

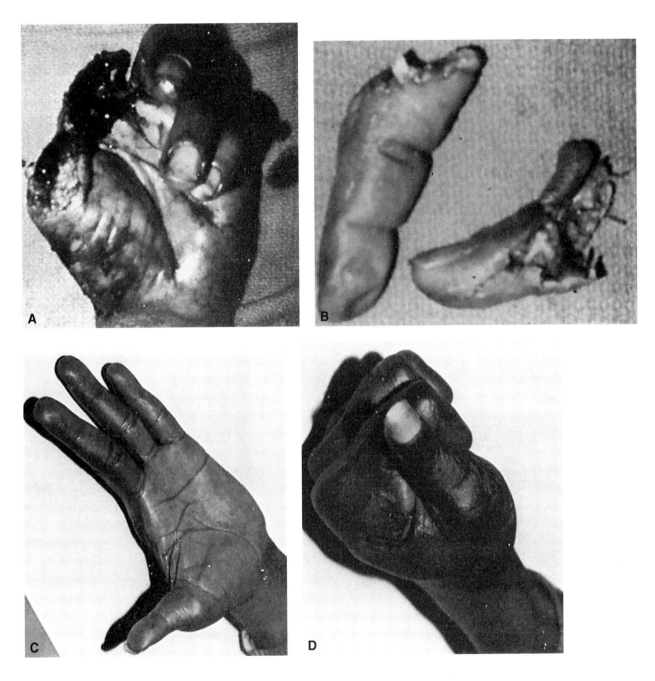

■ FIGURE 52–5

Replantation involving transposition of digits. **A,** Amputation of thumb and index finger. **B,** Amputated thumb unsuitable for replantation. Index finger replanted to thumb position. **C, D, and**

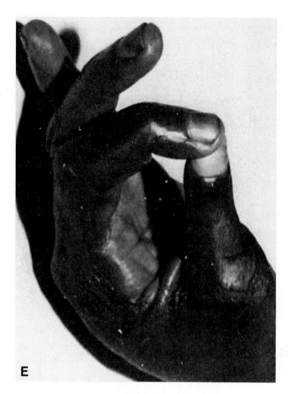

able synthetic sutures or 4–0 wire is used for tenorrhaphy. When technically feasible, the digital flexor sheath is repaired with 5–0 or 6–0 nonabsorbable suture, usually nylon.

A flexor digitorum profundus tendon injured distal to the flexor digitorum superficialis insertion near the distal interphalangeal joint is reattached with a pullout wire. For injuries over the middle phalanx the distal tendon stump is tenodesed to bone or tendon sheath.

In the digits our practice is to repair the arteries first. This allows evaluation of the adequacy of flow across the anastomosis and through the digit before proceeding with the replantation. If veins are repaired first, arterial anastomosis is necessary to determine whether blood will flow through the digit and across the venous anastomosis. Performing arterial repair first allows the dorsal veins to fill and helps identify the vein most suitable for repair.

After all arteries and veins have been identified and marked with sutures, mobilize them by dissecting them free from the surrounding tissues using gentle and meticulous technique. Transect small side branches and tributaries using 9–0 suture ligatures or bipolar electrocautery, depending on the size of the branch. This mobilization will aid in a tension-free anastomosis. Once the vessels have been mobilized, the size of the gap between the vessel ends will determine whether the anastomoses can be accomplished without additional bone shortening or the use of an interpositional vein graft. Vessel tension is evaluated with the digit in nearly full extension. If the vessel approximator holds the vessel ends together, of if the two 9–0 or 10–0 sutures can be placed without vessel separation, usually a successful anastomosis can be accomplished. Use magnification, including the operating microscope, to examine the vessel wall. If evidence of thrombosis in the wall is found or if the intima has been damaged, excise the damaged segment. If an avulsion appears to have caused the intima to be pulled out of the vessel ("telescoped"), excise that portion of the vessel as well. After all damaged vessel is excised, re-examine the gap between the vessel ends to determine if a direct anastomosis is still feasible. With the tourniquet deflated, ascertain that there is pulsatile flow from the proximal end of the artery.

After vessel preparation is completed, anastomose the vessels in the order noted above. Attempt to repair both digital arteries and as many veins as possible, preferably two veins for each artery. Use small vessel-approximating clips on the digital vessels. Similar clips are available for the larger vessels. Keep in mind the length of time these clips are in place, especially on small (1 mm) vessels; time elapsed should be kept to a minimum, preferably less than 30 minutes. After the vascular clips are released, bathe the vessel in lidocaine or bupivacaine to minimize spasm.

For digital vessels use 10–0 or 11–0 monofilament suture. Most digital arteries require six to eight sutures; digital veins require 8 to 10 sutures, and sometimes more. Expect a small amount of blood leakage; this usually stops in a few minutes. If spasm is encountered, the application of warm saline, topical lidocaine, papaverine, reserpine, and magnesium sulfate may help to relieve the spasm.

Vessel debridement may leave a gap too large to be corrected by simple end-to-end repair. Techniques such as interpositional grafting with arterial segments and reversed segments of vein, vein harvesting and shifting in the injured digit, and the transposition of arterial and venous pedicles from adjacent, uninjured digits are then indicated. Vein grafts usually are harvested from unsalvageable amputated parts, the dorsum of the hand or forearm, and from the foot. In some situations, a single vein graft anastomosed to a single digital artery proximally may be attached to two digital arteries distally, using side-to-end anastomoses or a Y configuration of the graft. When vein grafts are used, care should be taken to maintain the proper (reversed) flow direction so that flow is not obstructed by valves. The harvested vein grafts should have approximately the same diameter as the recipient vessel.

Using the operating microscope, locate and examine the nerve ends, which were identified in the initial dissection of the digits. Gently dissect the nerves free of the surrounding connective tissue and mobilize them so they can be repaired without excessive tension. Occasionally it may be necessary to transect small branches to provide sufficient mobilization. Once the proximal and distal ends of the nerve have been mobilized, inspect them using the operating microscope or magnifying loupes and trim minimal amounts of nerve from each end to allow identification of good fascicles. If the injury has been sharp, the nerves are repaired primarily. Use two to four epineurial stitches of 9–0 or 10–0 monofilament nylon suture to carefully align and approximate the fascicles.

Because of the additional operating time required for nerve grafting and the uncertainty regarding the extent of intraneural injury, primary nerve grafting usually is not done. Instead, suture the ends of the avulsed or crushed nerve together with an 8-0 mattress suture, anticipating later nerve exploration, debridement, repair, or grafting. As an alternative, if the nerve ends cannot be brought together, secure them to the adjacent soft tissues so that they can be easily identified and mobilized later for nerve grafting.

When multiple digits have been amputated, an attempt is made to save all fingers. Skeletal fixation is accomplished for all amputated parts, then tendon followed by vessel repair is done on all digits. Usually, the repair is done from the radial side of the hand proceeding to the ulnar side with the surgeon seated on the axillary side of the arm. As as alternative, replantation of the central digit followed by the radial and ulnar digits with the surgeon alternating sides allows easier access to the digits.

After all structures have been repaired, close the skin primarily if the procedure has been completed promptly, if no excessive swelling is present, and if the skin edges can be approximated without tension. Some areas may be left open to heal by secondary intention or to be covered with skin grafts. Nerves, vessels, bone, joints, and tendons should not be exposed if the wounds are left open. Satisfactory alternatives include closure with Z-plasties; local rotation of skin; remote, two-stage pedicle flaps; single-stage transfer of composite tissue (free flaps); and split-thickness skin grafts. In our experience, primary remote pedicle flaps and free flaps have not been needed. A combination of skin flap rotation, split-thickness skin graft, and leaving the wound partially open has been satisfactory.

Apply medicated gauze to the skin wounds, and use a bulky dressing to cover the dorsal and palmar surfaces. Fluffed cotton or synthetic material provides a soft and gently conforming dressing. Moisten the padding with physiologic saline or Ringer's lactate

■ FIGURE 52–6
Replantation bandage.
Bulky bandage, well-pad-
ded with soft, non-
compressing cotton, sup-
ported with plaster splint.
Replanted digits exposed
for monitoring. (From
Wright PE II, Jobe MT:
Microsurgery. In: Cren-
shaw AH (ed): Camp-
bell's Operative Orthopaedics, 8th ed, St. Louis:
Mosby-Year Book, 1992.)

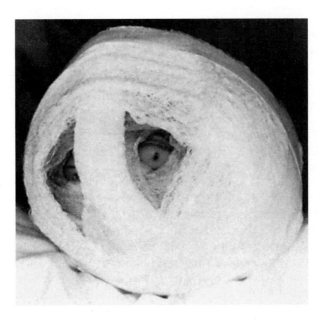

solution to allow blood to be absorbed into the bandage more readily and permit the
bandage to conform more easily to the contours of the part. Avoid localized pressure at
all times.

The part is adequately padded and a short-arm dorsal plaster splint is applied to support
the fingers, hand, and wrist. A palmar splint may be added for additional support. Tightness or constriction is avoided when securing the bandage. The fingertips and small areas
of skin are left exposed for evaluation of the circulation (Fig. 52–6). The wrist is slightly
flexed, as are the metacarpophalangeal and interphalangeal joints. During the first week,
the bandage is moistened with physiologic solution every 8 hours to prevent dried blood
from forming circumferential crusts that might have a constricting effect. Although early
and frequent dressing changes may be necessary for the evaluation of the circulation or
to determine the source and extent of any bleeding, our policy has been to delay the initial
dressing change for about 1 week in uncomplicated replantations. This decreases the risk of
disturbing the fragile vascular anastomoses and lessens the chance of stimulating vascular
spasm.

Postoperative management should include a comfortably warm room and sufficient
analgesic medication and sedation for the patient to minimize emotional distress. The
replanted part is positioned with the hand at heart level as long as the appearance of the
part is satisfactory. If the replanted part appears congested and cyanotic, elevation on
several pillows may be helpful. If the part becomes pale, positioning the part below the
level of the heart may improve arterial flow. Depending on the extent of the injury, the
patient usually is kept at bed rest except for bathroom activities for the first 3 to 7 days.
Generally, the more extensive the injury, the slower the mobilization.

Avoidance of smoking by the patient and visitors, and abstinence from caffeine-con-
taining beverages are measures that help to prevent vasospasm in the early postoperative
period. Vasospasm related to pain and emotional distress may be prevented or minimized
through the use of appropriate narcotic analgesics and sedative medication such as chlorpromazine.

It is our practice to use dextran, 500 ml every 24 hours (100 ml/kg/day in children) for
3 days, combined with aspirin 600 mg twice daily for 5 to 7 days. After hospital discharge,
aspirin is continued for another 2 weeks. Smoking and caffeine are not allowed for approximately 1 month.

Various anticoagulants, including heparin, low molecular weight dextran, aspirin, dipy-
ridamole, and coumadin have been used.[12] The use of heparin has been advocated for
patients believed to be at high risk for thrombosis, especially those with extensive crushing

or avulsing injuries, poor flow from the cut ends of vessels before anastomosis, poor or equivocal flow across completed anastomoses, and replantations in small children. Appropriate dosages should be individualized for each patient. Antibiotics usually are given for 1 week after surgery.

Nerve blocks are beneficial in the postoperative period to prevent vasospasm. If small Silastic catheters are left adjacent to the median and ulnar nerves, 4 to 5 ml of bupivacaine 0.25% injected every 6 to 8 hours may be sufficient. Stellate ganglion sympathetic blocks or axillary brachial plexus blocks with bupivacaine can be done once or twice daily if necessary.

In the immediate postoperative period, skin color, turgor, and temperature should be carefully monitored. If digital probes can be easily added, pulse oximetry also may be helpful.

Although the clinical determination of the color, capillary refilling, temperature, and turgor is easily made, there is room for error because of the subjective nature of these factors, especially color and temperature. This combined with the possibility that considerable ischemic injury may occur before clear clinical signs are present has led to the development and use of a variety of mechanical monitoring devices and techniques, including ultrasonic and laser Doppler probes, plethysmography, skin temperature probes, transcutaneous oxygen tension measurements, hydrogen washout techniques, and skin fluorescence measurements.

Both the Doppler probe and plethysmographic techniques are reasonably accurate indicators of arterial flow; however, they are not as accurate in evaluating venous flow. The use of skin temperature monitoring probes presently is a simple and reliable adjunct to the clinical evaluations. With separate temperature probes attached to the revascularized tissue, adjacent normal tissue, and the dressing, relative and absolute changes in the temperature can be monitored constantly. A drop in the temperature of the replanted digit below 30° C or a fall of more than 2° to 3° C below a normal digit is considered a sign of circulatory compromise.

The work of Smith and co-authors[33] and Matsen and co-authors[24] indicates that the transcutaneous oxygen measurements show changes in oxygen tension several hours before the onset of clinical signs of ischemia and before temperature changes occur. This and other techniques hold promise for the development of monitoring techniques with increasing sensitivity.

■ REHABILITATION

The specific rehabilitation program for each patient depends on many factors, especially the patient's needs and motivation and the extent of injury to the part. Generally, no attempt is made to begin significant movement of bone, joint, or tendon for the first 3 weeks after replantation. Then, depending on the extent of injury, most replantation patients are treated in a manner similar to most patients with combined tendon, bone, and nerve injuries. After the first 3 weeks, most patients are encouraged to participate in a graduated program of active exercises at 3 weeks, active-assistive, and protected passive stretching and range of motion exercises supplemented by appropriate dynamic and static bracing and splinting, which gradually progresses from 3 to 4 weeks, extending for 4 to 6 months. Splinting is modified to assist with mobilization of joints and protection of tenorrhaphies and bone fixation. Resistive exercises begin at approximately 4 to 6 weeks.

■ TECHNICAL ALTERNATIVES

If the amputated part has been avulsed or if significant crushing makes the extent of intraneural injury unclear, consider primary nerve grafting or mark the cut ends of the nerve with sutures for later identification. Although time-consuming, if nerve grafting is elected, trim the nerve ends proximally and distally so that normal-appearing nerve can be identified. Harvest nerve grafts from unreplantable parts, the lateral antebrachial cutaneous nerve, or the sural nerve. Insert the nerve graft with the finger in nearly full extension, and secure it with monofilament 9–0 or 10–0 nylon interrupted suture.

If the replanted part demonstrates signs of inadequate circulation, prompt evaluation and management of the problem might allow salvage of a part that would otherwise be lost. Mechanical monitors of skin temperature, oxygen tension, hydrogen, and fluorescein dilution often detect significant changes in blood flow before clinically apparent ischemic changes develop. If the part is cool and has developed the pallor and loss of turgor consistent with arterial insufficiency or if it is cyanotic, congested, and turgid consistent with venous obstruction, several measures can be helpful in relieving the problem before the patient is taken to the operating room for exploration.

Medical-grade leeches, *Hirudo medicinalis,* are effective in relieving venous congestion; however, they may be a source of infection and should not be used in the presence of nonviable tissue. If arterial insufficiency is suspected, placing the part in a dependent position may be beneficial. Splints and dressings are loosened or removed to ensure that nothing is causing direct pressure on the vessels and that nothing is constricting the limb. Using gentle digital pressure, the arteries are lightly "milked" from proximally to distally and the veins from distally to proximally.

In distal injuries, if Silastic catheters have been left adjacent to the median or ulnar nerves, 4 to 5 ml of 0.25% bupivacaine are injected. Stellate ganglion sympathetic blocks and brachial plexus blocks also may be useful, especially in patients with troublesome vessel spasm. Although it is not part of our usual routine, many surgeons with extensive experience find it useful to administer heparin intravenously as a bolus of 3000 to 5000 units when attempting to salvage a failing replanted part.

If the replanted part does not respond to these measures, the surgeon must decide, based on his knowledge of the injury and his experience, whether returning to the operating room to explore the vessels is worthwhile. This decision should be made promptly, once definite signs of impaired circulation are evident. Reoperation is more likely to be successful if done within 4 to 6 hours of the development of signs of ischemia.

Although circulatory compromise related to the vessel repairs is the most pressing complication after replantation, other complications that occur in the early postreplantation period include bleeding, skin necrosis, and infection.

Excessive bleeding may be from vessels that have not been cauterized, or it may be caused by anticoagulant therapy. Significant skin necrosis usually occurs after closure of skin that initially appears viable but later undergoes necrotic changes resulting from the initial injury. Additional debridement and secondary closure with local flaps or skin grafts may be required. Significant sepsis is rare after replantation and usually can be satisfactorily managed with appropriate systemic antibiotics and wound debridement and drainage as needed.

Although the clinical signs may indicate whether the problem is arterial or venous, once the decision to reoperate is made, all anastomoses are evaluated. First, inspect the arterial anastomoses to determine patency. If one or more arterial anastomoses are not patent, excise the anastomoses, ensure that there is adequate pulsatile flow proximally, and repair the vessels. If proximal flow is inadequate or the proximal artery appears excessively damaged, dissect more proximally, find good artery, and interpose a reversed segment of vein graft. Similar problems may be encountered in the distal arteries. If good arterial trunks cannot be found, search for other arteries to substitute. Repair any vein graft as needed. Assess the arterial flow and perfusion distally, as well as the appearance of the part. Next, inspect all venous anastomoses to assess patency. If flow cannot be restored despite all efforts, consider reamputation.

If on initial inspection all arterial anastomoses are patent and none appear to have spasm, torsion, pressure, or thrombosis proximally or distally, attention should next be directed to the veins. If all venous anastomoses are patent, the veins proximal and distal to the anastomoses should be inspected to exclude compression, torsion, and thrombosis. If areas of thrombosis are found, excise those segments and either repair the vessel end to end or interpose vein grafts. If the venous anastomoses are found to be obstructed by thrombi, excise and repair them either end to end or with vein grafts. Next evaluate arterial and venous flow and the appearance of the part. If all available and suitable veins have been located, repaired, or grafted and satisfactory flow cannot be restored, consider reamputation. For digital injuries, techniques such as pulp incisions and wedge excision of the nail to allow venous oozing may allow sufficient flow to persist long enough for a digit to survive. In such patients, hemoglobin and hematocrit levels should be monitored closely so that blood volume loss may be corrected promptly.

In 15 large series, reporting almost 2,000 digital replantations, the average survival rate was 80%, with a range from 68% to 94%.[4,7,9–11,13,21,32,34–37,41,45]

■ OUTCOMES

However, success of digital replantation is better measured by the extent of return of useful function than by survival statistics. It also is more meaningful to compare function of the replanted part with amputation stump closure or prosthetic function at the level in question.

Different grading systems, based on factors such as ability to return to work, return of muscle function, range of motion, sensibility, ability to perform activities of daily living, and patient satisfaction, are used by most authors to evaluate function after replantation.[6,23,25,31,44] Tamai[34,35] reported 72% excellent and good results, and Wang and co-authors[42] found 62% to "have practically recovered their function." Berger and co-authors[3] found that 78% of their patients were able to integrate the replanted part into their usual activities for a successful functional result. Satisfactory function is reported in 62% to nearly 80% of replanted parts when patients who had replantation were compared with a group of patients who had amputations closed at similar levels.[14,18,26,33,39] Grip strength was found to be better in patients who had replanted thumbs and in those with replanted multiple digits.[14]

Goldner and co-authors[9] reported an average of 90° range of motion of the proximal interphalangeal joint in their patients, Hamilton and co-authors[10] reported ranges of motion from 30° to 70°, and Urbaniak and co-authors[41] reported 82° of motion after replantations distal to the flexor digitorum superficialis insertion and 35° in those more proximal.

Some generalizations apply to most, but not all, replantation patients. Patient satisfaction with replantation is high, and most would undergo replantation again. Most workers are able to return to some form of work. Our experience also suggests that the more proximal the injury, the less likely is the patient to be able to return to his former employment in a reasonable period of time. Some are able to return to work in the first 2 to 3 weeks, whereas others take 1.5 to 2 years; some never return to work. Goldner and co-authors[9] and Urbaniak and co-authors[41] reported return to work in approximately 6 weeks in their patients, while Kleinert and co-authors[17,18] and Schlenker and co-authors[32] reported that the average time before return to work was 7 months.

Almost all replantation patients experience cold intolerance.[1,19,27–29] Although it may take 2 years or more to improve, cold intolerance alone usually is not incapacitating. Most replantation patients regain protective sensibility; however, two-point discrimination, especially in more proximal injuries, rarely is less than 10 mm. Useful two-point discrimination has been reported in approximately 60% to 90% of replanted digits.[8–10,21,40,41] Goldner and co-authors[9] reported an average two-point discrimination of 10 mm; Urbaniak and co-authors,[39,41] 11.7 mm; and McLeod and co-authors[21] and Hamilton and co-authors,[10] 9 mm. Return of fine tactile discrimination is unusual. Residual limitation of movement is common, especially if a joint has been injured and if the flexor tendon injury in the hand lies between the metacarpophalangeal and proximal interphalangeal joints.

The age of the patient, the level of the injury, and the mechanism of injury have an effect on the functional results of digital replantations. The more distal the injury, the sharper the injuring mechanism, and the younger the patient, the better the prognosis. This probably is due to nerve regeneration and the return of sensibility and motor function.

Later complications, such as nonunion and malunion of bones, tendon adherence, joint stiffness, and delay in return of nerve function, usually can be managed with the usual techniques appropriate to these problems. For nonunion and malunion, bone grafts and internal fixation may be required. Tendon adhesions with loss of excursion may require tendolysis, and in some situations, tendon grafting as one- or two-stage procedures. Stiff joints may require capsulotomy, or if sufficient damage has occurred, interposition arthroplasty may salvage motion in selected patients. If a primary neurorrhaphy fails to show return of function in a reasonable length of time, or if the nerves are not repaired as part of the original replantation, re-exploration and repair or interpositional nerve grafting may be necessary. The nature and timing of specific reconstructive procedures depend on the individual patient's problems and needs and the judgment and experience of the surgeon.

References

1. Backman C, Nyström A, Backman C: Cold-induced arterial spasm after digital amputation. J Hand Surg, 1991; 16B:378–381.
2. Baker GL, Kleinert JM: Microvascular digit transposition following a two-digit amputation in an infant. J Reconstr Microsurg, 1992; 8:23–29.
3. Berger A, Millesi H, Mandl H, Freilingr G: Replantation and revascularization of amputated parts of extremities: a three-year report from the Viennese replantation team. Clin Orthop, 1978; 133:212–214.
4. Biemer E: Vein grafts in microvascular surgery. Br J Plast Surg, 1977; 30:197–199.
5. Buncke HJ Jr, Schulz WP: Experimental digital amputation and reimplantation. Plast Reconstr Surg, 1965; 36:62–70.
6. Burton RI: Problems in the evaluation of results from replantation surgery. Orthop Clin North Am, 1981; 12:909–927.
7. Gelberman RH, Urbaniak JR, Bright DS, Levin LS: Digital sensibility following replantation. J Hand Surg, 1978; 3:313–319.
8. Glickman LT, Mackinnon SE: Sensory recovery following digital replantation. Microsurgery, 1990; 11:236–242.
9. Goldner RD, Stevanoic MV, Nunley JA, Urbaniak JR: Digital replantation at the level of distal interphalangeal joint and the distal phalanx. J Hand Surg, 1989; 14A:214–220.
10. Hamilton RB, O'Brien BM, Morrison WA, MacLeod AM: Replantation and revascularisation of digits. Surg Gynecol Obstet, 1980; 151:508–512.
11. Horn JS: The reattachment of severed extremities. In: Apley AG (ed): Recent Advances in Orthopaedics, Edinburgh: Churchill Livingstone, 1969:49–78.
12. Idler RS, Steichen JB: Complications of replantation surgery. Hand Clin, 1992; 8:427–452.
13. Ikuta Y: Microvascular surgery, Hiroshima: Lens Press, 1975:42.
14. Jones JM, Schenck RR, Chesney RB: Digital replantation and amputation: comparison of function. J Hand Surg, 1982; 7:183–189.
15. Kay S, Werntz J, Wolff TW: Ring avulsion injuries: classification and prognosis. J Hand Surg, 1989; 14A:204–213.
16. Kleinert HE, Kasdan ML: Restoration of blood flow in upper extremity injuries. J Trauma, 1963; 3:461–474.
17. Kleinert HE, Juhala CA, Tsai T-M, Van Beek A: Digital replantation: selection, technique, and results. Orthop Clin North Am, 1977; 8:309–318.
18. Kleinert HE, Kutz JE, Atasoy E, et al: Proceedings: replantation of nonviable digits: ten years experience. J Bone Joint Surg, 1974; 56A:1092.
19. Koman LA, Nunley JA: Thermoregulatory control after upper extremity replantation. J Hand Surg, 1986; 11A:548–552.
20. Komatsu S, Tamai S: Successful replantation of a completely cut-off thumb: case report. Plast Reconstr Surg, 1968; 42:374–377.
21. MacLeod AM, O'Brien BM, Morrison WA: Digital replantation: clinical experiences. Clin Orthop, 1978; 133:26–34.
22. Malt RA, McKhann CF: Replantation of severed arms. JAMA, 1964; 189:716–722.
23. Malt RA, Remensnyder JP, Harris WH: Long-term utility of replanted arms. Ann Surg, 1972; 176:334–342.
24. Matsen FA III, Bach AW, Wyss CR, Simmons CW: Transcutaneous PO2: a potential monitor of the status of replanted limb parts. Plast Reconstr Surg, 1980; 65:732–740.
25. Milroy BC, Sackelarious RP, Lendvay PG, Baldwin MRA, McGlynn M: Classification and evaluation of the functional results of replanted parts of the hand at the Prince of Wales Hospital and the Prince of Wales Children's Hospital: 1984 to 1988. World J Surg, 1991; 15: 446–451.
26. Morrison WA, O'Brien BM, MacLeod AM: Digital replantation and revascularization: a long term review of one hundred cases. Hand, 1978; 10:125–134.

27. Nunley JA, Penny WH III, Woodbury MA, Koman LA: Quantitative analysis of cold stress performance after digital replantation. J Orthop Res, 1990; 8:94–100.

28. Nyström A, Backman C, Backman C, et al: Digital amputation, replantation, and cold intolerance. J Reconstr Microsurgery, 1991; 7:175–178.

29. Nyström A, Backman C, Backman C: Effects of cold exposure on the circulation of replanted fingers during the early postoperative period. J Hand Surg, 1991; 16A:1041–1045.

30. O'Brien BMcC, Miller GDH: Digital attachment and revascularization. J Bone Joint Surg, 1973; 55A:714–724.

31. Russell RC, O'Brien BM, Morrison WA, Pamamull G, MacLeod A: The late functional results of upper limb revascularization and replantation. J Hand Surg, 1984; 9A:623–633.

32. Schlenker JD, Kleinert HE, Tsai T: Methods and results of replantation following traumatic amputations of the thumb in sixty-four patients. J Hand Surg, 1980; 5:63–70.

33. Smith AR, Sonneveld GJ, Kort WJ, van der Meulen JC: Clinical application of transcutaneous oxygen measurements in replantation surgery and free tissue transfer. J Hand Surg, 1983; 8: 139–145.

34. Tamai S: Digit replantation: analysis of 163 replantations in an 11-year period. Clin Plast Surg, 1978; 5:195–209.

35. Tamai S: Twenty years' experience of limb replantation: review of 293 upper extremity replants. J Hand Surg, 1982; 7:549–556.

36. Tatsumi Y, Tamai S, Komatsu S, et al: Functional recovery following digit replantation. In Proceedings of the 17th Annual Meeting, Japanese Soceity for Surgery of the Hand, Tokyo, May, 1974.

37. Tsai T-M: Experimental and clinical application of microvascular surgery. Ann Surg, 1975; 2: 169–177.

38. Urbaniak JR: Replantation of amputated hands and digits. AAOS Instr Course Lect, 1978; 27: 15–26.

39. Urbaniak JR: Results of sensibility recovery in 100 replanted digits, International Hand Surgery Congress, Melbourne, Australia, 1979.

40. Urbaniak JR, Evans JP, Bright DS: Microvascular management of ring avulsion injuries. J Hand Surg, 1981; 6:25–30.

41. Urbaniak JR, Roth JH, Nunley JA, et al: The results of replantation after amputation of a single finger. J Bone Joint Surg, 1985; 67A:611–619.

42. Wang S-H, Young K-F, Wei J-N: Replantation of severed limbs-clinical analysis of 91 cases. J Hand Surg, 1981; 6:311–318.

43. Ward WA, Tsai T-M, Breidenbach W: Per primam thumb replantation for all patients with traumatic amputations. Clin Orthop, 1991; 266:90–95.

44. Weiland AJ, Villarreal-Rios A, Kleinert HE, et al: Replantation of digits and hands: analysis of surgical techniques and functional results in 71 patients with 86 replantations. J Hand Surg, 1977; 2:1–12.

45. Yamano T: Replantation of the amputated distal part of the fingers. J Hand Surg, 1985; 10A: 211–218.

JOHN A. MCFADDEN
LEONARD GORDON

53

Thumb Replantation

■ HISTORY OF THE
TECHNIQUE

The functional importance of the thumb cannot be understated, and its restoration after traumatic loss has long been a goal of hand surgeons. Its unique combination of strength, sensibility, and wide range of motion makes the thumb the single-most important digit. Loss of the thumb, in fact, results in a 40% loss of hand function by some estimates.[9] It has been stated that the combination of a truly opposable thumb and human intelligence has allowed man to master his surroundings. The desire by surgeons to restore a sensate and agile thumb in cases of amputation has driven the development of this technique as an improvement over replacement of the thumb with distant tissues.

Before the advent of modern microsurgery, attempts at replantation of amputated parts were disappointing. Failure was the rule with early attempts at replantation, regardless of the level. This was due to an inadequate understanding of microvascular repair and the lack of adequate technology. Buncke and Schulz reported successful amputation and replantation of the thumb and index finger in rhesus monkeys.[1] The small size of the vessels to be repaired required a specially constructed suture, which was made by "metallizing" the end of a single strand of nylon suture measuring 10 μm in diameter. Appropriatly sized vascular clamps and forceps also were custom made for this procedure. Clearly, an emphasis was placed on improving the technology to achieve the goal of successful replantation. Although the success rate was low, this experiment helped to usher in the clinical era of replantation. Before this report in 1965, replantation of completely severed parts had only been successful for distal amputations that healed as composite grafts.[9]

Komatsu and Tamai[5] reported the first successful replantation of the thumb in 1968. This operation was performed using 7-0 braided silk and 8-0 nylon suture for the microanastomosis under magnifications of 10× to 16×. Snyder reported an account of a similar successful case in 1972.[9] In this report, however, only the digital artery was repaired and 7-0 nylon sutures were used. Veins, nerves, and the flexor tendon were not repaired, and the patient was given heparin and allowed to bleed through loosely approximated wounds. The replanted part survived and Snyder concluded that venous repair was not only unnecessary but was probably detrimental. Chow and Schlenker reported separate series of thumb replantations in 1979 and 1980, respectively.[2,7] Both of these reports emphasized the importance of repair of all vital structures including arteries, veins, and nerves and confirmed the efficacy of thumb replantation.

■ INDICATIONS AND
CONTRAINDICATIONS

Replantation of the thumb is generally indicated when the condition of the amputated part does not preclude reattachment for technical reasons and the general condition of the patient does not prohibit a potentially lengthy operation. The level of amputation must be considered. The more proximal the amputation, the stronger the indications are for replantation. Some individuals may function adequately after thumb amputation at or distal to the interphalangeal joint. This is somewhat unpredictable, however, and function and appearance are far better when the pulp and nailbed are preserved.[4] Amputation injuries that destroy the interphalangeal joint surfaces can be treated by joint fusion; the thumb will still have good function and range of motion even without motion at the interphalangeal joint. Avulsion injuries of the thumb have been successfully replanted and should be considered provided that the neurovascular pedicle has not been avulsed from the part.[10] Occasionally, the decision to proceed with replantation must be made in the operating room upon examination of the artery and vein of the amputated part under magnification. For successful replantation, there must to be a remaining portion of grossly uninjured artery and vein in the severed part.

Contraindications to thumb replantation are few. These may include severe crush or multiple level amputation, pre-existing neurologic injury or disease (i.e., no useful thumb function before injury), or life-threatening concomitant injury. Co-existing vascular disease, cigarette smoking, and diabetes mellitus may result in a higher failure rate but are not considered contraindications to replantation. Also, advanced age must be considered in light of the patient's overall condition. It is not unreasonable to replant the thumb in an active and otherwise healthy older person.

Under regional block, the patient may become uncomfortable and restless at some point during the procedure, so we recommend general endotracheal anesthesia. General anesthesia also has the advantage of simplifying the harvest of vein grafts from the lower extremity. The procedure is done under tourniquet control with an indwelling urinary catheter in place.

■ SURGICAL TECHNIQUES

The following anatomic features must be kept in mind when preparing for the replantation. The thumb lies in a plane that is oriented 90° in relation to the fingers. Its palmar surface is viewed best with the hand in extreme supination, but this position makes exposure for repair of the digital arteries and nerves difficult. Arterial reconstruction is often best performed with the hand in the pronated position using a dorsal approach.

The thumb has radial and ulnar neurovascular bundles and several dorsal veins. The *ulnar digital artery* is the dominant vessel and should be repaired if at all possible. If it is severely damaged distally, however, the radial vessel may be used in its place, although it is much smaller. The digital arteries of the thumb arise from the *first palmar metacarpal artery* (also known as the princeps pollicis artery) near the level of the metacarpophalangeal (MP) joint. The first palmar metacarpal artery is the first branch of the radial artery, arising near the point where the latter passes between the two heads of the first dorsal interosseous muscle.[3] Immediately after its origin from the radial artery, the first palmar metacarpal artery lies on the palmar surface of the first dorsal interosseous muscle with the opponens radially and the oblique head of the adductor ulnarly. The artery then passes dorsal to the deep head of the flexor pollicis brevis and then divides into the ulnar and radial digital arteries deep to the flexor pollicis longus tendon. This point of division is proximal to the level of the A1 pulley so that the origin of the digital artery is deep to the flexor tendon at this point. The ulnar digital artery emerges from deep to the flexor pollicis longus tendon on the ulnar side and travels parallel to the tendon from this point to its distal termination. The radial digital artery follows a similar course paralleling the tendon on the radial side.[3]

There are significant variations in this anatomy. In 20% of hands, the division of the first palmar metacarpal artery into the proper digital arteries to the thumb may be distal to the insertion of the adductor. Thus, it remains deep to the flexor pollicis longus tendon until approximately the distal side of the A1 pulley. Additionally, there are frequent contributions from the first palmar branch of the radial artery, the first dorsal metacarpal artery, and terminal branches of the superficial palmar arch.[3] In 50% of the population, the first palmar metacarpal artery also supplies the radial digital artery to the index finger, and in 75% it is the terminal blood supply to the thumb.[5] A thorough understanding of the arterial anatomy, especially that of the first palmar metacarpal artery in the thumb–index web space, will simplify the replantation procedure.

If possible, two surgical teams work simultaneously to shorten the length of the operation. Operative time also can be saved by bringing the amputated part to the operating room ahead of the patient and completing its dissection before the patient is ready. Dissection of the amputated part is done on a separate sterile operating table, that is set up in the corner of the operating room, away from other activities. We use a separate "tagging set" to prepare the amputated part. This consists of basic instruments including a scalpel, fine skin hooks and forceps, and microsurgical instruments, including jeweler's forceps and curved adventitia scissors. A 6-0 silk suture is cut into short lengths and pre-tied into

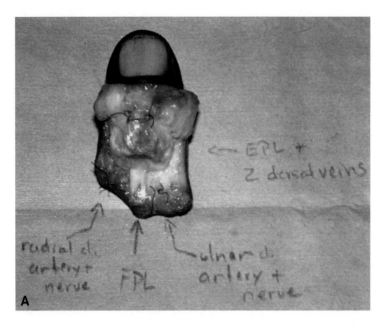

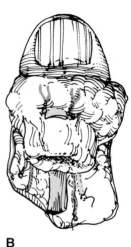

loops and set aside for easy tagging of the appropriate structures. This instrument set-up allows preparation of the amputated part to proceed as the patient is being readied by the anesthesiologist.

After the amputated thumb has been carefully debrided of devitalized and foreign material, two longitudinal skin incisions are made just dorsal to the midaxial line. This incision will usually be just dorsal to or sometimes into the substance of Cleland's ligament. Fine skin hooks are used to retract the palmar skin, and Cleland's ligaments are sharply divided. The neurovascular bundles are usually readily visible just underneath the ligament. Each nerve and vessel is tagged with 6-0 silk suture for later identification. The dorsal flap of skin is gently everted by carefully dissecting superficial to the epitenon of the extensor tendon. One or more suitable dorsal veins are identified, dissected to the point where the first uninjured tributary is encountered, and tagged with 6-0 silk suture (Fig. 53–1A). The flexor pollicis longus tendon is the last structure to be tagged; we use a suture of 3-0 nylon placed in modified Kessler fashion. The end of the tendon is sharply trimmed using a new scalpel blade and a tongue depressor, but care is taken to avoid excessive shortening of the tendon. In cases where there is segmental loss of the flexor tendon, we usually will not do a primary tendon graft, unless the injury is exceptionally clean. This is generally not the case. Delayed tendon reconstruction under these circumstances is preferable when there is associated crush and contamination. Next, the bone end is prepared for osteosynthesis. Some degree of shortening is usually required to match the bone length to the soft tissue defect to allow repair of arteries, veins, and nerves, without the need for grafting. Additionally, some degree of comminution and bone loss is usually present, and good cortical contact cannot be obtained without some debridement of the bone ends. The degree of shortening required is usually less than 1 cm. We use a microsagittal saw to perform a transverse osteotomy of the bone ends. A rubber dam is fashioned from a piece of glove rubber so that the bone end can protrude through the hole and the soft tissues can be protected from the saw blade. If there is excessive bone loss due to comminution, but the soft tissue is adequate to maintain more length than the bony defect allows, consideration is given for iliac crest bone grafting or maintaining the length with an external fixator for delayed bone grafting. Finally, the prepared part is wrapped in moist gauze and placed on ice.

The second operating team exsanguinates the injured limb by applying an Esmarch bandage and inflating the tourniquet. All wounds are irrigated with at least 1 L of sterile saline. Devitalized tissue and foreign material are debrided.

For amputations distal to the MP flexion crease, the proximal ends of the digital vessels and nerves are approached through a standard Bruner zig-zag incision and tagged with 6-0 silk suture. The arteries are dissected proximally to the point where they appear uninjured. For amputations that are at or proximal to the MP crease, exposure of the proximal digital artery may be difficult because of its position deep to the flexor pollicis longus tendon. Under these circumstances, we find it easier to use an interposition vein graft on the amputated part and anastomose this to a donor artery on the dorsum of the hand. This method also prevents having to keep the hand in an extremely supinated position during arterial repair. Next, a suitable dorsal vein is identified. If the veins draining the thumb have been extensively damaged, a dorsal vein overlying the index metacarpal can be mobilized and transferred over to reach the replanted thumb. This is done through a longitudinal incision directly over the index metacarpal. The incision is made just through the dermis and then the skin elevated in the subdermal plane so that injury to the veins which are just deep to this point is avoided. Once the radial and ulnar skin edges are elevated, and a suitable dorsal vein identified, the vein is ligated as distally as possible and elevated from its bed by ligating tributaries with 8-0 or 9-0 nylon sutures. Once adequate length is obtained a subcutaneous tunnel is created between the wound made for harvesting the vein and the amputation wound. The vein is then carefully passed through this tunnel to avoid kinking, traction, or torsion. Enough length can usually be obtained with this technique to obviate the need for a vein graft. The flexor pollicis longus tendon is then prepared. Its proximal end can often be retrieved with a tendon-passing clamp, but if it has retracted into the wrist, an incision is made in the distal volar forearm and the tendon identified. The tendon is then passed through the fibro-osseous tunnel using a red rubber catheter as a guide. The catheter is passed from the distal side of the fibrosseous tunnel, under the thenar musculature and into the distal volar forearm. A 3-0 nylon suture is then placed in the proximal tendon end in a modified Kessler fashion and the ends of the suture tied through a hole in the end of the red rubber catheter allowing enough length on the suture so that it can be used for tenorrhaphy once passed through the canal. The catheter is then withdrawn and the proximal tendon end delivered into the amputation stump. A Keith needle can then be used to transfix the flexor pollicis longus tendon temporarily while a tension-free tenorrhaphy is performed. The bone end is then prepared for osteosynthesis. This is done in a fashion similar to that described for the amputation part. The rubber dam and a microsagittal saw are again used to prepare the bone end.

Early in the operation, the surgeon should decide whether an interposition vein graft will be needed for arterial reconstruction. It must be remembered that the exposure for microsurgical repair can be very difficult. When the amputation is fairly distal and clean-cut, a direct repair of the ulnar digital artery can sometimes be performed with the hand in pronation. Otherwise, a vein graft must be anastomosed to the distal end of the artery on the amputated part before proceeding with the replantation.[7] The other indications for vein grafting include crush or avulsion of the artery, which preclude an end-to-end repair of uninjured vessel. It is critical to perform the distal vein graft anastomosis before the osteosynthesis, as this task becomes very difficult afterward (Fig. 53–1B).

We routinely use two methods of osteosynthesis: crossed Kirschner wiring and intraosseous wiring. Crossed Kirschner wiring is the simplest means of obtaining bone fixation. First, two wires are placed in the amputated part, one longitudinally and the other obliquely. The thumb is reattached by driving the longitudinal wire into the proximal bone fragment. Rotation is corrected so that the thumb is at a 90° angle in relation to the plane of the fingers, and the oblique wire is advanced. This method has a disadvantage in that the wires interfere with tendon gliding and joint motion, and is more suitable for cases in which joint fusion will be performed.

Intraosseous wiring also provides good fixation but does not interfere with early postoperative motion. Proper rotational alignment is the one challenging part to this technique. First the amputation part is tentatively aligned with the amputation stump so that the surgeon can assess the adequacy of bone contact and alignment. A marking pen is then used to mark the bone on the proximal and distal fragment at the 12-o'clock position, or mid-dorsal line, and in the midaxial line on the radial side. Again, a rubber dam is used to protect soft tissues on the amputation stump and on the amputated part. Next, 0.45 Kirschner wires are drilled in a dorsal-to-volar direction using the mid-dorsal mark as a reference point. The wire is thus passed from the 12-o'clock to the 6-o'clock position if one is viewing the bone end on. The wire is then removed and a hole drilled from the radial midaxial border to the ulnar midaxial border, so that the wire is passed from the 3-o'clock to the 9-o'clock position and then removed. This procedure is done on both the proximal and distal fragment so that the alignment of the holes is matched. Two 24-gauge stainless steel wires are passed through the proximal and distal holes and tightened so that fixation consists of two crossed loops of wire that compress the fragments and control rotation. The knots in the wire are oriented so that one is palmar and the other is radial. As they are progressively tightened down, rotation is rechecked to make sure alignment is adequate. The twisted ends of the wire are then cut short and buried so that the ends do not protrude and impair tendon gliding.

We do not use plates or interfragmentary screws because the comminution usually present makes these devices impractical on a routine basis.

If the interphalangeal joint can be preserved, repair of the flexor pollicis longus tendon is necessary. We use a Tajima suture of 3-0 nylon. The 3-0 nylon suture is placed in the proximal and distal tendon stumps in a fashion similar to the modified Kessler technique but are then tied so that the two knots are buried within the tendon ends. A running 6-0 nylon is used for an epitendonous repair. The extensor tendon is then repaired with interrupted horizontal mattress sutures of 3-0 or 4-0 nylon.

In those cases that do not require an interposition vein graft, the ulnar digital artery is repaired primarily. This repair is done with the hand in pronation using standard microvascular technique and 10-0 nylon suture. In many cases, however, arterial reconstruction requires vein grafting. By this time, graft anastomosis to the amputated thumb already has been performed. Anastomosis of the proximal end of the graft is performed to either the first palmar metacarpal artery or the radial artery, depending on the extent of injury. The first palmar metacarpal artery is exposed through an incision on the dorsum of the thumb-index web space. The dissection is then carried over the distal edge of and onto the palmar surface of the adductor pollicis muscle. The first palmar metacarpal artery can be seen lying on the surface of the adductor at this point. If the amputation injury does not involve the artery at this point, and the condition and length of the first palmar metacarpal artery are adequate, then a repair can be done to the artery at this level. If, however, the surgeon finds himself operating "in a hole," a decision should be made to repair the proximal end of the graft to the radial artery at the anatomic snuff box or to the first dorsal metacarpal artery at its origin from the radial artery if it is of appropriate size (Fig. 53–3A).

As a general rule, we usually do not repair the radial digital artery. This is because the ulnar digital artery is dominant and in most cases is adequate to reperfuse the thumb. Repair of the radial digital artery can be performed, however, with the hand in supination at the time the radial digital nerve is repaired providing that the vessel is in adequate condition for anastomosis.

Once the arterial repair has been completed, the digital nerves are repaired using 9-0 nylon suture. The ulnar digital nerve can usually be repaired with the hand pronated, approaching the thumb from the ulnar side. The radial digital nerve can then be coapted while the hand is placed in full supination for a brief period of time. At this point, the volar wounds are closed loosely with 5-0 nylon suture.

Next, one or more dorsal veins are repaired. If more than one good vein is available, multiple venorrhaphies should be performed. These repairs are done in an end-to-end fashion with 10-0 nylon suture. With adequate mobilization of the recipient vein, a primary anastomosis can usually be made, but the surgeon should not hesitate to use a vein graft. Segmental loss of the dorsal vein or crush injury requiring debridement of the veins may preclude anastomosis without a vein graft. Under these circumstances, we use a vein

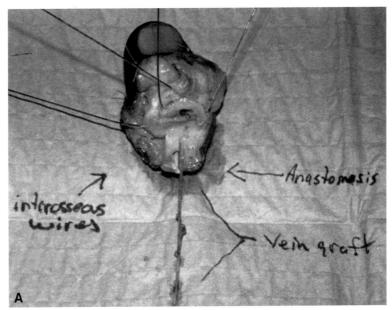

A

A and B, The amputated part just before reattachment. Crossed interosseous wires have been placed and a reversed interposition vein graft has been anastomosed to the ulnar digital artery.

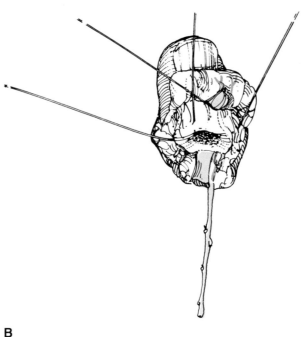

B

harvested from the dorsum of the foot that is of appropriate size. It is essential that the injured ends of the veins be debrided back to where uninjured tributaries are encountered and that the anastomosis be tension free. The other alternative as previously mentioned is a transfer of a dorsal vein from the index metacarpal.

The tourniquet is deflated, and all clamps are removed. Patency tests are done to confirm flow across the microanastomosis. If the thumb does not immediately become pink, patience is advised; reperfusion of the amputated part will usually occur after a 15-minute period in which warm soaks are applied.

The skin incisions are loosely closed with nylon suture. It is preferable to leave areas of the wound open or use small skin grafts than to risk a tight closure that may lead to venous congestion. Split-thickness skin graft can be harvested from the volar forearm and applied to these open wounds. Occasionally, an exposed neurovascular bundle will be

■ FIGURE 53-3
A and B, The dorsal approach to arterial reconstruction. The vein graft has previously been anastomosed to the amputated part. With the hand pronated, the proximal anastomosis is made to the radial artery. In the photograph, the vascular clamps have been removed and the proximal and distal anastomoses are highlighted by background material.

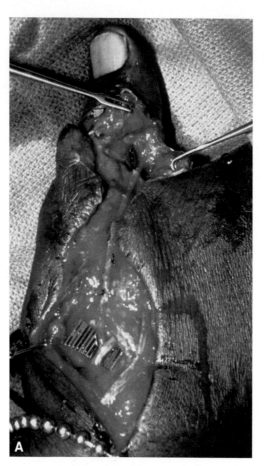

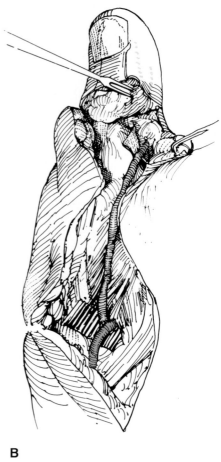

present in the base of this wound and it has been our experience that skin grafts applied over these will heal adequately.

Postoperative care includes application of a dressing of petrolatum gauze, followed by a well-padded soft dressing, loosely applied cotton, and a thumb spica forearm splint. The patient is kept under close observation in a warm environment with the hand well elevated. Tobacco, caffeine, and other vasoconstricting substances are avoided for 1 month postoperatively.

Pain control is provided by a patient-controlled analgesia infusion pump with morphine. This allows the patient to self-dose pain medication. This is usually only necessary for the first 24 to 48 hours, and then oral narcotic analgesics are administered. Oral intake is not permitted for the first 24 hours in the event that emergency re-exploration for microvascular failure is required. Intravenous crystalloid fluids are administered at 1.25 to 1.5 times maintenance values. After the 24-hour period has passed and the risks of microvascular failure decreases, the patient is given a regular diet and the crystalloid fluids are decreased to keep the venous access, usually by the third day.

An intraoperative anticoagulation protocol is initiated that consists of either low molecular weight dextran or systemic heparin. The dose of anticoagulant depends on the weight of the patient. For a 70 kg person, 30 ml/hr of intravenous Dextran is administered after a loading dose of 500 ml. Heparin is generally given as a loading dose of 5000 units followed by a continuous infusion of 800 to 1000 units/hr while adjusting the partial thromboplastin time to 1.5 times the control. Systemic anticoagulation is discontinued on the seventh postoperative day and 325 mg of aspirin is given daily for 1 month. Systemic anticoagulants have not been shown conclusively to improve the survival rate of replanted digits. Therefore, their adverse side effects should be considered on an individual basis.

Monitoring of the replanted part is done by clinical observation. Color, turgor, and capillary refill are monitored at least every 30 minutes for the first 6 hours, and then every 2 hours thereafter for the first day. After this time, observations are made every 2 to 4 hours. By the seventh postoperative day, the risk of microvascular failure is slight, and hospital observation can be discontinued. We do not routinely use surface temperature probes or plethysmography because these modalities have not been superior to clinical observation.

Rehabilitation of the replanted thumb begins after approximately 5 days. A dorsal blocking splint is fitted for continuous wear; the hand is positioned with the wrist in neutral or slight flexion, the interphalangeal and MP joints in 15° of flexion, and the thumb palmarly abducted. The program for passive and active motion must be individualized, but it essentially follows the modified Duran protocol for flexor pollicis longus rehabilitation.

■ REHABILITATION

From about day 6 through week 4, passive exercises are performed every 2 hours during the day; the interphalangeal and MP joints are put through individual and composite flexion and extension within the confines of the splint. Active flexion and extension are initiated at week 5, and as much range of motion as possible is recovered during the next 3 weeks. The splint is discontinued at week 6. Strengthening exercises are initiated at week 8, and recovery usually plateaus at about 12 weeks.

There are a variety of technical alternatives to thumb replantation which will be addressed in separate chapters. These range from the simple web space deepening to toe-to-thumb transfers. Our choice for thumb reconstruction is a great toe-to-thumb transfer in cases where there is insufficient remaining length for pinch and opposition following failed replantation or a nonreplantable amputation of the thumb. Index finger pollicization also provides a very functional reconstruction but does not provide pinch or grip strength that is as strong as that following great toe-to-hand transfers. Distraction lengthening and web space deepening are useful when little extra length is needed to improve overall function and in low demand situations. We have largely abandoned techniques to create a "post" such as a radial forearm or groin flap over a bone graft strut because of unacceptable appearance and motion and poor sensibility.

■ TECHNICAL ALTERNATIVES

A number of technical pitfalls can be avoided by careful attention to detail. One common technical error is rotational malalignment of the replanted part. This can be avoided by aligning anatomic landmarks such as the flexor tendon sheath and by marking the bone before drilling. Many different methods of osteosynthesis have been described for use during replantation. We find that the crossed interosseous wires allow for easy correction of rotational malalignment as the wires are tightened. Microvascular thrombosis is the most problematic complication. The temptation to repair damaged vessels to avoid the need for vein grafts should be avoided. The vessels to be repaired should be debrided to the point where they appear to be uninjured. Once the debridement has been accomplished, the need for a vein graft is assessed. Ultimately, the use of vein grafts, when required, will save a great deal of trouble compared with emergency reoperation for microvascular failure. Similarly, tension in the skin closure must be avoided as this leads to slowing of venous return and venous microvascular thrombosis. An immense degree of swelling can follow digital ischemia and allowance for this can be made by leaving one or both midlateral incisions open.

Attention to postoperative care is as important as the conduct of surgery. Thrombosis can occur from a dressing that is too tight or from blood which has dried and formed a constricting cast around the arm. We use a loosely applied Jones-type dressing consisting of a thick layer of cotton covered by a plaster splint and stockinette wrap. Ace wraps should be avoided. Allowing the hand to fall into a dependent position during the early postoperative period can cause enough venous stasis to result in thrombosis. The replanted part should be kept above the level of the heart for at least 1 week after surgery.

Survival occurs in 72% to 100% of replanted thumbs, depending upon the age of the

■ OUTCOMES

patient and the mechanism of injury. Remarkably, even thumbs that have been crushed or avulsed can be successfully replanted using vein grafts to bypass the zone of injury.[10]

Functional results vary with the precise anatomy of the injury. In a series of 30 replants reported by Chow and co-authors,[2] of the 82% of cases that survived, good circumduction, opposition, and key pinch were reported in all. Even the patients with a fused interphalangeal joint or very little motion had no more than a 20% difference in pinch strength between their two hands. Sensibility recovery was good; temperature sensation and light touch were restored, and two-point discrimination averaged 5 mm. Causalgia did not develop in any patient, although some patients had transient cold intolerance and hyperesthesia.

The experience of Schlenker and co-authors[7] is similar. Most of their 64 patients were satisfied with the result and returned to work, and at least half recovered good sensibility. The older patients had a significantly higher rate of unsatisfactory outcomes.

Because the thumb is unique in its ability to oppose the other fingers, the degree of hand function restored by its replantation is dramatic. Although the patient's age, occupation, and level and extent of injury can influence the outcome of surgery considerably, the results of this operation are usually good.

References

1. Buncke HJ Jr, Schulz WP: Experimental digital amputation and replantation. Plast Reconstr Surg, 1965; 36:62–70.
2. Chow JA, Bilos ZJ, Chunprapaph B: Thirty thumb replantations. Plast Reconstr Surg, 1979; 64:626–630.
3. Earley MJ: The arterial supply of the thumb, first web space, and index finger and its surgical application. J Hand Surg, 1986; 11B:163–174.
4. Gordon L: Microsurgical reconstruction of the extremities: indications, technique, and postoperative care. New York: Springer-Verlag, 1988, 163–164.
5. Komatsu S, Tamai S: Successful replantation of a completely cut-off thumb. Plast Reconstr Surg, 1968; 42:374–377.
6. Parks BJ, Arbelaez J, Homer RL: Medical and surgical importance of the arterial blood supply of the thumb. J Hand Surg, 1978; 3:383–385.
7. Schlenker JD, Kleinert HE, Tsai T: Methods and results of replantation following traumatic amputation of the thumb in sixty-four patients. J Hand Surg, 1980; 5:63–70.
8. Shafiroff BB, Palmer AK: Simplified techniques for replantation of the thumb. J Hand Surg, 1991; 6:623–624.
9. Snyder CC, Stevenson RM, Browne EZ: Successful replantation of a totally severed thumb. Plast Reconstr Surg, 1972; 50:553–559.
10. Vlastou C, Earle S: Avulsion injuries of the thumb. J Hand Surg, 1986; 11A:51–56.

54

Replantation of the Hand

The introduction of the operating microscope by Jacobson and Suarez in 1960,[10] together with the refinement of microsurgical instruments and the availability of small suture material, all were factors that enabled surgeons to successfully anastomose blood vessels with 1 mm of diameter or less. In 1962, Malt and McKhann[17] reported a successful complete arm replantation. In 1965, Kleinert and Kasden[13] reported successful digital vessel anastomosis in a devascularized thumb. In 1968, Komatsu and Tamai[14] reported successful replantation of a completely amputated thumb. The first successful hand replantation was reported by Chen[2] at the Sixth People's Hospital in China in 1963.

The technique of replantation and the development of replantation teams and microsurgical laboratories were well established in the 1970s.[1,4,16,19,25,27,32] During the 1980s, the technique was refined, and indications for replantation were developed.[2,6,8,9,11,15,21,24,26,28,29,31] Reports on replantations not only addressed the success rate, but also the functional outcome. Early on, the tendency was to delay nerve and tendon repair for several months after skeletal stabilization and restoration of vascular flow. It was found later that the second reconstructive procedure was troublesome because of excessive scarring and the possibility of further vascular damage.[25] At the present time, all structures are repaired at the time of the replantation.

The majority of published reports address digital or thumb replantation, with hand replantations being included. Tamai reported on 293 upper extremity replants, 15 of which involved the hand, 6 of which were completely amputated.[24] Many factors have helped improve the success rate of hand replantations. Patient selection and the development of the technique for microvascular anastomosis are the main factors. The key points in microvascular anastomosis are: minimal stripping of the adventicia, frequent intraluminal irrigation with diluted heparinized solution, interrupted sutures, proper needle insertion, and nonabsorbable suture material of the correct size.[25] Proper handling of the vessels both proximally and distally and the liberal use of vein grafts also are key factors.

■ HISTORY OF THE TECHNIQUE

Hand amputations occur at two levels—transcarpal and transmetacarpal. Transmetacarpal amputations may be total, with the hand and thumb as one or two units, or partial with an intact thumb (Fig. 54–1). A hand with partial recovery of function is far superior to a prosthetic replacement; therefore, every attempt should be made to salvage an amputated hand. Absolute indications for hand replantation are: clean cut guillotine-like amputations with minimum crushing or avulsion, partial hand amputations with an intact thumb, transcarpal amputations, relatively short ischemia time (fewer than 6 hours of warm ischemia time or 9 to 10 hours of cold ischemia time), and amputations in children. Appropriate management of the amputated hand is essential for successful replantation. The hand should be kept in a saline-filled plastic bag that is secured tightly and placed in a large container filled with crushed ice. At no time should the ice touch the hand. The goal is to keep the amputated hand at a temperature of 4°C. Other centers prefer to wrap the hand in gauze, place the hand in a sealed bag, and place the bag in ice.[2,12,19] An experimental study showed, however, that there was no difference between these two methods as long as the body part was not frozen.[30] Incompletely amputated hands with a soft tissue pedicle are difficult to cool and should be transported to the replantation center as soon as possible. These amputations, especially if the nerves or the tendons are intact, are strongly indicated for revascularization mainly because the functional outcome is usually quite good.

■ INDICATIONS AND CONTRAINDICATIONS

■ FIGURE 54-1
Three hand amputations to illustrate the level of injury: **A,** transcarpal; **B,** total transmetacarpal; **C,** partial transmetacarpal.

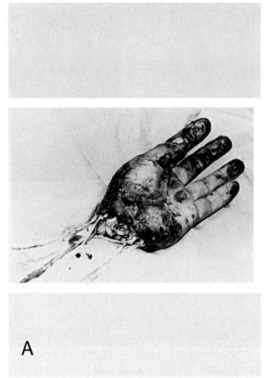
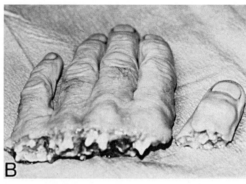
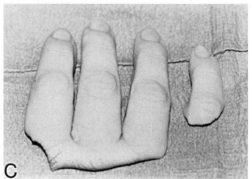

Contraindications for hand replantation are: severe crushing or avulsion that have produced a mangled hand, multilevel injuries, evidence of severe bruising, streaking or hemorrhage in the tissue of the amputated hand, inappropriate preparation of the amputated hand with freezing of the tissues or prolonged warm ischemia (more than 9 to 10 hours), or the presence of severe arteriosclerosis or other associated medical problems in the elderly. Self-inflicted amputations in the mentally unstable are not uncommon and should be considered for replantation. Many of these patients regret the injury and should undergo psychiatric evaluation after the replantation.

Of the contraindications mentioned above, the mangled hand is an absolute contraindication for replantation, as the injury usually covers a large area, and it becomes technically impossible to revascularize the hand. Other contraindications mentioned are relative, and it is my recommendation that if there is any chance of re-establishing blood flow to an amputated hand, it should be done. Under these circumstances, quick skeletal fixation followed by arterial anastomosis is performed. If vascular flow is re-established, then the procedure is completed, and, if not, then it is terminated.

■ SURGICAL
TECHNIQUE

I prefer general anesthesia, which allows proper positioning of the extremity on the hand table and adequate relaxation by the patient. It is possible, however, to perform the procedure under long-acting axillary block anesthesia using bupivicaine.[1] However, the patient may become uncomfortable during the procedure, and excessive movement may interfere with the surgeon's ability to perform the microvascular and the microneural repair. A Foley catheter should be inserted to monitor urine output. While the patient is being worked up and prepared for surgery, the surgeon takes the hand to the operating room for preparation. The hand is sterilized in a large basin containing a mixture of saline and betadine, where it is scrubbed with a sponge for a period of 5 minutes. It is unwise to use a brush for fear of further injury to the structures. The hand is then transported to a sterile field for examination under the microscope. A separate set of instruments is used for this portion of the procedure. The radial and ulnar arteries, at least four dorsal veins and the median, ulnar, and superficial radial nerves are identified and trimmed to normal

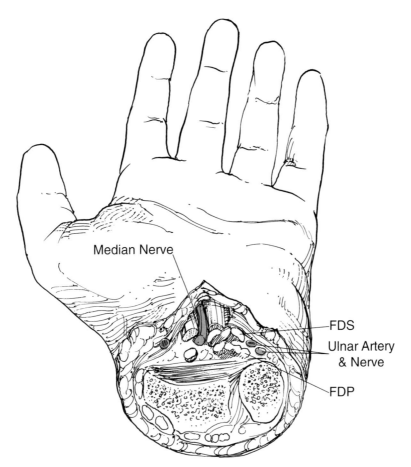

Median Nerve

FDS

Ulnar Artery & Nerve

FDP

■ FIGURE 54-2
In a hand amputated at
the transcarpal level, a
carpal tunnel release al-
lows identification of the
contents of the tunnel.

appearing tissue and tagged with 9-0 nylon sutures using the operating microscope. The radial and ulnar arteries are gently irrigated with heparinized saline. Avulsed tendons are debrided, and a carpal tunnel release is completed if necessary to identify the distal median nerve and flexor tendons (Fig. 54–2). A release of Guyon's canal also may be necessary to identify the distal ulnar nerve and artery. Similarly, a separate incision in the anatomic snuff box may be needed to identify the distal radial artery. Dorsal veins are looked for on the radial and mid-dorsal aspect of the hand. The dorsal veins are usually easily identifiable by retracting the dorsal skin distally and locating them in the subcutaneous tissues. After the hand is sterilized and the structures are identified, it is then transferred back to a sterile container filled with saline, which is placed in a basin filled with ice.

After anesthesia is administered and the hand is prepared, a tourniquet is applied to the arm, and the surgery is begun. I recommend that debridement, bone fixation, and tendon repair be completed with the tourniquet deflated. A pressure of 250 mmHg in adults and between 170 and 200 mmHg in children is recommended. The tourniquet is usually inflated before vascular repair, after elevating the arm. Exsanguination is not done. The following steps are followed.

1. Wound debridement. Adequate debridement of devitalized and dirty tissues in the amputated hand and in the stump is essential. All devitalized tissue and foreign material must be removed. Any muscle crushed at the site of the amputation should be debrided. The intrinsic muscles are debrided from the hand at the transmetacarpal level as they may be a source of infection. Tendons are left intact. One should, however, not be too aggressive in removing skin, and the pulse lavage can be used to clean the wound with care being taken to protect the vessels and nerves.

2. Skeletal fixation. Bone shortening for approximately 1 to 1.5 cm, using a rongeur, at

the metacarpal level is performed. For transcarpal amputations, shortening is done by performing a proximal row carpectomy. If the amputation is at the distal forearm, then a rongeur or a power saw is used to shorten the bone. The type of fixation depends on the level of amputation. For amputations of the distal forearm, I prefer plates and screws. A T-plate or a 3.5-mm Dynamic Compression Plate on the radius and a 3.5-mm Dynamic Compression Plate on the ulna are appropriate. If there is significant bone loss in the ulna (more than 1.5 cm) then only the radius is fixed (Fig. 54–3). For transcarpal amputations, following proximal row carpectomy, cross-Kirschner wire fixation using 0.62-inch K-wires is satisfactory. I do not recommend primary wrist arthrodesis, as this procedure will add time to the surgery. At the metacarpal level, intramedullary Kirschner-wire fixation, using 0.45-inch wires applied in a retrograde manner, is used (Fig. 54–4). It is essential to check the digits for rotational alignment, and any malalignment must be corrected at this time.

3. Extensor tendon repair. This is done using a modified Kessler suture of 4-0 Ethibond (No. B557, Ethicon, Inc., Somerville, NJ) and a running epitendonous suture of 5-0 Ethibond (No. X870, Ethicon, Inc., Somerville, NJ).

All extensor tendons including the extensor indicis proprius and extensor digiti minimi should be repaired. Wrist extensors also are repaired. Reconstruction of the extensor retinaculum is completed by repairing it or by using local tissue for augmentation. This is done to prevent bow stringing of the extensor tendons.

4. Flexor tendon repair. All flexor tendons are repaired. A volar incision in the stump is recommended for visualization of the proximal flexor tendons. This is a curved incision with its apex proximal ulnar to distal radial (Fig. 54–5). This is usually the same incision used to expose the arteries in the stump. A modified Kessler stitch of 4-0 Ethibond, and a running epitendonous 5-0 Ethibond suture is used for each tendon. I recommend repairing the palmaris longus, because it can function as a thumb abductor and may help improve thumb function before median nerve recovery.

5. Vein repair. I prefer to do the vein repairs before the arterial repairs. This reduces the amount of swelling and bleeding that always occurs after clamp release following the arterial repair. This also may help lessen the potential for no reflow phenomenon. At the

■ FIGURE 54–3
The radiograph on the left shows a hand that was incompletely amputated at the distal forearm. The radius was fixed with a T plate, but the ulna was not fixed because of bone loss. On the right, the radius is healed 6 months later.

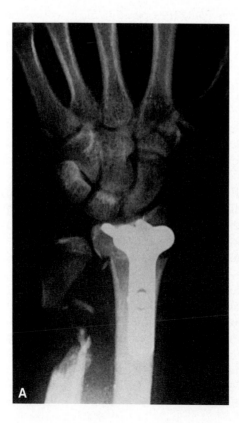
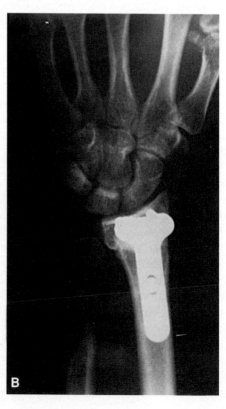

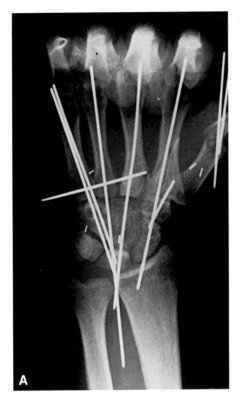
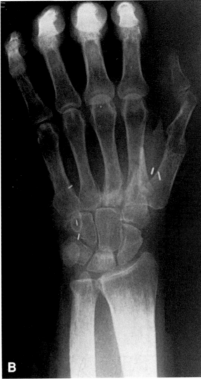

A

B

■ FIGURE 54-4
The radiograph on the left shows intramedullary wire fixation of a hand that was completely amputated at the metacarpal level and it shows primary arthrodesis of the thumb metacarpophalangeal joint. On the right, healing of the fractures and joint is demonstrated.

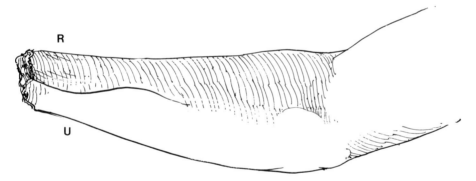

R

U

■ FIGURE 54-5
A volar forearm incision is used to explore the structures in the amputation stump.

level of the wrist, it is easy to find large veins that can be repaired successfully. The veins are usually found on the radial and mid-dorsal aspects of the hand. I recommend repairing at least four veins. The veins should be debrided to healthy tissue before repair.

6. Arterial repair. A volar curved incision may be needed for exposure. This is the same incision that is used to expose the proximal flexor tendons. The proximal radial and ulnar arteries are identified in the stump and trimmed until normal, healthy arteries are obtained. It is important that no injury to the intima is present before the anastomosis and that bleeding from the proximal end of the artery should be uninterrupted with a good head of pressure. This is determined by deflating the tourniquet. The bleeding from the proximal end of the artery should be sustained and projectile in nature. It is absolutely essential that normal arteries in the stump and the amputated hand be anastomosed to each other. Before the anastomosis, a vessel clamp is applied to the proximal end of the artery and left in situ for approximately 5 minutes. Upon release of the vessel clamp, the proximal artery should maintain a sustained, projectile flow; otherwise, there is an injury proximally in the forearm in the form of spasm or thrombosis and one then has to resect more artery proximally until normal artery with a projectile, sustained flow is obtained.

If the artery appears normal but there is still inadequate flow, then a No. 3 Fogarty catheter (size 3FR, No. EMB-080-3F, Applied Vascular, Laguna Hills, CA) is inserted to remove any clots that may be present proximally. The Fogarty catheter should not be used until all other methods have been exhausted. For the metacarpal amputation, if the level of amputation is at the base of the thumb, then only the ulnar artery constituting the superficial palmar arch, is reconstructed. At this level, the radial artery dives deep into the palm, and it becomes difficult to find the distal end. If thumb perfusion is inadequate and the distal stump of the radial artery cannot be found, then a vein graft can be applied from the radial artery proximally to the thumb ulnar digital artery distally. At the midpalm, arterial reconstruction becomes more difficult as the superficial palmar arch divides into many common digital branches. The principle here is to anastomose branches from the superficial arch proximally to the common digital artery to the index and long finger and the common digital artery to the ring and little fingers distally. If the thumb also is amputated, a branch from either palmar arch proximally should be anastomosed to the ulnar digital artery of the thumb (Fig. 54–6). Arterial repair is done under no tension otherwise a vein graft must be used. Tension at the anastomosis can be assessed by applying an 9-0 nylon suture. If the arterial ends stay together and do not tear, then the tension is acceptable. The artery with the better head of pressure, and least trauma, should be repaired first. At the carpal level, I prefer to repair both radial and ulnar arteries; however, if a vein graft is needed, then it is applied only to one artery, preferably the ulnar artery. If, after vein grafting, perfusion to all the fingers is adequate, then additional arterial repairs are unnecessary. If, however, perfusion is inadequate to a part of the hand, then the other artery must be repaired. In crush or avulsion injuries, 500 ml of Dextran 40 (10% Dextran 40 in 0.9% sodium chloride injection, Kendal McGraw Lab. Inc., Irvine, CA) should be given at completion of the vascular anastomosis.

Vein grafts are absolutely necessary in avulsion injuries. They also are used in children commonly, as bone shortening is not advisable. Vein grafts are taken from the same or

■ FIGURE 54–6
A diagram of the preferred method for vascular reconstruction at the transmetacarpal level. The solid lines indicate priority anastomoses for reconstruction and the dotted lines indicate additional repairs.

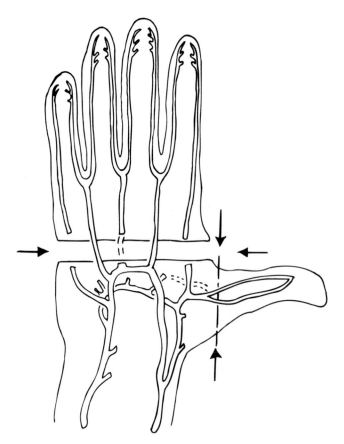

opposite volar forearm and are used to bridge defects in both arteries and veins. In my experience, vein grafts are used in approximately 50% of all replantations. The vein graft is harvested by making an incision directly over the vein to be used and after blunt dissection in the subcutaneous fat, the vein is identified and is dissected both proximally and distally. The branches are coagulated using bipolar coagulation or ties of 5-0 catgut suture (5-0 Chromic, No. U-202H, Ethicon, Inc., Somerville, NJ).

The distance to be bridged is measured to determine the length of the vein graft needed. It should be noted that the vein will recoil after being removed from its bed and become shorter. Accordingly, I harvest a piece of vein that is approximately 1.5 times the length of the defect. A vessel clamp is applied to the proximal end of the vein before it is removed. The vessel clamp is left on the vein until it is ready to be used. This method will allow proper reversal of the vein graft when it is used to bridge an arterial defect. I use 3.5 × loop magnification to harvest the vein graft. The vein is kept in a sterile specimen container filled with a small amount of heparinized saline. When applied to the recipient vessel, the vein is oriented so that blood flow is toward the end of the vein that was previously clamped. The vein graft should be dilated if the recipient vessel is larger. The proximal anastomosis is completed first, and the arterial clamp is released to allow blood to flow into the vein graft. This allows the vein graft to stretch and dilate and determines the proper length needed before it is anastomosed to the distal artery.

7. Nerve repair. The median and ulnar nerves and the superficial radial nerve are identified in the stump and in the amputated hand and an epineural repair is performed. Minimal trimming of the nerve ends is done. It is essential that nerve ends are properly oriented at the time of repair to assure the most optimal sensory and motor recovery. If end-to-end repair is not possible, then I reconstruct the nerve with a sural nerve graft 5 to 6 months after replantation.

I prefer to do the debridement, bony fixation, and tendon repair under no tourniquet control. The tourniquet is used at the time of the vessel repair. However, after 2 hours, it should be released and removed from the arm. The procedure should be continued using vascular clamps. Repeated application of the tourniquet may result in stagnation of blood at the repair site, which might lead to thrombosis.[7] It may take 5 to 10 minutes for reflow to occur in the replanted hand. Both arterial and venous repairs are inspected for patency before skin closure. As a general rule, if the replanted hand has the same color and capillary refill as the unaffected hand, then it is a sign of successful replantation. If no reflow occurs, then the vascular anastomosis should be explored. I prefer to explore both the venous and arterial anastomoses. Fasciotomy and release of intrinsic compartments should be done through two dorsal incisions if there is excessive swelling of the hand.

8. Skin closure. The skin is sutured loosely, and any tension overlying the vessel repair, particularly the veins, should be avoided. If tension is excessive, then a split-thickness skin graft obtained from the thigh should be used to cover the anastomosis. After loose approximation of the skin edges, a sterile dressing consisting of a layer of Xeroform gauze directly over the incisions and gauze fluffs covering the incision and in between the fingers, followed by a 4-inch Kurlex bandage, is applied. A well-padded dorsal plaster splint is applied and extends to the level of the distal interphalangeal joints. The splint should not touch the skin directly. The thumb is kept in abduction by applying several layers of gauze fluffs in the first web. The hand is kept slightly above the level of the heart, and the patient is transported to the intensive care unit. Excessive elevation is not advisable.

The patient is kept in the intensive care unit for approximately 48 hours for close monitoring. The room temperature must be kept at approximately 75°F. Skin temperature, color, capillary refill, and turgor are the main clinical parameters monitored. These are recorded every 2 hours in the first 48 hours after replantation. Skin temperature greater than 30°C or no less than 2°C different from the normal hand is desirable. There are many instruments and techniques available for monitoring of the replantation[26]; however, I firmly believe that accurate clinical observation is most essential. Five grains of aspirin are given rectally in the recovery room and then daily orally when the patient is allowed to eat. I do not recommend the use of heparin or dextran in the postoperative period.

Adequate hydration is essential, and this is monitored by the patient's urinary output. At least 50 ml of urine per hour should be obtained. In the first 24 hours after surgery, the patient is given 125 ml of intravenous fluid an hour and nothing by mouth. This is done in preparation for general anesthesia if vascular exploration is required. Vasoconstrictive agents such as caffeine and tobacco are prohibited, and no smoking is allowed in the room. We usually advise the patient to avoid these agents completely for at least 3 weeks after replantation, and the patient is advised to permanently stop smoking.

Replantation failure in the early postoperative period usually is due to thrombosis of the arteries and possibly the veins or both.[18] If there are signs of arterial insufficiency, as indicated by capillary refill more than 2 seconds, discoloration of the hand and loss of turgor, or drop of temperature below 30°C or 2°C less than the normal hand, then the patient should be taken immediately to the operating room for exploration of vascular anastomosis. Vein grafts are usually needed for arterial reconstruction. Venous insufficiency, as indicated by very brisk capillary refill, engorgement of the hand and bluish discoloration, is treated by a return to the operating room to look for more veins to repair or the application of medicinal leeches (Hirudo medicinalis, Leeches, USA, Westbury, NY). If leeches are to be used, then one leech every 4 to 6 hours should be applied for a total period of 48 hours. The first dressing is left on for 1 week, and the patient usually is discharged 3 to 5 days after the procedure.

■ TECHNICAL ALTERNATIVES

The alternatives to the surgical technique described above apply to skeletal fixation, arterial and venous repair, and nerve repair.

The goal in skeletal fixation is to obtain rigid, rapid fixation. In the distal forearm, crossed Kirschner wires or a Rush rod can be used. I believe, however, that plate fixation will produce a more rigid, stable fixation, which will allow bony union to occur in a short period of time. Intramedullary fixation may lead to nonunion. In transcarpal amputation, I recommend proximal row carpectomy. Wrist arthrodesis can be considered as an alternative; however, this procedure is time-consuming, and prolonged immobilization is required. Additionally, an iliac bone graft may be needed, which would further prolong the operative procedure. At the metacarpal level, I recommend retrograde Kirschner wire fixation. Plate fixation at the midmetacarpal level may be used. However, this will take much longer to perform than will retrograde intramedullary wire fixation. Both will produce a stable fixation.

I recommended that the veins be done before the arteries. This is done mainly to reduce the swelling that occurs after the arterial repair, and there is recent evidence that this may help avoid the no reflow phenomenon. Only if there is prolonged warm ischemia or there is a question about the suitability of the amputated hand for replantation do I recommend performing arterial repair first. Other authors recommend doing the arterial repair first and releasing the clamps in an attempt to visualize the bleeding veins. I find that to be unnecessary, however, as, at this level, the veins are easily identified. An alternative donor for vein graft is the lesser saphenous vein. This vein is much thicker than the arteries at the wrist and the palm level, and discrepancy in size may produce a problem.

In avulsion injuries, with segmental loss of the nerves, one may consider primary nerve grafting. I have no experience with primary nerve grafting, as this may prolong the surgical procedure and should be considered only if one of the two major nerves, the median or the ulnar, need grafting.

The use of postoperative anticoagulants varies among authors. My recommendation is to use only aspirin, as heparin or dextran may produce excessive bleeding. Careful selection of the patient, the nature of the injury, and the microvascular technique are most essential in the success of the replantation.

A potential pitfall in hand replantation is the failure to assess adequately the extent of the vascular damage. It is possible to assume that bleeding from the proximal artery is an indication that this artery is healthy. I stress that only normal vessels proximally to normal vessels distally should be anastomosed. Projectile sustained flow from the proximal artery should be obtained before the anastomosis. Upon release after 5 minutes of a vascular clamp from the proximal artery, the flow should maintain its character; otherwise, there is a problem proximally that should be corrected. If the vessel wall appears unusually thin and tears easily, that usually means that the muscularis has stripped off the intima, which will predispose to failure of the anastomosis.

Repeated applications of the tourniquet can produce vascular stasis and should be avoided. The tourniquet should be removed after 2 hours, completing the procedure using vascular clamps. Tight closure of the skin may produce thrombosis of the arteries and veins.

■ REHABILITATION

The first dressing change is done approximately 1 week postoperatively. Care should be taken to gently remove any dressing adherent to the incision, and excessive pulling is discouraged. If necessary, warm saline may be used to gently tease the Xeroform gauze off the skin. A new dressing and splint are applied, and these are changed again in 2 weeks. Gentle, passive range of motion of the fingers and the thumb may be started a few days after surgery in a cooperative patient. Three weeks from the time of surgery, the sutures are removed and active range of motion of the digits is started. Skin necrosis at the site of attachment is not uncommon, and scabs are left to separate spontaneously. Splinting of the wrist is continued for an additional 4 weeks in transcarpal amputations, at which time the transfixing pins across the carpus are removed and active range of motion of the wrist is started. In transmetacarpal amputations, the metacarpal pins are removed when bony union is evident on radiographs. This usually is the case approximately 8 to 10 weeks after the replantation. The therapy program is begun 3 weeks postoperatively and is progressed from active range of motion to active assistive and then passive range of motion exercises. Passive range of motion and dynamic splinting for contractures are started 6 weeks postoperatively. Secondary surgical procedures, such as nerve grafting or tenolysis, are done 6 months postoperatively.

■ OUTCOMES

The reported survival rate after digital and hand replantations vary from 69 to 87%.[11,16,19,20,22,24,32] A survival rate of 100% for hand amputations was reported by Tamai. In that report, replantations of six of six completely amputated hands and nine of nine incompletely amputated hands were successful. Survival rates in clean amputations are

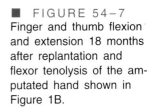

■ FIGURE 54–7
Finger and thumb flexion and extension 18 months after replantation and flexor tenolysis of the amputated hand shown in Figure 1B.

■ FIGURE 54-8
Finger and thumb flexion
and extension 2 years
after replantation of the
hand shown in Figure
1A. Notice the lack of intrinsic recovery.

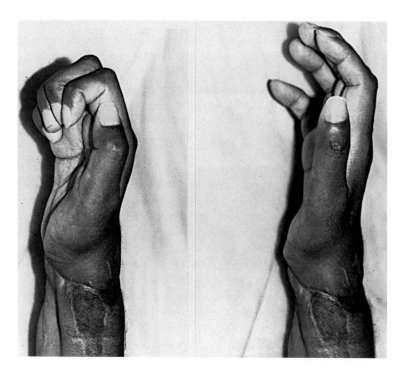

much higher, with reports of more than 80%, compared with avulsions and crush injuries, with reports between 20 and 50%.[20,22,32] Functional outcomes address cold intolerance, nerve recovery, recovery of motion, patient satisfaction, and ability to return to work. Cold intolerance is almost always present after hand replantations and is expected to last for approximately 2 years.[20,22,26] None of the patients report normal sensation after hand replantations. Recovery of light touch is expected and reports on recovery of two-point discrimination indicate less than 10 mm in 50% of patients.[16,19,20,22] Recovery of motion is expected to be approximately 50% of the normal, uninvolved side.[24,26] Recovery of motion at the transcarpal amputation level is much better than at the transmetacarpal level (Fig. 54–7). Patient satisfaction is quite high and is usually greater than 90%. The cosmetic appearance is much preferred to prosthetic replacement.[24,26] Return to work is at 3 to 4 months after replantation[11]; however, job modification may occur. Reporting on 293 upper extremity replants, Tamai found that excellent and good results were obtained in 63% of hand replantations compared with 50% of forearm amputations and 75% of digital replantations. Secondary surgery is often required after hand replantations, and in Tamai's series 43 procedures were done for 15 successful hand replantations. The majority of these procedures were done for tendon and nerve reconstruction, with flexor tendon procedures being the most used.

The outcome in my own cases is similar to what is reported in the literature. In avulsion injuries, intrinsic recovery is poor and opponensplasty may be needed to enhance the function of the hand (Fig. 54–8).

References

1. Bright DS: Microsurgical techniques in vessel and nerve repair. AAOS Instructional Course Lectures, 1978; 27:1–15.
2. Buncke HJ, Alpert BS, Johnson-Giebink R: Digital replantation. Surg Clin North Am, 1981; 61: 383–394.
3. Caffee HH: Improved exposure for arterial repair in thumb replantation. J Hand Surg, 1985; 10A:416.
4. Chow JA, Bilos ZJ, Chunprapaph, B: Thirty thumb replantations. Plastic Reconstruct Surg, 1979; 64:626–630.

5. Dell PC, Seaber AV, Urbaniak JR: The effect of systemic acidosis on perfusion of replanted extremities. J Hand Surg, 1980; 5:433–442.

6. Earley MJ, Watson JS: Twenty four thumb replantations. J Hand Surg, 1984; 9B:98–102.

7. Fahmy HWM, Moneim MS: The effect of prolonged blood stasis on a microarterial repair. J Reconstruct Microsurg, 1988; 4:139–142.

8. Goldner RD: Postoperative management. Hand Clin, 1985; 1(2):205–215.

9. Hamilton RB, O'Brien BM, Morrison A, MacLeod AM: Survival factors in replantation and revascularization of the amputated thumb—10 years experience. Scand J Plast Reconstr Surg, 1984; 18:163–173.

10. Jacobson JH and Suarez CL: Microsurgery and anastomosis of the small vessels. Surgical Forum, 1960; 11:243.

11. Jones JM, Schenck RR, Chesney RB: Digital replantation and amputation—Comparison of function. J Hand Surg, 1982; 7:183–189.

12. Kleinert HE, Juhala CA, Tsai T-M, Van Beek A: Digital replantation—selection, technique, and results. Ortho Clin North Am, 1977; 309–318.

13. Kleinert HE, Kasdan ML. Anastomosis of digital vessels. J Kentucky Med Assoc, 1965; 63:106.

14. Komatsu S, Tamai S: Successful replantation of a completely cut-off thumb. Case report. Plast Reconstr Surg, 1968; 42:374–377.

15. Lobay GW, Moysa GL: Primary neurovascular. Bundle transfer in the management of avulsed thumbs. J Hand Surg, 1981; 6:31–34.

16. MacLeod AM, O'Brien BM, Morrison WA: Digital replantation: clinical experiences. Clin Orthop Rel Res, 1978; 133:26–34.

17. Malt RA, McKhann CF: Replantation of severed arms. JAMA, 1964; 189:716–722.

18. Moneim MS, Chacon NE: Salvage of replanted parts of the upper extremity. J Bone Joint Surg, 1985; 67A:880–883.

19. Morrison WA, O'Brien BM, MacLeod AM: Evaluation of digital replantation—A review of 100 cases. Orthop Clin North Am, 1977; 295–308.

20. Morrison WA, O'Brien BM, MacLeod AM: Digital replantation and revascularisation, a long term review of one hundred cases. Hand, 1978; 10:125–134.

21. Nunley JA: Microscopes and microinstruments. Hand Clin, 1985; 1:197–204.

22. Schlenker JD, Kleinert HE, Tsai, T-M: Methods and results of replantation following traumatic amputation of the thumb in sixty-four patients. J Hand Surg, 1980; 5:63–70.

23. Shafiroff BB, Palmer AK: Simplified technique for replantation of the thumb. J Hand Surg, 1981; 6:623–624.

24. Tamai S: Twenty years' experience of limb replantation—Review of 293 upper extremity replants. J Hand Surg, 1982; 7:549–556.

25. Tamai S, Hori Y, Tatsumi Y, et al: Microvascular anastomosis and its application on the replantation of amputated digits and hands. Clin Orthop Rel Res, 1978; 133:106–121.

26. Urbaniak JR: Replantation. In: Green DP: Operative Hand Surgery, Vol. 2, 2nd Ed, New York: Churchill Livingstone, 1988:1105–1126.

27. Urbaniak JR: Replantation of amputed hands and digits. AAOS Instructional Course Lectures, 1978; 27:15–26.

28. Urbaniak JR, Evans JP, Bright DS: Microvascular management of ring avulsion injuries. J Hand Surg, 1981; 6:25–30.

29. Urbaniak JR, Roth JH, Nunley JA, Goldner RD, Koman LA: The results of replantation after amputation of a single finger. J Bone Joint Surg, 1985; 67A:611–619.

30. VanGiesen PJ, Seaber AV, Urbaniak JR: Storage of amputated parts prior to replantation—An experimental study with rabbit ears. J Hand Surg, 1983; 8:60–65.

31. Vlastou C, Earle S: Avulsion injuries of the thumb. J Hand Surg, 1986; 11A:51–56.

32. Weiland AJ, Villarreal-Rios A, Kleinert HE, Kutz J, Atasoy E, Lister G: Replantation of digits and hands: Analysis of surgical techniques and functional results in 71 patients with 86 replantations. J Hand Surg, 1977; 2:1–12.

33. Yamano Y: Replantation of the amputated distal part of the fingers. J Hand Surg, 1985; 10A: 211–218.

PART
IX

Drainage of Infections

LEWIS H. OSTER, JR.

55

Paronychia

Aggressive treatment of hand infection has been advocated since Kanavel's original descriptive, which states, "It is wise, generally, to be on the side of radicalism, since otherwise a secondary operation may become necessary."[9] Kanavel advocated that the incision for drainage should extend slightly beyond the edge of the indurated area. He believed this would provide sufficient drainage to the advancing margin of the infection. Very little has changed in the treatment of paronychia since Kanavel's description early in this century. Outlined in this chapter is the minimally modified version of his original description.

A paronychia is a subcuticular abscess in the eponychial and paronychial fold usually caused by *Staphyloccoccus aureus* (Fig. 55–1). Symptoms will include erythema, edema, tenderness, and occasionally fluctuance at the paronychial fold. Physical findings include fluctuance and point tenderness in proximity to the nail fold. Palpation of fluctuance can be difficult because of the low volume of purulence that can be present.

Surgical indications vary with the severity of infection. Simple infections in which loculated pus is located dorsal to the nail plate can be treated with eponychial elevation. If pus is located deep to the nail plate, the outer third of the nail is removed. More severe infections involving the subcutaneous tissue require that an incision be made in the nail fold.[3,14] The eponychial incision is indicated when an abscess cavity is present. The incision opens the cavity to the surface. When the entire eponychia is involved, the proximal nail plate is removed, and incisions are made on each side of the eponychial fold. This is occasionally referred to as a horseshoe abscess or run around abscess and is a rare finding.

Chronic paronychia present differently than acute paronychia; there is generally less erythema and rarely fluctuance palpated. Chronic paronychia is characterized by indurated eponychium with recurrent episodes of acute inflammation and drainage.[2] Chronic paronychia generally involves a chronic fungal infection. The cultured pathogen is *Candida albicans* in 95% of cases.[1,4,5] Tuberculosis and syphilis also have been identified as pathogens in chronic paronychia.[13,14,15] Individuals at risk for the development of chronic paronychia are those who have diabetes mellitus and those who are exposed to a wet environment. Conservative treatment includes vasodilators and oral and topical antibacterial and antifungal agents.[2] These treatment modalities have had minimal effectiveness. Conversely, the surgical technique of eponychial marsupialization has been highly effective.[10] Surgical treatment is indicated for all diagnosed chronic paronychia.

Certain antomic structures are relevant to the surgical treatment of paronychia. These structures include the nailplate, which rests on an epithelial matrix. The matrix is divided into the sterile and germinal layers. The germinal matrix is comprised of a fold in which the nail plate is positioned centrally. The eponychium is the soft tissue that overlies the germinal matrix. This structure is sometimes referred to as the eponychial fold.[17]

For anesthesia, digital block is instilled in the affected finger. The eponychial fold is gently elevated from the nail plate using a dental probe, freer elevator, or no. 11 scalpel blade. The pus will express onto the surface of the nail plate. Cultures should then be obtained. Care is taken not to damage the germinal matrix. This is best accomplished by keeping the flat part of the surgical instrument parallel and flush against the nail plate (Fig. 55–2). A gauze wick is inserted into the nail fold.

In more severe infections, a diagonal incision is made perpendicular to the edge of the

■ FIGURE 55–1
A diagram of a paronychia, with an abscess between the eponychial fold and the nail plate.

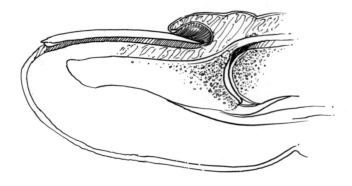

■ FIGURE 55–2
Surgical treatment of a single paronychia requires elevation of the eponychial fold.

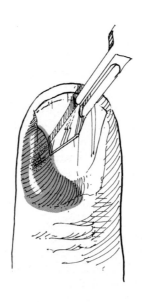

■ FIGURE 55–3
A, In more severe infections, a diagonal incision is centered over the paronychia. **B,** If the abscess has dissected under the nail plate, the outer third is removed.

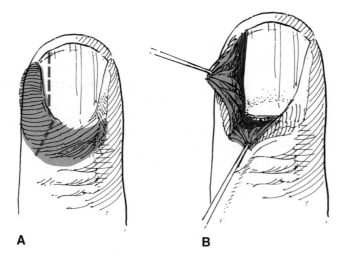

A   B

nail fold (Fig. 55–3A). A gauze wick can then be placed in the wound. When pus is present under the nail plate, the outer third of the plate is removed (Fig. 55–3B).

In the rare circumstance of horseshoe abscess, bilateral diagonal incisions are made (Fig. 55–4). The flap of the dorsal fold is elevated. The proximal third of the plate is discarded, preserving the distal nail plate if possible. A fine mesh gauze wick is placed under the

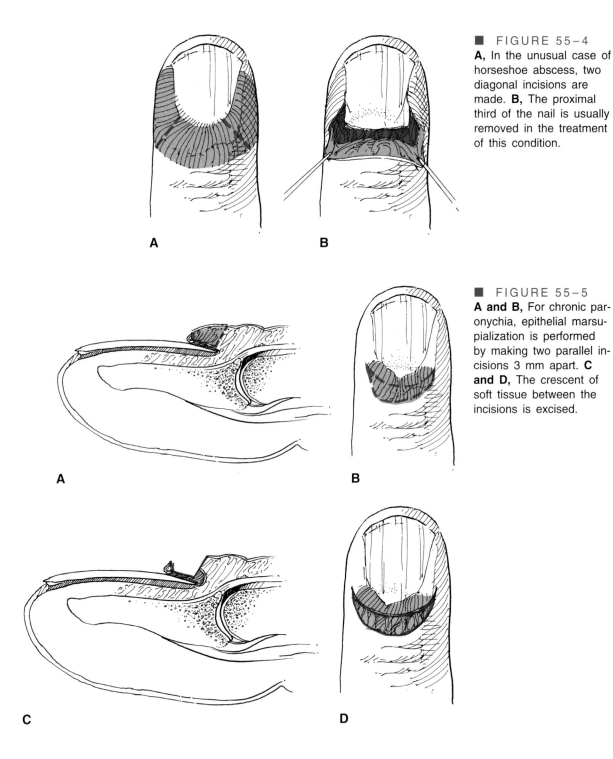

A, In the unusual case of horseshoe abscess, two diagonal incisions are made. **B,** The proximal third of the nail is usually removed in the treatment of this condition.

A and B, For chronic paronychia, epithelial marsupialization is performed by making two parallel incisions 3 mm apart. **C and D,** The crescent of soft tissue between the incisions is excised.

now elevated dorsal flap of the nail fold, and the wick is placed to promote drainage and early adherence.

For chronic infections, epithelial marsupialization is performed by making two incisions parallel to the dorsal edge of the nail fold. The distance between the incisions should be approximately 3 mm (Fig. 55–5A). The 3-mm wide crescent should be excised to include the tissue down to the germinal matrix[6,10] (Figs. 55-5B and 55-5C). Others advocate not excising the subcutaneous fat and removing the nail plate.[2]

Postoperative care of the acute and chronic paronychia encompasses treatment with appropriate antibiotics based on microbiologic tests. The wound should be examined within 48 hours, and, at that time, intermittent soaks of full strength hydrogen peroxide are initiated at least twice a day. Other solutions that can be used for soaking include betadine, chlorahexaphine, and water.

■ TECHNICAL
ALTERNATIVES

Alternative incisions include longitudinal incisions parallel to the nail sulcus. A major pitfall of these incisions is the complication of skin bridge necrosis and subsequent nail deformities secondary to skin adhesions to the nail fold. The skin bridge is the skin that lies between the diagonal incisions. This pitfall is best avoided by the use of diagonal incisions, which leaves a broad base to the skin flap.

A common pitfall in the management of paronychia concerns the diagnosis itself. An acute paronychia is easily confused with a viral infection—herpetic whitlow. The distinguishing symptom of herpetic whitlow is tingling and/or burning of the digital phalanx. After exposure, vesicles may form on an erythematous base for 7 to 10 days. The vesicles may appear honeycombed and hemorrhagic. Surgical intervention in the treatment of herpetic whitlow is contraindicated, as the infection is self-limiting in 2 to 3 weeks.[8,12] Kaposi's sarcoma, leukemia acutis, and subungual malignant melanoma also masquerade as chronic paronychia.[7,11,16]

■ REHABILITATION

Patients are seen at 48 and 72 hours after surgery. At that point, their dressing and packing are removed. A regimen of daily soaks is administered until healing is complete, and the infection has resolved. The patient continues a course of 10 to 14 days of antibiotic therapy based on culture sensitivities. For chronic infections, antifungal steroid ointment is applied to the nail bed. Once the nail is removed, antifungal steroid ointment such as 3% Vioform (iodochlorhydroxyquin) in Mycolog (nystatin, neomycin sulfate, gramicidin, and triamcilonone acetate) is applied to the nail bed for several weeks.[3]

■ OUTCOMES

Early treatment of acute paronychia results in complete resolution of symptoms. Good cosmetic results can be expected. Chronic paronychia has a very low rate of recurrence when marsupialization is performed with nail plate removal.[2]

References

1. Baran R, Bureau H: Surgical treatment of recalcitrant chronic paronychias of the fingers. J Dermatol Surg Oncol, 1981; 7:106–107.
2. Bednar MS, Lane LB: Eponychial marsupialization and nail removal for surgical treatment of chronic paronychia. J Hand Surg, 1991; 16A:314–317.
3. Canales FL, Newmeyer WL, Kilgore ES: The treatment of felons and paronychias. Hand Clinics, 1989; 5:525–523.
4. Chow E, Goh CL: Epidemiology of chronic paronychia in a skin hospital in Singapore. Inter Nat J Derm, 1991; 30:795–798.
5. Daniel CR: Paronychia. Derm Clinics, 1985; 3:461–464.
6. Hausman MR, Lisser SP: Hand infections. Ortho Clinics No Amer, 1992; 12:171–185.
7. High DA, Luscombe HA, Kauh YC: Leukemia cutis masquerading as chronic paronychia. Internat J Derm, 1985; No 9, 24:595–597.
8. Hurst LC, Gluck R, Sampson SP, Down A: Herpetic whitlow with bacterial abscess. J Hand Surg, 1991; 311–314.
9. Kanavel AB: Infections of the Hand. A guide to the surgical treatment of acute and chronic suppurative processes in the fingers, hand, and forearm. Philadelphia: 7th Ed. Lea & Febiger, 1943.
10. Keyser JJ, Eaton RG: Surgical cure of chronic paronychia by eponychial marsupialization. Plast Reconstr Surg; 58:66–70.
11. Keith JE, Shaw Wilgis EF: Kaposi's sarcoma in the hand of an AIDS patient. J Hand Surg, 1986; 11A:410–413.
12. Klotz RW: Herpetic whitlow: An occupational hazard. J Amer Assoc Nur Anesth, 1990; 58: 8–15.
13. O'Donnell TF, Jurgenson PF, Weyerich NF: An occupational hazard—Tuberculous paronychia. Arch Surg, 1971; 103:757–758.

14. Siegel DB, Gelberman RH: Infections of the hand. Ortho Clin North Am, 1988; 19:779–789.
15. Starzycki Z: Primary syphilis of the fingers. Br J Vener Dis, 1983; 59:169–171.
16. Ware JW: Sub-ungual malignant malanoma presenting as sub-acute paronychia following trauma. Hand, 1977; 9:49–51.
17. Zook EG, van Beck AH, Russell RC: Anatomy and physiology of the perionychium: a review of the literature and anatomical study. J Hand Surg, 1986; 6:518–536.

$$\overline{56}$$

Felons

■ HISTORY OF THE TECHNIQUE

Kanavel's original recommendations concerning felons are of significant importance in the discussion of this topic. He believed that the anatomy of the distal phalanx was unique and best described as a "closed sac" of fat separated by septae of connective tissue. Subcutaneous glands lying in the columns of fat presented a portal of entry for bacteria (Fig. 56–1).[4] The keys to diagnosis were severe, throbbing pain, tenderness, erythema, and swelling of the distal phalanx.

Kanavel recommended immediate incision once the diagnosis is made. The "incision should be made as soon as the edema restricted to the distal phalanx has proceeded to a degree causing hardness, but not necessarily the board-like feeling characteristic of pus in other subcutaneous areas." He noted that patients typically had diffuse involvement of the digital pulp. However, he did recognize that at times a well-localized area of the pulp was amenable to an incision directly over this area. Most often when there is no localization of the process, the incision "should be made somewhat to the side, and not in the median line, as is unfortunately frequently done."[4]

There continues to be controversy concerning the specific incision used. As alluded to by Kanavel, the criteria used in choosing the appropriate incision are not always obvious.

■ INDICATIONS AND CONTRAINDICATIONS

The digital pulp is a specialized connective tissue framework, isolated and different from the rest of the finger. Multiple trabeculae divide the pulp of the distal phalanx into a latticework, the interstices of which are filled by eccrine sweat glands and fat globules. The sweat glands open into the epidermis, thus providing a portal of entry into the volar fat pad. A history of penetrating trauma to the distal finger is usually obtainable, although the inciting event may have been so inconsequential that it has been forgotten. Wooden splinters, glass slivers, or minor cuts are common predisposing causes. Felons also can be iatrogenically induced, as in the case of "fingerstick felons," which follow the repeated trauma of fingerstick blood tests. The organism most frequently responsible for felons is *Staphylococcus aureus*, although infections caused by gram-negative organisms also have been reported.[2] These anatomic and pathophysiologic concepts are presently the basis for indicating and planning the decompression for felons.

Indications for surgical treatment of felons are predicated on distinguishing this entity from other maladies involving the digital pulp. Felons are clinically characterized by exquisite tenderness, erythema, digital pulp swelling, and severe throbbing pain.[4,8] Often, the pain is severe enough to prevent sleep. An early cellulitic process of the digital pulp may be empirically treatable with antistaphyloccoccal antibiotics. However, if there is no clinical resolution within 24 to 48 hours, re-evaluation for the presence of a felon is mandatory.[8] Differentiating a felon from a Herpetic whitelow is important because surgical treatment of the latter is contraindicated. Suppurative flexor tenosynovitis involves the entire digit with redness, swelling, and painful range of motion, rather than findings confined to the digital pulp only. Surgical treatment for this particular condition will be thoroughly discussed elsewhere in this text.

■ SURGICAL TECHNIQUES

As in all surgical procedures for infections in the hand and upper extremity, adequate anesthesia and a bloodless operative field are mandatory. These requisites can be achieved in a number of different ways. Digital block anesthesia is an alternative, although at times less reliable. Anesthesia via intravenous regional technique or wrist block technique are

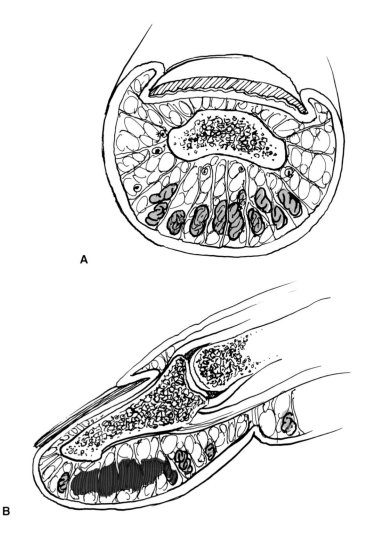

■ FIGURE 56–1
A, Normal crossectional
anatomy of digital pulp.
B, Sagittal plane view of
pathoanatomy of felon.

A

B

good alternatives. A general anesthetic may be necessary for the treatment of children. Tourniquet control is best achieved with an arm tourniquet set 100 to 150 mmHg above the patient's systolic blood pressure. Digital tourniquet control with rubber tubing may be used, although this is less reliable.

The placement and type of skin incision used is the most controversial issue in the treatment of felons.[2] In the most frequent case of diffuse involvement of the digital pulp, a high lateral incision just inferior (1 to 3 mm) to the lateral border of the nailplate and well distal to the distal interphalangeal joint flexion crease is recommended. (Fig. 56–2). This incision is best made on the nonoppositional surface of the digit involved. That is, the ulnar border of the index, long, and ring digits and the radial border of the thumb and small digits.[2,6,8]

The deeper structures at risk include the digital artery and nerve, the flexor tendon sheath, and the nail bed.[5] The majority of the terminal branches and arborization of the digital neurovascular structures are palmar to the incision. Therefore, this incision preserves digital tip sensibility and is unlikely to induce soft tissue avascular necrosis. However, patients may note numbness along the lateral border of the nail just dorsal to the incision, probably due to sectioning of a dorsal branch of the trifurcation of the digital nerve. The flexor tendon sheath is proximal to the recommended incision.[2] However, surgical dissection proximal to the midportion of the diaphysis of the distal phalanx could possibly result in penetration of the flexor tendon sheath with the subsequent development

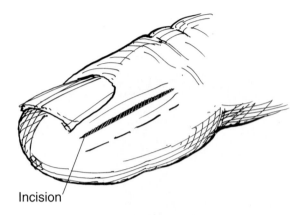

Incision

of suppurative flexor tenosynovitis. Injury to the nail bed would be unlikely unless the plane of dissection deviated dorsally.

Loupe magnification is helpful during dissection. After the skin is incised, care should be taken to avoid terminal branches of the digital nerve. Sharp dissection with a scalpel across the fibrous septae is performed until the abscess cavity is encountered (Fig. 56–3). If pus is encountered, aerobic and anaeorbic cultures and gram stains should be obtained. The extent of the abscess cavity should be assessed. This can be performed with a blunt narrow dental probe. Care should be taken to dissect toward the volar margin of the distal phalanx. Blunt dissection is usually required to separate the fibrous septae. Dissection of soft tissue should cease before penetration of the opposite side of the digital pulp is reached. The wound is left open and should be gently packed with sterile gauze, Vaseline gauze, bismuth impregnated gauze (Xeroform gauze), or some authorities recommend a thick layer of zinc oxide.[5] The goal of these dressing materials is to allow further drainage in the first 24 to 48 hours after surgery. The digit and wrist should be immobilized and elevated for 24 to 48 hours.[2] Oral cephalosporin should be given for 10 to 14 days. Antibiotic coverage may need to be modified depending on operative culture results.[7,11]

■ TECHNICAL ALTERNATIVES

If the felon can be unequivocally localized or a sinus tract is present, a small linear incision, oriented in the long axis of the digit, directly over the focus of presentation can be effective.[1,5,8] Some authorities believe that this incision should be used for all felons because the potential for digital nerve injury is lower.[5] A potential pitfall is mistaking a bleb of pus beneath the epidermis as the primary focus of the abscess. Inadequate drainage could result. Opponents to this philosophy believe that a palmar digital pulp scar may lead to tip insensibility and the risk of inadvertant damage to the digital flexor tendon sheath is high.[4] The alternatives of the "fishmouth," "lateral hockey stick," "bilateral midlateral" incisions are mentioned only for historic interest. These techniques led to an unacceptable number of complications including instability of the soft tissue of the digital pulp, insensibility, hypertrophic scar formation, and digital pulp necrosis with subsequent compromised digital function.[2,4,5,8]

Caution should be taken in the diabetic and immunocompromised patient with regard to selection of antiobiotic medication. These individuals are susceptible to gram-negative, anaeorobic bacteria, as well as more unusual opportunistic pathogens.[3,11]

■ REHABILITATION

Dressing changes three times a day with any one of a number of dressing materials (sterile gauze, bismuth-impregnated gauze, zinc oxide) should begin 1 to 2 days after surgery. Digital active range of motion exercises beginning in conjunction with dressing changes are usually all that is necessary to achieve the goals of normal preoperative range of motion. These exercises can usually be started 1 to 2 days after surgery, provided there has been resolution of signs of persistent soft tissue infection. Persistant distal interphalangeal joint stiffness may indicate articular involvement (septic arthritis). This condition

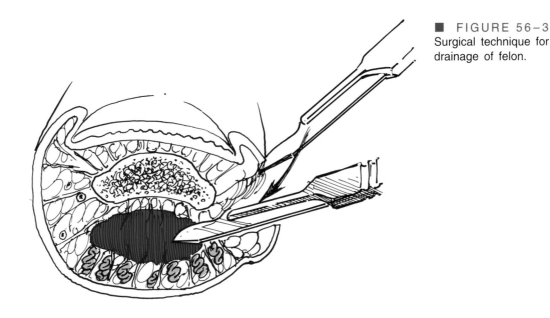

■ FIGURE 56–3
Surgical technique for
drainage of felon.

could have predated the operative treatment, thus indicating a missed diagnosis, or it could occur secondary to inadvertant penetration of this joint during the procedure.

Bolton[1] reported on 50 unselected cases of felons treated by incision or incision and intramuscular penicillin (10 to 14 days). He reported average healing times from 11.5 to 35 days, depending on the severity of the initial infection. Koch[6] also noted that most patients had "some limitation of movement of the terminal interphalangeal joint at the time of discharge from the clinic," five patients had a tender scar, and none developed "causalgia." Robins[9] noted an average healing time after incision of 10.5 to 30 days. He stressed the prolongation of healing and the increased incidence of complications when patients were encountered late in the course of the infection. They reviewed 18 of 33 of patients with established osteomyelitis at the time of initial presentation. Only two patients in the group were completely satisfied. Complaints included poor cosmesis, tender scars, limited range of motion, and one patient who went on to subsequent amputation. Scott[10] reported on 347 patients treated surgically for felons. Fifty-six percent of these cases healed in an average of 11 days, while 44% took an average of 34 days to heal. This points out that more longstanding infections (i.e., those with draining sinus tracts, osteomyelitis) are likely to have protracted courses until healing is achieved. They also noted the importance of thorough debridement to facilitate early healing. More recently, Kilgore[5] reported excellent functional results using the palmar midline incision technique; however, no specific series of patients or objective criteria were noted.

There is a relative paucity of follow-up studies on the treatment of felons. Definite conclusions with regard to different surgical techniques, specific type and duration of antibiotic therapy, duration and type of immobilization, and rehabilitation, will only be reached by prospective studies.

■ OUTCOMES

References

1. Bolton H, Fowler PJ, Jepson RP: Natural history and treatment of pulp space infection and osteomyelitis of the terminal phalanx. J Bone Joint Surg, 1949; 31B:499–504.
2. Canales FL, Newmeyer, WL, Kelgore ES: The treatment of felons and paronychias. Hand Clin, 1989; 5:515–523.
3. Glass KD: Factors related to the resolution of treated hand infections. J Hand Surg, 1982; 7: 388–394.
4. Kanavel AB: Infections of the Hand, 6th Ed, Philadelphia: Lea and Febiger, 1933:157–166.
5. Kilgore ES, Brown LG, Newmeyer WL, Graham WP, Davis TS: Treatment of felons. Am J Surg, 1975; 130:194–198.

6. Koch, SL: Infections of the fingers and palm. Pennsyl Med J, 1937; 40:597–604.
7. Leddy JP: Infections of the upper extremity. J Hand Surg, Vol. 1986; 11A:294–297.
8. Linscheid RL, Dobyns JH: Common and uncommon infections of the Hand Orthop Clin North Am, 1975; 6:1063–1104.
9. Robins RH: Infections of the hand. J Bone Joint Surg, 1952; 34B:567–580.
10. Scott JC: Results of treatment of infections of the hand. J Bone Joint Surg, 1952; 34B:581–587.
11. Stern PJ, Staneck JL, McDonough JJ, Neale HW, Tyler G: Established hand infection: A controlled, prospective study. J Hand Surg, 1983; 8:553–559.

DALE R. WHEELER

57

Suppurative Flexor Tenosynovitis

Infections involving the digital flexor sheath occur in a closed space and require prompt recognition and treatment to avoid flexor tendon adhesions, rupture, and necrosis. As is true of other closed space infections, the treatment of choice is surgical drainage and lavage. However, because of the anatomic location, the choice of surgical approach, whether by open drainage of the entire flexor sheath or by closed sheath irrigation, is important to achieve a speedy recovery and to diminish postoperative morbidity.[1]

Irrigation of the flexor tendon sheath using a catheter was described by Dickson-Wright in 1943.[2] A ureteric catheter was inserted through the opened wound, the sheath was flushed, and then 1 to 2 ml penicillin were instilled. The catheter remained in for daily instillation of penicillin. Before this case report was published in the proceedings of the Royal College of Medicine, Kanavel[8] had advocated open surgical drainage of the entire flexor sheath accomplished by an incision on the border of the digit and volar to the nerve and vessel. He described opening the sheath from the level of the distal interphalangeal joint to the digital web proximally. Unonius[15] described catheter irrigation from a single exposure, postoperative irrigation with saline, and instillation of penicillin. In 1978 Neviaser[11] reported on a study of 20 patients treated with closed sheath irrigation. He advocated this technique because it resulted in a rapid return of function and minimal morbidity. Others report comparative success with similar types of limited open sheath irrigation.[7,13]

■ HISTORY OF THE TECHNIQUE

Surgical drainage of the flexor tendon sheath is indicated in patients who have full-blown pictures of flexor sheath infection or in those who do not clearly respond rapidly to nonsurgical management of the early presenting flexor sheath infection. Kanavel[8] described the classic signs of flexor sheath infection. He characterized the digit as being in a semiflexed position, with tenderness over the digital flexor sheath, symmetric swelling of the digit, and significant pain on passive extension (Fig. 57–1). There is frequently a history of minor trauma and a puncture wound. Other causes include extension from other digital infections such as a felon or septic interphalangeal (IP) joint and occasionally hematogenous etiologies.[10]

The surgeon should maintain a high index of suspicion when assessing a patient with possible digital sheath infection. This infection is typically not accompanied by a significantly elevated temperature or leukocyte count. The diagnosis must be made predominantly on history and physical examination. The presentation may be atypical. One or more of Kanavel's classic signs may be absent in diabetic patients who have significant peripheral neuropathy, in patients partially treated with antibiotics, or in patients who take steroids or are otherwise immunocompromised.[14] The host response in such patients may be suppressed, resulting in less swelling and pain.

Occasionally, in addition to the history and physical examination, the flexor sheath is aspirated to obtain material for gram stain and culture for identification of the appropriate antibiotic therapy. Typically, it is better to err on the side of surgical drainage because it causes minimal morbidity and forestalls the complications associated with missed infections.

■ INDICATIONS AND CONTRAINDICATIONS

The initial management of a patient who presents fewer than 24 to 48 hours after onset of symptoms can include aspiration of the sheath, as mentioned previously, followed by

■ SURGICAL TECHNIQUES

463

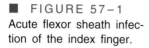

■ FIGURE 57–1
Acute flexor sheath infection of the index finger.

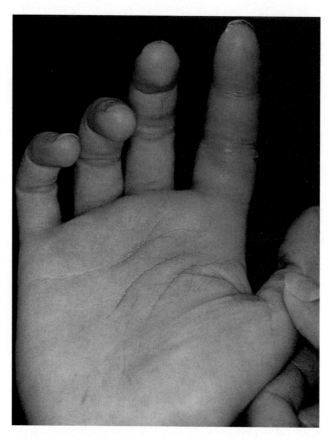

full hand and wrist splinting and appropriate broad spectrum antibiotic coverage. If prompt improvement is observed clinically, this may be all that is required. If patients present later, after onset of symptoms with established infections, or if they do not respond rapidly to nonoperative care, surgical drainage is indicated.

Digital or wrist block anesthesia is not satisfactory because it usually requires injection into areas that are edematous or erythematous. Intravenous regional blocks, which require exsanguination, may spread the infection and therefore should not be used. The preferred method is either axillary or general anesthesia. In the presence of axillary lymphadenopathy, general anesthesia is recommended as long as other health factors do not contraindicate this technique. The arm is elevated for several minutes for gravity exsanguination, and then the tourniquet is inflated.

The important surface landmarks to remember in this technique include the location of the neurovascular bundles in the digit, which lie palmar to the midaxial line and the location of the proximal extent of the flexor tendon sheath at the proximal aspect of the A-1 pulley, which is approximately at the level of the proximal palmar crease for the index, slightly more distal for the middle and at the level of the distal palmar crease for the ring and small finger. The proximal location of the flexor pollicis longus tendon is identified by the visible overlying flexor carpi radialis tendon and its sheath. The flexor tendon sheath is comprised of a membranous portion, a thin double-walled synovial tube (made up of visceral and parietal layers) joined at each end forming a closed space, and a retinacular portion, the pulley system.[3] The membranous portion begins at the metacarpal neck proximal to the A-1 pulley and ends at the distal interphalangeal (DIP) joint. The parietal layer is reinforced by bands of collagen representing the annular and cruciform pulleys. Typically, the thumb flexor sheath connects to the radial bursa and the small finger to the ulnar bursa, both of which extend proximal to the carpal tunnel.[3,10,12] There may be a connection that would permit the spread of infection from radial to ulnar bursae through the potential space of Parona posterior to the flexor digitorum profundus and anterior to the pronator quadratus. When a hand is being evaluated for the presence of flexor sheath infection of the thumb or small finger, particular attention should be directed to these areas about the wrist as well as the digits.

The surgical technique begins with two incisions and is similar for all fingers.[11,12] The proximal incision overlies the proximal extent of the flexor tendon sheath. Either a short transverse or zig-zag incision is made about the distal palmar crease for the middle, ring, and small fingers and over the proximal palmar crease for the index finger (Fig. 57–2). The radial and ulnar neurovascular bundles are identified and retracted and the flexor tendon sheath is exposed proximal to the A-1 pulley. The incision must provide adequate exposure of the flexor tendon sheath and avoid injury to the adjacent neurovascular bundles.

The distal incision is then made in the midaxial line of the digit at approximately the level of the DIP joint. The digital neurovascular bundle is retracted in a palmar direction. Dissection then extends directly to the flexor tendon sheath in the midaxial line. This provides exposure of the flexor tendon sheath distal to the A-4 pulley. Preferably the distal incision should be made on the ulnar aspect of the index, middle, and ring finger to place the incision and any area of potential postoperative tenderness away from the opposable pinch surface (Fig. 57–3). On the small finger, the radial side is preferred because the ulnar border is frequently involved with touch. The distal incision for drainage may incorporate a traumatic wound if present.

Proximally, the sheath is opened and cultures obtained. A portion of the sheath is excised to allow access to the flexor sheath and provide drainage. A window is made in the sheath distal to the A-4 pulley to provide outflow by excising a portion of the C-3 pulley. After both proximal and distal incisions have been made, the sheath is irrigated with a standard 2-inch 16- or 18-gauge angiocatheter (or longer central line catheter) with the trochar removed and inserted from the proximal incision carefully 2 to 3 cm distally into the sheath. The catheter is typically placed volar to the tendons inside the sheath. The sheath is then irrigated with a 10-ml syringe of normal saline until clear fluid is obtained at the

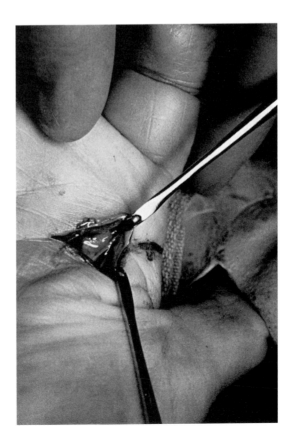

■ FIGURE 57–2
Proximal exposure for the index finger.

■ FIGURE 57–3
A distal, midaxial ulnar incision at the distal interphalangeal joint level of
the ring finger.

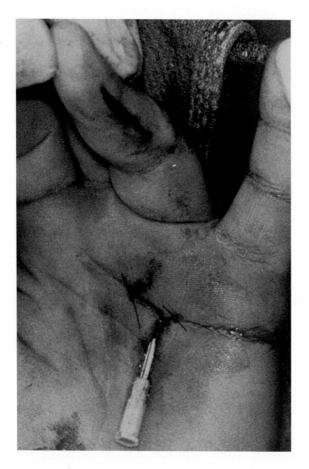

distal site. If resistance is encountered when attempting to irrigate the sheath, the catheter should be removed to assess whether it has been kinked and then repositioned in the flexor sheath. A new catheter may need to be used if the catheter is crimped. One should continue to adjust this catheter position until easy irritation is possible. Resistance will also be encountered if you have not made an adequate window distally for egress of fluid and this area should also be re-examined. The catheter is then carefully sutured to the skin to maintain its position and is connected to sterile intravenous tubing. The catheter retention suture must not occlude the lumen. The palmar wound is closed around the catheter and the distal wound is left open to maintain egress through the sheath window (Figure 57–4). A drain is typically not needed in the distal wound. The integrity of the sheath irrigation system should again be checked with the hand and fingers in the postoperative immobilization position to assure that easy flow will occur postoperatively.

When using this technique for the thumb, the distal incision should be made on the radial side to avoid the pinch surface, and the proximal exposure should be made using a short longitudinal incision just ulnar to the flexor carpi radialis (FCR) tendon two centimeters proximal to the wrist flexion crease. The FCR tendon is retracted radially and the digital flexors ulnarly to expose flexor pollicis longus (FPL). A catheter is inserted through the proximal incision into the FPL sheath and radial bursa. The catheter is irrigated until clear fluid flows from the distal incision.[12] The proximal incision should not extend distal to the wrist flexion crease to avoid the palmar cutaneous branch of the median nerve. The surgeon should look for this branch if the incision is extended distally.

The small finger flexor tendon sheath is sometimes in continuity with the ulnar bursa so that swelling and tenderness may extend into the carpal tunnel and proximally. Patients with this anatomic configuration may show symptoms of median nerve compression, and the index, middle, and ring fingers may assume a painful semiflexed position.[14]

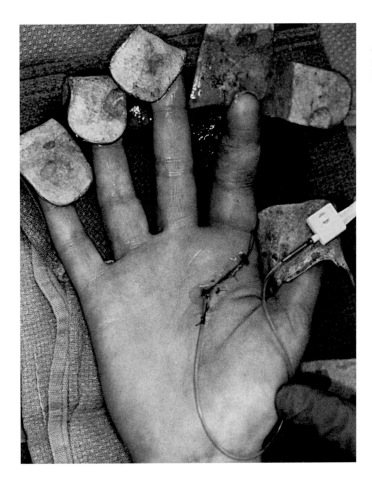

If this is the circumstance, the typical incisions are made for the small finger distally at the DIP joint and proximally at the level of the distal palmar crease. If there appears to be extension of the infection proximally, the ulnar bursa is identified proximal to the wrist. An incision is made on the ulnar aspect of the distal forearm, radial to the flexor carpi ulnaris and ulnar neurovascular bundle. The forearm fascia is opened and the ulnar bursa is identified and opened. The ulnar bursa is thoroughly irrigated through this exposure. In addition, a catheter is inserted through the palm wound and directed proximally along the small finger flexor tendon sheath. The ulnar bursa is then irrigated in a distal to proximal fashion, establishing outflow at the wrist level. This proximal forearm wound is left open and two-catheter irrigation system is utilized, one extending from the palm into the digit and one directed proximally.[12] A drain is inserted into the forearm wound to assure adequate outflow and to prevent accumulation of fluid in the carpal tunnel or distal forearm.

In the presence of severe infection and swelling involving the ulnar or radial bursa, the transverse carpal ligament may need to be released completely to decompress the median nerve and to allow adequate irrigation and debridement of this region as well as the space of Parona. The transverse carpal ligament should be released if there is evidence of increased pressure in the carpal canal due to accumulation of pus or need for debridement of infected tenosynovium.

The hand and forearm are then wrapped with a bulky dressing, supported with a resting splint, and elevated. Care should be taken while dressing the hand and forearm to maintain the digital position in which good digital irrigation was obtained. Postoperatively, the sheath should be continuously irrigated with 25 to 50 ml saline an hour using an I0-Vac pump or intermittently irrigated every 1 to 2 hours with 50 ml of fluid. Strict sterility of the catheter irrigation system must be maintained. Satisfactory flow of the irrigant should be possible as long as attention has been paid intraoperatively to catheter position and adequate distal sheath opening. If difficulties are encountered in the postoperative period, digital position may be altered in an attempt to improve flow. Reposition of the catheter is typically not possible due to issues of sterility. Occasionally flow can be re-established by a flush of irrigation utilizing a Heparin flush. If flow ceases and cannot be re-established, the catheter is removed and the patient begun on a program of therapy and soaks and is watched closely for signs of pus accumulation or worsening flexor sheath symptoms.

■ TECHNICAL ALTERNATIVES

An alternative treatment for flexor tendon sheath infection is by open technique involving an extensive surgical exposure of the digital flexor sheath. A variety of techniques have been described.[4,6,10] A midlateral digital incision is made on the ulnar side of the index, middle, and ring finger and the radial side of the small finger and thumb. The dissection is similar to that for the distal closed sheath irrigation extending dorsal to the neurovascular bundle and exposing the length of the flexor tendon sheath from the proximal aspect of the proximal phalanx distally to the DIP joint. A proximal incision is made over the palmar crease to expose and irrigate the tendon sheath proximal to the A-1 pulley. Additionally, debridement of the flexor tendon sheath is possible, but care is taken to preserve the pulleys, especially A-2 and A-4. The midlateral wound is left open, and postoperatively the splints are placed and the patient is given antibiotics. After 24 to 48 hours, the patient begins a directed therapy program using early range of motion techniques and soaks, which allow the wounds to heal by secondary intention. This extensive exposure may be necessary for those patients presenting late with frank infection to allow debridement of infected and ruptured necrotic flexor tendons. These patients are not indicated for drainage alone because the retained avascular necrotic tendon will be a source of continued sepsis.

Failure to provide adequate drainage and irrigation at the time of surgery is a potential problem in performing closed flexor sheath procedures. Before the patient leaves the operating room suite, the surgeon should ensure that good flow has been obtained so that the irrigation system continues to flush the tendon sheath postoperatively and fluid does not accumulate in the finger or hand. The forearm, wrist, and digits are immobilized postoperatively with the wrist in 20° of dorsiflexion and the digits in the functional position. Initially, all digits are included in this splint, which is well-padded and bulky in the region of the palm and digits. Some patients will experience discomfort during attempts at sheath irrigation. This is more problematic with intermittent irrigation than with continuous irrigation. In these circumstances, the digit should be examined to assure that fluid is not accumulating in the palm or digit. If this is not the problem and good flow is possible, local anesthetic can be mixed with the irrigant before intermittent irrigation. Use of regional or digital nerve blocks is not advised because of similar concerns as with the choice of operative anesthesia.

A second potential complication arises if the surgeon fails to recognize the primary focus of the infection and does not provide adequate treatment or drainage of the infected area. For example, if a septic proximal interphalangeal (PIP) joint becomes a flexor sheath infection, and if the primary site of infection is not adequately treated, cartilage loss and joint stiffness occur and osteomyelitis may result.

The locations of the surgical incisions, especially distally, are of importance to avoid potential areas of scarring that may be problematic. Typically, the pinch surfaces of the index, middle, and ring fingers are on the radial side, and the thumb and small finger contact areas are on the ulnar side.

The most important potential pitfall is a failure to recognize a flexor sheath infection in its early presentation. A high index of suspicion should be maintained, especially for those patients whose treatment included only oral antibiotics or those systemically ill patients, both of which may have been blunted clinical signs. As a consequence, when the surgeon sees the patient for the first time, the presentation may be atypical. In this situation, the surgeon should err on the side of surgical drainage, basing his or her judgements on knowledge of the patient's health status and prior treatment. As stated previously, tendon sheath aspiration can be an important adjunct to this decision making process.

Irrigation should continue for approximately 48 hours. If, after that length of time, the finger is significantly improved and swelling and pain have decreased, the catheter is removed, and the patient begins a directed therapy program of active and passive range of motion. Appropriate intravenous antibiotic coverage is continued for an additional 48 hours. If the clinical course shows continued improvement, the patient is discharged on oral antibiotics and directed therapy.

Therapy generally continues for 3 to 6 weeks after discharge from the hospital. A resting splint is frequently used in the initial phase after postoperative dressing removal. This is usually a hand-based resting splint with MP joint maximally flexed and IP joints extended and may include the wrist in cases where infection was established proximal to the wrist as well as in the digit. Therapy progress will need to be monitored closely as patients may have varying degrees of difficulty with digital flexion and digital extension such that creative and alternate splinting may be necessary including dynamic assisted extension and dynamic assisted flexion splinting in the recovery phase. Patients are released to full activities when wounds are closed and swelling has resolved and does not recur with activity. Digital range of motion should have recovered to a satisfactory functional degree and the patient should not be experiencing discomfort with use.

■ REHABILITATION

When the infection is recognized and treated early, treatment by closed tendon sheath irrigation can produce good results. Of Neviaser's 20 patients,[11] 18 recovered full range of motion within 1 week of treatment, and the other 2 achieved 255° and 245° of total active motion. Results in the presence of concomitant joint infections are less satisfactory, as might be expected. In a report of 85 digits, Freeland and co-authors[5] achieved good results in 74%, fair results in 13%, and poor results in 13%. The criteria used for this result classification was as described by Flynn[4] in 1955 with good results having 30° or less flexion contracture at the PIP joint, 90° of active PIP joint flexion or greater and the tip touched or nearly touched the palm in flexion. The fair results had greater than 30° of flexion contracture but 45° of further active PIP joint flexion and the tip came to within 2 cm of the palm. Poor results had less than 45° active PIP joint flexion and the digit did not reach within 2 cm of the palm. Nearly 25% had concomitant PIP or IP joint sepsis, and in these patients there was a longer delay before seeking treatment and less favorable overall outcome. There is a lack of information regarding correlation between infecting organism and expected outcome. The stage of presentation and other concomitant patient health factors are clearly related to outcome. If the patient has a flexor tendon that has already become necrotic or has an established joint infection, a poorer functional outcome can be expected. Delay in presentation or failure to recognize flexor sheath infections early are particularly detrimental. Patient health factors such as poorly controlled diabetes also typically result in a poorer outcome and require close attention to patient response to assure a satisfactorily improving course after initial irrigation and debridement.[9]

■ OUTCOMES

References

1. Delsignore JL, Ritland D, Becker DR, Watson HK: Continuous catheter irrigation for the treatment of suppurative flexor tenosynovitis. Conn Med, 1986; 50:503–506.
2. Dickson-Wright A: Tendon sheath infection. Proc R Soc Med, 1944;37:504.
3. Doyle JR: Anatomy of the finger flexor tendon sheath and pulley system. J Hand Surg, 1988; 13A:473–484.
4. Flynn JE: Acute suppurative tenosynovitis. In: Hand Surgery, 3rd Ed, Baltimore: Williams and Wilkins, 1982:696–706.
5. Freeland AE, Burkhalter, WE, Mann RJ: Functional treatment of acute suppurative digital tenosynovitis. Orthop Trans, 1981; 5:113–114.
6. Grinnel RS: Acute suppurative tenosynovitis of the flexor tendon sheaths of the hand. Ann Surg, 1936; 105:97–119.

7. Juliano PJ, Eglseder WA: Limited open-tendon-sheath irrigation in the treatment of pyogenic flexor tenosynovitis. Ortho Rev, 1991; 20:1065–1069.
8. Kanavel AB: Infections of the Hand: A Guide to the Surgical Treatment of Acute and Chronic Suppurative Processes in the Fingers, Hand, and Forearm, 7th Ed, Philadelphia: Lea and Febiger, 1939.
9. Maloon S, de Beer JdeV, Opitz M, Singer M: Acute flexor tendon sheath infections. J Hand Surg, 1990; 15A:474–477.
10. Mann RJ: Tenosynovitis. In: Infections of the Hand, Philadelphia: Lea and Febiger, 1988: 31–43.
11. Neviaser RJ: Closed tendon sheath irrigation for pyogenic flexor tenosynovitis. J Hand Surg, 1978; 3:462–466.
12. Neviaser RJ, Gunther SF: Tenosynovial infections in the hand—diagnosis and management. I: Acute pyogenic tenosynovitis of the hand. AAOS Instr Course Lectures, 1980; 29:108–117.
13. Pollen AG: Acute infection of the tendon sheaths. The Hand, 1974; 6:21–25.
14. Pollen AG: Acute tendon sheath infections. In: Lamb DW, Hooper G, Kuczynski K (eds): The Practice of Hand Surgery. 2nd Ed, Oxford: Blackwell Scientific Publications, 1989:606–612.
15. Unonius E: Local penicillin treatment of suppurative infection in the tendon sheath. Acta Chir Scand, 1947; 95:532–540.

58

RONALD J. MANN,
WILLIAM F. BLAIR

Septic Arthritis of the Wrist

Septic arthritis of the wrist presents a challenge in both diagnosis and treatment. Although septic arthritis in general is not uncommon, septic arthritis of the wrist itself is unusual. It is usually both acute and suppurative and results when pathogenic bacteria are introduced into the joint or as a local manifestation of bacterermia.

Septic arthritis of the wrist does not have a predilection for a specific age group, and it crosses racial and sexual boundaries. When it does occur in children, it is relatively unusual. Wilson and co-authors described one case of septic arthritis of the wrist in a series of 61 children and Speiser described it in one of 86. There are no substantial data to suggest that the relative occurrence is actually any greater.[4]

Septic arthritis of the wrist involves adults more than adolescents or children. Three major groups can be identified: those patients with unremarkable medical histories before an episode of wrist trauma, older patients in general, and patients with a predisposing medical condition. Trauma is a common etiologic factor. Blunt trauma to adjacent periarticular tissues, violation of the joint capsule by puncture wounds, and extension of a local hand infections can be causative. Rarely human, dog, or cat bites of the wrist have been causative factors.

Nongonococcal bacterial arthritis is an increasingly common problem in elderly patients. In a summary of 89 elderly patients with bacterial arthritis, the average age was 70.3 years.[4] Although the knee, hip, and shoulder were the most commonly involved joints,[1,8] infections in the wrist do occur. Vincent described 2 wrists in 21 (10%) septic joints in a group of elderly patients.[7] Although elderly patients may be predisposed to septic arthritis, a study by Ho suggests that prevalence of septic arthritis does not increase with age. In 37 septic joints in a population with an age range of 23 to 89 years, 3 of 37 (8%) infected joints were wrists.[5]

There is an increased incidence of septic arthritis, including the wrist, in the rheumatoid population. This increased incidence is caused by a variety of factors, including steroid injections, general debilitation, and immunosuppression secondary to medical treatment. This is an especially serious complication in rheumatoid arthritis and related disorders.[2,6] Other disorders that predispose to septic arthritis include diabetes mellitus, cirrhosis, chronic renal failure, and malignancy. Subacute bacterial endocarditis with secondary septic arthritis of the wrist also has been reported in patients undergoing parental antibiotic therapy.

Although much is known clinically about septic arthritis of the wrist, little is written about the technical aspects of surgically treating this condition. Most authors have recommended a dorsal approach, but the historic basis for this recommendation is not defined. We describe a standard dorsal approach for draining a septic wrist, with an emphasis on technical details.

■ HISTORY OF THE TECHNIQUE

■ INDICATIONS AND CONTRAINDICATIONS

A careful physical examination and diagnostic work-up must be done to differentiate septic arthritis from cellulitis of the hand and other conditions that can present with an inflamed wrist joint. The differential diagnosis of any painful wrist in the patient with an increased sedimentation rate should include the following: gout and pseudogout, acute rheumatic fever, a flare-up of rheumatoid arthritis, nonspecific synovitis, serum sickness, Reiter's syndrome, psoriatic arthritis, systemic lupus erythematosis, sarcoidosis, and ankylosing spondylitis. Septic arthritis of the wrist also can occur concurrently with any of these disorders. Tuberculosis and atypical mycobacterial infections can cause granulomatous wrist joint arthritis, which may be suppurative but tends to be chronic and indolent. Acute inflammation of the wrist mimicking septic arthritis can occur as an immunologic reaction to a distant foci of infection. This postinfectious wrist joint arthritis has been reported in association with internal infections, brucellosis, and micoplasma or urogenital infections. The arthritis may present acutely, causing effusion and local inflammation, but laboratory data often reflect a nonsuppurative and culture-negative effusion. The inflammation is usually transient and resolves as the underlying cause is effectively treated.

Patients with a septic wrist experience progressive pain, decreasing range of motion through the wrist, and swelling of both the hand and wrist. Pertinent physical findings include swelling and tenderness. Erythema and local warmth are not always present. Signs localize dorsally even in cases in which inoculation occurred through a volar injury. Fluctuance on palpation is a rare presentation. Most wrists are held in slight flexion. Severe pain results from all motion through the wrist joint, especially extension, although localization of the pain is sometimes difficult.

Careful physical examination of the wrist and hand can provide a great deal of useful information. The wrist should be gently and securely stabilized at 5 to 10° of dorsiflexion (Fig. 58–1) while fully ranging the metacarpophalangeal joints (Fig. 58–2). This maneuver may be performed without causing discomfort in the patient with septic arthritis of the wrist, but in the presence of other inflammatory lesions of the hand it causes great pain. Radiographs are of little help early in the course of wrist sepsis. A radiographic feature noted occasionally is capsular distention of soft tissues on the lateral projection (Fig. 58–3).

The importance of the diagnostic wrist aspiration cannot be stressed enough. The dorsal approach is used with an 18-gauge needle introduced through the sterilized skin (Fig. 58–4). The possible information that can be obtained from a gram stain and culture of the wrist aspirate outweighs the risk of introducing infection into the joint. Bacteria noted on gram stain are an invaluable diagnostic aid. The presence of bacteria on a gram stain from a wrist aspirate is pathognomonic for septic arthritis. Another diagnostic aid that has been suggested to be of some value is the nitroblue tetrazolium test. An increased number of tagged synovial cells will appear in the joints of patients with septic arthritis.

The indication for surgically draining a septic wrist begins with an index of suspicion, a supportive history, and a positive physical examination. Erythrocyte sedimentation rates (ESRs) are elevated above normal in all patients, but peripheral leucocytosis occurs in less than half. In acute septic arthritis radiographs are nondiagnostic, revealing only soft tissue swelling over the dorsal aspect of the wrist and hand in the majority of cases. Patients

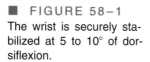

■ FIGURE 58–1
The wrist is securely stabilized at 5 to 10° of dorsiflexion.

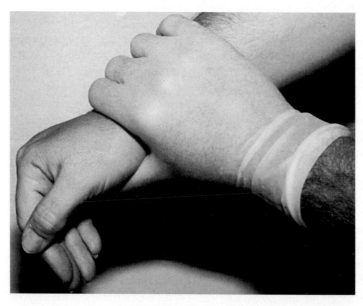

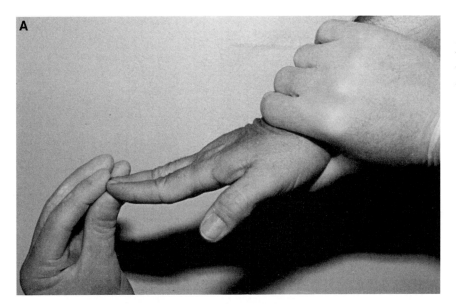

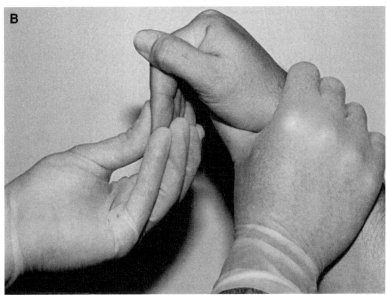

■ FIGURE 58–2
A and B, Manipulation of the MP joints while the wrist is held in 5 to 10° dorsiflexion is painless.

with bacteria present on gram stains of synovial fluid aspirates have septic arthritis and prompt arthrotomy and drainage are indicated. However, not all patients with septic arthritis of the wrist will have a positive gram stain. The anatomic basis for this observation is not clear. It is conceivable that septic arthritis could involve the radiocarpal joint and not the midcarpal joint, or the midcarpal joint and not the radiocarpal joint, especially in young patients who normally have a low prevalence of interosseous ligament performations. If one joint only is involved, false-negative aspirations would be a clinical possibility.

This operation is best performed under general anesthesia, although an axillary block can be used if the ipsilateral axillary nodes are nonpalpable and the axilla is nontender. The extremity is exsanguinated by elevation only, and not with the use of a compression wrap. An arm tourniquet is then inflated.

A dorsal, longitudinal incision is made just ulnar to Listers tubercle, between the third and fourth extensor compartments (Fig. 58–5). The incision is approximately 4 cm in length, with 1 cm of the incision proximal to Listers tubercle and 3 cm distal. The incision is carried through the skin and subcutaneous tissues to the extensor retinaculum. The

■ SURGICAL TECHNIQUE

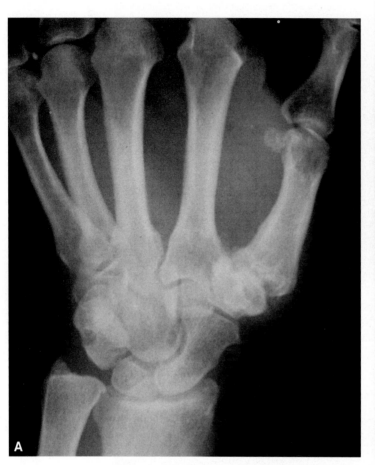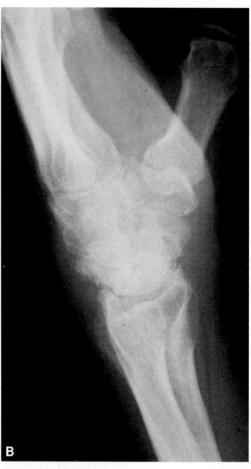

■ FIGURE 58-3
A and B, PA and lateral radiographs show soft tissue swelling without bone or joint changes.

distal aspect of the retinaculum is incised perpendicular to its fibers, just to the ulnar aspect of the third dorsal compartment. The attachment of the wrist capsule to the distal aspect of the radius is identified. A longitudinal incision is then placed in the wrist capsule, for a distance of approximately 3 cm. Any pus obtained from the joint should be sent for cultures. The proximal aspect of the capsule is then released from the distal aspect of the radius. A limited subperiosteal dissection is then performed under the radial aspect of the fourth compartment. The capsule is elevated from the underlying carpal bones using horizontal cuts with a scalpel. The proximal release will be from the dorsal aspect of the scaphoid and the lunate and from the capitate more distally.

The wrist capsule is then retracted to allow irrigation and inspection of the wrist joint. Repeat irrigation may be necessary to clear the joint. The wrist is then distracted by grasping the patient's index and long fingers and pulling distally. The wrist is passively moved and the joints inspected. The radiocarpal joint is located and inspected. After identification of the radialcarpal joint, the midcarpal joint more distally is also located and inspected.

The capsule itself is not excised, though the underlying synovial tissue should be identified, dissected from the undersurface of the capsule, and excised along the margins of the incised capsule. A narrow gauze strip soaked with Betadine (Purdue Frederick Co., Norwalk, CT) is then placed loosely into the wound, although the gauze should not be used as a packing. A compression dressing incorporating a volar plaster splint is then applied and the tourniquet is released.

The patient is placed on parenteral broad-spectrum antibiotics postoperatively. Dressing

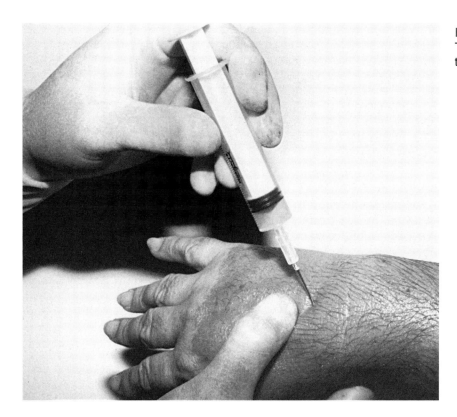

■ FIGURE 58–4
The technique for aspiration of the wrist joint.

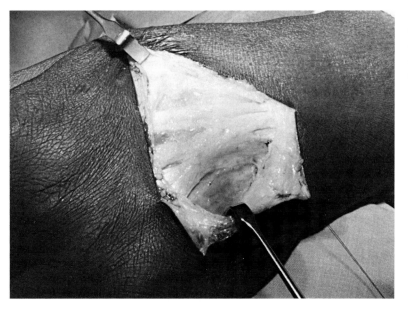

■ FIGURE 58–5
The surgical approach to the septic wrist joint between the third and fourth extensor compartments.

changes are started the following day and continued daily thereafter. When sensitivities return, the patient is placed on an organism-specific antibiotic.

Although drainage of the pus from a septic joint is a widely recognized principle of management, the choice of methods is controversial. For the hip and sacroiliac joints, where access with a needle is recognizably difficult, surgical drainage is widely accepted. The role of repeated needle aspiration to achieve joint drainage has advocates in essentially all other joints, including the wrist. Although needle aspiration of the wrist seems intuitively to be technically easy there are numerous practical problems. The anatomy of the

■ TECHNICAL
ALTERNATIVES

tendons, nerves, and vessels about the wrist leave the dorsal approach most practical. Identification of key landmarks, though, is sometimes difficult in a swollen and tender wrist. In addition, the palmar tilt of the distal radius sometimes makes introduction of a needle into the radiocarpal joint from the dorsal aspect of the wrist difficult in the best of circumstances. It also is difficult to introduce a needle into a septic wrist without passing through the third and fourth extensor compartments, risking their inoculation. It also is difficult to determine whether the needle has entered the radiocarpal or the mid carpal joint, unless the initial aspiration and all subsequent aspirations are done under fluoroscopic control. Because of the numerous potential problems associated with repeat aspirations, it is our opinion that surgical drainage is more effective and poses less risk of inadequate drainage.

Alternative incisions to access the wrist joint could be used. For example, the incisions could be placed on either the radial or ulnar aspects of the wrist. These alternative approaches would be more difficult and risk injury to the superficial radial nerve or the dorsal branch of the ulnar nerve. The dorsal approach could go directly through the fourth compartment, although there would be an increased chance of tendon adhesions and decreased extensor tendon motion postoperatively. The dorsal approach could go directly through the third compartment releasing the extensor pollicis longus tendon and letting it displace radially. This is an acceptable technical alternative, and is an approach that is often used in the course of other wrist operations. However, dissection far enough proximally to mobilize the extensor pollicis longus tendon is rarely needed to adequately drain an infected wrist.

A final aspect of the operation that could be approached differently is that relating to postoperative wound management. The wound could be closed primarily or it could be closed over passive or active drains. Primary closure does risk the chance of the reaccumulation of pus. The use of passive or active drains makes postoperative management more intensive, and the presence of the drains can interfere with attempts to obtain early range of motion.

■ REHABILITATION

The rehabilitation after this operation is usually relatively straightforward. Approximately 3 days after surgery, the compression dressings are progressively debulked. When the patient's wrist has become minimally painful during motion, the volar splint is discontinued. Progressive, active and gentle passive range of motion exercises are encouraged through 3 weeks. At that time, strengthening exercises can begin.

The wound itself is addressed using daily dressing changes. The wound will gradually contract and epithelialize. When the cavity has granulated, the gauze packing is discontinued, and topical dressing only are used. All dressings are discontinued when the wound has epithelialized. At that time the patient can also begin immersing the hand and wrist in water.

The return to limited activities of daily living usually occurs at approximately 2 weeks. By 4 weeks, the patient is usually returned to unrestricted activities of daily living. Return to unrestricted work related activities may require 6 to 8 weeks.

■ OUTCOMES

The results of the operative treatment of this specific condition are not especially well-documented in the literature. The results may be a function of the patient's underlying condition and general disability, the time to diagnosis, and the initiation of appropriate treatment, more than any other issues. In the debilitated patient with underlying medical problems, motion often seems to be limited, and function is further compromised. In an otherwise healthy patient, prompt diagnosis and appropriate surgical treatment in respect to range of motion, return of function, and the absence of the development of osteoarthritis.

References

1. Cooper C, Cawley MID: Bacterial arthritis in the elderly. Gerontology, 1986; 32:222–227.
2. Gardner GC, Weisman MH: Pyarthrosis in patients with rheumatoid arthritis: A report of 13 cases and a review of the literature from the past 40 years. Am J Med, 1990; 88:503–511.

3. Goldberg DL: Infectious arthritis complicating rheumatoid arthritis and other chronic rheumatic disorders. Arthritis Rheum, 1989; 32:496–502.

4. Ho G: Bacterial arthritis. In: McCarty DJ, Koopman WJ (eds): Arthritis and Allied Conditions, Philadelphia: Lea and Febiger, 1993:2003–2023.

5. Ho G, Su EY: Therapy of septic arthritis. JAMA, 1982; 247:797–800.

6. Speiser JC, Moore IL, Osborn TG, Weiss TD, Zuckner J: Changing trends in pediatric septic arthritis. Semin Arthritis Rheum, 1985; 15:132–138.

7. Vincent GM, Amirault JD: Septic arthritis in the elderly. Clin Ortho Rel Res, 1990; 251:241–245.

8. Wilkens RF, Healey LA, Decker JL: Acute infectious arthritis in the aged and chronically ill. Arch Intern Med, 1960; 106:354–364.

9. Wilson NIL, Di Paola M: Acute septic arthritis in infancy and childhood: 10 years' experience. J Bone Joint Surg, 1986; 68B:584–587.

Reconstruction

PART

I

Skin and Fascia

RICHARD L. UHL

59

Z-Plasty Techniques

The use of two triangular transposition flaps to reorient tissue displaced by scar contracture was described by Horner in 1837 and by Denonvilliers in 1854.[2,3,11] McCurdy first used the term "Z-incision" in 1904, and, later, in 1913, used "Z-plastic surgery."[3,7] Once the geometry of the transposition was examined, it became apparent that this technique could be used to lengthen scar contractures and reorient the scar lines.[6,10] Because scar tissue behaves differently after it has been reoriented, scarred tissue itself could be used in the flaps.[5] Although the flap angles are usually symmetric, techniques have evolved using flaps with different tip angles.[9]

Z-plasty is used in the hand to lengthen contractures that are spanning joints and restricting motion. In addition to the classic single Z-plasty, variations that are useful in hand surgery include multiple Z-plasties,[16] the four-flap Z-plasty for web deepening,[18] and the double opposing Z-plasty (butterfly flap) for partial syndactyly.[17]

Several goals can be accomplished by rearranging tissue using the Z-plasty technique: (1) lengthening of contracted scar, (2) rearrangement of scar lines into a more favorable orientation, (3) rearranging tissue to return it to a more normal position after scar contracture, and (4) deepening of a web space.[8] In addition, rearranging an adherent scar with a Z-plasty allows the subcutaneous tissue of the flap to cover underlying tendons and nerves, preventing adhesions along a length of scar.

Once a scar becomes troublesome, revision of the wound should be delayed until the scar has matured, which takes approximately 6 months. There is little to be gained by earlier intervention and, by waiting, the surrounding skin becomes more supple, which allows better flap mobility.[4] Ideally, surgical wounds in which scarring problems are anticipated should be closed using Z-plasty(ies) primarily, obviating the need for secondary reconstruction.

Z-plasty would be contraindicated in areas where there is insufficient tissue for transfer, or in cases where the tissue is so thickly and widely scarred that transposition would not be possible.

Z-plasty in the hand is best performed under regional or general anesthesia. Infiltration of local anesthetic in the area to be rearranged will make flap rotation more difficult.

The essence of the surgical technique for Z-plasty is the planning of the flaps. In the classic description of the Z-plasty, all three limbs are of equal length and form a 60° angle with each other (Figs. 59-1A and 59-1B). The two side limbs are parallel to each other.[13,14] This geometry will result in an approximately 75% increase in the length of the central limb and also will result in a 75% shortening of the transverse line.[16] While this shortening is rarely a problem in areas of redundant, mobile skin (forearm, neck, face), it may present a problem in the hand and fingers (Fig. 59–2A).[16] One alternative is to use an angle less than 60°. Assuming, however, that the directions of the scar and of the flexion crease are perpendicular, lowering the 60° angle will result in one of two situations. If the limbs are kept equal, they will not end at the transverse line or, if the central limb is made longer than the side limbs, the tips will have difficulty reaching all the way across. Decreasing the angle also increases the possibility of tip necrosis. In practice, an angle of 45° to 60° is usually used, with the central limb being somewhat longer when the lower angle is used.

■ FIGURE 59–1
A, The classic Z-plasty. Notice that all three limbs are 60° to each other and that all three limbs are the same length. **B,** After transposition, the length gained along the central limb is lost along the transverse axis. In the classic Z-plasty, the amount gained is approximately 75%.

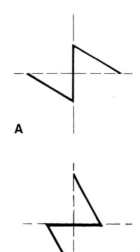

■ FIGURE 59–2
A, Diagram of a finger, showing the direction of a contracture, which crosses several flexion creases. Any length gained along the contracture will have to come from the sides of the fingers. Note also the neutral lines, drawn diagonally from the dorsal aspect of the flexion creases. **B,** Z-plasties have been drawn at each flexion crease. Note that the side limbs start on the crease.

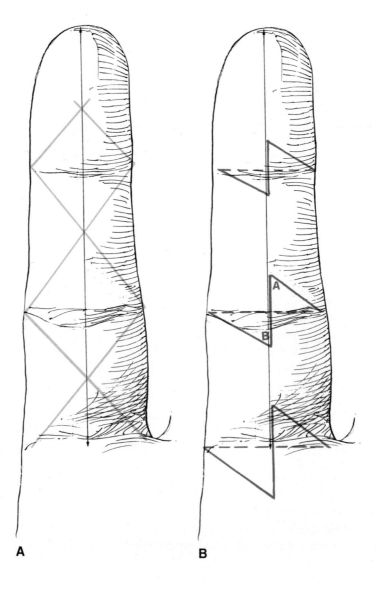

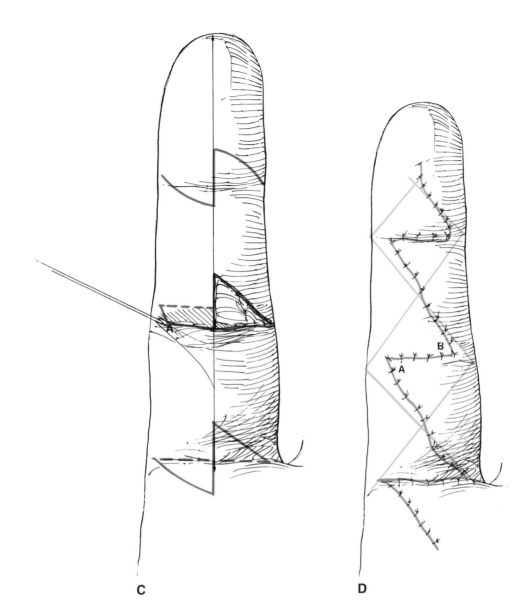

■ FIGURE 59–2
(continued)
C, The first side is cut
and mobilized and is
being transposed to con-
firm the mobility and de-
gree of coverage. Always
handle the tips gently,
using a skin hook. **D,**
The appearance after
transposition of all three
Z-plasties. Notice that the
vertical contracture has
been changed to lines
along the flexion creases
and to lines approximat-
ing Bruner's lines (neutral
lines).

C   D

Both the direction of the contracture and of neighboring flexion creases are considered when planning a Z-plasty in the hand. Most contractures are perpendicular (or approaching perpendicular) to the normal flexion creases of the hand. Contractures in this direction will be the most restrictive. Neutral lines are lines of skin that do not undergo a change in length with motion. In the finger, the diagonal lines (Bruner's lines) running from the dorsal aspect of the flexion creases represent such lines (Fig. 59–2A).[1] Scars in the direction of the neutral lines will be the least restrictive. The Z-plasty should be designed so that, once transposed, the incision lines lie along the neutral lines and flexion creases.

Marking a line along the scar and along the flexion crease(s) is the first step in planning (Figs. 59-2B and 59-3A). By starting each side limb of the Z-plasty on the line marked along the flexion crease, the final transverse portion of the incision, once transposed, will lie along the flexion crease (Figs. 59-2B and 59-3B).[13,15] After the flaps have been drawn and checked, the central limb and one of the side limbs are incised. While gently holding the tip with a small hook, the flap should be elevated with the subcutaneous tissue, carefully avoiding underlying neurovascular structures.[7] Thinning the flap while elevating it should not be done, as this will disrupt the blood supply and will lead to necrosis of the

■ FIGURE 59-3

A, A 58-year-old woman with recurrent median neuropathy. The scar from her previous decompression (marked with dots) crossed the wrist crease (dashes) perpendicularly. The nerve was adherent to the scar at the wrist. **B,** After opening along the original incision and freeing the nerve and tendon from the scar, Z-plasty flaps are designed to reorient the scar and to cover the nerve with the subcutaneous tissue of the flaps instead of the scar itself.

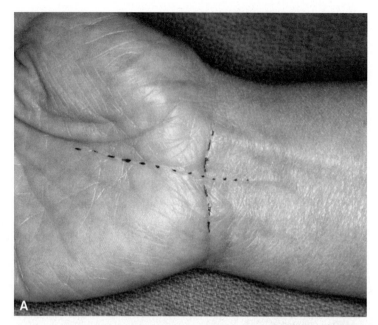

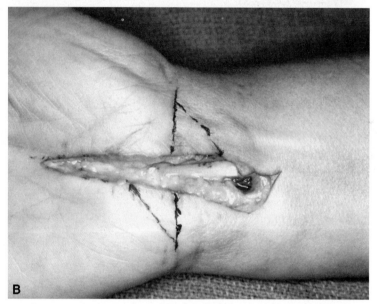

tip. Once elevated, the flap is mobilized at its base until the tip can be brought over into the transposed position. The coverage obtained and its relation to the other flap can then be confirmed and any necessary modifications made before the second flap is incised (Figs. 59-2C and 59-3C).[1,13] Once cut, the second flap is elevated in the identical manner. The two flaps are then transposed and sutured into place (Fig. 59–2D). If done under tourniquet, the tourniquet should be released before bandaging to assure the viability of the flap tips. If the tips cannot reach to the end without blanching, then they can be sutured short of the end in a V-Y fashion (which will somewhat compromise the amount of scar lengthening and scar alignment, but is preferable to tip necrosis) (Figs. 59-4A and 59-4B).

Multiple Z-plasties are used when several flexion creases must be crossed (Fig. 2), or when the amount of scar lengthening required exceeds the amount of tissue available along the transverse line. When using multiple Z-plasties, the gain in length is the sum of the length gained for each, but the narrowing of the transverse dimension is not additive. Thus, using four smaller Z-plasties in place of one large one will give the same increase

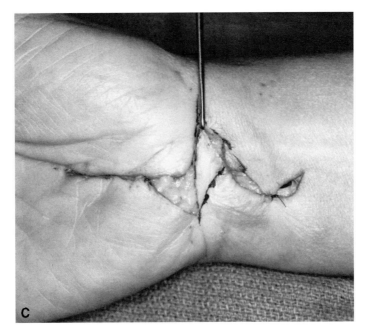

■ FIGURE 59–3
(continued)
C, The first flap is mobilized and held with a skin hook in the transposed position over the other, uncut flap to check mobility and coverage.

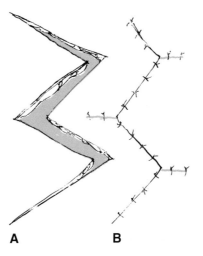

■ FIGURE 59–4
A, Problem: The tips don't quite reach. **B,** Solution: Use a V-Y configuration to "give back" some of the length gained by the Z-plasty to protect the tips.

in length along the central limb, but only require one quarter the amount of shortening along the transverse line.

When planning a Z-plasty closure after fasciectomy for Dupuytren's disease, it is sometimes helpful to choose the direction of the Z based on the condition of the skin. Areas where the skin is thinner should be used for the proximally based flap. The more robust skin is used for the distally based flap, which requires retrograde blood flow.[1]

A hypertrophic scar can be excised before flap transposition (Fig. 59–5A). The defect, if closed, would form a line that would correspond to the central limb. One or several Z-plasties can be designed along the scar line to change the direction in line with established tissue planes (Figs. 59-5B and 59-5C).

After the flaps are sutured in place, a dry sterile bulky dressing is applied. Occasionally, if the contracture involved a joint, a splint is used to maintain the correction.

Once the flaps are planned and the first side cut, there may be insufficient tissue laxity to allow full transposition. Especially in the hand, the amount of shortening that can be tolerated is limited, often less than the theoretical 75% required for the 60° classic flap

■ TECHNICAL
ALTERNATIVES

■ FIGURE 59–5

A, This 64-year-old woman has a thick, painful scar on the volar surface of her wrist following trapeziectomy and ligament reconstruction. She has pain with wrist extension and thenar paresthesias. **B,** The scar is marked for excision, and multiple Z-plasties. Both the palmar cutaneous nerve and the flexor carpi radialis tendon (that remained) were firmly adherent to the scar. **C,** The appearance of the wound 3 months after scar revision with multiple Z-plasties. The palmar cutaneous nerve recovered after neurolysis and coverage with the flaps. This patient went to therapy for 8 weeks for scar massage, elastomer mold, desensitization, and ultrasound.

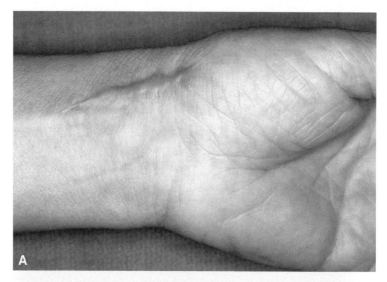

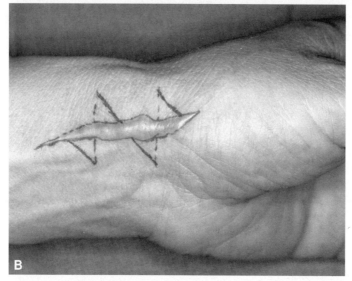

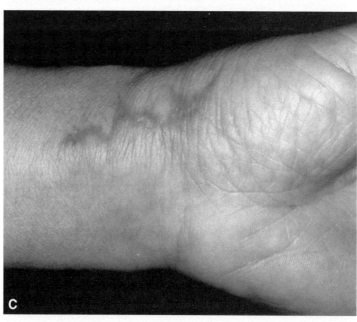

angle. By transposing the first flap before cutting the second, modifications can be made. It is better to lose some length than to put too much tension on the flap tips. If tip necrosis develops, it is often superficial and should be treated with local wound care.

Other flaps, such as rotation flaps and rhomboid flaps, are better suited for filling tissue defects.[13] Y-V advancement flaps can be used to lengthen but are not useful when the contracture is a straight line.[12]

The hand is rested in a bulky postoperative dressing for 5 to 7 days to allow the flaps to heal. After that, gentle active range of motion exercises are started. Sutures are usually removed at 2 weeks, and scar mobilization techniques and desensitization are started under the supervision of a hand therapist. If scar formation is abundant, then more aggressive techniques, such as elastomer molds and ultrasound, are started at 4 to 6 weeks postoperatively. Full scar maturation takes 4 to 6 months, and patients are encouraged to continue massage to soften and mobilize the healing scar during this time.

■ REHABILITATION

Whether congenital or acquired, scars and contractures of the hand limit motion and function. Tissue rearrangement using Z-plasty can relax contractures and rearrange scars to improve both the appearance and function of the reconstructed hand. Z-plasty can readily be combined with other reconstructive procedures, especially in more complex conditions. If basic principles are applied, the improvement obtained following Z-plasty is predictable and reliable.

■ OUTCOMES

References

1. Beasley RW: Hand Injuries. Philadelphia: W.B. Saunders 1981:76–80.
2. Borges AF: The enigma of Serre's "Z-plasty" technique. Plast Reconstr Surg, 1985; 76: 472–474.
3. Borges AF, Gibson T: The original Z-plasty. Br J Plastic Surg, 1973; 26:235–236.
4. Davis JS: Present evaluation of the merit of the Z-plastic operation. Plast Reconstr Surg, 1946; 1:26–38.
5. Davis JS: The relaxation of scar contractures by means of the Z- or the reversed Z-type incision stessing the use of scar infiltrated tissues. Ann Surg, 1931; 94:871–884.
6. Davis JS, Kitlowski EA: The theory and practical use of the Z-incision for the relief of scar contractures. Ann Surg, 1939; 109:1001–1015.
7. Davis WE, Boyd JH: Z-plasty. Otolaryngol Clin North Am, 1990; 23:875–887.
8. Furnas DW: The four fundamental functions of the Z-plasty. Arch Surg, 1985; 96:458–463.
9. Furnas DW: Transposition of the skew Z-plasty. Br J Plastic Surg, 1966; 19:88–89.
10. Furnas DW: The tetrahedral Z-plasty. Plast Reconstr Surg, 1965; 35:291–302.
11. Ivy RH: Who originated the Z-plasty? Plast Reconstr Surg, 1971; 47:67–72.
12. King EW, Bass DM, Watson HK: Treatment of Dupuytren's contracture by extensive fasciectomy through multiple Y-V plasty incisions: Short term evaluation of 170 consecutive operations. J Hand Surg, 1979; 4:234–241.
13. Lister GD: Skin Flaps. In: Green DP (ed): Operative Hand Surgery, 3rd Ed, New York: Churchill Livingstone, 1992:1741–1822.
14. McGregor IA: The theoretic basis of the Z-plasty. Br J Plastic Surg, 1957; 9:256–259.
15. McGregor IA: The Z-plasty. Br J Plastic Surg, 1966; 19:82–87.
16. McGregor IA: The Z-plasty in hand surgery. J Bone Joint Surg, 1967; 49B:448–457.
17. Shaw DT, Li CS, Richey DG, Nahigian SH. The interdigital butterfly flap in the hand (the double-opposing Z-plasty). J Bone Joint Surg, 1973; 55A:1677–1679.
18. Woolf RM, Broadbent TR: The four-flap Z-plasty. Plast Reconstr Surg, 1972; 49:48–51.

60

Four-Flap Transposition for the First Web Space

■ HISTORY OF THE TECHNIQUE

Jackson indicates that Berger provided the first description of the four-flap Z-plasty in 1904 in the German literature.[5] Most authorities, however, have credited Limberg with the most important original contributions related to this technique.[3,7,11] Limberg published his original descriptions in 1929 and 1946 in the Russian literature and then in 1966 in the English language.[6,11] In 1962, Iselin reported the first application of this method to correction of contracture of the thumb web space.[11] Later, in 1972, Woolf and Broadbert described a similar technique for correcting contractures of the web spaces of the hand, including the thumb.[11] These authors and many others have shown through clinical experience, experimental studies, and mathematical formulae that the amount of lengthening from a Z-plasty increases as the tip angle of the Z-plasty increases, but that the ease of transposition of a Z-plasty flap decreases as the tip angle increases.[1,9] Limberg and others each developed large, wide-angle Z-plasty flaps that they then bisected into two separate flaps each. This maneuver converts a two-flap Z-plasty into a four-flap design. The four-flap design provides a maximum gain in length consistent with the size of the initial flaps but allows easier rotation because of the smaller flaps created by subdividing each large flap (Fig. 60–1).

■ INDICATIONS AND CONTRAINDICATIONS

The four-flap Z-plasty procedure is indicated for mild to moderate web space contracture of the thumb caused by a linear scar tethering the thumb to the index finger. The linear scar should be located at the free edge of the web and should be discrete and well defined. The four-flap Z-plasty procedure is also indicated for deepening a shallow web. This situation is often encountered following partial thumb amputation or in congenital anomalies such as mild thumb hypoplasia.[2,10] The procedure is contraindicated if the web contracture is caused by a loss of skin on the dorsal or palmar surfaces of the web, scarring of the dorsal or palmar surfaces of the web space, and in the presence of a severe contracture associated with significant damage to the underlying fascia and muscles of the first web space.[8]

■ SURGICAL TECHNIQUES

The procedure may be completed under general or regional anesthesia. The patient is placed in the supine position, and an appropriate anesthetic is administered. A tourniquet is applied about the proximal arm, and the affected extremity is prepared and draped in the usual fashion. The surgeon should pay particular attention to the width of the web space and should carefully identify the junction of the free edge of the web with the thumb and index fingers. The approximate location of the radial proper digital nerve to the index finger and the ulnar proper digital nerve to the thumb also should be identified.

The skin incisions are marked with a marking pencil. A ruler or caliper is used to assure that the limbs of the proposed incisions are of equal length. Calipers provide the quickest and most accurate method to locate the six critical points in the design of the four-flap Z-plasty.[7] The initial skin marking is made on the free edge of the web. This line must not extend onto the ulnar border of the thumb or the radial border of the index finger. The calipers or a ruler is then used to measure the length of this limb because its length determines the lengths of all other incisions. Two equilateral 90° flaps are now designed by extending one end of the web incision at a 90° angle over the dorsum of the

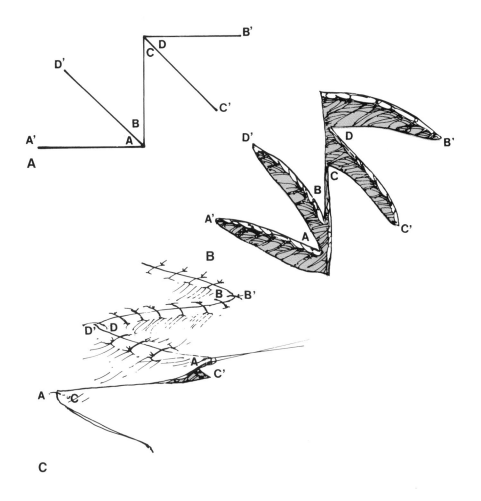

■ FIGURE 60–1

A, A four-flap Z-plasty constructed by bisecting the two flaps of a standard 90° design. This design combines the theoretical gain in length of a 90° degree Z-plasty with the ease in transposition of the smaller 45° degree angle flaps. All limbs have the same length. A caliper provides the quickest and most accurate method to locate the six critical points in the design and to assure that all limbs are equal in length. Each of the flaps may be labeled consecutively with letters or numbers to avoid confusion during the transposition phase of the operation. The correct arrangement of the four flaps relative to one another following transposition is then recorded and used as a reference. **B,** The borders of each flap are incised and the flaps are elevated and mobilized in the subcutaneous plane. **C,** The flaps are transposed and sutured into place as indicated.

web space adjacent to the index finger and the other end over the palmar surface adjacent to the ulnar border of the thumb (Fig. 60–2A, lines 2 to 3 and 1 to 4). Each of these 90° angle flaps is now bisected by a line that is equal in length to all of the others (Fig. 60–2A, lines 2 to 5 and 1 to 6). The caliper or a ruler is then used to confirm that all limbs are equal in length. For the surgeon who is relatively inexperienced with this procedure, each of the flaps should be labeled consecutively with letters or numbers to avoid confusion during the transposition phase of the operation (Fig. 60–2A, flaps A, B, C, and D). The arrangement of the four flaps relative to one another following transposition is then recorded and used as a reference. However, once the surgeon is familiar with the principles of this operation, this step is unnecessary. After the skin incisions are marked appropriately, the limb is exsanguinated and the tourniquet inflated.

The initial incision is made along the apex of the web (Fig. 60–2A, lines 1 to 2). The scar is included in the sides of flaps B and C and carried with each of these flaps. The 45°

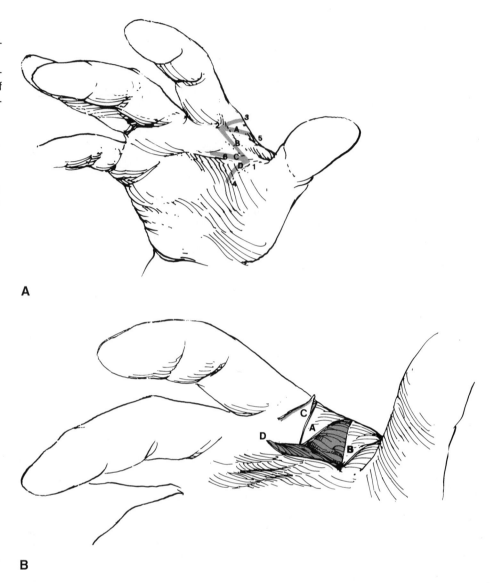

■ FIGURE 60–2
A, A four-flap Z-plasty designed on the first web. Note that line 1 to 2 is located on the free edge of the web and does not extend onto the border of the adjacent digits. Lines 2 to 3 and 1 to 4 are located on the dorsal and palmar surfaces of the web, respectively, and do not extend onto the adjacent digits. **B,** The borders of each flap are incised and the flaps are elevated, mobilized, and transposed.

A

B

angled incision should then be incised on the palmar and dorsal surfaces of the web (Fig 60–2A, lines 2 to 5 and 1 to 6) followed by the 90° angle incisions (Fig. 60–2A, lines 2 to 3 and 1 to 4) to create flaps B and C and then A and D (Fig. 60–2). The surgeon should take particular care to avoid the radial proper digital nerve to the index finger during development and mobilization of flap C and the ulnar proper digital nerve to the thumb during development and mobilization of flap D. Depending on the size of these flaps, these structures may be at risk for injury during this part of the procedure.

The flaps are elevated in the subcutaneous plane and retracted. Elevation of the flaps will reveal fascial bands at the apex of the web which contribute to the contracture. These are now released. After the flaps are elevated and the fascial bands are divided, the surgeon should assess thumb abduction. If it is still restricted, then the fascia of the first dorsal interosseus muscle is incised and the origin of this muscle is reflected from the thumb metacarpal. At the proximal aspect of the web, the surgeon must take care to identify and avoid injury to the palmar branch of the radial artery and during division of the dorsal interosseus fascia care must be taken to avoid injury to the first dorsal metacarpal artery. After release of all constricting structures, the surgeon should consider pinning the thumb in abduction. If the contracture is mild, pin fixation is unnecessary. More moderate contractures may require pin fixation to prevent recurrence of adduction postoperatively. The tourniquet is deflated and hemostasis achieved with pressure and electrocautery. The flaps are then transposed as illustrated and sutured into place using 5-0 nylon sutures (Fig. 60–2B). A soft dressing, consisting of a nonadherent gauze and 4 × 4s, should be placed in the web space to maintain even compression on all skin margins and to assist in appropriate positioning of the thumb in palmar abduction and pronation. A plaster thumb spica splint is then applied to maintain thumb abduction. The interphalangeal joint is left free for unrestricted motion.

A common pitfall encountered with four-flap transposition for the first web space is the use of this procedure in inappropriate clinical circumstances. Z-plasties designed on webs create flaps that lie on two different planes. These planes form an angle ("peak angle") where they meet at the free edge of the web. When the flaps are transposed, the web is obliterated and lengthening occurs along the previous free edge of the web. The amount of lengthening that occurs for any flap angle is determined by the peak angle but is always less than the amount predicted mathematically.[4] Although the four-flap Z-plasty provides a deeper web space, it will not overcome a severe adduction contracture and therefore is not indicated for this condition. The procedure also is contraindicated in the presence of diffuse scarring extending onto the dorsal or volar surfaces of the thumb web space. Scarring or injury to these tissues limits transposition of the flaps and threatens flap viability. Contractures caused by skin loss also will lead to disappointing results when this procedure is applied.

Errors in the design of a four-flap Z-plasty also may lead to problems with this procedure. If the incision along the free edge of the web is extended onto the border of the index finger or thumb, the flaps will be too large and will not transpose without excessive tension. Excessive tension will cause flap ischemia and necrosis. The surgeon also should ensure that the tip angles are not too narrow. This means that the initial design must be at least 90° as described, so that the tip angles of the bisected flaps are 45° each. Failure to maintain at least 45° tip angles also may lead to tip necrosis and postoperative scarring. This problem may be avoided by designing a four-flap z-plasty with 120° flaps each bisected into 60° angle flaps. This design provides an increase in the theoretical lengthening but requires smaller flaps to avoid encroachment onto the borders of the thumb and index fingers.

A final pitfall relates to failure to identify and protect the regional digital nerves or vessels. Unrecognized injury to these structures will lead to sensory loss and hematoma formation.

Alternative procedures that may be used for the contracted first web space include the single standard 60° Z-plasty, free skin grafts, local flaps including dorsal transposition, and advancement flaps and distant flaps. The single Z-plasty will produce a deeper web than the four-flap Z-plasty and effectively converts the thumb web space into a cleft. However little lengthening is achieved when a single, 60° Z-plasty is transposed on the thumb web.[3] Free skin grafts may be indicated if scarring is extensive and local transposition flaps of the Z-plasty variety are contraindicated. If scarring is extensive or if the contracture is severe, then local transposition flaps from the dorsum of the hand or thumb will provide more suitable skin to the deficient first web space and provide more acceptable and effective abduction. Dorsal advancement flaps may also be applied and, in the case of severe deficiency, distant pedicle or free flaps may be the most appropriate alternative.

■ TECHNICAL ALTERNATIVES

The thumb is immobilized in abduction for approximately 10 to 14 days after the procedure, at which time sutures are removed. If the thumb was pinned in abduction, then the pin is removed 2 to 3 weeks postoperatively and a range of motion exercise program begun. Static orthoplast splinting is continued for a variable length of time in between exercise periods, depending on the degree, cause, and severity of the initial contracture.

■ REHABILITATION

■ OUTCOMES

No objective or quantifiable outcome measures relative to the four-flap Z-plasty procedure are reported in the literature. However, all reports conclude that when appropriately indicated this procedure provides improvement in the breadth and depth of the first web space.

References

1. Converse JM: General Principles. In: Converse JM (ed): Reconstructive Plastic Surgery, Philadelphia: W. B. Saunders, 1977:58–61
2. Dobyns JH, Wood VE, Bayne LG: Congenital Hand Anomalies. In: Green DP (ed): Operative Hand Surgery. New York: Churchill Livingstone, 1993:355.
3. Furnas DW: The tetrahedral z-plasty. Plast Reconstr Surg, 1965; 35:291–301.
4. Furnas DW, Fischer GW: The z-plasty: Biomechanics and mathematics. Br J Plast Surg, 1971; 24:144–160.
5. Jackson IT: Local Flaps in Head and Neck Reconstruction. St. Louis: C. V. Mosby Co, 1985:27.
6. Limberg AA: Design of local flaps. In: Gibson T (ed): Modern Trends in Plastic Surgery, London: Butterworth, 1966:38.
7. Lister GD, Milward TM: Skin contractures of the first web space. Transactions of the Sixth International Congress of Plastic and Reconstuctive Surgery, 1976:594–604.
8. Littler JW: Principles of Reconstructive Surgery of the Hand. In: Converse JM (ed): Reconstructive Plastic Surgery, Philadelphia: W. B. Saunders, 1977:3119–3124.
9. McGregor IA: The theoretical basis of the Z-plasty. Br J Plast Surg, 1957; 9:256–259.
10. Strickland JW, Kleinman W: Thumb Reconstruction. In: Green, DP (ed): Operative Hand Surgery, New York: Churchill Livingstone, 1993:2091–2093.
11. Woolf RM, Broadbert TR: The four-flap Z-plasty. Plast Reconstr Surg, 1972; 49:48–51.

PETER E.
BENTIVEGNA
GRAHAM D. LISTER

61

Dorsal Transposition Flap for the First Web Space

Brand[2] reconstructed first web space contractures in patients with leprosy with dorsal transposition flaps from the index finger. Flatt and Wood[5] found multiple transposition flaps useful in congenital deformities, and Brown[3] used proximal based dorsal web skin as a rectangular transposition flap to release syndactylies. The dorsal thumb transposition flap, which is the subject of this chapter, was first described in recent English-language literature by Strauch.[13]

■ HISTORY OF THE
TECHNIQUE

Contracture of the first web space occurs in congenital differences including arthrogryposis, type II thumb hypoplasia, radial polydactyly, and cleft hand, but most cases are acquired, resulting from trauma, especially burn injuries. It is a disabling deformity, for the normal first web space is essential for normal grasp and pinch. Incorrect immobilization of the thumb after injury to the hand or thumb is the most common secondary cause of the deformity (Littler). If the thumb is incorrectly positioned in adduction and supination, the carpometacarpal joint will stiffen, and the skin, fascia, and musculature, primarily the adductor pollicis and first dorsal interosseous, will contract. The consequence is an adduction and supination contracture of the thumb, which comes to lie in the same plane as the digits.

Release of the acquired contracture requires, apart from division of the skin, removal of the shortened fascia, often release of one head each of the adductor, and the interosseous from the third and first metacarpals, respectively, and sometimes of the capsule of the basilar joint of the thumb. Normal thumb abduction is approximately 60° and, once that has been achieved, a significant skin defect remains. These defects tend to be smaller in disuse contractures, intermediate with isolated burn scar contracture and small tumors, but can be large with heavy burn scar contractures extending to the palm and dorsum of the hand. The full surgical armamentarium, from Z-plasty, local and regional flaps, to distant pedicle and free flaps, must be available to reconstruct all of these deformities. The essential specific prerequisite of the selected flap is that it is adequate but does not overfill, and thereby obstruct, the first web space. Provided it is unscarred, the dorsum of the thumb provides ideal material.

■ INDICATIONS AND CONTRAINDICATIONS

The theory and practice of transposition flaps has been described.[9] When a dorsal thumb transposition flap (Fig. 61–1) is intended, the skin release is done through an incision placed 5 to 10 mm radial to the thenar crease in the adult hand. It starts at Kaplan's cardinal line on the palmar surface and passes around the web margin to end at a corresponding point midway between the first and second metacarpals. This also is the proximal point on the ulnar limb of the flap design. The radial limb has its proximal point at the same level on the radial side of the first metacarpal, at the junction of palmar and dorsal skin. From this latter point, around which the flap will pivot, the distance over the web space margin to the palmar end of the releasing incision is measured with a piece of suture held between two hemostats. This distance corresponds to the theoretical length required of the flap. This can never be achieved, as it is longer than the thumb itself! This discrepancy is overcome by three facts: the pivot point will move with the flap (Fig. 61–1B); the resultant web will be deeper than the natural one; and the flap skin is somewhat elastic. All three

■ SURGICAL TECHNIQUE

■ FIGURE 61–1
A, A dorsal transposition
flap has been designed
for release of the first
web space in this arthro-
grypotic hand. **B,** The
pivot point will move, enabling flap movement.

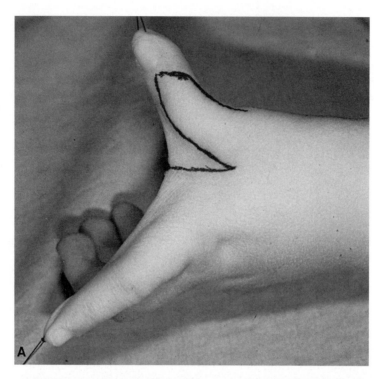

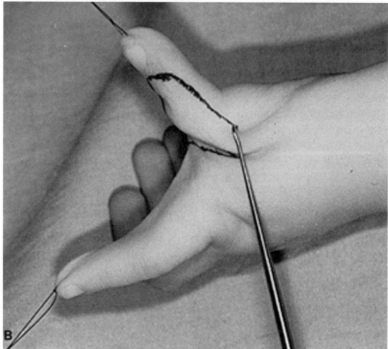

serve to make adequate a flap the distal point of which is placed midway between the
interphalangeal joint of the thumb and the nail fold.

An alternative design places the releasing incision much closer to the thumb, in which
case the ulnar limb of the flap commences at that point at which the releasing incision
crosses the web. The flap is elevated at the level of the epitenon of the thumb extensors,
taking with it branches of the superficial radial nerve and the dorsal veins. After the flap
has been raised and the contents of the web completely released, abduction should be

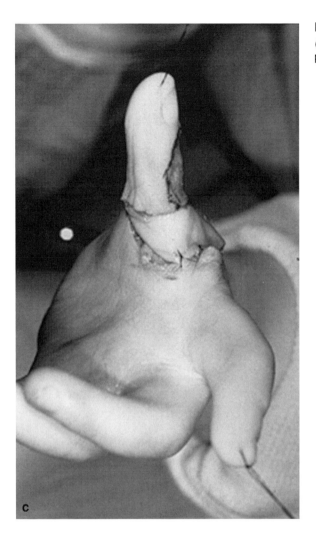

■ FIGURE 61-1
(continued) **C,** The flap
placed in position.[8]

maintained by use of a Kirschner wire bent into one of various configurations, V-shaped,[14] gamma shaped,[1] or a W, which has been our preference. Whatever the shape, the wire is set into the opposing cortices of the first and second metacarpals. At this time, additional procedures such as opponensplasty may be performed, partly through the exposure provided by these incisions. When an opponensplasty is done simultaneously, the abduction should be maintained by a percutanteous pin, which is more easily removed, allowing for ranging protocols to begin. In releasing the web muscles, care should be taken to avoid the princeps pollicis artery, which often lies deep to the first dorsal interosseous muscle, and the deep motor branch of the ulnar nerve and deep palmar arch, which lie at the proximal end of the adductor origin. Complete release may require division of the arteria radialis indicis, should it exert any traction on the princeps pollicis, from which it arises.

Once the flap has been sutured into position, the secondary defect is closed with a template fashioned full-thickness skin graft sewn with a 5-0 chromic running horizontal mattress suture to ensure edge to edge approximation (Fig. 61–2). A nonadherent dressing with antibiotic ointment and soft dressings are applied beneath an abduction splint immobilizing the interphalangeal and metacarpophalangeal joints in adults and an above elbow cast in children. A bolus dressing is unnecessary since the graft is applied to a convex surface. The flap and graft are left, especially in children, for 3 weeks. At that time, a first web space abduction splint is fashioned allowing IP joint motion for a total of 6 weeks. This splint can be worn at night thereafter until scar maturation occurs between 6 months and 1 year.

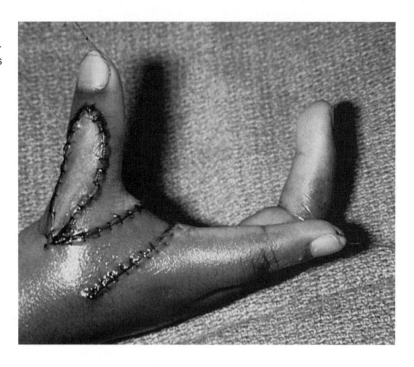

■ FIGURE 61-2
Another dorsal flap in position with a full thickness skin graft on the secondary defect.[8]

■ TECHNICAL ALTERNATIVES

Lesser first web space contractures can be released with two, three or four flap local transposition designs.

For substantial defects, multiple dorsal transposition flaps[5] may be raised and used for congenital or amputation cases where thumb dorsal skin is not present or appropriate. These have the advantage of primary closure but leave the dorsum of the hand and forearm with large scars that may hypertrophy.

Index finger skin, whether dorsal[11,12] or dorsal radial[10] has advantages that are similar to the thumb. However, postoperative range of motion of the donor digit is more essential than in the thumb, involving as it does the proximal interphalangeal and metacarpophalangeal joints of the index finger. Furthermore, the torsion required at the base of the index flap is much greater, potentially increasing ischemic complications. The thumb flap falls easily into the widened space created by release of the thumb into abduction.

The problems associated with the dorsal thumb flap are few, being more likely in the release of the web and in the preparation, application, and immobilization of the graft on the secondary defect.

■ REHABILITATION

The most common complication of any contracture release is differing degrees of recurrence. Internal splinting of the first web space may be helpful but more important is the continuous splintage of the thumb in abduction and supination for a full 6 weeks after which night splinting should be continued for 6 months to 1 year. The thumb may be flexed once the skin graft has taken. This can be done as early as 1 week after split-thickness skin grafts as used in burn centers or as late as 3 weeks after full-thickness grafts. At 6 weeks, simple transmetacarpal K wires are removed, and full thumb range of motion commenced with splinting at night. Internal splints are used for severe contractures and are usually permanent. If their removal is elected, this is done in the operating suite. In the pediatric population, the use of chromic sutures is kinder and gentler and permits uninterrupted casting.

■ OUTCOMES

In many cases, the tip of the transposition flap has poor circulation and may indeed go on to necrosis. This can be minimized by sequential excision of the tip intraoperatively until good bleeding is encountered. The resulting defect is closed with skin graft or by direct closure of that part of the releasing incision. In practice, the perfusion is difficult to assess, and any resulting necrosis is so minimal as to cause only insignificant additional scarring.

The efficacy of the dorsal transposition flap is such that alternative flaps are only indicated where the dorsum of the thumb is scarred.

References

1. Araico JL, Valdes JL, Ortiz JM: An internal wire splint for adduction contracture of the thumb. Plast Reconstr Surg, 1971; 48:339–342.
2. Brand P: Hand Reconstruction in Leprosy. British Surgical Practice—Surgical Progress. Butterworth, 1954:117–130.
3. Brown EZ Jr: Dorsal rectangular skin flap for web space reconstruction. In: Strauch B, Vasconez LO, Hall-Findley EJ (eds): Encyclopedia of Flaps, Boston: Little Brown, 1990: 1023–1025.
4. Brown PW: Adduction-flexion contracture of the thumb. Clin Orthop Rel Res, 1992; 88: 161–168.
5. Flatt AE, Wood BE: Multiple dorsal rotation flaps for the hand thumb web contractures. Plast Reconstr Surg, 1970; 45:258–262.
6. Herrick RT, Lister GD: Control of first web space contracture including a review of the literature and a tabulation of opponensplasty technique. Hand, 1977; 9:253–264.
7. Lister GD, Milward TM: Skin contracture of the first web space. In: Transactions of the Sixth International Congress of Plastic and Reconstructive Surgery, Paris: Masson, 1976.
8. Lister GD: Skin Flaps. In: Green DP (ed): Operative Hand Surgery, 3rd Ed, New York: Churchill Livingstone: 1741–1822.
9. Lister GD: The theory of the transposition flap and its practical application in the hand. Clin Plast Surg, 1981; 8:115–127.
10. Rae PS, Pho RWH: The radial transposition flap—a useful composite flap. Hand 1983; 15: 96–102.
11. Sandzen SC Jr: Dorsal pedicle flap for resurfacing a moderate thumb index web contracture release. J Hand Surg, 1982; 7:21–24.
12. Spinner M: Fashioned transpositional flap for soft tissue adduction contracture of the thumb. Plast Reconstr Surg, 1969; 44:345–348.
13. Strauch B: Dorsal thumb flap for release of adduction of the first web space. Bull Hosp Joint Dis, 1975; 36:34–39.
14. Littler JW: The prevention and correction of adduction of the thumb. Clin Orthop, 1959; 13: 182–192

EDWARD DIAO
OSAMU SOEJIMA

62

Butterfly Flaps for the Finger Webs

■ HISTORY OF THE TECHNIQUE

The normal digital web space is composed of dorsal skin sloping in a gentle fashion from a dorsal-proximal location between the metacarpal heads to a volar-distal location approximately halfway between the metacarpophalangeal (MP) joint and the proximal interphalangeal (PIP) joint. This normal anatomy can be altered in congenital anomalies or certain acquired conditions, such as with dorsal hand burns. Congenital deficiencies of soft tissue, or acquired scars can bridge across the natural concavity between the meta-carpal heads and create a syndactyly. In acquired syndactylies, dorsal webs can be pulled distally by contraction producing dorsal hooding with resultant cosmetic problems and functional abnormalities. In its milder forms, these syndactylies have primarily cosmetic consequences and function is minimally affected.

The most traditional early method for recession of a web space was the Z-plasty. Furnas and Fischer[2] determined that a single Z-plasty effaces a web more efficiently than a series of smaller Z-plasties. The peak angle of the web determines whether any given Z-plasty, regardless of tip angle, can be closed without tension or distortion. They determined that a simple Z-plasty can be used for only minor degrees of web deepening; the resultant reconstruction tended to be a V-shaped commissure. Woolf and Broadbent[6] used a modification of the Z-plasty techniques with the four-flap Z-plasty, which resulted in a more rounded commissure. However, it also was most useful for only minor degrees of webbing (Fig. 62–1). Shaw and co-authors[4] described a more useful technique for interdigital web recession, the double opposing Z-plasty or so-called "butterfly flap" in 1972 (Fig. 62–2). It provides a broad dorsal flap with a wide distal edge, to give width and laxity to the commissure and a more satisfactory width and depth to the web reconstruction. Its several variations, including the three flap web-plasty are described here.

■ INDICATIONS AND CONTRAINDICATIONS

Butterfly flaps, including the original descriptions by Shaw and co-authors[4,5] and its variations are applicable to incomplete syndactylies, congenital or acquired, that have the distal edge of the web located proximal to the (PIP) joint. These techniques use excess distal skin to restore a normal commissure without the need for a skin graft. These flaps can be reversed to release dorsal adduction contractions that may result from dorsal hand burns with subsequent dorsal scar hooding, provided the palmar tissue is relatively preserved.

For both congenital syndactylies and acquired dorsal adduction contractures, these butterfly flap reconstructions can establish a web that is normal in function and appearance. The resultant webs have a U or rectangular shape and are relatively broad, as in the normal digital web, with a gentle palmar inclination to the dorsal surface. These reconstructions can efficiently transfer the excess soft tissue to the lateral surfaces of the digits and a more proximally advanced web, without the need for skin grafts, provided the edge of the abnormally advanced flap lies proximal to the level of the PIP joint.

If the amount of redundant tissue between two adjacent fingers is minimal, or the affected web is at or beyond the level of the PIP joint, the technique of butterfly flaps will be insufficient to provide adequate inter-digital soft tissue for web reconstruction. In these cases, the more traditional volar and dorsal matching longitudinal Z-plasties, followed by opposing palmar and dorsal triangles or a dorsal rectangular flap with supplemental

500

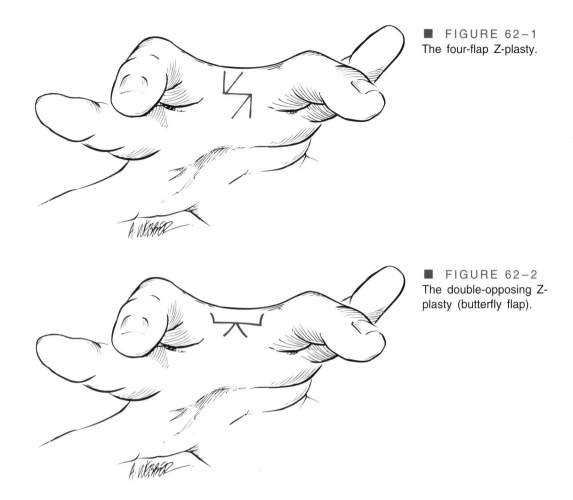

skin grafting will be more appropriate. If the deficiencies are great, full-thickness skin grafting of an entire surface of a released digit and reconstructed web may be required to bring sufficient soft tissue to the reconstruction.

Thumb web contractures are best handled by a large single Z-plasty, or a four-flap Z-plasty, as opposed to these techniques.

The butterfly flap Z-plasty can be performed with a wrist block or an axillary block in adults or with general anesthesia in children. Intravenous regional Bier block is a less satisfactory anesthetic choice as the opportunity to deflate the tourniquet to assess perfusion of the flaps prior to insetting is not possible without concomitant loss of anesthesia.

■ SURGICAL TECHNIQUES

The concept behind the butterfly flap and its variations is the use of two opposing Z-plasties in contrast to two in-line Z-plasties (Fig. 62–3). A pair of opposing Z-plasties points lateralward, creating a common dorsal pedicle from the two dorsal halves of each Z-plasty, thus providing a broad dorsal flap with an elongated distal edge, which is moved palmarward and proximally to create a commissure of sufficient width and slope.

There are several variations of the basic butterfly flap. In one, the flap described in the 1973 article by Shaw and co-authors[5] uses the inverted wide angle V on the palmar aspect. An alternate incision described is an inverted Y incision. This alteration causes a blunting of the tips of the palmar halves of each Z-plasty and can avoid a problem of flap tip necrosis if the skin is abnormal. Moreover, it can provide a greater amount of skin that can be transposed onto the sides of the digits. A third alternative, the three-flap Z-plasty, has been described in which the palmar flap is divided into two triangles via a Z-flap.[3]

For the butterfly flap with the palmar V incision, the original butterfly flap described by Shaw and co-authors,[4] it is best to draw the incisions with a marking pen or methylene

■ FIGURE 62–3
The Double-opposing Z-plasty. **A,** A pair of opposing Z-plasties creating a common dorsal pedicle from the two dorsal halves of each Z-plasty. **B,** Two in-line Z-plasties do not create a broad dorsal flap.

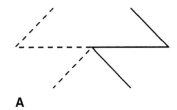

A

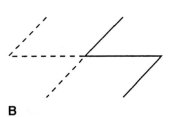

B

■ FIGURE 62–4
Butterfly flap with palmar V incision inscribed.

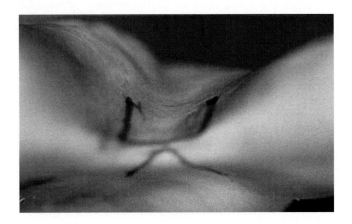

blue; the skin flap should be carefully marked with a straight edge and protractor or goniometer (Fig. 62–4). The most satisfactory result will be obtained if the angles of all flaps are at 60° and if the limbs are of equal length. In this instance, the double opposing Z-plasties are essentially two single Z-plasties with a common dorsal pedicle resulting from the two dorsal halves of each Z-plasty, and each side of the Z-plasty should be drawn with a strict adherence to the principles of equal angles, 60°, and equal limb lengths. This will result in lengthening along the span of the web of approximately 70% of its original dimension (Fig. 62–5). The width of the common dorsal pedicle should span the width of the contracted web, and one should try not to go beyond these points to the lateral aspects of the digits. After Esmark tourniquet exsanguination and either forearm or upper arm tourniquet elevation, the skin flaps are incised with a No. 15 blade (Fig. 62–6). Total division of flaps through skin and subcutaneous tissue is performed. Care is taken to preserve the underlying neurovascular bundles. Thereafter, dissecting scissors are used to free up the skin flaps so that they may be freely transposed. The lateral palmar triangles are rotated dorsally and sutured along the lines of the origin of the common dorsal pedicle. After this is done, the common dorsal pedicle is then advanced distally and sutured down against the wide central palmar V. I use 5-0 nylon sutures or 5-0 or 6-0 plain gut sutures in selected patients and pediatric patients (Fig. 62–7).

The butterfly flap with palmar Y incision is similar to the butterfly flap with a palmar V incision. However, instead of an inverted V incision, an inverted Y incision is planned on the palmar aspect (Fig. 62–8). This causes a blunting of the tips of the palmar portions of each Z-plasty with broader flaps to rotate laterally and dorsally. The result is that a

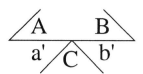 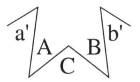

■ FIGURE 62–5
Diagram of double-opposing Z-plasty butterfly flap.

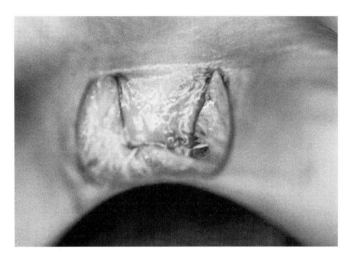

■ FIGURE 62–6
Intraoperative photograph after incisions have been made.

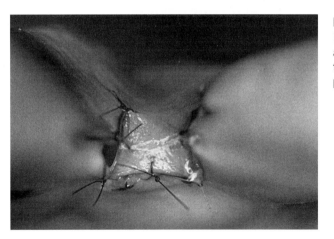

■ FIGURE 62–7
Intraoperative photograph after flaps have been rotated and sutured in place.

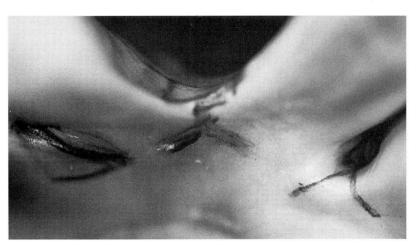

■ FIGURE 62–8
Butterfly flap with palmar Y incision outlined on skin.

greater amount of skin can be transposed onto the sides of the fingers. Additional advantages of this flap are more natural mating of the dorsal pedicle to the more broad palmar V which can be created when a Y-shaped incision is used. To accommodate the increased amount of skin that can be transposed, the angles of the common dorsal flap can be increased from 60° at the corners so that they can approach 90° at the corners with adequate primary closure of the defect (Fig. 62–9). The overall length of the dorsal flap should be equal to the overall length of the palmar inverted Y flap. The skin flaps are dissected in a similar fashion to the previous description after their inscription, exsanguination and tourniquet elevation, and flap division with scalpel (Fig. 62–10). The flaps are rotated in place and inset similarly with 5-0 nylon or 5-0 or 6-0 plain gut sutures (Fig. 62–11).

■ FIGURE 62–9
Diagram of the butterfly flap with an inverted Y incision.

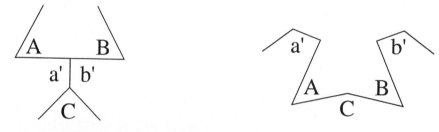

■ FIGURE 62–10
Butterfly flap with inverted Y incision after skin incisions have been made.

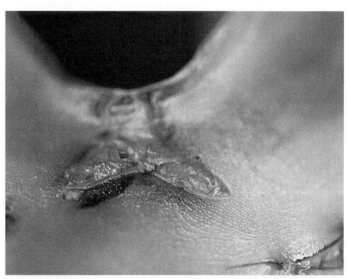

■ FIGURE 62–11
Butterfly flap with palmar Y incision after flaps have been rotated and sutured in place.

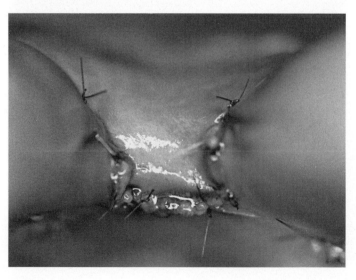

A variant of the butterfly flaps of Shaw is the three-flap web-plasty.[3] In this procedure, a rectangular or near-rectangular dorsal web incision is made. The dimensions of the dorsal flap are determined by the goals of the reconstruction. The width is generally determined by the width of the distal web, and the length determined by the distance between the leading edge of the existing web and the desired palmar extent of the recessed web. Optimal length:width ratio is 1:1; however, ratios of 1.5:1 can successfully be closed, providing the elasticity of the skin is relatively normal. After outlining the dorsal flap, a mirror image rectangle of equal dimensions is drawn on the palmar surface, and a diagonal drawn between either of the two corners then divides this rectangular area into two equal triangles, with lateral pedicles (Fig. 62–12). Incision of the flaps are made with a No. 15 blade, taking care to preserve the proximal base for the dorsal flap and the lateral bases for the two triangular flaps. Scissor dissection is performed, with the preservation of subcutaneous tissue with the skin flaps to preserve blood supply. The triangular flaps are then rotated laterally and dorsally, and their corners secured to the origin of the dorsal rectangular flap (Fig. 62–13). Then, the dorsal rectangular flap is advanced palmarward and sutured in place (Fig. 62–14). For dorsal adduction contractures, particularly those that are secondary to dorsal burns, the dorsal and palmar flaps can be reversed, with the rectangular flaps outlined on normal palmar web skin and the triangular flaps drawn on the dorsal scar hood. This scheme is more desirable as the more normal palmar skin is then used to resurface the depth of the reconstructed web, with the more abnormal scarred skin used to resurface the lateral aspects of the web. In these cases, certainly one should avoid exceeding a 1:1 length:width ratio, and if necessary, use small supplemental skin grafts.

It is recommended with these flaps, as in all flap reconstructions, that adequate vascularity to the tips of the flaps be determined before insetting. Therefore, the tourniquet should

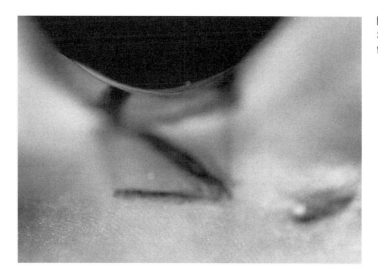

■ FIGURE 62–12
Skin inscribed for three-flap web-plasty.

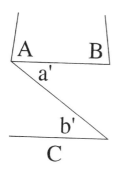
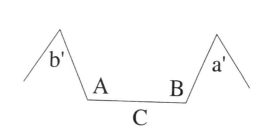

■ FIGURE 62–13
Diagram of the three-flap web-plasty.

■ FIGURE 62–14
Three-flap web-plasty
after flaps have been ro-
tated and sutured in
place.

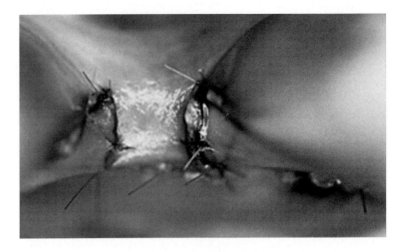

■ FIGURE 62–14
Three-flap web-plasty after flaps have been rotated and sutured in place.

be deflated and the vascularity of the tips of flaps ascertained before their insetting. Once vascularity has been determined to be adequate, insetting can be performed. After insetting of flaps, the hand is cleaned, and nonadherent gauze is cut to fit the web space precisely. Then saline-moistened cotton balls are placed to provide firm even pressure to the flaps. Interdigital gauze sponges are placed, followed by loose cotton rolled gauze. An elastic bandage or bias cut stockinette overwrap is applied and reinforced with tape. The patient is instructed to keep the hand elevated for the first 48 hours after surgery. Dressings are changed after 1 week, and sutures are removed after 2 weeks. Formal hand therapy or splinting is generally unnecessary but can be instituted for selected patients.

■ TECHNICAL ALTERNATIVES

Difficulties encountered with this procedure include circulatory compromise of the flaps, failure of the palmar recipient site to widen appropriately to receive the dorsal flap, difficulty in handling and suturing the small palmar flaps, and insufficient size of the small flaps relative to the defects on the sides of the fingers. Circulatory compromise can be avoided by making sure the flaps have a wide base and that the tips do not have an angle of less than 45°. If one attempts to create flaps of acute angles in damaged skin, the tips of the flaps may not survive. Deflation of the tourniquet after the flaps are created but before they are inset is helpful to evaluate circulation to each flap. If the flap tips are not getting sufficient circulation, they can be trimmed back before insetting to avoid future suture line breakdown.

In the butterfly flap with a palmar V incision, the palmar recipient site may not widen sufficiently to achieve full web release and accept the dorsal flap. A modification of this procedure using a palmar inverted Y incision will produce palmar flaps that can provide better coverage of the fingers yet may still be inadequate if the soft tissue webs are extensive. The palmar Z incision of the three-flap Z-plasty may provide further improved coverage, if the web tissue is sufficiently supple and mobile. In cases of severe contraction, augmentation of these flap reconstructions by small interposed skin grafts, or alternatively, the use of larger regional skin grafts for an entire digital surface may be appropriate.

When dissecting the flaps, one must take care to preserve the neurovascular bundles. In general, the neurovascular bundles lie more proximally in the web than where the reconstruction is being performed. However, acquired syndactylies with scarring can alter the normal anatomy and advance neurovascular bundles distally; in these cases, care must be taken in identifying and preserving them. In no instance should the proximal dissection for the web reconstruction be performed more proximal than the level of the lumbrical canal fascia as this would result in a constricted, V-shaped web, which will originate too proximally in the hand.

■ REHABILITATION

Generally, digital mobilization occurs easily after skin incisions are healed and sutures removed at 2 weeks, or dissolve; supervised hand therapy for mobilization and progressive resistance exercises are optional. In the pediatric patient, functional activities are generally instituted at this time. Intrinsic contractures can occur if mobilization is delayed for whatever reason, and in these cases, intrinsic stretch with MP joint hyperextension, and digital PIP flexion, as well as radial and ulnar deviation at the MP joints should be instituted.

For incomplete syndactylies where the contracted web level is proximal to the PIP joint, and where there is by palpation some redundant skin for the web reconstruction, the methods described here will provide excellent results. It is our impression that modest contractures can be handled easily by the butterfly flap with a palmar inverted V incision. Indeed, any of the three techniques described here will work well. More severe contractures with greater skin deficiencies will have more satisfactory reconstructions using the modified incision with a palmar inverted Y, or with the three-flap web Z-plasty.[1,3] We believe that of the three methods, the three-flap Z-plasty is the best when more aggressive rearrangement of soft tissue is required.

Ostrowski and co-authors[3] described their experience with more than 100 webs treated with three-flap web-plasty. Eighty-five percent were performed for incomplete congenital syndactylies, and 15% were treated for dorsal adduction contractures. None of the congenital syndactylies have required revisions (follow-up period, 6 months to 10 years), and none of the dorsal adduction contractures have required revisions (follow-up period, 6 months to 3 years). Even when there were minor residual skin defects when the guidelines were exceeded, patients healed without the need for secondary or revision surgery. Our own experience with the three-flap web-plasty supports these observations.

■ OUTCOMES

References

1. Flatt AE: The Care of Congenital Hand Anomalies, St. Louis: CV Mosby, 1977:186–189.
2. Furnas DW, Fischer GW: The Z-plasty: Biomechanics and mathematics. Br J Plast Surg, 1971; 24:144–160.
3. Ostrowski DM, Feagin CA, Gould JS: A three-flap web-plasty for release of short congenital syndactyly and dorsal adduction contracture. J Hand Surg, 1991; 16A:634–641.
4. Shaw DT, Li CS, Richey DG, Nahigian SH: Interdigital butterfly flap (The double opposing Z-plasty). Handchirurgie, 1972; 4:41–43.
5. Shaw DT, Li CS, Richey DG, Nahigian SH: Interdigital butterfly flap in the hand (The double opposing Z-plasty). J Bone Joint Surg, 1973; 55A:1677–1679.
6. Woolf RM, Broadbent TR: The four-flap Z-plasty. Plast Reconstr Surg, 1972; 49:48–51.

JOHN D. LUBAHN

63

Dupuytren's Fasciectomy: Open Palm Technique

■ HISTORY OF THE TECHNIQUE

Credit for the development of the open palm technique in Dupuytren's disease is due the man who earned the eponym, Baron Guillaume Dupuytren. Dupuytren's original description of treatment of the disease in 1833 involved surgical principles such as transverse incisions, division of the fascial bands responsible for the contracture, splinting of the fingers in extension for 4 weeks after the operation, and leaving the wounds open, thus allowing them to heal by secondary intent. In 1964, 134 years later, McCash[12] once again described this innovative approach. He recommended removal of only diseased fascia. Normal fascia was left intact to cover the common digital nerves and prevent the hypersensitivity seen with more radical fasciectomy. McCash clearly described the advantages of this technique to be skin closure without tension, prevention of hematomas and infection, and improved wound healing.

McCash also advised that the finger dissection be carried no farther distally than the proximal interphalangeal (PIP) joint, leaving the PIP joint contracted. For those patients who desired a completely straight finger, the intricate and dangerous dissection could be performed at a later date using digital block anesthesia. Currently, with loupe magnification of $3.5\times$ or greater, finger dissection may be extended beyond the PIP joint. Often, a contracture will extend to the lateral digital sheet or Grayson's ligaments at the level of the middle phalanx. This dissection can be performed while the neurovascular bundle is fully protected. Z-plasties can be fashioned into the incision to facilitate closure while leaving the transverse limbs open.

■ INDICATIONS AND CONTRAINDICATIONS

Indications for surgical treatment in Dupuytren's contracture vary widely, depending on the stage of presentation of the disease and the functional demands of the patient. For example, steroid injection may suffice in patients in the early stages who present with a small tender nodule or minimal metacarpophalangeal (MP) joint flexion contracture. Once an MP joint flexion contracture has progressed and the patient is unable to fully extend the palm on a flat surface, open palmar fasciectomy may be considered. This decision may be further supported if the contracture interferes with vocational or avocational interests or basic daily activities, such as putting on a glove. The procedure must be explained in detail in advance as certain individuals may have difficulty with an open wound and daily dressing changes. Patients generally tolerate the procedure well and are less likely to have problems with hematoma, infection, or significant pain on passive extension of the digit than with the wound closed.

Relative contraindications for surgery may include anyone with a strong "Dupuytren's diathesis," which is a term used by Hueston[7] to describe a subcategory of this disease that occurs in young people with a strong family history of Dupuytren's. Usually both hands are involved and knuckle pads (Fig. 63–1) may be present as well as Peyronie's and Ledderhose's disease. Knuckle pads are a benign proliferation of fibrous tissue over the dorsum of the PIP joint and do not interfere with function. Peyronie's disease involves the penis, and Ledderhose's results in lesions on the plantar surface of the foot but does not cause contracture of the toes. Patients who have Dupuytren's diathesis are more likely to develop recurrent disease after surgery to the hands. Depending on a patient's functional level and extent of disease, this risk may be a relative contraindication. A history

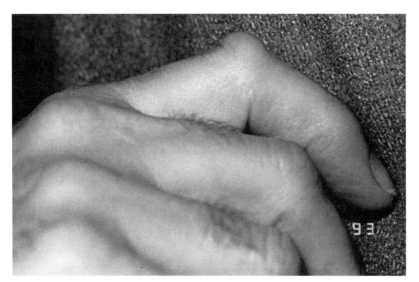

■ FIGURE 63-1
Garrod's knuckle pads, commonly seen in Dupuytren's disease, frequently recur if removed surgically.

of tuberculosis, seizures, excessive alcohol consumption, or acquired immunodeficiency syndrome (AIDS) also are relative contraindications. While alcohol consumption can be tempered, tuberculosis cured, and seizure disorders controlled, a person with AIDS is probably not a good candidate for fasciectomy, unless severe disability exists. However, a positive serology without signs of AIDS is another matter. The patient who is HIV-positive is a candidate for surgical fasciectomy if hand function is compromised to the extent that the patient is unable to care for daily needs or if vocational and avocational function is compromised.

Contraindications would include inability to tolerate a regional or general anesthetic because of severe underlying cardiovascular disease, bleeding diathesis, or other serious medical conditions.

Axillary block is the preferred anesthesia for Dupuytren's fasciectomy, although general anesthesia or Bier block may be suitable alternatives. While certain patients may tolerate a complete single digital fasciectomy under wrist block or local anesthesia, the majority will experience tourniquet pain and require its deflation. Loss of tourniquet control makes the dissection exceedingly difficult.

Because Dupuytren's disease is a contracture of the fascia of the palm and digits, surgical treatment requires the surgeon to have a thorough understanding of both normal and abnormal anatomy. The palmar fascia, or palmar aponeurosis, consists of a triangular-shaped section of fascia in the palm which is continuous with the palmaris longus, when present, in the forearm and extends with the base of its triangular shape distally toward the fingers. It is comprised of the four longitudinal bands, one corresponding to each individual digital ray. The ligaments of Legueu and Juvara originate from the undersurface of the palmar fascia and insert on the fascia of the intrinsic muscles. All of the palmar fascia is relatively adherent to the overlying palmar skin through thick, fibrous septae. Two additional clinically pertinent fascial elements in the palm include the superficial transverse metacarpal ligament, which is located at the fascial level beneath the distal palmar skin crease and the natatory ligaments that pass side-to-side in the web space with some fibers extending distally onto the finger (Fig. 63–2).

Important fascial structures on the finger include Cleland's and Grayson's ligaments, and the lateral digital sheet of Gosset (Fig. 63–3). These are neatly organized fascial bands with Cleland's ligament lying dorsal to the neurovascular bundle, running in an oblique direction and extending from the phalanx to the skin. Grayson's ligament is noted immediately volar or palmar to the neurovascular bundle and runs transversely from the skin to

■ SURGICAL
TECHNIQUES

■ FIGURE 63–2
The palmar aponeurosis
with the superficial transverse metacarpal liga-
ment and the palmar apo-
neurosis divided into four
longitudinal bands to
each finger.

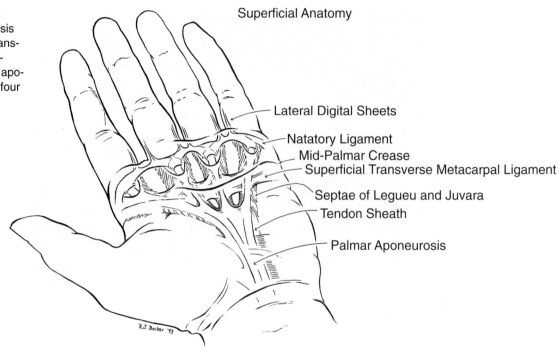

Superficial Anatomy

Lateral Digital Sheets

Natatory Ligament
Mid-Palmar Crease
Superficial Transverse Metacarpal Ligament

Septae of Legueu and Juvara
Tendon Sheath

Palmar Aponeurosis

R.J. Becker '93

■ FIGURE 63–3
A cross section through
the distal third of the
proximal phalanx showing
Cleland's ligament run-
ning dorsally and
obliquely from the proxi-
mal phalanx to the skin,
Grayson's ligament run-
ning more transversely
from the flexor sheath to
the skin, the lateral digital
sheet and the contents of
this "tunnel," the digital
artery and nerve.

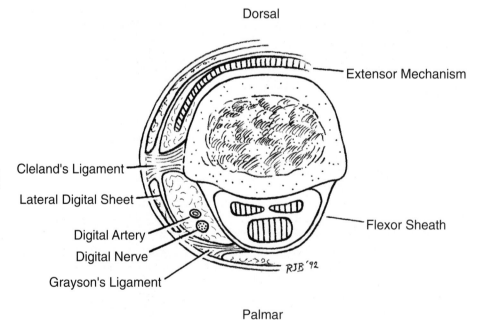

Dorsal

Extensor Mechanism

Cleland's Ligament

Lateral Digital Sheet

Digital Artery

Digital Nerve

Grayson's Ligament

Flexor Sheath

RJB '92

Palmar

the flexor sheath. Finally, the lateral digital sheet, described by Gosset,[5] runs superficially to the neurovascular bundle on both the radial or ulnar sides of the finger.

According to Skoog,[20] the superficial transverse metacarpal ligament is never involved in Dupuytren's contracture. While usually the case, it has been the author's experience that it may be involved on rare occasions. McFarlane[13] has reported that the superficial transverse metacarpal ligament may be involved where diseased fascia enters the thumb web and attaches to the skin at the base of the thumb. The natatory ligament, as well, may be involved and contributes to the "spiral cord." According to Luck,[11] abnormal fascial tissue is referred to as a cord and normal fascial structures, where appropriate, as a band. The pretendinous bands of the palmar aponeurosis become pretendinous cords in Dupuytren's disease and extend directly onto the finger through either a central cord, lateral cord through the natatory cord, or around the neurovascular bundle as a spiral cord. These lateral cords may be a combination of diseased fascia in Cleland's ligaments, Grayson's ligaments, or the lateral digital sheet.

The abnormal anatomy in Dupuytren's disease is represented by changes in previously normal structures. For example, the pretendinous band evolves into the pretendinous cord. As this extends toward the finger, the spiral band contracts beneath the neurovascular bundle, pulling it toward the midline and creating a "spiral cord." Watson and Paul[21] refute the term "spiral cord" as a misnomer assigned to the diseased bifurcating ends of the pretendinous bands or spiral bands (Fig. 63–4). A "spiral cord" continues distally joining the lateral digital sheet and Grayson's ligaments over the PIP joint. The natatory cord may be involved, as well, and contribute to contracture of the neurovascular bundle

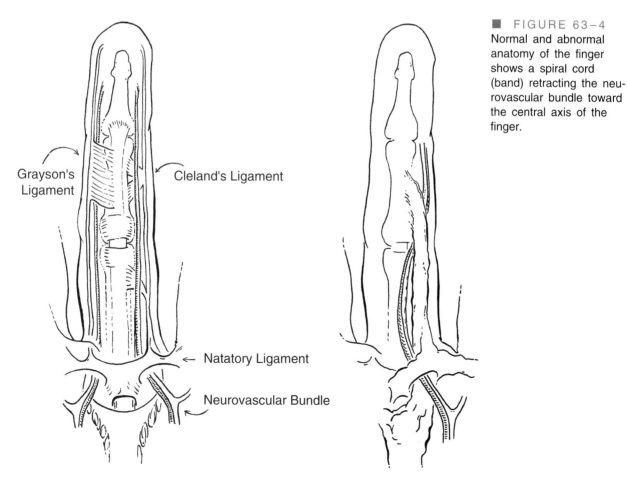

■ FIGURE 63–4
Normal and abnormal anatomy of the finger shows a spiral cord (band) retracting the neurovascular bundle toward the central axis of the finger.

Grayson's Ligament

Cleland's Ligament

Natatory Ligament

Neurovascular Bundle

A. Normal Anatomy

B. Spiral Cord

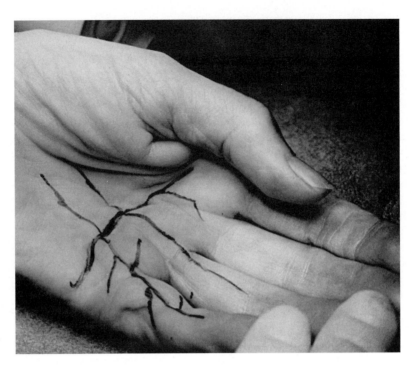

■ FIGURE 63–5
The author's preferred surgical approach for a hand with three rays involved. A transverse incision in the distal palm with extensions onto each finger. The long finger has MP involvement only and a Brunner type incision is used. For the ring and small fingers with more extensive involvement, essentially a longitudinal incision which is broken up into Z-plasties has been designed. When these Z-plasties are closed, the transverse limb is left open to allow drainage and prevent hematoma formation.

toward the midline. The dorsal most fascial structure of the finger, Cleland's ligament, like the superficial transverse metacarpal ligament is not believed to be involved in Dupuytren's disease.

A transverse incision is made in the distal palmar crease (Fig. 63–5). Extensions are outlined proximally and distally either in a straight-line fashion as shown in the ring finger and with projected Z-plasty as shown in the small finger, or in an oblique fashion, as shown in the long finger (Brunner-type).[1] The latter incision may be more effective when the disease is less severe and the contracture at the MP or PIP joint lends itself to VY closure.[9] The advantage of the longitudinal incision is that it may be broken up into multiple Z-plasties. In general, a classic 60° Z-plasty is preferred, with the central member consisting of a fixed length longitudinally. The two limbs then extend at 60° angles from this longitudinal cord or central member and must be equal in length. When closed, the 60° Z-plasty allows a theoretical 75% gain. This calculation is based on geometric principles. Skin has the potential for plastic deformation and, in reality, the gain and length may be more or less than the 75% calculation.[6]

Exposure of the underlying diseased fascia begins proximally with extension of the incision toward the distal palm. Normal fascia is located at the distal margin of the transverse carpal ligament. Skin incisions are reflected radially and ulnarward with the majority of the dissection performed with a No. 15 blade. Diseased fascia is carefully separated from the skin. In areas of dense adhesion between the skin and the underlying diseased palmar fascia, a segment of skin may be excised. The junction of diseased and normal fascia is isolated, usually near the distal extent of the transverse carpal ligament. Diseased fascia is reflected distally with a knife and held with a small Kocher or Alice clamp (Fig. 63–6). More blunt dissection using a Steven's (or other) tenotomy scissor is then begun, identifying the common neurovascular bundles within the lumbrical canals on both sides of the flexor tendon sheath. Skin hooks held by an assistant or attached to a small hand table via elastic straps may facilitate exposure. A small, sterile, rubber band or vessel loop is placed around the common digital nerve or artery as the normal vessel or nerve passes into the diseased fascia. At the level of the distal palmar crease, the surgeon must look for the presence of a spiral cord of diseased fascia which will displace the neurovascular bundle to a subcutaneous position. Short and Watson[19] have described a "soft pulpy mass" between the distal palmar crease and the proximal flexion crease of the finger,

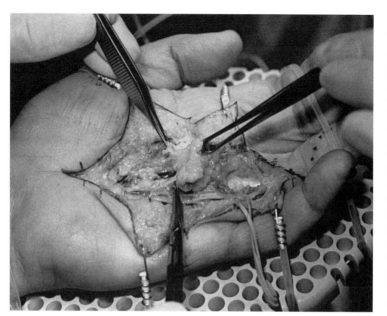

■ FIGURE 63-6
With the palm open, the diseased fascia has been surgically mobilized in the proximal palm. Peripheral dissection has exposed the common digital arteries and nerves proximally and the proper digital vessels distally. Dissection is being continued from known anatomy into the area of involved tissue for removal of the remaining fascial attachments, in this case to the underlying intrinsic muscles through the diseased ligaments of Legueu and Juvara.

which, if present, should alert the surgeon to the presence of the nerve lying subcutaneously. Proximal to distal dissection with continuous visualization of the nerve is imperative. The spiral cord may extend to the level of the middle phalanx, intertwining with Grayson's ligament and the lateral digital sheet (Figs. 63-3 and 63-4). Dissection through this complex region requires localization and protection of the neurovascular bundle at all times. Division of the diseased cord with small scissors may be difficult because of dense adhesions between the diseased fascia and skin, as well as the underlying flexor sheath. As long as the nerve or artery is directly visualized and protected, little risk exists in using a knife for dissection, particularly for dividing the diseased fascia from the base of the middle or proximal phalanx and the flexor sheath.

Transverse limbs of the Z-plasty over the finger are best outlined before the surgical incision at that level. The proper digital neurovascular bundles must be identified proximally, and then the proposed Z-plasty flap(s) at the base of the finger or over the proximal interphalangeal joint can be mobilized. In general, a 60° Z-plasty with the limbs between 5 and 10 mm in length is sufficient. The entire segment of diseased fascia for the involved ray is removed in one segment, with release of its most distal attachment. The tourniquet is usually deflated and hemostasis obtained before wound closure. The transverse limb of the Z-plasty over the PIP joint is left open. This allows the PIP joint more active and passive extension and drainage from beneath the flaps. The Z-plasty and remaining skin closure is usually accomplished with 5-0 nylon sutures in a horizontal or vertical mattress fashion. The transverse incision in the distal palm or distal palmar crease is left open and covered with Owens gauze. A bulky dressing, of longitudinally applied 4″ × 4″ gauze loosely wrapped with a 3″ Kling, and a dorsal plaster splint are applied. The patient is allowed active extension of the fingers against the splint as soon as the axillary block loses its effectiveness or the patient awakens from general anesthesia (Fig. 63–7). The dressing is changed within 48 to 72 hours, and the patient is instructed in local wound care consisting of dressing changes one to two times per day and gentle washing of the wound margins with a mild soap or half-strength peroxide. The patient is advised not to soak the hand, but that limited amounts of water for cleansing may be beneficial. The sutures are removed between 7 and 14 days—usually half the sutures are removed on day 7 and the remainder on day 14. Dressing changes of the palmar wound are continued until it is healed. This usually occurs between 2 and 3 weeks after surgery. A splint that holds the MP joint or joints in full extension is worn at night. With single digital ray involvement, a dorsal alumafoam splint with a Velcro strap may be used to hold the finger in extension

■ FIGURE 63–7
Splint to immobilize the hand for the first 24 to 48 hours, padded on the palm with absorbent 4″ × 4″ gauze and a dorsal splint allowing finger flexion.

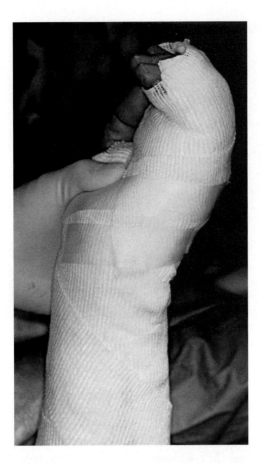

(Fig. 63–8A). Orthoplast splintage is more effective when multiple digits have been released (Fig. 63–8B). The patient is instructed to wear the splint at night and between 4 and 6 hours per day for 3 months. The frequency of postoperative visits depends on the patient's clinical progress. If inflammation in the palm and a tendency toward recurrent contracture exists, it may be necessary for the patient to wear the splint at night until the scar is soft and the finger can easily be fully extended.

■ TECHNICAL ALTERNATIVES

Today, with a severe flexion contracture of the metacarpophalangeal joint, several options exist to facilitate closure. Free skin grafts on the palm have been advocated, however, they cannot be directly applied to the flexor tendon sheath. Grafts are vulnerable to serous effusion, hematoma, and marginal viability of the flaps in the palm to which they must be sewn. Incisions may be closed with Z-plasty, a transposition flap from the dorsum of the hand, or a fillet flap from the dorsum of the hand when a finger has been amputated. Finally, the palm of the hand may simply be closed with the finger(s) in flexion, anticipating that full extension of the fingers will return with therapy, after the wound has healed.

The most appropriate surgical alternative to open palm technique is skin closure by VY flap.[9] This may be perfectly acceptable and may allow closure without tension when the contracture is minimal and involves only one digit. For contracture of more than one digit, the open palm technique is preferable. Good results have been described by Moermans with full-thickness skin grafting of segmental aponeurectomy.[16]

As with any surgical approach for Dupuytren's disease, the potential pitfalls include nerve or artery damage, hematoma, and flap necrosis. While nerve and artery damage should be avoidable with careful dissection and protection of the neurovascular bundle during the procedure, correction of a severe contracture may stretch the nerve to the extent sensation is lost or compromised. Correction also may embarrass the circulation, and tissue loss can occur.

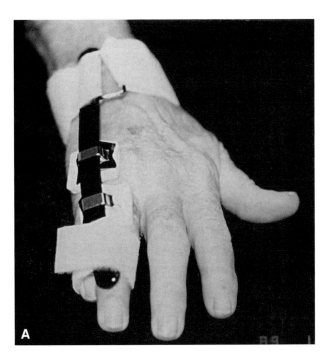

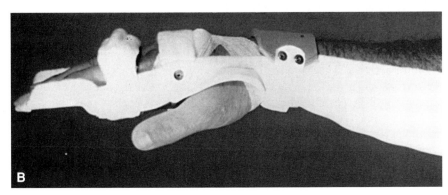

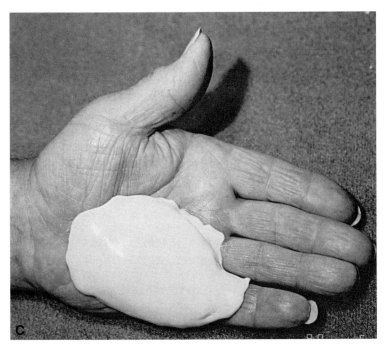

■ FIGURE 63–8

A, An alumafoam spring splint is ideal for single ray involvement. **B,** A palmar, forearm-based Neoprene splint maintaining the fingers extended in multiple digit involvement. **C,** Elastomer applied to a thickened area of scar along the ulnar side of the hand to prevent edema and improve early motion.

The open wound will prevent hematoma formation in the palm. Tight closure of incisions on the finger should be avoided. Also, failure to obtain hemostasis, resulting in hematoma on the finger could necessitate return to the operating room for evacuation and result in loss of digital flexion. Flap necrosis may be prevented by minimizing skin dissection and careful planning of the incision.

In the short term, patients with pre-existing contractures, those with a stronger diathesis, and others for unknown reasons, may develop a red painful palm as the wound heals. McFarlane[14] noted that some authors consider this to be a form of reflex sympathetic dystrophy. When this occurs, continued therapy to prevent edema and joint contracture, as well as regular use of nonsteroidal medication or, occasionally, a steroid injection, are crucial in maintaining joint motion, preventing secondary contracture, and minimizing pain and morbidity.

Reflex sympathetic dystrophy is an uncommon postoperative problem but may occur in 4% of males and 8% of females.[15] The longer a dystrophy goes undiagnosed and treatment is delayed, the worse the surgical outcome.

■ REHABILITATION

Many patients do not require hand therapy. When they do, the goal of postoperative rehabilitation is to maintain full motion in the individual fingers of the hand and prevent recurrent contracture at the MP or PIP joint. This is accomplished with a rigorous active range of motion program and night splintage, combined with frequent dressing changes. The wound must be closely observed for any problems such as increasing pain, swelling, and dysesthesia, which may herald the onset of a minor causalgia or reflex sympathetic dystrophy. With these early signs, a more intensive therapy program should be instituted.

In cases where therapy is required early for pain, swelling, and limited motion, the therapist should assist the patient in daily dressing care and see the patient regularly to monitor active and passive joint motion. In general, a thermoplast splint is formed on the first or second postoperative day and holds the metacarpal and proximal interphalangeal joints in full extension. The splint should be worn at all times when the patient is not engaged in active flexion and removed for active therapy sessions. When contracture recurs early, the splint should be worn for between 3 and 6 months or until such time as the fingers may be held in full extension and the scar begins to soften. Occasionally, dynamic extension splints may be used in patients with weak extension. Coban and otoform are helpful in minimizing swelling and erythema.

Finally, early communication via written prescription or verbal exchange between surgeon and therapist is important to establish clear goals. The patient and therapist must have a clear understanding of the expectations of the surgeon based on the operative findings and procedure. A good example of this is the PIP flexion contracture, which is common in the small finger, and if 30° or less may not have been released intraoperatively. Therapy should not attempt to correct this.

■ OUTCOMES

The most significant benefit of the open palm technique in improving outcome in the surgical treatment of Dupuytren's contracture is seen in the immediate postoperative period. Patients may fully extend the involved finger or fingers without tension on the palmar wound. This allows better active and passive extension of the MP joint and PIP joints, with no tension and secondary discomfort at the suture line. Complications, such as hematoma and persistent edema, are likewise eliminated by allowing immediate drainage of blood and serous fluid.

Gonzales[4] reports virtually all patients who are followed longer than ten years develop Dupuytren's disease once again in some area of the hand. Schneider and co-authors[18] confirm a low complication rate in the immediate postoperative period, e.g., no wound hematomas, wound infections, or skin sloughs in 49 hands. In six of their patients, edema, increasing pain, and signs of reflex sympathetic dystrophy developed, which were treated with hand therapy. Their transverse palmar wounds healed between 3 and 5 weeks. Whereas the overall follow-up was good, recurrent contracture developed in 34% of their patients, and 48% had extension of the disease or new disease in the operated hand. Kelly and co-authors[8] reviewed 254 hands of 213 patients treated with the open palm technique between 1977 and the present. They report a 75% recurrence rate after 27 months. Twenty-one percent of their patients required revision surgery by 70 months after surgery.

In a comparative study[10] that reviewed the open and closed palm technique, total active motion measurement of involved rays was better in the group treated with the open palm technique than in the group treated with the closed technique. Even more striking was the complication rate, which was 19% in the group of patients whose palmar wounds were closed versus 8% in those with the transverse incision in the palm left open.

Recurrent PIP joint contracture of the proximal interphalangeal joint with dermal and fascial involvement presents a significant challenge. In many patients, the contracture is functional, and as long as it does not interfere with vocational and avocational needs and activities of daily living, observation or perhaps steroid injection may be the most reasonable course to follow. Particularly in PIP joint contractures, surgical release is fraught with complications such as neurapraxia or actual damage to the radial or ulnar digital nerve or artery. Maintaining the finger in full extension either with splintage or Kirshner wire at the PIP joint may itself compromise circulation to the tip of the finger. In certain isolated circumstances, proximal interphalangeal joint fusion, arthroplasty, or amputation through the proximal phalanx may be the treatment of choice for the affected individual. Ray amputation is rarely necessary. The factor most likely to predict recurrence of disease is the patient's genetic predisposition, which is beyond the surgeon's control. However, limited, open fasciectomy with careful surgical technique will preserve the remaining palmar fascia anatomy of the palm, decrease associated morbidity, and lead to a more satisfactory result.

References

1. Bruner JM: The zig-zag volar-digital incision for flexor-tendon surgery. Plast Reconstr Surg, 1967; 40:571–574.
2. Gonzalez F, Watson HK. Simultaneous carpal tunnel release and Dupuytren's fasciectomy. J Hand Surg, 1991; 16B:175–178.
3. Gonzales RI: Open Fasciectomy in Full Thickness Skin Graft in a Correction of Digital Flexion Deformity. In: Hueston JT, Tubiana R (eds): Dupuytren's Disease, 2nd Ed, Edinburgh: Churchill Livingstone, 1985:158–163.
4. Gonzales RI: Recurrence and extension. In: McFarlane RM, McGourther DA, Flint MH (eds): Dupuytren's Disease. Biology and Treatment (The Hand and Upper Limb Series), Edinburgh: Churchill Livingstone, 1985:385.
5. Gosset J: Dupuytren's Disease, 2nd Ed, G.E.M. Monograph, 1985:18.
6. Grabb WC, Smith JW: Plastic Surgery, 4th Ed, Boston: Little, Brown, 1991:71–72.
7. Hueston JT: Dupuytren's Contracture, Edinburgh: Churchill Livingstone, 1963.
8. Kelly JJ, Peimer CA, Moy OJ, Wheeler DR: Late results of McCash fasciectomy for Dupuytren's disease (abstract). American Society for Surgery of the Hand 48th Annual Meeting, 1993:81.
9. King EW, Bass DN, Watson HK: Treatment of Dupuytren's contracture by extensive fasciectomy through multiple Y-V plasty incisions: Short-term evaluation of 170 consecutive operations. J Hand Surg, 1979; 4:234–241.
10. Lubahn JD, Lister GD, Wolfe T: Fasciectomy and Dupuytren's disease: A comparison between the open-palm technique and wound closure. J Hand Surg, 1984; 9A:53–58.
11. Luck JV: Dupuytren's contracture: A new concept of the pathogenesis correlated with surgical management. J Bone Joint Surg, 1959; 41A:635–664.
12. McCash CR: The open palm technique in Dupuytren's contracture. Br J Plast Surg, 1964; 17:271–280.
13. McFarlane RM: Dupuytren's Contracture. Green's Operative Hand Surgery, 2nd Ed, 1988:554.
14. McFarlane RM: Green's Operative Hand Surgery, 3rd Ed, 1993:568.
15. McFarlane RM, Botz JS: The results of treatment. In: McFarlane RM, McGourther DA, Flint MH (eds): Dupuytren's Disease. Biology and Treatment (The Hand and Upper Limb Series), Edinburgh: Churchill Livingstone, 1990:387–412.
16. Moermans JP: Segmental aponeurectomy in Dupuytren's disease. J Hand Surg, 1991; 16B:243–254.

17. Nissenbaum M, Kleinert HE: Treatment considerations in carpal tunnel syndrome with coexistent Dupuytren's disease. J Hand Surg, 1980; 5:544–547.
18. Schneider LH, Hankin FM, Eisenberg T: Surgery of Dupuytren's disease. A review of the open palm method. J Hand Surg, 1986; 11A:23–27.
19. Short WH, Watson HK: Prediction of the spiral nerve in Dupuytren's contracture. J Hand Surg, 1982; 7:84–86.
20. Skoog T: The transverse elements of the palmar aponeurosis in Dupuytren's contracture. Their pathological and surgical significance. Scand J Reconstr Surg, 1967; 1:51–63.
21. Watson HK, Paul H Jr: Pathologic anatomy. Hand Clin, 1991; 7:661–668.

LAWRENCE COLWYN
HURST

64

Dupuytren's Fasciectomy: Zig-Zag Plasty Technique

In 1614, Plater published the earliest known description of Dupuytren's disease in his manuscript Observations. Despite the 1777 description and fasciotomy by the English surgeon, Cline, and the early work of Sir Ashley Cooper, the eponym credits Baron Dupuytren because of his 1830 lectures and use of open fasciectomy. His notoriety was driven by the very active French medical journals of his time.[5] Historically, numerous skin incisions have been used for the surgical correction of Dupuytren's contractures.[4,13] Current methods use various transverse incisions, longitudinal incisions with Z-plasties, and zig-zag incisions to expose the diseased fascia. Then a partially or completely regional fasciectomy is done to remove the pathologic cords.

■ HISTORY OF THE
TECHNIQUE

The operative goals for Dupuytren's fasciectomies are excision of the grossly pathologic palmar aponeurosis, correction of joint contractures, preservation of the digital arteries and nerves, preservation of uninvolved skin, maintaining flexion, and minimizing the chances of recurrence. The zig-zag plasty fasciectomy is an effective method for achieving these goals, but no surgical procedure can cure Dupuytren's disease. Clinical indications for surgical treatment include a positive tabletop test, metacarpophalangeal (MP) joint contractures greater than 30°, or proximal interphalangeal (PIP) joint contractures greater than 30°. The tabletop test is positive when the patient can no longer place the palm and the fingers simultaneous on the same flat surface. These clinical indications are only guidelines. Before recommending surgery, the surgeon must review the potential complications, the patient's functional needs, and other medical problems. The possibility of digit loss must be discussed frankly in cases with previous neurovascular injury or severe recurrent disease. Surgical treatment may not always be in the patient's best interest. Conversely, those patients who are simply nervous about surgery must understand that prolonged observation usually results in worse contractures that are less amenable to surgical correction. A nodule alone is not an indication for surgery. However, the surgeon should consider the extremely rare possibility of fibrosarcoma in the young patient with severe pain, particularly night pain, who does not have classic early nodular formation.[7,9,15]

■ INDICATIONS AND
CONTRAINDICATIONS

The operation is done under axillary block or general anesthesia. The arm is exsanguinated, and a tourniquet is inflated to an appropriate pressure.

The three-part incision (I, II, and III) for the zig-zag plasties fasciectomy for pretendinous-central cords involving both the ring and small fingers are shown in Figure 64–1. Each part is first designed with a methylin-blue marking pen. The outlined incisions in the proximal and distal palm can be designed before the dissection begins. The digital design beyond the first finger crease should be finalized after the proximal dissection and release of the MP joint contractures. This allows a more realistic understanding of the digital skin contours.

In the proximal palm (zig-zag plasty part I), the incision can be made longitudinally with its distal end perpendicular to the distal palmar crease. While using loupe magnification, a no. 15 blade is used to elevate the two flaps on either side of this longitudinal part I incision. Note the short perpendicular distance from the cord to the fold in the elevated

■ SURGICAL
TECHNIQUES

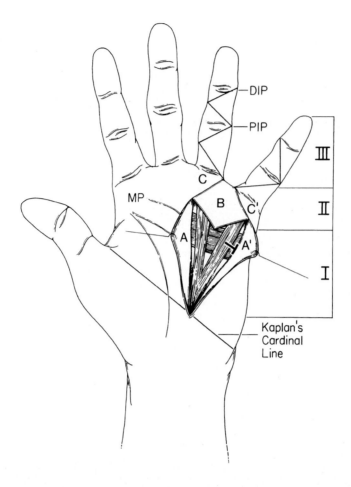

■ FIGURE 64–1

The zig-zag plasty incisions, parts I, II, and III, for pretendinous-central cords involving the left ring and small fingers. Palmar flaps are open and retracted. Notice the short perpendicular distance from the fold in the flap to the center of the cord. A and A′ = part I, proximal palmar flaps. B = web-based distal palmar flap. C and C′ = first triangular flaps of the ring and little digits, respectively. The small finger has one oblique incision between each transverse crease and the ring has two incisions between each.

flap (Fig. 64–1). Although they are not thick like the pretendinous cords, the transverse aponeurotic bands (superficial transverse intermetacarpal ligaments) do shorten and proximally the pretendinous cords adhere to each other at the level of the superficial vascular arch. The proximity of the pretendinous cords means that the distal apices of the part I (Fig. 64–1: A, A′) must be elevated only 1 to 2 cm to expose the ring and small finger pretendinous cords, the intervening transverse aponeurotic bands, the transverse bands radial to the ring finger pretendinous cords, and the transverse bands ulnar to the small finger cord.

Part II of the zig-zag plasty is opened next. Opening the radial and ulnar apices of this distally based flap must be performed meticulously because of the intimate relations of the digital nerves to the pathologic tissue and the possibility of a spiral cord. The spiral cord can bring the digital nerve superficial to the aponeurosis, immediately under the dermis. With significant proximal interphalangeal contractures, the risk of superficial volar displacement of the digital nerve is greatest at the junction of parts II and III of the zig-zag plasty fasciectomy. The spiral cord also can push the digital nerve and artery to the center of the flexor tendon sheath.

When there are two adjacent pretendinous-central cords, the web portion of part II of the zig-zag plasty dissection is a distally based flap (Fig. 64–1: B). This is a very resilient flap because of the proximity of the digital arteries, the dorsal digital arteries that traverse the web, and the terminal portions of the dorsal metacarpal arteries. With the fingers contracted and the web narrowed by the natatory ligament or spiral band involvement, the flap base appears narrow. However, the flap's width at the base is usually equal to at least 50% of the distance between the web and the palmar crease. The flap has a thick layer of subcutaneous web fat that does not need to be hinged distally on the web base to fully visualize the neurovascular bundles and dissect the combined pretendinous-central cords. The localization of the artery and nerve can be done through the flap's subcutaneous tissues without fully mobilizing them. Even lifting the adherent skin off the cord does not usually necessitate full mobilization of the web flap. The visualization of the neurovascular bundle also is enhanced by mobilizing the first triangular flaps of the fingers (Fig. 64–1: C, C').

Part III of the zig-zag plasty opens the finger from the first flexion crease to the distal end of the cord. Extending the zig-zag plasty beyond the pathologic tissue is unnecessary; however, caution is appropriate at the PIP joint flexion crease. Here, the central cord usually splits to either side of the flexor sheath and attaches to the base of the middle phalanx. It is not advisable to dissect under the distal skin and blindly snip the last attachments of the cord. Instead, extend the incision distally. These last attachments are in immediate proximity to the neurovascular bundle.

The design of the zig-zag flaps in part III can be made from two different basic designs. One choice is the Littler-Bruner design.[13] For example, in the fifth finger, this incision goes from the radial midlateral edge of the first flexion crease to the ulnar midlateral edge of the PIP joint flexion crease (Fig. 64–1: small finger).[2,11] The angle of these incisions should be carefully judged. The angle between the digital flexion crease and the incision should not exceed 45°. When the finger is contracted, the perpendicular distance from the first digital flexion crease to the second digital flexion crease will appear short. In my hand, this distance at the midvolar line is 7 to 10 mm. with the PIP joint flexed 45° and the MP joint flexed 45°. If the MP joint is flexed 70° and the PIP joint flexed 90°, this perpendicular distance shortens to 5 mm. When the finger extends fully, this midvolar distance is 15 mm. In Dupuytren's disease, the skin conforms to this fixed shortened posture, but there is no true skin loss and coverage will usually be adequate after the flexion contracture is corrected. This apparent skin shortage means that if the limbs of the zig-zag incisions are not made obliquely enough or are started too close to the volar midline or do not go from the proximal midlateral point to the distal midlateral point, the incision will be too longitudinal when the finger is straightened. At the time of closure, the zig-zag incisions that are too straight can be helped by doing V-Y advancements at the apices of each flap. Bedeschi has also shown that the transverse limbs of the V-Y can be left open and the flaps not advanced.[13] This also will be a helpful maneuver on those occasions when flap edges need to be trimmed or when the positioning needs to be adjusted to account for longitudinal displacement of the original oblique incisions. Leaving the transverse limb open also avoids excessive advancement, which can cause a digital tourniquet effect and troublesome postoperative swelling. Sometimes, the digit must be temporarily positioned in a flexed posture to avoid tension on the sutures. This positioning is easily overcome by postoperative splinting.

The second choice for the finger flaps is to include both limbs of the zig-zag plasty incisions between the first and second digital flexion creases and a second set of limbs between the second and third digital flexion creases (Fig. 64–1: ring finger). Again, the incisions start and stop at the midlateral line.

Regardless of the zig-zag plasty design choice, try to divide excessively soft or adherent thin skin so that it becomes the edges of two different flaps. Do not design flaps so that adherent thin areas become the base of a flap. Do not put an excessively soft skin pit or skin fold that is likely to "buttonhole" in the base of the flap. Try to put the incision through the middle of these easily damaged areas. The digital flap incisions are made with a no. 15 blade but mobilized with the scalpel, the Littler scissors, and the curved iris scissors as indicated by the difficulty and type of dissection. The Littler scissors spreads the fatty tissues well but for lifting adherent skin off the pathologic cord, dissection is done with a scalpel or a very sharp curved iris scissors. Before mobilizing the flaps, always locate the neurovascular bundle by dissecting them in the opened proximal parts of the zig-zag plasty. Next, dissect the part of the flap that has good subcutaneous fatty tissues and then mobilize the adherent areas of the flap. Once the flaps are safely mobilized, use retention sutures to keep the flaps retracted. These flaps should contain as much subcutaneous tissue as possible to enhance flap survival and postoperative skin quality. If the pathologic tissue is adherent to the skin or if vertical cords go up to the skin, then the diseased tissue must be excised to prevent recurrence. In recurrent cases do not hesitate to remove skin and apply split-thickness skin grafts, especially in young patients. In older patients, whose digits stiffen easily, the open palm technique is used with the zig-zag plasty instead of skin grafts.

Once the incision is designed and parts I and II of the zig-zag plasty are opened, the cord is dissected in a proximal to distal direction. If the skin is not adherent and there are no clinical signs of a spiral cord,[13,20] then the whole incision of the zig-zag plasty, parts I, II, and III, can be opened safely at once. If there is any chance of a spiral cord involvement such as a significant PIP joint contracture, then parts I and II are opened first to allow proximal neurovascular localization at the difficult area of the first digital crease.

The proximal cord dissection is started at the level of the superficial vascular arch or just proximal to it at the junction of the longitudinal incision and Kaplan's cardinal line (Fig. 64–2). Once the skin flaps are elevated and retracted, the pretendinous cords and the transverse aponeurotic bands are exposed. Usually, there is a small triangle devoid of fascia between the proximal edge of the transverse bands and the two cords. The cord dissection is initiated with a fine tipped mosquito clamp, which is put through the transverse bands at the ulnar side of the small finger's cord to spread the tissues (Fig. 64–2: A)

■ FIGURE 64–2
Zig-zag plasty incisions open and two pretendinous-central cords exposed. A clamp is passed from A under the cords to B to protect underlying structures while cords are cut. Point C locates the median nerve motor branch. Notice Kaplan's line from the first web to the hook of the hamate.

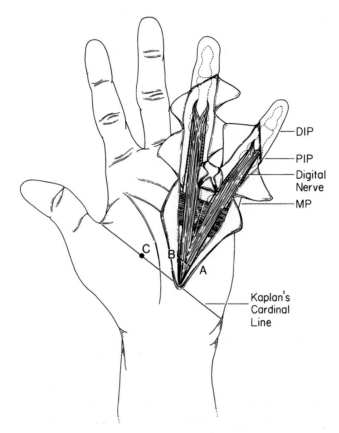

DIP

PIP

Digital Nerve

MP

Kaplan's Cardinal Line

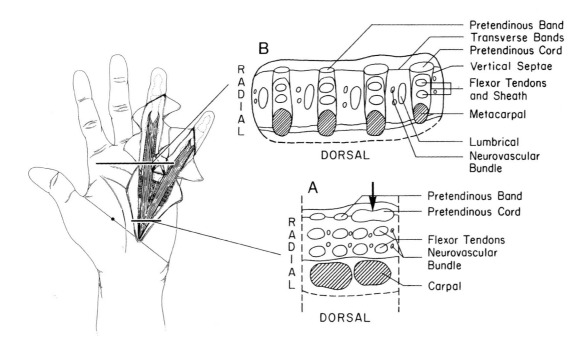

■ FIGURE 64-3

A, Cross-sectional anatomy is shown at the level of Kaplan's line (just proximal to the superficial vascular arch). The arrow shows the point where the two adherent cords must be split apart before the ring and small cords can be separately dissected. **B,** Cross-sectional anatomy at the level of the MP joints. Notice the small pretendinous bands superficial to the index and long flexor tendons and the larger pathologic cords volar to the ring and small flexor tendons. Notice the vertical bands of Legueu and Juvara.

and expose the superficial vascular arch, the common digital artery and/or the fifth flexor sheath. A little more spreading will allow the dorsal extent of the cord to be determined and separated from the underlying tissues. Next, the clamp is passed under the cord until the tip appears radial to the ring finger's cord (Fig. 64-2: B). The clamp then pulls the cord volarly toward the surgeon. A scalpel is now used to cut the stem of the pretendinous cords. With cords to the index and long fingers, the close proximity of the median motor branch which pierces the aponeurosis here should be noted (Fig. 64-2: C). After the cord's stem is cut, hold the proximal end with the hemostat and pull it distally.

Understanding the cross-sectional anatomy of the palm both proximally at Kaplan's line and distally at the MP joint level will facilitate the next part of the dissection (Fig. 64-3: inserts A, B). The radial and ulnar transverse aponeurotic bands must be cut next. At the most proximal point, the two pretendinous cords to the ring and small fingers will be connected with no transverse aponeurotic bands between them. To separate them, a mosquito clamp is passed under the more distal transverse bands to protect the neurovascular bundles while these transverse bands are cut. The clamp is then advanced proximally under the connected cord stems. A scalpel then splits the stem area longitudinally (Fig. 64-3A: arrow). This establishes two independent pretendinous cords, one to the ring and one to the small finger. Now each pathologic cord is dissected separately. Some surgeons recommend preserving the transverse aponeurotic bands, but this is not necessary.

Next, the cord is raised off the proximal portion of the flexor sheath, and any remaining attachments are cut. Dissecting farther distally, the flexor sheath's A-1 pulley is quickly reached. A pretendinous cord may initially appear attached to the A-1 pulley, but the scissors can be introduced between the cord and the flexor sheath. This potential space exists because the flexor sheath does not become involved in Dupuytren's disease. The spreading of the scissors blades in this space will be resisted by the vertical bands of aponeurotic tissue. These vertical bands, septae of Legueu and Juvara (Fig. 64–3B) join the sides of the combined pretendinous-central cord at the point where the transverse aponeurotic bands also attach to the cord. The exact anatomy and terminology of the vertical bands and the web space fascial coalescence is controversial.[13,17] The vertical bands then pass dorsally away from the surgeon along the sides of the flexor sheath and attach to the deep transverse fibers adjacent to the metacarpal neck. These vertical bands must be isolated and cut after visualizing the digital nerves and arteries. While using loupe magnification, the neurovascular bundle is exposed by spreading the adjacent fatty tissues with the Littler scissors. Most of this dissection occurs in the area of the web flap (Fig. 64–1: part II) but still does not require full mobilization of the flap. Meyerding finger retractors or Ragnell retractors are used to gently retract the neurovascular bundles. Next the surgeon spreads between the radial vertical band and the flexor sheath and between the vertical band and the radially located small finger lumbrical muscle. Once the lumbrical is freed, it is retracted with the radial neurovascular bundle. Next pull the cord distally and toward the surgeon. Put one blade of the scissors between the vertical band and the flexor sheath and the other blade radial to the vertical band keeping both blades as dorsally as possible but in sight while cutting the band. Sometimes the vertical bands or spiral bands that have been forced into a vertical attitude go distally to the level of the A-1 pulley. Do not cut the more distal vertical bands until further neurovascular bundle localization and retraction has been done. At this point, the combined pretendinous-central cord has been dissected into the finger and is now called a central cord. The central cord develops in the absence of a pre-existing anatomic fibrous band. The cord should now be free to the distal end of the A-2 pulley of the flexor tendon sheath.[12]

Some combined pretendinous-central cords in patients with early disease and MP joint contractures alone will end in the subcutaneous tissue over the proximal phalanx near the junction of the A-1 and A-2 pulley. If there is a PIP contracture, however, the central cord will extend past the PIP joint to the base of the middle phalanx. In this case the central cord will frequently split at the PIP joint level and go between the neurovascular bundles and the flexor sheath to attach to the periosteum of the middle phalanx. Sometimes the split central cord divides a second time so that the radial limb or the ulnar limb of the cord actually has two separate parts. One part may go between the sheath and the neurovascular bundle while the second part goes to the side of the neurovascular bundle and attaches to the dorsal lateral skin. In this retrovascular area, one may even find involvement of the transverse retinacular ligament. The final removal of the central cord at this distal attachment must be done delicately with the neurovascular structures well visualized to avoid nerve injury, vascular spasm, or damage.

After the cord material has been removed from the small finger, an identical dissection starting proximally at the level of the superficial arch is used to remove the combined pretendinous-central cord from the ring finger. Once this has been completed, then the next step is to deflate the tourniquet. If the dissection is unlikely to be completed in 2 hours, stop at 1.5 hours, and release the tourniquet for 15 minutes. Then reinflate the tourniquet for an additional hour. Once the tourniquet is let down, vascular staining sometimes makes dissection more difficult so try to fit each digit's dissection into a 1.5 hour tourniquet time. Before deflating the tourniquet, apply warm saline soaked sponges to the wound. The warm saline is a very efficient way to break vasospasm and make the fingers pink almost instantaneously. Next, a temporary pressure dressing is kept on the dissected area while the hyperemic phase passes. Then any excessive bleeding is carefully controlled with a delicate bipolar cautery. Cauterize carefully to avoid damage to the digital artery or nerve. Most bleeders will stop with a slightly longer period of gentle pressure. Next, the wound is irrigated with saline and the vascular supply to the flaps is carefully assessed. If any of the flap tips are still white at this point, consider removing a bit of the tip and adding a V-Y advancement for that flap. If tension complicates tip advancement, the transverse limbs of the V-Y can be left open.[13] Similarly, V-Y adjustments may be necessary if any of the flap limbs has become too longitudinal after correction of the joint contractures.

Following skin flap assessment, a small soft suction drain is placed in the wound and the closure is done. The tourniquet is reinflated if needed. Before closure carefully examine the A-1 pulleys. If there is any sign of an associated triggering, release the A-1 pulleys. Next the skin incisions are sutured with interrupted 5-O simple nylon sutures and a compressive dressing is applied. A piece of sterile foam rubber in the dressing is a useful splint that will not become rigid if it gets blood soaked. In older patients where skin may be deficient, the zig-zag plasty can easily be left open at the junction of parts I and II. This allows the web area to move distally and the longitudinal incisional area to move proximally. This procedure leaves a typical open palm transverse elliptical defect which will heal in 4 to 6 weeks with daily dressing changes and soaks.

For simple regional fasciectomies done with the zig-zag plasty technique, outpatient surgery is usually appropriate. The suction drain is removed before discharge from the ambulatory surgery center or at an early follow-up visit. Older patients with significant medical problems are hospitalized for 48 hours with the hand elevated and the suction drain in place for 36 to 48 hours. If the palm is left open, a drain is not needed. During hospitalization prophylactic intravenous antibiotics are given to diabetic patients, to patients with skin grafts, and to patients with recurrent Dupuytren's disease.

The fascial dissection technique above will vary considerably when other pathologic cords are present. Efficient dissection of these cords requires a careful review of the anatomy of the palmar aponeurosis (Fig. 64–4) and the pathoanatomy of the abductor digiti minimi cord, the spiral cord, the lateral cord, the retrovascular cord, the natatory cord,

■ TECHNICAL ALTERNATIVES

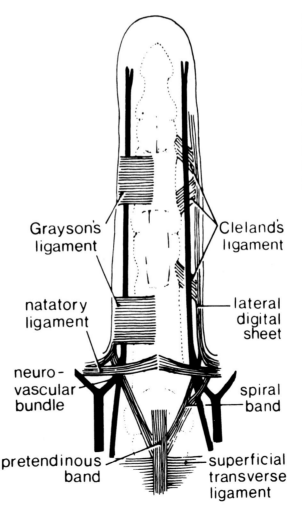

■ FIGURE 64–4
Normal fascial structures that can become involved in the various pathologic cords of Dupuytren's disease. (From McFarlane RM: Patterns of the diseased fascia in the fingers in Dupuytren's contracture. Plast Reconstr Surg, 1974; 54:31. Reprinted with permission.)

■ FIGURE 64–5
Five pathologic cords that
can develop in the digit
with Dupuytren's disease.
(From Chui HP, McFar-
lane RM: Pathogenesis of
Dupuytren's contracture:
A correlative clinical-path-
ological study. J Hand
Surg, 1978; 3:1–10. Re-
printed with permission.)

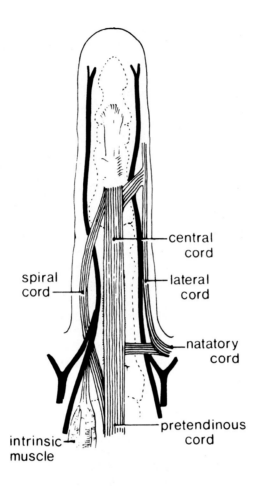

the isolated digital cord, or the first web's intercommisural cords (Figs. 64-5, 64-6).[1,10,12,13,16–19,21] The abductor digiti minimi cord will extend from the abductor digiti minimi's musculotendinous junction or tendon to the ulnar side of the base of the middle phalanx.[1,21] Adherence to the lateral skin is also common between the origin and insertion point. A spiral cord develops from the pretendinous aponeurosis, the spiral bands, the lateral digital sheaths, and Grayson's ligament, and usually connects to the middle phalanx (Fig. 64–5).[12] The only part of the web space fascial coalescence not involved in the spiral cord is the natatory ligament.[17] The spiral cord's presence is difficult to predict preoperatively, but this cord is common with significant PIP joint contractures. A spiral cord always puts the neurovascular bundle at risk because the bundle passes superficial to the cord and then immediately dives around and dorsal to the cord to reach its anatomic midlateral position at the PIP joint. Dissection of this cord actually reveals a spiraling neurovascular bundle and a straight "spiral" cord. As the PIP contracture increases, the spiral cord will push the bundle volarly toward the midline and proximally toward the first flexion crease. A lateral cord starts in the lateral digital sheath. It can involve the spiral band and natatory ligaments. Usually it does not trouble the bundle. It can go as far distal as the distal interphalangeal joint. A retrovascular cord involves longitudinal fibers dorsal to the bundle. This cord is commonly seen in combination with other cords. A natatory cord involves those aponeurotic bands that go from midvolar subcutaneous tissue through the web to the adjacent digit's midvolar subcutaneous tissue superficial to the A-2 and A-1 pulleys' junction. The intercommisural cords of the first web involve pathologic changes in the pretendinous band (radial longitudinal fiber), superficial transverse fibers of the palm (proximal transverse commissural ligament), and the first web natatory ligaments (Grapow's ligament).[13,19]

When dissecting the abductor digiti minimi cords, the ulnar neurovascular bundle must

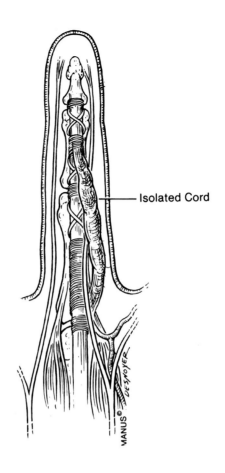

Isolated Cord

■ FIGURE 64–6

Strickland's isolated digital cord, which involves the lateral digital sheath and Grayson's ligaments. It starts on the periosteum of the proximal phalanx or intrinsic's musculotendinous junction and goes to the base of the middle phalanx. Like the spiral cord, it starts volar to the neurovascular bundle, twists around the bundle, and ends dorsal to it. (From Strickland JW, Basset RL: The isolated digital cord in Dupuytren's contractures: Anatomy and clinical significance. J Hand Surg, 1985; 10A:118–124. Reprinted with permission.)

be carefully protected because this cord can act like a spiral band. The nerve may spiral dorsal to the abductor digiti minimi cord or spiral through it. Also terminal portions of the dorsal ulnar sensory nerve may be closely applied to the dorsal lateral aspects of an abductor digiti quinti cord. When dissecting spiral cords, the preservation of the neurovascular bundle is challenging. Both the cord and the bundle may have to be dissected in a proximal to distal direction and from a distal to proximal direction. The cord may have to be divided at the point where the bundle twists around it and dissected in both directions. Alternatively the spiral cord may be dissected free from the neurovascular bundle and pulled from under these structures. This maneuver unwraps the cord from the neurovascular bundle. Gentle pulling on the neurovascular bundle with a delicate nerve hook can help locate the bundle distal to the point of the spiral. When dissecting natatory cords, which often go from one digit to another through the web, the bifurcation of the vessels and nerves will have to be completely localized while preserving the web fat. The natatory cord will frequently have to be dissected from two separate starting points in each digit. Eventually it can be pulled through the web into one digit and removed. When dissecting the commisural cords in the first web, special attention must be given to the index radial neurovascular bundle and the digital nerves of the thumb. A first web Z-plasty or skin graft is often needed. A more detailed discussion of the techniques for dissecting these cords and other combinations of cords is beyond the scope of this manuscript but more information can be found in the works of Barton, Hall-Finlay, Landsmeer, McFarlane, McGrouther, Stack, Tubiana, and White.[1,10,13,16–21]

As noted earlier, there are numerous alternative incisions for dissecting Dupuytren's disease. Currently, other common techniques are the open palm technique and the longitudinal incision with postfasciectomy Z-plasties. Hueston and others claim that the advantages of the longitudinal incision are preservation of the skin by incising the skin on the summit of the cord, good exposure of the neurovascular bundle, preservation of the flexor sheath, and volar digital skin lengthening because of the Z-plasty flaps.[8] One may argue that the zig-zag plasty technique provides simular advantages. Other useful techniques, especially in recurrent disease and in young patients with a severe diathesis, are limited fasciectomy with skin grafting and dermofasciectomy.[13]

A useful adjunct to fasciectomy is a soft tissue release of the severely contracted PIP joint. If a flexion contracture greater than 30° is left after complete regional fasciectomy, then releasing the PIP joint in a sequential manner as described by Curtis may improve the residual contracture.[3] Other adjunct procedures included PIP joint arthrodeses, PIP joint arthroplasties, and, in rare cases, amputations. In recurrent cases, particularly in young patients with recurrent disease, skin excision, and replacement with split-thickness skin graft is frequently needed. Although it is claimed that split-thickness skin graft will prevent recurrence, this is not always true.

In all surgery, even with meticulous care and excellent surgical technique, complications will occur. Potential complications seen after fasciectomies are flap necrosis, hematoma, infection, nerve injury, vascular injury, which sometimes results in loss of digits, loss of grip, recurrence, disease extension, or reflex sympathetic dystrophy. Plan ahead to avoid these complications, and warn your patients of these potential problems.

■ REHABILITATION

Postoperative hand therapy is a final important adjunct. Our center routinely uses the hand therapists to make a static night-time extension splinting and to teach the patient the postoperative exercises. Night splints are used for 4 months. Splints are modified as the finger straightens. Earlier gentle active and passive range of motion exercises with intrinsic and joint blocking exercises are encouraged. The therapist goal is to rapidly achieve full active flexion and to obtain, if possible, active extension equal to the surgical correction. Daily soaks or whirlpool, edema control, and vitamin E wound massage also are useful. As soon as the patient can do the therapy independently, the visits to the therapist are discontinued. Prolonged immobilization is not needed for healing after the zig-zag plasty fasciectomies. Continuous passive motion machines are not helpful.[14]

■ OUTCOMES

Early results of Dupuytren's surgery, regardless of the technique used, are generally good, and function is improved. Those patients with only MP joint contractures are often very happy. However, PIP joint contractures are rarely corrected to a truly normal range of motion, although significant improvement is initially achieved. The propensity for better results at the MP joint and poorer results at the PIP joint has been noted by McFarlane who reported only 75% improvement at the interphalangeal joint with only 20% perfect results and 25% of these contractures made worse. Those interphalangeal contractures that started at less than 30° did the worst in McFarlane's series.[13] Strickland's data further emphasize the difficulty of "curing" the PIP joint contracture. His long-term results (>5 years) showed an average PIP correction of only 15° (32% improvement).[18] If these same digits had been left untreated, their final deformity and loss of function would be severe and worse than the operative result. Ultimately, recurrence in the original operative area or the extension of the disease to previously "normal" parts of the hand are the rule not the exception. Fortunately, it is only a small group, the young patient with a strong diathesis, that will need multiple repeat operations. Long-term studies show recurrent rates ranging from 26 to 80%.[6,13] The surgeon must always remember and inform his patient before surgery that the surgery cannot cure Dupuytren's disease.

References

1. Barton N: Dupuytren's disease arising from the abductor digiti minimi. JHS, 1984; 9B:265.
2. Bruner J: Surgical exposure of flexor tendons in the hand. Ann R Coll Surg Engl, 1973; 53: 84–94.
3. Curtis R: Volar Capsulectomy of the Proximal Interphalangeal Joint. In: Hueston J, Tubiana R (eds): Dupuytren's Disease, New York: Grune and Stratton, 1974:135–137.
4. Elliot D: The early history of contracture of the palmar fascia. JHS, 1989; 14B:25–31.
5. Elliot D: The early history of contracture of the palmar fascia. Part 1. JHS, 1988; 13-B:246–253.
6. Hakstian R: Late Results of Extensive Fasciectomy. In: Hueston J, Tubiana R (eds): Dupuytren's Disease, New York: Grune and Stratton, 1974:79–83.
7. Hill N, Hurst L: Dupuytren's contracture. Hand Clinics, 1989; 5:349–357.
8. Hueston J: Dupuytren's Contracture. In: Converse J, McCarthy J, Littler J, (eds): Reconstructive Plastic Surgery, 2nd Ed, Philadelphia: W.B. Saunders Company, 1977: 3403–3427.
9. Hurst L, Badalamente M: Dupuytren's Contracture. In: Dee R, Hurst L, Mango E (eds): Principles of Orthopaedic Practice, New York: McGraw Hill, 1989:775–779.
10. Landsmeer J: Pathoanatomy of Dupuytren's Contracture. In: Atlas of Anatomy of the Hand, Edinburgh: Churchill Livingstone, 1976.
11. Littler J: Principles of reconstructive surgery of the hand. In: Converse J (ed): Reconstructive Plastic Surgery, Philadelphia: W.B. Saunders, 1977:3102–3153.
12. McFarlane R: Patterns of the diseased fascia in the fingers in Dupuytren's contracture. Plast Reconstr Surg, 1974; 54:31–44.
13. McFarlane R, McGrouther D, Flint M: Dupuytren's Disease Biology and Treatment, 1st Ed, Edinburgh: Churchill Livingstone, 1990:127–135, 155–167, 172–176, 205–210, 295–386.
14. Sampson S, Badalamente M, Hurst L, et al: The use of a passive motion machine in the postoperative rehabilitation of Dupuytren's disease. JHS, 1992; 17A:333–338.
15. Smith A: Diagnosis and indications for surgical treatment. Hand Clinics, 1991; 7:635–642.
16. Stack H: The Palmar Fascia. Edinburgh: Churchill Livingstone, 1973.
17. Strickland J, Leibovic S: Anatomy and pathogenesis of the digital cords and nodules. Hand Clinics, 1991; 7:645–657.
18. Strickland JW, Steichen JB: Difficult Problems in Hand Surgery. St. Louis: C.V. Mosby, 1982: 414–418.
19. Tubiana R, Simmons B, DeFrenne H. Location of Dupuytren's disease on the radial aspect of the hand. Clin Orthop Rel Res, 1982; 168:222–229.
20. Watson J. Fasciotomy and Z-plasty in the management of Dupuytren's contracture. Br J Plast Surg, 1984; 37:67.
21. White S. Anatomy of the palmar fascia on the ulnar border of the hand. J Hand Surg, 1984; 9B:50–56.

PART

II

Ligament Reconstruction

65

JOHN WIGHT
DURHAM

Thumb Metacarpophalangeal Ulnar Collateral Ligament Repair with Local Tissues

Chronic instability of the ligaments on the ulnar side of the thumb metacarpophalangeal (MP) joint was first described by Milch in 1926.[10] In 1955, Campbell noted the presence of chronic ulnar collateral ligament (UCL) instability in Scottish gamekeepers whose method of killing wounded rabbits placed stress on this ligamentous apparatus.[3] Since then, the term gamekeeper's thumb has been applied to chronic UCL instability of the thumb MP joint. Chronic UCL instability has been treated by casting,[4,7] tendon grafting,[2,13,17,18] tendon transfers,[6,9,12,13,15] and the use of local tissues.[4,5,11,14,17,18]

A technique using local tissues to reconstruct the UCL was first described by Milch, who performed a capsulorrhaphy in one patient.[10] Moberg and Stener described a similar procedure in which a proximally based flap of ulnar capsule was advanced with pullout wires into the base of the proximal phalanx.[11] Since then, several authors have recommended treating this lesion with primary repair and capsulorrhaphy.[4,18] The results following these procedures have not been critically reviewed, and the techniques are poorly described. We present a detailed and standardized technique of capsulorrhaphy for chronic ulnar collateral instability of the thumb MP joint.

■ HISTORY OF THE TECHNIQUE

The indications for reconstruction of chronic UCL instability in the thumb MP joint are pain or loss of function with UCL laxity. Laxity can be demonstrated by clinical stress testing or stress radiographs of the MP joint. Contraindications to reconstruction include the presence of arthritic changes in the MP joint or underlying inflammatory conditions such as rheumatoid arthritis.

■ INDICATIONS AND CONTRAINDICATIONS

The procedure can be performed under regional block or general anesthesia. A pneumatic tourniquet is placed on the upper arm over soft roll. The arm is exsanguinated and the tourniquet is inflated before making the incision. The skin incision is centered over the ulnar aspect of the thumb MP joint. It should begin distally in the midlateral position, curve gently over the MP joint, and then continue proximally just ulnar to the extensor pollicis longus (EPL) tendon (Fig. 65–1). The incision is carried down through skin and subcutaneous tissues, and care is taken to protect the branches of the superficial radial nerve. Skin flaps are elevated dorsally and volarly and held back with retraction sutures. This exposes the EPL, the extensor hood, and the adductor aponeurosis. At this point, a mass of scar tissue consisting of the proximally reflected UCL stump may be present at the proximal edge of the adductor aponeurosis. When present, this tissue consists of the retracted ulnar collateral ligament and represents a Stener's lesion (Fig. 65–2). The extensor hood is incised longitudinally just ulnar to the EPL tendon. The EPL tendon is reflected and retracted radially, preserving the underlying dorsal MP joint capsule. The adductor and its aponeurosis are reflected volarly exposing the ulnar aspect of the MP joint (Fig. 65–3). The dorsal capsule of the MP joint is incised transversely to the midline dorsally. This allows visualization of the interior of the MP joint. The joint is inspected, and any marginal osteophytes on the metacarpal or proximal phalanx are removed with a small rongeur. The specific reconstructive technique depends on the pathoanatomy observed

■ SURGICAL TECHNIQUES

■ **FIGURE 65–1**
The incision begins distally in the midlateral position of the ulnar aspect of the thumb. It curves gently over the joint and then runs proximally just ulnar to the EPL tendon.

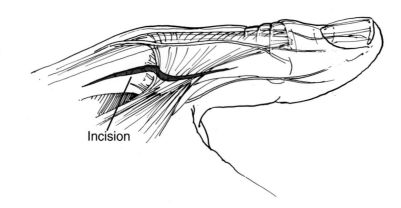

Incision

■ **FIGURE 65–2**
In a Stener's lesion, the distally ruptured UCL is folded under the adductor aponeurosis. The two ends of the ligament are thus held apart preventing primary healing.

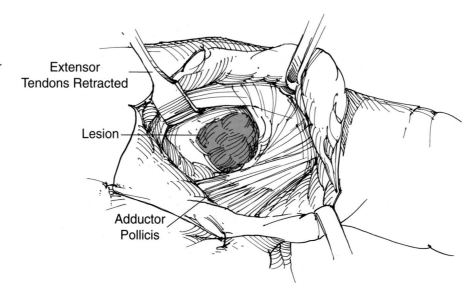

Extensor
Tendons Retracted

Lesion

Adductor
Pollicis

■ **FIGURE 65–3**
The adductor tendon is incised from its attachment to the extensor hood. Reflecting the tendon volarly exposes the ulnar aspect of the MP joint and the torn UCL.

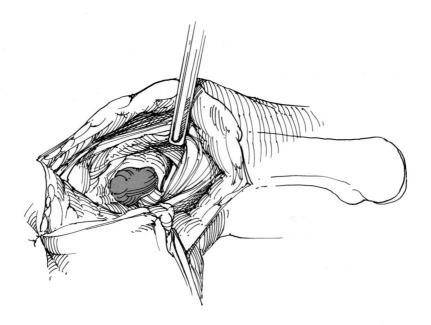

at time of surgery. In the case of an attenuated ligament or midsubstance tear, the ligament can be repaired in a pants over vest fashion using interrupted 4-0 Prolene sutures. More commonly, the ligament is avulsed distally and in this case is repaired with a pullout suture. In this technique, a proximally based flap of tissue is sharply fashioned from the scarred ligament and capsule. The flap is elevated from the ulnar aspect of the metacarpal head enough to allow advancement to the volar ulnar corner of the proximal phalanx. Care must be taken to avoid detachment of the ligament's proximal origin. A 3-0 Prolene suture is woven through the flap for future placement into drill holes in the proximal phalanx. The volar ulnar corner of the proximal phalanx is cleaned of soft tissue and scarified with a curette. A 0.045 K-wire is then used to drill two parallel holes, which are directed distally and obliquely from the prepared corner of the phalanx out the radial aspect of the phalanx. Each suture end in the fashioned ligament is threaded onto a Keith needle. The two Keith needles are then placed into the drill holes at the proximal volar-ulnar corner of the proximal phalanx. The Keith needles are pulled through the drill holes bringing the suture out through the skin on the radial side of the proximal phalanx. The suture ends are temporarily held in clamps. The thumb MP joint is then held in neutral flexion and slight ulnar deviation as a 0.045 K-wire is driven across the MP joint, transfixing it in the reduced position. The suture ends are passed through a small piece of foam and then through the holes of a button. This provides some protective padding for the skin beneath the button. The pull-through suture is then tied down over the button (Fig. 65–4). The distal-volar aspect of the reconstructed ligament is then sutured with 4-0 Prolene to the ulnar aspect of the volar plate. Finally the dorsal capsule is imbricated with 4-0 Dexon to prevent volar subluxation of the joint. In the unusual circumstance in which the collateral ligament is avulsed from the metacarpal, a distally based flap can be fashioned from the scarred ligament and capsule. Sutures placed in this flap are passed through drill holes

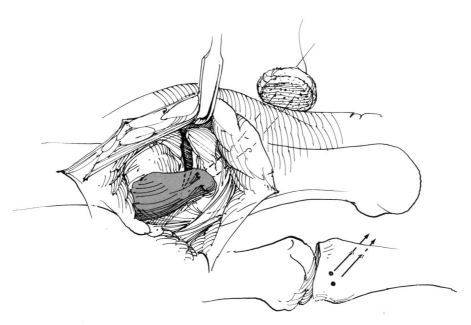

■ FIGURE 65–4
The sutures in the fashioned ligament are passed through the drill holes in the proximal phalanx to exit the radial aspect of the thumb and are tied over a padded button.

beginning at the site of origin of the ligament on the metacarpal head and exit the radial aspect of the metacarpal. They are tied over a button as described above.

Closure is performed by reapproximating the adductor aponeurosis to the extensor hood using 4-0 Prolene. Knots should be inverted to avoid subdermal prominence. The skin is closed with interrupted simple and horizontal mattress sutures using 5-0 nylon. The transarticular wire is bent, cut, and left outside the skin for simple removal in the clinic. After application of a dressing, the hand is immobilized in a radial gutter thumb spica splint. After 7 to 10 days, the sutures are removed, and the hand is placed in a short arm thumb spica cast.

■ TECHNICAL ALTERNATIVES

There are a variety of technical alternatives to the described technique. They can be classified as either static or dynamic ligament reconstructions. Static reconstructions include free tendon grafts and tendon transpositions. Strandell used a palmaris longus tendon graft. He passed this through dorsovolar drill holes on the ulnar aspects of the metacarpal head and proximal phalanx and crossed the ends in a figure-of-eight over the ulnar side of the MP joint.[18] Osterman used a similar technique in 11 of his 16 patients with chronic instability.[13] Smith also recommended use of a palmaris longus tendon graft for chronic reconstructions. In his procedure, the graft is passed through a hole beginning at the normal insertion of the UCL on the proximal phalanx and exits the radial aspect of the phalanx. It is held there with a pullout suture. The proximal stump of the graft is woven into the UCL remnant, which remains attached to the metacarpal.[17] A more complex reconstruction using a PL tendon graft has been described by Breek.[2]

Other authors have described tendon transpositions using the extensor pollicis brevis (EPB),[18] the abductor pollicis longus,[5] and the palmaris longus.[8] In these techniques, the distal insertion of the tendon is left undisturbed. The tendon is mobilized and transected proximally. The free end is passed distally to the level of the MP joint, passed through a drill hole in the metacarpal neck, and then used to reconstruct the UCL.

Kaplan was the first to use a dynamic transfer in two patients with long-term UCL instability. His patients had recurrent instability after primary repair of the ligaments. In his procedure, after reefing the adductor aponeurosis, the extensor indicis proprius is released from its distal insertion, passed subcutaneously to the level of the thumb MP joint, and sutured to the adductor aponeurosis.[6] Neviaser described a procedure that included repair of the UCL and advancement of the adductor aponeurosis distally into a drill hole in the proximal-volar aspect of the proximal phalanx.[12] McCue and Osterman have reported good results using this technique.[9,13] Sakellerides treated 100 patients with dynamic transfer of the EPB. In this technique, an extension of the EPB tendon is passed through a drill hole in the base of the proximal phalanx that begins dorsally and exits at the site of the normal insertion of the UCL. It is then pulled proximally and sutured to the proximal stump of the torn UCL.[15]

Most authors agree that MP joint fusion should be reserved for joints that have failed reconstruction or for joints that are arthritic at presentation. Reikeras however found the incidence of recurrent instability to be 50% in his patients following UCL reconstruction and suggested that chronic UCL laxity is best treated with an arthrodesis.[14]

The potential pitfalls in the described technique are common to all soft tissue reconstructions of the UCL. Possible complications of the procedure include damage to the superficial sensory branches of the radial nerve during the approach or during pin placement, pin tract infections, and failure to achieve an accurate reduction of the MP joint. Damage to the sensory nerves is avoided by meticulous dissection during exposure and careful retraction of the skin flaps during the procedure. Suturing the skin flaps back with 4-0 nylon sutures can minimize repetitive handling of the nerve and other soft tissues. Pin tract infections have been described but are often easily treated with a short course of oral antibiotics.[1] Pins left out through the skin should be well padded before placement of the splint or cast. The skin around the pins should be released with small incisions to prevent pressure necrosis of the surrounding skin. The MP joint must be accurately reduced when placing the transarticular K-wire. It is recommended that the MP joint be placed in slight ulnar deviation at this time. It also must be remembered that ulnar instability is often associated with a palmar subluxation, producing a supination deformity of the joint. This palmar and supination subluxation, if present, must be reduced before transfixing the joint. This can usually be done visually but if any doubt remains, intraoperative films can be helpful. Failure to imbricate the dorsal MP joint capsule or to suture the volar plate to the reconstructed ligament can predispose the joint to recurrent palmar subluxation.

Rehabilitation begins 4 weeks after surgery, when the short-arm thumb spica cast is removed. At this time, the transarticular K-wire and pull-through suture are removed. The patient is given a hand-based thumb spica splint, which is removed three times daily for thumb active range of motion exercises. Two months after surgery, the splint is used for protective purposes only and, at 3 months, the patient is released to normal activities.

■ REHABILITATION

Excellent results have been described in most patients with acute UCL tears treated with direct suture repair or with the pullout suture technique.[7,9,13] The results after similar repair of chronic UCL instability are less well defined. Moberg and Stener reported excellent stability in 13 of 14 patients using a pullout wire technique, but their group included patients with both acute injuries and chronic instabilities.[11] Other authors have reported poor success after primary ligament repair for chronic UCL instability. The number of patients in these studies, however, is small, and the techniques used are not clearly described.[5,14,17]

■ OUTCOMES

Good to excellent results have been reported in the majority of patients treated for chronic laxity with free tendon grafts,[2,13,17,18] tendon transpositions,[5,8,18] and tendon transfers.[6,9,12,13,15] These results are often reported only in terms of stability and subjective improvement. Osterman has performed the most critical analysis to date of patients treated for UCL instability. Sixteen patients with acute tears (group I) were treated by primary repair of the torn ligament or bony avulsion using a pullout wire technique. At a mean of 21 months follow-up, these patients had stable repairs with nearly normal grip and pinch strengths and a mean range of motion in the operated thumb that was equal to 84% of their normal thumbs. Sixteen other patients with chronic instability were divided into three subgroups. Group II patients were treated with adductor advancement, group III with tendon graft reconstruction, and group IV with a combination of the two. Excellent stability was obtained in most patients regardless of the technique. Grip strengths were nearly normal in all three groups. Thumb range of motion was better in group II patients (74% of normal) compared with group III and IV patients (64% and 66%, respectively). Pinch strengths were better in group IV patients (90% of normal) compared with patients in groups II and III (81% and 84%, respectively). These reconstructive procedures gave equally functional results with small clinical differences.[13] The procedure described in this chapter appears to provide results that are comparable to those in Osterman's groups II, III, and IV. Although this technique uses only local tissues, its successful application requires careful attention to technical details.

References

1. Arnold DM, Cooney WP, Wood MB: Surgical management of chronic ulnar collateral ligament insufficiency of the thumb metacarpophalangeal joint. Orth Rev, 1992; 21:583–588.
2. Breek JC, Tan AM, VanThiel TH.PH, Daantje CRE: Free tendon grafting to repair the metacarpophalangeal joint of the thumb. Surgical techniques and a review of 70 patients. J Bone Joint Surg, 1989; 71B:383–387.
3. Campbell CS: Gamekeeper's Thumb. J Bone Joint Surg, 1955; 37B:148–149.
4. Coonrad RN, Goldner JL: A study of the pathological findings and treatment in soft-tissue injury of the thumb metacarpophalangeal joint. J. Bone Joint Surg, 1968; 50A:439–451.
5. Frykman G, Johansson O: Surgical repair of rupture of the ulnar collateral ligament of the meracarpophalangeal joint of the thumb. Acta Chir Scand, 1956; 112:58–64.
6. Kaplan EB: The pathology and treatment of radial subluxation of the thumb with ulnar displacement of the head of the first metacarpal. J Bone Joint Surg, 1961; 43A:541–546.

7. Kessler I: Complete avulsion of the ulnar collateral ligament of the metacarpophalangeal joint of the thumb. Clin Orthop, 1961; 29:196–200.
8. Lamb DW, Angarita G: Ulnar instability of the metacarpophalangeal joint of the thumb. J Hand Surg, 1985; 10B:113–114.
9. McCue FC, Hakala MW, Andrews JR, Gieck JH: Ulnar collateral ligament injuries of the thumb in athletes. J Sports Med, 1974; 2:70–80.
10. Milch H: Recurrent dislocation of the thumb. Capsulorrhaphy. Am J Surg, 1929; 6:237–239.
11. Moberg E, Stener B: Injuries to the ligaments of the thumb and fingers. Diagnosis, treatment, and prognosis. Acta Chir Scand, 1953; 106:166–186.
12. Neviaser RJ, Wilson JN, Lievano A: Rupture of the ulnar collateral ligament of the thumb (gamekeeper's thumb). Correction by dynamic repair. J Bone Joint Surg, 1971; 53A:1357–1364.
13. Osterman AL, Hayken GD, Bora FWM: A quantitative evaluation of thumb function after ulnar collateral repair and reconstruction. J Trauma, 1981; 21:854–861.
14. Reikeras O, Kvarnes L: Rupture of the ulnar ligament of the metacarpophalangeal joint of the thumb. Arch Orthop Trauma Surg, 1982; 100:175–177.
15. Sakellarides HT: The surgical treatment of old injuries of the collateral ligaments of the MP joint of the thumb using the extensor pollicis brevis tendon (a long-term follow-up of 100 cases). Bull Hosp Joint Dis Orthop Inst, 1984; 44:449–458.
16. Stener B: Displacement of the ruptured ulnar collateral ligament of the metacarpophalangeal joint of the thumb. A clinical and anatomical study. J Bone Joint Surg, 1962; 44B:869–879.
17. Smith RJ: Post-traumatic instability of the metacarpophalangeal joint of the thumb. J Bone Joint Surg, 1977; 59A:14–21.
18. Strandell G: Total rupture of the ulnar collateral ligament of the metacarpophalangeal joint of the thumb. Results in 35 cases. Acta Chir Scand, 1959; 118:72–80.

OWEN J. MOY

66

Thumb Metacarpophalangeal Ulnar Collateral Ligament Repair with Tendon Graft

The term gamekeeper's thumb originally described a chronic laxity secondary to repetitive stress sustained by Scottish gamekeepers when breaking the necks of wounded hares. It has since become synonymous with both acute and chronic ulnar collateral ligament injuries of the metacarpophalangeal (MP) joint of the thumb.[2] Although the literature clearly supports the utility of direct repair of acute injuries, the treatment of chronic ulnar collateral ligament incompetence remains unsettled. Many techniques have been described, all of which, reportedly, provide satisfactory results.

■ HISTORY OF THE TECHNIQUE

Anatomically, the thumb MP joint is a multiaxial diarthrodial joint capable not only of flexion and extension, but also of adduction, abduction, and circumduction. Its stability is dependent on both static and dynamic structures, the origins and insertions of which are in the area immediately surrounding the joint. The joint is supported by the palmar plate, which originates from the metacarpal recess and extends to the volar proximal portion of the proximal phalanx. Although the proximal third of the plate is thin, the distal portion becomes progressively thicker. The collateral ligament system (both radial and ulnar) is composed of two intimately associated, although anatomically distinct, ligaments. The origin of the collateral ligament proper is at the level of the metacarpal head. The ligament moves in a distal palmar direction to insert at the lateral tubercle of the proximal phalanx. The accessory collateral ligament is superficial and palmar to the collateral ligament proper. Although sharing a common origin, the accessory collateral ligament inserts into the volar plate. Biomechanically, these ligaments provide complementary support to the MP joint. If the joint is extended, the collateral ligament proper is relaxed and the accessory collateral ligament is taut. With joint flexion, the collateral ligament is taut, and the accessory collateral ligament is relaxed. These structures and their inter-relationship are the basis for the static stability of the MP joint.

On the ulnar side, the adductor pollicis functions as the primary dynamic stabilizer of the MP joint. Its tendon inserts into the ulnar sesamoid, the lateral tubercle of the proximal phalanx, and, to a lesser degree, the dorsal expansion. The approximate contribution of each of the stabilizing structures has been delineated, in part, by Coonrad and Boldner.[4] They have found from their examination of fresh cadaveric specimens that partial instability of the MP joint occurs with disruption of the ulnar collateral ligament and adductor aponeurosis. Total instability results from disruption of the ulnar collateral ligament, a portion of the volar capsule, and the adductor pollicis aponeurosis.

The incidence of ruptures to the ulnar collateral ligament is 10 times that of ruptures to the radial collateral ligament.[9,10] This variation can be attributed to the critical role of the ulnar collateral ligament in providing stability during pinch and gripping types of functions. Cooney and Chao have shown that the actual forces impacting upon the metacarpophalangeal joint are three to four times the actual applied force.[3] Therefore, with a key pinch of 10 kg, the amount of force that dynamic and static stabilizers must resist can be as great as 40 kg.

Although the treatment of chronic ulnar collateral ligament injuries is controversial, the mechanism of injury is not. The ulnar collateral ligament and various combinations of the accessory collateral ligament, volar plate, and, at times, the dorsal expansion tear secondary to a hyperabduction force. As the MP joint flexes, the dorsal expansion is translated in a distal direction, allowing exposure of a distally detached ulnar collateral ligament from beneath the extensor expansion. As the MP joint extends, the collateral ligament may lie superficial to the interposed dorsal expansion, thus creating the Stenner lesion.[16] Other mechanisms of injury, which are more the exception than the rule, involve disruption of the extensor mechanism with subluxation of the extensor pollicis longus in a radial direction.[7]

If examined initially by a physician for whom this is not an area of expertise, an acute ulnar collateral ligament injury can be undiagnosed and untreated. Patients with such untreated injuries present later with a history of chronic pain and instability. It is generally accepted that ruptures occurring more than 3 weeks previously are not amenable to direct repair. The evaluation of a patient who presents with a chronic injury is not dissimilar to that of an acutely injured patient. The physician must ascertain the degree of discomfort, loss of strength, and instability. Unfortunately, there is no consensus on the optimum method for determining the degree of instability.

Some authors[5,15] have advocated applying radial stress to the MP joint while it is in extension. Smith[15] has recommended that in the extended position, radial deviation in excess of 45° is an indication of disruption of the ulnar collateral ligament. Other authors[13] have advocated that the MP joint be stressed in a flexed position so that the ulnar collateral ligament is stretched to maximum tension. This helps to relax the volar plate and affords an isolated examination of the ligament. In an effort to reconcile this discrepancy, Osterman, Dray and Eaton have recommended evaluation in extension as well as in flexion.[5,12] Instability is defined as radial deviation greater than 40° in extension or 20° in flexion.[12] Other useful criteria and methods of evaluation of suspected ligament incompetence include radiographic findings of a displaced rotated fracture, volar subluxation of the proximal phalanx greater than 3 mm in relation to the metacarpal head, and arthrographic evaluation of the MP joint and concomitant leak of dye from the capsule.

Various methods of ulnar collateral ligament reconstruction using tendon grafts have been described as early as 1955.[1,2,5,6,8,14,17] The sources of donor graft include, but are not limited to, palmaris longus, extensor tendons to the toe, fascia-lata, and abductor pollicis longus. The technique described by Smith,[15] using a palmaris longus tendon graft with some modification, is my preferred method.

In his review of 86 patients with collateral ligament instability of the thumb MP joint, Smith identified 66 patients with ulnar instability. Of those, 52 underwent surgical repair. Those patients with injuries of 3 weeks' duration or longer required ligamentous reconstruction. Using his technique, all but two patients returned to full activity. On average, patients experienced a 20 to 30° loss of motion at the MP and interphalangeal (IP) joints of the thumb.[15]

This technique has provided excellent results, and I have adopted only two modifications. These modifications pertain to the drill hole in the proximal phalanx and the point of terminal attachment of the tendon graft. The modifications are discussed further in the surgical techniques section.

■ INDICATIONS AND
CONTRAINDICATIONS

The indications for this operation are persistent pain, instability as defined by Osterman,[12] decreased strength, and local tenderness following an abduction injury to the thumb of more than 3 weeks' duration. Injuries that are diagnosed before 3 weeks can be treated with exploration and direct repair. With rare exception, maintenance of mobility at the MP joint is preferred. Therefore, soft tissue reconstruction would be my first choice in treating the chronic injury, although the surgeon's preference is most often based on previous training or personal bias.

Specific contraindications to soft tissue reconstruction would be the presence of degenerative arthritis on the preoperative radiographs. In such cases, arthrodesis of the MP joint should be considered. In the rare case where early arthritic changes are noted intraoperatively, one will need to decide on whether to proceed with soft tissue reconstruction or an arthrodesis. In this case, the specific occupation and needs of the patient must be taken into consideration. In those patients involved in heavy labor, arthrodesis would be favored. In all other circumstances, I would continue to favor a soft tissue reconstruction. A careful preoperative conference is recommended so that the possible change in treatment plan has been fully discussed with the patient. An additional contraindication to a soft tissue reconstruction would be an irreducible MP joint subluxation. In such cases, arthrodesis is preferred.

Using regional anesthesia, such as an axillary block, a lazy-S type incision approximately 3.5 cm in length is made centered at the ulnar aspect of the MP joint. While developing dorsal and volar flaps, it is essential that the sensory branches of the radial nerve be identified, mobilized, and gently retracted from the line of the incision. Injury to these small branches either by a sharp transection or contusion secondary to excessive retraction can result in problematic hyperpathia in the postoperative period. Following development of the flaps, the ulnar aspect of the dorsal expansion can be visualized. Careful inspection of the region may reveal a Stenner lesion, where the proximal aspect of the dorsal expansion is interposed between the avulsed collateral ligament and the underlying joint.

A midaxial incision is then made through the dorsal expansion, and dorsal and volar flaps are developed. These flaps are gently retracted in their respective directions, allowing exposure of the underlying metacarpophalangeal joint. The ulnar collateral ligament is typically found at its metacarpal head origin and noted to be retracted sufficiently to prevent direct repair. In the case of a small bony avulsion fracture, which does not involve a significant portion of the articular surface, the bony fragment should be excised. The ulnar base of the proximal phalanx is then exposed and, using a 2.7-mm drill, a drill hole is made in an ulnar to radial direction volar to the midaxial plane of the proximal phalanx (Fig. 66–1). The drill hole originally described by Smith involves penetration of both ulnar and radial cortices. A suggested modification would be to preserve the radial cortex, leaving it intact to provide a bony buttress and surface area to which the tendon graft can be secured.

A palmaris longus tendon graft is then obtained through two or more 1-cm transverse skin incisions commencing at the distal wrist crease and moving in a proximal direction over the course of the tendon. If palmaris longus is not present, additional sources include

■ SURGICAL TECHNIQUES

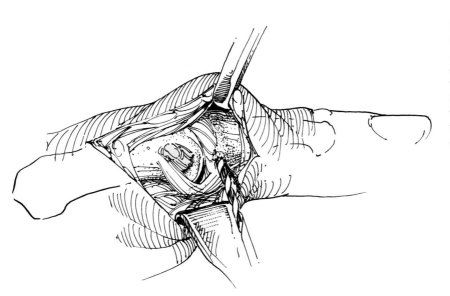

■ FIGURE 66–1
Lateral view of MP joint. Notice the residual ulnar collateral ligament attached at the metacarpal head. The drill hole in the proximal phalanx is volar to the midaxial line of the phalanx.

one of the toe extensors or a longitudinal portion of the flexor carpi radialis tendon. Once fully harvested, a pull-out stitch of 2-0 Prolene is placed at one end of the tendon graft. Using two Keith needles, the suture is fed through the drill hole exiting through the radial cortex and soft tissue of the proximal phalanx. This suture is then secured over a button (Fig. 66–2). The remaining free portion of the graft is brought proximal to the level of the residual ligamentous stump.

The method selected to secure the tendon graft to this area depends on the amount of residual collateral ligament. Ideally, there is sufficient residual ligament to make two small parallel longitudinal incisions in the remnant collateral ligament through which the graft can be passed. An alternate approach is to make a transverse incision at the base of the ligament and, again, weave the tendon graft through this incision site back onto itself. If the ligamentous tissue is inadequate, two small drill holes can be made in the 2- and 5-o'clock positions. The two holes are connected within the medullary canal and the tendon graft is threaded through them. Extreme care must be exercised to avoid fracture through the section of cortical bone that lies between the drill holes. The MP joint is reduced and the tendon graft is secured to the remnant collateral ligament (Fig. 66–3). The remaining distal portion of the graft is brought back to the level of the proximal phalangeal drill hole. Smith emphasized that the end of the tendon graft should lie parallel, volar and adjacent to the portion of the graft coming from the phalangeal drill hole. I attempt to secure the free end of the graft into the volar plate using a 4-0 braded nonabsorbable suture. If this is not feasible, then the technique described by Smith is used (Fig 66-4). Securing the graft to the volar plate provides additional support to the proximal phalanx and minimizes any tendency toward volar subluxation. The dorsal expansion is repaired in a side-to-side fashion once again using a 4-0 braided nonabsorbable suture. If the expansion was noted to be lax during the initial approach, a vest-over-pants repair can be performed in order to increase stability. Skin closure is attained with a 4-0 monofilament nonabsorbable suture (nylon).

■ TECHNICAL ALTERNATIVES AND PITFALLS

The surgical technique as described above is demanding, and attention to detail is critical. Special attention should be given to the placement of the phalangeal drill hole. It is critical for the drill hole to be located volar to the midaxial line of the phalanx. Placement of this hole ultimately assists in preventing volar subluxation of the joint. Attachment of the terminal end of the tendon graft to the volar plate is also important in providing support to prevent volar subluxation of the joint. It also should be reiterated that when drill holes in the metacarpal are necessary, extreme care must be exercised to prevent disruption of the cortical bone between the drill holes in order to prevent pullout of the tendon graft.

Other techniques also use tendon graft. Although the basic premise of each of these procedures is similar, the major difference is in the manner in which the tendon graft is secured to the bony and residual ligamentous structures. Authors such as Eaton have recommended small drill holes in both the base of the proximal phalanx and metacarpal

■ FIGURE 66–2
PA view of the MP joint. The drill hole does not penetrate the radial cortex of the proximal phalanx providing additional bony buttress for the tendon graft. The graft has been passed into the drill hole and a pullout suture is tied over a button on the radial aspect of the thumb.

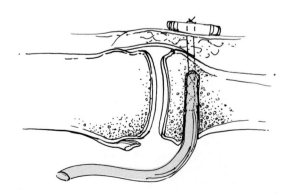

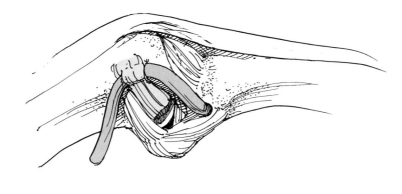

■ FIGURE 66-3
Lateral view of the MP joint. The tendon graft has been directed proximally and passed through the ulnar collateral stump.

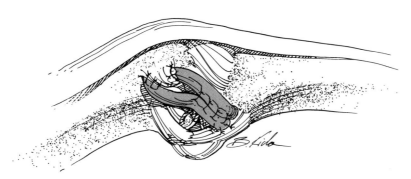

■ FIGURE 66-4
Lateral view of the MP joint. Distally, the free end of the tendon graft has been sutured to the volar plate. Additional sutures secure the tendon graft in a side-to-side fashion as well as to the ulnar collateral ligament.

head located at the 2- and 5-o'clock positions. A tunnel is then developed between the drill holes through which the tendon graft can be passed. Other techniques have been described, although with little attention to the orientation of tendon graft in relation to the original collateral ligament. There are no data collectively comparing these techniques, although various authors all report satisfactory results. Other soft tissue options for reconstructing the unstable MP joint include adductor pollicis brevis advancement and the use of local tissue.

Arthrodesis also can be used to reconstruct the chronically unstable MP joint. The normal range of motion of the MP joint has been defined as flexion of 10 to 100° with an average of 75°, extension ranging from 0 to 90° with an average of 20°, and abduction and adduction with a range of 0 to 20° with an average of 10°.[4] Arthrodesis of the MP joint results in loss of such mobility. Nevertheless, an arthrodesed MP joint provides reliable pain relief and stability.

■ REHABILITATION

Postoperatively, the patient is placed in a plaster radial thumb splint. Care should be taken to avoid placing the thumb in full opposition, which will stress the repair. After 2 weeks, the patient returns for suture removal and reapplication of a similar forearm based radial thumb splint, which includes the IP joint. This splint is maintained until the fourth postoperative week at which time the patient is seen by a hand therapist who fabricates a hand-based radial thumb splint with the IP joint free. The patient then begins isolated active and active-assisted MP and IP flexion and extension. Opposition of the fifth metacarpal head as well as circumduction exercises at the carpometacarpal joint also are performed. During this time, passive stretching is avoided as is resistive pinching and lateral stress to the MP joint. At 6 weeks after surgery, the splint is worn only when outdoors and in crowds. Therapy at this time consists of gentle passive thumb flexion. A flexion cuff may be added to assist in regaining MP flexion if necessary. The patient also is allowed to start light pinch strengthening. Once again, no lateral stress to the MP joint is allowed nor is heavy pinching activity. At weeks 8 through 12, the splint is discontinued, and the patient is allowed to increase resistive pinch strengthening. The patient also is allowed to return to sporting and work activities. Throughout the rehabilitation period, the patient is seen by a hand therapist on a regular schedule.

■ OUTCOMES

Osterman and associates[12] attempted to compare collateral ligament reconstruction using tendon graft to adductor advancement as described by Neviaser.[11] Both techniques provide adequate pinch strength; adductor advancement achieved 85% of the contralateral side whereas the free tendon graft method achieved 81%. Range of motion was 65% of the contralateral side for the adductor advancement group and 78% of the contralateral side for the free graft group. These authors suggest that a combination of tendon graft and adductor advancement should be considered for patients involved in physically demanding vocations.

The surgical options available for the treatment of chronic ulnar collateral instability of the thumb MP joint are numerous. Despite this, there are no objective data strongly favoring any one given technique. Free tendon grafts as described by Smith have proven to be a viable alternative. I have found this technique useful in the patient who does not exhibit overt arthritis or irreducible joint subluxation. The minor modifications to this technique described in this chapter are used to provide additional support for the tendon graft as well as the MP joint. This technique can result in an average loss of 20 to 30° of motion of the MP joint of the thumb.[15] Despite this loss of motion, all patients have been able to return to their normal occupational and recreational activities with little if any impediment. If it is believed that additional support and strength are required but arthrodesis is not desired, one can then consider the recommendation of Osterman and co-authors, who suggest that the free tendon graft be combined with an adductor advancement.

■ ACKNOWLEDGMENTS

The author would like to thank Frances S. Sherwin, Assistant Dean, School of Health Related Professions, University at Buffalo, for editorial assistance.

References
1. Alldred AJ: Rupture of the collateral ligament of the metacarpophalangeal joint of the thumb. J Bone Joint Surg, 1955; 37B:443–445.
2. Campbell CS: Gamekeeper's thumb. J Bone Joint Surg, 1955; 37B:148–149.
3. Cooney WP, Chow EYS: Biomechanical analysis of static forces in the thumb during hand function. J Bone Surg, 1977; 59A:27–36.
4. Coonrad RW, Coldner JL: A study of the pathological findings and treatment in soft tissue injury of the thumb metacarpophalangeal. J Bone Joint Surg, 1968; 50A:439–451.
5. Dray GJ, Eaton RG: Dislocations and Ligament Injuries in the Digits. In: Green's Operative Hand Surgery 3rd ed., New York, Churchill Livingstone, 1993, pp. 782–783.
6. Frykman G, Johansson O: Surgical repair of rupture of the ulnar collateral ligament of the metacarpophalangeal joint of the thumb. Acta Chir Scand, 1956; 112:58–64.
7. Kaplan EB: The pathology and treatment of radial subluxation of the thumb and ulnar displacement of the head of the first metacarpal. J Bone Joint Surg, 1961; 53A:541–546.
8. Lamb DW, Angarita G: Ulnar instability of the metacarpophalangeal joint of thumb. H Hand Surg, 1985; 10B:113.
9. Moberg E, Stenner B: Injuries to the ligaments of the thumb and fingers: Diagnosis, treatment and prognosis. Acta Chir Scand, 1953; 106:166–186.
10. Moberg E: Fracture and ligamentous injuries of the thumb and fingers. Surg Clin North Am, 1960; 40:297–309.
11. Neviaser RJ, Wilson JN, Lievano A: Rupture of the ulnar collateral ligament of the thumb (gamekeeper's thumb). J Bone Joint Surg, 1971; 53A:1357–1364.
12. Osterman AL, Hayken GD, Bora Jr FW: A quantitative evaluation of thumb function after ulnar collateral repair and reconstruction. J Trauma, 1981; 21:854–861.
13. Palmer AK, Louis DS: Assessing ulnar instability of the metacarpophalangeal joint of the thumb. J Hand Surg, 1978; 3A:542–546.
14. Sakellarides HT, DeWeese JW: Instability of the metacarpophalangeal joint of the thumb. Reconstruction of the collateral ligament using extensor pollicis brevis tendon. J Bone Joint Surg, 1976; 58A:106–112.

15. Smith RJ: Post-traumatic instability of the metacarpophalangeal joint of the thumb. J Bone Joint Surg, 1977; 59A:14–21.
16. Stenner B: Displacement of the ruptured ulnar collateral ligament of the metacarpophalangeal joint of the thumb. A clinical and anatomic study. J Bone Joint Surg, 1962; 44B:869–879.
17. Strandell G: Total rupture of the ulnar collateral ligament of the metacarpophalangeal joint of the thumb. Results of surgery in 35 cases. Acta Chir Scand, 1959; 118:72–80.

67

Rotary Subluxation of the Scaphoid

The scaphoid, as an intercalated segment in a three-link system composed of the radius, the scaphoid, and the two radialmost distal carpal row bones (trapezium and trapezoid), is inherently unstable.[2,8,14] Devoid of tendinous attachments, the scaphoid is stabilized only by the ligaments from the contiguous bones.[2,3] Due to its obliqueness with respect to the long axis of the forearm, the scaphoid has a natural tendency to collapse into flexion and pronation under compressive force.[8] The lunate, by contrast, has a tendency to extend and supinate by virtue of its volar wedge-shaped configuration.[8] The pronation-flexion tendency of the scaphoid is resisted by the supination-extension moment transmitted by the lunate via the scapholunate membrane and ligaments (palmar and dorsal).[14] According to this concept, the integrity of the scapholunate membrane and ligaments appears crucial in maintaining a normal intrinsic balance of the proximal row.[2,3,10,14]

A complete disruption of the scapholunate ligament usually occurs as a consequence of a hyperextension or torsional injury to the wrist.[3,14] When these ligaments are torn, the compressive forces across the wrist induce a structural alteration of the mechanical arrangement of the bones of the carpus, especially those of the proximal row.[8,10] The scaphoid rotates into flexion and pronation around the obliquely oriented radioscaphocapitate ligament, while the lunate follows its natural tendency toward extension and supination. As a consequence, a gap between the two bones is created resulting in an obvious articular incongruency.

The symptoms of a scapholunate dissociation vary markedly, depending on the magnitude and extent of the associated injuries, as well as on the time since the accident.[3,14] Weakness of grasp, limited motion, and swelling and point tenderness over the dorsal aspect of the scapholunate interval are frequent findings. Pain is common and may be aggravated by heavy use, sometimes coinciding with a snapping or clicking sensation with movement.

Radiographic findings indicating the presence of a rotary subluxation of the scaphoid include: on the anteroposterior view, a diastasis between the proximal pole of the scaphoid and the lunate, further accentuated by fist compression, and a foreshortened scaphoid with the typical "ring" sign (Fig. 67–1A); on the lateral view, a horizontal scaphoid relative to the radius, a scapholunate angle greater than 80°, and a dorsally subluxed capitate relative to an abnormally extended lunate.[10,14] (Fig. 67–1B). Comparative views of the contralateral normal wrist may help to confirm the diagnosis, allowing a better assessment of the amount of carpal malalignment.

Partial scapholunate ligament tears may cause substantial discomfort but plain radiographs appear completely normal. In these "dynamic instability"[15] cases, cineradiography may be helpful by showing abnormal motion between the scaphoid and lunate. Arthrograms also may be useful. Detection of dye leaking from the radiocarpal into the midcarpal joint (or vice versa) is an indirect sign of this pathology.[3,10,14]

Although in acute cases of a scapholunate dissociation a closed reduction and percutaneous pinning of the joint may produce acceptable results,[3,11] the overall experience tends to indicate that an early surgical repair of the disrupted ligaments is a more reliable procedure.[5,9,10,14] Experimental studies have shown that the key structures ensuring stability of the joint are the dorsal and proximal portions of the scapholunate membrane, includ-

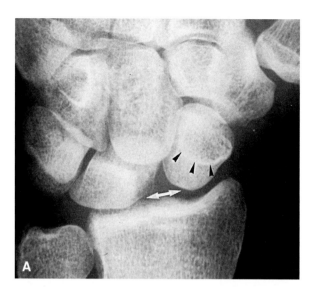

■ FIGURE 67–1
A, PA radiograph of a
wrist showing rotary
scaphoid subluxation. Key
features are: (1) widening
of the scapholunate
space (white arrows); (2)
foreshortening of the
scaphoid; and (3) the cortical "ring" sign (black arrows) representing the axially projected scaphoid
tuberosity. **B,** Lateral radiograph shows the verti-
calized orientation of the
scaphoid and an in-
creased scapholunate
angle.

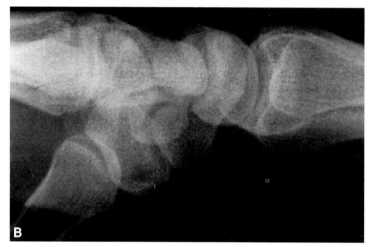

ing the dorsal scapholunate ligament.[3,8] Secondary constraints are the palmar scaphotrapezial-trapezoidal ligamentous complex and the controversial radioscapholunate
ligament.[4,14] Different ligamentoplasties using strips of adjacent tendons threaded through
drill holes in the involved carpal bones have been tried.[3,11] The results of such technically
demanding procedures, however, have been quite unreliable.[5] By contrast, reattachment
of the dorsal and proximal portions of the scapholunate interosseous membrane through
transosseous sutures, as suggested by Linscheid[10] and Lavernia and co-authors,[9] augmented with a dorsal capsulodesis, as described by Blatt,[1] has consistently given better
results.[9,10]

The surgical procedure discussed hereafter appears specially indicated in acute (up to
6 weeks) disruptions of the scapholunate supporting ligaments with demonstrable, dynamic or static, rotatory subluxation of the scaphoid. Chronic scapholunate instabilities
may be treated with this technique only if: (1) the malalignment is easily correctable by
manipulation, (2) adequate ligament tissue is still available, and (3) there are no local
arthritic changes at the radioscaphoid or midcarpal joints. Dynamic scapholunate instabilities secondary to partial tears of the scapholunate membrane, especially those affecting
the dorsal ligaments, also may be treated by this surgical procedure.

Stabilization of the wrist by ligament reconstruction is contraindicated in the following
situations: (1) uncorrectable or difficult to reduce scapholunate dissociations, (2) instabili-

■ INDICATIONS AND
CONTRAINDICATIONS

■ SURGICAL
TECHNIQUES

ties associated with local arthritic changes, and (3) late instabilities without adequate, available ligament remnants. Eventually, this technique also would be contraindicated in patients with a physically demanding occupation, requiring a forceful hand.

Surgery is always performed under axillary block anesthesia. The limb is exsanguinated with the use of an Esmarch bandage, and tourniquet control is used. A 6-cm longitudinal straight or slightly S-shaped skin incision over the dorsum of the wrist, centered on the scapholunate interval, is used in this procedure. The scapholunate joint is palpable in a small hollow located just distal and ulnar to Lister's tubercle. The superficial sensory branches of the radial and ulnar nerves are carefully preserved during the approach. All vessels crossing the operative field are cauterized or ligated.

The second to the fourth extensor compartments are identified by dissecting immediately on the plane of the extensor retinaculum. The subcutaneous tissue is raised with both flaps, keeping them full-thickness. The extensor retinaculum is incised over the extensor pollicis longus tendon (third compartment) and the extensor carpi radialis brevis and longus tendons (second compartment) (Fig. 67–2A). The tendons are removed from their compartments and retracted in a radial direction (Fig. 67–2B). The periostium on the floor of the third compartment is incised longitudinally. The incision is extended distally opening the capsule in line with the direction of the third compartment until the midcarpal joint is exposed. Another capsular incision parallel to the previous one is placed 1 cm radially in line with the second extensor compartment. A third transverse incision, approximately 1.5 cm distal to the dorsal rim of the radius, is made uniting the two previous

■ FIGURE 67–2
Surgical repair of a complete scapholunate ligamentous disruption. **A,** Dorsal incision. Exposure of the extensor retinaculum. Opening of the second and third extensor compartments.

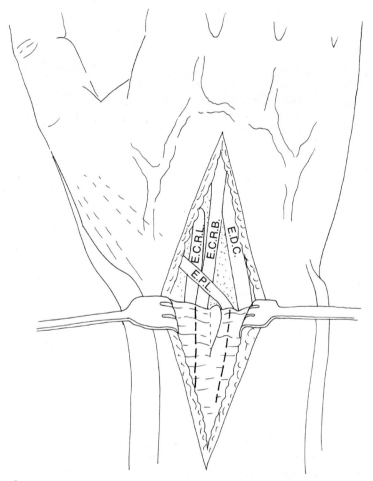

A

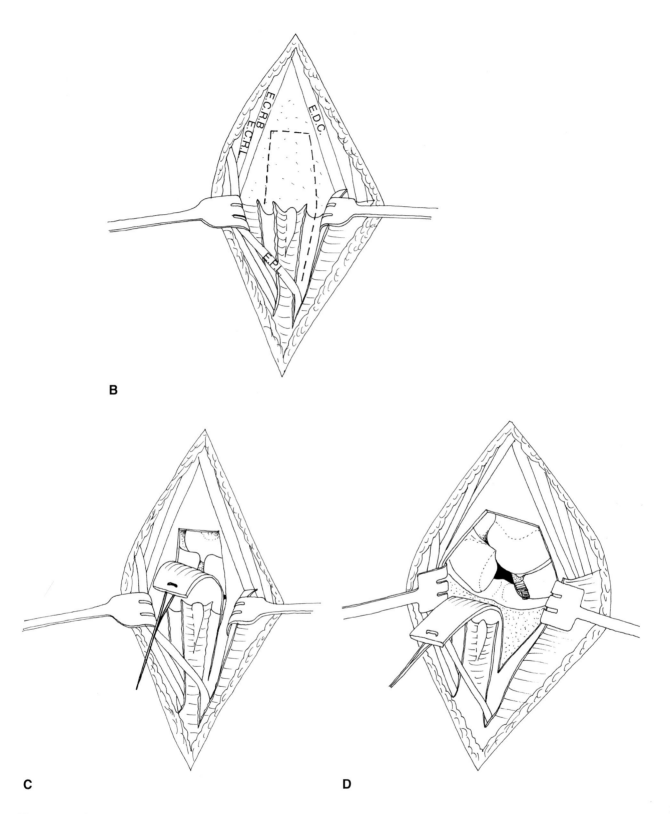

■ FIGURE 67–2
(continued)
B, The dorsal capsule is opened creating a proximal based capsular flap of dimensions 1.5 × 1 cm. The roof of the third compartment also is incised. **C,** The capsular flap is elevated, and the dorsal aspect of the scaphoid uncovered. **D,** To maximize exposure, the periostium under the fourth compartment is elevated and the radialmost fibers of the dorsal radiocarpal ligament are detached.

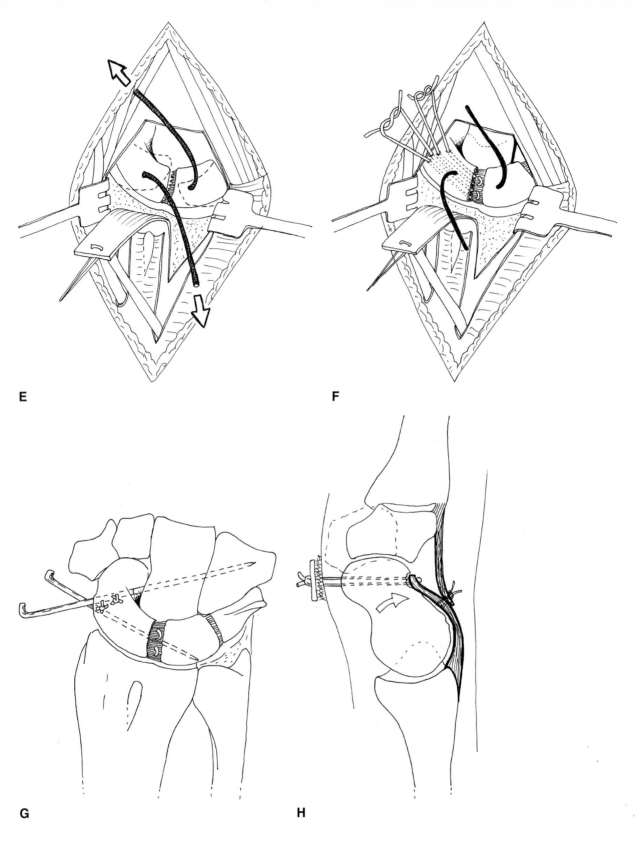

E

F

G

H

■ FIGURE 67–2

(continued) **E,** Two Kirschner wires inserted in each bone are used to mobilize and reduce the carpal malalignment. Arrows represent the direction toward which the wires need to be pulled in order to achieve reduction. **F,** Transosseous nonabsorbable sutures passed through the remnants of the scapholunate membrane and ligaments are tied while the reduction is maintained with the two "joy stick" wires. **G,** Two additional Kirschner wires transfixing the scapholunate and scaphocapitate joints are inserted to prevent motion during ligament healing. **H,** Schematic representation of the dorsal capsulodesis. The proximally based flap is tightly attached to a roughened area on the dorsum of the scaphoid by means of transosseous sutures tied over a button on the palm. The remaining capsule is sutured overlapping the flap.

incisions. The three incisions result in a 1-cm wide, proximally based, radiocarpal capsular flap, which is carefully elevated from the underlying, often protruding, proximal pole of the scaphoid (Fig. 67–2C).

The ulnar border of the incision on the periostium of the third compartment is elevated with an osteotome. By keeping the dissection in a subperiostal plane, the so-called infratendinous retinaculum is separated from the radius. In this way, the fourth extensor compartment containing the extensor digitorum communis tendons need not to be violated.[11] The capsule covering the dorsal aspect of the lunate is dettached from the bone and elevated in continuity with the periosteal flap of the distal radius. For a better exposure, the radialmost fibers of the dorsal radiocarpal ligament have to be detached from the dorsal rim of the radius. The exposure should be wide enough to visualize the scaphoid, the lunate, the lunotriquetral joint, and the head of the capitate (Fig. 67–2D).

Two Kirschner wires are inserted in a dorsopalmar direction into the scaphoid and lunate and used as "joy sticks" to manipulate the two bones. A complete realignment of the scapholunocapitate joints should be easily obtained by pulling proximally and ulnarly on the scaphoid wire, and distally and radially on the lunate wire (Fig. 67–2E). At this point, and depending on the presence or absence of cartilage wear, and on the difficulties found to correct the deformity, the final decision as to continue with the repair technique or to choose other alternatives is made. Usually the scapholunate membrane and ligaments appear avulsed from the scaphoid and remain attached to the lunate often with part of the scaphoid articular cartilage. It is not unusual, however, that the dorsal scapholunate ligament appears avulsed from the lunate keeping an osteochondral fragment with it. In the first situation, we will proceed as follows.

The wrist is fully flexed. The proximal rim of the scaphoid is freshened using a small rongeur. Four drill holes are made obliquely in the scaphoid from the denuded proximal rim to the dorsolateral aspect of the waist of the scaphoid, just distal to the styloid process of the radius (Fig. 67–2F). Horizontal mattress sutures of nonabsorbable material (0-Prolene) are passed through the remnants of the scapholunate membrane and dorsal ligament and threaded through the drill holes using Keith needles. The wrist is then extended, the bones are reduced using the two K-wires, and the sutures are tied (Fig. 67–2G). If there is a dorsal fragment avulsed from the lunate and yet still attached to the dorsal scapholunate ligament, the fracture bed is freshened and the fragment is secured with a small screw or two 1.5-mm K-wires. Before removing the two "joy stick" wires, the reduction is further stabilized with two 1.5-mm K-wires introduced percutaneously through the snuff box, transfixing the scapholunate and the scaphocapitate joints (Fig. 67–3).

At this stage, the radiocarpal stability should be tested by gently applying an ulnar translocating force to the carpus. If abnormal ulnar translation of the lunate is observed (scapholunate dissociation type B, according to Taleisnik,[14]) either an augmentation of the attenuated radiocarpal ligaments, as described by Rayhack and co-authors,[13] or a radiolunate arthrodesis may be indicated.[14] If even mild laxity is observed, the reduced lunate is stabilized in a slightly overcorrected position by means of another 1.5-mm K-wire transfixing the radiocarpal joint. Intraoperative radiographs to confirm the correction of the instability pattern are obtained at this point.

To further stabilize the scaphoid, a dorsal capsulodesis is performed as follows. The dorsal margin of the distal articular surface of the scaphoid is exposed and a narrow groove along the dorsolateral aspect of the bone is excavated with a small rongeur. Drill holes are made from that groove to the palmar tuberosity of the scaphoid. The previously prepared proximally based dorsal capsular flap is tightly attached to that hollow by means of one pullout suture (0-Prolene) passed through the drilled holes and tied over a button on the palmar aspect of the wrist (Fig. 67–2H). The capsule distal to the flap is overlapped and sutured to the flap. The rest of the capsule is sutured side to side to it. The tendons are replaced to their corresponding compartments and the extensor retinaculum repaired anatomically with small absorbable sutures. The wound is finally closed and drained, and a bulky compression dressing with a palmar and dorsal splint is applied with the wrist in neutral position.

■ FIGURE 67–3
Immediate postoperative
radiograph, following
open reduction and liga-
ment reconstruction,
showing percutaneous
Kirschner wire fixation
and anatomic reduction.

■ FIGURE 67–3
Immediate postoperative
radiograph, following
open reduction and liga-
ment reconstruction,
showing percutaneous
Kirschner wire fixation
and anatomic reduction.

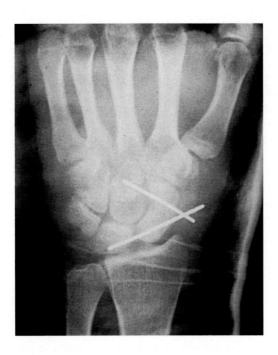

■ TECHNICAL
ALTERNATIVES

It is important to note that with the surgical technique described here only part of the injuries responsible for the subluxation of the scaphoid are addressed. As noted by Drewniany and co-authors,[4] in some instances the palmar and distal stabilizing structures (scaphotrapezial-trapezoidal and scaphocapite ligaments) may play an important stabilizing role requiring additional surgery. We add a palmar scaphotrapezial capsular plication to the procedure when the scaphocapitate angle is larger than 80° or the patient has hyperlax joints. Before closing the dorsal capsulodesis, the scaphoid tuberosity is exposed through a short S-shaped palmar incision. The flexor carpi radialis tendon sheath adjacent to the scaphoid is opened from proximal to distal to the level of the trapezial ridge. The palmar and medial aspect of the scaphotrapezial capsule, which contains the medial part of the scaphotrapezial-trapezoidal ligaments and the lateral insertion of the scaphocapite ligament, is detached from the scaphoid. The sutures from the dorsal capsulodesis are then passed through the predrilled holes and used to reinsert the capsule more proximally and laterally over the scaphoid tuberosity.

One common shortcoming of the procedure is to fashion the dorsal capsular flap too short to reach the scaphoid distal to its midaxis of rotation. It is important to note that the more distal the dorsal flap is inserted, the more effective will be its role as a checkrein preventing palmarflexion of the scaphoid. It is critical, therefore, to design a capsular flap at least 1.5 cm long and 1 cm wide to maximize the capsulodesis effect.

Failure to fully correct the scaphoid and lunate malposition is another common shortcoming of the procedure. Only with an anatomically reduced joint can the scapholunate ligaments be reapproximated closely enough to allow them to heal. Suboptimal reductions very seldom result in re-establishing solid ligamentous connections between the two bones. We recommend using an image intensifier when manipulating the two "joy stick" wires to determine whether the malaligned bones can be fully corrected and to know how much force and exactly in what direction the wires need to be pulled to achieve this. If the deformity cannot be reduced anatomically or the ligament remnants do not allow a strong repair, we advise against this procedure because early recurrence of the instability is likely.[11] Cases that cannot be successfully completed using this technique may be candidates for either a limited intercarpal fusion (scaphotrapezial-trapezoidal[15] or scaphocapitate[12] or a proximal row carpectomy.[7]) In chronic scapholunate instabilities with degenerative changes at the radioscaphoid and lunocapitate articulations, the so-called SLAC wrist, a "four corner" (lunate-capitate-hamate-triquetrum) arthrodesis plus resection of the scaphoid may be indicated.[16]

After the operation, the extremity is elevated for 3 to 5 days by use of an arm sling. Drains are removed at 24 hours, and a long arm thumb spica cast with the forearm slightly pronated is applied 5 days after surgery. During this time, active motion of the shoulder and fingers is encouraged. The above elbow immobilization is continued for 4 weeks and is followed by a below-elbow thumb spica cast for an additional 4 weeks. Both the K-wires and the pullout sutures are removed at this time. An additional 1 month of immobilization with a protective splint made of thermoplastic material is usually recommended, although this should be removed twice a day to start progressive active unresisted range of motion exercises, always under the supervision of a therapist. At this stage the patient and the therapist should be cautioned against trying to quickly regain a full range of motion through passive motion exercises, for they may stretch out the repaired ligaments. At 12 weeks postoperatively isometric strengthening exercises of the wrist motors are initiated. Supervised therapy usually continues until the end of the fourth month. No stressful activities of normal work or sport should be permitted before 6 months after surgery.

■ REHABILITATION

The only series of patients with a scapholunate dissociation treated by means of direct repair, without augmenting the repair with a tenodesis, has been recently reported by Lavernia and co-authors.[9] At an average follow-up of 3 years, pain was absent or significantly reduced in 20 of the 21 patients treated with this technique. All patients had regained a nearly normal grip strength, and wrist motion was full except for flexion that was reduced an average of 17°. Radiographs demonstrated only minimal degenerative changes in 3 of the 21 patients, and the condition had not progressed to an advanced collapse pattern. Based on their experience the authors stated that "open reduction with direct scapholunate interosseous membrane and dorsal ligamentous repair, with or without a dorsal capsulodesis, should be considered as the treatment of choice for the majority of these patients."[9]

■ OUTCOMES

References

1. Blatt G: Capsulodesis in reconstructive hand surgery: dorsal capsulodesis for the unstable scaphoid and volar capsulodesis following excision of the distal ulna. Hand Clinics, 1987; 3: 81–102.
2. Cooney WP, Linscheid RL, Dobyns JH: Ligament repair and reconstruction. In: Neviaser RJ (ed): Controversies in Hand Surgery, New York: Churchill Livingstone, 1990:125–145.
3. Dobyns JH, Linscheid RL, Chao EYS, Weber ER, Swanson GE: Traumatic instability of the wrist. AAOS Instructional Course Lecture, 1975; 24:182–199.
4. Drewniany JJ, Palmer AK, Flatt AE: The scaphotrapezial ligament complex: An anatomic and biomechanical study. J Hand Surg, 1985; 10A:492–498.
5. Glickel SZ, Millender LH: Ligamentous reconstruction for chronic intercarpal instability. J Hand Surg, 1984; 9A:514–527.
6. Goldner JL: Treatment of carpal instability without joint fusion-current assessment. J Hand Surg, 1982; 7:325–326.
7. Inglis AE, Jones EC: Proximal row carpectomy for diastasis of the proximal carpal row. J Bone Joint Surg, 1977; 59A:460–463.
8. Kauer JMG: The mechanism of the carpal joint. Clin Orthop Rel Res, 1986; 202:16–26.
9. Lavernia CJ, Cohen MS, Taleisnik J: Treatment of scapholunate dissociation by ligamentous repair and capsulodesis. J Hand Surg, 1992; 17A:354–359.
10. Linscheid RL: Scapholunate ligamentous instabilities (dissociations, subdislocations, dislocations). Ann Chir Main, 1984; 3:323–330.
11. Palmer AK, Dobyns JH, Linscheid RL: Management of posttraumatic instability of the wrist secondary to ligament rupture. J Hand Surg, 1978; 3:507–532.
12. Pisano SM, Peimer CA, Wheeler DA, Sherwin FS: Scaphocapitate intercarpal arthrodesis. J Hand Surg, 1991; 16A:328–333.

13. Rayhack JM, Linscheid RL, Dobyns JH, Smith JH: Postraumatic ulnar translation of the carpus. J Hand Surg, 1987; 12A:180–189.

14. Taleisnik J: Carpal instability. Current concepts review. J Bone Joint Surg, 1988; 70A: 1262–1267.

15. Watson HK, Ryu J, Akelman E: Limited triscaphoid intercarpal arthrodesis for rotatory subluxation of the scaphoid. J Bone Joint Surg, 1986; 68A:345–349.

16. Watson HK, Ballet FL: The SLAC wrist: scapholunate advanced collapse pattern of degenerative arthritis. J Hand Surg, 1984; 9A:358–365.

17. Weil C, Ruby LK: The dorsal approach to the wrist revisited. J Hand Surg, 1986; 11A: 911–912.

Repair of Chronic Peripheral Tears/Avulsions of the Triangular Fibrocartilage

Despite our increasing knowledge of the structural anatomy and vascularity of the triangular fibrocartilage (TFC) of the wrist, it remains difficult to understand the mechanisms of injury to this highly specialized intrinsic stabilizer of the distal radioulnar and ulnocarpal joints (Fig. 68–1). Traditional orthopaedic teaching suggests a tightening of the dorsal distal radioulnar ligaments in pronation and, conversely, a tightening of the palmar distal radioulnar ligaments in supination. In 1985, however, af Ekenstam[3] published a revolutionary work based on static TFC load studies in cadavers. The central articular disc of the TFC was sacrificed in each cadaver wrist, and tensile changes in the vascularized fibrous dorsal and palmar radioulnar ligaments were observed in pronation and supination. af Ekenstam showed that in full pronation the distal pole of the ulna translates dorsally at the sigmoid notch, increasing tension throughout the palmar limbus of the triangular fibrocartilage. He theorized that palmar destabilizing injuries to the TFC probably resulted from a loaded hyperpronation mechanism. Conversely, the dorsal limbus of the TFC was observed to tighten in supination, as the pole of the ulna translated palmarly along the sigmoid notch. Hypersupination injuries could therefore be expected to result in dorsal destabilizing TFC tears. af Ekenstam's 1985 observations seemed to refute traditional orthopaedic teaching regarding the restraining capacity of the triangular fibrocartilage.

In 1991, however, work generated in the Mayo Clinic Biomechanics Laboratory by Shuind and co-authors[12] directly contradicted af Ekenstam's findings. Using stereophotogrammetric techniques, and without sacrifice of the central articular disc, these researchers demonstrated precisely that in pronation the dorsal vascularized fibrous portion of the TFC tightens; in supination the palmar limbus tightens. Their findings reinforced traditional teaching regarding the joint-stabilizing capacity of the TFC.

Over the past decade, it has been clinically well-established that most peripheral injuries of the TFC occur in the medial or dorsomedial region. Tissue in this area is well-vascularized, with potential for biologic repair after injury. Since most patients with peripheral injury to the TFC historically report loaded hyperpronation as the mechanism of injury, these observations seem to clinically corroborate the laboratory findings of Shuind and co-authors.[12]

I hypothesized in 1985 that destabilizing peripheral injuries of the TFC within its well-vascularized fibrous portion might be amenable to direct open primary repair, even if chronic; and if, following the repair, the tissue was properly immobilized and given adequate time for healing and rehabilitation, its functional capacity as an intrinsic stabilizer might be restored, thus relieving chronic pain. A prospective study of the surgical application of this approach to chronic peripheral TFC injuries was begun that year. Preliminary results of the first 11 patients, treated after a mean time from injury to surgery of 32 months, were published in 1991.[5] Early data, based on follow-up time of more than 1 year, strongly suggested that the torn periphery of the TFC was amenable to surgical repair, and that chronic pain associated with inadequate primary treatment of the lesion could be eliminated or reduced in most patients. Sixteen patients with Palmer Class IB

■ HISTORY OF THE TECHNIQUE

■ FIGURE 68–1
The vascularized portions of the triangular fibrocartilage complex (TFC) are the dorsal 20%, the palmar 20%, and the medial origin at the sulcus of the distal ulna. With the ulnocarpal ligaments, the TFC is the primary intrinsic stabilizer of the distal radioulnar joint, allowing rotation through the full prosupination arc, while limiting the extent of palmar translation of the ulna in supination, and dorsal translation of the ulna in pronation.

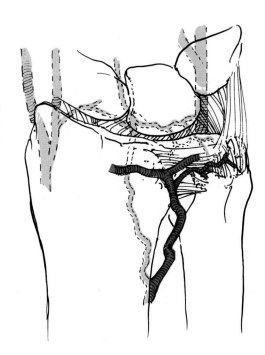

TFC lesions[9] have been treated to date. The data continue to support the role of surgical reattachment of the traumatically avulsed TFC to the fovea at the base of the distal ulna. The technique described in this chapter is effective in re-establishing the normal support system so critical for the ulnar-sided wrist mechanics.

■ INDICATIONS AND CONTRAINDICATIONS

The usefulness of the procedure for chronic ulnar-sided wrist pain is based on the surgeon's clear understanding of destabilizing and nondestabilizing injuries of the TFC. Tears along the peripheral, well-vascularized margins of the TFC or avulsions from its peripheral attachment to the fovea result in a compromise to normal DRUJ mechanics and are associated with pain. The instability may be severe and result in a chronic palmar DRUJ dislocation. More often the instability is less dramatic, manifesting itself as a subtle "piano key" sign or slightly increased DRUJ laxity (relative to the contralateral normal wrist).

To employ the open technique of reattachment or direct TFC repair, a definitive diagnosis must be made preoperatively. Large tears can now be visualized in some centers by noninvasive magnetic resonance imaging. But even with excellent equipment and an experienced radiologist, the incidence of false negative reports still remains very high. Arthroscopic examination, in contrast, has proved 100% accurate in identifying these chronic lesions. The most recent 12 of the 16 patients who have undergone open TFC repair had accurate preoperative positive arthroscopic identification of both magnitude and location of the tear. Direct visualization of the source of the patient's chronic ulnar-sided wrist pain affords the surgeon the opportunity to plan the open procedure for a later date and to discuss the arthroscopic findings and proposed reconstruction at length with the patient before the actual procedure is performed. I strongly recommend diagnostic arthroscopy be performed before using this operative technique.

Diagnostic arthroscopy also enables the surgeon to rule out certain TFC pathology in which this operation is contraindicated. Injuries to the hypovascular articular disc[9]—the central portion of the TFC—by their nature are not amenable to direct surgical repair. Arthroscopic identification of these central nondestabilizing lesions allows the surgeon to definitively debride the injured tissues using arthroscopic instruments only. Identification of lesions other than chronic peripheral detachments or tears of the TFC (e.g., lunatotriquetral ligament tears or central TFC lesions) does not obviate the need for the open operation discussed in this chapter. The surgeon must exercise clinical judgment in determining the need for any procedures in addition to the restoration of intrinsic stability to the DRUJ by peripheral TFC repair or reattachment. Although the presence of multiple lesions is relatively uncommon, I have performed the operation in association with ulna shortening osteotomy (in the presence of ulna positive variance), and lunatotriquetral arthrodesis (in the presence of chronic painful lunatotriquetral instability). Presence of even minor arthritic changes in either the DRUJ or the ulnocarpal joint is also a strict contraindication for the technique of open repair. Alternative salvage procedures should be sought by the surgeon.

The surgical approach to repair of chronic peripheral avulsions of the TFC is dorsoulnar, through a utilitarian incision 6 cm in length (Fig. 68–2). The procedure is performed under axillary regional anesthesia; preoperative prophylactic antibiotics are administered intravenously. The incision parallels the dorsal sensory branch of the ulnar nerve and affords access to the retinaculum of the extensor tendons, proximal to the transverse retinacular branch of the nerve.[8] A radially based "tongue" of retinaculum is raised from the margin of the flexor carpi ulnaris to be used at the close of the procedure to restabilize the extensor carpi ulnaris tendon in its normal dorsoulnar position. Elevation of the retinacular flap exposes the tendons of the fifth and sixth dorsal compartments, which can be retracted to allow access to the dorsal ulnocarpal capsule. Finger-traps and 14 lb of longitudinal traction are used for the exposure. An inverted "T"-shaped ulnocarpal capsulotomy is made, the stem of which lies between the troughs of the fifth and sixth compartments. The transverse limb of the "T" is made at the distal margin of the TFC, with care being taken to avoid further iatrogenic injury.

Once the capsular flaps are dissected free and retracted, visualization of the ulnocarpal joint and the entire TFC complex is facilitated by use of the finger-traps and distraction counterweights. Visibility is maximized by using a Freer elevator, gently introduced as a

■ SURGICAL
TECHNIQUES

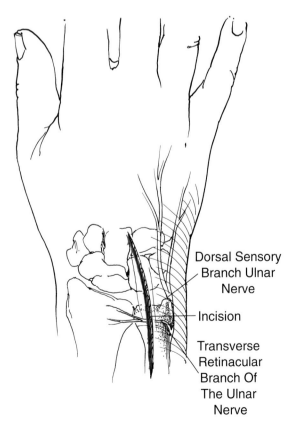

■ FIGURE 68–2
The skin incision for open repair of dorsomedial or medial TFC avulsions is utilitarian, and parallels the fibers of the dorsal branch of the ulnar nerve, to minimize the risk of injury to this vital structure.

Dorsal Sensory
Branch Ulnar
Nerve

Incision

Transverse
Retinacular
Branch Of
The Ulnar
Nerve

lever between the lunate and spherical fossa of the radius. A double-pronged skin hook can be used as a retractor along the dorsal distal TFC limbus, everting the tissue and facilitating a full view of the damaged area. The avulsed or torn periphery of the TFC (usually medial, or dorsomedial) can then be debrided of fibrotic matter and granulation tissue using curettes and rongeurs. Differentiation of the firm consistency of normal TFC tissue from softer, yellowish and hyperemic fibrotic granulation tissue is not difficult. Small fractures of the distal styloid not amenable to internal fixation can be debrided along with the granulation tissue (Fig. 68–3). A trough is then created along the sulcus at the base of the styloid, exposing cancellous bone; this preparation is performed at the site of avulsion or tear of the TFC. Two parallel holes are made with an 0.045 Kirschner wire, separated by 8 to 10 mm. The K-wires enter the medial cortex of the ulna and exit within the trough at the base of the styloid. Three nonabsorbable, braided nylon sutures (3-0 Surgilon) are then individually passed through one of these two holes, through the vascularized periphery of the TFC, along the margin of the tear (Fig. 68–4). Once it has been well-anchored, these three sutures are individually passed through the second paralleling hole (drilled with the 0.045 K-wire), and out through the medial cortex of the ulna (Fig. 68–3).

Before anchoring the loose TFC securely to the prepared trough, two 0.062 K-wires are introduced percutaneously through the medial border of the ulna into the radius, securing the seat of the ulna in its midposition at the sigmoid notch (Fig. 68–5); care must be taken to avoid violation of the DRUJ itself by K-wire placement. With stability of the forearm assured, the avulsed portion of the TFC can be anchored to the ulna, tying the three nonabsorbable sutures across the medial cortex of the ulna as tightly as possible (Fig. 68–6). Normal tension of the TFC in midposition is thus restored.

The dorsal capsule of the ulnocarpal joint is then carefully repaired with inverted 3-0 Surgilon sutures, leaving the transverse limb of the inverted "T" open. The long retinacular flap, designed at the start of the procedure, is passed deep to the extensor carpi ulnaris.

■ FIGURE 68–3
Debridement of chronic exuberant granulation and fibrous connective tissue from the injured periphery of the TFC facilitates creation of a cancellous trough at the fovea, or sulcus, at the base of the ulna styloid. Two parallel holes are made through the base of the styloid into the trough, using 0.045 Kirschner wires. The three retaining sutures securing the TFC are passed through these holes, to be securely anchored to the ulna.

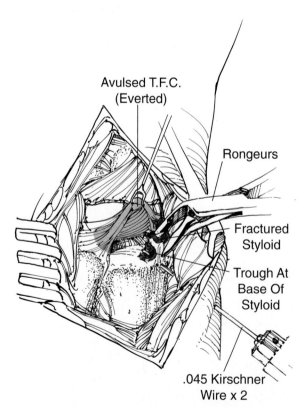

Avulsed T.F.C.
(Everted)

Rongeurs

Fractured
Styloid

Trough At
Base Of
Styloid

.045 Kirschner
Wire x 2

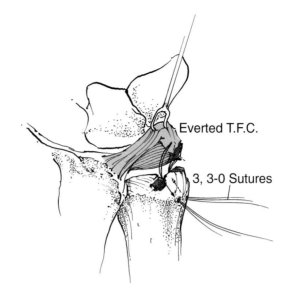

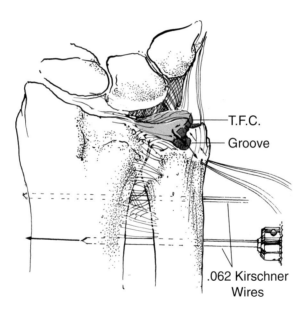

■ FIGURE 68-4
Three 3-0 nonabsorbable sutures are placed through the retracted medial TFC and passed through drill holes at the medial base of the ulna styloid.

■ FIGURE 68-5
Before tightly suturing the TFC to the prepared trough, the distal radioulnar relationship is secured by two percutaneous 0.062 Kirschner wires placed through the ulna into the radius in neutral position. Care must be exercised to avoid injury to the DRUJ. These K-wires are left in place for 6 weeks.

It is then looped back radially and distally, and anchored to the distal retinaculum as a sling for the ECU (Figs. 68-7A and 68-7B).

Chronic ulnocarpal pain resulting from inadequate treatment of destabilizing injuries to the TFC profoundly affects a patient's activities of daily living and his capacity for gainful employment. In the past, patients with gross distal radioulnar instability might have been surgically treated by one of the many free- or attached-tendon reconstructions available at the time, performed in an effort to add stability to an unstable distal radioulnar relationship. Most of these reconstructions have been abandoned, because of exceedingly high failure rates; in the face of persistent pain, most patients eventually underwent Darrach distal ulna resection. Only Hui and Linscheid's[6] ulnotriquetral augmentation tenodesis, using a 50% distally based portion of the flexor carpi ulnaris, has stood the test of time. Their technique remains an effective part of the hand surgeon's armamentarium in

■ TECHNICAL ALTERNATIVES

■ FIGURE 68–6
With the radioulnar relationship secured by two 0.062 Kirschner wires, the TFC is secured as tightly as possible to the trough by tying the three 3-0 nonabsorbable sutures across the medial cortical bridge of ulna.

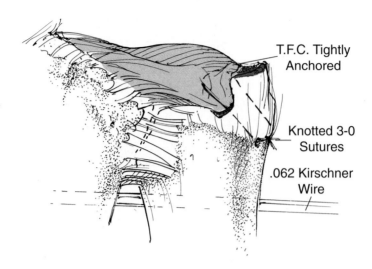

T.F.C. Tightly Anchored

Knotted 3-0 Sutures

.062 Kirschner Wire

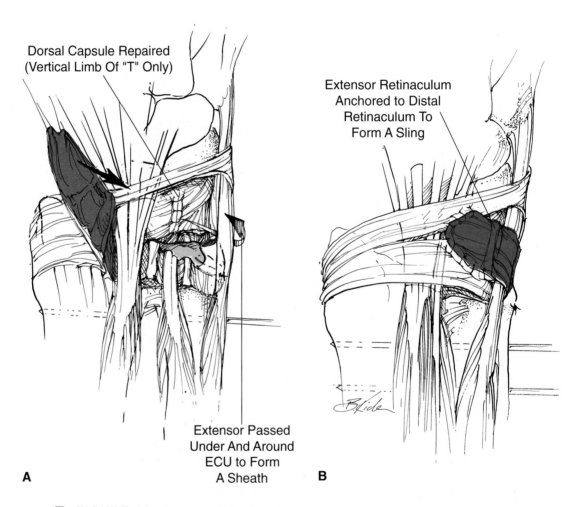

Dorsal Capsule Repaired (Vertical Limb Of "T" Only)

Extensor Retinaculum Anchored to Distal Retinaculum To Form A Sling

Extensor Passed Under And Around ECU to Form A Sheath

A

B

■ FIGURE 68–7
A, The radial-based tongue of retinaculum, prepared during the initial dissection, is used to support the extensor carpi ulnaris at the close of the procedure. The retinaculum is passed deep to the ECU, then brought back distally and radially **(B)** to be sutured to the distal donor retinaculum, creating a dorsal sling for the tendon.

managing severe chronic dorsal ulna "winging," or recurrent dorsal dislocation of the distal ulna in the absence of either bony pathology, or arthritic changes at the DRUJ.

Until recently, injury to the TFC at its peripheral attachment has been poorly understood, with regard to mechanism of injury, relation to ulna variance, and treatment potential. Imbriglia and Boland[7] studied avulsion injuries of the TFC in the area of its dorsal ligamentous attachment to the ulna; excision of the articular disc was recommended as treatment.

Hagert[4] reported good results with direct repair of the TFC in 10 patients with rheumatoid arthritis with DRUJ instability secondary to peripheral separation; none of his patients had DRUJ articular cartilage destruction. Functional demands of Hagert's rheumatoid population were considerably different from a population of patients with traumatic TFC separation; nevertheless, his technique of repair is innovative and worthy of consideration. Dameron[2] recommended direct surgical repair of acute injuries to the periphery of the TFC, but has suggested that all chronic injuries be treated by Darrach resection of the distal ulna.

A criticism of the open technique of direct surgical repair or reattachment of the TFC along its well-vascularized periphery has been the potential to iatrogenically damage the intrinsic stabilizer of the DRUJ, in a manner worse than the initial injury itself. The details of this operative procedure are demanding; performing the technique well requires a high level of understanding of wrist pathophysiology and pathomechanics and considerable experience in wrist surgery. To reduce the real risk of further destabilizing the distal radioulnar joint, a small number of investigators have been active in designing instruments, which may allow predictable repair of peripheral avulsion injuries to the TFC using arthroscopic techniques. At the time of this writing, however, experience remains quite limited, equipment is commercially unavailable, and the usefulness of the arthroscopic approach has not yet been completely assessed.

Major pitfalls in performing the open technique of TFC repair as described in this chapter are as follows.

A. Failure to accurately anchor the DRUJ in a "neutral rotation" position with percutaneous K-wires; malposition will affect the tension of the repaired TFC in extremes of prosupination, leading to persistent painful instability.

B. Closure of the transverse limb of the inverted "T" ulnocarpal capsulotomy; a dorsal capsulodesis may result, limiting flexion of the wrist and compromising the rehabilitation potential of the patient.

C. Performing the operation in the presence of ulna positive variance, without giving consideration to ulna shortening osteotomy and compression plating.

D. Failure to recognize associated injuries to adjacent tissues, leading to persistent wrist morbidity and compromised function, in spite of a technically well-executed operation.

E. Injury to the transverse retinacular branch of the dorsal branch of the ulnar nerve; painful neuromas in this area are very difficult to treat.

F. Failure to initially elevate a dorsal retinacular flap of length sufficient to serve as a sling for the ECU; medial detachment must be from the flexor carpi ulnaris.

■ REHABILITATION

Postoperative care consists of 2 weeks of immobilization in a long-arm, plaster-reinforced dressing with the elbow at 90°. After suture removal at 2 weeks, a circular long-arm cast is applied. At 6 weeks, the percutaneous 0.062 K-wires used to fix the distal radioulnar joint are removed. A short-arm circular cast is applied for an additional 5 to 6 weeks, after which time full prosupination activities can begin. The services of a highly skilled hand therapist are critical in attaining the maximum rehabilitation potential of each patient. The therapy prescription consists of active, active-assisted, and full passive range-of-motion exercises, beginning immediately upon removal of the short-arm cast. Interval thermoplastic splinting between exercises and at night continues for 4 weeks, after which time resistive strengthening exercises can begin. The goals of the rehabilitation program are for the patient to achieve full forearm prosupination, full wrist flexion/extension, and normal strength. While a plateau of recovery may take 12 to 18 months, supervised therapy continues until the end of the sixth postoperative month, with a gradual increase in the interval between visits. At 6 months, each patient is encouraged to continue his therapy at home, until a maximum state of improvement is achieved.

■ OUTCOMES

Sixteen consecutive procedures with follow-up adequate to assess long-term results have been performed using the technique described above. Each patient in the series could be classified as Palmer Class IB.[9] Preoperative, zero rotation posteroanterior radiographs of the injured wrists revealed an average ulnar variance of −0.2 mm. Considering the normal variance to be −2.0 mm,[10,11] the data suggest an average thinner-than-normal TFC in this group. Other plain films were noncontributory, except where concomitant bony injury or gross deformity were present. Five patients had ulna styloid fracture nonunions, classified as Palmar Class IB with styloid fracture.[9] Patients with styloid fractures amenable to open reduction and internal fixation were not included in the series.

Twelve of the 16 patients underwent preoperative videoarthrography, the majority with the three-compartment injection technique described by Zinberg and co-authors.[15] While a slight irregularity of the peripheral margin of the TFC was suggested in some of the studies, a clearly demonstrable fenestration was only found in two. I believe that the presence of fibrotic material and granulation tissue precludes the expected diagnostic flow of contrast material in most cases, leading to the high incidence of false negative studies. Three-phase scintigraphy was performed in eight cases and found to be of only marginal usefulness. Bone scanning was of no value in establishing the definitive diagnosis needed to plan this procedure. Similarly, comparative computerized tomographic scanning through the transverse plane of the wrist (at the level of the DRUJ) served only to corroborate those instabilities more easily demonstrable on physical examination. Magnetic resonance imaging, which has recently been shown to have potential for further development as a noninvasive investigative tool for injuries of the TFC, was not used in the work-up of this patient population. High cost, a high percentage of false-negative responses,[13] and the effectiveness of alternative diagnostic tools all preclude its routine use for this type of wrist pathology.

Only arthroscopy has proved to be consistently useful, allowing the surgeon direct image-enhanced visualization of TFC pathology. A definitive diagnosis was made in the twelve most recent consecutive cases in this series, using a 2.7-mm, 25° angled arthroscope and chip camera, introduced in each case through the dorsal 3–4 portal, with egress established in the 6U portal by a Wolf-Vorhees needle. In every patient, a traumatic tear of either the medial or dorsomedial border of the TFC could be visualized, and the definitive diagnosis made. Loss of normal tension or consistency of the entire TFC on ballottement of the central articular disc (using an arthroscopic probe introduced separately through the 4–5 portal) also was a consistent finding in each of the 12 arthroscopically examined patients. Normally, the TFC has a resilience or "spring" when ballotted. I have observed this to be a consistent finding, and refer to it as the "trampoline effect" (Fig. 68–8A and 68-8B). Patients in whom a chronic traumatic separation or avulsion of the periphery of the TFC is identified have decreased spring when the articular disc is ballotted: a loss of the "trampoline effect." In each of the 12 consecutive patients in whom arthroscopic examination was performed, the "trampoline effect" was absent; instead, ballottement elicited a soft, wave-like response from the tissue. Each of these patients was amenable to open surgical repair.

At final follow-up, the average postoperative grip strength (Jamar Dynamometer, third position) measured 87% of the opposite side. Despite what has been criticized by some as an unnecessarily prolonged period of immobilization after surgery, the final average extension/flexion arc was 96%, radial/ulnar deviation 97%, and prosupination 99%, compared with the opposite normal limb. Of 11 patients who have benefited by open repair of the TFC, 5 are completely pain-free, while 6 are essentially pain-free; patients in the latter group experience only mild discomfort with heavy use. Three patients have continued to have functionally incapacitating pain after their TFC repairs, each requiring a salvage procedure.

The rationale for repair of destabilizing peripheral tears of the TFC comes from careful

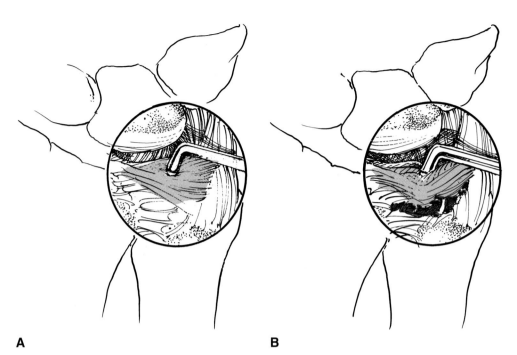

A   **B**

■ FIGURE 68–8

A, Normal tension or resiliency of the TFC results in a "trampoline effect" on ballottement of the articular disc with an arthroscopic probe. **B,** Separation of the peripheral anchor of the TFC at the fovea of the ulna results in a softness or sponginess of this usually tense, resilient structure causing a loss of the "trampoline effect."

study of the similarities between the vascular supply to the meniscus of the knee, and the microcirculation to the TFC. In 1986, Thiru-Pathi and co-authors[14] reported their results of injection studies of the wrist, which demonstrated a 15 to 20% dorsal and palmar vessel penetration of the substance of the articular disc, supplied by dorsal and palmar TFC vessels, respectively, both originating from the anterior interosseous artery (Fig. 68–1). In 1991, Bednar and co-authors[1] again studied the fine details of the microcirculation of the human articular disc using tissue cleaning (Spalteholz) techniques. They found that the triangular fibrocartilage of the wrist is supplied by "small vessels that penetrate . . . in a radial fashion from the palmar, ulnar, and dorsal attachments of the joint capsule and supply the peripheral 10% to 40%." At the same time that Bednar and co-authors[1] suggested (based on their experimental data) that tears in the periphery of the TFC might have blood supply sufficient to "mount a reparative response and, in theory, be repaired," the clinical population of patients presented in this chapter were being studied long-term. The results presented here clearly support Bednar and his co-workers' conclusions.

The patient population presented in this ongoing clinical study all had chronic traumatic avulsion injuries of the TFC from the area of the fovea or sulcus at the base of the distal ulna. In each, the tear was in the well-vascularized periphery of the TFC and was believed to be amenable to surgical repair. Chronic pain was reduced or eliminated in most cases. The results clearly indicate that an aggressive effort to reattach or repair the avulsed TFC to its site of origin should be made by the surgeon, after a definitive diagnosis has been established. Because the reparative potential in this area is high, I believe that surgical restoration of normal intrinsic support and kinematics at the ulnar aspect of the wrist and distal radioulnar joint can be realized using this method.

References

1. Bednar MS, Arnoczky SP, Weiland AJ: The microvasculature of the triangular fibrocartilage complex: its clinical significance. J Hand Surg, 1991; 16A:1101–1105.
2. Dameron TB: Traumatic dislocation of the distal radioulnar joint. Clin Orthop, 1972; 83: 55–63.
3. Ekenstam FW af, Hagert CG: Anatomical studies on the geometry and stability of the distal radio ulnar joint. Scand J Plast Reconstr Surg, 1985; 19:17–25.
4. Hagert CG: The distal radioulnar joint in relation to the whole forearm. Clin Ortho Rel Res, 1992; 275:56–64.

5. Hermansdorfer JD, Kleinman WB: Management of chronic peripheral tears of the triangular fibrocartilage complex. J Hand Surg, 1991; 16A:340–346.

6. Hui FC, Linscheid RL: Ulnotriquetral augmentation tenodesis: A reconstructive procedure for dorsal subluxation of the distal radioulnar joint. J Hand Surg, 1982; 7:230–236.

7. Imbriglia JE, Boland DS: Tears of the articular disc of the triangular fibrocartilage complex: results of excision of the articular disc. J Hand Surg, 1983; 8:620.

8. Lourie GM, Kleinman WB: The transverse radioulnar sensory branch from the dorsal sensory ulnar nerve: its clinical and anatomical significance. Presented Wednesday, October 2, 1991 at the 46th annual meeting of the American Society for Surgery of the Hand. Orlando, Florida.

9. Palmer AK: Triangular fibrocartilage complex lesions: a classification. J Hand Surg, 1989; 14A:594–606.

10. Palmer AK, Glisson RR, Werner FW: Ulnar variance determination. J Hand Surg, 1982; 7: 376–379.

11. Palmer AK, Glisson RR, Werner FW: Relationship between ulnar variance and triangular fibrocartilage complex thickness. J Hand Surg, 1984; 9A:681–683.

12. Shuind F, An KN, Berglund L, Rey R, Cooney WP, Linscheid RL, Chao EYS: The distal radioulnar ligaments: a biomechanical study. J Hand Surg, 1991; 16A:1106–1114.

13. Skahen JR III, Palmer AK, Levinsohn EM, Buckingham SC, Szeverenyi NM: Magnetic resonance imaging of the triangular fibrocartilage complex. J Hand Surg, 1990; 15A:552–557.

14. Thiru-pathi RG, Ferlic DC, Clayton ML, McClure DC: Arterial anatomy of the triangular fibrocartilage of the wrist and its surgical significance. J Hand Surg, 1986; 11A:258–263.

15. Zinberg EM, Palmer AK, Coren AB, Levinsohn EM: The triple-injection wrist arthrogram. J Hand Surg, 1988; 13A:803–809.

PART
III

Tendon Reconstruction

69

JACK L. GREIDER, JR.

Trigger Thumb and Finger Release

Stenosing tenosynovitis of the flexor tendons in the palm, frequently referred to as trigger thumb or finger, is a common clinical problem that can arise from a wide variety of causes. The majority of cases can be thought of as either primary or secondary in origin. The primary type is often seen in women between 40 and 60 years of age. The secondary type is associated with diseases that generally affect connective tissue such as diabetes, rheumatoid arthritis, gout, amyloidosis, and the mucopolysaccharidoses.[6]

The condition was first described by Notta in 1850.[19] Early treatments included observation, passive stretching and splinting, roentgen therapy, and steroid injections in varying combinations. Schönborn, in 1889, is credited with the first operative treatment on triggering digits by splitting the fibrous tendon sheath. Although a number of early reports advocate surgical treatment, the authors failed to specify the exact placement of their incisions and the extent of their digital sheath release. Fahey and Bollinger in 1954 advocated a transverse incision at the metacarpal phalangeal flexion crease for trigger thumb.[4] For trigger fingers, they suggested either transverse incisions paralleling the distal palmar crease or longitudinal incisions parallel to the creases often seen just proximal to the long and ring fingers. They described excision of the "thickened digital fibrous sheath," but make no mention as to the extent of this resection. Subsequent descriptions of the operative technique include variations on these incisions as well as "closed" subcutaneous techniques. Some more recent reports have further refined the operative techniques and the indications for the use of steroid injections in trigger digits.

Although there is some question as to the pathogenesis of primary triggering of digits, recent investigations point to frictional and compressive forces at the first annular pulley of the flexor tendon sheath. These biomechanical factors may cause a fibrocartilaginous metaplasia which may produce a decrease in the caliber of the flexor sheath resulting in a local constriction of the flexor tendons.[14] This is believed to produce a "bunching up" of the collagen arrangement comprising the deep flexor tendon producing a frequently seen nodule. It is this discrepancy between the cross sectional area of the first annular pulley and the flexor tendons that gives rise to the patient's symptoms. These can vary from a sluggish or slow flexion or extension of the digit, commonly seen just after arising, to a catching or triggering and, finally, to a digit that may be "locked" either in flexion or extension. Any of these stages may or may not be accompanied by discomfort or pain that is frequently centered about the annular portion of the entrance to the flexor sheath, but may be directed to the proximal interphalangeal joint of the finger or the interphalangeal joint of the thumb giving rise to occasional diagnostic confusion.

■ HISTORY OF THE TECHNIQUE

Most authors have suggested nonoperative treatment for the freshly diagnosed triggering digit.[5,6,13] Activity modification, systemic anti-inflammatory medications, and splinting may be considered in the patient with rather short duration of symptoms and minimal, if any, triggering. An injection of corticosteroid with or without added local anesthetic in the flexor sheath is the most frequently considered primary treatment. Relief of symptoms after injections varies widely from the low 40% to the mid 90% range depending on the severity of symptoms.[5,9,12,13]

Frieberg and co-authors[5] have studied the outcome of trigger digits treated nonopera-

■ INDICATIONS AND CONTRAINDICATIONS

tively with steroid injections. They distinguished two types, nodular and diffuse, on the basis of palpation of the digital sheath at the proximal annular pulley. A discreet well-defined nodule earned the nodular designation while a more generalized swelling was termed diffuse. They concluded that the nodular form of the disease responded well (93%) to steroid injections and suggested a series of two before advocating surgical release. The diffuse type, on the basis of their poor response (48%), were better served by an initial surgical release, or perhaps a trial injection offered for temporary relief of symptoms while awaiting surgery. I believe that if this distinction can be made on examination that the above treatment plan is to be recommended regardless of the duration of symptoms or the presence or absence of pain. My approach to noncongenital triggering digits in which the triggering can be actively overcome without assistance is to encourage the patient to undergo a series of two properly placed injections over a three week period. Patients with a history of diabetes, chronic renal failure, carpal tunnel syndrome, Dupuytren's disease, DeQuervain's syndrome or severe osteoarthritis respond poorly to the injections and I treat these, as suggested above, as I would the diffuse trigger digit.

Unless the patient experiences painful triggering with activities or during sleep, I do not use extension splints. The digit that is "locked" in flexion or extension and cannot be mobilized requires operative release.

Contraindications to injections or oral anti-inflammatory medications would include sensitivity to any of the materials or the presence of an infection. In particular, mycobacterial infections can mimic stenosing tenosynovitis. Neurilemmomas, flexor ganglions, and intratendinous tumors should be considered. Intrinsic joint problems including loose bodies, marginal osteophytes and ridges in the metacarpal head, impinging or entrapped sesamoid, and metacarpal head fractures should be excluded by a careful history and examination. Radiographic and special imaging may be required in specific cases. Periarticular causes of trigger digits such as volar plate avulsion and entrapment, collateral ligament and capsular tears, and partial lacerations of the flexor tendons and sheath would not be expected to respond to nonoperative treatments.

■ SURGICAL TECHNIQUES

Direct injection of a local anesthetic is the preferred technique for release of trigger fingers and thumb. A short-acting anesthetic such as lidocaine without epinephrine can be used alone or mixed with a longer acting anesthetic such as bupivacaine for postoperative pain control. Two to three milliliters are generally sufficient and are injected directly in the skin in the center line of each digit over the first annular pulley. One to two milliliters are injected beneath the skin and an additional 1 ml is placed in the flexor sheath.

An upper arm or forearm pneumatic tourniquet may be used. I prefer the forearm tourniquet placed just below the elbow crease as it seems to be better tolerated and simplifies the skin preparation and draping.

Pertinent surface anatomy centers about the metacarpophalangeal (MP) flexion crease of the thumb and the proximal and distal transverse creases in the palm. The proximal annular portion of the flexor sheath of the thumb begins directly beneath the MP flexion crease. In the small, ring, and long fingers, it coincides with the distal transverse palmar crease and in the index finger with the proximal transverse crease.

Skin incisions have generally been described as being placed within or parallel to the skin creases, slightly oblique to the creases or longitudinal, always centering on the origin of the flexor tendon sheath.[6,7,16] Experience with these has led me to the use of an alternate incision, which I believe makes direct visualization of the deeper structures easier and which does not seem to add to postoperative morbidity. This consists of a 90° chevron or V-shaped incision with the apex centered approximately 0.5 cm distal to the origin of the flexor sheath and with legs approximately 12 mm in length. The apex is centered approximately 5 mm to either the radial or ulnar side of the midline of the digit or flexor tendon and the legs can open out either in a radial or ulnar direction (Fig. 69–1). In the thumb the apex is at the MP joint flexion crease (Fig. 69–2).

Following anesthesia, skin preparation, marking of the appropriate incision and exsanguination and elevation of the tourniquet, an incision is made through the skin only. The

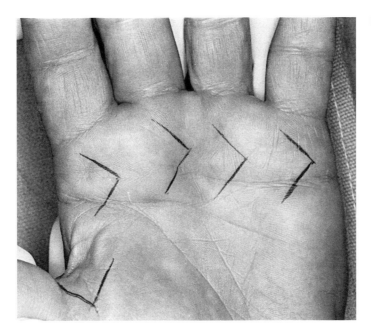

Chevron-shaped incisions can be placed over the first annular pulley in the palm for trigger finger or thumb release.

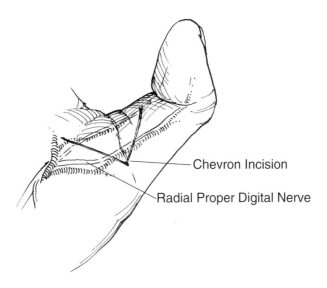

Chevron Incision

Radial Proper Digital Nerve

In the thumb, the apex of the incision is at the MP joint flexion crease.

subcutaneous tissue is grasped with a fine tooth forceps in the area just beneath the skin at the apex of the triangle and a no. 15 blade is used to divide the fibrous bands anchoring the skin to the deep structures of the palm. With traction on the forceps pulling upward, the vertically oriented septae are divided by "pushing" the blade toward the extended midline of the digit. Dissecting scissors can be placed directly in line with the sheath and a spreading motion will clear any remaining soft tissues. At this point, two small vein retractors can be placed on the sheath and traction on these away from the midline will expose the sheath clearly while protecting the neurovascular structures that lie to either side of the sheath and parallel to it (Fig. 69–3). Special care must be taken in the thumb for the radial digital nerve courses obliquely over the tendon sheath just beneath the dermis.[6,8] Here the skin only is incised and gentle traction can be provided using a pick-up or fine skin hook to pull the skin away from the deeper structures while entering the tissue just beneath it. Once again the scissors can be placed directly along the flexor sheath and spread carefully to divide the soft tissues. The retractors can then be placed directly on the sheath to provide visualization of the first annular pulley (Fig. 69–4). Small bleeders

■ FIGURE 69–3
Retraction, including the
use of vein retractors,
should expose the flexor
sheath while protecting
the neurovascular bun-
dles.

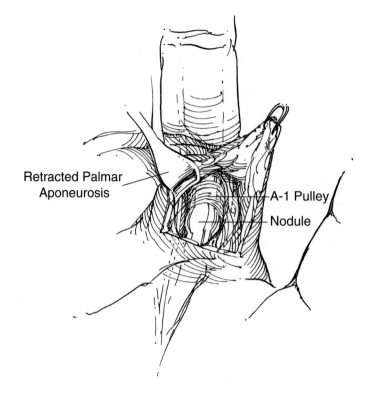

Retracted Palmar
Aponeurosis

A-1 Pulley

Nodule

■ FIGURE 69–4
Similar retraction is used
in the thumb, after care-
ful identification and protection of the radial
proper digital nerve.

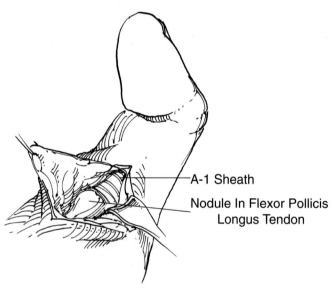

A-1 Sheath

Nodule In Flexor Pollicis
Longus Tendon

can be electrocoagulated with fine-tipped bipolar forceps without damaging the surrounding tissues.

At this point, the origin of the flexor sheath, the first annular pulley, is visualized and
is divided using a no. 15 blade (Fig. 69–3). Alternatively, some surgeons prefer to use a
no. 11 blade slipped just underneath the sheath and passed from a proximal to distal
direction. Small curved dissecting scissors can also be used, although the sheath may be
quite thickened and difficult to cut with the scissors alone. Only the first annular pulley
should be divided and in the adult this is generally 1.0 to 1.5 cm in length (Fig. 69–5).
The free margins of the annular pulley are retracted, and the flexor tendons are inspected
(Fig. 69–6).

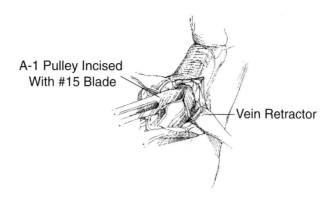

The first annular pulley is divided in the thumb.

A-1 Pulley Incised
With #15 Blade

Vein Retractor

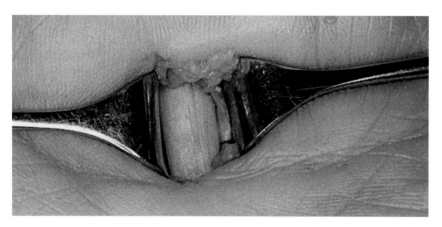

The free margins of the annular pulley are retracted, and the flexor tendons are inspected.

At this point, the patient is asked to flex and extend the digit fully and, if triggering has been present preoperatively, this should be relieved. Patients are sometimes reluctant to fully flex the digit and assistance may be provided until they are able to achieve active flexion equal to that obtained passively. This demonstration can frequently help to motivate those who would otherwise be slow in recovering their motion postoperatively. Occasionally, the local synovium is found to be hypertrophic and can be removed. If triggering is still present the tendons can be gently lifted with the tip of the scissors for closer inspection. The decussation of the superficial flexor may be stenotic about the deep flexor. Passively, flexing the finger and longitudinally dividing, thereby extending, the decussation 1.0 cm from proximally to distal with the scissors or blade can relieve the problem. If it does not, one slip of the superficial flexor may be resected. Should triggering persist, the problem may reside distal to the second annular pulley and the incision can be extended distally in a zig-zag or Bruner fashion to expose this area. If a nodule is found in the flexor tendon at this level a reduction tenoplasty may be performed, as described by Seradge and Kleinert, by excising the nodule through a longitudinal incision and repairing the tendon with a running 7-0 suture.[15]

Closure is accomplished with a nonabsorbable monofilament suture of 4-0 or 5-0. I prefer the smaller diameter and use a reverse cutting needle such as a PC-3. An apical stitch is placed first and the remainder of the incision is closed with vertical mattress or simple stitches. A soft dressing is applied with a layer of nonadherent gauze followed by doubled over 4 × 4 gauze sponges along the transverse palmar creases or over the flexion crease of the thumb. Fluffed sponges are placed between the fingers and secured by a gauze wrap. The day after surgery, patients are encouraged to change the dressing to a small coverage for the wound only and to begin exercising the fingers through a full range of motion. If they experience difficulty achieving a full range of motion by the third day, they are instructed to return for therapy, otherwise they are seen in 10 days for suture removal.

■ TECHNICAL ALTERNATIVES

Alternative methods of release fall into two categories, open and closed. The closed techniques where the annular pulley is released percutaneously without visualization of the pulley have been described and are worthy of note.[10,11,17] These employ a very fine-tipped blade or angiocath needle with or without a gentle curve. These techniques can certainly be successful with practice by the technically proficient in releasing the annular pulley. They all suffer, however, from a lack of visualization of the sheath and surrounding vulnerable structures, particularly in the thumb with the proximity of the radial digital nerve to the sheath. Damage to the flexor tendons themselves and incomplete release would also be more likely to occur in a "blind" procedure. Although the advantage of minimal soft tissue dissection is attractive, accepting even a slight increase in morbidity would seem to be unwarranted. In the open category, the differences generally involve the type and direction of incision. If one could imagine a compass rose sitting over the proximal angular pulley virtually every direction of incising the skin has been used with some success. Common variations include incisions placed parallel to or in the transverse palmar creases, longitudinally directly over the flexor sheath, and obliquely in the secondary flexion creases sometimes found at the base of the long and ring fingers. I have used all of the above incisions without problems, with the exception of the longitudinal approach. Caution should be exercised in crossing the transverse creases with incision at an angle greater than 45°, as scar hypertrophy may result.

Pitfalls in operative technique can occur in several areas. The vulnerability of the radial digital nerve in the thumb during closed techniques has been noted. During open release, care must be given to incising the skin only with the scalpel blade spreading the subcutaneous tissues bluntly with the dissecting scissors and retracting them allowing direct visualization of the flexor sheath. The first annular portion of the flexor sheath is released in trigger digits without continuing into the second annular pulley which may lead to reduced flexion and, particularly in the index finger, potential ulnar drift.[2] In patient's with rheumatoid arthritis, triggering usually results from a proliferative synovitis, usually with a discrepancy between active and passive motion. Should steroid injection fail in these patients, a flexor tenosynovectomy with preservation of the proximal annular pulley is advised to prevent increasing deforming forces on the digits thereby initiating or increasing ulnar drift. Further decompression of the flexor sheath can be obtained by resecting one slip of the superficial flexor.

■ REHABILITATION

Instructions to the patient on dressing changes, wound care, and motion commencing the day after surgery comprise the rehabilitation program in the vast majority of instances. Formal therapy for tender scars or contractures is sometimes necessary. The objective is relief of triggering and discomfort along with restoration of full motion without contractures. Follow-up care for 2 to 4 weeks is sufficient for most patients.

■ OUTCOMES

Among surgical procedures, the release of trigger digits has a gratifyingly high incidence of success with minimal incidence of complications. In a survey to which 177 members of the American Society for Surgery of the Hand (ASSH) responded, a full recovery was anticipated in almost 90% of patients, while modest limitation was noted in less than 3%. Return to limited use was estimated to occur in 94% of patients within 1 to 3 weeks while maximum recovery occurred at 6 to 12 weeks.[1] Complications can include recurrent triggering, fibrous nodule formation beneath the scar, damage to digital nerves, scar tenderness, joint stiffness, and infection.[3,6,18] Bow stringing of the flexor tendon and ulnar drift, particularly in the index finger and in patients with rheumatoid arthritis, has been mentioned as a consequence of releasing more than the first annular pulley.[2] The incidence of all complications by 177 respondents in the ASSH survey was 0% according to 27% of surgeons, less than 5% by 60%, and greater than 5% in the remainder. In my experience, the most frequently seen postoperative problems are scar tenderness and mild flexion contractures at the proximal interphalangeal joint. Scar massage and time generally take care of the tenderness, however, the flexion contractures can be rather resistant to treatment and generally require prolonged dynamic extension splinting. This may require 4 to 6 months before the tissues "settle down." People with a tendency to fibrosis seem a bit more prone to these problems specifically young women with diabetes, those with multiple trigger fingers, Dupuytren's disease, and "knuckle pads" over the proximal interphalangeal joints.

References

1. American Society for Surgery of the Hand: Hand Surgery Questionnaire. Trigger Finger Release, 1988; 127–128B.
2. Burton RI, Littler JW: Tendon entrapment syndrome of first extensor compartment (de Quervain's disorder). Curr Probl Surg, 1975; 12:32–34.
3. Carrozzella J, Stern PJ, Von Kuster, LC: Transection of radial digital nerve of the thumb during trigger release. J Hand Surg, 1989; 14A:198–200.
4. Fahey JJ, Bollinger JA: Trigger finger in adults and children. J Bone Joint Surg, 1954; 36: 1200–1218.
5. Freiberg A, Mulholland RS, Levine R: Nonoperative treatment of trigger fingers and thumbs. J Hand Surg, 1989; 14A-3:553–558.
6. Froimson A: Tenosynovitis and tennis elbow (DeQuervain's Disease). Operative Hand Surgery, 1988; 53:2117–2134.
7. Ger E, Kupcha P, Ger D: The management of trigger thumb in children. J Hand Surg, 1991; 16A-5:944–947.
8. Hirasawa Y, Sakakida K, Tokioka, T, Ohta Y: An Investigation of the Digital Nerves of the Thumb. Clin Ortho Rel Res, 1985; 198:191–196.
9. Kamhin J, Engel M, Heim M: The fate of injected trigger fingers. Hand, 1983; 15-2:218–20.
10. Lorthioir J: Surgical Treatment of Trigger-Finger by a Subcutaneous Method. J Bone Joint Surg, 1958; 40A-4:793–795.
11. Lyu, SR: Closed division of the flexor tendon sheath for trigger finger. J Bone Joint Surg, 1992; 74B-3:418–420.
12. Marks MR, Gunther SF: Efficacy of cortisone injection in treatment of trigger fingers and thumbs. J Hand Surg, 1989; 14A-4:722–727.
13. Rhoades C, Gelberman H, Manjarris JF: Stenosing Tenosynovitis of the Fingers and Thumbs. Clin Ortho Rel Res, 1984; 190:236–238.
14. Sampson SP, Badalamente MA, Hurst LC, Seidmean J: Pathobiology of the human A1 pulley in trigger finger. J Hand Surg, 1991; 16A-4:714–720.
15. Seradge H, Kleinert H: Reduction flexor tenoplasty. J Hand Surg, 1981; 6:543–544.
16. Stefanich RJ, Peimer CA: Longitudinal incision for trigger finger release. J Hand Surg, 1989; 14A-2:316–317.
17. Tanaka J, Muraji M, Negoro J, Yamashita J, Nakano T, Nakano: Subcutaneous release of trigger thumb and fingers in 210 fingers. J Hand Surg, 1990; 15B-4:463–465.
18. Thorpe AP: Results of Surgery for Trigger Finger. J Hand Surg, 1988; 13B-2:199–201.
19. Weibly A: Trigger finger. Acta Orthop Scand, 1970; 41:419–427.

70

De Quervain's Release

■ HISTORY OF THE
TECHNIQUE

Recognition of tenosynovitis of the first dorsal compartment of the wrist, which contains the tendons of the abductor pollicis longus and extensor pollicis brevis, has been attributed to the Swiss surgeon Fritz de Quervain.[6] The entity is frequently encountered in clinical practice. It results from sustained or repetitive strains in the tendons of the fibro-osseous sheath as they move through variable angles over the radial styloid fulcrum. These abnormal biomechanical factors result in a tenosynovitis and corresponding pain on the dorsoradial aspect of the wrist.[7]

The basis for operative treatment has been the seemingly simple release of the constricting extensor retinaculum as described by De Quervain[6] and subsequently modified to include removal of a longitudinal strip or complete removal of the entire tendon sheath fascia.[7,11,12] Finkelstein described simple incision of the sheath although most of his case reports described a microscopic examination of presumably excised tissue. He recommended excision of the sheath when it was very thickened and cartilaginous in consistency.[7] Radical sheath excision has been advocated as the procedure of choice although subsequent reports of tendon subluxation would appear to obviate its recommendation in the routine case.

■ INDICATIONS AND
CONTRAINDICATIONS

Pain over the dorsoradial wrist is the paramount complaint. This may radiate distally over the dorsum of the thumb and proximally over the radial forearm in the distribution of the abductor pollicis longus and extensor pollicis brevis musculotendinous units. There is frequently loss of function of the wrist and thumb with an inability to work, especially if duties require firm pinch or complex thumb motions.

The Finkelstein test is the sine qua non of de Quervain's tenosynovitis and is ascribed to Eichoff (1927) by Finkelstein as thus: "If one places the thumb within the hand and holds it tightly with the other fingers, and then bends the hand severely in ulnar abduction, an intense pain is experienced on the styloid process of the radius, exactly at the place where the tendon sheath takes its course."[7] Immediate and typically severe pain is elicited; indeed, patient rapport may be strained by callous provocation during this part of the examination. Palpation may elicit tenderness over the radial styloid. Ganglion cysts or crepitus are less frequently encountered, but the sheath may be thickened with subsequent triggering, especially of the extensor pollicis brevis.[18,20]

Nonoperative treatment measures include a splint incorporating the thumb and wrist. Splint wear decreases strain in the inflamed tendons and requires the patient to alter his or her activities. Oral analgesics and nonsteroidal anti-inflammatory drugs may be helpful in very early and mild cases if used in conjunction with the splint. Local cortisone solution (usually mixed with local anesthetic) injected into the compartment can be very effective, providing relief to approximately 60% of individuals[21] after a single injection and up to 90% after multiple injections although recurrences may occur.[2,8] Complications of injections are few. Steroid injections can result in dermal atrophy, blanching of pigmented skin, and local fat necrosis. The defect can be quite noticeable and cosmeticly objectionable. This complication may be partly obviated by injection of the solution within the sheath, rather than into the subcutaneous tissues. Ruptures of tendons in the nonrheumatoid hand after cortisone injections have been rarely reported.[2,14,17] Few data are available concerning the effectiveness of the transcutaneous delivery of steroids with or without other therapeutic modalities.

Differential or concurrent diagnoses include thumb basilar joint arthritis, arthritis among the articulations of the scaphoid, trapezium and trapezoid, scaphoid fracture, intersection syndrome, or cheiralgia paresthetica among other radial wrist based disorders. Carpal tunnel syndrome, trigger finger (stenosing tenosynovitis), lateral epicondylitis, or rheumatoid arthritis may be associated diagnoses.

Local anesthetic is infiltrated into the subcutaneous tissues deep to the incision site. The incision is preferably transverse or short oblique over the first dorsal compartment 1 cm proximal to the tip of the radial styloid and approximately 2 to 3 cm in length (Fig. 70–1). Active extension and abduction of the thumb helps to identify the appropriate dorsoradial position. Upper arm tourniquet control of bleeding is well tolerated for the length of this procedure. The initial incision is carefully made through the skin only. The remainder of the dissection to the extensor retinaculum is made longitudinally by blunt dissection using a fine hemostat or tenotomy scissors to obviate injury to the veins and especially the superficial sensory branches of the radial nerve (Fig. 70–2). The branches must be carefully and lightly retracted but not dissected unnecessarily out of their protective adipose tissue bed. The proximal and distal edges of the first dorsal compartment retinaculum can be visualized in this manner by alternately retracting distally and then proximally. This exposure technique facilitates complete release of the retinaculum. A scalpel is used to sharply divide the retinaculum longitudinally, in a distal to proximal direction (Fig. 70–3).

■ SURGICAL TECHNIQUES

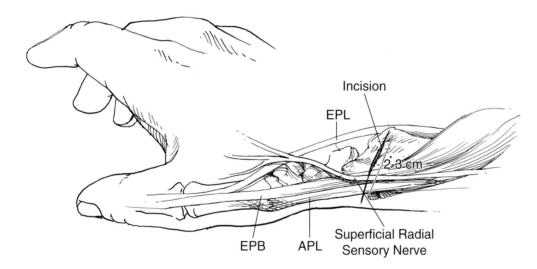

■ FIGURE 70–1
Palpation of the radial styloid and the actively extended tendons of the first dorsal compartment assist identification of the appropriate location for the skin incision.

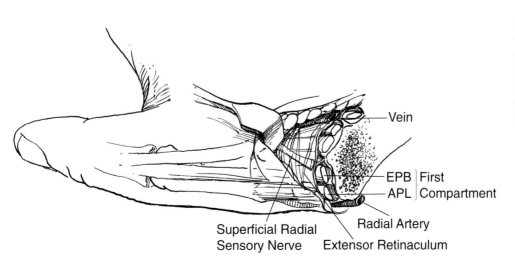

■ FIGURE 70–2
The subcutaneous neurovascular structures are bluntly retracted to expose the proximal and distal edges of the retinaculum.

■ FIGURE 70–3
The retinaculum is sharply incised longitudinally and the tendons of the abductor pollicis longus and extensor pollicis brevis are positively identified, sometimes necessitating exploration dorso ulnarly to ensure complete release of the extensor pollicis brevis.

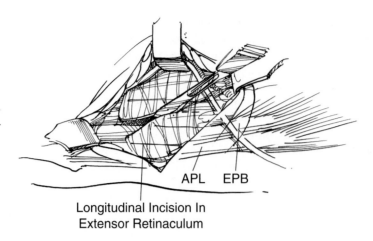

Longitudinal Incision In
Extensor Retinaculum

■ FIGURE 70–4
Multiple structures found within the first dorsal compartment may include multiple slips of abductor pollicis longus which are larger and relatively flatter, and one slip of extensor pollicis brevis, which is rounder and smaller and may be separated from the abductor pollicis longus by a septum.

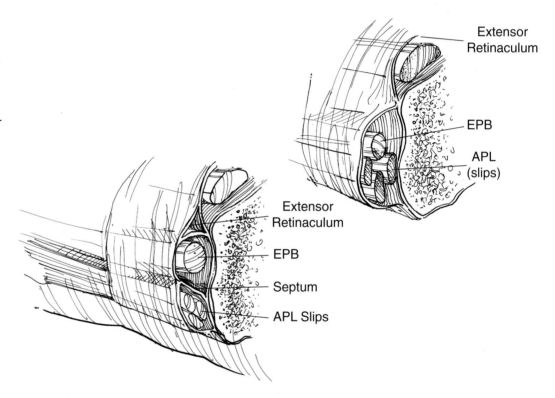

Gentle traction is applied by a hemostat or vascular loop to the tendons within the sheath for identification. The abductor pollicis longus produces abduction and extension of the first metacarpal. The extensor pollicis brevis extends the proximal phalanx (Fig. 70–4). Extension of the interphalangeal joint also may occur when the extensor pollicis brevis has a tendinous insertion into the distal phalanx and the thumb is simultaneously abducted during testing of this muscle. When only the tendon slips of the abductor pollicis longus are identified or if any doubt exists regarding identification of the tendons, exploration is warranted to rule out a separate compartment for the extensor pollicis brevis. If present, the fibrous septum may be excised. Further active and passive motion of the thumb and wrist assist in tendon identification.[1]

After releasing the tourniquet and obtaining hemostasis by electrocautery, closure is accomplished by interrupted plain catgut subcutaneous and fine nylon vertical mattress skin closures. A sterile bulky dressing is applied to additionally obviate the development of a subcutaneous hematoma.

Gentle range of motion exercises alternating with thumb spica splint immobilization may be encouraged initially and progressed after sutures are removed at 7 to 10 days postoperatively.

Regional or general anesthesia may be indicated in special circumstances. Because local tourniquet tolerance is seldom a problem local anesthetic offers the most expedient post anesthetic recovery. A transverse or oblique incision is preferred, as a longitudinal surgical incision is prone to develop hypertrophic and contracted unsightly scarring. An oblique or zigzag incision allows a more extensile exposure than the transverse incision without compromising the natural skin creases. A prior cortisone injection outside of the sheath may have resulted in blanching of the skin or fat necrosis with thinning of the subcutaneous tissue,[14] increasing the vulnerability of vital structures. The superficial sensory branches of the radial nerve, which may be multiple after bifurcations, are particularly vulnerable to injury.[1,3,12] Overly enthusiastic dissection of its branches is not necessary and may result in a symptomatic neurapraxia with a temporary sensory deficit or postoperative perineural adhesions.

A palmarly based flap of retinaculum to prevent tendon subluxation has been recommended[5] but is typically not necessary if the thumb is immobilized postoperatively. However, routine excision of a retinacular segment may result in tendon subluxation and should be avoided unless judiciously excised with a ganglion within its substance. The uncommon tendon subluxation has been treated by sheath reconstruction using the extensor retinaculum or brachioradialis.[15,19] An oblique enlargement of the retinaculum removes constricting forces but obviates gross tendon subluxation.[10]

Continued complaints may be expected if tendons within the first dorsal compartment have been incompletely released. The extensor pollicis brevis in particular resides in an anatomically distinct compartment in 11 to 40% of specimens and may be disconcertingly absent in 2% of individuals.[9,12,13,21] The tendon itself is rounder and smaller than the abductor pollicis longus, which may have multiple slips. Care should be taken to avoid violation of the extensor carpi radialis longus tendon by overly enthusiastic dissection in a dorsoulnar direction.

Splint immobilization protects the wrist and thumb, moderating postoperative pain. Early gentle thumb and wrist range of motion with restricted grasping and pinching are allowed until sutures are removed at 7 to 10 days. A progressive program of stretching and demonstration of protective techniques may be incorporated into a work hardening program, especially if the onset of the initial tenosynovitis was work-related. A formal hand therapy program is not needed for most patients, especially when compensability is not an issue.

Although seemingly straightforward, the treatment of de Quervain's tenosynovitis is not innocuous in the experience of most hand surgeons.[3,4,8] Transient complications such as radial paresthesias, scar tenderness, local infection, and adhesions are frequently encountered and require careful postoperative follow-up. Reflex sympathetic dystrophy, radial nerve laceration, and neuromata are fortunately rare disorders, but do necessitate an obviously more prolonged course of postoperative treatment and hand therapy. Return to sedentary work or light duty activities can be accomplished within 2 weeks postoperatively as long as there is some modification of duties to prevent excessive pinching or repetitive thumb motions. Medium to heavy work duties are seldom tolerated before 6 weeks after surgery and even then a permanent alteration of some aspect of the job may be necessary.[16]

References

1. Alegado RB, Meals RA: An unusual complication following surgical treatment of DeQuervain's disease. J Hand Surgery, 1979; 4:185–186.
2. Anderson BC, Manthey R, Brouns MC: Treatment of DeQuervain's tenosynovitis with

corticosteroids. A prospective study of the response to local injection. Arthr Rheum, 1991; 34: 793–798.

3. Arons MS: De Quervain's release in working women: A report of failures, complications & associated diagnoses. J Hand Surg, 1987; 12:540–544.

4. Belsole RJ: DeQuervain's tenosynovitis—diagnostic and operative complications. Orthopedic, 1981; 4:899–903.

5. Burton RI, Littler JW: Tendon entrapment syndrome of first extensor compartment (DeQuervain's disorder). Curr Prob Surg, 1975; 12:32–34.

6. DeQuervain F: Ueber eine Form von chronischer Tendovaginitis. Cor.—Bl. f. schweiz Aerzte (Basel), 1895; 25:389–394.

7. Finkelstein H: Stenosing tendovaginitis at the radial styloid process. J Bone Joint Surg, 1930; 12:509–540.

8. Harvey FJ, Harvey PM, Horsley MW: DeQuervain's disease: surgical or nonsurgical treatment. J Hand Surg, 1990; 15:83–87.

9. Jackson WT, Viegas SF, Coon TM, Stimpson KD, Frogameni AD, Simpson JM: Anatomical variations in the first extensor compartment of the wrist: a clinical and anatomical study. J Bone Joint Surg, 1986; 68A:923–926.

10. Kapandji AI: Enlargement plasty of the radio-styloid tunnel in the treatment of DeQuervain's tenosynovitis. Annales de Chirurgie de la Main et du Membre Superieur, 1990; 9:42–46.

11. Keon-Cohen B: DeQuervain's Disease. J Bone Joint Surg, 1951; 33B:96–99.

12. Leao Luiz: DeQuervain's Disease; a clinical and anatomical study. J Bone Joint Surg, 1958; 40A:1063–1070.

13. Leslie BM, Ericson WB Jr, Morehead JR: Incidence of a septum within the first dorsal compartment of the wrist. J Hand Surg, 1990; 15A:88–91.

14. McGrath MH: Local steroid therapy in the hand. J Hand Surg, 1984; 9A:915–921.

15. McMahon M, Craig SM, Posner MA: Tendon subluxation after DeQuervain's release: treatment by brachioradialis flap. J Hand Surg, 1991; 16:30–32.

16. Minamikawa Y, Peimer CA, Cox WL, Sherwin FS: DeQuervain's syndrome: surgical & anatomical studies of the fibro-osseous canal. Orthopedics, 1991; 14:545–549.

17. Stanley D, Conolly WB: Iatrogenic injection injuries of the hand and upper limb. J Hand Surg, 1992; 17B:442–446.

18. Viegas S: Trigger thumb of DeQuervain's Disease. J Hand Surg, 1986; 11A:235–237.

19. White GM, Wieland AJ: Symptomatic palmar tendon subluxation after surgical release for DeQuervain's disease: A case report. J Hand Surg, 1984; 9A:704–706.

20. Witczak JW, Masear VR, Meyer RD: Triggering of the thumb with DeQuervain's stenosing tendovaginitis. J Hand Surg, 1990; 15A:265–268.

21. Witt J, Pess G, Gelberman RA: Treatment of DeQuervain's tenosynovitis. A prospective study of the results of injection of steroids and immobilization in a splint. J Bone Joint Surg, 1991; 73A:219–222.

GARY R. KUZMA

71

Extensor Tendon Grafts in Zones 1 to 4

Injuries to the extensor mechanism over the dorsum of the finger from the tip to the level of the metacarpophalangeal joint are commonly encountered in hand surgery.[2] The extensor tendon in zone 1 through zone 4 is thin and is balanced by multiple connections between intrinsic and extrinsic components. The extensor hood mechanism virtually surrounds the proximal phalanx and injury at this level rarely disrupts the extensor mechanism completely.

From zone 1 over the distal interphalangeal joint (DIP) joint to zone 3 over the proximal interphalangeal (PIP) joint, the extensor tendon is smaller and more vulnerable to complete disruption. The treatment of acute injury in these zones is straightforward and generally yields acceptable results. Those injuries with loss of tendon substance, e.g. Doyle type 3 mallet injury, that are neglected or inadequately treated can result in imbalance of the extensor mechanism. Loss of conjoint tendon continuity in zones 1 or 2 results in increased tensile forces in the medial oblique fibers of the lateral bands to the central slip. This force hyperextends the PIP joint while allowing the unopposed flexion force of the flexor digitorum profundus at the DIP joint. These two deforming forces eventuate in the characteristic swan-neck deformity of the finger.[4,10]

A similar loss of continuity of the central slip at zone 3 also produces an extensor hood imbalance. In this situation, the force of the central slip is transferred to the intact lateral bands via the lateral slips of the central tendon. Forces are then concentrated on DIP joint extension by both intrinsic and extrinsic motor units. Unchecked this will progress to hyperextension of the DIP joint and flexion of the PIP joint as changes in the retaining ligaments of the extensor hood occur. This Boutonniere deformity may be either supple or fixed.[4,10]

■ HISTORY OF THE TECHNIQUE

The treatment of acute injury to the extensor tendons in zones 1 to 4 is presented in part II. The technique of primary grafting is most commonly reserved for reconstructive procedures. I personally have used the technique in the acute situation where there has been loss of tendon substance and skin coverage can be provided with local flap coverage. This allows single stage reconstruction of the hood (Fig. 71–1). More commonly, skin coverage is provided initially, and tendon grafting is performed at a secondary stage.

If primary treatment is unsuccessful or the patient does not seek medical attention, delayed reconstruction with a tendon graft may be considered. Grafting also may have an important role in the reconstructive treatment of burns involving the extensor mechanism.[7]

The prerequisites for primary extensor tendon reconstruction with tendon grafts are the same for any primary tendon grafting procedure.[10] Passive range of motion must be complete or acceptable and joints supple. The skin must be adequate and abundant enough to allow joint flexion. Tissue equilibrium may require 6 to 8 weeks after the initial injury to stabilize. Sensation in the reconstructed finger must be adequate; preferably at least one digital nerve should be intact. Intrinsic muscles must be functioning.

As important to extensor function as skin coverage is bone coverage. The bone must

■ INDICATIONS AND CONTRAINDICATIONS

■ FIGURE 71–1
A 20-year-old man experienced this grinder injury to his index finger with loss of skin and the terminal slip. Repair was provided with a primary flap and graft using half of the radial lateral band.

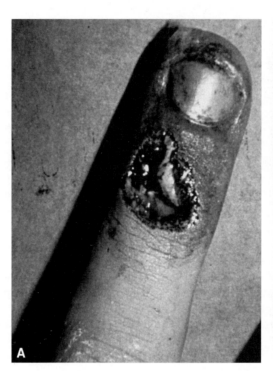

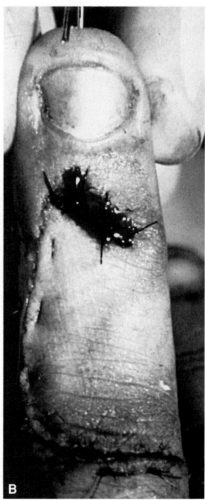

have intact dorsal periosteum to allow adequate tendon glide and excursion. In cases with loss of skin, flap reconstruction may be necessary to provide adequate tissue depth for this purpose. Preparatory splinting to relieve joint contracture must be complete and joint motion free and full.

Where joints have been exposed, the risk of infection should be minimized by adequate initial treatment. No infection should be present. If initial injury has resulted in or primary treatment has not prevented an infection, it must be adequately treated and eradicated. The tissues must then be allowed time to mature and reach equilibrium. In this situation several months of waiting may be required. The existence of a joint infection is an absolute contraindication to proceeding with this operation.

■ SURGICAL TECHNIQUES

The selection of donor tendon is dependent on the recipient tendon, in this case a thin, small sheet of tendinous expanse. As a consequence, only a portion of palmaris longus, the thickness of a no. 1 catgut suture, a slip of the extensor digitorum communis of the ring or the extensor digiti quinti have been recommended. I also have used the radial half of the radial lateral band for graft.

The procedure can be done under regional anesthesia. However, some benefit may be gained by using local anesthesia to allow mobility and to more accurately assess balance of the extensor components intraoperatively. A bloodless field and loupe magnification facilitate the procedure.

Basically there are two techniques that will be reviewed in this chapter. The first repair technique presented is useful for reconstruction in zones 1 and 2.[4–6,8,9] The second technique is used for zones 3 and 4 extensor tendon primary graft reconstructions.[1,3–10]

The extensor mechanism is approached through a dorsal hockey stick incision with a transverse limb over the DIP joint and a longitudinal limb proceeding proximally along the lateral border of the digit to the level of the PIP joint. This flap is elevated to expose the scarred extensor mechanism. The adhesions to the tendon are lysed. This scar to the terminal stump may be preserved or excised depending on its nature.

The graft is harvested from the palmaris longus via small transverse incisions over the desired length. This can be done with a wire used like a cheese cutter or by partial incision and stripping with a tendon passer. The length of the tendon graft needed is best appreciated by proceeding with the dissection of the site to be grafted until the scar and tendon are prepared. The diameter of the graft is equivalent to a large suture only. If the finger extensor is used, transverse or straight incisions may be utilized. The entire slip, unless very narrow, should not be harvested. The stump is repaired to an adjoining tendon slip to prevent any extensor lag to the donor finger. The lateral band portion can only be used in the situation where a small graft is necessary because adequate lateral band length may not be available. The length of the graft necessary varies between 7 and 10 cm. The donor site is closed in the usual manner.

If adequate tendon remains attached to the dorsal rim of the distal phalanx, this may be used for the distal anchor of the tendon graft. The graft can be threaded onto a free needle as if a suture. The needle should be small, round and fully curved with a large eye trochar point, and heavy body (Ferg ½ Tapper—244222). Alternatively, or if there is no adequate stump remaining, the tendon graft can be anchored through a drill or burr hole in the distal phalanx. Great care must be exercised during this step to maintain an adequate bone bridge and to avoid injury to the proximal nail matrix. The graft is passed with the aid of a fine wire of 30 or 32 gauge folded over the tendon end. This is folded over on itself to form a U. It is passed through the drill hole. The graft is put into the closed end of the U which is squeezed over the graft. The wire is then pulled through the drill hole.

The two graft ends are then brought back over the joint. It is woven through the scar, if retained, and then woven separately into each sound lateral band tendon, with each end of the graft woven separately into each good lateral band. The tension is adjusted to maintain the desired position of the distal interphalangeal joint. The position desired is comparable to the position of the adjacent fingers when the wrist is placed in flexion and extension. The graft is then fixed in this position with figure of 8, 4-0 nonabsorbable suture (Fig. 71–2). The scar in the tendon gap does not have to be removed. The proper tension is necessary so that flexion and extension is obtained at follow-up, and the graft does not tear loose. The triangular ligament is reconstructed by suturing the proximal portion of the graft together.

I prefer to protect the repair by transfixing the DIP joint in full extension with a 0.028 K-wire at this point. The skin is closed following hemostasis. This is done using 5-0 nylon horizontal mattress sutures. A compressive dressing and splint is then applied.

Surgical preparation of the patient up to the point of surgical incision is the same for grafting in zones 3 and 4 as for grafting in zones 1 and 2. The incision is an S-shaped dorsal incision beginning over the middle phalanx distally. The distal limb can be radial or ulnar. It is then carried transversely across the PIP joint to the opposite side of the finger over the proximal phalanx. The flaps are then deepened taking care to protect the underlying extensor hood.

The components of the extensor hood and scar in the intervening gap are isolated. The adhesions to the functional tendon are lysed. The lateral band may have to be mobilized from the sides of the PIP joint.

The distal attachment for the graft is again prepared first. Similar to the attachment

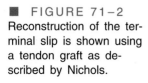

■ FIGURE 71–2
Reconstruction of the terminal slip is shown using a tendon graft as described by Nichols.

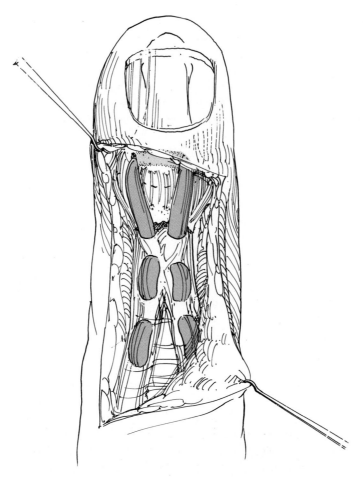

of the graft at the DIP joint, the fixation to the base of the middle phalanx may be through a drill hole or into the remnant of the central slip if it is substantial enough to accept a pass of the graft.

The proximal limbs of the graft are then woven through the scar or the remaining normal central tendon (Fig. 71–3). This is done again with the use of the free needle. The graft is woven in a criss-cross manner into the substance of the remaining central tendon. The lateral bands are not included in the repair and are not drawn over the dorsum of the PIP joint. Tension is adjusted as described for zones 1 and 2. The graft is sutured with 4-0 nonabsorbable suture. The integrity of the repair is confirmed and the PIP joint is transfixed in full extension with a 0.035 K-wire to protect the reconstruction. Hemostasis is confirmed and skin closure performed with horizontal mattress suture of 5-0 nylon (Fig. 71–3).

The reconstruction is dressed and splinted with the wrist in extension. Splinting should also support the PIP joint, but the DIP joint need not be included.

■ REHABILITATION

Pins are maintained for 3 weeks and are then removed. Full-time joint support is maintained for 3 more weeks with either static (zones 1 and 2) or dynamic splinting (zones 3 and 4). After this period, the splint is weaned over a 3-week period. This is accomplished by allowing full activity for 4 hours a day for 1 week, then 8 hours a day for 1 week, and then using the splint at night only. This allows a gradual resumption of force and

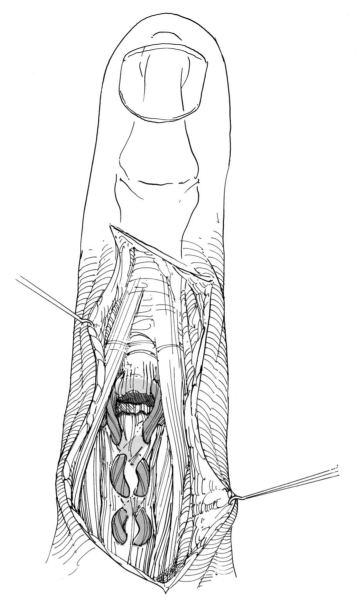

■ FIGURE 71–3
Nichols' technique for reconstruction of the central
slip using tendon graft is
schematically depicted.

increasing activity to be applied to the reconstruction. PIP joint protection in the weaning period can be provided by using a finger-based dynamic extension splint. These splints should allow freedom of movement of the PIP joint when treating zones 1 and 2 reconstructions while the DIP joint is not immobilized when rehabilitating zones 3 and 4 reconstructions.

■ OUTCOMES

There are a few outcomes reports to rely on when considering the functional results of the extensor tendon grafting procedures. Consequentially, the ability to compare the results of grafting with other methods is virtually impossible. Nichols reported the use of tendon grafts for extensor tendon reconstruction in 12 cases but classifies results only as good or poor. There was only one poor result due to recurrence of the original deformity. This was due to an infection destroying the graft. My own experience with this approach to tendon reconstruction is also limited. My results using grafts however have matched those results of other reconstructive procedures (Fig. 71–4).

■ FIGURE 71–4

The range of flexion and extension at 3 months after reconstruction of the terminal slip using the grafting technique in the patient shown in Figure 1.

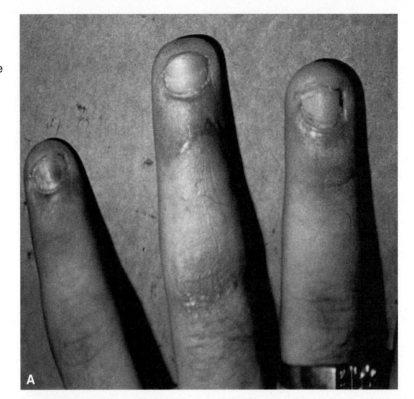

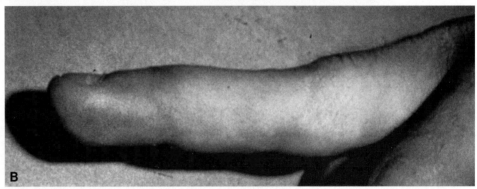

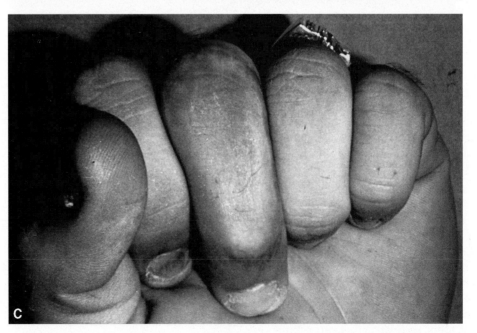

References

1. Aiche A, Barsky AS, Weiner DL: Prevention of the boutonniere deformity. Plastic Reconstructive Surgery, 1970; 46:164–167.
2. Blair WF, Steyers CM: Extensor tendon injuries. Orth Clin North Am, 1992; 23:141–148.
3. Fowler SB: Editorial: The management of tendon injuries. J Bone Joint Surg, 1959; 41A:5 79–80.
4. Littler JW: The digital extensor-flexor system. In: Converse JM (ed): Reconstructive Plastic Surgery, Philadelphia: W.B. Saunders 1977:3166–3214.
5. Lluch AL, Maddew JW: Tendon ruptures of the upper extremity. In: Jupiter J (ed): Flynn's Hand Surgery, Baltimore: Williams and Wilkins, 1991:262–282.
6. Nichols HM: Repair of extensor tendon insertions in the fingers. J Bone Joint Surg, 1951; 33A: 836–841.
7. Rico AA, Tolguin DH, Vecilla LR, del Rio JL: Tendon reconstruction for post burn boutonniere deformity. J Hand Surgery, 1992; 17A:862–867.
8. Tubiana R: Surgical repair of the extensor apparatus of the finger. Surg Clin North Am, 1968; 48:1015–1031.
9. Van Der Meulen JC: The treatment of prolapsed and collapse of the proximal interphalangeal joint. Hand, 1972; 4:154–162.
10. Zancolli EA: Pathology of the extensor apparatus of the finger. In: Zancolli EA (ed): Structural and Dynamic Basis of Hand Surgery, Philadelphia: J.B. Lippincott, 1979:64–105.

$$\overline{72}$$

Primary Extensor Grafts in Zones 5 to 7

Injuries to the dorsum of the hand and wrist in zones 5, 6, 7, or zones 3, 4, and 5 of the thumb can require more than a simple repair of the transected extensor tendons. The loss of tendon substance may prevent primary approximation of the tendon ends. Some of the causes that have been associated with spontaneous rupture and associated loss of substance of extensor tendons are tuberculosis, rheumatoid arthritis, Colles' fracture, occupation, positive ulnar variance, Madelung's deformity, osteoarthritis of the wrist, and rotational trauma. Other injuries that may result in tendon substance loss are third degree burns to the dorsum of the hand, severe infections with tissue loss, abrasions of the skin, subcutaneous tissues and tendons, crush injuries with tissue necrosis, degloving injuries, neglected lacerations, and subcutaneous extravasation of caustic intravenous solutions.

After laceration or rupture, myostatic contracture also can impair direct approximation. Irreversible myostatic contracture can develop as early as 10 days (personal experience) or as late as 48 months after injury.[4,7,10] With the loss of tendon substance or myostatic contracture, a tendon graft may be warranted. As early as 1956, Bunnell advocated the use of grafts to treat extensors tendon deficits.[4] He used photographs to document results in the extensor digitorum communis, abductor pollicis longus, extensor pollicis brevis, extensor carpi ulnaris, extensor digiti quinti proprius, extensor indicis proprius, and extensor pollicis longus.[4]

■ INDICATIONS AND
CONTRAINDICATIONS

The use of tendon grafts to bridge deficits in zones 5, 6, 7 for the hand and wrist, and zones 3, 4, and 5 for the thumb is an effective way of restoring function to the injured hand.[9] The operation is simple enough, provided the basic principles of hand surgery are met before restoration of full finger and thumb extension and flexion and the ability to make a full strong fist. The tendon graft must be placed in a healthy environment of skin and subcutaneous tissue. In post-traumatic conditions, extensor tendon reconstruction may have to be done after or concurrently with coverage. The intercalated graft must glide without adhesions, be held in place by the retinacular system, and be attached to a muscle-tendon unit that is strong enough to move the joint it is supposed to act upon. Any associated unstable fractures must be stabilized before the tendon operation. Infections, burns, or disease processes must be controlled or eliminated before performing the tendon graft surgery. The metacarpophalangeal (MP) joints must remain supple, and they should be splinted as close to 90° as possible to keep the collateral ligaments properly stretched. It may be necessary to pin the MP joints with 0.45 K wires if the position of function cannot be maintained until the tendon grafts are used.

■ SURGICAL
TECHNIQUES

Quality soft tissue coverage on the dorsum of the hand is a prerequisite of primary extensor tendon reconstruction. However, it is not within the scope of this chapter to discuss the details of the many flaps that can be used to cover deficits in the dorsum of the hand. Sometimes the area of deficit will be too large to take advantage of local tissue transfer. The distant flaps of skin and subcutaneous tissue have included the upper arm, thorax, abdomen, flank and groin. One advantage of these flaps is that the injured dorsum of the hand can be transported to the donor site. Although these distant flaps tend to be more bulky than local tissue, they provide similar tissue for further procedures. Disadvantages include the following: (1) they will require at least two procedures, one to inset the flap and another to separate it from the donor site when mature; (2) the mobility of the MP joints may be compromised especially in older individuals; (3) they leave a donor scar; (4) they are dependent and cause edema; and (5) they will most likely need debulking surgery at a later date.

There are numerous potential sources of donor tendon for grafting. The palmaris longus, the ulnar half of the extensor digiti quinti proprius, the ulnar slip(s) of the abductor pollicis longus, the extensor indicis proprius and the flexor digitorum superficialis are the local tendon graft sources in the hand and forearm, mentioned in order of preference. The palmaris longus is present in 85% of the population and, if present, can easily be palpated. It can provide up to 16 cm of tendon graft. The extensor digiti quinti proprius always has two tendon slips. Through small step-cut incisions on the dorsum of the hand, including the portion under the fifth dorsal compartment, the ulnar half can provide up to 12 cm of tendon graft with no residual extension deficit to the fifth MP joint. The dorsal sensory branch of the ulnar nerve crosses the tendon approximately 1 centimeter distal to the ulnar styloid and must not be injured. The abductor pollicis longus can have as many as seven extra tendon slips.[13] The radial-most slip is the largest and inserts at the base of the first metacarpal. The other slips insert into the thenar muscles at the base of the thumb and can be taken by elevating flaps through a transverse incision just distal to the radial styloid. Care should be taken to avoid injuring the superficial branch of the radial nerve which is located just on top of the tendon. The extra slips can provide up to 8 cm of graft if the first dorsal compartment is released. There is no deficit to the hand if these slips are taken.

The plantaris tendon, the long extensors of the toes, the independent fifth toe extensor[1] and the tensor fascia lata are potential sources of tendon graft from the lower extremity.

Except for tensor fascia lata, all the tendon grafts mentioned above should be sutured to the distal tendon end using the Kessler single or double knot grasping suture.[8] A 4-0 nonabsorbable-type suture should be used for the distal repair. The repair should be reinforced with a running 6-0 atraumatic epitenon suture. The Halstead[17] running suture not only everts the epitenon but adds strength to the repair. A noncutting needle should be used for the epitenon repair so as not to fray the tendon graft and tendon ends. If the distal repair is over the MP joints where the distal tendons may be more flat, then two figure-of-eight type sutures with an atraumatic 4-0 nonabsorbable braided suture should be used. The proximal repairs should be completed last. Before suturing the proximal ends of the tendon, graft, the wrist should be placed in as much dorsiflexion as possible, with the MP joints in maximum flexion, as wrist tenodesis will help extend the MP joints.

When both repairs are finished, the tourniquet should be released and the wrist flexed and extended to see that wrist tenodesis will flex and extend the digits. Meticulous hemostasis should be achieved and the wound closed.

Xeroform or Adaptic dressings are placed over the incisions so the two or three sterile 4- × 4-inch gauze dressings will not stick to the wound. Then, a 3-inch sterile Webril should be wrapped smoothly around the forearm, wrist and fingers; four sets of plaster slabs, with each set containing five 3- × 15-inch slabs, are then wet, and each set of five is applied individually, two on the dorsum and two on the palmar side of the extremity, leaving just the fingertips exposed. Next, one layer of wet 3-inch Kling is wrapped around the plaster to hold it in place. The cut end can be secured to the plaster with a small 3- × 3-inch "patch" of one layer of plaster. Since the grafts were placed with the wrist in dorsiflexion and the MP joints in maximum flexion, the wet slabs can be molded into the position of function, with the wrist in about 30° of dorsiflexion and the MP joints at about 70°. Care should be taken so the dorsal and palmar slabs do not touch on the ulnar or radial side. This is very important because if the patient experiences undue postoperative pain, the dressing may have become a constricting tourniquet, and it can be easily split down either side to relieve pressure. In this case, even the soft Webril should be split. Once split, an Ace wrap can be gently applied to hold the slabs together. Patients are seen in the office 3 to 4 days after surgery for application of postoperative dynamic extension splints.

Frequently, the nature of the injury to the dorsum of the hand is such that primary insertion of Silastic rods at the time of flap coverage may be necessary. They are placed under the flap using the same principles as for reconstructive flexor tendon surgery. After 3 months, the rods are replaced with the tendon grafts. Stern and co-authors[16] described such a case; however, the traditional treatment for these contaminated, devitalized wounds is to debride them until the base can accept a flap without the danger of infection.

It may be more prudent to place the rods under the flap once the flap has been detached from the donor site. This requires a different technique. Once the flap has matured on the dorsum of the hand, small incisions are made over the MP joints that are missing tendons. Then a blunt hemostat is passed from distal to proximal under the flap to the area of the proximal cut end of the tendon. A separate tunnel is then made for each Silastic rod. The Silastic rods are sutured to the distal cut ends of the extensor tendons with two to three figure-of-eight sutures, using a 4-0 braided nonabsorbable suture. The proximal ends are left free next to the tendon, which will motor the grafts. Next the wounds are closed and a soft dressing is applied. Postoperatively, the MP joints must be kept supple.

After 3 months, tendon grafts replace the Silastic rods. In this case, the tendon grafts should be longer than the Silastic rods because the proximal ends will have to be brought together and woven to the motor unit. Therefore, a palmaris longus, independent fifth toe extensor or plantaris tendon are the best sources for the longer tendon grafts demanded by this situation. The extensor carpi radialis brevis, brachioradialis, pronator teres and flexor digitorum superficialis can all be used to motor the extensor digitorum communis.

Additionally, the suture technique is different. The distal anastomosis are sutured to the distal tendon with two or three figure-of-eight nonabsorbable 4-0 braided sutures using an atraumatic needle. The second dorsal compartment is opened, exposing the extensor carpi radialis longus and brevis. The extensor carpi radialis brevis, to be used as a motor, is taken from the base of the third metacarpal. Each tendon graft is woven through the distal tendon once (Fig. 72–1). Tension is placed by placing the wrist in 30° of dorsiflex-

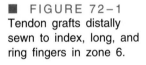
■ FIGURE 72–1
Tendon grafts distally sewn to index, long, and ring fingers in zone 6.

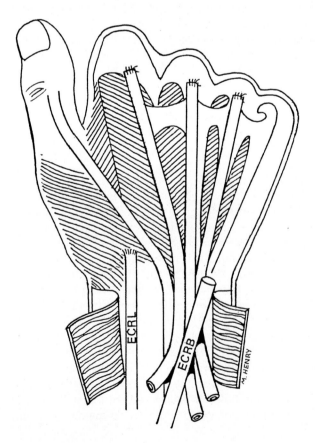

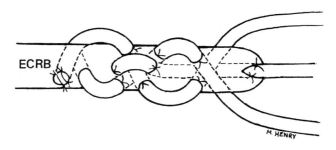

■ FIGURE 72–2
Tendon grafts woven to extensor carpi radialis brevis motor.

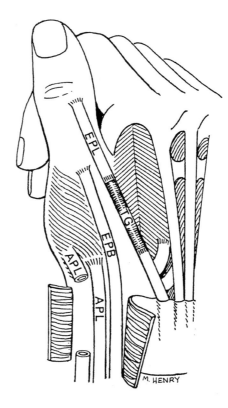

■ FIGURE 72–3
Diagram of a 3-cm abductor pollicis longus ulnar slip, used as a tendon graft for the patient in Figure 72–2.

ion with the MP joints at 0° of flexion. Each of the grafts is secured to the extensor carpi radialis brevis with nonabsorbable 4-0 braided sutures. The remainder of the tendon grafts are woven in different planes two more times and then secured with sutures (Fig. 72–2). Next the wounds are closed. Plaster slabs, as previously mentioned, are applied on the dorsum and palmar sides of the forearm, hand, and fingers, on top of sterile dressing and Webril. The fingers are placed in extension at the level of the MP joints with the wrist in dorsiflexion.

Rupture of the extensor pollicis longus had been associated with multiple etiologies,[12,14] and treatment of the extensor pollicis longus with tendon grafts is well documented.[2,4,10,11] In spontaneous ruptures of the extensor pollicis longus and delayed repairs of lacerations, myostatic contracture will occur. I personally have attempted to repair a simple laceration of the extensor pollicis longus at 12 days after injury in zone 3 and failed to approximate the proximal end, which was found in zone 4, to the distal end, which was found in zone 3. A 3-cm tendon graft obtained from the ulnar side of the abductor pollicis longus was sutured to the proximal and distal ends of the tendon (Figs. 72–3 and 72–4). A dynamic extension splint was used for 4 weeks, starting 2 days after the repair.

If the initial cause of the rupture was the result of a previous Colles' fracture, then Lister's tubercle should be rongeured smooth and a pulley reconstructed using the exten-

■ FIGURE 72–4
A, B, Three months after
extensor pollicis longus
repair with a tendon graft
shows good extension
and flexion of the thumb
interphalangeal joint.

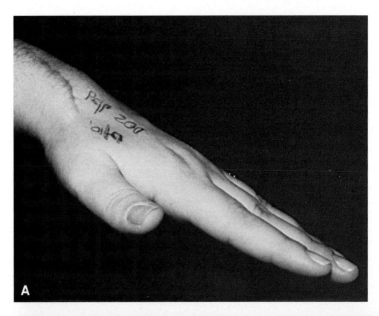

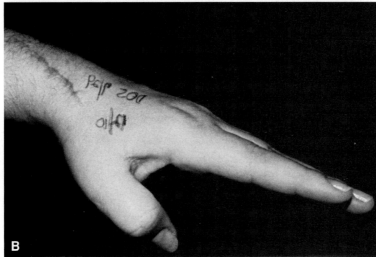

sor retinaculum as described by Saffar and co-authors.[15] The interphalangeal joint of the
thumb's capacity for hyperextension, with the wrist in complete extension, is the test for
a good result.

■ REHABILITATION

Postoperative rehabilitation of all of these repairs has been done with static extension
splinting.[4,7,10] The rehabilitation of extensor tendon injuries to the proximal extensor zones
5 to 7 in the fingers, hand, and wrist, and zones 3 to 5 in the thumb, without grafts, has
been achieved successfully with dynamic extension splinting.[3,5] Chow and co-authors not
only demonstrated that the rehabilitation of extensor tendons with controlled mobilization
gave better results and returned patients to work earlier, but they also showed how controlled mobilization can be successfully used with flexor tendon grafts.[5,6] Extensor tendon
grafts to the proximal zones can be successfully treated by using the 12-week protocol
shown in Table 1. The use of tendon grafts will usually leave a greater extensor lag at the
time the dynamic splint is removed. With time, usually 6 months, the residual extensor
lag is minimal to zero.

■ OUTCOMES

Results of tendon grafts to extensor tendons all have been reported in the literature as
good to excellent. Bunnell provided excellent documentation of results.[4,9] The restoration

TABLE 72-1 EXTENSOR TENDON REHABILITATION PROTOCOL ZONES 4-7

MP Degrees of Active Flexion

WEEK				
1	30			
2		45		
3			60	
4				90
5	Remove splint and begin gentle active flexion.			
6	Remove splint and begin gentle active flexion.			
7	Use of hand for ADL's, no resistance or heavy lifting.			
8	Use of hand for ADL's, no resistance or heavy lifting.			

* After eight weeks—unlimited use of the hand at day 56—Grip Strength Measurement.

of individual extensor tendon function is achieved. However, there are no reported series of tendon grafts in any of the extensor zones that are supported by statistically proven outcomes. From my own experience, an intercalated tendon graft, placed appropriately and followed with good rehabilitation, will yield good function of the repaired extensor tendon.

References

1. Aulicino PL, Ainsworth SR, Parker M: The independent long extensor tendon of the fifth toe as a source of tendon grafts for the hand. J Hand Surg, 1989; 72A:395–396.
2. Boyes JH: Rupture of tendons. Report of four cases of latent rupture of the tendon of the extensor pollicis longus. West J Surg Gyn Obstet, 1935; 43:442–445.
3. Browne EZ, Ribik CA: Early dynamic splinting for extensor tendon injuries. J Hand Surg, 1989; 14A:72–76.
4. Bunnell S. In: Boyes JH (ed): Tendons. In: Surgery of the Hand, 4th ed, Philadelphia: J.B. Lippincott, 1956:459–463.
5. Chow JA, Thomes LJ, Dovelle S, et al. A comparison of results of extensor tendon repair followed by early controlled mobilization vs. static immobilization. J Hand Surg, 1989; 14B:18–20.
6. Chow JA, Thomes LJ, Dovelle S, et al. Controlled mobilization rehabilitation after flexor repair and grafting. J Bone Joint Surg, 1988; 70B:591–595.
7. Hamlin C, Littler WJ. Restoration of the extensor pollicis longus tendon by an intercalated graft. J Bone Joint Surg, 1977; 59A:412–414.
8. Kessler I. The grasping technique for tendon repair. Hand, 1979; 5:253.
9. Kleinert HE, Shepel S, Gill T. Flexor tendon injuries. Surg Clin North Am, 1981; 61:267–280.
10. Magnell TD, Pochron DD, Condit DP. The intercalated graft for treatment of extensor pollicis longus tendon rupture. J Hand Surg, 1988; 13A:105–109.
11. Mason ML. Rupture of tendons of the hand. Surg Gyn Obstet, 1950; 50:611–24.
12. Moore T. Spontaneous rupture of extensor pollicis longus tendon associated with Colles' fracture. Br J Surg, 1936; 23:721–726.
13. Muchart RD. Stenosing tenovaginitis of abductor pollicis longus and abductor pollicis brevis at the radial styloid (DeQuervain's disease). Clin Orthop
14. Redden JF. Closed acute traumatic rupture of extensor pollicis tendon—a report of two cases. Hand, 1976; 8:173–175.
15. Saffar P, Fakhoury B. Secondary repair of the extensor pollicis longus. Ann de Chir de la Main, 1987; 6:225–229.
16. Stern PJ, Amin AK, Neale HW. Early joint and tendon reconstruction for a degloving injury to the dorsum of the hand. Plast Reconst Surg, 1983; 72:395–396.
17. Wade PJF, Wetherell RG, Amis AA. Flexor tendon repair: significant gain in strength from the Halsted peripheral suture technique. J Hand Surg, 1989; 14B:232–235.

MARY LYNN
NEWPORT

73

Staged Extensor Grafts in Zones 5 to 8

■ HISTORY OF THE TECHNIQUE

The hand that requires staged extensor tendon reconstruction has been subjected to a catastrophic injury—one in which there has been a significant injury to or loss of skin and tendon, periosteum and bone, and possibly neurovascular structures. These injuries occur as a result of burns, manufacturing or farm implement mishaps, motor vehicle accidents in civilian life, or shrapnel wounds and high-velocity missile injuries during wartime. Little has been written concerning staged extensor tendon repair.[1,6] Engel first introduced the concept of staged reconstruction for extensor injuries in 1977.[1] This was a result of treating several wartime injuries and was conceived as a direct corollary of staged flexor reconstruction. In fact, Schneider, involved with the development of staged flexor reconstruction,[4] discussed staged extensor reconstruction as well in 1982.[6] Until the widespread acceptance of silicone rubber tendon spacers, most attention after severe extensor injury was directed toward tenolysis or direct tendon grafting with often poor, but accepted, functional results.

Tendon transfers have been a long proven and reliable method for treating extensor loss. They will continue to be a cornerstone of treatment when applicable, but circumstances can mandate more complex, staged reconstruction to provide an adequate foundation for extensor tendon gliding and reconstruction.

■ INDICATIONS AND CONTRAINDICATIONS

There are three basic circumstances under which staged extensor tendon reconstruction can be performed. The most common is as a two-stage procedure performed long after the initial trauma. Skin and fractures would now be well-healed, and there would be insufficient extensor function. Here tenolysis has failed or is believed to be inappropriate because of a large area of skin adherence or known extensor loss. If the skin is durable and believed to have good capacity for tendon gliding, tunneling for each silicone rod can be performed. If the skin is of poor quality, it must be replaced with flap coverage during the first reconstructive phase. Silicone rods are placed under the flap during this phase. In rare circumstances, there will be adequate motors capable of transfer but a poor bed. Here tunneling with placement of a silicone rod or flap coverage with silicone rod(s) can be performed in preparation for tendon transfer. The last circumstance used for staged grafting is in the acutely injured hand, where fractures are stabilized and silicone rods are placed under a flap or repaired skin during treatment of the initial trauma in preparation for subsequent tendon grafting.

The principles of staged extensor grafting are similar to those for flexor grafting. First, one must be dealing with a well-vascularized hand, which has at least protective sensibility. Second, bony stability must be achieved through rigidly fixed or healed metacarpal and/or phalangeal fractures. Third, skin coverage must be adequate to allow tendon gliding. This is usually not a significant problem for staged flexor grafting, as this procedure is usually performed because of a scarred flexor sheath and not because of poor skin coverage. In reconstructive hand surgery, however, it is not uncommon to encounter a patient previously treated for severe injuries to the dorsum of the hand by split-thickness skin grafting, with extensor tendons intact or missing. The patient now has thin but reasonably stable skin overlying the dorsum of the hand, but no extensor function. Extensor tenolysis under such circumstances should be considered, especially if there appears to be only one involved tendon or a small area of tendon adhesion. Larger areas of adherence are seldom effectively treated with tenolysis. Thickly grafted areas may be amenable to tunneling and insertion of silicone rods to produce a pseudosheath, but most often this skin should be replaced with a flap capable of better tendon gliding.[2] Lastly, joint mobility should be sufficient enough that restored extensor function will be useful. This may require capsulotomy, collateral ligament excision, or silicone joint replacement for badly destroyed joints.

After the preceding criteria for staged reconstruction have been met, the decision can then be made to embark on the first stage of this rather arduous task. The patient must be able to tolerate medically and, more importantly, psychologically at least two and perhaps more surgical procedures, all of which require significant investment of time and effort in postoperative physical therapy regimens.

In the subacutely injured hand, there should be no evidence of infection, all fractures should be healed, and all joints should be made as supple as possible through therapy.

Once the first stage has been completed, the second stage should be performed when all wounds are completely healed and mature (usually 2 to 3 months), there is adequate motion obtained in interphalangeal (IP) and metacarpophalangeal (MP) joints through surgery and/or therapy, and all fractures appear to be healed or healing. Staged reconstruction should be abandoned or delayed at this point if sufficient joint motion has not been obtained to warrant extensor grafting or, as has been reported, the pseudosheath produced by the silicone rod has itself reconstituted extensor function and a graft is not necessary.

This operation can be done under axillary block or general anesthesia. Under tourniquet control, all scarred, inadequate skin should be sharply excised over the dorsum of the hand in areas that require reconstruction. Periosteum should be left intact if possible. Badly scarred extensor tendons, if present, should be left undisturbed to allow a good gliding surface volar to the tendon grafts, rather than leave raw bone adjacent to the tendon rods. All related procedures should be performed at this time, including hardware removal if indicated, correction of fracture malunion or nonunion, joint mobilization procedures, and silicone joint replacement. Proximal motors should be identified in the most proximal aspect of the wound. If these have been injured and have retracted, they should be placed on maximal stretch and anchored to surrounding soft tissue. If potential motors have not been previously injured, they should be left undisturbed. Flap coverage should be extended proximally if necessary to insure adequate gliding of the proximal suture line. The skin on the dorsum of the forearm, if intact, should be incised longitudinally to identify and deal appropriately with potential motors.

The choice of coverage depends on many factors including the patient's age, joint stiffness, size of defect, and the microvascular expertise of the surgeon. The flap chosen should allow IP and MP joint motion at the outset.[5] The flap should then be inset after silicone rods have been placed over each appropriate metacarpal (Fig. 73–1A and 73-1B). The rods should be 3 or 4 mm in diameter, depending on the size of the hand. They should reach from the distal aspect of extensor tendon loss to 4 to 6 cm proximal to the wrist or several centimeters proximal to the available motor. The rods should be sutured to the distalmost intact portion of the extensor tendon or into the dorsal hood over the MP joint with a nonabsorbable suture such as 4-0 Prolene in a figure-of-eight fashion. If the dorsal hood is thin or attenuated, the rod can be anchored into MP capsule if necessary. If extensor loss extends onto the proximal phalanx, the rod should also extend this far distally and should be sutured to that remnant. The proximal end of the rod(s) should be proximal to the new flap and left free. This will usually be proximal to the extensor retinaculum, if still present. If the retinaculum is present and capable of accomodating rod gliding, it should be preserved. Rods should pass under the retinaculum and into the distal forearm. If the retinaculum is not present, it should not be reconstructed. Wrist motion should be evaluated to make certain that the free edge of the rod does not move distal to the proximal margin of the flap. If this occurs, the rod can ultimately protrude through the flap suture

■ SURGICAL TECHNIQUES

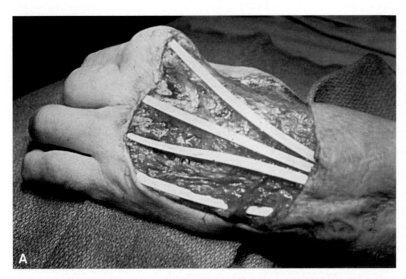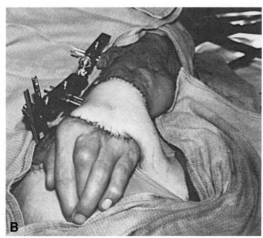

■ FIGURE 73–1

A and B, 24-year-old man who had lost all skin and extensor tendons in the dorsum of hand and forearm in a cotton gin accident. After several debridements, all wounds were covered with split-thickness skin grafts. Extensor reconstruction began 2 years after the initial injury with arthroplasty of the long finger MP joint, silicone rods for the extensors of all fingers, and a groin flap for coverage. A free flap was not possible secondary to loss of veins on the dorsum of the hand and forearm.

line. The rods should glide freely with wrist and MP joint motion. A passive or suction drain under the flap should be used to decrease the risk of hematoma formation. A large, bulky compressive dressing with the wrist in neutral position and the fingers in a safe position should be applied. Finger mobilization should begin as soon as possible after the viability of the flap is assured. This usually begins within a few days after surgery. Wrist motion usually is possible within the first week, depending on flap choice. After adequate maturation of the flap, the hand and wrist are left free or in a dynamic radial nerve splint. Passive wrist and finger range of motion exercises are performed several times hourly.

For the patient who does not need flap coverage, a transverse incision approximately one centimeter proximal to the most prominent aspect of the metacarpal head(s) should be made over the affected fingers, as for MP joint replacements. The dorsal hood over the metacarpal head should be identified. A longitudinal incision should be made overlying the extensor retinaculum. Possible motors for later tendon grafts should be identified and anchored on maximal stretch if necessary. Intact potential motors should be identified but left undisturbed. The appropriate number of subcutaneous tunnels are then made with blunt dissection using a hemostat passed from the proximal wound into the distal wound. The appropriate number and size of silicone rods are inserted and anchored distally into the dorsal hood. These are left free proximally and should extend 4 to 6 cm proximal to the retinaculum. The hand is dressed as above.

For the hand where a gliding tunnel is needed in preparation for a tendon transfer, a sequence as above takes place. The distal transverse incision is made over the metacarpal head(s). The proximal incision should again be over the extensor retinaculum. An appropriate tunnel is bluntly dissected and an appropriate silicone rod inserted. It is attached distally to normal tendon or to dorsal hood and left free proximal to the retinaculum.

In the acutely injured hand with extensor loss, reconstruction can begin immediately if the hand is well perfused, meticulous debridement has been performed and there seems little likelihood of infection, and all fractures have been rigidly stabilized. It is extremely important in the acute situation to identify all potential motors and anchor them on maximal stretch. Here silicone rods can be inserted at the time of skin or flap coverage or after three to four weeks of flap maturation. They are sutured to the distal-most remnant of extensor tendon or to the dorsal hood as above.

The pseudosheaths surrounding the silastic rods generally mature after 2 to 3 months.[2,3] A reasonably reliable indicator of maturation is softening and decreasing erythema at the suture lines. After adequate maturation of flap skin margins and pseudosheath, the proximal and distal skin margins are raised and the appropriate number of grafts brought through the pseudosheaths. Grafts are generally obtained from the plantaris or from the extensor digitorum longus of the second through fifth toes. The tendon graft is attached to the distal or proximal end of the silicone rod and brought into the opposite wound. The modified Kessler or Bunnell technique should be used at the distal suture line into extensor tendon remnant or directly into the dorsal extensor mechanism. Stout nonabsorbable suture material, such as 4-0 Prolene, should be used. Proximally, the appropriate motor is held on maximum stretch and each extensor graft woven into the recipient by the Pulvertaft method with at least two and, preferably three passes. Again, material such as 4-0 Prolene should be used at each point of tendon crossing. The MP joints should be held in 0° flexion and the wrist held in 30° of extension while the grafts are sutured in place. A full, flexed fist with the wrist in approximately 30° extension must be possible at the conclusion of graft suturing. In addition, wrist flexion should bring the MP joints into full extension and wrist extension should produce near full MP joint flexion. If multiple grafts are used, each should be checked as above before the next is placed. This is easily done by placing only one suture in the proximal Pulvertaft weave until proper tension is achieved. After all grafts have been positioned, the tension on all should be rechecked.

Postoperatively, the hand is wrapped in a bulky compressive bandage. The wrist is held statically in 30° of extension and the MP joints in 0° extension, allowing free IP joint motion. Once wounds are stable, usually in 3 to 5 days, a smaller static splint or a dynamic extensor outrigger can be applied. Dynamic splinting is probably preferable. It has been most useful in improving results after primary extensor repair by allowing immediate postoperative gliding of the tendon and it is reasonable to presume it should be most beneficial under grafting circumstances.

The technical alternatives available after extensor tendon loss in zones 5 to 8 are limited. A wrist fusion should be considered in someone unable to undergo or cooperate with a two-stage reconstruction. By arthrodesing the wrist in extension, the hand and wrist are stabilized on the forearm and the hand intrinsics provide finger, but not MP joint function. A spring-loaded splint, which includes the MP joint, is another effective substitution for lost extensors. Intact flexor tendons still function appropriately and the splint returns the wrist and MP joints to a resting, extended position. This is the same splint used for radial nerve palsy. Obviously, neither alternative provides all components for fully effective wrist and finger extension, but may be quite suitable and beneficial for a badly damaged hand where a prolonged two-stage procedure is deemed undesirable or inappropriate.

■ TECHNICAL ALTERNATIVES

Other potential alternatives include use of a silicone rod tunneled under skin of marginal gliding potential for use with later tendon graft, bioprosthesis, or tendon transfer. This would most likely be considered for smaller areas of tendon and skin injury, and would be performed with the knowledge that failure may well occur but could be salvaged with flap reconstruction. Bioprostheses are occasionally used, especially if suitable donors are unavailable or undesirable, but there has not been enough clinical research concerning them to justify their use when tendons of the extensor digitorum longus are adequate.[7] Another potential but not yet well-explored avenue of treatment includes composite grafting of toe extensor tendons and dorsal foot skin as a microvascular free flap based on the dorsalis pedis artery.[2]

Surgical pitfalls accompanying this operation for two-stage extensor tendon reconstruction are numerous. The most common problem is not adequately reconstructing or rehabilitating joints aggressively enough during and after the first stage of reconstruction. It is imperative to achieve as great an arc of motion as possible to help the pseudosheaths mature and provide a skeleton mobile enough to benefit from extensor grafting. Postoperative rehabilitation must be aggressive and unremitting.

Another pitfall during the first stage of reconstruction involves inflammation or infection of the rods. Infection can occur but, as with flexor tendon reconstruction, inflammation presenting as swelling, erythema, and mild or modest pain is far more common. Such a situation is treated with rest, elevation, and careful observation. Once the inflammation recedes, joint motion is gently resumed. Another rod problem can occur when the rod protrudes through the proximal or distal flap or skin suture line. There often is a zone of tenuous skin next to the flap, commonly over the MP joints. Postoperative motion then erodes this tenuous area and the rod protrudes through the suture line. There can be serous drainage or even infection under these circumstances. If the wound cannot quickly be treated and closure obtained with local wound care and decreased motion, the rod should be removed. Two tendon grafts can then be brought down another tunnel during the second stage of reconstruction. Finally, the tunnel must be mature enough to allow good gliding of the tendon graft. This takes a number of months. While no length of time is absolutely reliable, 2 months seems to be the minimum and 3 or 4 months seems best. The wound margins should no longer be swollen, firm, or erythematous.

The last surgical pitfall is one that occurs in all tendon reconstruction, namely, securing the graft under inappropriate tension. In hands already severely injured, it may be particularly difficult to find and maintain appropriate graft tension. The large number of tendon grafts usually used in these circumstances also increases the difficulty of placing each at the appropriate tension. While time-consuming and often frustrating, meticulous attention must be paid to this issue at the second reconstructive step to prevent complications. Even under the best circumstances further intervention, either by graft tenolysis or by shortening the graft, is not uncommon.

■ REHABILITATION

Rehabilitation is, of necessity, a two-stage program. The first stage, after implantation of the silicone rods, must take into account all other aspects of that first stage. Motion must be started as soon as soft tissue healing and bone and joint stability allow. As previously mentioned, this is crucial from the standpoint of overall hand function and pseudosheath formation. Joint range of motion usually begins gently 3 or 4 days after surgery and progressively increases as soft tissue healing allows, usually with full range of motion permitted within the first 2 weeks after surgery.

After extensor tendon grafting is performed during the second reconstructive stage, the hand is removed from the bulky dressing on the third postoperative day. A dynamic extensor outrigger splint made of a thermoplastic is applied. The wrist should be placed in approximately 30° of extension. The MP joints are held in approximately 15° of flexion by a dorsal hood (Fig. 73–2A and 73–2B). The finger IP joints are held in full extension by rubber bands. Exercises are done hourly. If the tendon repair sites are believed to be adequate, 60 to 70° of MP flexion within the splint is allowed. If the repair is tenuous, a volar block can be added to the splint to limit MP flexion as necessary. The dynamic extensor outrigger can be changed to a static splint holding the wrist in 30° extension and MP and IP joints in full extension for bedtime use. Full-time static splinting after tendon grafting can be used but is less likely to allow final full gliding of the tendon grafts within their tunnels and therefore should be avoided if possible. Full-time splinting, either static or dynamic, continues for approximately 6 weeks. Active range of motion is then instituted. Full activities, including heavy lifting, are generally possible 3 to 4 months after tendon grafting.

■ OUTCOMES

The outcome of staged reconstruction for extensor tendon loss is obviously most dependent on the severity of the initial injury. Joint destruction or flexor injury may significantly reduce the quality of result, as measured in joint range of motion. The function of these severely injured hands, however, can be significantly improved by extensor reconstruction if that improves the position of the functional arc of motion.

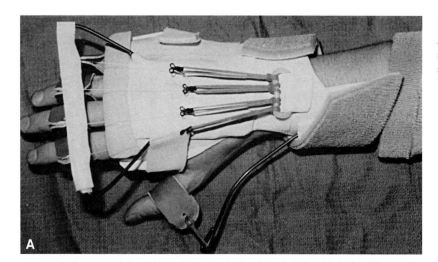

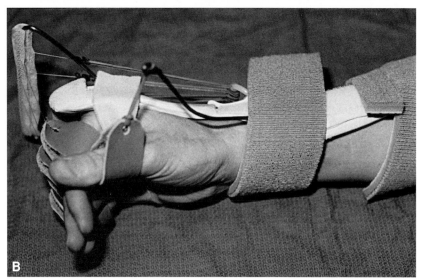

■ FIGURE 73–2

A and B, Dynamic extension outrigger for extensor tendon injuries.

Little has been written concerning the quantitative results of extensor injury, although qualitative results have been described as good.[1,6] Gabel and co-authors, using relatively strict grading criteria, found 44% good or excellent results after traditional two-stage extensor tendon reconstruction, 25% fair results, and 31% poor results in 32 digits. Results were significantly influenced by concomitant MP joint injury, with only one of nine such digits having a good result and the remaining eight fair or poor[3] (presented by Gabel GT, Nunley JA, and Urbaniak JR at the American Society for Surgery of the Hand, Kansas City, MO, 1993).

The ultimate goal of staged extensor reconstruction in zones 5 to 8 is to restore or improve function in, by definition, a badly injured hand. While results may not be quantitatively spectacular, the qualitative results are often gratifying and worth the tremendous investment required.

References

1. Engle J, Tsur C, Farine I, Horoshowsky H: Dorsal silicone rods in the primary care of war injuries. Hand, 1977; 9:153–156.
2. Hentz VR, Pearl RM: Hand reconstruction following avulsion of all dorsal soft tissues. Ann Chir Main, 1987; 6:31–37.
3. Hunter JM, Salisbury RE: Flexor tendon reconstruction in severely damaged hands. A two-

stage procedure using a silicone-dacron reinforced gliding prosthesis prior to tendon grafting. J Bone Joint Surg, 1971; 53A:829–858.

4. Hunter JM, Schneider LH: Staged tendon reconstruction. In: American Academy of Orthopaedic Surgeons Instructional Course Lectures; 26:134–144, 1977.

5. Muhlbauer W, Herndl E, Stock W: The forearm flap. Plast and Recon Surg, 1982; 70:336–344.

6. Schneider LH: Reconstruction in chronic extensor tendon problems. In: Strickland, JW, Steichen, JB (eds): Difficult problems in hand surgery. St. Louis: The CV Mosby Company, 1982:47–53.

7. Smith DJ Jr., Jones CS, Hull M, Robson MC, Kleinert HE: Bioprosthesis in hand surgery. J Surg Res, 1986; 41:378–387.

74

GUY D. FOULKES

Conjoint Tendon Advancement for Mallet Deformity

Surgical reconstruction of the chronic mallet finger is problematic. In 1930, Mason[9] advocated operative reapproximation of the proximal terminal tendon to the distal terminal tendon stump and capsule for patients who had failed conservative therapy. He credited Kanavel with the concept of a step-cut recession of the terminal tendon. After World War II, Pulvertaft[13] demonstrated "remarkable" results following shortening of the dorsal expansion. In 1957, Pratt and co-authors[12] suggested an "internal splint" consisting of a Kirschner wire crossing both interphalangeal joints: the proximal interphalangeal (PIP) joint was thus held in 60° of flexion and the distal interphalangeal (DIP) joint in "slight hyperextension" for 4 to 5 weeks. Although these authors claimed successful resolution of the mallet finger in 75 consecutive cases, no mention is made of the results in the PIP joint using this technique. Kaplan[7] later condemned flexion of the PIP joint, preferring a joint held in "moderate extension."

Although a host of surgical interventions have been proposed,[6–13] Garberman and co-authors[5] have demonstrated that splintage is effective, even in patients who seek treatment after as many as 17 weeks.

Doyle[3] has classified mallet fingers as follows:

Type I: Closed injury with loss of tendon continuity with or without a small avulsion fracture.

Type II: Laceration of the terminal or conjoint tendon.

Type III: Deep abrasion with loss of skin, subcutaneous tissue, and tendon.

Type IV: (A) Transepiphyseal fracture in children; (B) Hyperflexion injury with 20 to 50% articular surface fracture; (C) Hyperextension injury with over 50% articular surface fracture and volar subluxation of the distal phalanx.

■ HISTORY OF THE TECHNIQUE

The indications for conjoint tendon advancement for chronic mallet finger are few. Even established mallet finger, whether due to late presentation or to failed attempts at conservative therapy, deserve consideration of splintage. I treat both acute and chronic mallet finger with a minimum of 6 weeks of continuous splinting of the DIP joint, followed by 2 weeks of night splinting. I generally prefer a dorsal alumifoam splint holding the DIP in slight hyperextension, but also have used the bulkier Stack splint, which only can achieve neutral extension. Meals has recently developed the Mallet Mender, a form-fitting, custom-molded orthosis (Figs. 74-1A to 74-1D).

Indications for conjoint tendon advancement in mallet finger include a symptomatic patient who has failed conservative therapy using the above regimen. Patients treated for a shorter period of time, or those with demonstrated noncompliance with splinting, constitute a relative if not absolute contraindication to operative intervention. I counsel my patients that a DIP fusion is the most reliable solution to the recalcitrant or recurrent mallet finger. Patients who have concomitant swan-neck deformity are best served by an oblique retinacular ligament reconstruction.[1] Dorsal skin loss or active infection are contraindications to surgical correction. Patients with Type III mallet fingers require a skin coverage procedure and DIP fusion, because the likelihood of regaining active gliding of the conjoint tendon under scar or graft is small and would require at least two separate procedures.

■ INDICATIONS AND CONTRAINDICATIONS

■ FIGURE 74–1
The Mallet Mender, a custom-molded orthosis designed by Roy A. Meals, M.D., and manufactured by George Tiemann & Company. This device is waterproof and can hold the DIP joint at any angle. After microwave heating in water **(A)**, the orthosis can be applied to fit the individual DIP joint **(B)**. Once cooled, the orthosis is form-fitting, low profile, and well-tolerated by the patient **(C and D)**.

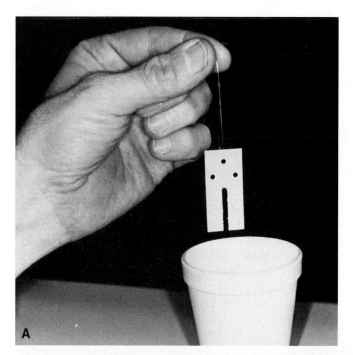

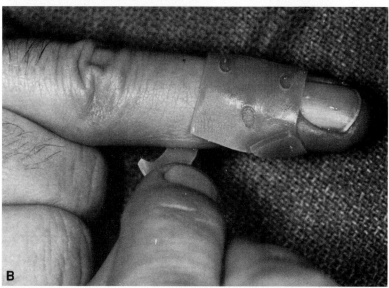

In summary, the *rare* patient to whom I offer conjoint tendon advancement should meet a number of rigid criteria, including a symptomatic mallet finger exceeding 30° of DIP flexion at maximal active extension. The digit should be passively correctable to at least neutral extension and free of swan-neck deformity. There should be normal skin over the DIP joint. The patient should have been compliant with, but failed, a previous adequate splinting regimen. Lastly, the patient should be offered DIP fusion as a therapeutic alternative, especially if the digit is the index or long finger.

■ SURGICAL
TECHNIQUES

Conjoint tendon advancement is performed with the patient in a supine position, using a standard hand table. I prefer intravenous regional (Bier block) anesthesia using a forearm tourniquet, but interdigital block using a 9:1 ratio of 1% plain lidocaine to sodium bicarbonate also is acceptable. Using the latter method, the surgeon should provide a dorsal infiltrative or "ring" block of 2 to 3 ml in addition to 3 to 4 ml in each interdigital space as an intermetacarpal block. Unanesthetized forearm tourniquets can be tolerated by most

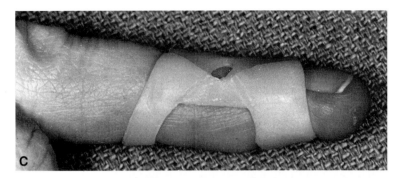

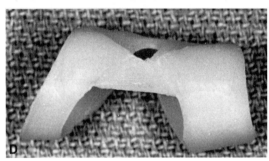

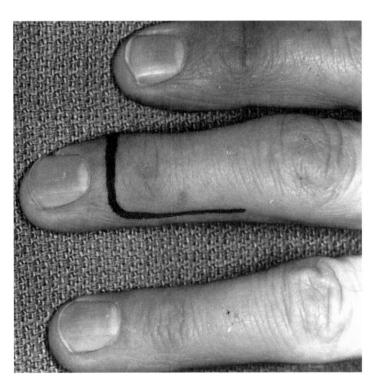

■ FIGURE 74-2
Skin incision for conjoint tendon advancement. Care should be taken to avoid the germinal matrix. The incision is on the ulnar aspect of the index, long, and ring finger and the radial aspect of the small finger.

patients for approximately 30 minutes. If a Penrose drain is used as a finger tourniquet, provide only as much pressure as required for hemostasis.

Using the dorsal distal interphalangeal creases as a guide, a transverse skin incision is created 7 mm proximal to the nail fold, extending from the radial to the ulnar midlateral line. The incision then turns 90° to continue proximally down the midlateral line for a distance of 3 cm (Fig. 74-2). The ulnar midlateral line is used for the index, long, and ring fingers because of its cosmetic advantage. The radial midlateral line should be used on the small finger, to protect the scar from repeated contact.

The neurovascular bundles are volar to this incision and should not be encountered.

The germinal matrix is at risk from either an excessively distal incision or overvigorous dissection or retraction. As the insertion of the terminal tendon is into the dorsal capsule and proximal dorsal lip of the distal phalanx, there should be no reason to dissect in the paronychial region.

A triangular flap is raised, reflected, and temporarily sutured to the contralateral skin. The operation is then modified according to the mechanism of injury (Doyle classification[3]) and operative findings.

If the tendon has *healed in a lengthened position* (Type I without fracture or Type II), the neotendon is resected and the two ends reapproximated with 4-0 nonabsorbable figure-of-eight sutures. Usually no more than 1 to 2 mm is resected[4] (Fig. 74–3A). The neotendon often has a characteristic, slightly translucent appearance without obvious longitudinal collagen fibers. Care should be taken to leave a distal stump, including the DIP joint capsule and lateral periosteal tissue. Although most texts depict the terminal tendon as a narrow, discrete structure, there is often a fan-like expansion of lateral fibers that insert onto the lateral aspects of the distal phalanx, which may be used for additional sutures if care is taken to preserve them (Fig. 74–3B). The dorsal capsule should be incised transversely. This allows inspection of the joint and use of the distal leaf of the capsule to reinforce the suture repair (Fig. 74–3A).

If the mallet is secondary to a *small avulsion fracture* (Type I with fracture), then the small flake of bone can be resected and the procedure is otherwise as described above.

If a large *intra-articular or epiphyseal dorsal fragment* is found (Type IV mallet), any angulation, translocation, or subluxation must first be corrected. This diagnosis should be apparent from the preoperative lateral radiograph and demands accurate reduction and pinning of the DIP joint under direct vision, flouroscopy, or intraoperative radiography. If the dorsal fragment constitutes more than 30% of the articular surface, an open reduction and internal fixation of the fragment to the distal phalanx is perfomed. After reflecting the dorsal fragment with the attached terminal tendon proximally, the cancellous surfaces are first freshened with a fine dental curette. A 26-gauge stainless steel pullout suture is passed through the fragment, and each end is routed around the distal phalanx, perpendicular to the fracture plane, and through the finger pulp to be tied over a padded button.

Skin closure with 5-0 nonabsorbable sutures and a light postoperative dressing allow placement of a volar splint with the DIP in 0° to 10° of hyperextension.

■ TECHNICAL
ALTERNATIVES

The extensor mechanism is an exquisitely balanced structure that appears deceptively simple. Its unique design allows semi-independent extension of three sequential joints

■ FIGURE 74–3
A, Lateral view of conjoint tendon advancement. One to two millimeters of resection will produce 20° to 40° of mallet correction. The distal joint capsule, shown in black, may be used to reinforce the distal stump of the terminal tendon. **B,** Dorsal view of conjoint tendon advancement. Dotted line illustrates initial incision in terminal tendon. Notice that lateral projections of terminal tendon are preserved so that additional sutures may be placed.

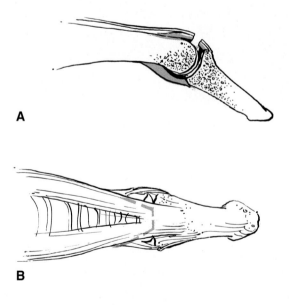

without the need for separate motors as seen on the flexor side of the digits.[1] The disadvantage to this harmonious interdependence is that imbalance at any joint may lead to late deformity of the other joints in the system. Each millimeter of excess length at the terminal tendon translates to 20° of mallet deformity.[2] Any surgeon attempting conjoint tendon advancement must carefully assess the clinical appearance and resting tone of *both* interphalangeal joints before skin closure.

Patients with mallet finger who will not or cannot wear a splint, such as surgeons or dentists, may be managed with an *internal splint,* that is, pinning the DIP joint in neutral for a period of 6 weeks. Pulp scarring or proximal pin migration may be handled by inserting the pin obliquely in the frontal plane as suggested by Tubiana.[14] Pin breakage is a recognized complication of this procedure and may require secondary arthrotomy.

■ REHABILITATION

Patients should be maintained in a volar DIP splint until the dorsal wound permits placement of a dorsal splint (usually when the skin sutures are removed at 10 to 14 days). The splint is continued for 6 weeks, followed by 2 weeks of night splinting. Active PIP motion should not be restricted by the postoperative dressing. Using cadavers, Dagum and Mahoney[2] have shown that motion of the PIP and MP joints have no effect on separation of the terminal tendon in experimental mallet finger, while wrist flexion can produce 0.9 mm of gap in the terminal tendon, which equates to approximately 20° of extensor lag. Failure to immobilize the wrist after mallet finger surgery may be one explanation for the residual postoperative extensor lag reported in many studies.[5,7,10,11]

Using microvascular injection techniques, Warren and co-authors[15] have shown that the area from 11 to 16 mm proximal to the insertion of the terminal tendon is essentially avascular. This may explain the common finding of Type I mallet injuries, especially in the elderly, following trivial or even unrecalled trauma. The biology of this situation can only be worsened through surgical attack, and these findings provide another strong impetus to exhaust conservative options before offering to the patient a surgical remedy.

■ OUTCOMES

No controlled study on conjoint tendon advancement for chronic mallet deformity exists. Garberman and co-authors[5] have shown that splinting is as effective for delayed (up to 17 weeks) as for acute (less than 2 weeks) cases of mallet finger. I believe that surgical rebalancing of the delicate extensor mechanism through chronically scarred tissue is a procedure fraught with difficulty and of uncertain benefit over nonoperative means. In the compliant, well-informed patient who meets all of the criteria presented earlier, however, some degree of functional and cosmetic improvement might be expected. Fortunately, most of the patients I see with chronic mallet finger fall into two main groups: young (post-traumatic) patients who have neglected therapy, and who respond well to a second trial of splinting, and the elderly (attritional rupture) patients, who are generally quite functional despite their deformity and thus not insistent about surgical correction.

References

1. Burton RI: Extensor tendons—Late reconstruction. In: Green DP (ed): Hand Surgery, New York: Churchill Livingstone, 1993:1955–1988.
2. Dagum AB, Mahoney JL: Effect of wrist position on extensor mechanism after disruption separation. J Hand Surg, 1994; 19A:584–589.
3. Doyle JR: Extensor tendons—Acute injuries. In: Green DP (ed): Hand Surgery, New York: Churchill Livingstone, 1993:1925–1954.
4. Elliot RA: Extensor tendon repair. In: McCarthy JG, May JW, Littler JW (eds): Plastic Surgery, Philadelphia: W.B. Saunders, 1990:4565–4592.
5. Garberman SF, Diao E, Peimer CA: Mallet finger:Results of early versus delayed closed treatment. J Hand Surg, 1994; 19A:850–852.
6. Grundberg AB, Reagan DS: Central slip tenotomy for chronic mallet finger deformity. J Hand Surg, 1987; 12A:545–547.
7. Kaplan EB: Anatomy, injuries and treatment of the extensor apparatus of the hand and digits. Clin Orthop, 1959; 13:24–40.

8. Lucas GL: Fowler central slip tenotomy for old mallet deformity. Plast Reconstr Surg, 1987; 80:92–94.

9. Mason ML: Rupture of tendons of the hand: with a study of the extensor tendon insertions in the fingers. Surg Gynecol Obstets, 1930; 50:611–624.

10. Nichols HM: Repair of extensor tendon insertions in the fingers. J Bone Joint Surg, 1951; 33A: 836–841.

11. Niechajev IA: Conservative and operative treatment of mallet finger. Plast Reconstr Surg, 1985; 76:580–585.

12. Pratt DR, Bunnell S, Howard LD: Mallet finger: classification and methods of treatment. Am J Surg, 1957; 93:573–579.

13. Pulvertaft RG: Tendon surgery in the hand. Proceedings of the British Orthopaedic Association, Spring Meeting, 1949. J Bone Joint Surg, 1949; 31B:477.

14. Tubiana R: Surgical repair of the extensor apparatus of the fingers. Surg Clin North Am, 1968 48: 1015–1031.

15. Warren RA, Kay NRM, Norris SH: The microvascular anatomy of the distal digital extensor tendon. J Hand Surg, 1988; 13B:161–163.

75

EDWARD C.
McELFRESH

Central Slip Advancement for Mobile Boutonniere Deformity

One of the earliest reports of the defect of the extensor mechanism, which has come to be known as the boutonniere deformity, was made by Hauck[6] in 1923. Mason[8] wrote in 1930 that a prompt repair of the extensor mechanism ruptured at the proximal interphalangeal joint should be performed with approximation of the lateral bands in the midline distal to the joint. Milch,[9] in 1931, referred to the injury as the "buttonholed" extensor mechanism injury where the central slip is ruptured along with the triangular ligament, allowing the lateral bands to subluxate volarly below the axis of the proximal interphalangeal (PIP) joint. This creates the "buttonhole" defect with the PIP joint protruding between the lateral bands. A characteristic finger deformity results, with the PIP joint flexed and the distal interphalangeal (DIP) joint extended.

Bunnell,[1] in 1942, described repair of the central slip using a figure-of-eight wire suture. In 1959, Kaplan[7] emphasized the importance of repairing as broad an area of the central slip as possible. Souter,[11] in 1962, reviewed the patients of Pulvertaft where the surgical repair had been performed with excision of the fibrous tissue in the area of the central slip and the lateral bands. Elliott[3] gave a detailed analysis of the surgical technique in 1970. Zancolli[13] later emphasized the importance of the release of the oblique fibers of the retinacular ligaments to mobilize the lateral bands. Rothwell[10] pointed out that flexion of the distal interphalangeal joint 45° when the lateral bands are realigned helps prevent loss of the flexion with the boutonniere repair. Grundberg[5] pointed out that you do not have to resect more than 3 mm when the central slip scar is excised.

■ HISTORY OF THE TECHNIQUE

Repair of the boutonniere by advancement of the central slip is indicated if conservative treatment of a mobile deformity fails. The proximal interphalangeal joint indeed must be truly mobile and passively fully extendable. Most boutonniere deformities respond to conservative splinting with minimal residuals. A radiograph showing a central slip avulsion with proximal migration of a bony fragment is an indication for an operative repair of the fracture. AP and lateral radiographs should show an adequate joint space without subluxation or deviation of the middle phalanx. The flexor tendons should be intact and functioning. Age plays a factor; the patient should be younger than 45 years old.

It is important that the boutonniere deformity is not due to joint deformity or the attrition abnormalities seen with rheumatoid arthritis, other collagen disorders, and burns.

The differential diagnosis includes the pseudoboutonniere deformity with joint contracture after avulsion of the proximal end of the volar plate with resultant scarring. Rupture of the A2 and A3 pulleys, as found in rock climbers, may be mistaken for a boutonniere deformity. Dupuytren's contracture in a finger also may present with digital deformity that is similar to a boutonniere.

■ INDICATIONS AND CONTRAINDICATIONS

The operative procedure is performed in the operating room under regional anesthesia. General anesthesia may be used if axillary block or Bier intravenous block is unacceptable. The incision is a dorsal lazy-S over the joint. This gives better exposure than a lazy-C, which theoretically causes less problems with venous drainage. After mobilization of the overlying skin and subcutaneous tissue, inspection of the dorsal apparatus will reveal scarring of the central slip and lateral subluxation of the lateral bands (Fig. 75–1). The

■ SURGICAL TECHNIQUES

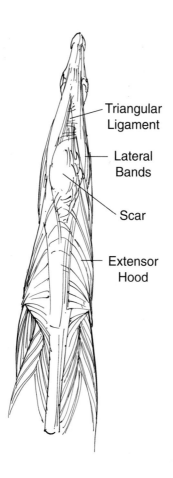

■ FIGURE 75–1
Boutonniere deformity with scarring of the central slip and lateral subluxation of the lateral bands.

Triangular Ligament

Lateral Bands

Scar

Extensor Hood

lateral bands are mobilized from their junction at the distal extent of the triangular ligament to the midportion of the proximal phalanx by releasing the more volar transverse retinacular fibers. The scar overlying the dorsum of the proximal interphalangeal joint is sectioned transversely preserving a cuff of tendon or scar attached to the middle phalanx. Incisions are made along the sides of the central slip, and it is mobilized proximally about half the length of the proximal phalanx (Fig. 75–2). The proximal interphalangeal joint is fixed in full extension by placing a 0.45-mm Kirschner wire obliquely across the joint being sure the pin is below the elevated lateral bands.

The mobilized central slip is advanced by firm traction on the excess scar. Excess scar is excised; usually this does not exceed 3 mm. Repair is performed with 3 or 4 interrupted 4-0 synthetic braided sutures. The knots are buried if possible (Fig. 75–3). A few sutures are then placed in each lateral side of the central slip and the medial edge of the lateral band while holding the distal interphalangeal joint in approximately 45° flexion. A few 4-0 or 5-0 synthetic braided sutures are then placed in the redundant triangular ligament or retinaculum to pull the lateral bands back into a normal position distal to the proximal interphalangeal joint (Fig. 75–4). The tourniquet is released and hemostasis is obtained.

The subcutaneous tissue is closed with interrupted 5-0 absorbable sutures. The skin is closed with interrupted 5-0 nylon sutures. The Kirschner wire is cut and a cap placed on the protruding pin. A dressing and a plaster gutter splint including the adjacent finger is applied holding the wrist in a neutral position and the metacarpophalangeal joint in 20 to 30° flexion. The distal interphalangeal joint is included in the plaster splint and flexed 45°.

■ TECHNICAL ALTERNATIVES

The surgeon must be sure that the patient has full passive extension of the proximal interphalangeal joint preoperatively or the outcome will most likely be less than desired.

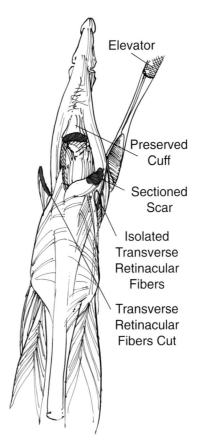

■ FIGURE 75-2
Resection of central slip scar and release of the transverse retinacular ligament.

Elevator

Preserved Cuff

Sectioned Scar

Isolated Transverse Retinacular Fibers

Transverse Retinacular Fibers Cut

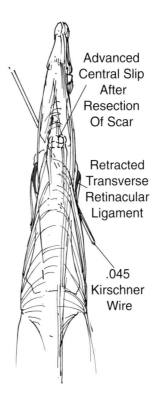

■ FIGURE 75-3
The proximal interphalangeal joint is pinned in extension beneath the lateral bands and the central slip is repaired.

Advanced Central Slip After Resection Of Scar

Retracted Transverse Retinacular Ligament

.045 Kirschner Wire

■ FIGURE 75–4
The lateral bands are brought back and sutured to the central slip. The defect in the triangular ligament is repaired.

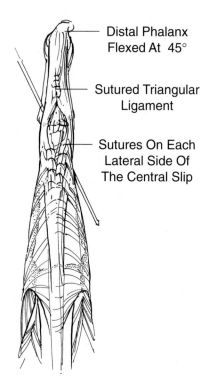

— Distal Phalanx
Flexed At 45°

— Sutured Triangular
Ligament

— Sutures On Each
Lateral Side Of
The Central Slip

Zancolli[13] believes that in cases with retinacular stiffness, the longitudinal cords need to be released by resecting the lateral half of the lateral bands at the level of the middle phalanx base for an approximate 1 cm distance, which effectively releases the oblique retinacular ligaments. If there is insufficient material into which to sew the central slip, small transverse drill holes can be made in the dorsal base of the middle phalanx to secure sutures. Some surgeons also will overlay the central slip rather than excising tissue. If the overlay technique is used, the 3-mm limit for advancement still applies. A terminal tendon release as advocated by Dolphin[2] or Fowler[4] may be more appropriate for the patient older than 45 years of age.

■ REHABILITATION

One week after surgery, mobilization of the distal interphalangeal joint, both actively and passively, is begun under the supervision of a hand therapist. The Kirschner wire through the proximal interphalangeal joint is left in place. The proximal joints at the wrist and metacarpophalangeal joints are mobilized passively. The finger is still splinted in a thermoplastic splint when exercises are not being performed. The splint holds the wrist in a neutral position and the metacarpophalangeal joint in 20° flexion, and includes the pinned proximal interphalangeal joint but leaves the distal interphalangeal joint free.

The Kirschner wire is removed at 6 weeks, and the hand therapist now assists with mobilization of the PIP joint. Active and passive flexion exercises are started and progressed to gentle resistive exercises. Often the PIP joint is mobilized by bending it over a wooden block. Between exercise periods, the PIP joint is splinted in extension for at least 3 more weeks; a spring splint is used during the daytime and a safety-pin splint at night. The hand therapist works with the patient as needed during the first 3 months after surgery.

The goal of hand therapy is to maintain the ability to extend the PIP joint, regain the flexion of the PIP joint, and have full mobilization of the PIP joint. Older patients have a tendency to develop residual stiffness, and Elliott[3] believes that the Kirschner wire should be removed 1 week earlier and hand therapy started if the patient is 45 years of age or older.

Souter[11] reported on 106 digits in 101 patients from Pulvertaft's clinic. These patients underwent a direct surgical repair of the central slip. Of the 60 patients with central slip rupture uncomplicated by fractures or tissue loss, only 14 (23%) obtained good or excellent results. Rothwell[10] and Grundberg[5] reported excellent or good results in 10 and 7 patients, respectively. The ages of the patients in these two series ranged from 11 to 51 years. Rothwell wrote in general terms and only described the two patients with good results. Grundberg did a more careful analysis in which he described each patient's range of motion and final outcome.

Credit should be given to Steichen and co-authors[12] for their thorough evaluation of 35 patients with surgical repair of the mobile boutonniere deformity. Their patients had the type of operation described in this chapter. With the initial evaluation, patients with a mild contracture of 0 to 30° achieved a 65% good or excellent result, patients with 31 to 60° achieved a 27% good or excellent result, and those with more than 60° achieved no good or excellent results. If passive motion was achieved before the operation, 59% had an excellent or good result, but if not, only 8% had an excellent or good result. Age also played a role. In patients younger than 21 years of age, 50% had excellent or good results; whereas only 33% of patients between 21 and 45 years of age had excellent or good results. In patients older than 45 years of age, there were no excellent results and only 20% had good results.

In conclusion, the mobile boutonniere deformity can be successfully treated surgically. The operation described in this chapter, which includes reattachment of the central slip and dorsal mobilization of the lateral bands, can provide very good to excellent results. It is important to splint an early deformity to avoid contracture, to obtain full passive motion preoperatively, and to give careful consideration before indicating this operation for the older patient.

References

1. Bunnell S: Surgery of intrinsic muscles of hand other than those producing opposition of the thumb. J Bone Joint Surg, 1942; 24:1–32.
2. Dolphin JA: Extensor tenotomy for chronic boutonniere deformity of the finger. J Bone Joint Surg, 1065; 47A:161–164.
3. Elliott RA Jr: Injuries to the extensor mechanism of the hand. Orthop Clin North Am, 1970; 1: 335–354.
4. Fowler SB: Extensor apparatus of the finger. J Bone Joint Surg, 1949; 31B:477.
5. Grundberg AB: Anatomic repair of boutonniere deformity. Clin Orthop Rel Res, 1980; 153: 226–229.
6. Hauck G: Die Ruptur die Dorsal Aponeurose am ersten Interphalangeal Gelenk, Zugleich eim Beitrag zur Anatomic und Physiologic der Dorsal Aponeurose. Arch F Klin Chir, 1923; 123:197–232.
7. Kaplan EB: Anatomy, injuries, and treatment of the extensor apparatus of the hand and digits. Clin Orthop Rel Res, 1959; 13:24–41.
8. Mason ML: Ruptures of tendons of the hand. Surg Gynecol Obstet, 1930; 50:611–624.
9. Milch H: Buttonhole rupture of the extensor tendon of the finger. Amer J Surg, 1931; 13: 244–245.
10. Rothwell AG: Repair of the established post traumatic boutonniere deformity. Hand, 1978; 10:241–245.
11. Souter WA: The boutonniere deformity. A review of 101 patients with division of the central slip of the extensor expansion of the fingers. J Bone Joint Surg, 1967; 49B:710–721.
12. Steichen JB, Strickland JW, Call WH, Powell SG: Results of surgical treatment of chronic boutonniere deformity: An analysis of prognostic factors. In: Strickland JW, Steicher JB (eds): Difficult Problems in Hand Surgery, St. Louis: CV Mosby, 1982:62–69.
13. Zancolli E: Structural and Dynamic Basis of Hand Surgery, 2nd ed, Philadelphia: JB Lippincott, 1979:79–92.

THOMAS R.
KIEFHABER

76

Conjoined Tendon Release for Boutonniere Deformity

■ HISTORY OF THE
TECHNIQUE

The boutonniere deformity is comprised of an extensor deficit at the proximal interphalangeal (PIP) joint and a hyperextension deformity of the distal interphalangeal (DIP) joint (Fig. 76–1). The deformity is always initiated by a disruption or attenuation of the central tendon over the PIP joint. The central tendon can be sharply divided by a laceration, ruptured by a hyperflexion injury, or attenuated by chronic synovitis. DIP hyperextension occurs as a secondary effect of the extensor apparatus imbalance. Disruption of the central tendon allows proximal migration of the lateral bands and concentration of all of the extensor force at the DIP joint. Additional tension is added to the terminal tendon by stretching of the palmarly subluxed lateral bands around the broad condyles of the proximal phalanx. In a chronic boutonniere deformity, the lateral bands become foreshortened and adherent in their subluxed position, further accentuating the DIP extension contracture (Fig. 76–2). The physician's attention is frequently directed to the flexed PIP joint but the loss of DIP flexion is often the patient's primary concern.

The terminal tendon tenotomy allows patients to regain DIP flexion by eliminating the hyperextension forces provided by the tightened lateral bands. After tenotomy, DIP extension is achieved through the static tenodesis effect of the oblique retinacular ligament. As a secondary effect of the tenotomy, the distal tether of the lateral bands is released allowing proximal migration of the entire extensor apparatus, subsequent tightening of the central tendon, and some improvement in the PIP extensor deficit.

Fowler is given credit for the original description of the terminal tendon tenotomy,[3,5,7,8] but Dolphin[3] provides the earliest written report of the technique. Fowler,[1] Dolphin,[3] Stern,[8] and Nalebuff[7] all have reported good clinical results after simple division of the terminal tendon proximal to the insertion of the oblique retinacular. Littler[5] modified the procedure by separating the insertion of the lumbrical tendon from the lateral band and preserving it with the oblique retinacular ligament. Tubiana[9] and Curtis[2] have both recommended lengthening of the terminal tendon as an alternative to complete division. Surgeons describing central tendon reconstructions have recognized the importance of restoring DIP flexion in addition to correcting the PIP extensor deficit and have recommended concurrent terminal tendon tenotomy or lengthening.[4,6] The simple terminal tendon tenotomy is effective and predictable and will be described in this chapter.

■ INDICATIONS AND
CONTRAINDICATIONS

Restoration of DIP flexion is the primary indication for terminal tendon tenotomy. Patients should be willing to accept the existing PIP extensor deficit and clearly understand that the purpose of the procedure is to improve DIP flexion. The procedure is most helpful after a traumatic disruption of the central tendon that has left the patient with a 30° or less PIP extensor deficit and an inability to attain full active and passive DIP flexion. Contraindications include radiographic evidence of significant damage to the DIP joint surface, secondary to post-traumatic or inflammatory arthritis, incompetence of the profundus tendon, or extensive soft tissue scarring over the DIP joint.

A small improvement in the PIP extensor deficit may be a secondary, although unpredictable, effect of the procedure and will only occur if the joint demonstrates full passive extension. The maximum expected correction of PIP extension by terminal tendon tenotomy is 20°.[2] Correction of larger deficits requires a formal reconstruction of the central tendon.

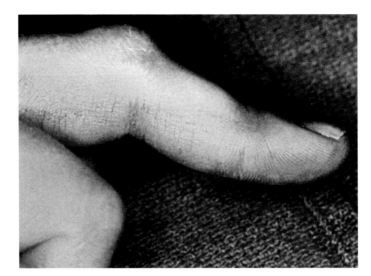

■ FIGURE 76-1

A typical boutonniere deformity is noted in this digit with an extensor deficit at the PIP joint and a hyperextension deformity of the DIP joint. The patient demonstrated full passive extension of the PIP joint but was limited to 5° of active DIP flexion.

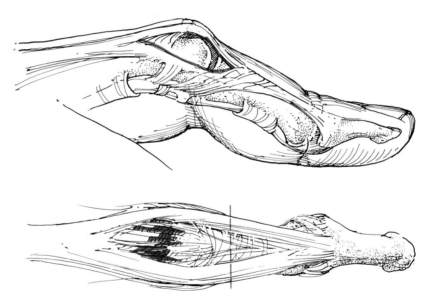

■ FIGURE 76-2

A and B, The boutonniere deformity is initiated by disruption of the central tendon and followed by palmar subluxation of the lateral bands. The increased tension in the lateral bands contributes to DIP hyperextension. In chronic deformities, DIP flexion is further limited by adhesions of the lateral bands and contracture of the oblique retinacular ligament.

■ SURGICAL TECHNIQUES

Terminal tendon tenotomy should be performed under local anesthesia so that active range of motion can be tested and full correction assured. A metacarpal block leaves the intrinsic musculature fully functional and is preferable to more proximal neuromuscular blockade. Intravenous sedation is used to calm the anxious patient.

After instillation of the anesthetic, the upper extremity is thoroughly scrubbed, prepared, and draped in the standard fashion. A Penrose drain applied to the base of the proximal phalanx is used as a tourniquet. A sterile pediatric tourniquet at the distal forearm is an alternative method of maintaining hemostasis although this device induces flexor spasm making assessment of finger extension difficult.

J-shaped[3] and longitudinal[4,8] incisions have been described, but we find that an oblique incision[9] provides excellent exposure to the extensor apparatus with a minimal amount of soft tissue dissection. The incision is centered over the proximal one half of the middle phalanx (Fig. 76–3). Small veins in the subcutaneous tissue are isolated and coagulated as the dissection proceeds down to the extensor apparatus. The lateral bands are identified

■ FIGURE 76–3
An oblique incision over
the proximal one half of
the middle phalanx is
used to expose the con-
joint lateral bands and
the triangular ligament.

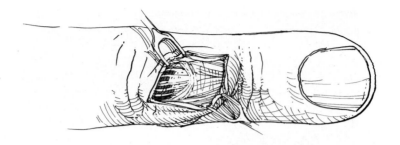

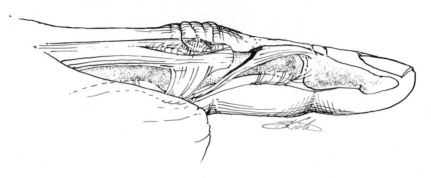

■ FIGURE 76–4

The tenotomy is performed just proximal to the point where the conjoint lateral bands unite to form the terminal tendon. It is important to preserve the oblique retinacular ligament and its insertion into the terminal tendon. The terminal tendon is liberated from the overpull of the lateral bands, allowing DIP flexion. The oblique retinacular ligament provides DIP extension through a static tenodesis effect. The tenotomy allows the entire extensor apparatus to migrate proximally concentrating its force on the elongated central tendon providing some improvement in PIP extension.

distal to the triangular ligament as they converge to form the conjoined terminal tendon. It is at this juncture that the tenotomy must be performed (Fig. 76–4). Before tendon division, the lateral bands and the conjoined terminal tendon are tenolysed. Care is taken to avoid damage to the underlying periosteum, as adhesions may form or an exostosis may develop. The tendon is elevated by a hemostat and a transverse or oblique tenotomy performed. Formal identification of the oblique retinacular ligament is not necessary, but the insertion into the terminal tendon must be preserved by performing the tenotomy in the most proximal aspect of the conjoined terminal tendon at the confluence of the lateral bands.

The tourniquet is released and active flexion tested. If the patient lacks active and passive DIP flexion, the DIP joint may be gently manipulated or a tenolysis and capsulotomy performed with care taken to maintain the insertion of the oblique retinacular ligament. Flexor tendon adhesions must be suspected and appropriately treated if passive mobility is restored but the patient is unable to demonstrate active flexion. After hemostasis is obtained and the wound is irrigated, skin closure is performed with 5-0 nylon horizontal mattress sutures, and a light dressing is applied.

■ TECHNICAL
ALTERNATIVES

After terminal tendon tenotomy, most patients will have no significant DIP extensor deficit and can be started on an immediate active range of motion program. An extensor deficit of greater than 10 to 15° should be treated by splinting the PIP and DIP joints in extension for 10 days. If the tenotomy was performed in the proper location, the extensor deficit will respond quickly to splinting, and no formal reconstruction will be necessary. Terminal tendon tenotomy performed distal to the insertion of the oblique retinacular ligament may result in an extensor deficit that is severe and refractory to splint treatment. Fusion of the DIP joint or spiral oblique retinacular ligament reconstruction using palmaris longus tendon graft,[9] may provide the only acceptable salvage solutions.

To more accurately control the lengthening of the terminal tendon, Tubiana[10] has recommended a V-shaped tenotomy that allows a tenorrhaphy in the lengthened position, and Curtis[2] has proposed a sliding lengthening and repair of the lateral bands. Although simple tenotomy of the terminal tendon lacks the aesthetic appeal of the more complex procedures, it is based on solid biomechanical principles and, if properly performed, has proven to be clinically successful. The additional surgery required to lengthen the terminal tendon and perform suture repair is probably unnecessary and may contribute to adhesion formation. Terminal tendon tenotomy has not been designed to correct PIP extensor deficits of greater than 20°. Surgeons should choose a procedure that addresses the central tendon attenuation if the primary goal is the restoration of PIP extension.

■ REHABILITATION

The desired result of terminal tendon tenotomy is improved DIP flexion, and most authors agree that this goal is most likely to be achieved with an immediate active range of motion program (Figs. 76-5 and 76-6). The DIP joint should only be splinted if a significant DIP extensor deficit develops. The operation also can result in improved active extension of the PIP joint (Fig. 76–6). Nalebuff[7] states that it is important to support the PIP joint in full extension with a dynamic extension splint that allows active DIP flexion, and Tubiana[10] recommends a static PIP extension splint for five weeks after surgery. PIP extension splinting has some theoretical advantages, but it has not proven to be necessary in the majority of patients.

Most patients can begin active flexion of the PIP and DIP joints on the day of surgery. Passive DIP flexion, with the PIP joint held in full extension, is encouraged at 10 to 14 days after surgery, but must be discontinued if a significant DIP extensor deficit develops. For the first 8 weeks, the surgeon and hand therapist should evaluate the patient's progress every 10 to 14 days and make appropriate changes to the therapy program.

■ OUTCOMES

Stern[8] reported the results of terminal tendon tenotomy in 13 patients with DIP hyperextension associated with traumatically acquired boutonniere deformities. All but one patient had a significant improvement in DIP flexion. Preoperative DIP motion was 10° of hyperextension to 10° of flexion. Post-tenotomy DIP flexion averaged 45°. A DIP extensor deficit of 5 to 10° was noted in four digits. Nalebuff[7] also reported a small number of

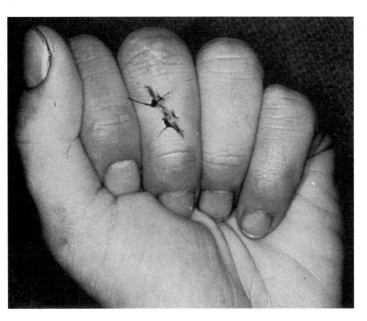

■ FIGURE 76–5
The tenotomy has allowed immediate restoration of near normal DIP flexion.

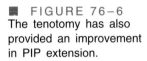

■ FIGURE 76-6
The tenotomy has also provided an improvement in PIP extension.

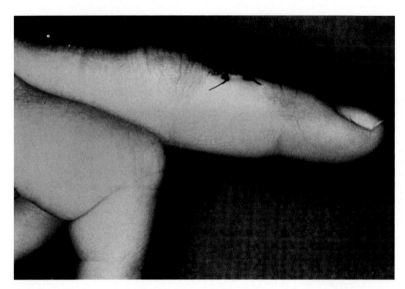

patients with a DIP extensor lag. Both authors state that patients were not bothered by the extensor lag and had significant functional improvement from the regained DIP flexion. PIP extension was only improved by 5° in 3 patients and by 15° in 1 patient.

For many patients with a boutonniere deformity, the loss of DIP flexion is the most disabling component. They complain of the inability to manipulate small objects with the tip of the finger and of grip weakness. A PIP extensor lag of 30° or less can be cosmetically objectionable but rarely results in a functional deficit.

Terminal tendon tenotomy does little to improve PIP extension, but effectively and predictably improves DIP flexion. This elegantly simple procedure is an excellent reconstructive option when the primary goal is to restore DIP flexion.

References

1. Burton RI: Extensor Tendons—Late Reconstruction. In: Green DP (ed), Operative Hand Surgery, New York: Churchill Livingstone, 1988:2073–2116.
2. Curtis RM, Reid RL, Provost JM: A staged technique for the repair of the traumatic boutonniere deformity. J Hand Surg, 1983; 8A:167–171.
3. Dolphin JA: Extensor tenotomy for chronic boutonniere deformity of the finger. J Bone Joint Surg, 1965; 47A:161–164.
4. Elliott, R.A. Boutonniere deformity. In: Cramer LM, Chase RA (eds), Symposium on the Hand, St. Louis: C.V. Mosby, 1971:42–56.
5. Littler JW, Eaton RG: Redistribution of forces in the correction of the boutonniere deformity. J Bone Joint Surg, 1967; 49A:1267–1274.
6. Matev I: Transposition, the lateral slips. Br J Plast Surg, 1964; 17:281–286.
7. Nalebuff EA, Millender LH: Surgical treatment of the boutonniere deformity in rheumatoid arthritis. Ortho Clin North Am, 1975; 6:753–763.
8. Stern PJ: Extensor tenotomy: a technique for correction of posttraumatic distal interphalangeal joint hyperextension deformity. J Hand Surg, 1989; 14A:546–549.
9. Thompson JS, Littler JW, Upton J: The spiral oblique retinacular ligament. J Hand Surg, 1978; 3A:482–487.
10. Tubiana R, Grossman JA: The management of chronic posttraumatic boutonniere deformity. Bull Hosp Jt Dis Orthop Inst, 1984; 44:542–551.

77

Oblique Retinacular Ligament Transfer for Swan Neck Deformity

Swan neck deformity may cause considerable functional impairment of a digit. Characterized by hyperextension of the proximal interphalangeal (PIP) joint and inability to fully extend the distal interphalangeal (DIP) joint, the swan neck deformity results from imbalance of the normally finely concatenated components of the extensor system. Causes include: (1) mallet deformity of the DIP joint with compensatory hyperextension of the PIP joint; (2) incompetence of the palmar plate of the PIP joint (primary or post-traumatic) with reciprocal inability to actively extend the DIP joint; (3) intrinsic muscle contracture due to spasticity or ischemia; or (4) the combination of factors created by systemic inflammatory disease (e.g., rheumatoid arthritis).

Several techniques have been described for correcting swan neck deformities. Some address primary pathology at the PIP joint and propose methods of restraining hyperextension of that joint. Portis[11] recommended reinsertion of the palmar plate into the base of the middle phalanx, and Adams[1] described a criss-cross free tendon graft on the palmar aspect of the PIP joint to block hyperextension. Superficialis hemitenodesis using one slip of the superficialis tendon fixed to bone at the base of the proximal phalanx was proposed by Littler,[8] and superficialis tenodesis in which both slips of the tendon were fixed by suture to the proximal phalanx at the junction of the middle and distal thirds was described by Swanson.[13] Bate,[2] and later Kleinert and Kasdan[7] recessed the collateral ligament of the PIP joint to correct palmar laxity.

The spiral oblique retinacular ligament reconstruction (SORL) is most appropriately discussed in the historic context of procedures described for correction of swan neck deformity resulting from a "mallet" deformity of the DIP with secondary hyperextension of the PIP joint. Pratt and co-workers[12] suggested shortening and repair of the terminal extensor tendon and fixation of the DIP joint. Fowler[5] divided the central tendon insertion on the dorsal aspect of the base of the middle phalanx to correct the mallet and rebalance the extensor mechanism. Nichols[10] reconstructed the extensor tendon insertion on the distal phalanx with a free tendon graft. Littler[9] used a volar slip of one lateral band passed beneath Cleland's ligaments at the PIP joint and fixed to the flexor tendon sheath to reconstruct the oblique retinacular ligament. Kilgore and Graham[6] modified this technique by proximal fixation to the intact part of the lateral band. Thompson and co-workers[14] described the technique of SORL reconstruction with a free tendon graft. It is this procedure that is the basis for this chapter.

The SORL reconstruction is primarily indicated for patients with swan neck deformity secondary to "mallet" injuries of the DIP joint with loss of active extension. The reconstruction restrains hyperextension of the PIP joint and extends the DIP joint by an active tenodesis, which recapitulates the function of the normal ORL. To be amenable to reconstruction, the deformity must be supple; rigidity is an absolute contraindication. In addition, swan neck deformity due solely to incompetence of the PIP palmar plate is a relative contraindication and is more appropriately treated by a procedure like the superficialis hemitenodesis, which addresses the primary pathology more selectively.

■ HISTORY OF THE TECHNIQUE

■ INDICATIONS AND CONTRAINDICATIONS

Swan neck deformities in patients with rheumatoid arthritis are multifactorial, and treatment must be tailored to the pathology. A possible indication for ORL reconstruction in the rheumatoid patient is a supple swan neck in the absence of significant pathology of the PIP or metacarpophalangeal joint or of the intrinsics. Even in this setting, in the patient with rheumatoid arthritis, it is significantly more likely that the transfer will not restore full extension of the DIP joint, although it will probably restrain hyperextension at the PIP joint. Furthermore, the transfer may attenuate over time. Swan neck deformities in patients with spasticity are most commonly due to laxity of the PIP volar plate and, therefore, treatable by the sturdier superficialis hemitenodesis rather than ORL reconstruction. However, due to the broad spectrum of deformities in spastic hands, treatment needs to be individualized.

■ SURGICAL
TECHNIQUES

Littler's technique of ORL reconstruction,[14] which is described in this section, has not been significantly modified since its description in 1978. My preference is to perform the procedure under axillary block anesthesia, which affords anesthesia of the hand and forearm and a prolonged period of tolerance of the tourniquet. General anesthesia would only be preferred in the setting of other procedures being done simultaneously.

The operation, as described in general terms, is done through several short longitudinally oriented incisions. The dorsum of the base of the distal phalanx is exposed through an ulnarly based hockey stick-shaped incision extending proximally across the DIP joint to the level of the distal third of the middle phalanx (Figs. 77-1 and 77-2). The tendon graft is routed along the ulnar aspect of the digit to the level of the PIP joint. A 1.5-cm longitudinal midaxial incision is centered over the ulnar side of the PIP joint. The graft passes to the radial side of the digit, where access is afforded by a 1.5-cm long midaxial incision. A gouge hole traverses the proximal phalangeal base and a small ulnar stab wound allows the gouge to exit percutaneously. The palmaris longus tendon when present is the preferred source of graft. As a rule, this can be harvested through two short transverse incisions at the distal wrist crease and musculotendinous junction.

■ FIGURE 77–1
A diagram of the operation primarily from the dorsal perspective shows the incisions and the course of the free tendon graft (a) including its emergence on the palmar aspect of the distal phalanx (b). Cross sections are shown at the PIP (c) and proximal phalangeal (d) levels. III = long finger; ul. = ulnar. Arabic numerals indicate the steps of passage of the graft. t.sh. = tendon sheath; ct. = central tendons.

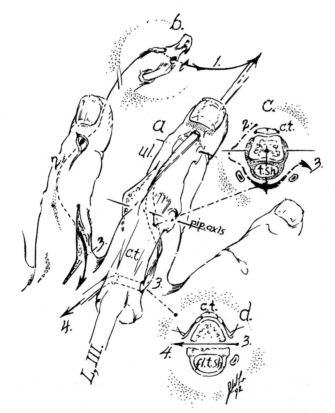

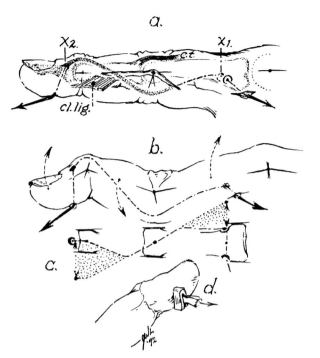

■ FIGURE 77–2
A diagram of the operation from the lateral aspect of the digit (a) shows the direction of pull on the phalanges when the graft is under tension (b). The graft spirals around the digit, a truncated cone. If the cone is flattened the course of the graft is a straight line (c). cl. lig. = Cleland's ligament; c.t. = central tendon; X 1 = point of fixation in proximal phalanx; X 2 = point of fixation in distal phalanx.

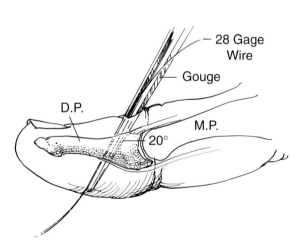

■ FIGURE 77–3
A hand-held gouge is used to make a dorso-palmar hole in the base of the distal phalanx. The slight distal inclination of the gouge avoids the subchondral bone.

More specifically, the SORL reconstruction is begun with the incision over the dorsal aspect of the base of the distal phalanx. A gouge hole is planned beginning approximately 3 mm distal to the articular surface of the distal phalanx between the extensor tubercle and the base of the germinal matrix nail, which must be identified and avoided. The hole in the distal phalanx is made with a hand-held gouge directed palmarly to exit in the midline of the base of the distal phalanx (Fig. 77–3). The hole must be in the midline to avoid injuring the neurovascular bundles and angled approximately 20° distally to avoid the subchondral bone. A small stab wound is made over the tip of the gouge palmarly. A 28-gauge stainless steel wire is passed along the concavity of the gouge facilitating its passage through the hole.

A 1.5-cm long midaxial incision is made on the ulnar side of the PIP joint. Care is taken to protect the dorsal branch of the ulnar digital nerve. Cleland's ligament is identified

■ FIGURE 77–4
A subcutaneous tunnel is made from the distal, dorsal incision to the midaxial incision on the ulnar side of the joint.

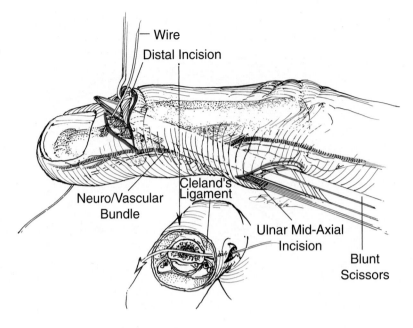

■ FIGURE 77–5
A transverse gouge hole is made in the metaphysis of the proximal phalanx from the radial to the ulnar side.

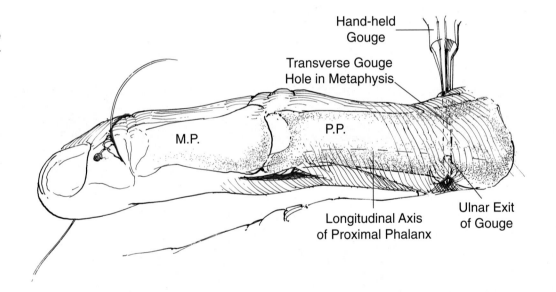

and the plane palmar to its fibers is developed with blunt dissection. The neurovascular bundle lies within this plane. A subcutaneous tunnel is then created between the distal dorsal incision and the ulnar midaxial incision (Fig. 77–4). This tunnel is superficial to the extensor mechanism and dorsal to Cleland's ligament until the level of the PIP joint where it is directed palmarward in the interval between the ulnar neurovascular bundle and the flexor tendon sheath. The dissection is carried obliquely and remains between the flexor sheath and neurovascular bundle. This ulnoradial oblique passage, superficial to the tendon sheath at the PIP level, is the crux of the operation making dorsal displacement of the graft impossible thereby preventing PIP hyperextension while extending the terminal phalanx. A second 28-gauge stainless steel wire may be placed along this soft tissue tunnel for later use to pass to the tendon graft which alternatively may be done with a small curved hemostat.

A longitudinal skin incision is made in the radial mid axial line over the metaphysis of the proximal phalanx. The lateral band is retracted dorsally. A transverse gouge hole is made in the metaphysis using progressively larger gouges (Fig. 77–5). The hole should be made slightly palmar to the longitudinal axis of the phalanx and directed absolutely transversely avoiding dorsal or palmar inclination. Another 28-gauge wire is placed through the gouge hole.

At this point in the procedure, the tendon graft is obtained. The palmaris longus is preferred when available. Alternatives would be the plantaris or a toe extensor.

The dorsal part of the wire previously placed in the distal phalanx is then secured with a knot around the distal end of the tendon graft. The cut tail of the wire is bent so that it lies parallel to the tendon, which is carefully drawn through the hole in the base of the distal phalanx from dorsal to palmar using a gentle, twisting motion rather than a forceful longitudinal pull. A few centimeters of tendon are left outside the skin palmarly. The second wire, which had been previously placed in the soft tissue tunnel, is secured to the proximal end of the tendon in the dorsal, distal wound. It is advanced through the soft tissue tunnel along the ulnar border of the middle phalanx, beneath Cleland's ligaments and in the interval between the neurovascular bundles and the flexor tendon sheath crossing from the ulnar to radial side of the digit. The wire, which had been placed in the transverse gouge hole in the proximal phalanx, is then tied around the proximal end of the graft, which is drawn through the proximal phalangeal hole from radial to ulnar where it is delivered percutaneously.

The tension on the tendon graft can be set either proximally or distally. It is easiest to fix the tendon proximally and then set the tension distally. For fixation, the tendon may be split longitudinally, and each of the two tails placed through the enlarged holes of a shirt button. The tendon ends are tied over the button and the knot secured with 3-0 or 4-0 braided synthetic suture or a hemoclip. An alternative to the shirt button is a rubber catheter with a hole in its center and Xeroform or felt padding beneath it. One limb of the split tendon is placed through the hole and tied to the other tail over the catheter and sutured. The correct tension is set by pulling the distal tendon end longitudinally until the PIP and DIP joints are fully extended (i.e., the graft is tight with the interphalangeal joints extended) (Figs. 77-6 and 77-7). The tendon may be fixed distally in the same manner as described above.

Wounds are sutured with interrupted simple or vertical mattress sutures of 5-0 nylon. A hand dressing is applied using fluffs in the web spaces on either side of the affected digit and in the first web. These are secured with kling gauze. A short arm cast is applied incorporating the involved digit if it is a border digit or the involved and the adjacent border digit if it is a central digit.

The SORL reconstruction is indicated in patients with swan neck deformity secondary to mallet deformity of the DIP joint. The SORL can be used to reconstruct swan necks of

■ TECHNICAL
ALTERNATIVES

■ FIGURE 77–6
The correct tension on the reconstruction is demonstrated by pulling the graft proximally and distally until the PIP and DIP joints are fully extended.

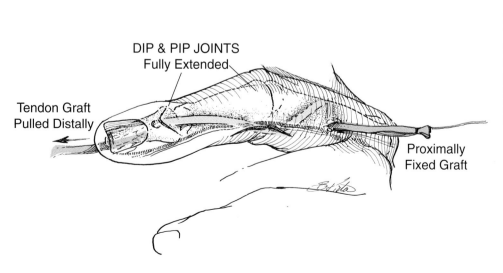

DIP & PIP JOINTS
Fully Extended

Tendon Graft
Pulled Distally

Proximally
Fixed Graft

A photograph of the graft in place with applied tension, before attachment proximally over a button.

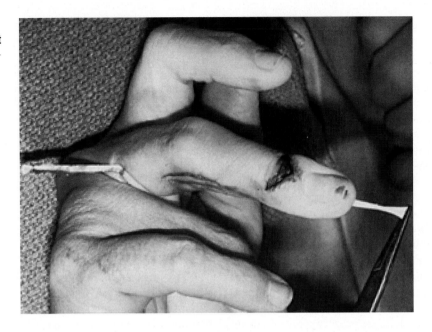

other etiologies but may represent "overkill" in these settings. An alternative to the SORL reconstruction is the ORL reconstruction using a segment of lateral band rather than a free tendon graft. This is useful when the terminal extensor is competent. Superficialis hemitenodesis is effective for reconstructing swan neck deformities due to incompetence of the palmar plate of the PIP joint. It will not restore active extension of the DIP joint. In Fowler's tenotomy, the central tendon at the base of the middle phalanx just proximal to its insertion is divided, allowing the lateral and oblique components of the extensor mechanism to extend the DIP joint. Alternatively, the fibrotic portion of the extensor tendon caused by rupture may be excised and the ends of the tendon reapproximated.

The SORL reconstruction has potential pitfalls. If the graft tension is set too tightly it can result in an inability to fully extend the PIP joint and hyperextension of the DIP joint. Specifically, a swan neck may be converted into a boutonniere deformity. It also is possible to fracture the proximal phalanx during the creation of the gouge hole. This is more likely to occur if the hole is either too dorsal or too volar within the metaphysis. A conceivable but unlikely pitfall is disruption of the proximal or distal tendon graft junctures. If the tendon is split longitudinally and tied in a knot, which is sutured it is highly unlikely for the juncture to dehisce.

Brief mention should be made of an alternative technique of distal tendon fixation described by Foucher.[3] He does not fix the tendon distally through bone. Rather, he passes it in the interval between the nail matrix and underlying periosteum of the distal phalanx; it is secured on the fingertip.

■ REHABILITATION

The SORL reconstruction is under tension in extension and relaxed in flexion of the interphalangeal joints. This provides the rationale for a therapy program, which allows relatively early flexion. The digit is immobilized in a cast for approximately 1 week with the PIP joint flexed to approximately 20° and the DIP extended to neutral. The cast can be removed at that point and a dorsal thermoplastic extension block splint applied. The involved digit can be blocked palmarly either with a Velcro strap or removable shell. Passive range of motion in flexion as well as gentle active range of motion including extension to the splint can be started at 1 week and performed 4 times a day. After 3 weeks, this splint can be eliminated and a simple aluminum dorsal extension block splint used for an additional 2 to 3 weeks. Beginning 1 month after surgery, the patient should attempt to gently and progressively extend the interphalangeal joints to neutral. Ideally, at 6 weeks, the digit can be fully extended and fully flexed. At 5 or 6 weeks after surgery, the stumps of tendon graft can be amputated at the level of the skin. The skin will close over the tendon. Dimpling of the skin may occur but is not a functional problem and rarely a significant cosmetic one.

Thompson and co-workers[14] described excellent results in a series of 10 patients. The average preoperative DIP extension lag was 54° and PIP hyperextension was 22°. Five of the ten patients had full extension of the PIP and DIP joints at follow-up. Two had 10° extension lags of the DIP joint and 1 had a 10° extension lag of the PIP joint. One patient had a 15° lag of the DIP and another a 15° lag of the PIP joint. There were no postoperative problems with the exit sites of the tendon grafts. One patient required lengthening of the reconstruction at a second procedure to correct hyperextension of the DIP joint. Girot and co-workers[4] reported results of the SORL reconstruction in 35 patients. There was complete correction of PIP hyperextension in 95% of the patients and correction of the DIP extension lag in 70%. My personal experience has, to a reasonable approximation, been similar to that described in the series cited above. The authors of the original paper have continued to do the operation in essentially the same manner as described with comparable results (personal communication).

■ OUTCOMES

This specific technique for oblique retinacular ligament reconstruction is demanding but the procedure elegantly restores normal function of the ORL, which is disrupted in soft tissue mallet and subsequent swan neck deformity. Complications are infrequent. Good results can be anticipated when the procedure is meticulously performed with particular attention directed toward placement of the gouge holes in the proximal and distal phalanges and on setting the tension of the graft.

I would like to acknowledge J. William Littler, M.D., for his expertise and generosity in rendering some of the drawings for this chapter.

■ ACKNOWLEDGMENT

References

1. Adams JP: Correction of chronic dorsal subluxation of the proximal interphalangeal joint by means of a criss-cross volar graft. J Bone Joint Surg, 1959; 41A:111–115.
2. Bate JT: An operation for the correction of locking of the proximal interphalangeal joint of the finger in hyperextension. J Bone Joint Surg, 1945; 27:142–144.
3. Foucher G. Personal communication, 1992.
4. Girot J, Marin-Braun F, Amend P, et al: L'operation de Littler (SORL-spiral oblique retinacular ligament) dans le traitment du "col-de-cyane." Ann Chir Main, 1988; 1:85–89.
5. Harris C: The Fowler operation for mallet finger. J Bone Joint Surg, 1966; 48A:613.
6. Kilgore ES, Graham WP: Operative treatment of swan neck deformity. Plast Reconstr Surg, 1967; 39:468–470.
7. Kleinert HE, Kasdan ML: Reconstruction of chronically subluxed proximal interphalangeal finger joint. J Bone Joint Surg, 1965; 47A:958–964.
8. Littler JW: The hand and wrist. In: Howorth MG (ed): Textbook of Orthopaedics, New York: D. F. Saunders, 1952:284.
9. Littler JW: Restoration of the oblique retinacular ligament for correcting hyperextension deformity of the proximal interphalangeal joint. GEM. No. 1, L'Expansion Editeur, 1966: 39–42.
10. Nichols HM: Repair of extensor tendon insertions in the fingers. J Bone Joint Surg, 1951; 33A: 836–841.
11. Portis RB: Hyperextensibility of the proximal interphalangeal joint of the finger following trauma. J Bone Joint Surg, 1954; 36A:1141–1146.
12. Pratt DR, Bunnell S, Howard LD Jr: Mallet finger classification and methods of treatment. Am J Surg, 1957; 93:573–579.
13. Swanson AB: Surgery of the hand in cerebral palsy and the swan neck deformity. J Bone Joint Surg, 1960; 42A:951–964.
14. Thompson JS, Littler JW, Upton J: The spiral oblique retinacular ligament (SORL). J Hand Surg, 1978; 3:482–487.

DUFFIELD ASHMEAD,
IV
O. ALLEN GUINN, III
H. KIRK WATSON

78

Primary Flexor Tendon Grafts of the Fingers

■ HISTORY OF THE
TECHNIQUE

Free tendon grafts are a well-established and widely accepted means of restoring digital flexion. At one time advocated in preference to direct suture, free grafts are now viewed as the treatment of choice in those circumstances where direct repair of the flexor tendon in zones 1 or 2 is not possible. While more complex cases will generally fare better with a staged reconstruction, conventional one stage grafting remains a viable and important technique.

The history of flexor tendon grafting has been well reported by Adamson and Wilson.[1] Scattered case reports of tendon autografts and xenografts appeared in the late nineteenth century. Erich Lexer is credited with the first published series in 1912, documenting the results of 10 patients who underwent primary flexor tendon grafting. The palmaris longus or toe extensor tendons were used as donors, and motion was initiated on the sixth postoperative day. Isolated replacement of the flexor digitorum profundis yielded a "good" result. In 1916, Leo Mayer published three articles that have become the basis of modern flexor tendon reconstruction. Included in these papers are detailed anatomic descriptions of the tendon and its surrounding structures, including the relevant blood supply. He stressed choosing an adequate muscle to serve as a motor and a direct attachment of the distal tendon graft to bone. He also advocated preservation of peritenon around flexor tendon grafts.

In January 1918, Sterling Bunnell reported a landmark study that reviewed the anatomy and physiology of tendons. He discussed the importance of peritenon and fat to the gliding mechanism and presented his atraumatic technique, including strict asepsis, a bloodless field, and gentle handling of tissues. He expressed a preference for using the palmaris longus as a donor and described a tendon stripper made from a modified cork borer. He recommended immobilization of the operated finger for 3 weeks followed by active motion. Mason and Allen would later reinforce this recommendation on the basis of tensile strength studies in 1941.[11]

Subsequent reports, including those by Pulvertaft,[15] Littler,[10] and Boyes and Stark,[3] presented large clinical series. Schemes of classifying outcome were developed, and prognostic factors associated with better results were identified. Basic science research, including that reported by Potenza,[13,14] Eichen and co-authors,[4] and Gelberman and co-authors[5–8] has focused on mechanisms of tendon healing, revascularization of tendon grafts, and the advisability of flexor sheath reconstruction. Recent clinical work has called into question the relative merits of early and late mobilization.[16] The degree to which adhesion formation is necessary for revascularization of the graft remains controversial; there is, however, no doubt that excessive adhesion formation restricts excursion and will lead to a mediocre result.

Pending more definitive research, flexor tendon grafting remains at least as much art as science. We present here one of many acceptable approaches. While we would readily acknowledge that our technical preferences and biases may not always be supported by the available literature, they are nonetheless approaches that have withstood the test of time, proving successful in our hands.

Briefly summarized, flexor tendon grafting should be considered in any patient for whom reconstruction by primary or delayed primary repair is not feasible. Typical indications would include segmental injuries with loss of tendon substance and cases in which primary repair has been sufficiently delayed (months) that direct approximation is no longer feasible. An additional indication, in our view, is a lacerated or avulsed profundus tendon, which recoils into the palm or distal forearm, disrupting the vincular blood supply. Even in the acute setting, this tendon has been largely devascularized, effectively becoming a free tendon graft in itself. In our view, this profundus is best replaced with a true graft of smaller caliber, rather than simply repaired. Both glide space within the sheath and nutrition, whether by synovial bathing or vascular ingrowth, are thus optimized. In addition, tenorrhaphy in zone 2 is avoided. Simple profundus laceration in zone 2, however, is no longer viewed as an indication for tendon grafting in the acute setting.

Results are best when preoperative soft tissues are supple and joint motion is maximal. Rarely will postoperative active motion match preoperative passive motion, much less exceed it. Relative contraindications include inadequate soft tissue coverage, skeletal instability, or fixed joint contractures. Marginally sensate or inadequately perfused digits usually will do poorly. Patient motivation is important. The ideal candidate for grafting is not only cooperative, but extremely motivated. While we have no strict age criteria, the very old and the very young are often better served by an alternative approach.

Results in free tendon grafting are technique-dependent. A regional (axillary or interscalene) anesthetic is acceptable, although we prefer general anesthesia. Tourniquet control is essential to ensure a bloodless field, and atraumatic technique is paramount. We are fanatical to the point of superstition when handling the graft itself.

For exposure of the flexor apparatus, we use a Brunner incision, modified as necessary to take into account existing wounds and scars. Triangular flaps are blunted somewhat at their tips to avoid local skin flap necrosis, and the incision apex at the proximal interphalangeal (PIP) joint should be placed ulnarly for the index finger (avoiding the lateral pinch contact surface) and radially for the little finger (avoiding the resting surface on the ulnar side of the hand). Skin flaps are elevated with subcutaneous tissue from the flexor sheath, exposing the entire length of the sheath from the distal phalanx to the midpalm (or distal forearm as necessary). Great care is taken to avoid injury to the neurovascular bundles.

The flexor sheath is carefully assessed for patency and scarring. We do not hesitate to resect cruciate and membranous portions of the sheath for better exposure, although we do not advocate extensive resection of the majority of the sheath as previously recommended by Bunnell. Conversely, we do not make any effort to reconstruct an intact sheath as proposed by Eichen. The A2 and A4 pulleys must be preserved. When these are inadequate, we prefer to proceed with a staged reconstruction using a silicone spacer or dynamic implant, rather than attempt extensive pulley reconstruction and flexor tendon grafting simultaneously. When sheath patency is poor, or the bed extensively scarred, we once again retreat to a staged approach.

Residual profundus tendon is resected proximally to the level of the midpalm, and distally, preserving 5 to 7 mm at the distal phalangeal insertion if possible. An intact sublimis is never sacrificed, and even sublimis remnants are generally left undisturbed rather than risk the creation of adhesions between the graft and broad surfaces of freshly dissected tissue.

Only after complete preparation of the recipient bed will the graft be harvested, although the donor site will have been carefully selected preoperatively. In our view, the ideal flexor tendon graft is of narrow caliber. Smaller tendons are more readily accommodated by the flexor sheath and presumably more readily nourished by synovial bathing and vascular ingrowth. Longitudinal splitting of larger tendons is not an option, given the raw tendon surface created by such a maneuver. The ipsilateral palmaris longus, when available, affords the convenience of a donor site within the same operative field. Our second choice is the contralateral palmaris longus. The tendon is identified and isolated through a distal transverse incision at the level of the wrist crease. With tension at this

■ INDICATIONS AND
CONTRAINDICATIONS

■ SURGICAL
TECHNIQUES

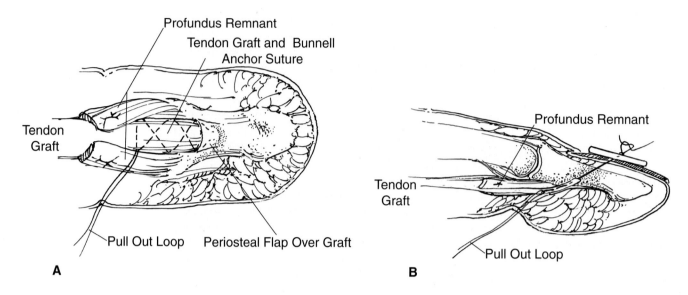

■ FIGURE 78–1

A and B, Our preferred distal insertion: A small osteal/periosteal flap is raised with a fine osteotome, creating a cancellous pocket. The graft is secured into this pocket with a Bunnell type hemisuture passed through the distal phalanx and tied over the nail. The profundus remnants on either side may be sutured to the graft for additional reinforcement. The pullout loop for the Bunnell suture is brought out midlaterally.

level, the proximal musculotendinous junction is readily palpable. A counter-incision at this level will allow proximal tenotomy and atraumatic retrieval of the graft.

Once harvested, grafts are handled as little as possible, using washed, gloved hands rather than moist sponges. We have traditionally dimmed overhead operating lights so as to minimize desiccation. Total graft exposure time may be decreased by placement of a hemitenorrhaphy suture in the tendon end before completion of harvest. The graft is placed immediately within a soft tissue environment, in this case the digital sheath. In the context of a preserved sublimis, we will generally thread the profundus through the chiasm, so as to "normalize" tendon inter-relationships. This is hardly essential, however, and the profundus can easily be threaded alongside the sublimis if passage through the chiasm is not readily accomplished.

The distal profundus insertion is usually performed first (Fig. 78–1A and 78-1B). Our preference is to longitudinally split and elevate the distal stump, exposing a small portion of the volar ridge of the distal phalanx. Using a small osteotome, a shallow pocket of exposed cancellous bone is created by raising a small bone flap. A 4.0 stainless steel pullout wire secured to the tendon by Bunnell suture is then readily drilled through the phalanx with a Keefe needle and tied over a button on the nail surface. The bony insertion is reinforced by suturing the distal profundus stump to the graft in zone 1. In younger, growing patients we avoid insertion into bone so as to prevent injury to the distal phalangeal physis by bony excavation. Instead we prefer a standard tenorrhaphy to the distal profundus stump (provided sufficient length is available).

After accomplishing the distal tenorrhaphy and threading the tendon through the flexor sheath, the proximal repair is performed. We have found a Pulvertaft weave to be ideal, as it allows infinitely fine adjustment of graft tension prior to placement of any sutures (Fig. 78–2). A weave also provides the advantage of considerable tensile strength at the time of mobilization. We will generally use a long-lasting but dissolvable suture such as PDS using a large number of interrupted stitches with very small "bites." In theory, these small sutures will readily share distractive tension with minimal tendon displacement. Under no circumstances should the lumbrical of the involved or adjacent digits be sutured

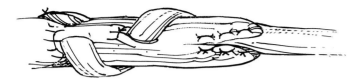

■ FIGURE 78-2

The proximal tenorrhaphy is generally performed as a tendon weave. The profundus stump is fish-mouthed and the proximal graft end buried to minimize exposed tendon. Multiple tiny sutures are used to secure the two tendons to each other at all points of interweave.

around the proximal repair site, as altered lumbrical tone may result in a "lumbrical finger" or quadregia effect.

Graft length is adjusted using the normal finger cascade as an indicator of tension. The digit is generally overcorrected (i.e., overflexed) to a minimal degree to allow for subsequent, gradual relaxation of any myostatic contracture.

Closure is completed with interrupted and running nylon in a single layer. A bulky compressive hand dressing is applied over Xeroform, incorporating a dorsal protective plaster splint.

The principle alternatives to primary (single stage) flexor tendon grafting are staged techniques using static or dynamic tendon spacers.[9] Although a permanent tendon prosthesis may ultimately provide an additional alternative, this remains a theoretical construct at present. Conditions favoring a staged approach would include significant scarring of the graft bed, unstable bony or articular injuries, and the need for concurrent pulley reconstruction. The latter two situations create conflicting rehabilitation goals of active mobilization for tendon gliding and protection of healing structural elements. Distal interphalangeal (DIP) joint fusion is a viable alternative to profundus grafting when sublimis function is intact. The result is predictable and, for selected patients and certain digits, may be preferable to the uncertainties and inconveniences of a complex procedure with extended postoperative rehabilitation. In digits further disabled by stiffness or neurovascular compromise, amputation may be a reasonable approach.

■ TECHNICAL ALTERNATIVES

Having chosen to proceed with primary flexor tendon grafting, there are a variety of procedural alternatives to the technique outlined above. Flexor sheath exposure may be accomplished from a lateral approach provided neurovascular bundles are carefully protected. There are a variety of tendon donor alternatives to the palmaris longus. In order of preference, these include the plantaris (providing a long graft of ideal caliber when present), the extensor indicis proprius, the extensor digiti minimi, or central toe extensors. A segment of flexor sublimis from the same digit (if nonfunctional) or an adjacent finger may be considered if the caliber is sufficiently fine. This donor site offers the advantage of being within the same operative field. There is also experimental evidence suggesting that "intrasynovial" donors may be preferable in terms of decreased adhesion formation.[5] Regardless of donor site, a tendon stripper is to be avoided as we believe it tends to traumatize the edges of the graft, with concomitant risk of adhesion formation. A vein stripper (without a sharpened ring) will facilitate harvest of the plantaris. The tendon may be threaded through the ring distally and the stripper gently advanced proximally to facilitate localization of the tendon within the calf, and its subsequent division through a solitary proximal incision.

There are myriad alternatives for the graft insertion at the distal phalanx. Most of these are perfectly acceptable. The only technique that we advise against is that in which the entire tendon is pulled through the distal pulp. Although this facilitates adjustment of tension, the technique produces an unacceptable degree of scarring on the touch surface of the digit.

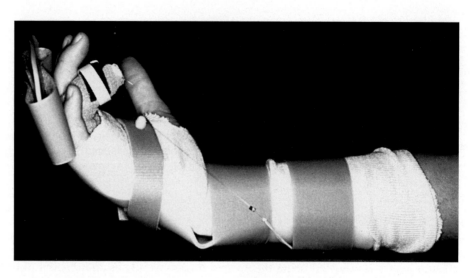

■ FIGURE 78–3
A dorsal splint is used for protective mobilization of the tendon graft. Wrist and MP joints are blocked in 35° of flexion; the IP joints are allowed full extension. Elastic traction is placed on the grafted digit via a palmar pulley to ensure full composite flexion. The patient is instructed in active extension, which is facilitated by release of the proximal elastic. A palmar strap splints fingers in IP extension at night.

■ REHABILITATION

Considerable controversy continues to surround postoperative rehabilitation of flexor tendon grafts. The goal in all cases is to strike a balance between protective immobilization (to avoid tenorrhaphy failure) and early mobilization (to minimize the formation of adhesions, which would limit excursion). Over time, we have become more aggressive, allowing earlier mobilization. Our current protocol is as follows.

Four to five days after surgery, the bulky dressing is removed, and the patient's hand is placed in a dorsal blocking splint with the wrist and metacarpophalangeal joints flexed at 35° and the PIP and DIP joints at full extension. Elastic traction is placed on the digit, using a palmar pulley (Fig. 78–3). The patient is instructed to actively extend the digit to the limit of the splint on an hourly basis. The elastic may be released at these times to facilitate full extension.

After 4 weeks, the splint is modified to a neutral wrist position and traction discontinued. Active flexion and extension are encouraged on an hourly basis, within the constraints and protection of the splint.

After 5 to 7 weeks, the splint is removed, and active motion is encouraged, supplemented by passive ranging as necessary to avoid flexion contracture. After 7 weeks, progressive resistive exercise is commenced. Our goal is to return the patient to a work setting within 10 to 12 weeks if possible. Range of motion should continue to improve for 1 year or more.

■ OUTCOMES

Results of flexor tendon grafting are reported and graded in a variety of schemes. Flexion lag from the pulp to the distal palmar crease, as popularized by Boyes,[2] is easily measured but fails to record any associated extensor lag. Total active motion fails to distinguish loss of motion before grafting from loss of motion at final outcome. Percent of preoperative passive motion achieved actively by tendon grafting provides a measure of graft "success," but is perhaps less relevant to actual function than simple measures of total active motion.

Recent large series of single stage flexor tendon grafting are lacking. Boyes and Stark[3] reported that in "good candidates," more than 60% of digits flexed to within 1.25 cm of the distal palmar crease. In McClinton and co-authors' experience,[11] almost 80% did so, with active DIP motion averaging 48°. Thompson[16] reports "good" to "excellent" results for 50% of a diverse series of flexor tendon grafts. Results are graded on the basis of total flexion, extensor lag, and pulp to distal palmar crease lags.

The most frequently encountered disappointment with primary flexor tendon grafting is poor range of motion. Both flexion and extension lags may result from excessive adhesion formation. Although surgical technique is certainly a contributing factor, other issues such as preoperative status of the digit and digital sheath, age, skin and soft tissue type, and concurrent digital nerve injuries play a role. In our experience, the most significant factor is usually the motivation of the patient and adherence to an aggressive rehabilitation protocol. When necessary, tenolysis may be undertaken 3 to 4 months after grafting.

Rupture of proximal or distal tenorrhaphy may occur occasionally. This is considerably less likely with tendon insertion into bone and tendon weave techniques than with traditional tendon suture. When it occurs early, it is usually due to technical failure; in the late setting (after 3 to 4 weeks), overly aggressive mobilization is usually to blame. Flexor tendon grafts will almost never rupture along their length, but rather at sites of repair.

Hematoma formation may be associated with poor operative hemostasis or development of bleeding at the time of early mobilization. The presence of blood at the graft site increases the formation of adhesions. A hemostatic bulky dressing is thus essential whether or not tourniquet is deflated for hemostasis intraoperatively. Iatrogenic injury to neurovascular structures may occur in previously injured and operated fingers. Inadequate preservation of flexor sheath structures will result in bowstringing of the flexor tendon and a resulting compromise of composite excursion. Infection is rare and generally responds well to antibiotic therapy.

References

1. Adamson JE, Wilson JN: The history of flexor-tendon grafting. J Bone Joint Surg, 1961; 43A: 709–716.
2. Boyes J: Evaluation of results of digital flexor tendon grafts. Am J Surg, 1955; 80:1116–1119.
3. Boyes JH, Stark HH: Flexor-tendon grafts in the fingers and thumb. J Bone Joint Surg, 1971; 53A:1332–1342.
4. Eiken O, Homberg J, Ekerot L, Salgeback S: Restoration of the digital tendon sheath. Scand J Plast Reconstr Surg, 1980; 14:89–97.
5. Gelberman RH, Chu CR, Williams CS, Seiler JG, Amiel D: Angiogenesis in healing autogenous flexor-tendon grafts. J Bone Joint Surg, 1992; 74A:1207–1216.
6. Gelberman RH, Khabie V, Cahill CJ: Revascularization of healing flexor tendons in the digital sheath. J Bone Joint Surg, 1991; 73A:868–881.
7. Gelberman RH, Woo SLY, Amiel D, Horibe S, Lee, D: Influences of flexor sheath continuity and early motion on tendon healing in dogs. J Hand Surg, 1990; 15A:69–77.
8. Gelberman RH, Vande Berg JS, Lundborg GN, Akeson WH: Flexor tendon healing and restoration of the gliding surface. J Bone Joint Surg, 1983; 65A:70–80.
9. Hunter JM: Staged flexor tendon reconstruction. J Hand Surg, 1983; 8:789–793.
10. Littler JW: Free tendon grafts in secondary flexor tendon repair. Am J Surg, 1947; 74:315–321.
11. Mason ML, Allen HS: The rate of healing of tendons: An experimental study of tensile strength. Ann Surg, 1941; 113–424.
12. McClinton MA, Curtis RM, Shaw Wilgis EF: One hundred tendon grafts for isolated flexor digitorum profundus injuries. J Hand Surg, 1982; 7:224–229.
13. Potenza AD: The healing of autogenous tendon grafts within the flexor digital sheath in dogs. J Bone Joint Surg, 1964; 46A:1462–1484.
14. Potenza AD: Philosophy of flexor tendon surgery. Orth Clin North Am, 1986; 17:349–352.
15. Pulvertaft RG: Tendon grafts for flexor tendon injuries in the fingers and thumb. J Bone Joint Surg, 1956; 38B:175–194.
16. Strickland JW: Biologic rationale, clinical application, and results of early motion following flexor tendon repair. J Hand Ther, 1989; 2:71–83.
17. Thompson RV: An evaluation of flexor tendon grafting. Br J Plast Surg, 1967; 20:21–44.

79

Staged Flexor Tendon Grafts

The idea of staged tendon reconstruction is credited to Leo Mayer, who, in 1936, used a rigid rod in the first stage of the procedure.[5] The use of a silicone rod was first reported by Bassett and Carroll in 1963.[1] It was further developed through the arduous efforts of James Hunter; his early results were reported in 1971,[4] and long-term follow-up was reported in 1981.[12] The concept of using silicone rods has been applied to flexor and extensor tendons as well as nerve reconstruction in the upper extremity. This procedure is most commonly used to reconstruct the flexor digitorum profundus and flexor pollicis longus tendons.

The implant that is used for staged tendon reconstruction is available in 3, 4, 5, or 6 mm widths with a thickness of 2 mm and length of 25 cm (Phoenix Bioengineering Inc., Bridgeport, PA). It is made with a core of polyester weaved tape, coated with barium-impregnated silicone elastomer. It can be obtained with or without a fixation plate, which accommodates a 2.0-mm cortical screw. The plate can be cut off if desired; the proximal end also can be cut to shorten the implant, without affecting its structural integrity. "Active" rods also are available, to allow proximal fixation to muscle, but these implants are still experimental and are not recommended for general use.

■ INDICATIONS AND
CONTRAINDICATIONS

Staged tendon reconstruction is a salvage procedure. It is indicated whenever simpler procedures are not feasible or have failed, such as a failed primary tendon repair or graft. Staged reconstruction also is indicated when scarring is expected in the flexor sheath as after a severe crushing injury, a comminuted fracture or infection, and whenever pulley reconstruction is necessary. Many of these conditions can be determined preoperatively; often, however, the decision cannot be made as to the best course of action until the digit is explored and the condition of the flexor sheath and tendons is observed directly.

Contraindications to this procedure are all relative. Poor patient compliance can be a significant factor leading to failure; this can be ascertained preoperatively when the patient is required to attend therapy for preconditioning. A stiff finger also is a relative contraindication, but this may be reversed by an intensive course of preoperative hand therapy. Neurovascular compromise may put the viability of a digit at risk and requires the weighing of the potential benefits of the procedure in view of risking loss of that digit. An intact superficialis tendon in an index or long finger is another situation where staged reconstruction may not improve the function of a digit a great deal, since both digits function very well without flexion at the distal interphalangeal (DIP) joint.

These indications and contraindications are never absolute. They must be weighed against the needs of the digit considered for reconstruction, the need of the hand, and the need of the patient who carries that digit.

■ SURGICAL
TECHNIQUES

Local anesthesia with intravenous sedation is preferred if there is a suspicion that a tenolysis may be all that is necessary to restore digit flexion. A Bier block is otherwise preferred for stage I, especially in the face of extensive scarring and the equally extensive dissection that is usually required. Stage II is best done under general anesthesia because a tendon graft is often necessary and may be taken from one or both lower extremities.

In stage I, a standard Bruner incision is performed on the palmar aspect of the hand. Prior incisional scars are incorporated as much as possible. Previous midaxial incision scars are ignored. Provisions are made for any necessary Z-plasties or scar revisions. The incision starts in the midline of the pulp and proceeds proximally to the distal edge of the transverse carpal ligament. The carpal tunnel is not opened unless absolutely necessary; this allows flexion of the wrist postoperatively without a concern for tendon bowstringing at the wrist. The incision parallels the thenar crease and crosses all other creases at acute angles. In the distal forearm, the incision is continued in consideration of the wrist flexion creases, slightly to the ulnar aspect of the palmaris longus tendon, or of the midline of the forearm if that tendon is not palpable. Deep dissection is carried out with great care to preserve neurovascular structures. The lumbrical muscles and all flexor tendons are also preserved, unless severely damaged and cannot be recovered by a tenolysis. The flexor sheath and all pulleys must be preserved.

Familiarity with the anatomy of the flexor sheath is essential to the successful reconstruction of flexor tendon function. The flexor profundus tendon owes its mechanical advantage to the pulley system that holds it near the axis of rotation of the joints. There are 5 annular pulleys. A1, A3, and A5 pulleys insert on the volar plates of the metacarpophalangeal (MP), proximal interphalangeal (PIP), and DIP joints, respectively. The A2 and A4 pulleys insert on the proximal and distal phalanges, and have been touted as the only important pulleys in a finger. All annular pulleys, however, are important in flexor tendon reconstruction.[12] The palmar aponeurosis pulley is proximal to A1 and is part of the palmar fascia; it can substitute for the function of A1 if it is intact.[3] The cruciform pulleys do not add to the mechanical integrity of the flexor sheath and may be excised if needed. The superficialis tendon insertion consists of two slips of tendon that encase the profundus tendon and thus provide it with some structural support inside the flexor sheath. An intact superficialis tendon also improves the result of staged flexor tendon reconstruction and should be preserved.[10,12] The thumb pulleys are similar, in that there is a pulley over the volar plate at the MP and interphalangeal (IP) joints. In addition, it has a significant oblique pulley on the proximal phalanx, which must be preserved to prevent bowstringing.

Once all deep structures have been dissected out the flexor sheath is opened between the annular pulleys, starting in the area of suspected injury. A flexor tenolysis is performed, and all scar tissue is excised from the sheath. A decision is made at this point whether to proceed with the staged reconstruction. It should be done if the sheath or tendon bed are markedly scarred, especially if this is associated with pulley deficiency. A pulley may be reconstructed alone and does not warrant a staged flexor tendon reconstruction in itself. Injured nerves are prepared for neurorrhaphy if needed. The actual nerve repair is usually done just before wound closure, to prevent undue tension on the nerve during the reconstruction.

The distal forearm part of the incision is opened. The tendons are identified, and traction is applied on them to determine the degree of function of these tendons. This usually will help in the decision of proceeding with further tenolysis or reconstruction. The carpal tunnel is not opened, unless there is scarring into it or a median neuropathy requires its release. Detailed notes should be made of each step of the procedure for later reference, at stage II.

When the decision is made to proceed with staged reconstruction, the flexor profundus tendon is tagged and sutured to a neighboring profundus tendon in the distal forearm (side to side, with a 3-0 braided polyester suture). This will prevent excessive pull on the lumbrical muscle origin with active flexion. A decision is made as to which muscle will be used eventually in the reconstruction, and its tendon is tagged with 4-0 silk. The original profundus muscle is usually the preferred choice. The profundus tendon is then excised from the flexor sheath. A 1-cm stump of tendon is left distally at its insertion in the distal phalanx. In the palm, the tendon is divided just distal to where the lumbrical muscle originates.

Portions of the superficialis tendon (distally based flaps or free grafts) may be used for pulley reconstruction if needed. If that tendon must be excised, it is first sutured to a neighboring superficialis tendon in the distal forearm to maintain the length of its musculotendinous unit and for later identification if it is to be used in stage II. It is then divided at Camper's chiasm and excised from the flexor sheath and palm. All bone and joint reconstruction is performed at this time; joint contractures are released, and necessary osteotomies are performed.

A tendon sizer is used to determine the appropriate size implant. (Tendon sizers are not available commercially. Such a set could be made with implants of various sizes, without fixation plate.)

The implant is inserted from distal to proximal (Fig. 79–1). It should be the widest implant to fit inside the sheath without binding at any pulley, especially A4. It is usually inserted through Camper's chiasm of the superficialis tendon, then between the profundus and superficialis tendons and muscles in the carpal tunnel and distal forearm. As an alternative, the implant may be passed alongside the superficialis tendon at the A3 and A4 pulleys, and in the forearm it may be passed deep to the profundus muscle mass. A proximal pocket is created with blunt finger dissection in the distal forearm, to allow proximal gliding of the implant, without buckling anywhere along its course. Pulley reconstruction is done at this point in time, with the sizer implant in place. Next, preparation of the distal phalanx is made for the distal fixation.

■ FIGURE 79–1

Insertion of a silicone rod through preserved or reconstructed pulleys and the carpal tunnel, from distal to proximal.

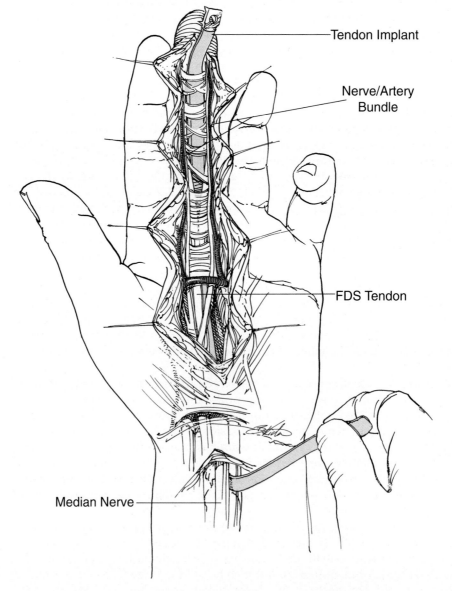

Tendon Implant

Nerve/Artery Bundle

FDS Tendon

Median Nerve

Whenever possible, distal plate fixation is preferred. The profundus tendon stump is elevated just enough to allow close approximation of the metallic plate against bone without impinging on the volar plate of the DIP joint. A hole is drilled at the base of the distal phalanx from palmar to dorsal with slight proximal angulation, using a 1.5-mm drill bit. Care is taken not to penetrate the joint or to injure the nail bed dorsally. Screw length may be ascertained with a depth gauge, and the hole may be tapped with a 2-mm tap.

The selected implant is now taken out of the package and soaked in antibiotic solution. The implant should be handled with blunt forceps only, and should not be allowed to touch skin, gloves, towels or any other source of particle contamination. It should be rinsed thoroughly if it does come in contact with any of these. The implant is inserted by holding the fixation plate above the wound, and by threading the silicone rod's proximal end through A5 pulley and from there on proximally. The distal end of the sizing implant may be loosely sutured to the proximal end of the final implant to help thread it into the flexor sheath. If the implant is excessively long, it is curled temporarily in the distal forearm.

Now the plate is secured to the distal phalanx with a 2.0-mm cortical screw (Fig. 79–2). The screw is tightened with the thumb and index finger only, while the plate is held with a Kelly clamp to prevent rotation. The stump of the profundus tendon is then folded back over the plate and screw. If the fixation is not found to be secure, for any reason, the plate may be cut off through the implant, and the latter is sutured under and to the profundus tendon stump with 4-0 or 3-0 polyester sutures (Fig. 79–3). Care is taken to insert the suture through the polyester core of the implant.

The implant is now located in the distal forearm; tension is applied and range of motion is observed. The fingertip should be brought to touch the distal palmar crease without undue tension. Failure to do so may be the result of joint stiffness or bowstringing of the implant. Appropriate measures are taken to correct this, such as joint release or further pulley reconstruction as needed. Once the desired range of motion is obtained, the digit and wrist are hyperextended simultaneously, pulling the implant distally, and the implant is cut approximately 3 cm proximal to the wrist flexion crease. This will ensure that the proximal end of the implant will not get caught at the level of the forearm incision in the postoperative period. Continuously using a no-touch technique, the proximal end of the implant is now embedded in the previously prepared pouch in the forearm.

The skin is closed in the digit first, using 4-0 nylon interrupted sutures. Passive range

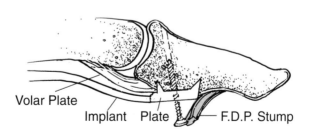

■ FIGURE 79–2
Application of a distal fixation plate. Care must be taken to preserve the A5 pulley and not to impinge on the volar plate. A distal stump of FDP tendon is used to cover the plate and screw.

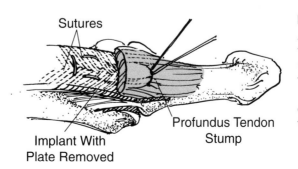

■ FIGURE 79–3
A silicone rod without a fixation plate may be used. It is anchored to the distal stump of the FDP tendon, with the end of the rod buried under the tendon.

of motion of the digit will now again confirm that the implant is gliding in the forearm without buckling. Finally, the forearm incision is closed. Silicone ribbon drains are left in all wounds, which are then covered by nonadhesive gauze and a bulky bandage. A dorsal splint is applied, maintaining the wrist in 20 to 30° of flexion, with the MP joints at 60 to 70°, and with the IP joints in neutral position.

During stage II, only the ends of the stage I incision need to be reopened. The pulp incision is opened to a level just proximal to the DIP flexion crease. Great care must be exercised in the process of the dissection not to injure the flexor sheath or pulleys. The distal forearm incision is reopened, for a length of 3 to 5 cm proximal to the wrist flexion crease.

The implant is identified at the wrist and tension is applied to it to determine the potential for active flexion that can be expected. Excessive scar tissue and sheath formation are excised in that location. A Kocher clamp is used to tag the implant and prevent premature distal pullout. The fixation plate is dissected distally, while again preserving the profundus tendon stump. The screw is removed, and a towel clip is passed through the screw hole for better purchase on the implant. The screw hole is enlarged with a Zuelzer bone awl, and a Keith needle is inserted through that hole in a distal direction, exiting in the center of the nail plate, using a hand drill.

A decision is made as to which musculotendinous unit will be used to motorize the digit using notes taken during stage I. If a tendon graft is necessary, the length needed is measured from the fingertip to the motor tendon, with the wrist and digit in a neutral position. The tendon graft is obtained from an appropriate site.[11] The palmaris longus is adequate most of the time, when available. A double length of tendon graft may be used if the graft is thin but long, as is common for the plantaris tendon. The graft is debrided of any residual muscle or excessive adventitia.

A grasping suture is inserted in the thin end of the tendon graft, using 4-0 Prolene suture. The suture is then tied loosely into the proximal end of the implant and the needle is cut off. The tendon graft is now threaded into the carpal tunnel and flexor sheath by pulling on the implant distally. Care is taken not to pull the proximal end of the graft out of sight at the wrist incision. The Prolene suture is threaded into the Keith needle and pulled distally through the nail. The tendon end is packed into the drill hole and the suture is tied over a button on the nail plate (Fig. 79–4). The profundus tendon stump is then sutured to the graft with two 4-0 polyester sutures. A gentle pull on the tendon graft proximally will confirm the adequacy of the distal anchor. A portion of the A5 pulley may be released if impingement is noted in that location. The digit incision is now closed with 4-0 nylon interrupted sutures.

Attention is next turned to the wrist incision. The tendon graft is sutured to the motor tendon with a single suture, using 2-0 polyester. Appropriate tension on the tendon graft is gauged by observing the normal flexion cascade posture of the fingers at rest, as well as with the wrist flexed and extended. Once the correct tension is obtained, the tendon graft is connected to the motor tendon with a Pulvertaft weave (Fig. 79–5). The wrist is flexed, and the digit is taken through a passive range of motion, to confirm that the tendon juncture glides smoothly in and out of the carpal tunnel.

■ FIGURE 79–4
The tendon graft is anchored distally into bone with a Prolene pullout suture, which is tied over a button on the nail; the tendon is also sutured under the FDP stump.

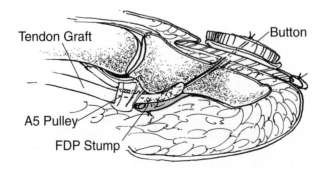

Tendon Graft   Button
A5 Pulley
FDP Stump

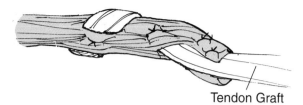

Tendon Graft

■ FIGURE 79–5
The tendon graft is sewn
to the motor tendon with
a Pulvertaft weave.

The wrist incision is closed with interrupted 4-0 nylon sutures. A 2-mm wide strip of Vaseline gauze is wrapped around the button to snug up the distal anchor and to prevent any impingement of the button of the dorsal skin (Fig. 79–4). A nail traction suture is inserted at the distal rim of the nail plate, with two loops of 4-0 nylon suture, without injuring the nailbed. Multiple silicone ribbon drains are left in both incisions which are then covered by nonadherent gauze, followed by a bulky bandage and a protective splint. The wrist is flexed to 30°, with the MP joints at 60° and IP joints free.

Technical pitfalls are numerous in such a demanding reconstruction. The silicone tendon implants are highly electrostatically unstable and can bind dust and debris. They should therefore be handled strictly with a no-touch technique and kept in an irrigation antibiotic solution, rather than on the instrument table. Care must be taken to prevent buckling of the implant when the digit is taken through a passive range of motion. At stage II, overzealous suturing of the tendon graft at either end can weaken the tendon to a point that would make tendon rupture unavoidable. Another difficult judgement issue is deciding the length of the tendon graft; a long graft will result in weak grip and a short tendon graft will produce a flexion contracture.

Most of these procedures are scheduled as "possible" staged flexor tendon reconstruction. This underlines the fact that alternate methods can sometimes effectively restore flexor tendon function.[8] Flexor tenolysis is the most satisfying of these procedures. A primary tendon graft can be performed if scarring is not extensive in the flexor sheath or, as an alternative, a superficialis tendon may be transferred with suture to the injured profundus tendon in the palm.[7] This also could be done in a more elaborate fashion, using the Paneva-Holevich staged tendon transfer.[6] Finally, consideration should be given to minimizing motion at the DIP joint with a partial flexion tenodesis or to an arthrodesis. A decision must be made as to whether PIP motion can be restored with any of the above surgical techniques, or even with staged tendon reconstruction. A capsulectomy or joint release may also be necessary, but when all else fails, an arthrodesis may salvage the digit.

■ TECHNICAL ALERNATIVES

Rehabilitation of a staged tendon reconstruction starts before surgery. The patient needs to undergo an extensive program of active and passive range of motion exercises, muscle strengthening, splinting of contracted joints, scar and edema control.

Hand therapy is started 3 days after stage I surgery. A resting splint is made, to be used mostly at night. The patient is instructed in wound care and edema control, as well as range of motion exercises with finger trapping. Unrestricted use of the hand is usually allowed, and close follow-up is needed to make sure any contractures are splinted out as soon as they occur.

Stage II is normally performed no sooner than 2 months after stage I. The patient returns to therapy the next day after surgery. The same splint used after stage I can be used at this time. The nail traction suture is connected to the distal forearm through a rubberband. The splint is worn full-time except when a tendon mobilization program is performed in therapy.[2] The rehabilitation is basically the same as used following flexor tendon repair. Close follow-up is again needed to make sure any contractures are splinted out as soon as they occur, especially at the DIP joint. Place-holds are started within the first 2 weeks. The splint is replaced by a wristlet at 3 to 4 weeks after surgery or sooner, if stiffness is noted. Active tendon gliding exercises are started at that time.[9] The rubberband and wrist-

■ REHABILITATION

let are discontinued at 5 to 6 weeks. The button and distal pullout suture are removed at 7 to 8 weeks. Unrestricted muscle strengthening is started 2 months after surgery, and heavy activity or sports are not allowed until 6 months after surgery.

■ OUTCOMES

Potential complications can be avoided by meticulous surgery and close monitoring of the rehabilitation program. Staged flexor tendon reconstructions have better results when performed in younger patients (age younger than 21 years). The outcome is worse if there are preoperative contractures or injury to the superficialis or lumbrical tendons. Injury to bone, joints, extensor tendons, or neurovascular bundles does not affect the outcome significantly. Revision surgery may be necessary in 1% of patients after stage I and in up to 33% of patients after stage II.[12]

Synovitis after stage I is usually due to implant contamination, buckling, or loosening of the distal anchor. It can usually be treated with rest and antibiotics. On rare occasions, the implant may need to be replaced, with thorough irrigation of the flexor sheath. Occasionally, stage II may be performed earlier if exploration is needed and the sheath appears to be adequate. Synovitis does not affect the final outcome.

The most dreaded complication after stage II is tendon rupture. This has occurred in 14% of 150 cases reviewed.[12] The rupture usually occurs at one end of the tendon graft, at a mean of 12 weeks after surgery. A prompt repair will salvage the graft. Adhesions requiring tenolysis occurred in 12% of cases in that series; they were all corrected successfully with the tenolysis.

The staged flexor tendon procedure failed in 16% of cases. These were salvaged with graft recession to a superficialis position, tenodesis, or arthrodesis. An amputation was done in 3% of cases as a last resort, because of multiple problems.

Staged tendon reconstruction using a silicone tendon implant is a salvage technique. It is technically demanding and labor intensive for all involved—patient, surgeon, and hand therapist. It requires at least two surgeries and many months of rehabilitation. With meticulous surgery and close monitoring, such a lengthy endeavor can be turned into a successful outcome. It can turn a flail digit that handicaps the hand into a powerful contributor to grip and hand function.

References

1. Bassett CAL, Carroll RE: Formation of tendon sheaths by silicone rod implants. Proceedings of the ASSH. J Bone Joint Surg, 1963; 45A:884.
2. Crosby C, Wehbé MA: Dynamic splinting after extensor tendon repair. Proceedings Am Soc Hand Therapists. J Hand Ther, 1991; 4:28.
3. Doyle JR: Anatomy and function of the palmar aponeurosis pulley. J Hand Surg, 1990; 15A: 78–82.
4. Hunter JM and Salisbury RE: Flexor-tendon reconstruction in severely damaged hands. A two-Stage procedure using a silicone-dacron reinforced gliding prosthesis prior to tendon grafting. J Bone Joint Surg, 1971; 53A:829–858.
5. Mayer L and Ransohoff N: Reconstruction of the digital tendon sheath. A contribution to the physiological method of repair of damaged finger tendons. J Bone Joint Surg, 1936; 18: 607–616.
6. Paneva-Holevich E: Two-Stage tenoplasty in injury of the flexor tendons of the hand. J Bone Joint Surg, 1969; 51A:21.
7. Schneider LH and Wehbé MA: Delayed repair of flexor profundus tendon in the palm (zone 3) with superficialis transfer. J Hand Surg, 1988; 13A:227–230.
8. Wehbé MA: Flexor tendon injury. Late solution. Hand Clinics, 1986; 2:133–137.
9. Wehbé MA: Tendon gliding exercises. Am J Occ Ther, 1987; 41:164–167.
10. Wehbé MA: Staged tendon reconstruction: Technique and rationale. In: Hunter JM, Schneider LH, Mackin EJ (eds): Tendon Surgery in the Hand, St. Louis: CV Mosby, 1987:260–264.
11. Wehbé MA: Tendon graft donor sites. J Hand Surg, 1992; 17A:1130–1132.
12. Wehbé MA, Hunter JM, Schneider LH and Goodwyn BL: Two-Stage flexor-tendon reconstruction. J Bone Joint Surg, 1986; 68A:752–763.

PART

IV

Tendon Transfers in Rheumatoid Arthritis

80

Extensor Carpi Radialis Longus to Extensor Carpi Ulnaris Transfer for Radial Deviation of the Wrist

Ulnar drift of the fingers is one of several debilitating deformities affecting the hands of patients with advanced rheumatoid arthritis. Using principles derived from Landsmeer's intercalated bone model, this deformity may result from abnormal posturing of the wrist and metacarpals.[4] Although differing in a number of respects from earlier theories, it is currently believed that one of the fundamental causes of this posturing is attenuation of the tendon of extensor carpi ulnaris and its supporting structures. This attenuation leads to a concurrent decrease in the ulnar deviation moment arm at the wrist and a reduction of the dorsal soft tissue suspension of the ulnar side of the wrist.[5,7] Consequently, there is a relative overpull of the radial wrist extensor tendons and a palmarward subluxation of the ulnar side of the wrist.[1] Combined, these factors posture the wrist and metacarpals in radial deviation, dorsiflexion, and supination. Attempting to maintain a mechanical equilibrium, the fingers would then be progressively positioned in a force-balancing posture of ulnar drift, defined as ulnar deviation, palmar flexion, and pronation.[6] Recurrence of ulnar drift after metacarpophalangeal arthroplasty may be due in part to a mechanical interdependence of the posture of the wrist and the fingers, particularly in those patients with untreated rheumatoid disease of the ipsilateral wrist. In an attempt to reduce the incidence of recurrence of ulnar drift by dynamically correcting the pathologic posturing of the wrist, Clayton and Ferlic developed the procedure of transferring the tendon of extensor carpi radialis longus (ECRL) to the tendon of extensor carpi ulnaris (ECU).[3]

■ HISTORY OF THE TECHNIQUE

The transfer of ECRL to ECU should be considered as a surgical option in any patient with an inflammatory arthropathy producing radial deviation and supination at the wrist and inability to actively ulnarly deviate the wrist. If ulnar drift of the fingers is present, the tendon transfer should be performed as a staged procedure before metacarpophalangeal joint arthroplasties or reconstructions. Additionally, ECRL to ECU transfer should be considered as a viable surgical option for post-traumatic ECU disruption in which direct repair is not possible.

Any condition in which the passive correction of a radially deviated wrist to a neutral position is not possible, such as severe arthropathy, ankylosis, or arthrodesis, is a contraindication to this tendon transfer. Similarly, any wrist already malpositioned in ulnar deviation, for whatever reason, would not be appropriate for the ECRL to ECU transfer. Finally, any neuromuscular condition leading to diminished activity of the extensor carpi radialis longus muscle precludes consideration for this transfer.

■ INDICATIONS AND CONTRAINDICATIONS

This procedure may be performed under pneumatic tourniquet control, using either regional or general anesthesia. The patient is placed in the supine position on the operating table, with careful attention directed at padding all potential pressure points. If a wrist capsulotomy is contemplated, I generally administer a dose of a first generation cephalosporin intravenously before exsanguination of the extremity and inflation of the tourni-

■ SURGICAL TECHNIQUES

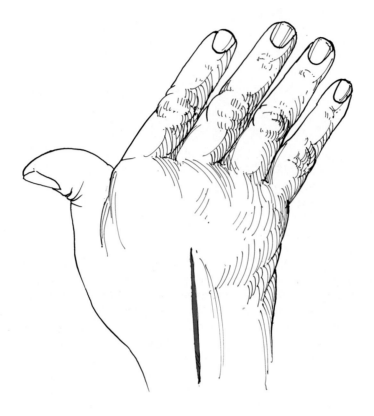

quet. A dorsal longitudinal skin incision is centered midway between the ulnar border of the head of the ulna and the radial styloid process. The length of the incision is 5 to 6 cm proximal and distal to the dorsal rim of the radius (Fig. 80–1). The skin and subcutaneous tissue are bluntly elevated as a single layer, with care exercised to protect the veins and nerves. It often is necessary to cauterize and divide several penetrating vessels to gain sufficient exposure of the deep fascia. The skin and subcutaneous tissue are gently retracted and held with self-retaining retractors. Once this is accomplished, the extensor retinaculum will be seen as a thickening of the deep fascia, approximately 3 cm wide, coursing obliquely from the distal aspect of the radius toward the ulnar border of the carpus.

Near the ulnar limit of the extensor retinaculum, the sixth extensor compartment is entered by incising the extensor retinaculum proximo-distally (Fig. 80–2). The superficial layer of the retinaculum is elevated as a radially based flap by dividing the deep fascia parallel to the proximal and distal margins of the retinaculum. The free ulnar edge of the retinaculum is elevated and retracted radially by placing two 2-0 sutures in the free corners of the retinaculum as retaining sutures. The tendon of ECU is now visible within the sixth compartment. A careful blunt dissection around the distal end of the tendon will demonstrate its broad insertion over the ulnar and somewhat dorsal aspect of the base of the fifth metacarpal. If ruptured, the distal end of the tendon will generally be found loosely adherent to the adventitial lining of this compartment. The distal end of the ECU tendon is gently freed from all adhesions. If minimal or no tenosynovitis is evident, there is no need to elevate the extensor retinaculum beyond the sixth extensor compartment. I find this, however, to be a rare situation. Therefore, the retinaculum is elevated as a single flap of tissue radially through each compartment, including the second extensor compartment. The septae between the third and fourth, fourth and fifth, and fifth and sixth compartments can be divided horizontally to allow this continuous elevation of the retinaculum. The septum between the second and third compartments, however, is a periosteal attachment of the extensor retinaculum into Lister's tubercle. Therefore, a sub-periosteal elevation of the retinaculum through this region is necessary to maintain its

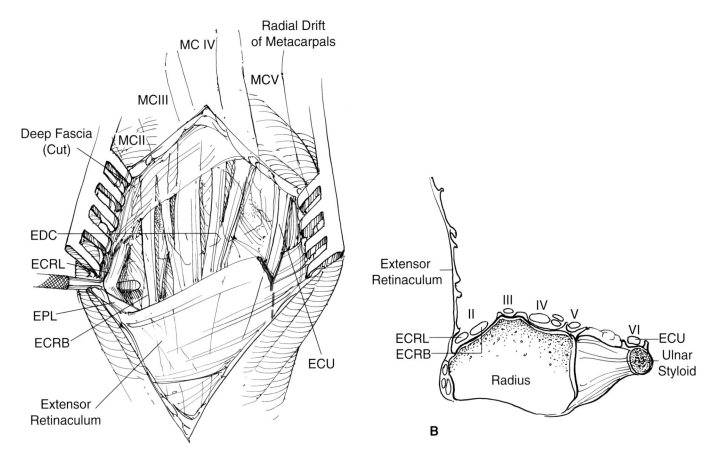

■ FIGURE 80–2
The key structures to identify are the tendons of extensor carpi radialis longus (ECRL) and extensor carpi ulnaris (ECU), attaching to the bases of the second and fifth metacarpals (MCII and MCV), respectively, and the extensor retinaculum. After dividing the insertion of ECRL into the second metacarpal (1), the tendon is passed proximally, under the extensor retinaculum. To expose the sixth extensor compartment, the extensor retinaculum is incised ulnarly and elevated on a continuous radial-based flap, using stay sutures placed in the free edge to maintain tension (2).

continuity. Unless obvious tenosynovitis is present, the first extensor compartment is left intact.

The tendon of ECRL is in the second extensor compartment, always radial to the tendon of extensor carpi radialis brevis, and inserts into the dorsoradial surface of the base of the second metacarpal. The base of the second metacarpal is palpated and cleared of all soft tissue except periosteum, carpometacarpal joint capsule, and the insertion of the ECRL tendon. Using a scalpel, the insertion is released as close to bone as possible. If the second extensor compartment has not been opened, a complete release of the tendon will allow only a minimal proximal retraction, as the vincular attachments within the second extensor compartment will continue to hold the tendon at length. Proximal to the extensor retinaculum, the deep fascia overlying the ECRL is incised, if not already done. Once the tendon of ECRL is identified, it is carefully isolated throughout its course in the second extensor compartment and proximally to the musculotendinous junction. The tendon is gently pulled proximally until it is free of attachment within the second extensor compartment. If an intra-articular procedure has been planned, it is carried out at this point, before the tendon transfer.

The retinaculum is repaired in one of two ways (Fig. 80–3). The first method is used if

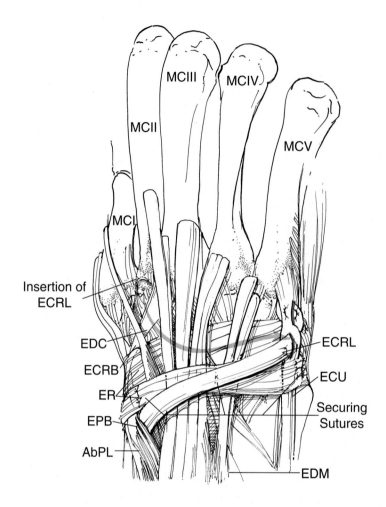

■ FIGURE 80–3

After delivering the divided tendon of extensor carpi radialis longus (ECRL) proximally through the extensor retinaculum (ER), the extensor retinaculum is repaired. The tendon of ECRL is passed ulnarly, superficial to the repaired extensor retinaculum, where it is interwoven with the tendon of extensor carpi ulnaris (ECU) through a series of perpendicular slits and secured with nonabsorbable sutures (3).

the retinaculum was elevated radially through the second compartment. Lister's tubercle is excised with a ronguer until the base of the tubercle is flush with the surrounding dorsal cortex of the distal radius. The retinaculum is divided in a fiber-splitting fashion into proximal and distal halves. The proximal half is placed superficial to the extensor tendons to reconstruct the retinaculum. The tendon of extensor pollicis longus is maintained superficial to the reconstructed retinaculum. The proximal half of the retinaculum is secured to the distal radius in the intervals between the second and third compartments and between the fourth and fifth compartments and just ulnar to the sixth compartment by passing two figure-of-eight 2-0 braided nonresorbable sutures through the retinaculum into the periosteum of the radius. Care should be taken to ensure that the extensor tendons glide easily through the reconstructed compartments. The distal half of the retinaculum is passed deep to the extensor tendons and secured to the dorsal wrist joint capsule with interrupted 2-0 braided nonresorbable sutures in a figure-of-eight fashion. The ulnar free edge of the retinaculum is specifically secured to the periosteum of the dorsal-ulnar base of the fifth metacarpal under tension to provide additional resistance to recurrent metacarpal flexion and carpal supination.

The second method of retinacular repair is used if only the sixth extensor compartment is opened. In this situation, the entire length of elevated extensor retinaculum is passed deep to the tendon of extensor carpi ulnaris, and is secured under tension to the dorsal-ulnar base of the fifth metacarpal with 2-0 braided nonresorbable sutures.

The free distal end of the tendon of ECRL is interwoven into the tendon of ECU, 1 cm proximal to its insertion into the base of the fifth metacarpal (Fig. 80–3). A 5-mm incision is made through the substance of the tendon with a scalpel, and the free cut end of the ECRL tendon is drawn through the slit. Tension is adjusted by pulling the tendon through the slit until the wrist is held in a neutral position. The transfer is secured with a figure-of-eight pass of 2-0 braided nonresorbable sutures through both tendons at the pass-through point. A second pass-through is made distal to the first pass-through, offset axially by 90°. Excess ECRL tendon is trimmed flush with ECU tendon. Care is taken to be certain that the tendon of ECRL is not kinked by overlying fascia, especially near its musculotendinous junction. The tourniquet is deflated, and hemostasis is obtained with pressue and electrocautery. The wound is closed over a small silicone drain with a few subcutaneous 4-0 resorbable sutures and 5-0 monofilament nonresorbable skin sutures place in a horizontal mattress fashion. A sterile dressing is applied, using Xeroform gauze, folded 4 × 4s over the wound, interdigital fluffed gauze, and padding for an anterior plaster splint, which holds the wrist in neutral deviation and approximately 20° of dorsiflexion. A more extensive plaster support may be necessary if the head of the ulna has been resected or if other reconstructive procedures were performed concurrently.

■ TECHNICAL ALTERNATIVES

There are no true alternatives to this procedure that have been described in the literature. A common pitfall is overzealous application of tension on the tendon of ECRL during the transfer, resulting in an unacceptably ulnarly deviated wrist. Further, this ulnar deviation of the wrist may indeed contribute to radial deviation of the fingers, through the same intercalated bone concept. Although this is seldom a functional impairment, the result is cosmetically objectionable. A second pitfall is to underestimate the degree of articular destruction in the wrist, which may interfere with the ability to restore proper alignment of the wrist. In this circumstance, treatment should be directed at the intra-articular pathology, with either an arthroplasty or arthrodesis procedure. Either technical error can contribute to the patient's sense of pain, instability, and limitation of function.

■ REHABILITATION

Immediately after surgery, the patient should be given active range of motion instructions for the fingers, forearm, elbow, and shoulder. At approximately 2 weeks, upon removal of sutures, a removeable splint is fabricated, again holding the wrist full-time in neutral deviation and approximately 20° of dorsiflexion. Three weeks after surgery, the patient is given careful instructions to begin progressive passive wrist range of motion exercises twice daily. At 6 weeks after surgery, active range of motion is initiated, with intermittent daytime and continuous night-time splint support continued for an additional month. It may be desirable to continue night-time splint use for an indeterminate time, but this is left to the surgeon's discretion.

■ OUTCOMES

In 1974, Clayton and Ferlic reported their results of ECRL to ECU tendon transfers in 14 hands in 10 patients with rheumatoid arthritis where an average reduction of wrist radial deviation of 15° was found.[3] In a similar study, Boyce and co-authors[2] found significant correction of resting wrist posture in 13 of 20 patients. Three patients were found to have no change postoperatively, and four patients experienced worsened radial deviation of the wrist after the transfer. In summary, I believe that the ECRL to ECU tendon transfer, if performed with careful technique and applied to patients meeting the appropriate indications, is a valuable and reliable procedure to correct deforming forces that may contribute to unacceptable initial correction or recurrent ulnar drift of the fingers.

References

1. Berger RA, Blair WF, Andrews JG: Resultant forces and angles of twist about the wrist after the ECRL to ECU tendon transfer. J Orthop Res, 1988; 6:443–451.

2. Boyce T, Youm Y, Sprague BL, Flatt AE: Clinical and experimental studies on the effect of extensor carpi radialis longus transfer in the rheumatoid hand. J Hand Surg, 1978; 3:390–394.
3. Clayton ML, Ferlic DC: Tendon transfer for radial rotation of the wrist in rheumatoid arthritis. Clin Orthop Rel Res, 1974; 100:176–185.
4. Landsmeer JMF: Studies in the anatomy of articulation. I. The equilibrium of the "intercalated" bone. Acta Morphol Neerl Scand, 1967; 3:287–303.
5. Pahle JA, Raunio P: The influence of wrist position on finger deviation in the rheumatoid hand: A clinical and radiographic study. J Bone Joint Surg, 1969; 51B:664–676.
6. Shapiro JS: A new factor in the etiology of ulnar drift. Clin Orthop Rel Res, 1970; 68:32–43.
7. Zancolli E: Structural and Dynamic Basis of Hand Surgery, Philadelphia, J.B. Lippincott, 1968:66.

HARRIS GELLMAN
MYLES J. COHEN

81

Extensor Indicis Proprius Transfer for Extensor Digitorum Communis and Extensor Digiti Quinti Minimi Rupture

Rupture of the extensor digiti quinti minimi (EDQM) and extensor digitorum communis (EDC) tendon in patients with rheumatoid arthritis is caused by attrition of the tendons over bony spurs, synovial invasion, or tendon ischemia.[7,9,12,15–18] Even if rupture has been relatively recent, end-to-end repair is seldom possible because of loss of tendon substance and shortening of the musculotendinous unit. For this reason, tendon transfer often is used to restore ring and small finger extension. A tendon transfer involves dividing the insertion of a musculotendinous unit and reinserting it into bone or another tendon while preserving the innervation and blood supply of the donor muscle.[14] If the rupture is many months old, the ruptured muscle may become contracted and lose much of its potential force and excursion. Therefore, when treating an old rupture, transfer is usually preferred to grafting.

In patients with rheumatoid arthritis, extensor tendon ruptures usually occur first on the ulnar side of the wrist secondary to synovitis of the radioulnar joint and dorsal subluxation of the ulna, resulting in rupture of extensor tendons to the fingers. EDQM and EDC ruptures of the fifth finger are probably the most common tendon ruptures in patients with rheumatoid arthritis. Patients rarely recall pain at the time of rupture. The first awareness by the patient that a tendon has ruptured is often the observation that one or more of the fingers cannot be extended.[4] The amount of extensor lag depends on whether both the EDQM and EDC tendons have been ruptured (Fig. 81–1). If repair or reconstruction is not done promptly, after a period of weeks to months, additional, more radial EDC tendons usually rupture.

The donor muscle used to reconstruct the EDQM and fifth finger EDC tendons should have adequate strength and excursion to restore a full arc of finger motion. The normal EDC excursion is approximately 5.0 cm.[14] The effective amplitude of a musculotendinous unit may be increased by the tenodesis effect of the wrist. Wrist motion can increase the effective amplitude of a transferred tendon, depending on the location of the transfer relative to the center of wrist rotation and the direction of wrist motion. The musculotendinous unit chosen for transfer should be both functional and expendable. In addition, transfers in which the function of the donor and recipient muscles are in-phase are much easier for patients to relearn than transfers that are out-of-phase.[4] In the older patient with rheumatoid arthritis, rehabilitation may take longer, and failures may be more frequent if retraining of the transferred muscle is required. The direction of transfer should, if possible, pass in a straight line from its origin to its insertion. If a tendon transfer must change direction, it should be passed around a smooth and stable pulley. After surgery, critical hand function should not be sacrificed as a result of the selected tendon transfer. The goal of tendon transfer is restoration of function, while not trading loss of one function for another.

The choice of transfer donor will differ depending on the number of EDC tendons that have ruptured. Although synovectomy and side-to-side suture to the adjacent, intact EDC

■ HISTORY OF THE TECHNIQUE

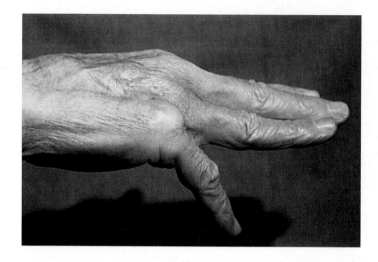

tendon can be performed, this will not restore independent finger extension. Additionally, if side-to-side suturing of the small finger extensor tendons to the ring finger EDC tendon is chosen as the method of treatment, care should be taken to ensure that the tension of the small finger extensor tendon is not excessive. If this occurs, the small finger will hyperextend and abduct with flexion of the wrist. To minimize problems with hyperextension and abduction of the small finger, as well as the loss of independent extension of the small finger, the extensor indicis proprius (EIP) transfer can be an excellent alternative for extensor tendon reconstruction.[8]

■ INDICATIONS AND CONTRAINDICATIONS

The EIP transfer is indicated for rupture of the EDQM tendon to the small finger or for combined EDQM rupture to the small finger and EDC tendon rupture to the ring and small fingers. When the extensor tendons to the long, ring, and small fingers have ruptured, transfer of the EIP tendon to the ring and small fingers combined with side-to-side suture of the long finger EDC to the index finger EDC also can be of value. The contraindications to the EIP to EDQM and EDC transfers should be considered carefully. Metacarpophalangeal (MP) joint and wrist synovitis should be under optimal medical control to minimize the possibility of attritional rupture to the transferred tendon. Also, other clinical possibilities that would explain the patient's inability to extend the MP joints of the small and ring fingers must be excluded. These possibilities include, first, subluxation of the extensor tendons. The tendons in the patient with rheumatoid arthritis can sublux to the ulnar side of the MP joint, coming to rest volar to the axis of rotation. The displaced tendons lose their mechanical advantage and can no longer initiate active extension. In contrast to extensor tendon rupture, these patients can usually maintain finger extension after the MP joint has been extended passively. A second cause for the inability to actively extend the MP joints is subluxation or dislocation of the metacarpophalangeal joints, often associated with flexion contractures. With dislocation, the fingers are typically positioned in flexion and ulnar deviation and are not easily or fully passively reducible. A third cause for inability to extend the fingers is posterior interosseous nerve palsy, usually secondary to proliferative synovitis at the elbow level.[3,10] Each of these three conditions are contraindications to the EIP to EDQM and EDC transfer; the conditions should be resolved before performing the described operation.

■ SURGICAL TECHNIQUES

The posture of the fingers as well as the passive range of motion should be observed before starting surgery. If rupture of the EDQM and EDC tendons is confirmed and other conditions are excluded, the operation is appropriate. The operation can be performed using either an axillary block or general anesthesia. The extremity is exsanguinated, and an arm tourniquet is inflated. A longitudinal incision is made along the axis of the fourth ray, allowing adequate exposure of the entire fourth and fifth extensor compartments (Fig.

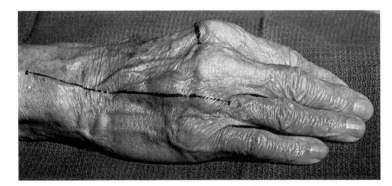

■ FIGURE 81–2
A longitudinal incision along the axis of the fourth ray exposes the fourth and fifth extensor compartments.

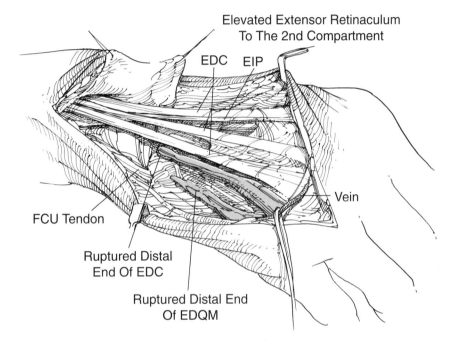

Elevated Extensor Retinaculum
To The 2nd Compartment

EDC   EIP

Vein

FCU Tendon

Ruptured Distal
End Of EDC

Ruptured Distal End
Of EDQM

■ FIGURE 81–3
Tenosynovectomy of the intact and ruptured tendons is completed before transfers.

81–2). These skin and subcutaneous tissues are mobilized from the extensor retinaculum. The retinaculum is elevated from the ulnar aspect of the wrist and mobilized to the second or to the first compartment, depending on the amount of synovitis present in those compartments. The dorsal fascia of the hand is divided longitudinally, as is the fascia over the distal aspect of the forearm. Once the ends of the ruptured tendons have been identified, synovectomy of the remaining intact tendons as well as the ruptured tendon ends is completed (Fig. 81–3). A longitudinal incision is made in the capsule over the distal aspect of the ulna. A synovectomy of the distal radioulnar joint and ulnocarpal joint is performed as indicated. Contouring or resection of the distal ulna is performed to remove rough edges, which may cause recurrent rupture. The capsule is then imbricated over the distal ulna and closed with a nonabsorbable suture. The EIP tendon is found ulnar and deep to the index EDC tendon. It is released distally just proximal to the insertion of the sagittal bands into the dorsal apparatus. This will minimize the chances of an extensor lag in the index finger, and patients will usually retain the ability to independently extend the index finger, even with the remaining fingers flexed.[2] The EIP tendon is then woven into the EDQM tendon using a Pulvertaft weave technique (Fig. 81–4). After placing the first stitch into the transfer site, passively flexing the wrist will allow an assessment of the tension by comparing the extension of the small finger with extension in the other fingers. Tension should be sufficient to maintain the fingers in full extension with the wrist in 20 to 30° of flexion, and the MP joints should assume a position of 20 to 30° of flexion with the wrist

■ FIGURE 81–4
The EIP tendon is woven
into the EDQM tendon
using a Pulvertaft weave
technique.

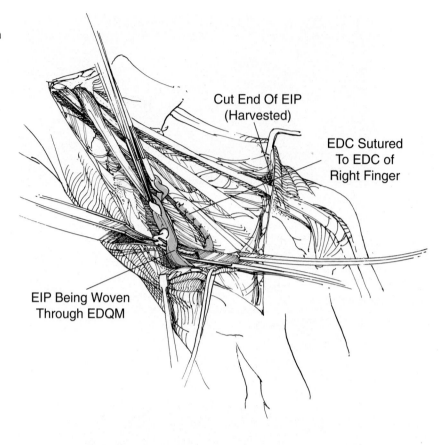

Cut End Of EIP
(Harvested)

EDC Sutured
To EDC of
Right Finger

EIP Being Woven
Through EDQM

■ FIGURE 81–5
The EDC tendon to the
small finger is then su-
tured securely to the
ulnar side of the EDC to
the ring finger.

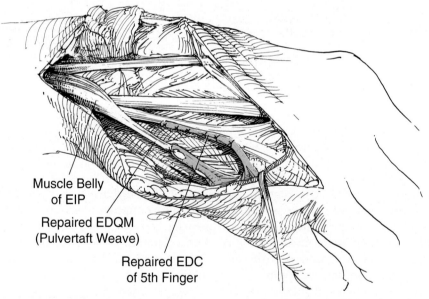

Muscle Belly
of EIP

Repaired EDQM
(Pulvertaft Weave)

Repaired EDC
of 5th Finger

in a neutral position. If the tension is judged to be appropriate, the weave, using two or three passes, is completed. If the tension is inappropriate, the temporary suture is removed, and the tension in the transfer is either increased or decreased depending on the intraoperative observations. Another trial suture is inserted, and the process is repeated. After the appropriate tension is selected, the weave is completed using a nonabsorbable suture material, preferably a size 4-0. The EDC tendon to the small finger is then sutured securely to the ulnar side of the EDC to the ring finger (Fig. 81–5) preferably with the knots deep. The extensor retinaculum is then transferred deep to the reconstructed extensor tendons at the wrist level to cover any exposed bone and the underlying wrist capsule. It is sutured along its ulnar boarder using 4-0 absorbable sutures. Similarly, the distal forearm fascia is closed, and the dorsal hand fascia is closed over the transfer site. The skin is closed with interrupted 5-0 nylon sutures. Small wick drains are inserted at the proximal and distal extent of the incision. A compression dressing with a volar plaster splint is applied. The dressings are changed and the drains are removed 24 hours after the operation. The sutures are removed 10 to 14 days after surgery.

An alternative to EIP transfer is transfer of the EDQM to the EDC tendon of the ring finger. However, this alternative may result in an abduction deformity of the small finger if not tensioned properly. When the EDQM tendon is ruptured and when there is attritional change in or rupture of the EDC tendon to ring finger a primary intercalary or bridge graft may be used to span the gap between the tendon ends.[1,5] A tendon graft requires transecting the donor tendon proximally and distally, temporarily devitalizing the tendon graft. For these reasons, tendon grafts are more likely to develop adhesions than tendon transfers.[6] Bora reported excellent results using palmaris longus tendon grafts to bridge extensor tendon defects after multiple tendon ruptures.[1] In the presence of an arthrodesed wrist or wrist with very limited active motion, the flexor digitorum superficialis transfer as described by Nalebuff and Patel may be effective.[13]

■ TECHNICAL ALTERNATIVES

The most common pitfall in EIP to EDQM and EDC transfer is incorrect tension. The best way to evaluate tension during surgery is to observe the amount of passive extension of the fingers with passive wrist flexion at the time of surgery. The surgeon should be readily willing to remove the temporary stitch and adjust the tension. If the procedure is done using peripheral nerve blocks and if the tourniquet time is minimal, the tension can be checked near the end of the procedure by having the patient actively flex and extend the fingers prior to wound closure.

Another potential error is allowing patients to move their tendon transfer too early after surgery. This can result in stretching or rupture of the transfer or graft, especially if the Pulvertaft weave is not tightly sewn. In contrast, the transfer can be immobilized for an excessively long period of time leading to limited transfer excursion, MP joint stiffness, and loss of motion.

Post-operatively a tendon transfer should be protected until the tendon juncture has healed and the tendon has revascularized. I usually immobilize the patients in a plaster cast or dynamic extension splint for a minimum of 3 weeks, but more commonly 4 weeks, and then start protected active motion. After immobilization, the patient is asked to move the hand actively and slowly through a full range of motion of the joints. The goal of therapy is to maximize active and passive motion, while protecting the tendon transfer. Patient education is very important to help prevent further loss of joint motion. The occupational therapist can make custom static and dynamic splints to assist in tendon and joint mobilization, as well as joint protection.

■ REHABILITATION

The endpoint of therapy comes when the patient has achieved a range of active finger extension as near full extension as is possible based on the patient's passive range of joint motion.

The use of the EIP transfer to restore finger extension after extensor tendon rupture to the ring and small fingers in patients with rheumatoid arthritis is a well-recognized operation. It is a viable option to transferring the EDC from the ring and small fingers into the EDC to the long finger, to intercalary free grafts, and to FDS transfer. In our experience, the EIP transfer is an effective and relatively predictable method for restoring finger extension when appropriately indicated. Transfer of the retinaculum under the reconstructed tendons is an important part of the operation, to minimize subsequent ruptures of the reconstructed tendon or previously involved extensor tendons to the more radial aspect of the dorsum of the wrist.[11] However, there is little documentation in the literature addressing the results of this operation in respect to finger motion, function, or patient

■ OUTCOMES

satisfactions; similarly the complication rates of this specific operation are not well defined. Nevertheless, this operation, when carefully performed and monitored in the postoperative period, can provide very gratifying results for the patient with rheumatoid arthritis.

References

1. Bora FW, Osterman AL, Thomas VJ, Maitin EC, Polineni S: The treatment of ruptures of multiple extensor tendons at wrist level by a free tendon graft in the rheumatoid patient. J Hand Surg, 1987; 12A:1038–1040.
2. Browne EZ, Teague MA, Synder CC: Prevention of extensor lag after indicis proprius tendon transfer. J Hand Surg, 1979; 4:168–172.
3. Chang LW, Gowans JD, Granger CV, Millender LH: Entrapment neuropathy of the posterior interosseous nerve, a complication of rheumatoid arthritis. Arthritis Rheum, 1972; 15:350–352.
4. Ehrlich GE, Peterson LT, Sokoloff L, Bunim JJ: Pathogenesis of rupture of extensor tendons at the wrist in rheumatoid arthritis. Arthritis Rheum, 1959; 2:332–346.
5. Feldon P, Millender LH, Nalebuff EA: Rheumatoid Arthritis in the Hand and Wrist. In: Green DP, Hotchkiss RN (eds): Operative Hand Surgery, New York: Churchill Livingstone, 1993:1587–1690.
6. Flatt AE: The Care of the Arthritic Hand, 4th Ed, St. Louis: C.V. Mosby Co., 1983; 123–130.
7. Goldner JL: Tendon transfers in rheumatoid arthritis. Orthop Clin North Am, 1974; 5: 425–444.
8. Leslie BM: Rheumatoid extensor tendon ruptures. Hand Clinics, 1989; 5:191–202.
9. Mannerfelt L, Norman O: Attrition ruptures of flexor tendons in rheumatoid arthritis caused by bony spurs in the carpal tunnel. J Bone Joint Surg, 1969; 51B:270–277.
10. Marmor L, Lawrence JF, Dubois EL: Posterior interosseous nerve palsy due to rheumatoid arthritis. J Bone Joint Surg, 1967; 49A:381–383.
11. Millender LH, Nalebuff EA, Albin R, Ream JR, Gordon M: Dorsal tenosynovectomy and tendon transfer in the rheumatoid hand. J Bone Joint Surg, 1974; 56A:601–610.
12. Nalebuff EA: The Recognition and Treatment of Tendon Ruptures in the Rheumatoid Hand. In: American Academy of Orthopaedic Surgeons, Symposium on Tendon Surgery in the Hand. St. Louis: C.V. Mosby, 1974:255–270.
13. Nalebuff EA, Patel MR: Flexor digitorum sublimus transfer for multiple extensor tendon ruptures in rheumatoid arthritis. Plast Reconstr Surg, 1973; 52:530–533.
14. Smith RJ, Hastings H: Principles of tendon transfer to the hand. AAOS Instr Course Lect, 1980; 29:129–152.
15. Straub LR: The rheumatoid hand. Clin Orthop 1959; 15:127–139.
16. Straub LR, Wilson EH Jr: Spontaneous rupture of extensor tendons in the hand associated with rheumatoid arthritis. J Bone Joint Surg, 1956; 38A:1208–1217.
17. Vaughan-Jackson OJ: Rupture of extensor tendons by attrition at the inferior radio-ulnar joint. Report of two cases. J Bone Joint Surg, 1948; 30B:528–530.
18. Vaughan-Jackson OJ: Attrition ruptures of tendons in the rheumatoid hand. J Bone Joint Surg, 1958; 40A:1431.

82

Extensor Indicis Proprius Transfer for Extensor Pollicis Longus Rupture

The extensor pollicis longus (EPL) tendon is commonly ruptured in the hand with rheumatoid arthritis (Fig. 82–1). It is often overlooked because the rupture is painless and there may be only a minimal functional deficit. There is minimal functional loss because the extensor pollicis brevis (EPB) often provides adequate extension of the metacarpophalangeal (MP) and interphalangeal (IP) joints.[2,4] Rupture of the EPL is usually due to rheumatoid synovitis within the closed sheath of the third dorsal compartment, with resultant impaired nutrition of the tendon. Mechanical attrition caused by the tendon rubbing on the roughened Lister's tubercle also may play a part, but rupture can occur from tenosynovitis alone.[2] Rupture of the EPL may present as a solitary lesion or be associated with rupture of all of the extensor tendons to the digits and wrist.

In the isolated case of EPL rupture, a number of alternatives for reconstruction are available, but a dorsal synovectomy with excision of bony prominences is necessary first, to prevent further tendon damage and rupture. It would be an unusual case in which direct suture alone would be a viable option,[13] although additional length could be obtained from rerouting the EPL out of its compartment and radial to Lister's tubercle. Therefore, a tendon transfer or a graft is almost always necessary.

Midgley[8] considers the extensor indicis proprius (EIP) the ideal motor because it is expendable, straight, synergistic, and subcutaneous.[5] Others also have recommended the EIP with satisfactory results.[9,12]

Millender and co-authors[9] reported on 12 patients with EIP transfer, 11 of whom showed active extension and ability to oppose the thumb to the little finger postoperatively if the carpometacarpal and MP joints were supple. The twelfth tendon reruptured, and at exploration the tendon was found to have ruptured proximal to the repair site and within the substance of the transferred EIP. They treated this with a bridge graft from the palmaris longus. In doing this transfer, they suture the EIP to the EPL and capsule at the MP joint, hoping to provide a stronger repair and prevent the adhesions that might occur at the suture site.

Clayton[3] reported on four EPL ruptures. One was repaired using the EPB and three with the EIP. Results of the thumb with the EPB were rated as good. Results of two with the EIP were excellent, and one was rated only as good because of limited motion.

Moore and co-authors[10] reported on 15 patients with rheumatoid arthritis or its variants. In 1 patient the palmaris longus was used, in 1 the extensor carpi radialis longus (ECRL) was used, and in 13 the EIP was transferred. No specific results were noted.

My preferred approach to the ruptured EPL is transfer of the EIP, but it must be kept in mind that in the patient with rheumatoid arthritis it is necessary to do a tenosynovectomy, dorsal retinaculum transfer, and bony debridement as well as the tendon reconstruction.

This transfer is indicated where the EPL is ruptured, the IP joint of the thumb is supple, and where the EIP is available to transfer.

Contraindications to this procedure are if the IP joint is stiff or has arthritic changes in

■ HISTORY OF THE TECHNIQUE

■ INDICATIONS AND CONTRAINDICATIONS

■ FIGURE 82–1
Photograph of a preoperative hand shows dorsal tenosynovitis and lack of extension of the interphalangeal joint of the thumb.

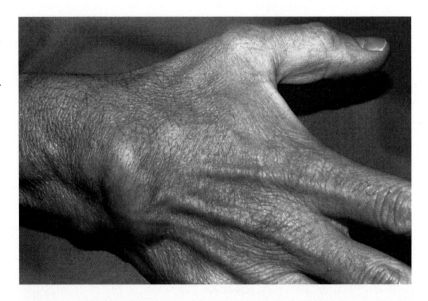

■ FIGURE 82–2
The ruptured EPL with tenosynovitis.

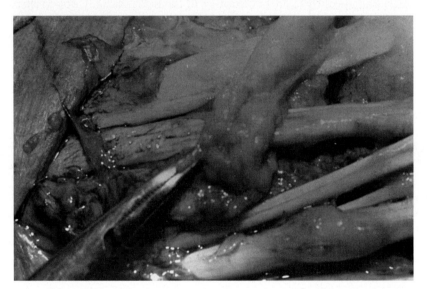

it. The joint would be best fused in these cases, and the tendon transfer would be superfluous. If the EIP is not available, this transfer is of course contraindicated. The EIP may have been used previously or if the finger extensors have also ruptured, the EIP may have been previously used or will be for motoring the fingers. If the common extensor to the index finger has ruptured, the EIP should not be used for a transfer.

■ SURGICAL
TECHNIQUES

General anesthesia or axillary block may be used. Often with the patient with rheumatoid arthritis, surgery other than this specific tendon transfer is performed simultaneously.

A straight midline incision is made over the dorsum of the wrist. The subcutaneous tissue is retracted with the skin in one layer. The dorsal retinaculum is reflected from the ulnar side through a longitudinal incision along the sixth dorsal compartment exposing the extensor tendons. A tenosynovectomy is performed, and the ruptured EPL is identified. Appropriate surgery to the distal radioulnar joint is performed as indicated. Bony prominences about Lister's tubercle are removed with rongeurs. The dorsal retinaculum is passed beneath the extensor tendons. The EIP is then harvested with a narrow strip of hood expansion by detaching it from the ulnar side of the extensor mechanism just proximal to the MP joint of the index finger. A deficit is created in the extensor mechanism which is closed with undyed 4-0 nonabsorbable suture; an extensor lag of the index finger PIP joint may develop if this is not done. This is due to the disruption of the stabilizing effects of the transverse laminae (components of the transverse fibers in the hood expansion that allow extensor forces to be transmitted to the lateral bands). If these fibers are intact, either the indicis proprius or the communis to the index finger can extend the finger properly.[1] The EIP is then attached with an in and out weave into the distal stump of the EPL starting proximally and going back through the EPL three times, and 3-0 nonabsorbable sutures are used to fix the transferred tendons. Excess tendon ends are trimmed (Figs. 82-2, 82-3, and 82-4).

Setting the tension is a critical aspect of this operation. One should error on the side of increased tension. Moore and co-workers[10] noted that they have never had a patient with an extension contracture, although an extensor lag is common. The tendon should be sutured with the MP joints of the thumb flexed, the wrist in slight extension, and maximal passive excursion of the transferred tendon.[10]

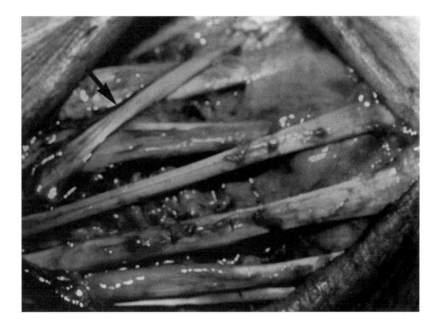

■ FIGURE 82-3
The EIP, which is indicated by the arrow, is transferred to the EPL.

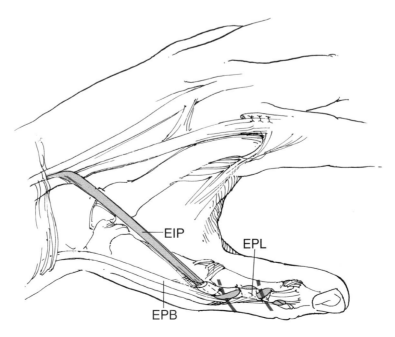

■ FIGURE 82-4
Method of tendon weave.

EIP

EPL

EPB

The wounds are closed, and thumb spica splints are applied with the thumb in extension.

■ TECHNICAL
ALTERNATIVES

A number of options have been proposed. Goldner,[5] and Hamlin and Littler[6] suggested using a free tendon graft (although Hamlin and Littler did not have any cases of rheumatoid arthritis in their series). Goldner also recommends transferring the brachioradialis. Goldner,[5] Pressly and Goldner,[11] and Straub and Wilson[14] suggest transferring the ECRL to the ruptured EPL.

Harrison and co-workers[7] recommended using the EPB. Their reasons for using this transfer were: (1) it preserves the EIP, which may be needed later to repair the finger extensors; (2) after this repair, extension of the thumb is in abduction rather than adduction; and (3) the operation is much easier to perform. They reported on 40 repairs in thumbs of patients with rheumatoid arthritis. Satisfactory results were obtained in all but one patient in whom the tendon ruptured again.

Shannon and co-workers[13] reported on 29 ruptures that were repaired with 20 EIP transfers, 8 ECRL transfers, and 1 EPB tenodesis. Only two patients were dissatisfied, both

■ FIGURE 82–5
A and B, Postoperative photographs of both hands show that the active range of motion of both thumbs is equal. The ruptured tendon was on the right thumb.

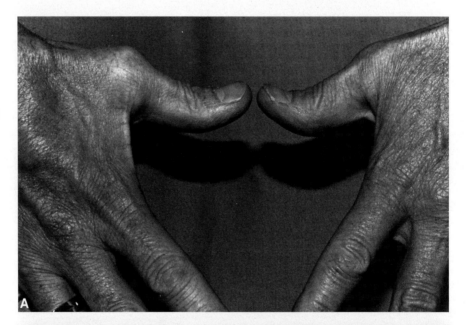

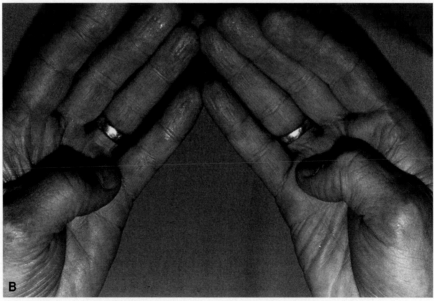

from the EIP group. Use of the ECRL provided extension equal to that achieved by an EIP transfer. There was a greater flexion deficit using the ECRL, but this was not considered a handicap by the patients and had the advantage of sparing the EIP for other tendon repairs. There were four failures due to rerupture, but two of the thumbs were still satisfactory because of EPB activity. Their recommendation was for the use of the ECRL. Others believe that because of the short excursion of the muscle of the ECRL, this transfer should rarely be used.[15] Other pitfalls that may occur are harvesting too much EIP so that the extensor mechanism over the index MP joint is compromised; likewise not taking enough tendon will force one to use an intercalated graft to compensate for the deficit or not being able to attach the tendon with a secure weave, thus not being able to start motion.

At 10 days, the dressings and sutures are removed, and a thumb spica cast is applied. Three weeks after surgery, the patient is seen by the hand therapist who fashions a removable, moulded splint with the thumb in extension. Active and passive exercises are started under the therapist's direction as well as instructing the patient on a home program. The splint is discontinued 6 weeks after surgery with unlimited use, although the exercise program continues until maximal range of motion and strength are obtained.

■ REHABILITATION

The results of the EIP transfer for rupture of the EPL in rheumatoid arthritis generally are good. Millender and co-workers[9] reported satisfactory results in 11 of 12 transfers, with 1 failure due to rupture. Clayton[3] had three EIP transfers, two were described as excellent, one only good because of limited motion.

My results have been quite favorable, making this transfer my procedure of choice for rupture of the EPL. I generally obtain active extension and opposition of the thumb if the basal joint, MP, and IP joints are supple (Figs. 82-5A and 82-5B).

■ OUTCOMES

References

1. Browne EZ, Teague MA, Snyder CC: Prevention of extensor lag after indicis proprius transfer. J Hand Surg, 1979; 4:168–172.
2. Clayton ML: Surgery of the thumb in rheumatoid arthritis. J Bone Joint Surg, 1962; 44A: 1376–1385.
3. Clayton ML: Surgical treatment at the wrist in rheumatoid arthritis. J Bone Joint Surg, 1965; 47A:741–750.
4. Ferlic DC: Management of the Rheumatoid Wrist. In: Clayton ML, Smyth CJ (eds): Surgery for Rheumatoid Arthritis. New York: Churchill Livingston, 1992:155–189.
5. Goldner JL: Tendon transfers in rheumatoid arthritis. Orthop Clin North Am, 1974; 5:425–444.
6. Hamlin C, Littler JW: Restoration of the extensor pollicis longus tendon by an intercalated graft. J Bone Joint Surg, 1977; 59A:412–414.
7. Harrison RD, Swannell AJ, Ansell BM: Repair of extensor pollicis longus using extensor pollicis brevis in rheumatoid arthritis. Annals Rheum Dis, 1972; 31:490–492.
8. Midgley RD: In: Creuss RL, Mitchell NS (eds): Soft tissue surgery of the rheumatoid hand. In: Surgery of Rheumatoid Arthritis. Philadelphia: J.B. Lippincott, 1971:159–163.
9. Millender LH, Nalebuff EA, Albin R, Ream JR, Gordon M: Dorsal tenosynovectomy and tendon transfer in the rheumatoid hand. J Bone Joint Surg, 1974; 56A:601–609.
10. Moore JR, Weiland AJ, Valdata L: Tendon ruptures in the rheumatoid hand: analysis of treatment and functional results in 60 patients. J Hand Surg, 1987; 12A:9–14.
11. Pressly JA, Goldner JL: Extensor pollicis longus rupture due to old fracture, collagen degeneration, or rheumatoid arthritis: analysis and treatment by transfer of the extensor carpi radialis longus. J Bone Joint Surg, 1974; 56A:1093.
12. Schnieder LH, Rosenstein RG: Restoration of extensor pollicis longus function by tendon transfer. Plast Reconstr Surg, 1983; 71:533–537.
13. Shannon FT, Barton NJ: Surgery for rupture of extensor tendons in rheumatoid arthritis. Hand, 1976; 8:279–286.
14. Straub LR, Wilson EH: Spontaneous rupture of extensor tendons in the hand associated with rheumatoid arthritis. J Bone Joint Surg, 1956; 38A:1208–1217.
15. Supple KM, Zvijac JE, Janecki CJ: Spontaneous, traumatic, nonrheumatic rupture of the extensor pollicis longus tendon: a case report. J Hand Surg, 1992; 17A:456–457.

GAIL MATTSON-
GATES, BRADFORD W.
EDGERTON

83

Flexor Digitorum Superficialis to Flexor Pollicis Longus Tendon Transfer for Flexor Pollicis Longus Rupture

■ HISTORY OF THE
TECHNIQUE

The sudden loss of the ability to flex the interphalangeal (IP) joint of the thumb is distressing and debilitating. In a patient with a diagnosis of rheumatoid arthritis, it is usually diagnostic of rupture of the flexor pollicis longus (FPL) tendon. Laine and Vainio[4] first described spontaneous ruptures of flexor tendons in rheumatoid disease. Mannerfelt and Lund[5] postulated that ruptures of the FPL are caused by erosion from volar bony spurs on the scaphoid or trapezium. Spicules from these carpal bones protrude through the volar carpal ligaments adjacent to the FPL tendon. Although the FPL is generally believed to rupture due to attrition in rheumatoid disease, direct synovial invasion into the tendon with resultant ischemia also may play a role by weakening the tendon.

Transfer of the flexor digitorum superficialis (FDS) from the ring finger to the distal portion of the FPL has widespread applications in hand surgery. Goldner[3] described the location of the typical rupture of the FPL in patients with rheumatoid arthritis as well as treatment alternatives. He mentions that the FDS of the ring finger to the FPL is a reliable treatment option, although the IP joint range of motion may be diminished. He briefly describes cutting the FDS tendon at the proximal crease of the ring finger, bringing it out at the volar surface of the wrist, and then passing it through the FPL canal once the FPL tendon has been removed. Schneider and Wiltshire[10] described the same transfer but provide more technical details. The technique we describe in this chapter is very similar to that described by Schneider and Wiltshire. In a more recent article, Ertel[2] mentions the FDS to FPL transfer as one of the options available to recreate thumb IP flexion. He gave no details on the technique. Instead, he emphasized the need to eliminate the bone spur in the carpal canal before tendon reconstruction. He illustrated a volar rotation flap he occasionally uses to close the defect left in the carpal floor once the spur has been removed.

■ INDICATIONS AND
CONTRAINDICATIONS

When a rheumatoid patient has a rupture of the FPL and desires reconstruction, transfer of the ring finger FDS is the most desirable procedure available. Although it might be feasible to restore the FPL muscle tendon unit with a tendon graft, unless this is accomplished within a couple of days of the rupture, the FPL muscle belly will undergo myostatic contracture and will lose the ability to provide full tendon excursion at the thumb IP joint. Generally, the delay in diagnosis and referral to a hand surgeon have precluded operating in this time period, and the FDS to FPL transfer remains the optimal surgical option.

The FDS to FPL transfer is indicated in rheumatoid patients with supple joints and a biomechanically stable thumb. These conditions are carefully considered during the preoperative evaluation. This evaluation should include: (1) careful physical examination of the thumb ray to assess the presence of arthritis, pain, and mobility in the carpometacarpal (CMC), metacarpophalangeal (MP), and IP joints; (2) careful examination of the tendons of the thumb and fingers to exclude the presence of either stenosing tenosynovitis of the thumb (which might also prevent IP flexion) and to exclude the presence of proliferative tenosynovitis of the fingers, which would preclude the ability to perform a transfer;

(3) careful neurologic examination to exclude an anterior interosseous nerve palsy that may be partial and only involve the FPL (this may require electromyographic study of the FPL and pronator quadratus); (4) radiographs of the hand and thumb, including carpal tunnel views, to look for bony spurs.

Assuming the diagnosis is correct, there exists a lengthy list of contraindications to this procedure. Significant pain or deformity of the wrist, thumb CMC joint, or thumb MP joint are conditions that would prevent an acceptable outcome. If the underlying problem in the wrist or thumb is correctable by arthroplasty or arthrodesis of the wrist, thumb CMC joint, or thumb MP joint, then a secondary FDS to FPL transfer may be considered. Other absolute contraindications include: (1) significant stiffness, pain, or deformity of the thumb IP joint; (2) swan neck deformity of the ring finger; (3) absence of function of the flexor digitorum profundus (FDP) to the ring finger; (4) significant proliferative tenosynovitis of the flexor tendons; (5) the presence or a history of ruptures of other flexor tendons in the operated hand; and (6) a patient who is poorly motivated, unwilling, or unable to cooperate in a 4-month period of rehabilitation and retraining. In the presence of an absolute contraindication, the reconstruction should not be performed, and an alternative should be considered (e.g., IP joint arthrodesis).

Before taking a patient to surgery, permission should be obtained to cover all potentialities. A carefully administered axillary block is the preferred anesthesia technique. Preoperative lateral cervical spine radiographs should be obtained in all rheumatoid patients to rule out C1–C2 subluxation that would make intubation extremely hazardous and contraindicated in the case of a failed axillary block. The possible need to extend the operation precludes the utility of the shorter-acting Bier block technique of intravenous anesthesia.

■ SURGICAL TECHNIQUES

The distal stump of the ruptured FPL tendon can usually be located at the volar thumb MP flexion crease as it emerges from between the two heads of the flexor pollicis brevis to enter the flexor tendon sheath of the thumb. Digital nerves and arteries to the thumb lie in proximity on each side of the FPL tendon.

The site of the rupture usually lies on the deep radial side of the carpal canal at its distal border. This is directly below the location of the recurrent motor branch of the median nerve to the thenar musculature and can be located on the surface at the midpoint of Kaplan's cardinal line.[9] Below this point lies the bony spur on the trapezium. The proximal stump of the FPL has usually retracted up to the level of the proximal wrist crease as it has no lumbrical muscle to hold it in the palm. If a cross-connection with the index finger FDP exists, it may be held more distally.

The point of decussation of the ring finger FDS is located at the palmar digital crease and is the most distal site that the FDS should be harvested. Understanding the surface anatomy of the structures that need to be exposed leads to the following skin incisions:

1. An ulnarly based zig-zag flap centered over the thumb MP flexion crease will expose the distal FPL tendon. This is performed first to confirm the diagnosis (Fig. 83–1).
2. A longitudinal incision to open the carpal tunnel is next performed in line with the fourth metacarpal to allow inspection of the flexor tendons and careful rerouting of the FDS tendon (Fig. 83–1).
3. After the decision to continue with a ring FDS transfer has been made, a separate longitudinal incision overlying the ring finger flexor tendon is performed from the distal palmar crease to the proximal digital crease to harvest the FDS tendon (Fig. 83–1).

To prevent injury to underlying structures in each incision, the surgeon should be aware of special anatomic relationships. The digital nerves and arteries to the thumb are in proximity to the FPL stump and must be identified and gently retracted. In the carpal canal, the thenar motor branch usually is located on the distal-radial side of the median nerve. An ulnarly based approach should avoid injury. The volar palmar arch and distal branches of the median nerve all lie superficially to the flexor tendons and must be protected. The ulnar communicating branch of the median nerve may be present in 80% of

The approaches for the FDS to FPL transfer use three incisions: (1) a zig-zag incision to expose the FPL distal stump; (2) a palmar incision to visualize the carpal canal and flexor tendons, and to identify the proximal FPL stump; and (3) a distal palmar incision to harvest the FDS tendon.

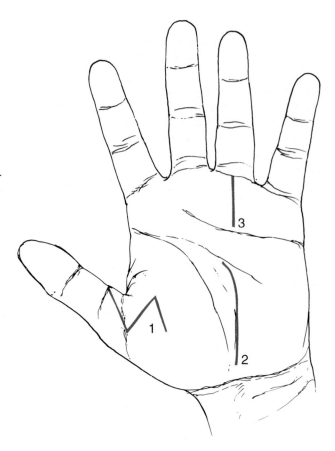

patients and should be sought and preserved.[6] In the distal palm, the digital nerves and vessels lie beside the tendon sheaths. They also should be identified and protected.

After exposure of the ruptured distal FPL stump at the MP joint level of the thumb, the other eight flexor tendons are carefully inspected through the carpal tunnel incision. If there is minimal synovitis and no other ruptures, the excursion of the FDP to the ring finger is tested. If the FDP produces full digital flexion, the FDS can be safely removed, and the third incision over the ring finger flexor tendons in the distal palm is made. If, for some reason, the ring FDS is not usable, the middle finger FDS may be substituted and the incision should thus be adjusted. A transverse incision in the tendon sheath between the A1 and A2 pulleys is made and the FDS is pulled into the wound, flexing the PIP joint. Each slip is divided at the decussation, leaving a 3-cm distal stump within the tendon sheath. The FDS is then brought into the carpal incision and freed proximally (often there are tendinous interconnections) (Fig. 83-2).

The floor of the carpal canal is inspected, and bony spicules on the scaphoid, trapezium, or base of the first metacarpal are carefully removed with a rongeur. If possible, the raw bone surfaces are covered with a flap of volar capsule as described by Ertel.[2]

A curved tendon passer is then passed retrograde from the thenar wound and used to grasp the cut end of the ring finger FDS tendon that is then positioned deep to the median nerve and FDS tendons to the index and middle fingers. The ring finger FDS tendon is repaired to the stump of the FPL at the base of the thumb crease. Tendon ends are sharply cut so that an end-to-end repair can be performed. The surgeon places a temporary stitch to determine the appropriate tension. The tendon repair is planned to lie within the soft thenar musculature. By moving the wrist, the tension of the repair is assessed. With the wrist in neutral position, the thumb IP joint should be flexed 30°. The IP joint should be fully extended when the wrist is flexed volarly. The tip of the thumb should flex to within 1 cm of the index finger as the wrist extends. During all movements of the wrist, the thumb

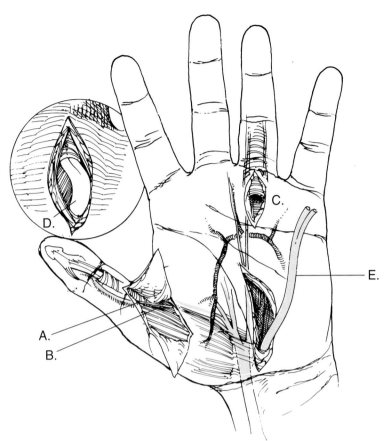

■ FIGURE 83–2
The three exposures re-
veal the anatomic struc-
tures important to com-
pleting the transfer: (a)
Distal stump of FPL; (b)
Neurovascular bundles;
(c) FDP tendon and neu-
rovascular bundles to ring
finger; (d) FDS tendon;
and (e) FDS tendon split-
ting into two slips, division of tendon was just
distal to this point.

metacarpal should be in 45° of palmar abduction. The end-to-end repair is completed with two core grasping sutures of 4–0 braided synthetic suture and a running 6–0 monofilament suture in the epitenon.

After tourniquet deflation, meticulous hemostasis is obtained, and all wounds are closed with 5–0 monofilament sutures placed in a vertical mattress fashion.

Gauze dressings are carefully molded to the hand, and a plaster splint is placed to hold the hand in a position to minimize tension on the tendon repair. The wrist is placed in 45° of flexion, the thumb is brought into full palmar abduction, and each joint of the thumb (CMC, MP, and IP) is placed in 30° of flexion.

In the rare case of early diagnosis of an FPL rupture, a short interposition tendon graft may be performed using the palmaris longus if available. This must be done before the proximal muscle belly has retracted and foreshortened (3 to 5 days). Interposition tendon grafting has the advantage of using the original motor and not disturbing another finger. It has the disadvantage of producing two tendon junctures that may form restrictive adhesions.

■ TECHNICAL
ALTERNATIVES

Some surgeons prefer to place the FDS tendon within the flexor tendon sheath of the thumb and affix it to the terminal phalanx. This will avoid creating a tendon juncture in the palm (potential adhesions or rupture) but has the disadvantage of violating the flexor tendon sheath in the thumb (more potential for restrictive adhesions). If there is adequate distal length in the ruptured FPL tendon, a proximal juncture is preferred. With a strong tendon repair and guarded therapy, the rupture rate should be acceptably low.

If exploration of the thenar wound reveals an intact FPL, the diagnosis is in error and the lack of IP joint flexion may be due to stenosing tenosynovitis or anterior interosseous nerve palsy. Release of the A1 pulley will correct the stenosing tenosynovitis, but exploration and decompression of the median nerve in the proximal forearm will be necessary to improve an anterior interosseous nerve palsy. (The surgeon should receive consent from the patient for these potential incisions.)

If exploration of the flexor tendons in the carpal canal reveals extensive proliferative synovitis, any attempt to transfer a weakened FDS should be abandoned, and a flexor tenosynovectomy of the fingers should be performed. If stabilization of the thumb IP joint is desired, an arthrodesis can be performed if patient consent has been received.

Proper care in the harvesting of the ring finger FDS tendon must be exercised along the guidelines proposed by North and Littler[8] to prevent PIP joint flexion contractures or swan neck deformities. These usually occur by attempting to harvest the FDS tendon too far distally. Correct routing of the transferred tendon in the carpal canal must be performed to pass it deep to the median nerve and prevent compression of the nerve. Preservation of all pulleys in the thumb is important to maximize the vectors that produce optimal thumb IP flexion, as emphasized by Apfelberg and co-authors.[1]

■ REHABILITATION

The procedure is usually performed on an outpatient basis. The patient is instructed to elevate his hand continuously for at least 1 week and is encouraged to move his shoulder, elbow, and fingers. All patients receive follow-up treatment from a hand therapist. The hand is immobilized in the plaster splint for 3 to 4 days. A guarded exercise program is then initiated with the thumb protected in a thermoplastic splint 24 hours a day. The therapist begins passive range of motion to all the thumb joints. The IP joint should be manipulated through a full range of motion with the MP joint blocked. At home, the patient begins active extension and passive flexion of the IP joint. At 4 weeks, the splint is modified to place the wrist at 0°. At 6 weeks, the patient begins strengthening exercises under the therapist's guidance. At 8 weeks, the splint is removed. Strengthening and gliding exercises can then take place without fear of rupture. Immobilization and protection of the transferred tendon may need to be continued for longer periods of time in patients taking oral corticosteroids. The cortical reorientation (using the ring FDS muscle to pull the thumb IP joint) may require months of hand therapy.

■ OUTCOMES

Very little has been written on the results of FDS to FPL transfer in rheumatoid patients. Mannerfelt[5] reported 21 of 25 cases of ruptured flexor tendons involving the FPL. FDS to FPL tendon transfer was mentioned as a therapeutic option but tabulation of their results was not given. Moore and co-authors[7] reported on five patients who underwent an FDS to FPL transfer. One developed carpal tunnel syndrome, but ultimately all did well. Overall, the patients received a score of 6 of 9 possible points. The exact range of motion was not reported.

Schneider and Wiltshire[10] reported on 14 patients with FDS to FPL transfer for irreparable FPL injuries. Two of these patients had rheumatoid arthritis. Eight patients had greater or equal to 60° of IP motion, 4 had 30° to 60°, 1 patient had less than 30°, and 1 had no motion. Pinch strength analysis showed four patients equal, four patients stronger, and six patients weaker than the contralateral side. They did not isolate their results in rheumatoid patients.

Although there are no studies available with sufficient numbers of patients to definitively evaluate the FDS to FPL transfer in rheumatoid patients, we have been very satisfied with this technique in the occasional patient with an isolated FPL rupture. It provides some motion and strength to the thumb IP joint with minimal risks. The ring finger functions very well using the FDP tendon alone. The operation itself is straightforward and can be done under a regional block in a relatively short period of time. Considering the benefits of preserving active thumb IP joint function, the FDS to FPL transfer should be the first line treatment in any suitable patient with an FPL rupture or laceration.

References

 1. Apfelberg DB, Maser MR, Lash H, Keoshian L: "I-P flexor lag" after thumb flexor reconstruction-causes and solution. Hand, 1980; 12:167–172.

2. Ertel AN: Flexor tendon ruptures in rheumatoid arthritis. Hand Clin, 1989; 5:177–190.
3. Goldner JL: Tendon transfers in rheumatoid arthritis. Orthop Clin North Am, 1975; 5: 425–444.
4. Laine VAI, Vainio K: Spontaneous ruptures of tendons in rheumatoid arthritis. Acta Orthop Scand, 1955; 24:250–257.
5. Mannerfelt L, Lund ON: Attrition ruptures of flexor tendons in rheumatoid arthritis caused by bony spurs in the carpal tunnel. J Bone Joint Surg, 1969; 51B:270–277.
6. Meals RA, Shaner M: Variations in digital sensory patterns: A study of the ulnar nerve-median nerve palmar communicating branch. J Hand Surg, 1983; 8:411–414.
7. Moore JR, Weiland AJ, Valdata L: Tendon ruptures in the rheumatoid hand: Analysis of treatment and functional results in 60 patients. J Hand Surg, 1987; 12A:9–14.
8. North ER, Littler JW: Transferring the flexor superficialis tendon: Technical considerations in the prevention of proximal interphalangeal joint disability. J Hand Surg, 1980; 5:498–501.
9. Riordan DC, Kaplan EB: Surface anatomy of the hand and wrist. In: Kaplan's Functional and Surgical Anatomy of the Hand, 3rd Ed, Morton Spinner. Philadelphia: J. B. Lippinicott, 1984: 353–360.
10. Schneider LH, Wiltshire D: Restoration of flexor pollicis longus function by flexor digitorum superficialis transfer. J Hand Surg, 1983; 8:98–101.

WILLIAM F. BLAIR

84

Crossed Intrinsic Transfers

Ulnar drift of the fingers is a common deformity in the hands of patients with rheumatoid arthritis. In rheumatoid arthritis, synovitis and attenuation of soft tissues in the wrist can lead to volar subluxation and ulnar translation of the carpal bones, which is characterized by radial deviation of the metacarpals. This orientation of the metacarpals is associated with soft tissue changes about the metacarpophalangeal (MP) joints. The soft tissue changes are secondary to synovitis that attenuates the extensor hoods, allowing ulnar subluxation of the extensor tendons, and flexor tenosynovitis that attenuates the flexor sheath allowing palmar and ulnar subluxation of the flexor tendons. The net affect of these tendon displacements is a moment at the MP joint, which rotates the proximal phalanx in an ulnar direction. This ulnar deviation or drift of the fingers completes the zigzag deformity characteristic of rheumatoid hand deformity.[2,5,9,12]

Of the dynamic tendon transfers available to treat ulnar drift of the fingers, crossed intrinsic transfers (CITs) were first used by Straub in 1966.[11] In this operation, the ulnar lateral bands from the index, long, and ring fingers were inserted into the radial aspect of the dorsal apparatus of the long, ring, and small fingers, respectively. A more complex operation, using a strip of the extensor digitorum communis and transfer of the intrinsic into holes in the proximal phalanx, was described by Harrison and co-authors.[7] Straub's operation was later modified by Flatt, who was concerned that the transfer into the dorsal apparatus would contribute to the development of swan-neck deformities in the recipient fingers.[4,6] This concern was based on observations of Straub's patients at follow-up, during a personal visit by Dr. Flatt to Dr. Straub's practice. Consequently, Flatt modified Straub's procedure and recommended insertion of the transfer into the radial collateral ligament of the MP joint of the recipient finger. Regardless of precisely where the transfer is inserted, the transfer itself is usually only one component of a complex soft tissue reconstruction about the MP joint. This concept is inherent in Wood's description of soft tissue reconstruction of the MP joint in rheumatoid arthritis.[13] Interestingly, Dr. Wood served his hand fellowship with Dr. Flatt, during which time he was introduced to the crossed intrinsic transfer procedure. The operation that I describe is essentially that of Flatt,[6] except that the transfer is usually inserted into the radial aspect of the dorsal apparatus, rather than routinely into the radial collateral ligament of the MP joint.

Crossed intrinsic transfers are indicated primarily in the care of patients with rheumatoid arthritis who have ulnar drift of the fingers (Fig. 84–1). The rate of progression of the drift and the magnitude of the deviation should be advanced enough to interfere with the patient's activities of daily living and work-related activities. Rapid progression of drift in a 6-month period of time or deviation of 30° or more will usually cause this degree of impairment. During physical examination, the ulnar deviation should be passively correctable to neutral, the proximal phalanges should not be subluxed palmarward on the metacarpal heads, and there should be no flexion contractures at the MP joints. Plain radiographs should demonstrate not more than minimal changes associated with rheumatoid arthritis in the MP joints. The wrist should be well aligned in the frontal plane, both on physical examination and in radiographs. This operation is best performed early in the course of the disease, before subluxation of the proximal phalanx or the development of MP joint flexion contractures.

Contraindications to CIT include ulnar drift that, despite meeting other criteria, is not

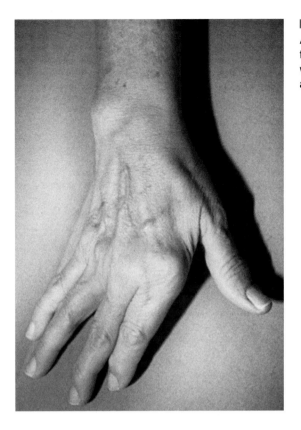

associated with a functional impairment for the patient. A zigzag collapse of the wrist, with palmar subluxation of the wrist and radial deviation of the metacarpals, is a contraindication to CIT. The wrist deformity should be corrected, either through bony procedures or an extensor carpi radialis longus to extensor carpi ulnaris transfer. Correction of wrist deformity should be done prior to the CIT transfer, either as a staged or during a combined procedure.

Advanced MP joint disease also is a contraindication to the operation. Unacceptable MP joint disease is characterized on physical examination by flexion contractures or irreducible palmar subluxation of the proximal phalanx and in radiographs by extensive erosions, joint space narrowing, and reactive subchondral bone. Reducible subluxation of the proximal phalanx is a relative although not absolute contraindication. Finger flexor or extensor tendon ruptures or tenosynovitis should be addressed before the CIT operation. The patient's general medical condition, motivation, and ability to meaningfully participate in a rehabilitation program should be assured before performing this operation.

The operation may be done under either axillary block or general anesthesia. A pneumatic tourniquet is applied about the upper arm. The arm is exsanguinated and the tourniquet is inflated. The initial approach is through a transverse skin incision 1 cm distal to the center of the prominence of the metacarpal heads, as defined with the MP joints slightly flexed. The skin incision is completed, and blunt dissection is then used to spread the skin and subcutaneous tissues apart. All veins in the depressions between the metacarpal heads should be carefully preserved. Some of the very small veins directly over the metacarpal heads may have to be electrically cauterized. The skin flaps are sewn proximally and distally with 4-0 nylon retention sutures. A longitudinal incision is made in the sagittal fibers of the dorsal apparatus, just to the radial side of the extensor digitorum communis (EDC) tendon. This release is usually carried to a point about 5 mm distal to the MP joint. The dorsal apparatus is bluntly dissected from the underlying dorsal capsule. When a significant amount of synovitis is present in the MP joint, a longitudinal incision is made

■ SURGICAL TECHNIQUES

in the dorsal capsule, and a synovectomy of the MP joint is completed. The extent of the synovectomy is governed by the dorsal approach; only the synovium that can be easily accessed is removed. Retractors are placed under the dorsal skin of each finger, the skin is elevated, and the ulnar "wing tendon" is identified. Beginning with the index finger, a longitudinal incision is made along the ulnar aspect of the EDC tendon to include the most proximal fibers of the sagittal bands, extending distally for approximately 2.5 cm; this incision is along the dorsal border of the "wing tendon." Distally the "wing tendon" narrows to become the lateral band; here it is transected transversely as far distally as the exposure allows. The tendon is mobilized from distally to proximally. Mobilization is accomplished by bluntly releasing all loose fibrous adhesions that are usually most apparent between the deep surface of the intrinsic tendon and MP joint capsule. This dissection is completed far enough proximally to include any adhesions to the intrinsic muscle itself. When satisfactorily completed gentle traction on the tendon should demonstrate 3 to 5 mm of free excursion. A tunnel is then bluntly dissected in the subcutaneous tissues deep in the web space between the fingers and the transfer is passed from the index finger to the radial aspect of the long finger (Fig. 84–2). The same procedure is then completed, moving the ulnar intrinsic from the long to the radial side of the ring finger, and moving the ulnar intrinsic from the ring finger to the radial side of the small finger (Fig. 84–3). Blunt dissection is then used to expose the abductor digiti quinti minimi (ADQM) tendon at the base of the small finger, and the medial-most fibers are isolated and divided.

If operative findings had previously indicated a synovectomy of the MP joint of the index finger, the radial collateral ligament insertion into the radial aspect of the second metacarpal is taken down using sharp dissection. The periosteum is stripped from the dorsal radial aspect of the second metacarpal, and it is roughened with a curet. A 3-0 Prolene suture is woven through the radial collateral ligament. An oblique hole is drilled in the distal metacarpal with a 0.035 K-wire from dorsal-ulnarly to volar-radially. A 22-gauge needle is passed from dorsally out the hole volarly. The deep end of the 3-0 Prolene

■ FIGURE 84–2
A diagram of each of the major steps taken to complete the crossed intrinsic transfers. 1, the ulnar intrinsic tendon is released and mobilized. 2, the tendon is transferred to the adjacent finger. 3, the transfer is usually sewn into the EDC tendon. 4, the most medial fibers of the ADQM are isolated and released. Inset: one technique for inserting the transfer into the EDC tendon.

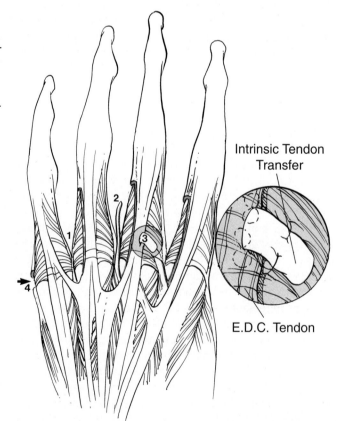

Intrinsic Tendon
Transfer

E.D.C. Tendon

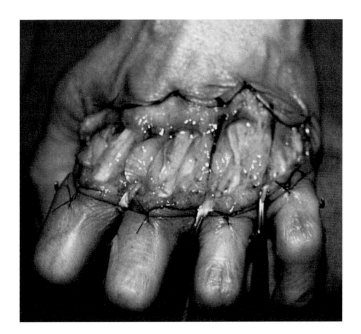

After releasing the intrinsic tendons, they are passed under the subcutaneous tissue to the radial aspect of the adjacent finger, and centralization of the EDC tendon is completed before intrinsic tendon insertion.

suture is passed up the needle. The needle is withdrawn, delivering the suture out the dorsal hole. The suture is placed in a clamp and set aside. The index finger is then held in full extension and slight radial deviation relative to the longitudinal axis of the metacarpal. The radial collateral ligament is reattached in a slightly advanced position by tying the 3-0 Prolene suture. The capsule, in those joints where it has been opened, is then trimmed and closed with interrupted 4-0 absorbable sutures. The EDC tendons of each finger are then centralized. This usually requires releasing the ulnar sagittal fibers until the EDC tendon can be easily and freely moved to a position that is centered over the metacarpal head. With the MP joint held in neutral alignment the radial sagittal fibers of the dorsal apparatus are repaired using a pants over vest suture of 4-0 Prolene, with the knot buried between the two layers of the dorsal apparatus. Three sutures are used over each MP joint. This repair will retain the EDC tendon in a centralized location.

The crossed intrinsic transfers are then completed, beginning with the long finger. The very end of the transfer is grasped with a hemostat, and tension is gently applied. If the excursion of the transfer along the radial aspect of the MP joint is adequate no further dissection is needed. If the excursion is not free, additional dissection and release of adhesions proximally may be required. The radial margin of the EDC tendon is then located. Two small parallel incisions are made in this tendon. The transfer is passed through the two incisions and back onto itself. Very gentle traction is applied, to snug the transfer, without displacing the dorsal apparatus radially. The tendon transfer is then sewn to the recipient tendon using two figure-of-eight stitches of a 4-0 nonabsorbable material. The transfer is then sewn back onto itself, if length permits, and additional stitches are added (Fig. 84-2, inset). The same procedure is repeated for the ring and small fingers. As each transfer is being inserted, the finger is positioned in neutral alignment relative to the longitudinal axis of the metacarpal, the MP joint is positioned at neutral, and the proximal interphalangeal (PIP) joint is allowed to assume a slightly flexed (20 to 30°) position. As each transfer is inserted, the alignment of each finger is reassessed and assured.

The tourniquet is then deflated and compression is applied for a few minutes. Hemostasis is confirmed and the skin is closed with interrupted horizontal and simple sutures of 5-0 nylon. The skin margins should not be inverted. Two small passive drains are inserted into the wound. A compression dressing with volar and dorsal splints is applied, holding the wrist in neutral and the fingers in neutral flexion-extension and deviation at the MP joints, and in slight flexion at the PIP and distal phalangeal (DIP) joints.

■ TECHNICAL
ALTERNATIVES

Historically a variety of different operations have been described to correct ulnar drift. Static operations include arthrodesis of the MP joint of the ring or small finger,[10] or cross-fusions of the ring and small finger proximal phalanges.[1] Operations using dynamic transfers have used extrinsic tendons or simple intrinsic releases. The primary extrinsic transfer for ulnar drift has used the extensor indicis proprius. The intrinsic release operation may be done alone or with EDC centralization over the MP joints.

The primary technical issue with the CIT operation has historically concerned the locus of transfer insertion. The operation that I have described inserts the transfer into the radial aspect to the dorsal apparatus. Flatt's alternative recommendation was to insert the transfer into the radial collateral ligament of the MP joint. We presently transfer into the dorsal apparatus as there has not been clear demonstration that transferring of the tendon into the dorsal apparatus increases the likelihood of the development of a swan-neck deformity. However, in patients with very lax PIP joints or with a predisposition to swan-neck deformity, Dr. Flatt has advised that it is best not to insert the transfer into the dorsal apparatus. With this I concur, and modify the operation to place the transfer into the radial collateral ligament of the MP joint.

A potential pitfall with this operation is a failure to release the ADQM tendon, predisposing to recurrent ulnar drift of the small finger. In contrast, excessive release of the lateral fibers of the ADQM tendon can inadvertently release the flexor digiti minimi, resulting in decreased postoperative flexion of the small finger MP joint. Failure to adequately and securely centralize the EDC tendons may allow recurrent ulnar subluxation, again predisposing to ulnar drift. It is also possible to insert the transfers under too much tension, resulting in radial deviation of all fingers, which is cosmetically disturbing, but rarely a functional impairment. Care should be taken to harvest the lateral band far enough distally. If it is too short, too much tension has to be imparted to the recipient dorsal apparatus to complete the transfer, resulting in radial displacement of the dorsal apparatus.

■ REHABILITATION

For approximately 5 to 7 days postoperatively, the patient is left in the plaster apposition splints, to maintain the wrist in neutral, the MP joints in neutral, and the fingers well aligned. As soon as local wound conditions permit, the patient is placed in a dynamic MP joint extension orthotic, using outriggers and rubber bands. In addition to routine flexion exercises in the splint, the patient is encouraged to remove the rubber bands at least three times a day to work fairly aggressively on active range of motion exercises, with an emphasis on MP joint flexion. Failure to initiate early active MP joint motion will contribute to MP joint stiffness following this operation. The patient continues to wear the splint for 3 weeks after surgery. At that time, the dynamic splint is discontinued and limited activities of daily living are allowed. The patient is encouraged to work regularly on active and passive ranges of motion for all joints of the operated fingers. If there is a tendency for recurrent ulnar drift, a static night splint holding the operated fingers in neutral is prescribed. Six weeks after surgery, unrestricted activities of daily living and household-related activities are allowed, and the patient is encouraged to begin active resisted exercises. Eight weeks after surgery, resumption of unrestricted activities is recommended, and at 3 months, the static splint is discontinued (Figs. 84-4A and 84-4B).[5]

■ OUTCOMES

Evaluations of the CIT operation have emphasized the following criteria: (1) correction and maintenance of correction of ulnar drift, (2) active ranges of MP joint motion, (3) active ranges of PIP and DIP joint motion, and (4) the development of postoperative swan-neck deformity.

That the CIT operation can effectively correct ulnar drift is fairly well established. Wood and co-authors[13] observed an average ulnar drift of 6° at 81 months postoperatively, and Oster and co-authors[8] observed an average of 5° at 12.7 years postoperatively. Although the magnitude of actual change in degrees of ulnar drift has not yet been documented, if preoperative ulnar drifts of about 30° for the patients in these studies is assumed, the improvement is substantial. That the correction in ulnar drift is maintained is also fairly well established. Oster and co-authors compared ulnar drift by finger in three groups of

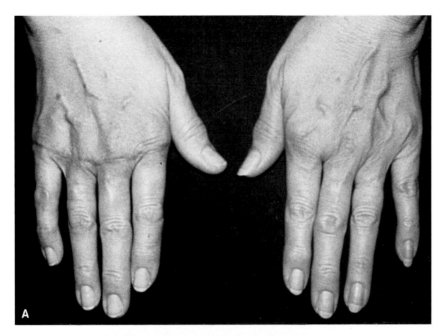

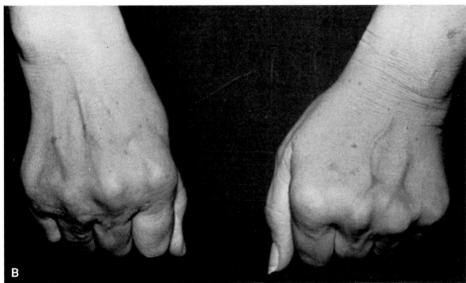

■ FIGURE 84-4
A, One year postoperatively, the patient's ulnar drift is well corrected. **B,** Although loss of MP active motion can be a limitation, good MP motion can be obtained.

patients followed for short, intermediate, and long terms, and found 7, 3, and 5° of drift, respectively. There were no significant differences among these groups, leading the authors to conclude that "the correction can be maintained over time."

Surgery of the magnitude inherent in the CIT operation in and around the MP joint has the potential to decrease active range of motion. Wood and co-authors[13] observed an average active MP motion of 56° at 81 months postoperatively, and Oster and co-authors[8] observed 47° at 12.7 years postoperatively. The extent to which these motions represent a change over preoperative motion was assessed by El-Gammel and Blair.[3] They observed an average loss of 18°. This tendency for MP joint active flexion to decrease after the CIT operation has led me to modify the postoperative management, allowing earlier, more aggressive active MP joint motion than previously.

A conceptual objection to the CIT operation concerns its effect on PIP and DIP joint motions. It is argued that increased tension in the dorsal apparatus of the recipient finger will decrease the ability of the PIP joint to flex. This issue was also addressed by El-Gammel and Blair,[3] who found a significant increase in PIP joint motion through 5 years postoperatively and a significant increase in DIP motion through 2 years postoperatively. These results suggest that release of the tight intrinsic tendon had a greater salubrious effect on PIP joint motion of the donor finger than insertion of the intrinsic into the dorsal apparatus of the recipient finger.

The development of swan-neck deformity has been and remains a concern. Oster and co-authors compared the development of swan-neck deformity in two groups of patients, one of which had the original transfer described by Straub and the other the modified transfer described by Flatt. Oster and co-authors[8] found swan-neck deformity in 25% of the fingers in the original group and in 16% of the modified group. Although the differences between the two groups were not statistically significant, it may be prudent to transfer into the radial collateral ligaments of fingers with a preexisting tendency for swan-neck deformity.

The CIT operation can play a significant role in the reconstruction of the rheumatoid hand. In the hand impaired by ulnar drift of approximately 30° or more, a technically well-performed CIT operation has the potential to correct ulnar drift, maintain that drift over time, and improve PIP joint and DIP joint ranges of motion. Potential problems include a tendency for active MP joint flexion to decrease postoperatively, a concern that must be addressed through increasingly early active MP joint motion during postoperative rehabilitation.

References

1. Backdahl RM, Myrin SO: Ulnar deviation of the fingers in rheumatoid arthritis and its surgical correction: a new operative method. Acta Chir Scand, 1961; 122:158–165.
2. Backhouse KM: The mechanics of normal digital control in the hand and an analysis of the ulnar drift of rheumatoid arthritis. Am R Coll Surg Engl, 1968; 43:154–173.
3. El-Gammal TA, Blair WF: Motion after metacarpophalangeal joint reconstruction in rheumatoid disease. J Hand Surg, 1993; 18A:504–511.
4. Ellison MR, Flatt AE, Kelly KJ: Ulnar drift of the fingers in rheumatoid disease: treatment by crossed intrinsic tendon transfer. J Bone Joint Surg, 1971; 53A:1061–1082.
5. Flatt AE: Some pathomechanics of ulnar drift. Plast Reconstr Surg, 1966; 37:295–303.
6. Flatt AE: The Care of the Rheumatoid Hand, 4th Ed, St. Louis: C.V. Mosby, 1983:277.
7. Harrison DH, Harrison SH, Smith P: Re-alignment procedure for ulnar drift of the metacarpophalangeal joint in rheumatoid arthritis. Hand, 1979; 11:163–168.
8. Oster LH, Blair WF, Steyers CM, Flatt AE: Crossed instrinsic transfer. J Hand Surg, 1989; 14A:963–971.
9. Straub LR: The etiology of finger deformities in the hand affected by rheumatoid arthritis. Bull Hosp Jt Dis Orthop Inst, 1960; 21:322–329.
10. Straub LR: Surgical rehabilitation of the hand and upper extremity in rheumatoid arthritis. Bull Rheum Dis, 1962; 12:265–268.
11. Straub LR: The intrinsic muscles in disease with particular reference to the rheumatoid hand. Dixieme Congress International de Chirurgie Orthopedique et de Traumatologie, 1966: 863–871.
12. Wise KS: Anatomy of the metacarpophalangeal joints with observations of the etiology of ulnar drift. J Bone Joint Surg, 1975; 57B:485–490.
13. Wood VE, Ichertz DR, Yahiku H: Soft tissue metacarpophalangeal reconstruction for treatment or rheumatoid hand deformity. J Hand Surg, 1989; 14A:163–174.

PART
V

Tendon Transfers in Nerve Palsy

ALLEN T. BISHOP,
JULIE A. KATARINCIC

85

Abductorplasty with Palmaris Longus to Abductor Pollicis Brevis

Carpal tunnel release for median nerve compression at the wrist is one of the most common surgeries performed in the musculoskeletal system. In hands with longstanding compression and significant thenar atrophy, little improvement in thumb opposition can be expected postoperatively.

The thumb is key in providing strength for prehensile pinch and grasp. Opposition is a complex motion involving abduction, flexion, and rotation of the carpometacarpal (CMC) joint and flexion and rotation of the metacarpophalangeal (MP) joint. Camitz in 1929 described transfer of the palmaris longus tendon to the abductor pollicis brevis (APB) insertion to provide immediate augmentation of thumb opposition in hands with weakness of the median innervated intrinsic muscles (Fig. 85–1).[3] The Camitz palmaris longus transfer actually augments palmar abduction, or antepulsion, more than opposition, which is a more complicated motion. Littler and Li in 1967 offered a review of the original technique.[7] In 1978, Braun reported on 28 cases using a palmaris longus transfer, with satisfactory results in all patients.[2]

Tendon transfers that are intended to provide full opposition must satisfy several requirements, including adequate strength, sufficient excursion, and proper orientation.[1,4] An ideal transfer should be in phase and be used for only one function. The palmaris longus (PL) transfer fulfills all but one of the above requirements. Its cross-sectional area and tension fraction are approximately equal to those of the APB.[1,4] Modest improvements in pinch and significant gains in abduction strength have been reported with this transfer. Tendon excursion is more than ample. Excursion is directly proportional to fiber length and measures 4.9 cm for PL compared with 3.6 cm for APB. Further, the PL is properly phased for pinch and probably plays a secondary role in opposition through its palmar fascial insertion.[5] With transfer of the PL to APB in cadaver specimens, 35° of palmar abduction, 48° of pronation, and 10° composite flexion could result.[4] The Camitz transfer does not, however, result in full opposition primarily because its orientation is radial to the ideal axis for opposition transfers. When the direction of pull is from the APB insertion toward the pisiform, which is an ideal axis approximating the orientation of APB fibers, relatively more flexion than abduction will occur, along with thumb pronation. The Camitz transfer results in more abduction with less pronation.

The Camitz PL opponensplasty is indicated primarily in severe compressive neuropathy of the median nerve at the carpal tunnel, at the time of median nerve decompression. Complaints of weakness of pinch and grasp due to paresis of median-innervated thenar muscles are the primary indications for the transfer. In low median nerve compression (carpal tunnel syndrome), the thenar muscles are generally weak but infrequently completely paralyzed. Such patients will demonstrate impaired opposition primarily due to weak palmar abduction of the thumb. With chronicity, significant thenar atrophy also will be noted. Because of the palmar abduction provided by the Camitz transfer described above, and because of the palmaris longus' accessibility in a standard carpal tunnel incision, the procedure is ideal for these individuals at the time of carpal tunnel release. In

■ HISTORY OF THE TECHNIQUE

■ INDICATIONS AND CONTRAINDICATIONS

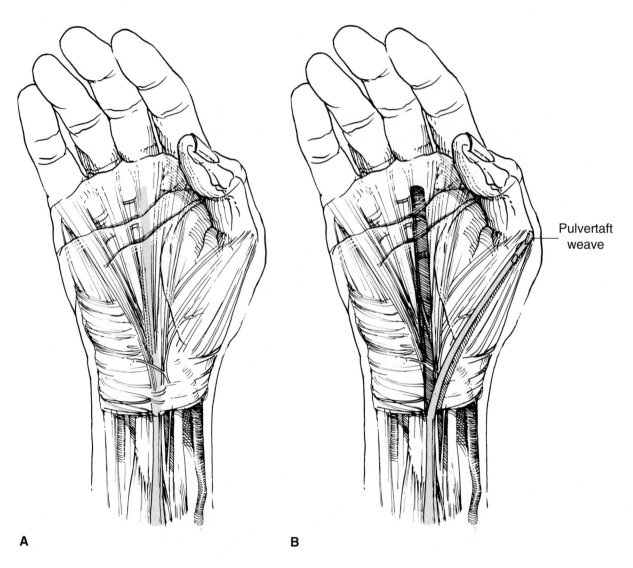

A   **B**

Pulvertaft
weave

■ FIGURE 85–1
The position of the palmaris longus tendon before **(A)** and after **(B)** surgical transfer.

carpal tunnel syndrome, 30% to 70% of hands may regain some thenar bulk and strength following nerve decompression, although recovery is unpredictable and prolonged.[8] Augmentation of weakened thenar muscles by the Camitz transfer will provide immediate improvement in all cases, and will function during the recovery of thenar function as an "internal splint" in those who subsequently recover.

Other indications include weakness following previous carpal tunnel release, in the absence of thenar muscle recovery, or after an injury to the recurrent branch of the median nerve in the palm. With complete paralysis and severe impairment of thumb pronation as well as abduction, however, other transfers with more appropriate vectors should be considered. These include the flexor digitorum superficialis, extensor indicis proprius or extensor digiti minimi, and abductor digiti minimi transfers described in standard texts.

Involvement of the thenar muscles should be demonstrable on physical examination by the presence of thenar muscle atrophy and weak opposition of the thumb and small finger. In addition, fasciculation potentials in the APB on preoperative electromyographic studies should be documented. Some carpal tunnel patients may have adequate opposition despite chronic median nerve compression, due either to mild impairment of the APB, opponens pollicis and superficial head of the flexor pollicis brevis, or a significant ulnar nerve contribution to normally median-innervated muscles. In a review of 1480 patients with carpal tunnel syndrome, Foucher found 6.6% of the patients had significant thenar atrophy with loss of thumb opposition by physical examination.[6] Eighty-eight of 98 of these patients underwent a PL transfer with their carpal tunnel release with 90.7% good results.

The only absolute contraindication to the Camitz transfer is absence of the muscle. Approximately 10% to 14% of the population does not have a palmaris longus. Its presence should be determined preoperatively, by asking the patient to simultaneously flex the wrist and oppose the thumb to the small finger. The tendon is visible and palpable ulnar to the flexor carpi radialis tendon with this maneuver.

The procedure is best performed under a regional anesthetic. A gently curved incision is made in the palm, parallel to and just ulnar to the thenar crease, approximately 4 cm in length. The incision is then extended obliquely across the proximal wrist crease up the forearm an additional 2 cm. Superficial dissection is carried down to the palmar fascia. The palmaris longus is then identified proximally in the wound. During the more proximal dissection, attention must be paid to the palmar cutaneous branch of the median nerve. This branch typically arises from the median nerve proximal to the wrist crease from its radial aspect, and lies immediately adjacent to the ulnar border of the flexor carpi radialis tendon. The palmaris longus must be prolonged distally using a centimeter-wide strip of palmar fascia, elevated to the midpalmar level to ensure adequate length. The tendon, together with its fascial prolongation is mobilized completely from all fascial connections and retracted proximally. At this point, a standard release of the transverse carpal ligament is performed.

Following carpal tunnel release, a second incision is then made over the radial aspect of the MP joint of the thumb. The incision should be approximately 2 cm long, slightly curved, at the radial palmar aspect of the distal first metacarpal. The abductor pollicis longus tendon is identified, inserting into the base of the proximal phalanx. The transferred palmaris longus will be sutured to the tendinous insertion of the abductor pollicis brevis.

A subcutaneous tunnel is then made from the wrist to the MP joint of the thumb (Fig. 85–2). The course of the tunnel should approximate that of the abductor pollicis brevis,

■ SURGICAL
TECHNIQUES

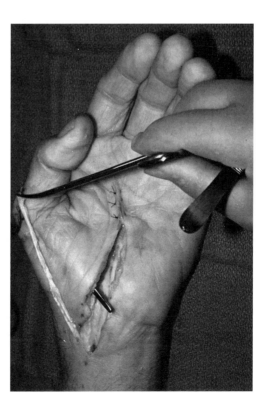

■ FIGURE 85–2
The subcutaneous tunnel for transferring the palmaris longus from the palm to the MP joint of the thumb.

■ FIGURE 85–3
The palmaris longus is
woven into the tendinous
portion of the abductor
pollicis brevis.

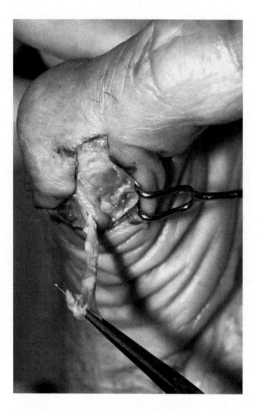

directed from the APB insertion towards the pisiform.[4] The palmaris longus is then passed through the tunnel. It is interwoven using a Pulvertaft weave and 3–0 nonabsorbable braided suture to the tendinous insertion of the abductor pollicis longus just proximal to the joint (Fig. 85–3). The tension in the PL should be set to allow full palmar abduction with the wrist in neutral but adduction into the palm when the wrist is flexed (Fig. 85–4).

At this point, the tourniquet is released and hemostasis is obtained. The wounds are then closed with interrupted sutures and a bulky, compressive hand dressing with a thumb spica splint is applied. A thumb spica cast is maintained for 4 to 5 weeks.

■ TECHNICAL
ALTERNATIVES

The classic opponensplasty described by Camitz using the palmaris longus primarily augments thumb abduction. Because opposition of the thumb is a complex motion involving multiple joints, and because the motion is a complex combination of flexion, pronation, and abduction, the Camitz transfer does not meet the full criteria as an opposition transfer. Cooney, in 1984, noted that compared with other standard transfers, the PL transfer was the least effective, supplying good abduction but weak opposition and flexion.[4] In cadaveric specimens, this transfer provided 35° of palmar abduction, 48° of rotation at the fingertip, and 10° of flexion. While it is sufficient for augmentation of weakened thenar muscles in carpal tunnel syndrome, and indeed preferred in this clinical setting because of its local availability, adequate strength and excursion, and normal phasic activity with opposition, it should not be used when complete thenar paralysis is present. This may be judged clinically by the amount of loss of pronation, compared with the opposite side. In these circumstances, other transfers with a line of pull at or distal to the pisiform should be considered, including the flexor digitorum superficialis, abductor digiti minimi, and extensor proprius transfers.

■ REHABILITATION

Patients are placed in a thumb spica splint postoperatively. The dressing is changed and the stitches removed approximately 10 days after surgery. A fiberglass thumb spica cast is then applied and continued for 4 weeks. The thumb is positioned in the cast in approximately 45° of palmar abduction. The wrist should be kept in a neutral position in the cast to avoid compromising the carpal tunnel release.

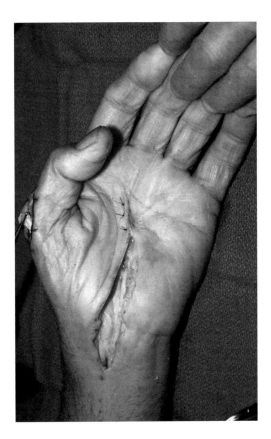

■ FIGURE 85–4
The tension in the trans-
fer is set by evaluating
the thumb position.

At 4 weeks after surgery, the patient is instructed, in a therapy program, on gentle active and passive range of motion of the thumb and wrist. The exercises are done hourly if possible. A thumb spica splint is fabricated for wear between exercises and at night. After 6 weeks, the splint is discontinued and the patient starts strengthening exercises.

Reports of outcomes from Camitz transfers have been sparse in the literature. The original reports of procedures provided no detailed results. Terrono in 1993 reported on 33 transfers performed for chronic median nerve compression. Twenty-six patients were followed for a mean of 17 months after the index procedure.[9] Satisfaction was achieved among 94% of patients because the function of their thumb was improved. In 1991, Foucher reported on the results of 73 Camitz transfers at an average follow-up of 38.7 months.[6] Good results were reported by 90.7% of his patients at final follow-up based on thumb motion. Foucher and co-authors believed they had obtained good antepulsion but no significant pronation.

■ OUTCOMES

We recently reviewed the results of 17 Camitz transfers at an average of 53 months after surgery. In 82% of patients, improved motion and strength were reported. Of these, less than half demonstrated any return of thenar muscle bulk or function. Significantly, strength of palmar abduction measured 102% of the involved side. In our patients, 93% returned to work, and 87% returned to all activities (Fig. 85–5).

Reported complications are rare but include scar tenderness, adhesions around the transfer, and thumb triggering. There have been no reported problems with the sacrifice of the palmaris longus itself.

Abductorplasty using the palmaris longus is an effective procedure when combined with a carpal tunnel release in the appropriate patient with thenar muscle atrophy. The palmaris longus provides the appropriate force vector and adequate excursion to provide opposition, with minimal morbidity related to the donor tendon. Complications are minimal, the procedure can be technically mastered, and results have been uniformly good.

■ FIGURE 85–5
Good postoperative
thumb abduction; the
functioning PL transfer is
seen on the palmar as-
pect of the wrist.

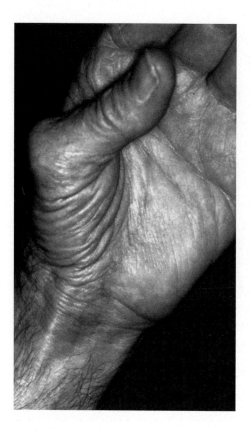

References

1. Brand PW: Relative tension and potential excursion of muscles in the forearm and hand. J Hand Surg, 1981; 6:209–219.
2. Braun RM: Palmaris longus tendon transfer for augmentation of the thenar musculature in low median nerve palsy. J Hand Surg, 1978; 3:488–491.
3. Camitz H: Surgical treatment of paralysis of opponens muscle of thumbs. Acta Chir Scandinavia, 1929; 65:77–81.
4. Cooney WP: Opposition of the thumb: An anatomic and biomechanical study of tendon transfers. J Hand Surg, 1984; 9A:777–786.
5. Fahrer M, Tubiana R: Palmaris longus, anteductor of the thumb. Hand, 1976; 8:287–289.
6. Foucher G, MC Sammut D, Marin Braun F, Michon J: Primary palmaris longus transfer as an opponensplasty in carpal tunnel release. J Hand Surg, 1991; 16B:56–60.
7. Littler JW, Malizos C, Li CS: Primary restoration of thumb opposition with median nerve decompression. Plast Reconstr Surg, 1967; 39:74–75.
8. Phalen GS: The carpal tunnel syndrome. Seventeen years' experience in diagnosis and treatment of six hundred fifty four cases. J Bone Joint Surg, 1966; 48A:211–228.
9. Terrono AL, Rose JH, Mulroy J, Millender LH: Camitz palmaris longus abductorplasty for severe thenar atrophy secondary to carpal tunnel syndrome. J Hand Surg, 1993; 18A:204–206.

MICHAEL JABLON

86

Opponensplasty with Ring Finger Flexor Digitorum Superficialis Tendon

Opposition of the thumb to the other digits is required for fine prehension. The hand functions of grasping and pinching are based on the ability to bring the thumb into opposition. Precision handling has been considered an advantage in our evolution.[12]

Opposition of the thumb is a composite motion that includes abduction of the first metacarpal, abduction of the proximal phalanx at the metacarpophalangeal (MP) joint, rotation of the metacarpal into pronation, and flexion of the metacarpal.[2]

The tip of the thumb moves through a large arc from the plane of the palm; it pronates to a position across from the fingers for tip-to-tip prehension. The motion occurs at the carpometacarpal and MP joints. The distal phalanx thumb nail plane pronates as there is angulatory motion at the carpometacarpal joint and pronatory motion at the MP joint. The metacarpal abducts from the plane of the palm.[8]

Median nerve palsy or the loss of the thenar muscle function due to direct injury will deprive the thumb of its ability to oppose. Restoration of opposition requires the presence of transferable functioning tendons and a thumb that has adequate mobility without contractures. Similarly, for adequate prehension with true pulp-to-pulp pinch, sensibility in the thumb and fingertips is required.

In 1918, Steindler[14] reported a tendon transfer using the flexor pollicis longus to restore thumb opposition. In this operation, the distal end of the tendon was split and rerouted through the flexor sheath on the radial side of the proximal phalanx. Surgical reconstruction for intrinsic thenar paralysis became popular with Thompson's modification of Royle's procedure.[15] In the original Royle procedure,[11] the sublimis of the ring finger was passed through the sheath of the flexor pollicis longus, similar to Steindler's description. Thompson's modification left the flexor digitorum superficialis tendon of the ring finger under the volar carpal ligament, and then brought the two slips out subcutaneously across the thenar eminence. One slip inserted onto the thumb distal to the MP joint and the other slip inserted proximal.

Bunnell,[3] in 1938, outlined the essential considerations for the choice of muscle and tendon, the construction of a pulley, the correct insertion of the transfer and the direction of the pull to achieve opposition of the thumb. Bunnell used the flexor digitorum superficialis of the ring finger. If the MP joint is stable, then any force duplicating the abductor pollicis brevis muscle will provide opposition.[9]

■ HISTORY OF THE TECHNIQUE

■ INDICATIONS AND CONTRAINDICATIONS

The indication for opponensplasty is the restoration of thumb opposition to the fingers for the fine prehension of pulp-to-pulp contact. Prerequisites include intact sensation, functioning extrinsic motors, and adequate thumb mobility. Injury to the median nerve may affect both motor and sensory function. Injury distal to the junction of the proximal and middle thirds of the forearm spare the innervation of the extrinsic motors, provided absence of concomitant anterior interosseous nerve injury. Nonetheless, median nerve repair to restore sensibility should precede an opponensplasty. Inadequate thumb mobility associated with first web space contractures requires correction before opponensplasty. Contractures in adduction or adduction-supination may require release of joints and intrinsic muscles. Local rotation flaps, Z-plasties, or distant flaps to enhance first web space mobility should precede opponensplasty. Adequate mobility includes basal thumb joint rotation, MP joint, and interphalangeal joint extension to allow for pulp-to-pulp pinch.

The contraindications to opponensplasty include anticipation of the complete return of intrinsic function, although early transfers may internally splint and minimize first web space contracture. The flexor digitorum superficialis transfers are contraindicated in patients with high median nerve injury, as reinnervation of the superficialis muscles may be inadequate to provide power. Severe local thumb or web space damage may preclude the achievement of adequate mobility. Interphalangeal or MP joint arthrodeses may be considered for damaged or contracted thumb joints. The correct choice of opponensplasty procedure depends on the patient's needs. The insensate thumb may benefit from a synergistic muscle transfer (extensor indicis proprius), which minimizes the retraining difficulties.[4] Patients with progressive or polyneuropathies require careful evaluation regarding selection of appropriate motors for transfer.

■ SURGICAL
TECHNIQUES

Opponensplasty by transfer of the flexor digitorum superficialis of the ring finger may be performed under axillary block anesthesia. Careful preoperative evaluation to assure independent function of the flexor digitorum superficialis of the ring finger should be performed. By holding the long and little fingers in extension and testing for active proximal interphalangeal (PIP) joint flexion of the ring finger, flexor digitorum superficialis tendon function is checked. After anesthesia has been administered and the extremity has been prepared and draped and a well-padded tourniquet has been applied, the surface anatomy is marked. A transverse incisional line is marked at the base of the ring finger just proximal to the skin crease at the proximal phalanx (Fig. 86–1). A gently curved incisional line is marked at the distal forearm starting at the center of the volar wrist crease and extending proximally 4 cm toward the flexor carpi ulnaris tendon. A third incisional line is drawn over the midaxial radial aspect of the first metacarpal neck and is extended distally and dorsally over the MP joint to the mid portion of the proximal phalanx of the thumb.

Next the extremity is elevated, exsanguinated, and the tourniquet appropriately inflated.

■ FIGURE 86–1
Surface anatomy is depicted as well as incisions for opponensplasty.

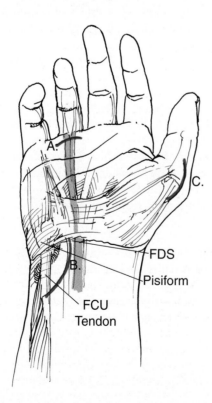

Harvesting the flexor digitorum superficialis from the base of the ring finger is performed by making the incision, then gently spreading the subcutaneous tissues and approaching the flexor tendon sheath in the midline of the ray. Distal extensions of the palmar fascia[12] may need to be divided. The digital nerves on both sides of the flexor tendon sheath should be identified and protected. A longitudinal incision is made in the flexor tendon sheath and a small curved retractor is placed under the flexor digitorum superficialis tendon. The retractor is pulled and the finger observed to assure the correct tendon has been selected. A small drain or vessel loop is then passed around the tendon and when tension is applied the finger will flex at the PIP joint. The tendon will later be harvested with the ring finger flexed. The tendon is harvested just proximal to the chiasm of Camper, which is retained in the digit.

The wrist-forearm incision is next performed. The flexor superficialis tendons are exposed at the distal forearm as is the flexor carpi ulnaris tendon throughout its distal 4 cm. The flexor digitorum superficialis of the ring finger may now be found at the wrist and gently retracted to confirm the correct tendon has been selected. The synovium surrounding the flexor digitorum superficialis may need to be freed. The tendon is then cut in the distal wound and delivered into the proximal wound.

The tendon is protected with a saline-soaked sponge to prevent drying. If difficulty is encountered in bringing the flexor digitorum superficialis proximally the carpal tunnel may be opened to free it from adjacent tendons. If performed with opening of the transverse carpal ligament, then repair of the palmar fascia[12] should be performed before passing the flexor digitorum superficialis tendon subcutaneously to protect the median nerve.

The pulley at the base of the pisiform is constructed from the flexor carpi ulnaris tendon (Fig. 86–2). The flexor carpi ulnaris must carefully be isolated to prevent damage to the ulnar neurovascular structures. The pulley is constructed by using half the thickness of the flexor carpi ulnaris tendon severed approximately 4 cm above its insertion and looped by suturing it to the pisiform ligamentous tissue. Without changing its original insertion,

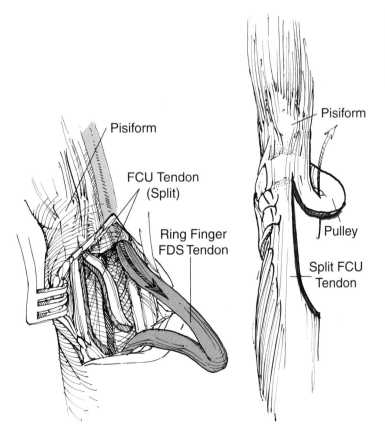

■ FIGURE 86–2
A pulley is constructed with a segment of the flexor carpi ulnaris tendon.

Pisiform

FCU Tendon (Split)

Ring Finger FDS Tendon

Pisiform

Pulley

Split FCU Tendon

the ulnar half is allowed to remain attached distally to the pisiform. The proximal end of the split radial half of the flexor carpi ulnaris tendon is brought through a small hole in the tendon distally near the tendon insertion on the pisiform. A loop is created, the diameter of which is maintained while suturing the tendon end. Care is used to avoid placing sutures into the pulley's opening. The looped flexor carpi ulnaris should be sutured with nonabsorbable material firmly to flexor carpi ulnaris tendon. Creation of the pulley will direct the tendon transfer pull toward the pisiform to angulate the thumb towards the ulna.

Next the incision on the thumb is made. The incision is performed with care to protect any distal twigs of the superficial radial nerve over the dorsum of the thumb. Attachment of the flexor digitorum superficialis to the thumb is an important part of the procedure. The flexor digitorum superficialis is brought through the pulley (Fig. 86–3). A subcutaneous tunnel is made by carefully advancing a hemostat through from the wrist wound to the thumb. Gently spreading the hemostat facilitates advancing the instrument. Use care to avoid injury to the palmar cutaneous nerve branch of the median nerve as it crosses the base of the thenar eminence.

The flexor digitorum superficialis is split into two slips once it is passed into the thumb wound. With the wrist flexed approximately 30° and the thumb placed and held in full abduction, the slips are sewn into place at sufficient tension to take up any remaining slack in the tendon transfer. An additional 1-cm advancement is recommended to adjust tension. One half of the split tendon is interwoven and sutured to the abductor pollicis brevis muscle and tendon, and the other half is sutured to the extensor pollicis longus tendon over the MP joint on the ulnar dorsal aspect (Fig. 86–4). This attachment provides rotation and an extensor moment at the MP joint.

Tension is tested before completing the suturing of the slips. The wrist is brought though a full range of motion. When the wrist is maximally extended the thumb should be brought into full opposition, and when the wrist is maximally flexed it should be possible to place the thumb into full adduction. If at maximal wrist extension the thumb is not fully opposed, then the tendon transfers need to be tightened. If at full flexion of the wrist, the thumb

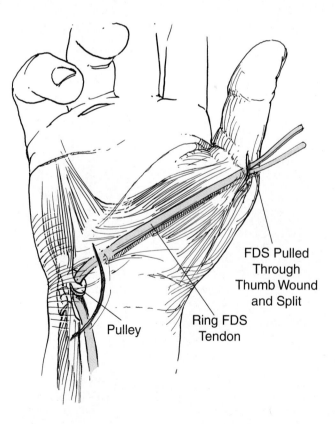

■ FIGURE 86–3
The direction of pull for the transferred flexor digitorum superficialis tendon is determined by pulley location.

FDS Pulled
Through
Thumb Wound
and Split

Ring FDS
Tendon

Pulley

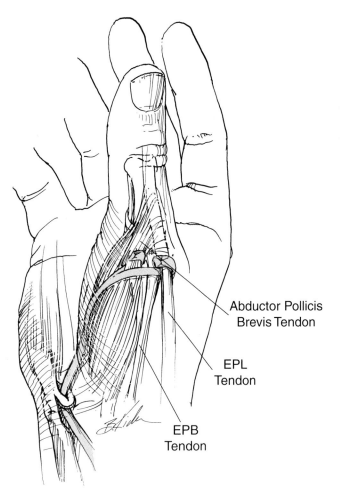

■ FIGURE 86–4
Riordan's distal attach-
ment technique for the
opponens transfer passes
one slip through the ab-
ductor pollicis brevis and
the other slip around the
extensor pollicis longus
tendon.

Abductor Pollicis
Brevis Tendon

EPL
Tendon

EPB
Tendon

cannot be fully adducted, then the tendon transfer needs to be lengthened. Testing the tension by placing one temporary suture into each slip to anchor it is advisable before cutting off the excess tendon length. Once appropriate tension has been satisfactorily achieved, the tourniquet is deflated and hemostasis obtained. Multiple sutures may be used with nonabsorbable material to anchor the tendon attachments. The wounds are closed with 6-0 nylon simple interrupted sutures and sterile dressings are applied. A splint is applied with the wrist flexed 30° and the thumb fully opposed. Avoid excessively bulky dressings. The patient's hand is then elevated to heart level with an arm elevator or sling bandage.

■ TECHNICAL
ALTERNATIVES

Other opposition transfers utilizing the flexor digitorum superficialis include those described by Brand, Krukenberg, Mayer, Bunnell, as well as Riordan's described above. Smith[12] summarized 23 opponensplasties. There are variations for the selections of motors, pulleys, and the methods of attachment to the thumb.

The Camitz procedure[5] is an especially worthwhile procedure. In this procedure, the palmaris longus is lengthened distally by harvesting palmar fascia. The tendon is then directed subcutaneously to the abductor pollicis brevis aponeurosis to act as a transfer. This transfer is particularly useful when combined with release of the transverse carpal ligament for severe carpal tunnel syndrome in which thenar atrophy has obviated thumb opposition.

Opponensplasty using extensor carpi radialis brevis, the extensor indicis proprius and the extensor digiti minimi as well as the abductor digiti minimi are alternatives depending on the presentation and needs of the individual patient. Burkhalter[4] favored the extensor indicis proprius opponensplasty because it is easily retrained and will not weaken flexion of the ring finger. This transfer is also suitable for high median nerve lesions. Eversmann[7] pointed out that a Silastic rod may be useful for the creation of a palmar tunnel when scarring is present. The rod should be placed approximately three months before the opponensplasty.

Other options for pulleys include Guyon's canal, the flexor carpi ulnaris itself, windows in the palmar fascia or the transverse carpal ligament, or the ulnar border of the palmaris longus. Bunnell favored a pulley near the pisiform to best direct the pull of the transfer.

Other methods[6] of attachment of the transfer to the thumb include Bunnell's direct method of insertion into the proximal phalanx at the dorsal ulnar border. Similar to Riordan's[10] technique, Brand's method interweaves one slip of tendon through the abductor pollicis brevis with the slip continuing to the extensor pollicis longus. The second slip in Brand's method is attached to the ulnar aspect of the adductor pollicis to rotate the thumb while providing stability of the metacarpophalangeal joint. For more severe presentations with extensive nerve, muscle or bone damage, tenodesis procedures or osteotomy and arthrodesis of the thumb may be considered.[7]

Complications of opponensplasty will occur when there is failure to achieve the necessary prerequisites of adequate motors, thumb mobility and sensation. Adhesions may develop requiring tenolysis or rerouting of the transfer. Inadequate rehabilitation may lead to contractures in the thumb or donor finger. If swan-neck deformity develops in the donor finger due to loss of its flexor digitorum superficialis, then correction may require suture of one slip of the remaining flexor digitorum superficialis to the proximal interphalangeal joint volar plate to prevent hyperextension.

■ REHABILITATION

The initial plaster splint applied in the operating room may be maintained through the first postoperative week. At the first dressing change a thermoplastic splint may be fabricated by the hand therapist. The wrist is maintained at 30° flexion with the thumb held in full opposition. At the fith week, the wrist may be brought to neutral while training is begun. A common cause of failure following opponensplasty is first web contracture which can be avoided by appropriate splinting.[1]

The postoperative rehabilitation[13] may be approached in three phases as follows: phase one—immobilization, phase two—the initiation of active motion, and phase three—strengthening and coordination training. Supervised hand therapy continues until the specific goals of restored opposition and pinch are achieved.

In phase one, immobilization is maintained 4 to 6 weeks to allow for healing of the juncture sites in soft tissues. Phase two is the initiation of active motion to minimize adhesions and scar formation to facilitate tendon gliding, while minimizing stress at the juncture sites. Special splints may be helpful. In phase three, strengthening and improvement of coordination are emphasized. The duration of therapy varies with the factors of patient motivation and the initial presentation.

■ OUTCOMES

If an opponensplasty is appropriately planned and takes into account the key factors of direction of pull and attachment of the transfer, then opposition should be attained. The prerequisites of adequate sensibility, mobility, and appropriate motor power must of course also be present. If the median nerve is injured at the wrist, then the abductor pollicis brevis, the opponens pollicis, and part of the flexor pollicis brevis are paralyzed. The adductor pollicis, the abductor pollicis longus, the flexor pollicis longus, and the extensor pollicis longus would still be functioning in such a case. If nerve repair does not provide return of opposition for this situation, then a strong motor with proper direction of pull and tendon insertion is required. The flexor digitorum superficialis of the ring finger transfer for thumb opposition is an appropriate choice. As a broad range of presenting findings may be present, a successful outcome is dependent on many factors. Currently, a quantitative outcome analysis for opponensplasty is not available.

References

1. Boyes JH: Bunnell's Surgery of the Hand, Philadelphia: J.B. Lippincott, 1970:488–501.
2. Brand PW: Medical Mechanics of the Hand, St. Louis: C.V. Mosby, 1985:154–155, 229.
3. Bunnell S: Opposition of the thumb. J Bone Joint Surg, 1938; 20:269–284.
4. Burkhalter WE: Median Nerve Palsy. In: Green DP (ed): Operative Hand Surgery, New York: Churchill Livingston, 1993:1419–1448.
5. Camitz H: Surgical treatment of paralysis of opponens muscle of thumb. Acta Chir Scand, 1929; 65:77.
6. Curtis RM: Opposition of the thumb. Orthop Clin North Am, 1974; 5:305–321.
7. Eversmann WW: Median Nerve Palsy. In: Gelberman RH (ed): Operative Nerve Repair and Reconstruction, Philadelphia: J.B. Lippincott, 1991:711–728.
8. Kaplan EB, Smith RJ: Kinesiology of the Hand and Wrist and Muscular Variations of the Hand and Forearm. In: Spinner M (ed): Kaplan's Functional and Surgical Anatomy of the Hand, Philadelphia, J.B. Lippincott, 1984:314–328.
9. Littler JW: Tendon transfers and arthrodesis in combined median and ulnar nerve paralysis. J Bone Joint Surg, 1949; 31A:225–234.
10. Riordan DC: Tendon transfers for nerve paralysis of the hand and wrist. Curr Pract Orthop Surg, 1964; 2:17.
11. Royle ND: An operation for paralysis of the intrinsic muscles of the hand. JAMA, 1938; 111:612.
12. Smith RJ: Tendon Transfers to Restore Thumb Opposition. In: Tendon Transfers of the Hand and Forearm, Boston: Little Brown, 1987:57–83.
13. Stanley BG: Preoperative and Postoperative Management of Tendon Transfers after Median Nerve Injury. In: Hunter JM, Schneider LH, Mackin EJ, Callahan AD (eds): Rehabilitation of the Hand. Surgery and Therapy, St. Louis: C.V. Mosby, 1990:705–713.
14. Steindler A: Orthopaedic operations on the hand. JAMA, 1918; 71:1288.
15. Thompson C: A modified operation for opponens paralysis. J Bone Joint Surg, 1942; 24:632–640.

PETER J. L. JEBSON
CURTIS M. STEYERS

87

Adductorplasty with the Extensor Carpi Radialis Brevis

■ HISTORY OF THE TECHNIQUE

Patients with ulnar nerve palsy have weakness of thumb adduction and pinch strength because the adductor pollicis and first dorsal interosseous muscles are paralyzed. Adduction is weakened by approximately 75% and pinch strength may be reduced by more than 80%.[3,15]

Many procedures have been described to restore thumb adduction; most were designed to restore balance and improve the appearance of the hand rather than to improve pinch and adduction strength. Many of these transfers improve stability and pinch to only 25% to 50% of normal.[3,15] In 1983, Smith[20] described a transfer of the extensor carpi radialis brevis (ECRB) to the adductor pollicis to restore thumb adduction and pinch. In his procedure, the ECRB is lengthened with a tendon graft, passed distally through the interspace between the second and third metacarpals deep to the adductor pollicis, and then sutured to the tendon of the adductor pollicis. Reconstruction with the ECRB adductorplasty has proven quite successful and is our preferred technique for restoration of power pinch.[12,18,20]

■ INDICATIONS AND CONTRAINDICATIONS

Adductorplasty with the ECRB is indicated in patients who are functionally impaired by weak thumb pinch caused by paralysis or absence of the adductor pollicis muscle. It is especially indicated in patients with weak pinch who also have sustained injuries to the digital flexor tendons or who have scarring on the palmar aspect of the hand or wrist. It also is indicated if additional tendon transfers using digital flexors are planned for reconstruction of other deformities (i.e., Zancolli "lasso" procedure for claw deformity).

Contraindications to the ECRB adductorplasty include weak power pinch without functional impairment, open wounds or infection in the operative area, a nonfunctioning or damaged extensor carpi radialis brevis muscle, and extensive first web space scarring or contracture. The thumb metacarpophalangeal (MP) joint must be stable and the radiocarpal and carpometacarpal joints mobile. In patients with combined median and ulnar nerve palsies, adductorplasty with the ECRB should not be performed unless an opposition transfer also is planned. The patient must be properly motivated to participate in the postoperative rehabilitation program.

■ SURGICAL TECHNIQUES

Adductorplasty with the ECRB may be performed under an axillary block or general anesthetic. The opposite arm or a lower extremity may need to be simultaneously prepared and draped, depending on the anticipated donor site for the tendon graft used to prolong the ECRB tendon. A pneumatic tourniquet is applied about the proximal arm over an appropriate layer of padding.

The extremity is exsanguinated, and the tourniquet is inflated. A 15- to 20-cm tendon graft is harvested first. The palmaris longus is the preferred tendon graft, and harvesting typically is done from the same extremity. If the palmaris longus is absent bilaterally, a plantaris tendon graft may be used. After the graft has been obtained and the harvest site incisions closed, the graft is wrapped and protected in saline-soaked gauze.

The ECRB is exposed through a 2- to 3-cm transverse incision on the dorsum of the wrist just proximal to the base of the third metacarpal. The ECRB is identified, isolated, and sharply transected just proximal to its insertion. A second transverse incision of similar

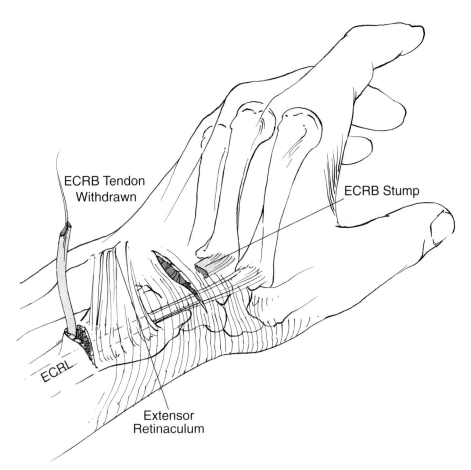

FIGURE 87–1
The ECRB is transected distally and delivered into the most proximal incision.

ECRB Tendon
Withdrawn

ECRB Stump

ECRL

Extensor
Retinaculum

length is made just proximal to the extensor retinaculum directly over the tendons of ECRB and extensor carpi radialis longus. Blunt dissection is used to identify and protect dorsal veins and branches of the superficial radial nerve. The ECRB is identified, isolated, and delivered into this wound and wrapped in a saline-soaked sponge (Fig. 87–1). A third 2- to 3-cm transverse incision is then made directly over the proximal aspect of the second intermetacarpal space. Blunt dissection allows exposure of the dorsal interosseous fascia, which is incised longitudinally to expose the interosseous muscles. A small portion of the interosseous muscle is excised to permit unhindered passage of the tendon graft. Careful blunt dissection is used to develop a pathway between the most proximal forearm incision and the incision over the second intermetacarpal space. The plane of dissection should be between the deep layer of subcutaneous fascia and the dorsal antebrachial fascia. A longitudinal incision is then made on the ulnar side of the MP joint of the thumb. Blunt dissection is used to expose the adductor pollicis insertion. Care must be taken to avoid injury to the adjacent branches of the superficial radial nerve. A curved hemostat or similar instrument is now passed through the second intermetacarpal space and directed toward the thumb MP joint in the interval between the adductor pollicis and the first metacarpal and first dorsal interosseous muscle. The tip of the instrument should lie just dorsal to the adductor tendon (Fig. 87–2). One end of the tendon graft is then sutured to the adductor pollicis by making a longitudinal split in the adductor tendon with a scalpel, passing the graft through this split, and suturing it to both the adductor and itself using several figure-of-eight sutures of a 3-0 nonabsorbable material. The free end of the graft is gently grasped with the hemostat, which is then withdrawn through the second intermetacarpal space. The hemostat is then placed in the most proximal transverse incision and is directed distally until the tip emerges in the incision overlying the second intermetacarpal space. The tendon graft is then gently grasped and delivered into the most proximal incision.

■ FIGURE 87–2
A curved hemostat is
passed through the sec-
ond intermetacarpal
space and directed to-
ward the thumb MP joint.
The instrument must
pass in the interval be-
tween the adductor pol-
licis and the index meta-
carpal and first dorsal
interosseous muscle.

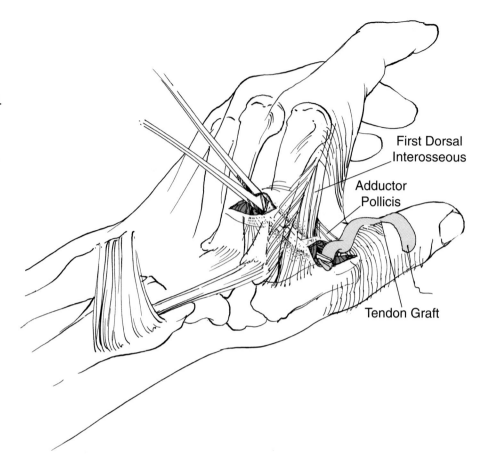

First Dorsal
Interosseous

Adductor
Pollicis

Tendon Graft

The hand is now positioned for suturing the tendon graft to the ECRB. The wrist is held in the neutral position and the thumb is placed slightly palmar to the index finger (Fig. 87–3). An assistant holds the hand in this position as the ECRB and tendon graft are joined using one Pulvertaft weave. A single 3-0 nonabsorbable suture is inserted. Graft length and tension are tested by passively dorsiflexing and palmar flexing the wrist. When the wrist is dorsiflexed, the thumb should fall into abduction. With the wrist palmar flexed, the thumb should lie firmly against the palm. Excessive tension on the juncture must be avoided. In patients with absent or nonfunctioning median nerve innervated thenar mus-cles, the graft should be made slightly longer so that the thumb is adjacent to the palm only when the wrist is palmar flexed. When the tension is appropriate, two additional weaves are completed, and excessive graft is excised. Two 3-0 nonabsorbable sutures are applied in a figure-of-eight technique to each weave. Compression is applied as the tourniquet is deflated. Hemostasis is obtained, and the skin is closed with alternating simple and horizontal mattress sutures of 5-0 nylon. Drains are used if necessary. A fore-arm-based plaster thumb spica splint is applied with the wrist in approximately 40° of dorsiflexion and the thumb in the neutral position.

■ TECHNICAL
ALTERNATIVES

Many procedures have been described to restore thumb adduction.[1,3,5,9,17,18,20,23] The extensor carpi radialis longus, brachioradialis, extensor indicis proprius, flexor digitorum superficialis of the ring finger (FDS), extensor digiti quinti, and abductor digiti minimi all have been used to restore thumb adduction. The donor tendon or tendon graft has been passed through the second and third intermetacarpal spaces, around the ulnar border of the forearm, and across the palm deep and superficial to the finger flexors.

The potential excursion of the extensor carpi radialis longus is considerably greater than the ECRB; however, this muscle cannot generate as much tension as the ECRB, and using

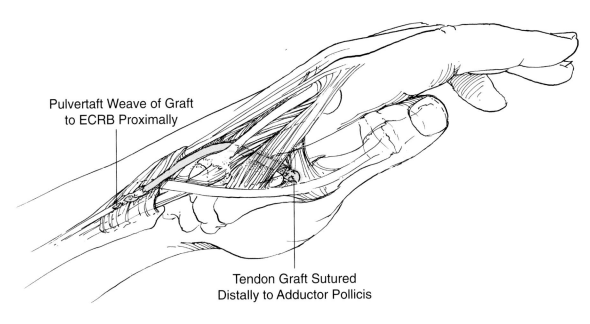

Pulvertaft Weave of Graft
to ECRB Proximally

Tendon Graft Sutured
Distally to Adductor Pollicis

■ FIGURE 87-3
The tendon graft is sutured proximally with the thumb held against the palmar surface of the index finger and the wrist held in the neutral position.

this muscle will eliminate the patient's ability to perform radial deviation of the wrist.[2] The brachioradialis, extensor indicis proprius, and extensor digiti quinti also have been used to restore adduction. Although these transfers can position the thumb in adduction, none of these muscles can generate enough tension to provide powerful pinch.[2] In addition, the abductor digiti minimi is unavailable in most patients with ulnar nerve lesions. Boyes'[1] technique for brachioradialis transfer involved passage of the free graft between the third and fourth metacarpals. Omer,[18,19] when performing an adductorplasty procedure with either the ECRB or brachioradialis, also prefers passage of the graft through the third intermetacarpal space. We, like Hastings and Davidson,[12] prefer passage between the second and third metacarpals as originally described by Smith.[20]

The ring finger FDS transfer to the adductor tubercle causes flexion and adduction of the thumb. Although this transfer does not require a tendon graft, the work capacity of the FDS is slightly less than that of the ECRB.[11] This transfer is contraindicated in a patient with a high ulnar nerve palsy or if there is scarring in the palm of the hand.

Thumb pinch also can be improved by arthrodesis of either the interphalangeal (IP) or MP joints, particularly if they are unstable. Interphalangeal joint arthrodesis prevents hyperflexion with power pinch and has been reported to increase pinch force by 2 pounds.[3] However, fine manipulative functions of the thumb may be impaired. Arthrodesis of the MP joint provides a 2- to 3-pound improvement in pinch strength and leaves the IP joint mobile.[12] Satisfactory results have been described with this approach, and patients indicate that preservation of IP joint motion is helpful for performing activities of daily living.[12]

The greatest technical challenge in the ECRB adductorplasty procedure is to suture the transferred muscle-tendon unit under the correct amount of tension. A graft that is too short and placed under too much tension will not permit adequate thumb abduction. Consequently, the patient will not be able to place the thumb around larger objects. Judging graft length and tension is even more difficult in patients who have additional palsies or absent muscles. An understanding of associated palsies and their deficits is necessary for the adductorplasty to be successful. Overcorrection and imbalance will occur if the "standard" adductorplasty technique is used in a patient with concomitant thenar paralysis. Less tension is required in this setting.

A potential pitfall of this operation is failure to provide stability to the index finger. A stable index finger is necessary for power pinch. Abduction of the index finger is provided by the first dorsal interosseous muscle, which, in the majority of patients, is innervated by the ulnar nerve. Loss of index finger abduction can be restored and pinch augmented via transfer of the accessory slip of the abductor pollicis longus, with a free tendon graft, to the tendon of the first dorsal interosseous muscle[16] or transfer of the extensor indicis proprius,[17] extensor pollicis brevis,[1,19] extensor digiti minimi,[23] FDS,[7,10] extensor carpi radialis longus,[9] or palmaris longus.[13] An additional potential pitfall is graft impingement at the intermetacarpal space. Care should be taken to release or remove any potentially impeding structures at the intermetacarpal interval and dorsal to the adductor pollicis muscle in the palm of the hand.

■ REHABILITATION

Ten days after surgery, skin sutures are removed. The hand is immobilized for an additional 2 weeks in a short arm thumb spica cast with the wrist in approximately 40° of dorsiflexion and the thumb in the neutral position. The cast is removed 3 weeks postoperatively, a hand-based opponens splint is applied, and the patient begins a supervised exercise program. The first phase of this program includes active range of motion of the wrist and fingers, active thumb abduction with the wrist in flexion and extension, and passive thumb adduction. The purpose of this phase of the program is to restore joint mobility and to avoid tendon adherence, especially in the intermetacarpal space. The splint is removed 6 weeks after surgery, and the exercise program is advanced to include active thumb adduction and progressive resistive exercises. Unrestricted activities are permitted 8 weeks after surgery.

■ OUTCOMES

Smith's[20] original description of the ECRB adductorplasty included 18 patients. Ten patients had low ulnar nerve palsy due to lacerations and three had high ulnar nerve palsy, two from lacerations and one from severe cubital tunnel syndrome. All patients underwent the adductorplasty procedure and seven also had a tendon transfer for index finger abduction. Of the 15 patients who had an ECRB adductorplasty for adductor avulsion or paralysis, only 1 was made worse by surgery. This patient had a combined median and ulnar nerve palsy and had previously undergone an extensor indicis proprius opposition transfer. After the adductorplasty, he had difficulty grasping objects because he could no longer fully abduct his thumb. The lack of complete thumb abduction was caused by a short tendon graft. The remaining 14 patients had significant improvement in their ability to use the thumb, and all were satisfied. Most patients returned to their original occupation. Pinch strength was restored to 50% of normal. The mean preoperative pulp-to-side pinch was 5.3 pounds and the postoperative value was 11 pounds. The significance and influence of concomitant procedures on functional abilities and pinch strength could not be determined because of the small number of patients.

Several patients had early limited thumb abduction that resolved with therapy. No patient had a loss of wrist motion or difficulty with phase conversion. Synovitis at the second intermetacarpal space that ultimately required a tenosynovectomy occurred in one patient. Of the three patients who underwent the adductorplasty for conditions other than paralysis or avulsion, all had complex deformities and deficiencies in the hand that made objective analysis of their outcomes impossible. Nevertheless, all three were functionally improved by surgery.

Hastings and Davidson[12] described their experience with the ECRB adductorplasty in eight patients. Six of these patients also had simultaneous thumb arthrodeses (three MP and three IP joints). Of these eight patients, only five were available for follow-up. Pinch strength improved from 6.9 pounds (33% normal) to 16.3 pounds (62% normal). The number of patients was too small to determine if significant differences existed among the various treatment groups and how concomitant arthrodeses and index finger abduction procedures influenced pinch strength. However, the authors noted that those patients who had an IP joint fusion had difficulty with fine manipulative thumb functions. They concluded that the ECRB adductorplasty combined with MP joint arthrodesis is the most effective procedure for restoring powerful pinch.

References

1. Boyes JH: Bunnell's Surgery of the Hand, 4h Ed, Philadelphia: J. B. Lippincott, 1964:515–518.
2. Brand PW, Beach RB, Thompson DE: Relative tension and potential excursion of muscles in the forearm and hand. J Hand Surg, 1981; 6:209–219.
3. Brown PW: Reconstruction for pinch in ulnar intrinsic palsy. Orthop Clin North Am, 1974; 5: 323–342.
4. Bruner JM: Tendon transfer to restore abduction of the index finger using the extensor pollicis brevis. Plast Reconstr Surg, 1948; 3:197–201.
5. Edgerton MT, Brand PW: Restoration of abduction and adduction to the unstable thumb in median and ulnar paralysis. Plast Reconst Surg, 1965; 36:150–164.
6. Froment J: La paralysie de l'adducteur du pouce et le signe de le préhension. Rev Neurol (Paris), 1914; 28:1236–1240.
7. Goldner JL: Deformities of the hand incidental to pathological changes of the extensor and intrinsic muscle mechanisms. J Bone Joint Surg, 1953; 35:115–131.
8. Goldner JL: Replacement of the function of the paralyzed adductor pollicis with the flexor digitorum sublimis—a ten-year review. J Bone Joint Surg, 1967; 49A:583–584.
9. Goldner JL: Tendon transfers for irreparable peripheral nerve injuries of the upper extremity. Orthop Clin North Amer, 1974; 5:343–375.
10. Graham WC, Riordan D: Sublimis transfer to restore abduction of index finger. Plast Reconstr Surg, 1947; 2:459–462.
11. Hamlin C, Littler JW: Restoration of power pinch. J Hand Surg, 1980; 5:396–401.
12. Hastings HH, Davidson S: Tendon transfers for ulnar nerve palsy. Evaluation of results and practical treatment considerations. Hand Clinics, 1988; 4:167–178.
13. Hirayama T, Atsuta Y, Takemitsu Y: Palmaris longus transfer for replacement of the first dorsal interosseous. J Hand Surg, 1986; 11B:31–34.
14. Littler JW: Tendon transfers and arthrodeses in combined median and ulnar nerve paralysis. J Bone Joint Surg, 1949; 31A:225–234.
15. Mannerfeldt L: Studies on the hand in ulnar nerve paralysis. A clinical-experimental investigation in normal and anomalous innervation. Acta Orthop Scand [Suppl], 1966; 87: 1–176.
16. Neviaser RJ, Wilson JN, Gardner MM: Abductor pollicis longus transfer for replacement of first dorsal interosseous. J Hand Surg, 1980; 5:53–57.
17. Omer GE: Tendon transfers in combined nerve lesions. Orthop Clin North Amer, 1974; 5: 377–387.
18. Omer GE: Reconstruction of a balanced thumb through tendon transfers. Clin Orthop, 1985; 195:104–116.
19. Omer GE: Ulnar nerve palsy. In: Green DP (ed): Operative Hand Surgery, 3rd Ed, New York: Churchill Livingstone, 1993;1458–1459.
20. Smith RJ: ECRB tendon transfer for thumb adduction. A study of power pinch. J Hand Surg, 1983; 8:4–15.
21. Solonen KA, Bakalim GE: Restoration of pinch grip in traumatic ulnar palsy. Hand, 1976; 8: 39–44.
22. Wright PE: Campbell's Operative Orthopaedics, 8th Ed, St. Louis: Mosby, 1992:3032.
23. Zweig J, Rosenthal S, Burns H: Transfer of the extensor digiti quinti to restore pinch in ulnar palsy of the hand. J Bone Joint Surg, 1972; 54A:51–59.

88

Intrinsic Transfers with the Extensor Indicis Proprius and the Extensor Digiti Minimi Tendons

■ HISTORY OF THE TECHNIQUE

Loss of intrinsic muscle function results in an imbalance of forces at all three joints of each finger.[6,14] The intrinsic muscles simultaneously flex the metacarpophalangeal (MP) joints and extend the interphalangeal (IP) joints. Clawing of the fingers results when the MP joints hyperextend from the unopposed action of the extrinsic extensors, and the IP joints cannot extend because of the paralysis of the intrinsic muscles. Clawing is an obvious deformity, but the serious defect is functional loss.[2] The grip strength of the hand after low ulnar and median nerve palsy is decreased as much as 80%.[9,15] The correction is an active flexor for the MP joint, which should be corrected very early in a high combined palsy.[6,7]

Ulnar palsy also results in loss of active lateral mobility with the fingers in extension, due to paralysis of the interossei and hypothenar muscles.[1,9,14] There may be a persistently abducted little finger, first described by Wartenberg,[9,14] secondary to paralysis of the third palmar interosseus muscle. When unopposed by this intrinsic muscle, the EDM abducts the little finger through its indirect insertion into the abductor tubercle on the proximal phalanx.[1]

There have been many procedures described to correct intrinsic muscle loss, and most of them have used the extrinsic muscles of the wrist or fingers as transfers, such as the extensor carpi radialis brevis or the flexor digitorum superficialis. These are relatively strong motors for intrinsic reconstruction. A single insertion of a strong muscle into one lateral band of a finger might cause significant lateral deviation and rotation of the finger on a long-term basis and also hyperextension at the proximal interphalangeal joint (PIP) in a mobile finger. The EIP and EDM have adequate but not excessive strength and a good excursion,[2] limiting their potential to cause deformity.

Riordan[13] states that Fowler developed a transfer in 1946 for intrinsic paralysis that utilized the extensor indicis proprius (EIP) and the extensor digiti minimi (EDM) tendons. Each tendon was split into two slips. The EIP was inserted into the radial oblique fibers of the extensor aponeurosis of the index and long fingers, while the EDM was inserted into the radial oblique fibers of the extensor aponeurosis of the ring and little fingers. Riordan modified the procedure, using a free tendon graft for the index and long fingers, with the EIP as the only motor for all four digits. To improve thumb-index pinch, Brand[2] modified the free tendon insertion for only the index finger by inserting the tendon into the ulnar oblique fibers of the extensor aponeurosis. Brooks and Jones[3] and Zancolli[17] modified the tendon insertion by threading the tendon slip into a pulley made in the distal part of the proximal annular ligament of the flexor tendon sheath, then turning the tendon slip proximally, and suturing it to itself. Burkhalter[4,5] used a distal bony attachment to the proximal phalanx of the intrinsic minus digit.

Fowler[13] used the EIP tendon slips for the radial side of the hand and the EDM tendon slips for the ulnar side of the hand. The EDM is often too short for the appropriate insertion or is missing. For that reason, I prefer the Riordan technique,[14] which uses only the EIP and free grafts.

If a patient is seen early after nerve injury, he must be instructed on passive range of motion exercises and the hand protected with dynamic splinting to replace the function of the lost intrinsic muscles. If a patient is seen late after a nerve injury and contractures have developed, then the contractures must be overcome and supple joints restored by appropriate traction splints, exercises, and hand therapy. Only after normal or nearly normal joint motion has been established should reconstructive procedures be done.[13]

An indication for the EIP transfer is an ulnar nerve palsy with claw deformity, in which case the EIP is transferred only to the ring and small fingers. The EIP transfer with an attached free tendon graft of palmaris longus or plantaris may be indicated in a combined median and ulnar nerve palsy with claw deformity of all four fingers. Although Fowler indicated a combined EIP and EDM transfer in this clinical situation, the EDM is often too short for the appropriate insertion. If the EIP remains the motor of choice, I recommend the Riordan technique utilizing only the EIP and free grafts.

A contraindication to using the EDM transfer is the presence of only one EDM slip or its developmental absence.

■ INDICATIONS AND CONTRAINDICATIONS

The EIP arises from the dorsal side of the ulna and the interosseous membrane. In the forearm, it is situated on the ulnar side of the extensor pollicis longus and is covered by the extensor digitorum communis (EDC). The muscle belly of the EIP usually extends more distally than the bellies of the EDC. The tendon of the EIP lies dorsal to the tendons of the EDC in the fourth compartment beneath the dorsal retinaculum of the wrist. The EIP is consistently present in humans.

The EDM arises in common with the EDC from the lateral condyle of the humerus, and the two muscles are intimately adherent until they terminate in tendons. The EDC has three or four bellies; when there are only three bellies, the ulnar one gives off tendons for both the ring and little fingers. The tendons of the EDC pass through the fourth compartment beneath the dorsal retinaculum to the back of the hand, where they are connected by oblique tendinous fasciculi termed junctura tendinum. The tendon of the EDM passes through the fifth compartment beneath the dorsal retinaculum to the dorsal aponeurosis of the little finger, and is usually double, taking the place of the tendon of the EDC to the little finger (Fig. 88–1). The tendon of the EDC to the little finger is significantly deficient or absent in up to 75% of humans.[12,16] The EDM cannot be wholly transferred if there is no active extension of the little finger through the EDC. The posterior interosseous nerve and the posterior interosseous artery supply both the EIP and the EDM.

The operation may be done under either axillary block or general anesthesia. A pneumatic tourniquet is applied about the upper arm. The arm is exsanguinated and the tourniquet is inflated approximately 75 mm above resting systolic pressure.

Through a longitudinal chevron incision over the dorsal aspect of the index MP joint, the tendons of the EDC and the EIP are identified. The tendon of the EIP inserts on the ulnar side of the dorsal aponeurosis (extensor hood) of the index finger. The EIP tendon can be increased a centimeter in length by parallel incisions along the sides of the tendon into the extensor hood mechanism. Nonabsorbable 4-0 sutures should be placed on the lateral sides of the incisions to control the edges of the extensor hood mechanism. The enlongated EIP tendon is excised from the extension hood, and the hood is meticulously repaired with interrupted sutures. The EIP tendon is grasped with a small clamp and pulled distally. The tented skin will indicate the proximal tendon, and a short transverse incision over the mid third of the second metacarpal may be necessary to free fibrous connections between the EIP and the juncturae tendinum. It is appropriate to make a 1.5 cm transverse incision distal to the dorsal retinaculum, and the EIP tendon is completely mobilized from the EDC tendon to the distal edge of the extensor retinaculum. Gentle traction on the EIP should demonstrate free excursion, and the approximate position of the tendon on the proximal edge of the extensor retinaculum. A 1.5 cm transverse incision

■ SURGICAL TECHNIQUES

■ FIGURE 88–1
Transfer of the EIP and/ or EDM for supple claw deformity of the hand. The EIP and EDM tendons are ulnar to the EDC tendons in their respective fingers.

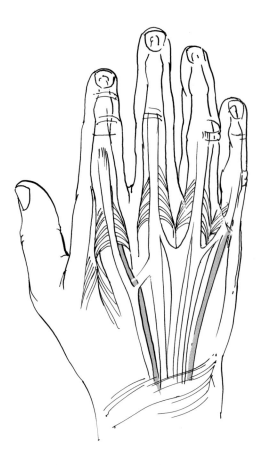

■ FIGURE 88–2
The EIP tendon is fully mobilized and prepared for transfer. Notice the repair of the extensor hood mechanism.

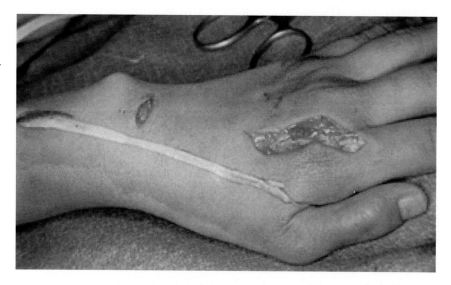

is made proximal to the extensor retinaculum and the EIP is mobilized into the forearm and delivered (Fig. 88–2). The EIP tendon is held in tension and split longitudinally into two slips.

If the diagnosis is isolated ulnar palsy, the operation is continued with the two EIP slips. If the diagnosis is combined median and ulnar palsy, the palmaris longus (PL) tendon is obtained. The distal portion of the PL is isolated through a transverse 2 cm incision proximal to the palmar crease. The PL tendon is mobilized to its musculotendinous junction through short transverse incisions. The freed PL tendon is woven into the EIP tendon proximally with 4-0 nonabsorbable sutures. The PL tendon is held in tension and split longitudinally into two slips, as the EIP tendon. This results in four slips, two from each tendon. The plantaris tendon may be used if the PL is absent.

A transverse incision is made just distal to the palmar creases. The neurovascular bundles and the flexor sheath are identified, as well as the deep transverse metacarpal ligament. A curved tendon passer is used to draw the tendon slips from the dorsal to the palmar wounds and volar to the deep transverse metacarpal ligament (Fig. 88–3). Usually, the two EIP slips are passed between the fourth and fifth metacarpals and the third and fourth metacarpals; the two PL slips are passed between the second and third metacarpals. The extensor aponeurosis is visualized through a midlateral longitudinal incision made over the radial aspect of the proximal phalanx of the long, ring, and little fingers; and over the ulnar aspect of the index finger. The tendon slips are passed distally and anterior to the deep transverse metacarpal ligament through the interdigital spaces to the oblique fibers, or lateral bands, of the dorsal aponeurosis (Fig. 88–4). The palmar incisions are closed.

While stabilizing the wrist in 45° of extension, and the MP joints in 60° of flexion, the tendon slips are attached with interrupted nonabsorable 4-0 sutures. The tension in the transfer should position the radial fingers in more extension, with the little finger in the most flexion.

All remaining surgical incisions are closed. The hand and forearm are placed in a bulky dressing. A "sugar-tong" plaster splint is applied that holds the wrist at 45° of extension and the MP joints in 60° of flexion.

In low ulnar palsy without evident clawing but persistent abduction of the little finger, a similar but alternative operation can be used. In this operation the EDM rather than the EIP is used as the motor. Through a longitudinal chevron incision over the dorsal aspect

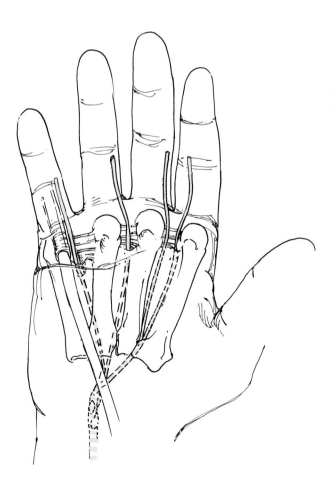

■ FIGURE 88–3
The four tails of the EIP and PL graft are passed from the dorsum of the hand between the metacarpals and volar to the intermetacarpal ligament.

■ FIGURE 88–4
The transferred tendons
are passed distally and
dorsally, between the fingers before attachment to
the lateral bands of the
dorsal aponeurosis.

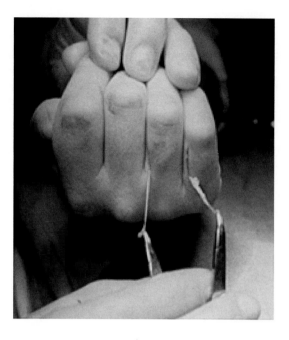

■ FIGURE 88–5
To correct abduction of
the little finger the ulnar
half of EDM is passed
volar to the intermetacarpal ligament and inserted
into the phalangeal at-
tachment of the MP col-
lateral ligament.

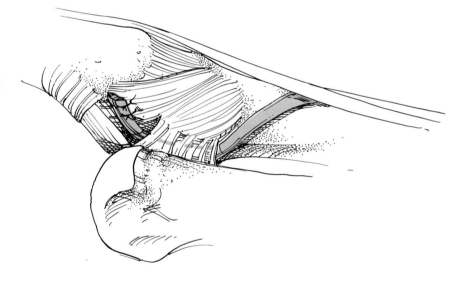

of the little MP joint, the tendons of the EDC and the EDM are identified. The ulnar of
the two EDM tendons is detached from the extensor hood distally and is dissected from
its companion tendon slip proximally to the distal edge of the extensor retinaculum.

A 2 cm oblique incision is made from the distal palmar crease overlying the MP joint
of the little finger to the proximal digital crease. The neurovascular bundle to the fourth
web space is retracted radialward to expose the deep transverse metacarpal ligament. A
curved tendon passer is used to draw the free EDM tendon slip from the dorsal to the
palmar wound between the fourth and fifth metacarpals. To correct abduction of the little
finger, the tendon is inserted into the phalangeal attachment of the radial collateral ligament (Fig. 88–5). If the finger is clawed as well as abducted, the A2 pulley of the flexor
sheath is identified, and a transverse slit is made in the vaginal ligament just distal to the
A2 pulley. The EDM slip is advanced through the slit, then turned back on itself (Fig.
88–6). The wrist is held at neutral and the MP joints in 20° of flexion while the tendon is
sutured. The incisions are closed, and the hand and forearm are placed in a bulky dressing.
A "sugar-tong" plaster splint is applied to immobilize the wrist in 30° of extension and
the MP joints in 30° of flexion.

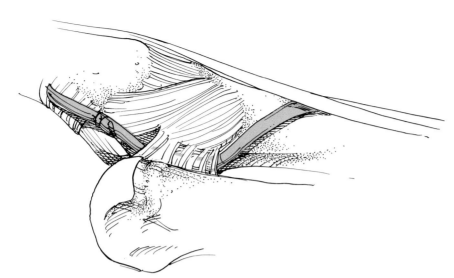

If the patient with supple fingers needs increased PIP extension with MP flexion, then transfers should extend to the lateral bands of the extensor mechanism.[15,16] Transfers to the proximal phalanx or to the proximal pulley will prevent the risk of overcorrection and swan-neck deformity.

MP flexion with power is better restored with the A2 pulley insertion, as described by Brooks[1,3] and Zancolli.[17] A transverse slit is made in the pulley; then each slip is passed into the flexor sheath and out distally through the slit and sutured back on itself with 4-0 nonabsorbable sutures. In this transfer, to identify the A2 pulley, an oblique incision is made from the distal palmar crease to the proximal digital crease over each digit, but the midlateral finger incision is not necessary.

Instead of looping the transferred tendon through the flexor tendon sheath pulley, it can be attached to a radially based flap of the flexor tendon sheath, as described by Brooks.[1] A radially based flap 7 to 8 mm wide is raised distal to the A1 pulley, and the tendon is sutured to the flap of the sheath and the adjacent periosteum of the proximal phalanx.

If the little finger is persistently abducted but not clawed, and the MP joint cannot be passively extended beyond neutral, the transferred tendon slip can be sutured into the phalangeal attachment of the radial collateral ligament of the MP joint of the little finger. Ranney[12] indicates that this attachment also restores the metacarpal arch; instability of the transverse metacarpal arch may contribute to recurrent clawing in ulnar play.[9–11]

When intrinsic transfer procedures are done with the EIP and EDM, both tendons should be harvested with maximum length because the slips are passed volar to the deep transverse metacarpal ligament, and advanced distally a distance of approximately 1 inch (2.5 cm). If these procedures are to succeed, the patient must demonstrate preoperatively an ability to obtain PIP extension with the MP joint stabilized in less than full extension.

Techniques using the EDM[18] or the EIP[7–9] for thumb-index pinch have not demonstrated adequate strength to indicate clinically improved function.

■ TECHNICAL ALTERNATIVES

The hand and forearm are initially immobilized in a bulky dressing and a "sugar-tong" splint that holds the fingers in 60° of flexion and the wrist in 45° of extension. This is followed by a circular short arm cast that extends beyond the distal palmar crease and immobilizes the MP joints in 60° of flexion and the wrist in 30° of extension for 3 weeks. The patient is encouraged to move the fingers to obtain full extension of the PIP joints and full flexion of the fingers to the distal palmar crease. Movement is evaluated periodically by a hand therapist, and supervised exercise is used as indicated.

After 3 weeks, the cast is removed, and an orthoplast dorsal splint is fitted that will hold the MP joints in 60° flexion and allow wrist motion. The splint is worn at least 3 weeks and can be worn up to 6 weeks to obtain full extension of the PIP joints and full flexion of the fingers to the distal palmar crease.

■ REHABILITATION

■ OUTCOMES

Cases with clawing deformity and loss of a normal flexion pattern in intrinsic minus fingers are difficult to measure for functional outcomes. Exact evaluation is difficult in these cases secondary to associated bone and soft-tissue injuries that interfer with function. Burkhalter[4] evaluated patients in three ways: (1) grip strength, (2) correction of clawing deformity, and (3) improved pattern of flexion for the fingers. Grip strength outcome will vary according to the level and extent of the nerve lesion. Burkhalter found 51 of 54 patients had successful loss of clawing deformity and an improved flexor pattern. Grip strength varied with the nerve loss: (1) in low ulnar palsy there was the least increase in grip strength, but measurable functional gain; (2) in high ulnar or median-ulnar palsy, there was a considerable increase in the relative grip strength, but minimal power for function.

In cases with a persistently abducted little finger in low ulnar palsy, Blacker[1] eliminated persistent abduction of the little finger in seven of eight patients. In the eighth patient, a flexion deformity resulted at the MP joint.

In a practical sense, intrinsic reconstruction corrects abnormal digital positions (clawing, abduction) and provides an improved pattern for digital flexion, but adds very little strength for improved functional activities.

References

1. Blacker GJ, Lister GD, Kleinert HE: The abducted little finger in low ulnar palsy. J Hand Surg, 1987; 1:190–196.
2. Brand PW: Tendon Transfers for Correction of Paralysis of Intrinsic Muscles of the Hand. In: Hunter JM, Schneider LH, Mackin EJ (eds): Tendon Surgery in the Hand, St. Louis: Mosby, 1987:439–449.
3. Brooks AL, Jones DS: A new intrinsic tendon transfer for the paralytic hand. J Bone Joint Surg, 1975; 57A:730.
4. Burkhalter WE: Restoration of power grip in ulnar nerve paralysis. Orthop Clin N Amer, 1974; 5:289–303.
5. Burkhalter WE, Strait JL: Metacarpophalangeal flexor replacement for intrinsic-muscle paralysis. J Bone Joint Surg, 1973; 55A:1667–1676.
6. Omer GE Jr: Evaluation and reconstruction of the forearm and hand after traumatic peripheral nerve injuries. J Bone Joint Surg, 1968; 50A:1454–1478.
7. Omer GE Jr: Tendon transfers in combined nerve lesions. Orthop Clin N Amer, 1974; 5: 377–387.
8. Omer GE Jr, Spinner M: Management of Peripheral Nerve Problems, Philadelphia: W.B. Saunders, 1980:817–846.
9. Omer GE Jr: The Palsied Hand. In: Evarts C Mc (ed): Surgery of the Musculoskeletal System, New York: Churchill Livingstone, 1990:849–878.
10. Omer GE Jr: Ulnar Nerve Palsy. In: Green DP (ed): Operative Hand Surgery, New York: Churchill Livingstone, 1993:1449–1466.
11. Omer GE Jr, Pierla-Cruz M: Complications of Peripheral Nerve Injuries. In: Epps CH Jr: Complications in Orthopaedic Surgery, Philadelphia: J.B. Lippincott, 1994:811–856.
12. Ranney DA: Reconstruction of the transverse metacarpal arch in ulnar palsy by transfer of the extensor digiti minimi. Plast Reconstr Surg, 1974; 52:406–412.
13. Riordan DC: Tendon transfers for nerve paralysis of the hand and wrist. Curr Pract Orthop Surg, 1964; 2:17–40.
14. Riordan DC: Tendon transplantation in median-nerve and ulnar-nerve paralysis. J Bone Joint Surg, 1953; 35A;312–320.
15. Smith RJ: Intrinsic Muscles of the Fingers: Function, Dysfunction, and Surgical Reconstruction. St. Louis, Mosby, AAOS Instructional Course Lectures, 1975; 24:200–220.
16. Smith RJ: Tendon Transfers of the Hand and Forearm. Boston, Little Brown, 1987:57–83.
17. Zancolli E: Structural and Dynamic Bases of Hand Surgery, 2nd Ed, Philadelphia: J.B. Lippincott, 1979:169–198.
18. Zweig J, Rosenthal S, Burns H: Transfer of the extensor digiti quinti to restore pinch in ulnar palsy of the hand. J Bone Joint Surg, 1972; 54A:51–59.

AMIT GUPTA
THOMAS W. WOLFF

89

Flexor Digitorum Sublimis Transfer to A1 Pulley for Claw Hand

Two major types of tendon transfers have evolved for the treatment of the claw hand deformity caused by intrinsic paralysis. In one type, the transferred motor actively extends the last two phalanges with digital extension and actively flexes the proximal phalanx with digital flexion. In the second type, the transferred motor prevents hyperextension of the metacarpophalangeal (MP) joint during digital extension and actively flexes this joint with digital flexion. By restricting MP joint extension, this transfer allows the extensor apparatus to extend the last two phalanges.

The first type of transfer was introduced in 1916 by Nissenbaum.[11] He used two strips from the entire length of the flexor digitorum sublimis (FDS) to the lateral bands of the extensor. These were routed dorsal to the deep transverse metacarpal ligament. Lexer[8] modified this technique using tendon grafts from the flexor sublimis in the palm to the extensor tendon placing the grafts through the lumbrical canals. In 1922, Stiles and Forrester-Brown[14] sutured the split flexor sublimis, routing each slip around the corresponding side of the finger to the extensor tendon. Bunnell[4] noted that he was unable to achieve useful results with the Stiles procedure. He refined the technique by altering the path of the FDS transfer in a way that provided a straight course for the tendon, good leverage, and an improved angle of approach. Bunnell achieved this by routing the transfer through the lumbrical canal. He advised suturing the transfer to the transverse fibers and lateral band to avoid the gliding surface of extensor tendons and to minimize adhesions. Similar transfers were later described by Fowler[6] and Brand.[1]

The second type of transfer has been accomplished by inserting the transferred FDS tendon into either the base of the proximal phalanx or the proximal aspect of the flexor tendon sheath. In 1964, Littler[9] suggested fixing tendinous strips harvested from the length of FDS to the base of the proximal phalanx. Littler believed this procedure to be simpler and more predictable than previous operations. Moreover, by actively flexing the MP joint, the procedure allowed the extrinsic extensors to extend the proximal interphalangeal (PIP) joint. A similar procedure was described by Burkhalter and Strait[5] in 1973. They attempted to provide flexor power to the proximal phalanx by transferring FDS strips to this bone; this was a modification of the Stiles-Bunnell operation, in which the strips of FDS tendon were transferred to the lateral band of the extensor tendon.

In 1975, Brookes and Jones[3] used the A2 pulley for insertion of their motor. This provides greater flexion power to the proximal phalanx, especially at initiation of flexion. In 1974, Zancolli[15] suggested transfer of motors, particularly FDS, to the A1 pulley. This transfer is called the "lasso" procedure because the FDS tendon is looped around the A1 pulley and then sutured to itself, thus "lassoing" the A1 pulley. Zancolli[16] makes a distinction between direct "lasso" in which the FDS is the motor and indirect "lasso" where, due to paralysis of the FDS, another forearm motor is prolonged by tendon grafts and transferred to the A1 or the FDS tendon, which "lassos" the A1 pulley and is motored by another forearm muscle.

Correction of claw hand by tendon transfer provides both a cosmetic and functional benefit to the patient. FDS transfer to the A1 pulley can be used to correct claw hand of

■ HISTORY OF THE TECHNIQUE

■ INDICATIONS AND CONTRAINDICATIONS

varying causes, including traumatic or compressive ulnar nerve palsy, combined ulnar and median nerve palsy, brachial plexus lesions, spinal cord lesions, Charcot-Marie-Tooth disease, or leprosy.

The need to correct claw hand is not merely a cosmetic consideration. Correction of the deformity attempts to restore the dynamic function arc of motion of the fingers by restructuring the proper sequence of digital flexion—MP joint flexion followed by synchronous flexion of interphalangeal joints, thus providing better distribution of forces in the hand.

A clinical approach to claw hand is germane to a discussion of the surgical procedure. Although it is possible to prevent or minimize claw hand deformity by proper splintage, the patient still has an intrinsicly weak hand with all the attendant problems of "rolling" flexion and weak inefficient grasp and tip-to-tip pinch. Therefore, tendon transfer may be necessary not merely to overcome the cosmetic problem but to correct the functional deficit.

The Bouvier test[16] is an important maneuver to differentiate the various types of claw hand. Results of this maneuver are positive when the patient is able to actively extend the proximal and distal interphalangeal joints when the MP joint is passively flexed. Patients who have a positive result with the Bouvier test are classified as having simple claw hands.

Patients with a negative Bouvier result may be of two types—those in whom the proximal and distal phalanges can be passively extended and those in whom these joints cannot be passively extended. The former situation occurs in long-standing claw hand where the central slip of the extensor tendon becomes elongated due to pressure over a flexed PIP joint. The latter situation arises in cases of adhesions of the long flexor tendon, shortening of long flexors due to Volkman's ischemic contracture, interphalangeal joint stiffness, and volar skin contracture at the PIP joint level.

It is therefore clear that every case of claw hand must be carefully assessed to identify other problems that must be addressed before treating claw hand by tendon transfers. The best indication of FDS transfer to A1 pulley will be in cases of simple claw hand with a positive Bouvier test.

The absolute contraindication to FDS to A1 pulley transfer is a complex claw hand with a negative Bouvier test. If the patient is unable to actively extend his PIP joint with passive flexion of the MP joint, then the attempt to correct the claw hand by actively flexing the MP joint by FDS to A1 pulley transfer will fail. In those situations, an active transfer to the lateral bands (like a Brand transfer) should be used to correct the claw hand.

The other absolute contraindication of this procedure is a fixed claw hand. Every attempt must be made to first mobilize the PIP and distal interphalangeal joints before doing this tendon transfer.

The relative contraindication to this transfer is in patients who require power grip. In these patients, a transfer that adds power to the hand like a Brand transfer should be done. Long-standing claw deformities also form a relative contraindication for this procedure as in situations where the extensor tendon may be stretched out, making it impossible for the patient to actively extend the PIP joint after the FDS to A1 pulley transfer.

■ SURGICAL TECHNIQUES

The surgery is performed under a brachial plexus block or general anesthesia. Local or wrist blocks are not satisfactory. We prefer a standard axillary block. An arm tourniquet is used. The hand and forearm are exsanguinated and the tourniquet elevated to 100 mm Hg above the patient's systolic pressure.

The A1 pulley is located beneath the distal palmar crease. Depending on the number of fingers to be operated, a transverse incision is made at the distal palmar crease. The length of the incision is approximately 1.5 cm. Proximal and distal flaps are carefully elevated avoiding the digital neurovascular bundles. The A1 pulley of each finger is exposed. The FDS tendon is isolated proximal to the A1 pulley with a tendon hook. A small curved hemostat is then introduced into the fibro-osseous tunnel beneath the proximal end of the A1 pulley and advanced to the interval to emerge between the A1 and A2 pulleys. The sheath is then opened at this interval, and a small (1 to 2 mm) longitudinal back cut is made distally on the radial or ulnar side of A2 pulley. This will give access to the FDS between the A1 and A2 and facilitate the delivery of the FDS tendon between the A1 and A2 pulleys. The FDS tendon, which already has split in two at this location, is isolated and delivered into the wound and divided. Both FDS slips are divided. The protection of FDP and delivery of the FDS can be facilitated by placing a tendon hook around the FDS tendon. Before division of the FDS tendon, 4-0 braided sutures are placed in each of the two proximal slips of the FDS to prevent its retraction under the A1 pulley (Fig. 89–1). The distal end is allowed to retract into the sheath. Care is taken to protect the profundus tendon throughout the procedure.

The proximal end of the cut FDS tendon is now looped over the A1 pulley and pulled to its maximum tension while the wrist and all finger joints are held in the neutral position (Fig. 89–2). The tendon is sutured to itself and to the A1 pulley. The ring finger MP joint should rest at 40° flexion and the small finger MP joint at 60° flexion with the wrist in neutral position. We use 4-0 braided suture material, using three sutures for the FDS itself and one or two sutures between the FDS and A1 pulley. Further proximally, the tendon

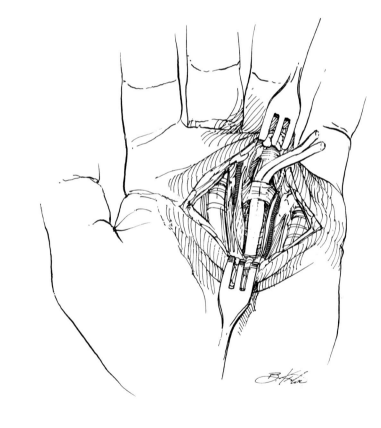

■ FIGURE 89–1
Delivery of FDS in the interval between A1 and A2 pulleys.

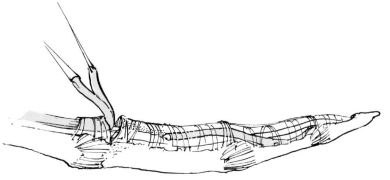

■ FIGURE 89–2
Division of two slips of FDS tendon with suture passing through each slip.

■ FIGURE 89–3
FDS to A1 pulley loop. FDS is sutured to itself and the A1 pulley. The finger should be in neutral extension, with the FDS pulled to maximum length.

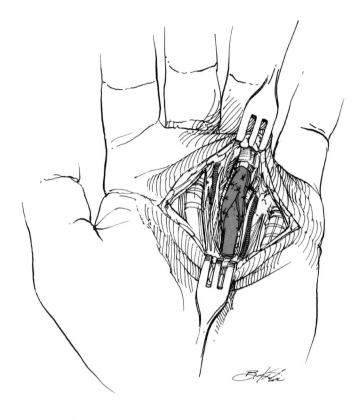

is again sutured to itself (Fig. 89–3). Tension is then tested by altering the position of the wrist and observing finger motion. With full wrist flexion, MP extension will occur (neutral to 20° MP flexion) along with interphalangeal extension (0° to 20° at PIP). Adjustment in the tightness of the transfer can be easily made at this stage by removing the applied sutures and resuturing. Hemostasis is obtained, and the tourniquet is deflated before skin closure. The wound is closed and dressings are applied. Drains are not necessary. Postoperative splintage consists of a dorsal splint that holds the MP joints immobilized in 40° flexion. Lateral edges of the splint are extended volarly to serve as flexion blocking for the MP joints. Thus, free active motion of the PIP joints is allowed but the MP joints are held in 30° flexion. Sutures are removed at 2 weeks, but immobilization is continued for 4 weeks. The interphalangeal joints are left free and active and passive motion is encouraged.

■ TECHNICAL ALTERNATIVES

Care must be taken to harvest the FDS tendon and not the FDP tendon.

In patients who have laxity of joints, particularly those of Asian nationality, removal of the FDS may result in hyperextension of the PIP joint or even swan neck deformity of the finger. To prevent this, one of the FDS slips may be left long and tenodesed to the floor of the fibrous flexor sheath with one suture.

In performing a four-tailed "lasso" where one FDS tendon is split into four parts, care must be taken to pass these tendon strips dorsal to the neurovascular bundles, otherwise there is a theoretical risk of compressing the neurovascular bundles. Injury to the digital neurovascular bundle can be avoided by staying in the midline of the finger.

Proper tensioning of the transfer is very important. If the transfer is too loose, it will not function in an effective manner and the claw finger will recur. Conversely, if the transfer is too tight, it will cause a flexion deformity of the MP joint.

Occasionally, the FDS to the small finger may be absent or abnormal. Preoperative examination is a clue to this abnormality. However, if such a finding is encountered at operation, the ring finger FDS may be transferred in a split fashion to the A1 pulley of both ring and small fingers.

The backcut in the A2 pulley should be minimal. It should not be made in the midline or this may result in some bowstringing of the FDP tendon.

If an FDS tendon is split and transferred to two or more fingers, a suture should be placed at the apex of the split to prevent proximal extension of this split. If one FDS tendon is split and transferred to two or more fingers, some of the flexor sheath may become overcrowded as they now contain their own FDS, FDP, and a transferred slip of FDS. Ensure that there is no triggering of the tendon before wound closure.

The technique described above is one of direct "lasso" procedure using a single FDS for the same finger. In cases where all FDS tendons are not available for transfer or some may have to be used for other transfers, a single FDS tendon (usually of the ring or middle finger) may be used and split into four tails to be "lassoed" around the A1 pulley of each finger. Each tail must be routed under the superficial palmar arch.

In situations where superficialis tendons are paralyzed, the "lasso" procedure can still be performed provided there are no adhesions of the superficialis tendons. A functioning motor unit will have to be transferred to the FDS in the forearm.

Another modification of the procedure is the transfer of FDS to the A2 pulley as proposed by Omer. According to Tsuge, this provides a stronger flexion force to the MP joint. This procedure may have to be done if the A1 pulley is thin or nonexistent, as may occasionally occur in the small finger.[7]

■ REHABILITATION

Postoperatively, the hand is placed in a dorsal block splint holding the MP joint in 40° flexion. This splint prevents any motion of the MP joints. Full active motion of the interphalangeal joints is permitted. This splint is continued for 4 weeks.

At this point, the splint is removed and the patient uses a dorsally based anti-claw splint that holds the MP joints in 40° flexion. Full active and passive flexion of the digit is permitted. This splint is worn for another 4 weeks, at which point full active motion and strengthening exercises are begun.

■ OUTCOMES

In selected cases, FDS transfer to A1 pulleys provides a predictable and long-lasting correction of clawing. Hastings and McCollan[7] found that FDS lasso to the A1 pulley successfully corrected claw deformity in 19 of 23 digits. This transfer does not add power to the hand but improves grip strength from the preoperative state by altering the arc of flexion. In the Hastings and McCollan[7] series, there was no significant improvement in grip strength. If power and grip improvement are the goals, this should not be a treatment of choice. Rather, a Brand transfer is preferred.

In a recent series,[7] all patients believed that their clumsiness was reduced but not eliminated. Manipulative skills were improved. All patients except 1 of 23 believed that they had improved function and would have the lasso operation performed again. Four digits showed mild swan neck deformity.

References

1. Brand PW: Paralytic claw hand. J Bone Joint Surg, 1958; 40B:618–632.
2. Brand PW: Tendon transfers for correction of paralysis of intrinsic muscles of the hand. In: Hunter JW, Schneider LH, Mackin EJ (eds): Tendon Surgery in the Hand, St. Louis: Mosby, 1987:439–499.
3. Brooks AL, Jones DS: A new intrinsic tendon transfer for the paralytic hand. J Bone Joint Surg, 1975; 57A:730.
4. Bunnell S: Surgery of the Hand, Philadelphia: JB Lippincott, 1944:366.
5. Burkhalter WL, Strait JL: Metacarpophalangeal flexor replacement for intrinsic muscle paralysis. J Bone Joint Surg, 1973; 55A:1667–1676.
6. Fowler SB: Discussion on the extensor apparatus of the finger. First Meeting of the American Society for Surgery of the Hand. J Bone Joint Surg, 1947:.
7. Hastings H II, McCollan SM: Flexor digitorum superficialis lasso tendon transfer in isolated ulnar nerve palsy: a functional evaluation. J Hand Surg, 1994; 19A:275–280.
8. Lexer E: Die Freien Transplantationen. Von Ferdinand Enke, Stuttgant, 19.

9. Littler JW: Restoration of power and stability in the partially paralyzed hand. In: Converse JM (ed): Reconstructive Plastic Surgery, Vol 6, Philadelphia: WB Saunders, 1977; 3266–3305.

10. Littler JW: On adaptability of man's hand. Hand, 1973; 5:187–191.

11. Nissenbaum A: Sehenplastik bei Ulnarislähmung. Zentralbl Chir, 1916:978–979.

12. Shah A: One in four flexor digitorum superficialis lasso for correction of claw deformity. J Hand Surg, 1985; 11B:404–406.

13. Smith RJ: Tendon Transfers of the Hand and Forearm, Boston: Little, Brown, 1987:103–134.

14. Stiles AJ, Forrester-Brown MF: Treatment of Injuries of the Peripheral Spinal Nerves, London: Henry Frowde, Hodder and Stoughton, 1922.

15. Zancolli EA: Corección de la Garza digital por parálisis intrinseca. La operación del "lazo". Acta Orthop Latino Americana, 1974; 1:65–72.

16. Zancolli EA: Structural and Dynamic Bases of Hand Surgery, 2nd Ed, Philadelphia: JB Lippincott, 1979; 174–188.

PART
VI

Compression
Neuropathy

RICHARD A. BROWN
RICHARD H.
GELBERMAN

90

Carpal Tunnel Release: Open Technique

Although Sir James Paget described a case of post-traumatic median nerve compression at the wrist in 1853, operative treatment for this condition was not performed until 1933 when Learmonth performed the first documented transverse carpal ligament release.[15,20] In 1947, Brain and associates reported the first detailed analysis of the clinical symptoms, physical findings, and pathophysiology of median nerve compression in the carpal tunnel. They recommended early operative release of the transverse carpal ligament for those patients with characteristic presentations.[1] In the 1950s and 1960s, Phalen's work popularized the diagnosis and treatment of carpal tunnel syndrome to the extent that it is currently the most widely recognized, frequently treated entrapment neuropathy.[5,21]

■ HISTORY OF THE
TECHNIQUE

The diagnosis of carpal tunnel syndrome is established on the basis of clinical history (pain, numbness, or paresthesias in the distribution of the median nerve) and physical findings (diminished sensibility, weakness, or positive provocative tests).[6,9,12] Diagnostic confirmation is obtained with electrophysiologic studies demonstrating abnormal values: distal motor latency values of greater than 4.5 msec or a difference in values between the affected hand and the unaffected hand of 1 msec or greater, or a sensory latency of greater than 3.5 msec, or 0.5 msec greater than the opposite side or both.[28] Nonoperative treatment measures such as splinting or steroid injections are used effectively in many cases. However, patients with severe symptoms; symptoms that are present for more than 1 year; weakness and constant numbness in the thumb, index, and long fingers; atrophy; or two-point discrimination greater than 6 mm frequently do not benefit from nonoperative measures.[6] Those individuals who fail nonoperative treatment and who fulfill the above subjective and objective criteria of established carpal tunnel syndrome are candidates for operative release of the transverse carpal ligament.

■ INDICATIONS AND
CONTRAINDICATIONS

There are no specific contraindications to performing carpal tunnel release when clinical and electrophysiologic data are consistent with the diagnosis. Patients who are pregnant usually experience resolution of their carpal tunnel syndromes by 6 weeks postpartum; therefore, operative release is not performed until this period has elapsed.[25] Patients with endocrinologic disorders (e.g., diabetes, hypothyroidism) are evaluated and treated medically before being considered for operative treatment. Similarly, when patients present with work-related symptoms, ergonomic adjustments in work schedules and at the work station are strongly recommended before indicating the operation.

Operative decompression of the carpal canal is performed with the patient in the supine position. A tourniquet is applied, and the arm is placed on a hand table with the forearm fully supinated. While general or local anesthesia is acceptable, we prefer intravenous regional anesthesia. The limb is exsanguinated with an Esmarch bandage and the tourniquet elevated to 250 mmHg. An injection of 40 to 50 ml of 0.5% lidocaine without epinephrine is administered. With the ring finger flexed to the palm, a dot is made with a skin marking pencil on the distal wrist crease in line with the ulnar aspect of the ring finger ray (Fig. 90–1). Neither the skin incision nor subsequent deeper dissection is carried lateral to the longitudinal plane created by this point and the ulnar aspect of the ring finger ray. The position of the recurrent motor branch of the median nerve is separately marked by

■ SURGICAL
TECHNIQUES

■ FIGURE 90–1
The lateral extent of the carpal tunnel incision is determined by placing a mark just proximal to the flexed ring finger along the proximal wrist crease.

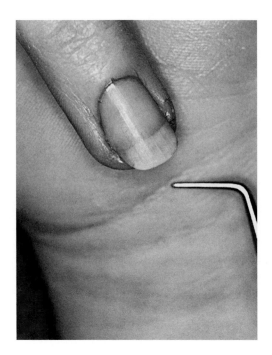

■ FIGURE 90–2
Kaplan's landmark, constructed by extending one line along the distal aspect of the abducted thumb and a second line proximally from the index-long web, localizes the motor branch of the median nerve. The superficial palmar arch is located along the oblique palmar arch.

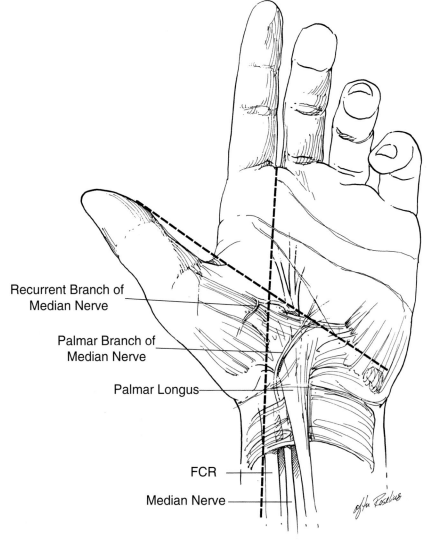

Recurrent Branch of Median Nerve

Palmar Branch of Median Nerve

Palmar Longus

FCR

Median Nerve

flexing the long finger to the thenar eminence (Fig. 90–2). The incision begins distally along Kaplan's oblique line just ulnar to the thenar crease.[11] This point marks the distal border of the transverse carpal ligament. It is extended proximally 2 mm ulnar to the thenar crease to the distal wrist crease at a point just ulnar to the longitudinal axis of the ring finger in the interval between the palmar cutaneous branches of the median and ulnar nerves (Figs. 90-3 and 90-4).[3,26] Under 3.5× loupe magnification, sharp dissection is carried down to the superficial palmar fascia, which is divided longitudinally. The skin edges and palmar fascia are retracted, exposing the transverse carpal ligament. The distinct proximal edge of the ligament is isolated at the level of the distal palmar crease (Fig. 90–5). The ligament is divided proximally by incising it longitudinally with a scalpel in line with the ring finger ray. This must be done with care as the median nerve may be directly under the ligament. The distal half of the transverse carpal ligament is divided in layers, using a combination of scalpel and scissor dissection. Particular care is taken as the adipose tissue surrounding the superficial palmar arch is approached (Fig. 90-6). The median nerve is observed beneath the lateral flap of the transverse carpal ligament and the motor branch at the distal radial aspect of the flap (Fig. 90–7).

Attention is then directed to the distal aspect of the antebrachial fascia. The palmar cutaneous branch of the median nerve is attached to the undersurface of the antebrachial fascia beneath the medial margin of the flexor carpi radialis; therefore, skin hooks are used to elevate the proximal edge of the incision and the antebrachial fascia is divided for 2 to 3 cm proximal to the transverse wrist crease along the ring finger axis (Fig. 90–8). Incising the fascia in this plane prevents inadvertent transection of the palmar cutaneous nerve. Finally the floor of the carpal canal is explored by retracting the flexor tendons radially. Neither tenolysis nor neurolysis are performed routinely.

The skin edges are infiltrated with 1% lidocaine without epinephrine, and the tourniquet is deflated. Hemostasis is obtained, and the skin is closed with 5-0 nylon mattress sutures. A bulky short-arm hand dressing is applied, with plaster splints maintaining the wrist in 30° extension.[8]

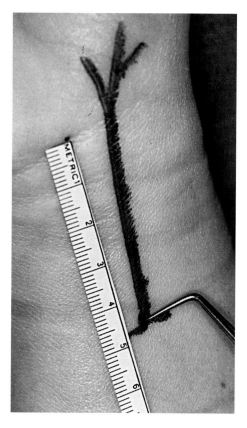

■ FIGURE 90–3
Location and distribution of the palmar cutaneous branch of the median nerve.

■ FIGURE 90–4
The incision parallels the thenar crease 2 mm ulnar to its border.

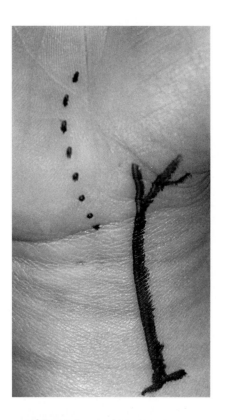

■ FIGURE 90–5
The proximal edge of the transverse carpal liga-ment is isolated.

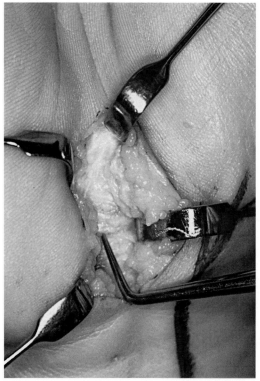

■ TECHNICAL
ALTERNATIVES

Eversmann recommends an incision that begins at the distal border of the transverse carpal ligament, follows the longitudinal crease of the palm, and crosses the base of the palm in a zigzag fashion ulnar to the longitudinal axis of the ring finger. The incision is continued proximally into the forearm for 3 cm. The antebrachial fascia is divided and the median nerve isolated and protected; subsequently, the transverse carpal ligament is

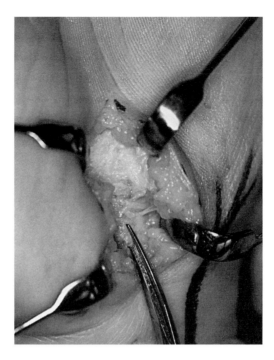

■ FIGURE 90-6
The transverse carpal ligament is incised distally to the level of the superficial palmar arch.

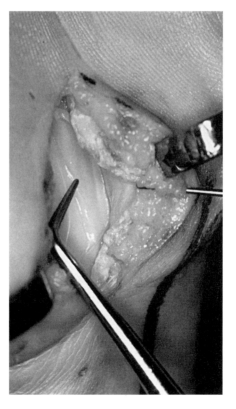

■ FIGURE 90-7
After division of the transverse carpal ligament, the median nerve is exposed.

divided. Special attention is directed toward identification and release of the motor branch of the median nerve.[4]

Others advocate incisions that parallel the thenar crease in a curvilinear or longitudinal fashion and cross the wrist crease obliquely or at 90° and extend proximally 1 to 3 cm. The antebrachial fascia and transverse carpal ligament are divided under direct vision.[8]

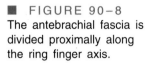

■ FIGURE 90–8
The antebrachial fascia is
divided proximally along
the ring finger axis.

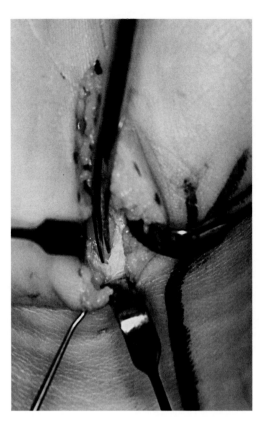

In cases of acute carpal tunnel syndrome, we recommend a departure from the standard operative technique. Instead, the incision is extended across the wrist crease in a curvilinear fashion and is then carried 4 cm proximally into the forearm. The antebrachial fascia is divided proximally and the median nerve is isolated as it emerges from the lateral border of the flexor digitorum superficialis. The fascia is divided in line with the ring finger axis. The transverse carpal ligament is approached and divided as described in the Surgical Technique section.[5]

Internal neurolysis of the median nerve has been previously recommended as an adjunct to transverse carpal ligament release. More recent studies indicate that this procedure does not improve patient outcomes and therefore is rarely indicated.[7,17,19,22]

Similarly, it has been shown that patients with concomitant distal median and ulnar nerve symptoms markedly improve after division of the transverse carpal ligament. Therefore, separate release of Guyon's canal is not recommended.[23]

The median nerve and nine flexor tendons course through the carpal canal. Spontaneous carpal tunnel syndrome is most frequently caused by nonspecific chronic tenosynovitis. Synovectomy is not performed unless there is evidence of invasive proliferative synovitis, such as that occurring with rheumatoid arthritis. When synovectomy is necessary, the operative approach described for use in acute carpal tunnel syndrome is used.[8]

The complication most commonly reported after open carpal tunnel release is transection of the palmar cutaneous branch of the median nerve.[16] Since Taleisnik's description of the course of this branch, the operative incision has been altered to avoid it.[26] Other complications associated with open carpal tunnel release include transection of the superficial palmar arch, the recurrent motor branch of the median nerve, the main trunk of the median nerve, flexor tendon bowstringing, adherence of the median nerve to the flexor tendons and the skin, wound hematoma, and infection. These complications occur relatively infrequently and can be avoided with careful attention to operative technique and postoperative wrist extension splinting.[13,14,16,18,27]

The postoperative dressing, splint, and sutures are removed 8 to 9 days after surgery. Patients are encouraged to use their hands as tolerated. Most can perform basic activities of daily living by 10 days and nearly all activities of daily living by 3 weeks after surgery. The timing for return to work is varied and dependent on many factors. Motivated individuals with jobs that do not require repetitive or stressful hand activities may return within a few days after surgery. Most individuals return to work in approximately 3 weeks. Those who are less motivated or have highly stressful and repetitive jobs may require 4 to 6 weeks before returning to work.

Hand therapy modalities are not routinely used. If swelling or stiffness of the fingers is present on the first postoperative visit, elastic finger wraps and instruction on supervised active and passive motion exercises can be very helpful.

■ REHABILITATION

Open carpal tunnel release has been the procedure of choice for relief of numbness and paresthesias in patients with median nerve compression at the wrist unresponsive to nonoperative measures. Previous studies have demonstrated that this operative procedure provides lasting alleviation of symptoms and patient satisfaction in more than 80% of cases.[2,13,21,23]

Recurrence is often traced to incomplete release of the transverse carpal ligament.[18] Although prolonged scar tenderness and loss of grip strength are the two most common postoperative complaints, complete resolution of these symptoms typically occurs within the 6-month period after surgery.[10,13,14]

■ OUTCOMES

References

1. Brain W, Wright A, Wilkinson M: Spontaneous compression of both median nerves in the carpal tunnel. Six cases treated surgically. Lancet, 1947; 1:277–282.
2. Cseuz K, Thomas J, Lambert E, Love J, Lipscomb P: Long-term results of operation for carpal tunnel syndrome. Mayo Clinic Proceedings, 1966; 41:232–241.
3. Engber W, Cmeiner J: Palmar cutaneous branch of the ulnar nerve. J Hand Surg, 1980; 5A: 26–29.
4. Eversmann W: Entrapment and compression neuropathies. In: Green D (ed): Operative Hand Surgery, 2nd Ed, New York: Churchill Livingstone, 1988:1423–1478.
5. Gelberman R: Acute carpal tunnel syndrome. In: Gelberman R (ed): Operative Nerve Repair and Reconstruction, Philadelphia: J.B. Lippincott, 1991:939–948.
6. Gelberman R, Aronson D, Weisman M. Carpal-tunnel syndrome: Results of a prospective trial of steroid injection and splinting. J Bone Joint Surg, 1980; 62-A:1181–1184.
7. Gelberman R, Pfeffer G, Galbraith R, Szabo R, Rydevick B, Dimick M: Results of treatment of severe carpal tunnel syndrome without neurolysis of the median nerve. J Bone Joint Surgery, 1987; 69A:896–903.
8. Gelberman R: Carpal tunnel release: Open Release of Transverse Carpal Ligament. In: Gelberman R (ed): Operative Nerve Repair and Reconstruction, Philadelphia: J. B. Lippincott, 1991:899–912.
9. Gellman H, Gelberman R, Tan A, Botte M: Carpal tunnel syndrome: An evaluation of the provocative diagnostic tests. J Bone Joint Surgery, 1986; 68A:735–737.
10. Gellman H, Kan D, Gee V, Kuschner S, Botte M: Analysis of pinch and grip strength after carpal tunnel release. J Hand Surgery, 1989; 14A:863–869.
11. Kaplan EB: Functional and Surgical Anatomy of the Hand, 2nd Ed, Philadelphia: J.B. Lippincott, 1965.
12. Koris M, Gelberman R, Duncan K, Boublik M, Smith B: Carpal tunnel syndrome: Evaluation of a quantitative provocational diagnostic test. Clin Orthop Rel Res, 1990; 251:157–161.
13. Kulick M, Gordillo G, Javidi T, Kilgore E, Newmeyer W: Long-term analysis of patients having surgical treatment for carpal tunnel syndrome. J Hand Surgery, 1986; 11A:59–66.
14. Kuschner S, Brien W, Johnson D, Gellman H: Complications associated with carpal tunnel release. Orthopedic Review, 1991; 20:346–351.
15. Learmonth J: The principle of decompression in the treatment of certain diseases of peripheral nerves. Surg Clinics North America, 1933; 13:905–913.
16. Louis D: Complications of carpal tunnel surgery. J Neurosurg, 1985; 62:352–356.
17. Lowry W, Follender A: Interfascicular neurolysis in the severe carpal tunnel syndrome: A

prospective, randomized, double-blind, controlled study. Clin Orthop Rel Res, 1988; 227: 251–254.

18. MacDonald R, Lichtman D, Hanlon J, Wilson J: Complications of surgical release for carpal tunnel syndrome. J Hand Surg, 1978; 3A:70–76.

19. Mackinnon S, McCabe S, Murray J, Szalai J, Kelly L, Novak C, Kin B, Burke G: Internal neurolysis fails to improve the results of primary carpal tunnel decompression. J Hand Surg, 1988; 16A:211–218.

20. Pfeffer G, Gelberman R, Boyes J, Rydevik B: The history of carpal tunnel syndrome. J Hand Surg, 1988; 13B:28–34.

21. Phalen G: The carpal tunnel syndrome. J Bone Joint Surg, 1966; 48A:211–228.

22. Rhoades C, Mowrey C, Gelberman R: Results of internal neurolysis of the median nerve for severe carpal tunnel syndrome. J Bone Joint Surg, 1985; 67A:253–256.

23. Shurr DG, Blair WF, Bassett G: Electromyographic changes after carpal tunnel release. J Hand Surg, 1986; 11A:876–880.

24. Silver M, Gelberman R, Gellman H, Rhoades C: Carpal tunnel syndrome: Associated abnormalities in ulnar nerve function and the effect of carpal tunnel release on these abnormalities. J Hand Surg, 1985; 10A:710–763.

25. Szabo R: Carpal Tunnel Syndrome—General. In: Gelberman R (ed): Operative Nerve Repair and Reconstruction. Philadelphia: J.B. Lippincott, 1991:869–888.

26. Taleisnik J: The palmar cutaneous branch of the median nerve and the approach to the carpal tunnel. An anatomical study. J Bone Joint Surg, 1973; 55A:1212–1217.

27. Urbaniak J: Complications of Treatment of Carpal Tunnel Syndrome. In: Gelberman R (ed): Operative Nerve Repair and Reconstruction. Philadelphia: J.B. Lippincott, 1991:967–979.

28. Van Beek A, Heyman P: Electrophysiologic Testing. In: Gelberman R (ed): Operative Nerve Repair and Reconstruction. Philadelphia: J.B. Lippincott, 1991:171–184.

91

Carpal Tunnel Release with the Agee Endoscope

The Agee Carpal Tunnel Release System was developed by John M. Agee, M.D., and Francis C. King in the Hand Biomechanics Lab, Sacramento, CA. Development was based on the hypothesis that a surgical approach combining endoscopic visualization of the transverse carpal ligament (TCL) with a limited incision would decrease postoperative morbidity.

Four prototypes and corresponding surgical techniques were developed using cadaver specimens (Fig. 91–1). Each technique used a single incision placed proximal to the glabrous skin of the palm and heel of the hand to help avoid a tender scar. A commercial device (3M Company, St. Paul, MN) was eventually derived from the January 1987 prototype shown in Figure 91–1. This device has a pistol grip, in which there is an integral trigger mechanism for blade elevation. The blade assembly features a rectangular window near the tip of its flat upper surface (Fig. 91–2). An endoscope permits visualization of the TCL and the point of entry of the blade into the ligament. By holding the viewing window and flat upper surface of the blade assembly snugly against the ligament, the median nerve and flexor tendons are excluded from the path of the blade.

The original commercial version of the Agee endoscope was removed from the market because of a problem with incomplete blade elevation secondary to an engineering problem with the push-rod. In consultation with the surgeons involved with the original clinical trial, a decision was made to remove the device from the market until the blade assembly had been redesigned to allow endoscopic visualization of the point of entry of the blade into the tissue. The device, with its point-of-entry design, was reintroduced into the market in June 1992.

■ HISTORY OF THE TECHNIQUE

The indications and contraindications for endoscopic TCL release have been enumerated by Agee and co-authors[1] and North.[4] Generally, endoscopic release of the TCL is indicated for those patients with idiopathic carpal tunnel syndrome (CTS). The syndrome should not be associated with or secondary to any other known pathology of the carpal tunnel. The technique should not be used for those patients with associated pathology requiring treatment by open surgical exposure.

Patients with severe idiopathic CTS and patients with associated diabetic peripheral neuropathy are not contraindicated for endoscopic TCL release. Some surgeons experienced with single-portal endoscopic carpal tunnel release have expanded their indications to include patients with severe CTS, as evidenced by thenar atrophy and sensory loss. Although not supported by data from a prospective study, their collective impression is that these patients can be treated successfully with endoscopic carpal tunnel release.

Patients with rheumatoid arthritis who have proliferative carpal tunnel synovitis should be treated with open release and synovectomy. Rheumatoid wrist subluxation or erosive disease of the carpal bones evident on carpal tunnel radiographs are additional contraindications. Similarly, CTS secondary to the crystalline deposits of gout requires open surgical debridement of the tophi combined with synovectomy. Additional contraindications include compromise of the digital flexor tendons as evidenced by palpable crepitation with finger motion, prior flexor tendon rupture, and prior carpal tunnel surgery. However, patients requiring tendon transfer to restore thumb opposition may benefit, as the path

■ INDICATIONS AND CONTRAINDICATIONS

■ FIGURE 91–1
Prototypes of the Agee
Carpal Tunnel Release
System. (Courtesy of
Hand Biomechanics Lab,
Inc., Sacramento, CA.)

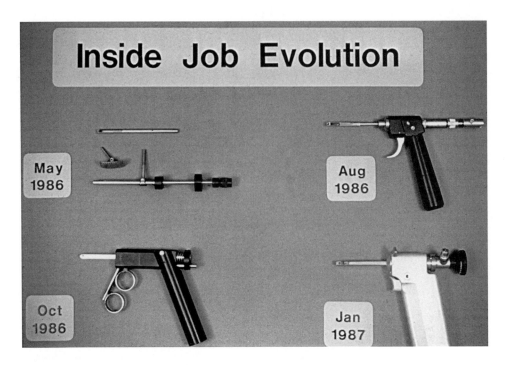

■ FIGURE 91–2
Blade assembly for the
Agee Carpal Tunnel Re-
lease System. (Courtesy
of 3M Surgical Products
Division, St. Paul, MN.)

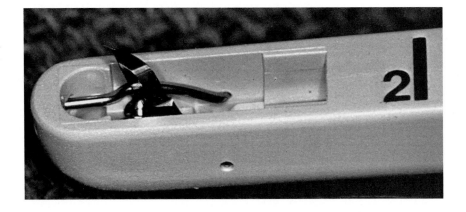

of the transferred tendon is not scarred by the incision of a traditional open carpal tunnel release.

All candidates for endoscopic release require preoperative wrist and carpal tunnel radiographs to rule out bony abnormalities of the carpal tunnel. Fracture, nonunion and congenital anomaly of the hook of the hamate are absolute contraindications. Fractures of the hook of the hamate may abrade or rupture the flexor tendons to the ulnar fingers and therefore require open surgical assessment and repair. More detailed knowledge of anatomical abnormalities associated with congenital anomalies is necessary before endoscopic TCL release can be recommended.

No data are available on the use of the endoscopic device for acute CTS, such as that occurring secondary to fractures of the distal radius. I have no experience using the device for CTS associated with acute fractures of the distal radius, and I am unaware of its use for that purpose. Carpal tunnel syndrome associated with a significant post-Colles' deformity of the distal radius has been treated successfully with this endoscopic technique. There also have been a few cases of CTS in patients with traumatic degenerative arthritis of the wrist that have been treated with this technique. Each surgeon's understanding of the etiology of CTS caused or aggravated by conditions such a malunited Colles' fracture or traumatic arthritis of the wrist should guide the treatment plan. These and other applications of carpal tunnel release should remain the responsibility of the surgeon if he chooses to use it for conditions other than idiopathic CTS for which no data base currently exists.

General or regional anesthesia is strongly recommended. After the surgeon has gained experience with the surgical technique with patients under general or regional anesthesia, the procedure can be performed using local anesthesia infiltrated at the site of the skin incision. Local anesthesia is used in conjunction with sedation as approximately 50% of the patients have significant pain during insertion of the blade assembly into the carpal tunnel or during incision of the TCL.

The surgeon should obtain hands-on training using fresh cadaver specimens and, when possible, perform endoscopic TCL releases with an experienced surgeon in attendance.

The endoscope, video camera, monitor, and light source should be checked, including white balance and focus, before the patient is given anesthesia. The ideal light intensity produces a texture or contour lighting of the collagen bundles in the ligament. Excessive light "bleeds" the detail from the video image. The arrangement of equipment in the surgical suite should offer the surgeon a view such that his gaze can easily shift from the patient's hand to the video monitor. Ambidextrous surgeons using the pistol grip device generally sit on the axillary side of the extremity when performing a left or right TCL release. Surgeons who prefer their right hand for the pistol grip sit on the axillary side for a right TCL release and on the cephalic side for a left TCL release. The surgeon and the patient must be prepared to abandon the endoscopic approach in favor of a conventional open carpal tunnel release if the normal anatomy of a TCL cannot be visualized clearly.

An alternate technique is to block the median nerve in the forearm just proximal to the ulnar bursa. Care should be taken to avoid injecting local anesthesia into this bursa as it will extend into the carpal tunnel and leak onto the lens of the endoscope and obscure visualization.

Key anatomic structures are diagrammed on the skin with a pen. These structures include the flexor carpi radialis and ulnaris tendons, the pisiform bone, and the hook of the hamate (Fig. 91–3). The skin incision is placed in a wrist flexion crease extending from the adjacent borders of the flexor carpi radialis and ulnaris tendons. With the patient's wrist slightly flexed, choose a wrist crease that separates the glabrous palmar skin from the "mobile" skin of the forearm. When choosing between two or more creases, use of the more proximal crease may be easier technically because of thinner subcutaneous fat.

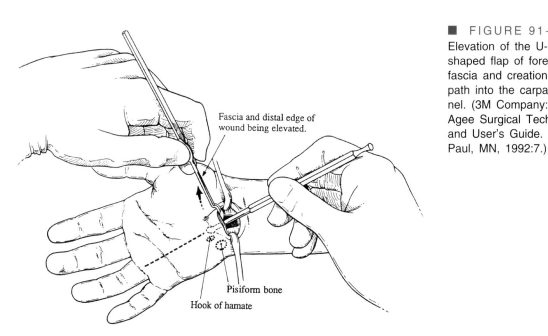

■ FIGURE 91–3
Elevation of the U-shaped flap of forearm fascia and creation of a path into the carpal tunnel. (3M Company: The Agee Surgical Technique and User's Guide. St. Paul, MN, 1992:7.)

Generally, the more distal incision is cosmetically superior. Mark the transverse skin incision and then draw a construction line from the middle of the proposed incision, which is halfway between the two wrist flexor tendons, to the palmar base of the ring finger. This line should pass just radial to the hook of the hamate.

The goal is to define endoscopically and to instrument a surgical plane extending from proximal to distal between the deep side of the TCL and the synovium surrounding the digital flexor tendons. If the surgeon is unable to identify an ulnar strip of TCL with a definite distal margin, which is characterized by a transition from ligament to fat, the procedure should be converted to a conventional open TCL release.

After exsanguination and under tourniquet control, make a 2- to 3-cm transverse skin incision between the flexor carpi radialis and ulnaris tendons, stopping short of the subcutaneous tissues and their cutaneous nerves. Use a spreading, longitudinal (blunt) dissection to protect the nerves and expose the forearm fascia. Create a U-shaped flap based distally on the TCL (Fig. 91–3). The median nerve is directly under the fascia at this level and care must be taken to protect it.

The forearm fascia is split proximal to the skin incision. Left undivided, the distal edge of this fascia forms a fulcrum that may angulate the nerve causing persistent or recurrent symptoms of median nerve compression. Bluntly dissect the soft tissues from the deep and superficial surfaces of the deep fascia proximal to the incision. Elevate the skin and subcutaneous tissue with a blunt right angle retractor. Under direct vision and using scissors, divide the deep fascia proximally for 3 to 5 cm.

Use a double skin hook to elevate the previously prepared distally based flap, then carefully dissect the synovium from the deep side of the flap creating a plane between the synovium and deep side of the TCL. With the wrist in slight extension, the synovium elevator, which is a probe with a miniature "spoon" tip, is used to complete separation of the ulnar bursa from the overlying ligament (Fig. 91–3). Separation of the bursa is complete when the tip of the elevator is palpable at the distal end of the carpal tunnel. Do not scrape the elevator side-to-side, as this may free the median nerve to interfere with the instrumentation.

The hamate finder, a thin, banana-shaped probe, is gently passed distally around the hook of the hamate until its curved tip can be palpated subcutaneously as it exits the distal tunnel (Fig. 91–4).

With the patient's wrist in slight extension, the blade assembly is passed down the ulnar

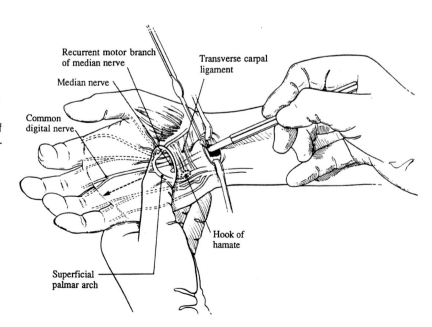

■ FIGURE 91–4
Preparation of a path for the blade assembly. Notice that the probe exits the distal carpal tunnel in a triangular area bordered by the ulnar half of the transverse carpal ligament, the superficial palmar arterial arch and the ulnar border of the median nerve. (3M Company: The Agee Surgical Technique and User's Guide. St. Paul, 1992:8; by permission.)

Recurrent motor branch of median nerve

Median nerve

Transverse carpal ligament

Common digital nerve

Hook of hamate

Superficial palmar arch

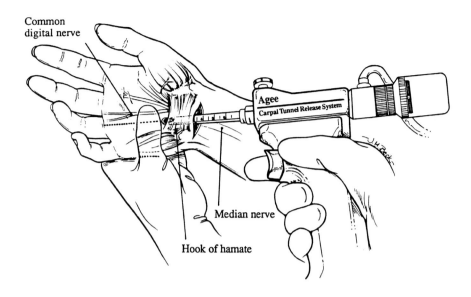

Common
digital nerve

Median nerve

Hook of hamate

■ FIGURE 91–5
Introduction of the blade
assembly into the carpal
tunnel. (3M Company:
The Agee Surgical Tech-
nique and User's Guide.
St. Paul, MN, 1992:9.)

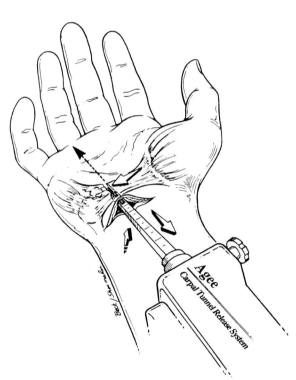

■ FIGURE 91–6
Steps to incise the transverse carpal ligament. 1,
aim at the ring finger; 2,
hug the hook of the ha-
mate; 3, apply upward
pressure on the blade as-
sembly to keep the win-
dow snug against the
transverse carpal liga-
ment; and 4, elevate the
blade and withdraw the
instrument. (3M Com-
pany: The Agee Surgical
Technique and User's
Guide. St. Paul, MN,
1992:12.)

side of the carpal tunnel while aiming at the ring finger (Fig. 91–5). The viewing window
of the blade assembly is pressed snugly against the deep side of the ligament. Proximal-
to-distal passes are used to view endoscopically and define a strip of TCL aligned with
the ring finger and adjacent to the hook of the hamate. In the central third of the tunnel,
palpation of the overlying tissues demonstrates the stability of the TCL as it receives a
firm, bony anchor from each "pillar" of the carpal tunnel; i.e., attachment to the scaphoid
and trapezium on the radial side and the pisiform and hook of the hamate on the ulnar
side. Distally, the ligament can be defined at its junction with the pad of fat by using the
opposite thumb to palpate the overlying soft tissues.

With endoscopic control, the blade is elevated to penetrate the distal ligament at its
junction with the fat pad. A final position check (Fig. 91–6) confirms alignment with the

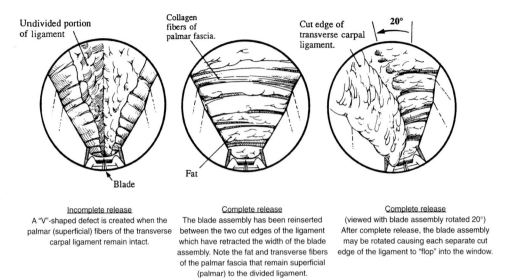

Incomplete release
A "V"-shaped defect is created when the palmar (superficial) fibers of the transverse carpal ligament remain intact.

Complete release
The blade assembly has been reinserted between the two cut edges of the ligament which have retracted the width of the blade assembly. Note the fat and transverse fibers of the palmar fascia that remain superficial (palmar) to the divided ligament.

Complete release
(viewed with blade assembly rotated 20°)
After complete release, the blade assembly may be rotated causing each separate cut edge of the ligament to "flop" into the window.

ring finger axis, an ulnar course hugging the hook of the hamate and snug apposition of the window against the TCL. The ligament is incised as the device is firmly but gently withdrawn.

With the blade retracted, the assembly is reinserted to inspect for completeness of ligament division. With incomplete division, a V-shaped defect is created with the palmar or superficial fibers of the ligament remaining intact (Fig. 91–7). Additional cuts are made with the window snugly applied to the ligament to avoid injury to the median nerve. With complete release, the two halves of the ligament retract, producing a trapezoidal defect capable of accepting the 5.6-mm width of the assembly (Fig. 91–7). Fat and transverse fibers of palmar fascia are visualized superficial to the transected ligament. Palpation of the overlying skin demonstrates the mobility of the soft tissues that are preserved superficial to the ligament. Completeness of ligament division is additionally assessed by palpating the more superficial course of the blade assembly, by feeling the reduced pressure inside the carpal tunnel as the blade assembly is reinserted and by direct vision using small right angle retractors.

With the endoscope repositioned at the distal end of the carpal tunnel, the tourniquet is deflated and the device is slowly withdrawn while inspecting for potentially troublesome bleeders. I prefer to use an intracuticular stitch with 4-0 or 5-0 monofilament steel and Steri-Strip reinforcement. By placing the incision in a wrist flexor crease between the glabrous skin on the heel of the hand and the mobile skin of the distal forearm, the scar matures to become essentially invisible.

■ TECHNICAL
ALTERNATIVES

Alternatives to the single-portal endoscopic technique described include two-portal endoscopic techniques,[2,7] the universal subcutaneous endoscope system,[5] and conventional open surgery techniques.[3,6]

To avoid potential complications, the surgeon must have in mind a complete three-dimensional picture of the anatomy and a clear concept of the path of the blade assembly. Preoperative planning should involve the operating room nurses and the anesthetist to discuss the optimal positioning of the patient with respect to the surgeon's control of the operative hand and his view of the video monitor. The surgeon should be able to hold his patient's hand comfortably while moving his gaze easily from the hand to the video monitor as needed. Endoscopic release of the carpal tunnel requires accurate visualization and incision of the TCL collagen bundles. "If you can't see, don't cut," is an appropriate motto to protect the patient.

Surgeons gaining experience with the procedure may benefit from my observation that patients with thin subcutaneous fat on the palmar side of the distal forearm are ideal candidates for the endoscopic procedure from a technical point of view.

The postoperative course of endoscopic TCL release patients is notable for its absence of complaints. Five years ago, I treated patients with 3 weeks of postoperative splinting with the wrist in extension and the thumb in opposition. That course of treatment has been modified and patients are now seldom splinted postoperatively. Each patient is instructed to avoid grasping with the wrist in a flexed position as this forces the digital flexor tendons into the cut edge of the ligament. Although patients are advised to avoid forceful gripping and lifting until soft tissue healing is complete in 6 to 8 weeks, the relative absence of pain and tenderness correlates with an earlier return to activities than the surgeon might expect. Patients do not require hand therapy.

■ REHABILITATION

In my practice, all patients are educated about the positive benefits of early return to gainful employment. Patients, including those compensated for being off work, can easily appreciate the gains in postoperative morbidity achieved by reducing operative trauma. I have observed that patients treated with endoscopic CTL release generally return to gainful employment sooner after surgery than patients treated with an open procedure. This observation supports data demonstrating that less postoperative loss of grip and pinch strength and less wound tenderness in the endoscopic patients are directly related to earlier return to work.[1] I am aware that many of the issues defining return to work will continue to be related to factors other than the surgical approach to a given patient.

In a prospective randomized multicenter study that compared open and endoscopic TCL releases, Agee and co-authors[1] reported statistically significant preservation of grip and pinch strength favoring the endoscopic approach during the first 3 postoperative weeks. Patients with endoscopic release returned to gainful employment sooner than those with open release (median time, 25.5 versus 46.5 days); when patients who received workmen's compensation were removed from the comparison groups, the group of patients treated by endoscopic TCL release returned to work 29 days sooner than the group treated with open TCL release (median time, 16.5 versus 45.5 days).

■ OUTCOMES

North and Green (personal communication) reported a 0.4% nerve injury rate and 0.12% vascular injury rate from TCL release by the "Agee" endoscope, based on a 350-surgeon survey of 2447 procedures. The original blade has been redesigned, and the new point-of-entry device allows direct visualization of the blade as the tissue is being transected. A customer acceptance trial of 1049 procedures performed in 63 centers in the United States, Canada, and Europe was performed with the newly designed device (3M Surgical Products Division, St. Paul, MN). In this trial, there were no confirmed device related complications involving transected nerves or arteries.

Endoscopic carpal tunnel release is a natural extension of less invasive surgery characterized by knee and other large joint arthroscopy. More recently, endoscopic abdominal procedures have altered traditional approaches to general and gynecological surgery. By leaving the overlying skin, subcutaneous fat, palmar fascia, and palmaris muscle intact, patients have been shown to return earlier to activities of daily living and gainful employment.[1]

References

1. Agee JM, McCarroll HR, Tortosa RD, Berry DA, Szabo RM, Peimer CA:Endoscopic release of the carpal tunnel: A randomized prospective multicenter study. J Hand Surg, 1992; 17A: 987–995.
2. Chow JCY: Endoscopic release of the carpal ligament: A new technique for carpal tunnel syndrome. Arthroscopy, 1989; 5:19–24.
3. Learmonth J: The principle of decompression in the treatment of certain diseases of peripheral nerves. Surg Clin North Am, 1993; 13:905–913.
4. North ER: Endoscopic carpal tunnel release. In: Gelberman RH (ed): Operative Nerve Repair and Reconstruction, Philadelphia: JB Lippincott Co, 1990:913–920.

5. Okutsu I, Ninomiya S, Takatori Y, Ugawa Y: Endoscopic management of carpal tunnel syndrome. Arthroscopy, 1989; 5:11–18.
6. Phalen G, Gardner W, LaLonde A. Neuropathy of the median nerve due to compression beneath the transverse carpal ligament. J Bone Joint Surg, 1950; 32A:109–112.
7. Resnick CT, Miller BW: Endoscopic carpal tunnel release using the subligamentous two-portal technique. Contemp Orthop, 1991; 22:269–277.

92

Carpal Tunnel Release with the Chow Endoscope

For the past decade, arthroscopy has become one of the most rapidly developing techniques in orthopaedic surgery. Despite the controversies that surrounded its introduction 20 years ago, surgical techniques such as the arthroscopic partial meniscectomy have now successfully replaced the conventional arthrotomy and total meniscectomy.

By using the minimally invasive concept of arthroscopy and current arthroscopic equipment advancements, I began to develop a technique in which the carpal ligament may be released for carpal tunnel syndrome without the large characteristic incision of the standard open procedure. The goals of this technique were to preserve the vital structures above the carpal ligament, decrease the postoperative pain and scarring, and minimize the loss of pinch and grip strength. By making the cut from inside the carpal canal, the carpal ligament is the first layer incised; therefore, the muscle fibers, superficial palmar fascia, vessels, and numerous variations of nerves and their cutaneous branches above the carpal ligament are preserved.

■ HISTORY OF THE TECHNIQUE

I believe all surgeons will agree that not all patients with carpal tunnel syndrome require surgery. Only the patients with long duration of symptoms, usually longer than 6 months, who fail to respond to conservative treatment will be considered for surgery. These patients usually have classic carpal tunnel syndrome, especially nocturnal symptoms: sensations of tingling and numbness in the long fingers, weakness in grip, a propensity to drop things, and occasional pain referred to the elbow and shoulder.[13–18] In my patients, results of a nerve conduction test (NCV) were positive in 91%. When the motor or sensory distal latency is more than 7.0 msec, there is definitely a strong indication for surgery. Obviously, the patient should be carefully examined to exclude the possibility of pronator teres compression syndrome, thoracic outlet syndrome, or cervical disc. Conservative treatment should include splinting, anti-inflammatory drugs, physical therapy, rest, alternative employment, etc.

The endoscopic procedure for the release of the carpal ligament for carpal tunnel syndrome is designed to release only the carpal ligament. It does not make it possible to examine the entire carpal canal; therefore, it is possible to miss a space occupying lesion. Fortunately, the occurrence of this has been rather low. Obviously, the endoscopic technique is not designed for neurolysis, tenosynovectomy, Z-plasty, or repair of the carpal ligament. If the surgeon believes that the patient will require an extensive neurolysis or tenosynovectomy, or suspects that there is a space occupying lesion in the carpal canal, endoscopic surgery should not be the procedure of choice. It also is not possible to release the Guyon's canal at the same time, as some surgeons prefer. An additional contraindication for using the Chow technique is that if full extension of the patient's wrist and fingers is limited, the chance of damaging the superficial palmar arch or distal structures is increased, and this procedure should not be done.[6–11,19,20]

■ INDICATIONS AND CONTRAINDICATIONS

Standard hand instrumentation is required. The routine set-up for arthroscopy, including the camera, video monitor, and a light source, is required. To perform the procedure, a special ECTRA System from Dyonics (Andover, MD) also is required. This system consists of a short 4-mm, 30° video endoscope with the lightpost on the same side of the

■ SURGICAL TECHNIQUES

direction of view, a slotted cannula, a ridged conical obturator, a curved blunt dissector, and a hand holder, probe, and straps. An ECTRA™ disposable kit of specially designed knives also is required. This consists of a probe knife, which can be used for forward cutting and as a probe/retractor because it is blunt on the top and back; a triangular knife, designed for making the incision in the center of the ligament; a retrograde knife, designed with the cutting edge on the axillary or center of the hook; a hand pad and swabs. With the input and assistance of a multicenter study group, a second generation of instrumentation has been under development. This instrumentation includes a removable handle to which numerous obturator tips can be attached. Depending on the surgeon's preference, a different tip can be attached and inserted with the slotted cannula. Currently, I use a curved, blunt, dissector/obturator combined as a single unit with the slotted cannula assembly. This enters the carpal canal a lot easier and decreases the chance of the slotted cannula/obturator being inserted above the carpal ligament.

A hand table is used for this operation. The surgeon and the assistant sit facing each other. Two television monitors are recommended so that both the surgeon and the assistant have a clear view of the procedure. A deflated pneumotourniquet is placed on the upper arm. The tourniquet is only used when there is uncontrolled venous bleeding.

In my first 100 cases, either a regional or general anesthetic was used. Since then it has been discovered that the procedure is tolerated fairly well with a local anesthetic. Up to now (1995), more than 1400 cases have been performed using a local anesthetic. The local anesthetic consists of 1% xylocaine without epinephrine, along with a general intravenous sedation of 1 to 2 mg of Versed (midazolam hydrochloride) and 200 μg of Alfenta (alfentanil hydrochloride), which is given to the patient just before the skin incision. If needed, an additional 100 μg of Alfenta may be given.

The location of the skin incision for the entry portal is determined in a standard manner. Using the proximal pole of the pisiform bone as a landmark and depending on the size

■ FIGURE 92–1
The entry portal is made using the proximal pole of the pisiform bone as a landmark and drawing a line approximately 1 to 1.5 cm radially. A second line is drawn 0.5 cm proximally from the end of the first line. The third line is drawn about 1 cm radially from the end of the second line. A small incision of about 1 cm is made for the entry portal.

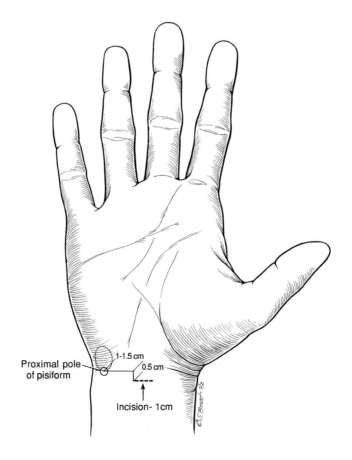

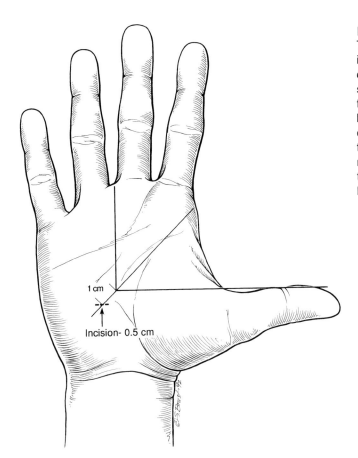

■ FIGURE 92–2
The exit portal is made in the palm surface, 0.5 cm in length, on the bisect line of the angle formed from the distal border of the fully abducted thumb and the third web space approximately 1 cm proximal to the junction of these lines.

1 cm

Incision- 0.5 cm

of the hand, a line is drawn approximately 1 to 1.5 cm radially. A second line is drawn 0.5 cm proximally from the end of the first line. The third line is drawn approximately 1 cm radially from the end of the second line. This represents the small incision, approximately 1 cm in length, for the entry portal (Fig. 92–1).

The opening for the exit portal is made in the palm surface, 0.5 cm in length, on the bisect line of the angle formed from the distal border of the fully abducted thumb and the third web space approximately 1 cm proximal to the junction of these lines (Fig. 92–2).

The entry portal is created first by using a hemostat with blunt dissection to open the subcutaneous tissue. The superficial vein and nerve are pushed away, and the antebrachial fascia is exposed. One should always remember that 18% of the variations of the nerve of Henle pass through this area and any cutting and coagulation should be avoided.[9] A longitudinal cut is then made through the fascia, cutting proximally and distally as far down as possible and using the skin's flexibility to cut down to the proximal edge of the carpal ligament. The distal edge of the entry portal skin incision is gently lifted with the small retractor which creates a small space, which can be seen between the carpal ligament and the ulnar bursa. A curved dissector, with the pointed side facing the carpal ligament, is then used to enter this space and push the ulnar bursa free from the bottom surface of the carpal ligament. The underside of the carpal ligament forms a slight, gently curved shape that can be felt with the curved dissector. When the dissector is maneuvered proximally and distally, a washboard or railroad track effect is felt from the transverse fibers of the carpal ligament. The tightness of the carpal ligament is tested by applying a lifting force to ensure that the dissector is beneath the carpal ligament and has not been inserted above it. Caution is used to be certain that the dissector and the trocar follow the long axis of the forearm.

The slotted cannula assembly is gently inserted into the space between the carpal ligament and the ulnar bursa, passing downward cautiously to avoid insertion above the carpal ligament. When the tip of the slotted cannula assembly touches the hook of hamate, the surgeon uses both hands to lift the patient's hand above the table. This is done by using one hand to hold the patient's fingers and the other hand to hold the slotted cannula assembly. The assistant then places the hand rest under the patient's hand. The patient's wrist and fingers are now gently hyperextended. The slotted cannula assembly is passed down and pointed towards the exit portal. Caution should be taken during the whole maneuver to ensure that the assembly follows the long axis of the forearm.

The second small incision is made in the palm surface. A specially designed depressor is used to push down the superficial palmar arch creating a vertical safety zone, and the trocar is pushed through this exit portal. The hand is stabilized in a special hand holder and the scope is inserted proximally into the cannula. A probe is inserted distally and the carpal ligament can be identified by the fibers that run transversely. If any other tissue (i.e., tendon, nerve) is caught between the trocar and the carpal ligament, the trocar should be removed and reinserted.

With the scope proximal in the tube and the probe distal, the distal edge of the carpal ligament is identified. This distal edge of the of the carpal ligament is a very important landmark; it not only can be seen but it can also be felt with the probe. It is important to remember that all of the important structures (i.e., superficial palmar arch, digital nerve, the sensory branch communication from the ulnar nerve to the median nerve) are located distal to the distal border of the carpal ligament. There might be a small fat pad covering the distal border of the carpal ligament and the probe can be used to dissect the fat pad away so that the distal edge can be identified. A sequence of cuts are then made to release the carpal ligament. The cuts begin by using the probe knife and cutting distally to proximally to release the distal edge of the carpal ligament (Fig. 92–3). By doing so, the important distal structures can be protected. The triangle knife is then inserted to cut through the midsection of the carpal ligament (Fig. 92–4). Next, the retrograde knife is positioned in this second cut and drawn distally to join the first cut (Fig. 92–5). A little "give" will be felt by the surgeon when the third cut enters the first cut. The retrograde knife should not be advanced farther to avoid injury to the important structures that are distal to the carpal ligament. This completes the release of the distal half of the carpal ligament. The scope is then removed from the proximal opening of the tube, inserted into the distal opening, and the instrument is brought in proximally. The uncut proximal section of the ligament is identified and the probe knife is used to release the proximal edge (Fig. 92–6). The retrograde knife is once again inserted into the midsection and drawn proximally to complete the release of the carpal ligament (Fig. 92–7). If any additional cuts are needed, the surgeon may choose the proper knife and proceed until satisfied. Because of the positioning of the slotted cannula, the tube will migrate toward the skin after the completed release of the carpal ligament; therefore, both edges of the cut carpal ligament will begin to disappear from the open slot. If both edges of the carpal ligament are still visible, it would indicate that there are still some additional fibers that needed to be released, and

■ FIGURE 92–3
The first cut is made by using the probe knife and cutting distally to proximally to release the distal edge of the carpal ligament.

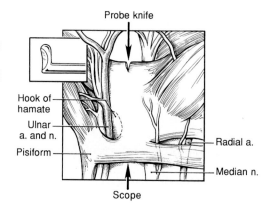

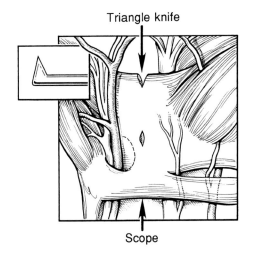

■ FIGURE 92–4
The triangle knife is then inserted to cut through the midsection of the carpal ligament.

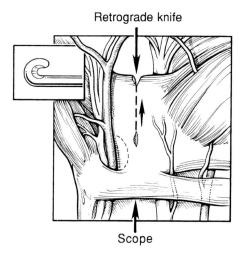

■ FIGURE 92–5
The retrograde knife is positioned in this second cut and drawn distally to join the first cut.

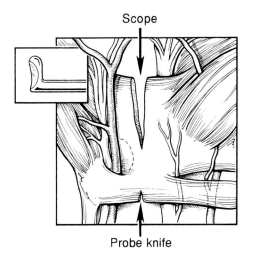

■ FIGURE 92–6
The scope is then removed from the proximal opening of the tube, inserted into the distal opening, and the instrument is brought in proximally. The uncut proximal section of the ligament is identified and the probe knife is used to release the proximal edge.

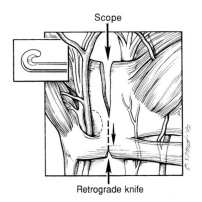

The retrograde knife is once again inserted into the midsection and drawn proximally to complete the release of the carpal ligament.

the surgeon should look for the incompletely released section of the carpal ligament. If the assistant fully abducts the thumb, the ligament will be pulled open and the unreleased fibers should be more visible and accessible. With a triangle knife, under full visualization and control, the surgeon should usually be able to cut one fiber at a time until the ligament is released completely. The trocar is then reinserted and the slotted cannula is removed from the hand.

There is rarely any bleeding and only one suture is required at each portal. A simple dressing is applied and no splint is necessary. Active movement is encouraged immediately after surgery and the sutures are usually removed in 1 week.[5]

■ TECHNICAL ALTERNATIVES

There are several single portal techniques for endoscopic release of the carpal ligament on the market that have been described by several other investigators. It is their opinion that, without the distal palmar portal, there will be no painful palm scar and the danger of injury to the superficial palmar arch, digital nerve, and other important distal structures will be avoided.[1,12] This has not been a problem in my experiences with the dual portal Chow technique. On the contrary, the additional portal allows for the security of using the slotted cannula and locks the instrumentation and tube in certain positions so that there is no chance of deviation or movement in the carpal canal. The additional portal also adds the safety factor of allowing the surgeon to not only see, but to palpate the carpal ligament as well. The surgical procedure and the cutting can be carried out in a more controlled fashion. The additional portal allows the surgery to be performed more easily and decreases the chance of complications or incomplete releases of the carpal ligament.

One of the most common mistakes is placing the entry portal too ulnarly; therefore, before making the skin incision, a three-point checklist is recommended. The first checkpoint is as follows: after using the sterilized marker to mark the entry and exit portals, the surgeon should be able to palpate the pulsations of the ulnar artery. This should be located ulnar to the entry portal. The second checkpoint is that, because of variations in hand size, the surgeon is advised not to use an exact measurement of 1 to 1.5 cm as described above. To measure the entry portal precisely 1 to 1.5 cm radially in a large hand will usually result in an ulnar placement of the entry portal; therefore, the second checkpoint to observe is that in most wrists the entry portal will be located approximately in the center of the total width of the wrist. If the palmaris longus is present, the entry portal should be slightly ulnar of the palmaris longus. The third checkpoint is that a line drawn from the entry to the exit portal should follow the long axis of the forearm. If the entry portal is placed ulnarly, not only is the ulnar neurovascular bundle endangered proximally but there is also danger distally to the superficial palmar arch, digital nerve, and median nerve.

Local anesthesia with intravenous sedation is recommended for this procedure. The advantage of using local anesthesia is that the surgeon can communicate with the patient, which also acts as a safety factor for the procedure if there is a variation of the nerves and vessels. The patient is able to relate to the surgeon any extreme discomfort. In this case, the procedure can either be altered or abandoned to avoid irreversible damage to the important normal structures of the hand.

By using a local anesthesia, after the procedure is complete, the surgeon also can examine the hand for any possible repairs or explorations that would be required. This could then be done under the same sterile setting without having to bring the patient back to surgery for another procedure.

I find that this is a relatively simple procedure if it is done correctly. The surgeon should not feel forced to complete an endoscopic release of the carpal ligament. If there are abnormalities of the muscles and tendons, or if clear identification of normal anatomical structures is not possible, the endoscopic technique should be abandoned and converted to the standard open procedure. In the case of a recurrent carpal tunnel syndrome where the patient has previously undergone a standard open procedure that resulted in a great deal of scar tissue in the wrist area, the original technique will be needed to ensure proper access to the carpal ligament.

This original technique consists of making the entry portal (1 cm in length) approximately 1 cm radially and 1 cm proximally from the proximal pole of the pisiform bone. By using a hemostat with blunt dissection to open the subcutaneous tissue, the superficial vein and nerve are pushed away, and the fascia is exposed. A longitudinal cut is then made through the fascia, cutting distally as far down as possible and using the skin's flexibility to cut down to the thick portion of the proximal edge of the carpal ligament. Using two blunt dissectors to find and retract the flexor tendons toward the radial side, the space between the ulnar neurovascular bundle and the flexor tendons is identified and a special trocar is inserted. By using the tip of the trocar, the surgeon can feel the base of the hook of hamate. Following the body of the hook of hamate, the trocar is lifted up and touches the under surface of the carpal ligament; the patient's fingers and wrist are placed in full extension, and the trocar is gently advanced distally, reaching the subcutaneous tissue of the palm and aiming towards the area of the exit portal. The flexor tendons are slipped out of the way and the trocar is placed beneath the carpal ligament. The second small incision is made in the palm surface as marked for the exit portal. A depressor is used to push down the superficial palmar arch creating a vertical safety zone, and the trocar is pushed through this exit portal. The rest of the procedure remains the same as described above.[2–4,21]

I always emphasize that a blind surgeon is never a good surgeon; therefore, if for any particular reason visualization is poor or if there is a tendon or any other structures appears on top of the slotted cannula and it is difficult to see the undersurface of the carpal ligament, the slotted cannula should either be reinserted or the endoscopic release should be abandoned and converted to the open conventional procedure. Surgeons who are interested in this technique should always remember that there is absolutely no shame in converting the endoscopic release of the carpal ligament to an open standard procedure. The patient should be informed prior to surgery that if, for any reason, the endoscopic release of the carpal ligament cannot be carried out, an open procedure will be performed.

■ REHABILITATION

Physical therapy is seldom necessary. Postoperatively, the patient is encouraged to move the hand, fingers, and wrist as much as possible. Generally, normal use of the hand is accomplished within 1 week. Squeezing a rubber ball or clay is encouraged to build up the strength of the hand. Direct pressure to the palm area and heavy lifting should be avoided for 2 to 3 weeks or until the discomfort disappears.

The majority of patients have been able to regain normal strength much sooner than patients who have had the standard open surgery. Occasionally, there is some swelling and soreness of the palm area when a patient uses the hand extensively or picks up heavy objects too soon after surgery. A course of fluid therapy is helpful to decrease this swelling, using 20-minute sessions daily for 1 to 2 weeks.

■ OUTCOMES

I began to perform this procedure in September 1987. In the first 3 years, 403 wrists, or 279 patients, underwent endoscopic release of the carpal ligament for carpal tunnel syndrome. The results of the study from this 3-year period were presented at the International Arthroscopic Annual Meeting in Toronto 1991. From the report at that time, there were no cases of permanent nerve damage, vascular complications, hematomas, infection, or recurrences. One patient had a temporary loss of interosseous muscle postoperatively, but recovered spontaneously in 4 weeks. After an endoscopic release, one patient went elsewhere to have the standard procedure performed because of persistent numbness at the tip of the index and middle fingers. Postoperatively, the majority of patients had little or no pain and were able to immediately begin active range of motion. Eight patients in the study were lost to follow-up. Of 395 patients, 129 (33%) were able to return to normal activities and work within 1 week after surgery; 229 (58%) of 395 were able to return within 2 weeks; 287 (73%) of 395 were able to return within 3 weeks; and 331 (84%) of 395 were able to return within 4 weeks.

Pinch and grip tests were performed before and after surgery, but because of a wide geographical distance, only 33% of patients were able to return for postoperative testing. Of the 96 patients tested within 24 hours, 4% regained 100% of their pinch and grip strength; 33% regained their normal pinch and grip strength within 1 week; 70% regained normal pinch and grip strength within 2 weeks; and 86% regained normal pinch and grip strength within 3 weeks. In this series, all patients who returned for testing regained normal pinch and grip strength within 5 weeks. Up to July 1995, more than 1400 cases of endoscopic release of the carpal ligament for carpal tunnel syndrome have been performed in Mt. Vernon, IL. The complication rate has been rather low, and the majority of patients are extremely pleased with the results. An analysis of the fourth and fifth years of experiences with this procedure is being done at the present time.

After 5 years of performing this procedure, I personally believe that this procedure can be performed safely and that the significant advantages include decreased postoperative pain, less scar formation, a much faster recovery of the pinch and grip strength than with the standard procedure, and, of course, a faster recovery for the patient.

■ ACKNOWLEDGMENTS   I would like to acknowledge my wife, Ada, and my two children, Jimmy and Jacqueline, for their support and assistance during the preparation for this chapter. I would also like to acknowledge the assistance of my staff members: Linda McLane, Clara Peters, and Conni Schauf, in preparing this chapter.

References

1. Agee JM, McCaroll HR Jr, Tortosa RD, Berry DA, Szabo RM, Peimer CA: Endoscopic release of the carpal tunnel: a randomized prospective multicenter study. J Hand Surg, 1992; 17A: 987–995.
2. Chow JCY: Endoscopic release of the carpal ligament: a new technique for carpal tunnel syndrome. Arthroscopy, 1989; 5:19–24.
3. Chow JCY: Endoscopic release of the carpal ligament: 22-month clinical results. Arthroscopy, 1990; 6:388–396.
4. Chow JCY: Endoscopic release of the carpal ligament: analysis of 300 cases. Presented at the 58th annual meeting of the American Academy of Orthopaedic Surgeons, Anaheim, CA, March 9, 1991.
5. Chow JCY: The Chow technique of endoscopic release of the carpal ligament for carpal tunnel syndrome: four years of clinical results. Arthroscopy, 1993; 9:301–314.
6. Gelberman RH, Pfeffer GB, Galbraith RT, Szabo RM, Rydevik B, Dimick M: Results of treatment of severe carpal tunnel syndrome without internal neurolysis of the median nerve. J Bone Joint Surg, 1987; 69:896–903.
7. Gelberman RJ, Hergenroeder PT, Hargens AR, Lundborg GN, Akeson WH: The carpal tunnel syndrome: a study of carpal canal pressures. J Bone Joint Surg, 1981; 63A:380–383.
8. Kerrigan JJ, Bertoni JM, Jaeger SH: Ganglion cysts and carpal tunnel syndrome. J Hand Surg, 1988; 13A:763–765.
9. Kleinert J: The nerve of Henle. J Hand Surg, 1190; 15A:784–788.
10. Kremchek TE, Kremchek EJ: Carpal tunnel syndrome caused by flexor tendon sheath lipoma. Orthop Rev, 1988; 17:1083.

11. Lowery WE, Follender AB: Interfascicular neurolysis in severe carpal tunnel syndrome: a prospective, randomized, double-blind, controlled study. Clin Orthop Rel Res, 1988; 227: 251–254.
12. Menon J: Endoscopic carpal tunnel release: preliminary report. Arthroscopy, 1994; 10:31–37.
13. Phalen GS: Spontaneous compress of the median nerve at the wrist. JAMA, 1951; 145: 1128–1133.
14. Phalen GS: The carpal tunnel syndrome: seventeen years experience in diagnosis and treatment of 654 hands. J Bone Joint Surg, 1966; 48A:211–228.
15. Phalen GS: The carpal tunnel syndrome: clinical evaluation of 598 hands. Clin Orthop Rel Res, 1972; 83:29–40.
16. Phalen GS, Gardner W, Lalonde A: Neuropathy of the median nerve due to compression beneath the transverse carpal ligament. J Bone Joint Surg, 1950; 32A:109–112.
17. Phalen GS, Kendrick J: Compression neuropathy of the median nerve in the carpal tunnel. JAMA, 1957; 164:523–530.
18. Phalen GS, Kendrick J, Rodriguez J: Lipomas of the upper extremity. Am J Surg, 1971; 121: 298–306.
19. Rhoades CE, Gelberman RH, Szabo RM, Botte M: The results of carpal tunnel release with and without neurolysis of the median nerve for severe carpal tunnel release. J Hand Surg, 1986; 11A:448.
20. Viegas SF, Pollard A, Kaminski K: Carpal arch alteration and related clinical status after endoscopic carpal tunnel release. J Hand Surg, 1992; 17A:1012–1016.
21. Whipple T (ed). Arthroscopy of the Wrist, Philadelphia, J.B. Lippincott, 1992, 157–169.

$\overline{93}$

Guyon's Canal Release

■ HISTORY OF THE
TECHNIQUE

Felix Guyon is given credit for the first description of the contents of the space that now bears his name.[6] Recent descriptions of this area have been made by McFarlane, Mayer, and Hugill,[13] and by Gross and Gelberman.[5] The anatomy as generally agreed upon by the aforementioned authors is depicted in Figure 93–1. The volar carpal ligament which is augmented by radially directed fibers of the flexor carpi ulnaris tendon forms the roof of the canal. The floor of the canal is formed by the transverse carpal ligament, which is confluent with the fibers of the piso-hamate ligament distally. The side walls are formed by the pisiform ulnarly and the hook of the hamate radially and distally. The superficial branch of the ulnar nerve passes through the canal and lies on the bellies of the abductor and the flexor digiti minimi muscles. The deep motor branch of the ulnar nerve passes over the piso-hamate ligament and between the fibrous arch formed by the abductor digiti minimi and the flexor digiti minimi muscles as they arise from the hook of the hamate.

Entrapment of the ulnar nerve at the level of Guyon's canal may be manifested by motor or sensory findings on physical examination, or a combination of both may be seen. Precise physical diagnosis demonstrating aberrant sensation in the ulnar nerve sensory distribution may be seen when there is isolated sensory nerve compression. When the motor branch alone is involved, weakness of the hypothenar muscles, the first dorsal interosseous, and the adduction and abduction functions of the interosseous muscles will be deficient. The combination of deficits will be found when both motor and sensory components of the ulnar nerve at this level are involved. Electroneuromyographic studies will further identify the precise nature of the lesion. Ulnar nerve compression in Guyon's canal may be caused by tumors such as synovial cysts, ganglions, lipomas, and giant cell tumors.[2,12,16] Intercarpal fractures and dislocations may likewise cause compression at this level.[7,19] Fractures of the hook of the hamate may cause coincident trauma to the ulnar nerve and are usually manifest by motor deficiency findings.[13] Aneurysms of the ulnar artery as well as thrombosis of the ulnar artery also may present with findings of ulnar neuropathy at this level.[9] Rarely, anomalous muscles may be associated with ulnar nerve compression.[10,15]

In 1908, Hunt[8] precisely described three patients with isolated entrapment of the motor branch of the ulnar nerve at the wrist. Subsequent reports of surgical decompression of this area have been made by multiple authors. Sir Herbert Seddon[16] was one of the first to describe surgical decompression of this area for four patients where carpal ganglia were responsible for motor paralysis. Brooks,[1] at the same time, reported four cases at the wrist. Neither of these authors, nor later reports by Dupont and co-authors,[3] Kleinert and Hayes,[11] or Shea and McClain[17] furnished a detailed operative exposure. The technique that I use is essentially that used by Gelberman.[4] Exactly who first used the incision is unclear from the literature.

■ INDICATIONS AND
CONTRAINDICATIONS

The major indication for decompression of Guyon's canal is the clinical demonstration of localized compression at this level, whether it be motor or sensory, or both. A major contraindication to decompression at this level is the routine release of the canal as part of carpal tunnel release in the absence of demonstrated nerve dysfunction, coincident with median nerve compression in the carpal tunnel. Carpal tunnel release as demonstrated by Richman and co-authors[14] changes the contour of Guyon's canal from triangular to ovoid, and effectively increases the volume of the space, thus effectively decompressing it. Silver and co-authors[18] also have shown this result after carpal tunnel release.

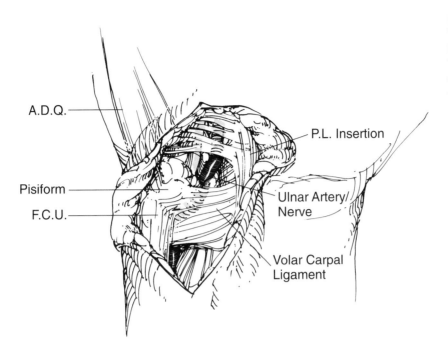

A.D.Q.

P.L. Insertion

Pisiform

F.C.U.

Ulnar Artery/
Nerve

Volar Carpal
Ligament

■ FIGURE 93-1
With the skin flaps mobi-
lized; the underlying
flexor carpi ulnaris tendon
and volar carpal ligament
are exposed.

In general, electrophysiologic documentation is sought before considering surgical decompression. Such corroboration is helpful in confirming the clinical diagnosis. In very
early cases of isolated sensory compression alone, results of these studies may be normal.
Surgical exploration in these circumstances will be based on the experience and confidence
of the surgeon. The presence of a mass, of course, would prompt exploration and biopsy.
Diabetic polyneuropathy or polyneuropathy from any other cause is not a contraindication
to exploration, especially when electrodiagnostic tests show superimposed local involvement. A patient so affected, however, should be advised that all of their symptoms may
not resolve because of the coexistence of a polyneuropathy.

Release of Guyon's canal can be done under local or regional anesthesia. It may be done
with a field block at the wrist. It may be done with an ulnar nerve block at the elbow, or
with intravenous regional or axillary block anesthesia. I prefer to use intravenous regional
anesthesia because it is relatively easy to effect and because it is predictable. Usually the
procedure can be accomplished in less than 1 hour. If it is anticipated that the procedure
will take longer, a method other than intravenous regional anesthesia would probably be
more appropriate.

The incision that is shown in Figure 93–2 is the one that I prefer for release at this level.
The zig-zag nature of the incision allows one to cross the wrist flexion crease obliquely.

It is best to begin the incision proximally and extend it distally. In this fashion, the ulnar
nerve can be identified immediately radial to the flexor carpi ulnaris tendon and it can
be protected through the entirety of the exposure by interposing an instrument such as
a hemostat or a pair of scissors superficial to the incising scalpel.

The incision of the skin and subcutaneous tissues exposes the underlying flexor carpi
ulnaris tendon and volar carpal ligament. The volar carpal ligament is incised, and the
flexor carpi ulnaris tendon is retracted ulnarly while protecting both the artery and the
nerve. When the palmaris brevis muscle is present, it is incised coincident with division
of the ligament. The ulnar nerve ultimately divides into a superficial sensory, or palmar
branch, and a deep motor branch. This division is not always constant and it may occur
at any level throughout the tunnel, but most consistently the division is in the midportion
of the tunnel. The superficial branches course distally on the surface of the hypothenar
muscles and the deep motor branch courses around the hook of the hamate to cross the

■ SURGICAL
TECHNIQUES

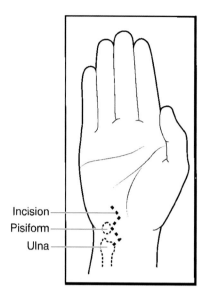

■ FIGURE 93-2
A zig-zag skin incision is used to approach Guyon's canal, to cross the wrist flexion crease obliquely.

Incision —
Pisiform —
Ulna —

■ FIGURE 93-3
Release of the volar carpal ligament exposes the contents of Guyon's canal.

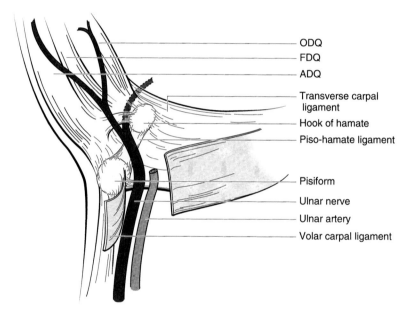

— ODQ
— FDQ
— ADQ
— Transverse carpal ligament
— Hook of hamate
— Piso-hamate ligament
— Pisiform
— Ulnar nerve
— Ulnar artery
— Volar carpal ligament

palm deeply in a radial direction, to ultimately innervate the interosseous muscles, the adductor pollicis and the deep head of the flexor pollicis brevis (Fig. 93–3). The artery remains superficial, also curving in a radial direction, and forms the superficial palmar arch. The piso-hamate ligament is inspected and any unusual findings such as ganglions or tumors may be appropriately dealt with. The proximal fibrous arch of origin of the hypothenar muscles is well developed in 40% of patients (according to Gross and Gelberman[5]). If the motor branch is compressed, then this fibrous arch should be released (Fig. 93–4). The motor branch courses between the hypothenar muscles in the interval between the abductor digiti minimi and the flexor digiti minimi muscles. After entering this interval, the nerve then courses through the opponens digiti minimi and crosses the palm. Careful inspection throughout the tunnel is performed after it has been unroofed. After complete inspection of the tunnel has been performed and appropriate treatment rendered for areas of compression, local anesthetic infiltration of the margins of the incision is performed. The pneumatic tourniquet is released and hemostasis is obtained. The skin only is closed at this point, and a soft dry sterile dressing is applied.

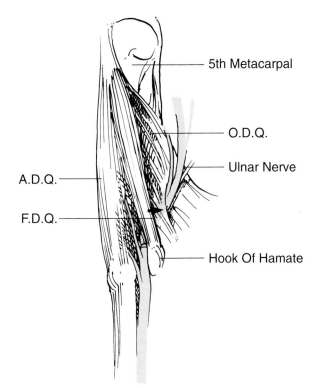

5th Metacarpal

O.D.Q.

Ulnar Nerve

A.D.Q.

F.D.Q.

Hook Of Hamate

■ FIGURE 93–4
If the motor branch is compressed as it enters the hypothenar muscles, the fibrous arch should be released.

This description of the operation to decompress Guyon's canal is fairly standard and straightforward; there are no notable alternatives to this technique. The surgeon should be aware of technical issues which could compromise results. On occasion an incision perpendicular to the wrist flexion crease will lead to a hypertrophic scar or become adherent to underlying structures, and for this reason I prefer to use the zig-zag incision. The nerve anatomy in this area is highly variable and must be approached cautiously. The motor branches to the hypothenar muscles, especially the abductor digiti minimi, may have a proximal origin and may course through Guyon's canal as a separate branch. Each nerve branch must be identified and protected in the course of the exposure and dissection. Also, the vascular anatomy can be quite complex with numerous small veins and arterial branches coursing through the canal. These vessels must be mobilized to allow access to the nerve branches. When cauterization is required, the vessels must be elevated to avoid thermal injury to the ulnar nerve and its branches. Technical modifications of the proposed technique may be required by masses and anomalous muscles in and around Guyon's canal. For ulnar neuropathy in the presence of a nonunion of the hook of the hamate, excision of the hook is the essential aspect of surgical treatment, with or without release of Guyon's canal. This incision may be extended proximally or distally as the need arises. The incision arises distal to the hook of the hamate and extends proximally to the radial side of the pisiform and then crosses the wrist crease obliquely for approximately 3 cm.

■ TECHNICAL ALTERNATIVES

Patients are given the opportunity to open and close their fingers immediately in the recovery room and are encouraged to use their hands for light activities. The sutures are removed after 2 weeks, and the patient is allowed to resume activities as soon as possible. In the absence of postoperative complications, an extensive rehabilitation program is not required for recovery from this surgery.

■ REHABILITATION

The literature is replete with reports of isolated cases of ulnar nerve compression at various levels throughout the canal. These reports suggest that the anticipated result from compression alone, be it motor, sensory, or combined, would be return of function. Unfor-

■ OUTCOMES

tunately, there is insufficient published data derived from large series of cases to give any meaningful interpretations. Gross and Gelberman have summarized the existing literature in their exhaustive review. It is presumed, however, that a compressive neuropathy of the ulnar nerve at Guyon's canal has an excellent chance for complete return of function if the lesion is treated early and all other factors are equal. It should be emphasized that there is no evidence that routine release of Guyon's canal enhances the outcome from conventional carpal tunnel release.

References

1. Brooks DM: Nerve compression by simple ganglia. J Bone Joint Surg, 1952; 34B:391–400.
2. Dell PC: Compression of the ulnar nerve at the wrist secondary to a rheumatoid synovial cyst: case report and review of the literature. J Hand Surg, 1979; 4A:468–473.
3. Dupont C, Cloutier GE, Prevost Y, et al: Ulnar-tunnel syndrome at the wrist. J Bone Joint Surg, 1965; 42A:757–761.
4. Gelberman RH: Ulnar tunnel syndrome. In: Gelberman RH (ed): Operative Nerve Repair and Reconstruction, Vol. II, Philadelphia: J.B. Lippincott, 1991:1131–1143.
5. Gross MS, Gelberman RH: The anatomy of the distal ulnar tunnel. Clin Orthop Rel Res, 1985; 196:238–246.
6. Guyon F: Note sur une disposition anatomique propre a la face anterieure de la region du poignet et non encore decrite par le docteur. Bull Soc Anat Paris, 1861; 6:184–186.
7. Howard FM: Ulnar nerve palsy in wrist fractures. J Bone Joint Surg, 1961; 43A:1197–1201.
8. Hunt JR: Occupational neuritis of the deep palmar branch of the ulnar nerve. J Nerv Ment Dis, 1908; 35:673–689.
9. Jackson JP: Traumatic thrombosis of the ulnar artery in the palm. J Bone Joint Surg, 1954; 36B:438–439.
10. Jeffery AK: Compression of the deep palmar branch of the ulnar nerve by an anomalous muscle. J Bone Joint Surg, 1971; 53B:718–723.
11. Kleinert HE, Hayes JW: Ulnar tunnel syndrome. Plast Reconstr Surg, 1971; 47:21–24.
12. Mackinnon SE, Dellon AL: Ulnar nerve entrapment at the wrist. In: Surgery of the Peripheral Nerves, New York: Thieme, 1988:197–216.
13. McFarlane RM, Mayer JR, Hugill JV: Further observations on the anatomy of the ulnar nerve at the wrist. Hand, 1976; 8:115–117.
14. Richman JA, Gelberman RH, Rydevik BL, et al: Carpal tunnel syndrome: Morphologic changes after release of the transverse carpal ligament. J Hand Surg, 1989; 14A:852–857.
15. Schjelderup H: Aberrant muscle in the hand causing ulnar nerve compression. J Bone Joint Surg, 1964; 46B:361.
16. Seddon HJ: Carpal ganglion as a cause of paralysis of the deep branch of the ulnar nerve. J Bone Joint Surg, 1952; 34B:386–390.
17. Shea JD, McClain EJ: Ulnar nerve compression syndromes at and below the wrist. J Bone Joint Surg, 1969; 51A:1095–1103.
18. Silver MA, Gelberman RH, Gellman H, Rhoades CE: Carpal tunnel syndrome: Associated abnormalities in ulnar nerve function and the effect of carpal tunnel release on these abnormalities. J Hand Surg, 1985; 10A:710–713.
19. Vance RM, Gelberman RH: Acute ulnar neuropathy with fractures at the wrist. J Bone Joint Surg, 1978; 60A:962–965.

94

Cubital Tunnel Release with Subcutaneous Transposition

The first documented report of ulnar nerve compression at the elbow was written by Panas in 1878.[24] Early reports focused on patients with post-traumatic cubitus valgus or osteophytes in the cubital tunnel causing friction and traction neuritis. The term "tardy ulnar nerve palsy" came into common usage given the extended time interval often observed between initial injury and presentation. Early treatment methods included supracondylar osteotomies of the distal humerus to correct cubitus valgus,[22] and deepening of the postcondylar groove.[8]

The first anterior transposition of the ulnar nerve is credited to Roux of Lausanne in 1897.[8] The first documented case of subcutaneous transposition in the United States was in a 28-year-old woman with post-traumatic ulnar nerve palsy, reported by B. F. Curtis in 1898.[7] On surgical exploration, the nerve was found "thickened for a distance of about an inch and a half, and to about twice its normal diameter." There was a "general increase of the fibrous tissue of the nerve. The nerve was split and stretched gently, and then removed from its exposed situation to a more protected part, i. e., to the front of the elbow. The result has been surprisingly satisfactory, so that she has been enabled to resume her long hours of writing without discomfort."

During this century, other surgical treatments have included in situ decompression reported by Osborne,[23] medial epicondylectomy described by King and Morgan,[16] intramuscular transposition and neurolysis introduced by Adson,[2] and submuscular transposition reported by Learmonth.[18]

Feindel and Stratford,[11,12] along with Osborne,[23] changed our conception of ulnar nerve palsy at the elbow to one of a compression neuropathy analagous to carpal tunnel syndrome at the wrist. These authors coined the term "cubital tunnel syndrome" in 1958.

■ HISTORY OF THE TECHNIQUE

Subcutaneous ulnar nerve transposition is the treatment of choice for patients with cubital tunnel syndrome that is unresponsive to conservative care. The syndrome is characterized by symptomatic ulnar nerve compression at the elbow and objective changes in nerve function.

Patients present with pain in the medial elbow or distally in the distribution of the ulnar nerve. Occasionally, the pain may radiate proximally. A combination of numbness, tingling, or coldness in the ring and small fingers, which may be intermittent and activity-related, often is described. Weakness and clumsiness manifested by dropping objects may be associated symptoms.

Objective findings of a mild degree include decreased light touch and vibration sense with a positive elbow flexion test and a positive Tinel's sign at the cubital tunnel. With moderate compression neuropathy abnormal two-point discrimination and measurable decreased grip strength are found. Severe ulnar neuropathy causes visible atrophy in the intrinsics of the hand. Electromyography and nerve conduction velocity studies may help rule out cervical radiculopathy, thoracic outlet syndrome, and compression of the ulnar nerve at Guyon's canal.

Patients who present for the first time with mild to moderate ulnar nerve compression[21] are indicated for a trial of nonoperative treatment. This may include a combination of splinting to avoid acute and repetitive elbow flexion, padding to avoid direct pressure on

■ INDICATIONS AND CONTRAINDICATIONS

the cubital tunnel, and education to change habitual elbow flexion postures at work or during sleep. Patients who have severe ulnar neuropathy are unlikely to gain significant relief from conservative treatment and are therefore considered surgical candidates initially.

Patients who are exposed to work- or sports-related activities that risk trauma to the nerve in a subcutaneous position anterior to the elbow are relatively contraindicated for this procedure. Those with previously failed decompression or transposition also are relatively contraindicated. Submuscular transposition is the recommended treatment for this group based on retrospective review of outcomes.[5,14,19,25] Unfortunately, other than the study by Campbell and co-authors,[6] in which Silastic strips were used to protect the nerve in a subcutaneous position, no studies have explored the efficacy of subcutaneous transposition as a revision procedure. The likelihood of symptomatic improvement after multiple previous procedures is very low; therefore, patients with this medical history are contraindicated for any further surgery.

■ SURGICAL
TECHNIQUES

General anesthesia is commonly used for this procedure, although axillary block may be used in select cases if it allows the surgeon to work from the middle third of the arm distally. As there is only room for one tourniquet above the surgical exposure, Bier block anesthesia is not recommended. The patient is placed in the supine position with the operative extremity abducted in supination on the hand table. A bump under the elbow may aid exposure, and loupe magnification is recommended.

Relevant topographic anatomy includes the medial epicondyle of the distal humerus and the olecranon process. Superficially, one to three variable branches of the medial antebrachial nerve's posterior division may cross the operative field from proximal anterior to distal posterior.[9]

Deep to the investing fascia of the arm at approximately the level of the midshaft of the humerus, the ulnar nerve pierces the medial intramuscular septum to enter the posterior compartment of the arm. It then passes distally between the medial head of the triceps and the medial intramuscular septum. At a level 8 cm proximal to the medial epicondyle, one may notice in a minority of patients the arcade of Struthers, which is thickened fascia and superficial fibers of the medial head of the triceps that covers the ulnar nerve.[3] In the posterior compartment, the nerve may be accompanied by small veins as well as by the superior ulnar collateral branch of the brachial artery, which becomes the posterior recurrent ulnar artery in the region of the cubital tunnel. This tunnel is formed by the postcondylar groove, which is bordered medially by the medial epicondyle and laterally by the olecranon, and by transverse fascial fibers connecting these latter two structures. The ulnar nerve gives off no branches to the arm and few articular branches to the elbow. Distal to the postcondylar groove the nerve courses beneath thickened transverse fascial fibers termed "Osborne's band" bridging the humeral and ulnar heads of the flexor carpi ulnaris (FCU). Significant motor branches to the FCU originate as the nerve courses deep in this muscular interval. For 5 cm distal to the medial epicondyle, one may see a thickened aponeurosis, which serves to augment the origin of the flexor digitorum communis, flexor digitorum superficialis, and flexor carpi ulnaris. This structure may be important in compressive neuropathy.[4] The ulnar nerve then runs down the medial side of the forearm on the flexor digitorum profundus and deep to the flexor carpi ulnaris.

The curvilinear skin incision is made longitudinally 8 cm proximal and 6 cm distal to the medial epicondyle directly over the cubital tunnel (Fig. 94–1). This is done to avoid scar formation directly over bony prominences as well as over the future sight of the nerve anteriorly. With branches of the medial antebrachial cutaneous nerve protected, the anterior flap is raised off of deep fascia 5 cm anterior to the medial epicondyle.

The ulnar nerve is gently dissected free from 8 cm proximal to 6 cm distal to the medial epicondyle. It is usually easily identified just as it enters the cubital tunnel, and this is a convenient location to begin the dissection. A vessel loop is passed around the nerve; it aids in circumferential dissection proximally. Small capsular branches of the nerve will have to be sacrificed. Complete excision of the medial intramuscular septum for 8 cm

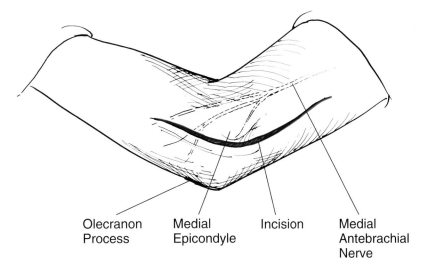

■ FIGURE 94–1
The curvilinear skin incision is made longitudinally between the medial epicondyle and the olecranon.

Olecranon
Process

Medial
Epicondyle

Incision

Medial
Antebrachial
Nerve

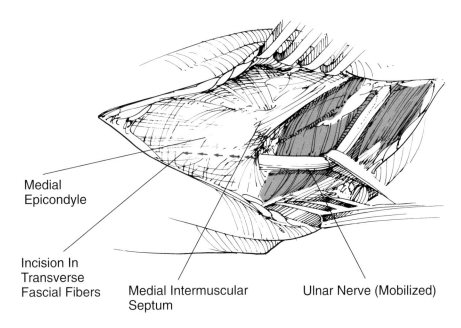

■ FIGURE 94–2
After mobilization of the nerve proximally, the transverse fascial fibers that form the roof of the cubital tunnel are divided.

Medial
Epicondyle

Incision In
Transverse
Fascial Fibers

Medial Intermuscular
Septum

Ulnar Nerve (Mobilized)

proximal to the medial epicondyle is necessary to prevent impingement. The arcade of Struthers, if present, must be released. The nerve must be dissected under direct vision to prevent damage to accompanying vessels, especially proximally where the temptation is to dissect beyond the limits of optimum exposure. The actual point at which the nerve courses from anterior to posterior through the septum will not be seen on this approach.

Distally the nerve is dissected free by incising the transverse fascial fibers that form the roof of the cubital tunnel (Fig. 94–2). Just distal to the cubital tunnel Osborne's band is divided sharply along with the superficial fascia for 6 cm distal to the medial epicondyle. The nerve is exposed by blunt dissection of muscle fibers in the interval between the humeral and ulnar heads of the FCU, taking care to protect motor branches (Fig. 94–3). A constricting flexor-pronator aponeurosis is released if present. External neurolysis is performed in areas of constriction or thickening.

With the elbow flexed ninety degrees, the nerve along with accompanying vessels is transposed 2 to 3 cm anterior to the medial epicondyle to lie directly on fascia (Fig. 94–4). The nerve should assume a gentle curve in its new bed, without kinking proximally or distally from the structures mentioned above. Flexion is maintained during closure of the

■ FIGURE 94–3
Distally, the transverse fibers that form an arch between the two heads of the flexor carpi ulnaris are also divided.

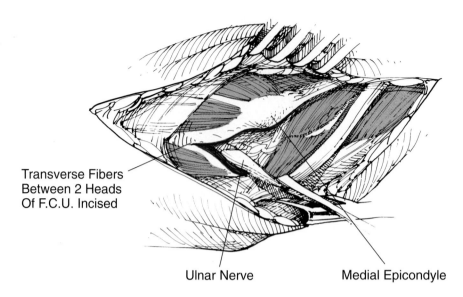

Transverse Fibers
Between 2 Heads
Of F.C.U. Incised

Ulnar Nerve   Medial Epicondyle

■ FIGURE 94–4
With the elbow flexed 90°, the ulnar nerve should rest in its anterior bed without tension or acute bends.

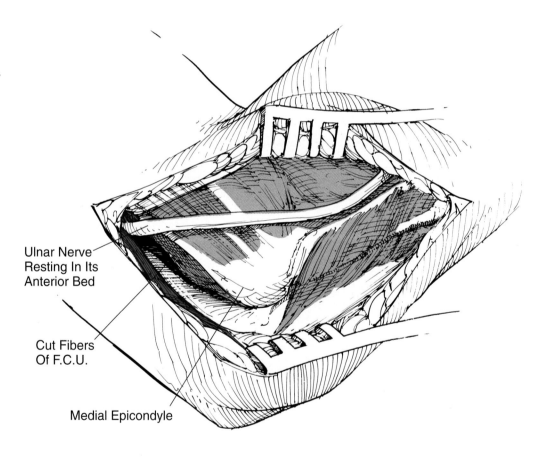

Ulnar Nerve
Resting In Its
Anterior Bed

Cut Fibers
Of F.C.U.

Medial Epicondyle

subcutaneous tissue with absorbable suture and the skin with interrupted nylon. A light bulky dressing is applied and the elbow is splinted in 90° of flexion for 10 to 14 days. This allows early soft tissue healing and helps to prevent return of the nerve to the cubital tunnel.

■ TECHNICAL
ALTERNATIVES

An acceptable alternative to the procedure described above is the addition of a carefully designed fascial sling to prevent posterior displacement of the ulnar nerve, similar to that described by Eaton and co-authors.[10] A strip of antebrachial fascia 2 cm wide and 2 cm long is raised at the medial epicondyle and reflected distal laterally. The fascial sling then passes posterior to the nerve and is sutured to the subcutaneous fat of the previously raised anterior flap. The use of sutures between antebrachial fascia and subcutaneous fat to prevent posterior migration is not advocated, due to the risk of creating a new site of compression.

Pitfalls of the procedure may be avoided by careful surgical technique. Injury to the posterior division of the medial antebrachial cutaneous nerve may result in hypesthesia, painful scar, or hyperalgesia.[9] The findings at reoperation for failed transposition[5,14,19,25] underscore the need for complete release of the arcade of Struthers, the cubital tunnel, Osborne's band over the entrance between the two heads of the flexor carpi ulnaris, and the deep flexor-pronator aponeurosis. The medial intramuscular septum must be completely excised, not just notched for the nerve to pass anteriorly. Symptomatic subluxation in and out of the cubital tunnel may be prevented by operative placement of the nerve far enough anteriorly coupled with adequate postoperative immobilization with the elbow in flexion. The option of a fascial sling may be considered, but this in itself may cause compression.

■ REHABILITATION

An advantage of subcutaneous transposition when compared with submuscular transposition is the earlier postoperative rehabilitation of the former group of patients. The elbow is splinted in 90° of flexion for 2 weeks. Passive motion is begun with early progression to active motion during the first week out of the splint. A goal of full elbow extension is emphasized. Resisted active motion and the use of the extremity in activities of daily living are encouraged during the fourth postoperative week. Most patients return to sedentary jobs during the fourth week or to heavy labor type jobs approximately 6 weeks after surgery.

■ OUTCOMES

Overall improvement may be expected in 70 to 93% of patients.[10,13,15,17,20] Improvement in preoperative pain has been reported in 50 to 100%, numbness in 55 to 90%, weakness in 50 to 83%, and atrophy in only 17 to 43% of patients. In general, patients with minimal involvement have the best prognosis, those with objective weakness and sensation are intermediate, and patients with preoperative atrophy can anticipate less improvement. Duration of symptoms seems important only if compression is severe. A study that compared decompression versus subcutaneous anterior transposition showed the latter procedure was better for improving paresthesias, weakness, and muscle wasting.[13] The one study that included a prospective randomized comparison of in situ release, subcutaneous transposition, and submuscular transposition failed to show a statistically significant advantage of either.[1]

References

1. Adelaar RS, Foster WC, McDowell C: The treatment of cubital tunnel syndrome. J Hand Surg, 1984; 9A:90–95.
2. Adson AL: The surgical treatment of progressive ulnar paralysis. Minn Med, 1918; 1:455.
3. AL-Qattan MM, Murray KA: The arcade of Struthers: an anatomic study. J Hand Surg, 1991; 16B:311.
4. Amadio PC, Beckenbaugh RD: Entrapment of the ulnar nerve by the deep flexor-pronator aponeurosis. J Hand Surg, 1986; 11A:83–87.
5. Broudy AS, Leffert RD, Smith RJ: Technical problems with ulnar nerve transposition at the elbow: findings and results of reoperation. J Hand Surg, 1978; 3:85–89.
6. Campbell JB, Post KD, Morantz RA: A technique for relief of motor and sensory deficits occurring after anterior ulnar transposition. J Neurosurg, 1974; 40:405–409.
7. Curtis BF: Traumatic ulnar neuritis—transplantation of the nerve. J Nerv Ment Dis, 1898; 25:480.
8. Davidson AJ, Horowitz MT: Late or tardy ulnar paralysis. J Bone Joint Surg, 1935; 17:844–856.
9. Dellon AL, Mackinnon SE: Injury to the medial antebrachial cutaneous nerve during cubital tunnel surgery. J Hand Surg, 1985; 10B:33–36.

10. Eaton RG, Crowe JF, Parkes JC III: Anterior transposition of the ulnar nerve using a non-compressing fasciodermal sling. J Bone Joint Surg, 1980; 62A:820–825.
11. Feindel W, Stratford J: Cubital tunnel compression in ulnar nerve palsy. Can Med Assoc J, 1958; 78:351–353.
12. Feindel W, Stratford J: The role of the cubital tunnel in tardy ulnar nerve palsy. Can J Surg, 1958; 1:287–300.
13. Foster RJ, Edshage S: Factors related to the outcome of surgically managed compressive ulnar neuropathy at the elbow level. J Hand Surg, 1981; 6:181–192.
14. Gabel GT, Amadio PC: Reoperations for failed decompression of the ulnar nerve in the region of the elbow. J Bone Joint Surg, 1990; 72A:213–219.
15. Kamhin M, Ganel A, Rosenberg B, Engel J: Anterior transposition of the ulnar nerve. Acta Orthop Scand, 1980; 51:475–478.
16. King T, Morgan FP: Treatment of traumatic ulnar neuritis. Aust NZ J Surg, 1950; 20:33–45.
17. Laha RK, Panchal PD: Surgical treatment of ulnar neuropathy. Surg Neurol, 1979; 11:393–398.
18. Learmouth JR: Technique for transplantation of the ulnar nerve. Surg Gynecol Obstet, 1942; 75:792–793.
19. Lluch AL: Ulnar nerve entrapment after anterior transposition at elbow. New York State Med J, 1975; 1:75–76.
20. Lugnegard H, Waldheim G, Wenberg G: Operative treatment of ulnar neuropathy in the elbow region. Acta Orthop Scand, 1977; 48:168–176.
21. MacKinnon SE, Dellon AC: Ulnar nerve entrapment at the elbow. In: Surgery of the Peripheral Nerve, New York: Thieme, 1988.
22. Mouchet A: Paralysies tardives du nerf cubital a la suite des fractures du condyle externe de l'humerus. J Chir (Paris), 1914; 12:437.
23. Osborne GV: Surgical treatment of tardy ulnar neuritis. J Bone Joint Surg, 1957; 39B:782.
24. Panas J: Sur une cause peu connue de paralysie du nerf cubital. Arch Gen Med, 1878; 2:5.
25. Rogers MR, Berfield TG, Aulicino PL: The failed ulnar nerve transposition, etiology and treatment. Clin Orthop Rel Res, 1991; 269:193–200.

95

Cubital Tunnel Release: Deep Transposition

In the early twentieth century, anterior subcutaneous and intramuscular transpositions of the ulnar nerve already were recognized as appropriate treatments for cubital tunnel syndrome. Submuscular transposition is a relative new treatment, having been first advocated in published form by Learmonth in 1942.[11] Learmonth stated in that article that he developed the technique by happenstance to accommodate a shortened ulnar nerve after neurorrhaphy.

Subsequent to Learmonth's work, submuscular transposition has been used and reported on by a number of authors. The critical anatomy has been better defined[3] with five main areas of potential compression identified: (1) the arcade of Struthers, (2) the medial intermuscular septum, (3) the medial epicondyle, (4) the cubital tunnel, and (5) the deep flexor pronator aponeurosis (Fig. 95–1). This additional detail not withstanding, little technical modification has been made to Learmonth's original description other than an emphasis on adequate distal dissection to ensure a smooth path for the nerve distally.[4,8]

■ HISTORY OF THE TECHNIQUE

Submuscular transposition of the ulnar nerve is theoretically indicated for any ulnar neuropathy at the level of the elbow. Practically speaking, however, it is only one of several options in the primary treatment of ulnar neuropathy in the region of the elbow. Submuscular transposition has greater perioperative morbidity than other options such as cubital tunnel release, subcutaneous transposition, medial epicondylectomy, and intramuscular transposition. Although there is some suggestion in some series that submuscular transposition has a slightly better outcome for primary ulnar nerve decompression at the elbow than some of the other options,[3,9,12–14] others suggest that each of these options provides relatively similar results in the primary treatment of ulnar neuropathy in the region of the elbow.[1] In my opinion, the primary reason for choosing submuscular transposition of the ulnar nerve for the treatment of primary ulnar neuropathy in the region of the elbow is therefore surgeon preference, which must be weighed against the increased cost and perioperative morbidity of this procedure. Typically, submuscular transposition requires an inpatient hospital stay and several months of postoperative rehabilitation to regain strength in the flexor pronator muscles. Most of the other options for treatment of ulnar neuropathy in the region of the elbow involve outpatient surgery and shorter rehabilitation times. Inasmuch as submuscular transposition cannot offer much in the way of advantage, and has some disadvantages in the treatment of primary ulnar neuropathy in the region of the elbow, I am less inclined to use this option in primary cases except in young, vigorous people such as athletes, and in a very thin individual in whom subcutaneous positioning of the ulnar nerve might render it particularly liable for repeat injury, even in an anterior location.

■ INDICATIONS AND CONTRAINDICATIONS

The strongest indication for submuscular transposition is in revision surgery for ulnar neuropathy in the region of the elbow. Submuscular transposition is the only revision procedure that has success rates in excess of 50%[5,7,15]; in fact, for the first or second reoperation, the success rate for submuscular transposition as a revision procedure is almost as great as the success rate for submuscular transposition as a primary procedure. The same cannot be said for any of the other treatment alternatives for ulnar neuropathy in the region of the elbow.

■ FIGURE 95-1
Areas of potential ulnar
nerve compression. (With
permission of Mayo Foun-
dation.)

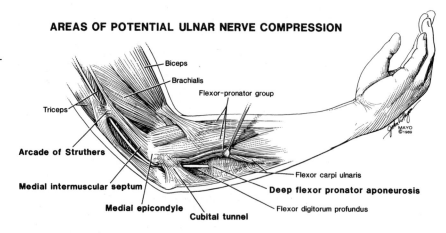

AREAS OF POTENTIAL ULNAR NERVE COMPRESSION

Biceps

Brachialis

Flexor-pronator group

Triceps

Arcade of Struthers

Medial intermuscular septum

Medial epicondyle

Cubital tunnel

Flexor carpi ulnaris

Deep flexor pronator aponeurosis

Flexor digitorum profundus

MAYO ©1989

■ SURGICAL
TECHNIQUES

Contraindications to submuscular transposition certainly exist. At least a relative contra-indication would be the presence of significant arthritic changes in the elbow, as loose bodies, osteophytes, and effusions might well distort the submuscular plane. Another relative contraindication is the multiply reoperated ulnar nerve. After two or three revisions, the likelihood of success from a fourth or fifth operation is extremely low. Finally, of course, it should go without saying that the surgeon must be quite clear that the diagnosis is ulnar neuropathy in the region of the elbow, before performing an operation designed to treat that problem. Well-localized physical findings should be the minimum requirement; an abnormal electromyographic study, if not mandatory, should certainly be an important additional piece of supporting evidence.

Because the operation extends quite proximal to the elbow, regional anesthesia often will be inappropriate. Furthermore, there is some concern, at least in some anesthesiologist's opinions, about the wisdom of blocking a nerve that already is demonstrably abnormal. For this reason, I usually perform submuscular transposition with a general anesthetic and, as mentioned previously, plan on an overnight hospital stay.

The medial epicondyle is the key landmark. The incision is typically extended at least 10 cm proximal and 5 to 6 cm distal to the medial epicondyle, to adequately visualize the arcade of Struthers proximally[2,3] and the deep flexor pronator aponeurosis[3,4] distally. The skin incision is made so that it does not overlie the medial epicondyle, and I prefer a more posterior route, raising a skin flap to get the anterior exposure that is necessary. It is important to look for branches of the medial cutaneous nerve of the arm and medial antebrachial cutaneous nerve of the forearm, which often cross the incision proximally and distally, respectively. These branches should be protected where at all possible. Sometimes that involves working underneath the branches if they cannot be elevated safely away. If, for reasons of surgical exposure, a nerve branch must be sacrificed, it should be trimmed well proximal so that the resulting neuroma does not lay in the suture line at the time of closure.

Once the skin and subcutaneous tissue are elevated, the ulnar nerve is identified just proximal to the medial epicondyle and traced proximally to the level of the arcade of Struthers (Fig. 95-2). The arcade is identified when superficial fascial fibers from the triceps are noted to be crossing to the medial intermuscular septum. The nerve is exposed by incising the fascia over it. The nerve is gently mobilized with its collateral vessels. The nerve can be protected and mobilized with a silicone rubber vessel loop. It is important to incise the arcade of Struthers and always completely excise the medial intermuscular septum (Fig. 95-3). Distally, there are a number of vessels which perforate the septum just above the medial epicondyle. It is important to cauterize these vessels as they are exposed, in order to avoid troublesome bleeding postoperatively.

The ulnar nerve is freed behind the medial epicondyle, through the cubital tunnel reti-

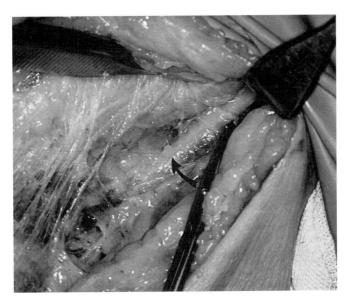

■ FIGURE 95-2
The ulnar nerve (arrow) should be freed well proximal to the medial intermuscular septum; crossing fibers from the triceps fascia to the intermuscular septum mark the arcade of Struthers.

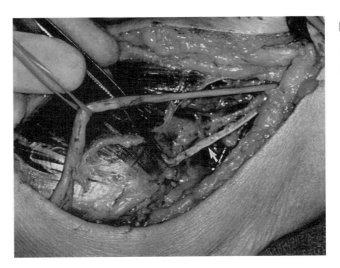

■ FIGURE 95-3
The medial intermuscular septum (arrow) should be excised completely.

naculum and between the two heads of the flexor carpi ulnaris. Care should be taken to identify the motor branches to the two heads of the flexor carpi ulnaris. Typically these are fairly readily seen. Usually the dissection in the flexor carpi ulnaris is done bluntly, and it is usually possible to identify the plane between the two heads of the flexor carpi ulnaris. A vessel loop can then be placed around the ulnar nerve distally so that circumferential dissection can continue around the nerve over the entire length of the dissection. At the most distal end of the incision, it is important to identify and divide the deep flexor pronator aponeurosis, to avoid later compression at that level.

The next step is to elevate the flexor pronator muscle group. This is done by raising the subcutaneous flap anteriorly and incising the fascia overlying the fat pad just proximal to the flexor pronator muscle group. The level of this fat pad varies from individual to individual, depending on how proximal on the humerus the flexor pronator muscle group arises.[6] Usually the median nerve can be readily visualized at the lateral most extent of the incision. Once the flexor pronator muscles are elevated down to the level of the medial epicondyle, an osteotome is used to elevate the flexor pronator muscles with some small flecks of bone. I believe that this may result in a more secure repair later.

Dissection continues distally, elevating the flexor pronator muscles off the ulna. This is not quite so satisfactory a surgical plane as it is proximally; muscle fibers must be carefully dissected from periosteum. Part of the flexor pronator origin includes the medial elbow ligaments. It is important when elevating the fibrous muscle origin distal to the elbow not to inadvertently incise the medial collateral ligaments of the elbow. Typically, there is a palpable ridge of fibrous tissue that binds the flexor pronator muscles to the proximal medial ulna. The more superficial part of this ridge includes muscle insertion fibers; the deep portion is the medial collateral ligament and therefore this ridge must be separated carefully. Two to three millimeters of thickness of the ligament should be left on the ulna. Usually, this is sufficient to preserve the integrity of the medial collateral ligament and yet maintain a smooth course for the transposed ulnar nerve. Dissection and elevation of the flexor pronator muscles continues distally for 5 to 6 cm from the medial epicondyle. Usually by this point the branch of the median nerve that enters the flexor pronator muscles has been encountered and should, of course, be carefully protected.

It is now time to consider submuscular transposition of the ulnar nerve. One benefit of submuscular transposition over subcutaneous transposition is that very little dissection of the nerve's blood supply is usually necessary. The ulnar nerve travels with the ulnar recurrent artery. Usually there are feeding vessels to the ulnar recurrent artery just proximal to the medial epicondyle and occasionally just distal as well. These feeding vessels need to be divided but otherwise the ulnar recurrent artery can usually be transposed with the ulnar nerve into the submuscular location as the nerve is really just being moved a few centimeters laterally. The total distance that the nerve has moved is much less than is usually the case with subcutaneous transposition. Despite this, because the nerve is so close to the axis of motion of the elbow joint in the submuscular position, usually a considerable amount of slack is generated in the nerve. The ulnar nerve should lie smoothly in its new bed, without any kinking (Fig. 95–4). If kinking does occur, it is usually distal, and further dissection of the flexor pronator muscles from the distal ulna is required. Once the ulnar nerve is transposed to the submuscular position, three small drill holes are made in the medial epicondyle. The flexor pronator muscle group can then be reattached with interrupted sutures of No. 2 Mersilene or similar nonabsorbable material. The knots are tied in the postepicondylar groove so that they are not prominent in the subcutaneous tissue. It is easier to reattach the flexor pronator origin with the elbow flexed and the forearm pronated, but after the sutures are tied, it should be possible to extend the elbow without any gapping or separation of the flexor pronator origin from the medial epicondyle. If gapping does occur, the sutures should be redone.

After the flexor pronator origin is reattached, I put gentle traction on the vessel loops proximally and distally around the ulnar nerve (Fig. 95–5). The nerve should easily glide in its new bed. If it does not, again, the cause should be investigated and the nerve freed until easy gliding is possible. The fascia over the flexor carpi ulnaris is not closed at this point. The tourniquet is deflated, and hemostasis is obtained. If dissection has been careful and proper hemostasis achieved during the dissection, the wound will be quite dry. In

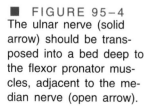

■ FIGURE 95–4
The ulnar nerve (solid arrow) should be transposed into a bed deep to the flexor pronator muscles, adjacent to the median nerve (open arrow).

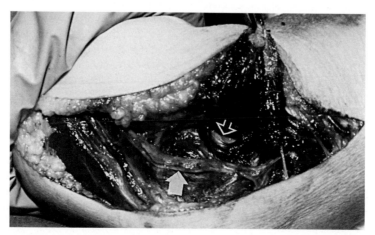

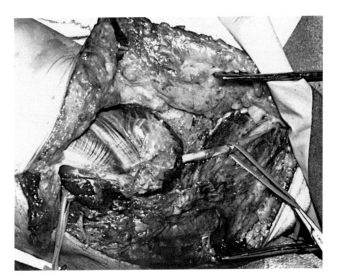

Once the nerve is transposed and the aponeurosis securely reattached, traction proximally and distally should show easy gliding of the nerve without kinking.

that case, the subcutaneous tissue is closed with 4-0 Vicryl sutures, and the skin usually is closed with a running subcuticular suture of 3-0 or 4-0 Prolene reinforced with Steristrips. If there is considerable oozing from the wound, every effort should be made to control it, as it will only contribute to perineural fibrosis. If there is any doubt or question, a suction drain should be left in the wound for 24 hours after surgery.

Once the wound is closed, the arm is immobilized in a posterior splint holding the elbow flexed 90° and the forearm pronated with the wrist in neutral position. This is maintained for 48 hours, after which the dressing is changed. If there is some question about patient cooperation, at this point a long-arm waterproof cast is applied with the elbow and forearm in the same position for 2 to 3 weeks and then range of motion exercises are begun. In a cooperative patient, an orthoplast splint will be fabricated and gentle motion exercises can begin as soon as the patient is comfortable.

The technique of submuscular transposition is relatively standard without any major variations among proponents. Most of the technical alternatives would therefore involve alternative surgical approaches such as cubital tunnel release, medical epicondylectomy, and the like. The only exception to this would be the recommendation by Mass and Silverbert[13] that the medial epicondyle be osteotomized and reattached with screw fixation postoperatively. Although I have no objection to this technique, it does seem technically a bit more complex than the procedure described above and adds at least the theoretical risk of epicondylar nonunion. I do not think that the additional strength of screw fixation over suture fixation is clinically important, as I have not hesitated to begin gentle mobilization exercises with suture fixation often using the technique described above.

The major pitfalls of submuscular transposition relate to three areas. First, cutaneous neuromata may be a problem as described above. Every effort must be made to carefully identify and protect cutaneous nerves. Second, if the flexor pronator muscle group is not elevated completely enough, the nerve could actually be placed in an intramuscular position or may not have enough freedom beneath the flexor pronator mass to glide smoothly. The flexor pronator muscle should be elevated sufficiently enough so that the entire flexor pronator origin can be lifted cleanly from the humerus and ulna exposing the median nerve. Probably the most common problem is distal kinking of the nerve, which is related to inadequate mobilization of the flexor pronator muscle mass from the ulna. It should be possible at the end of the procedure to place the surgeon's finger along side the ulnar nerve in the transposed position after the flexor pronator origin has been reattached to the medial epicondyle; furthermore, the examining finger in this location should not feel tightly compressed either proximally or distally even with the elbow extended and the

■ TECHNICAL ALTERNATIVES

■ FIGURE 95–6
An examining finger
should fit easily adjacent
to the nerve, beneath the
reattached flexor pronator
muscles.

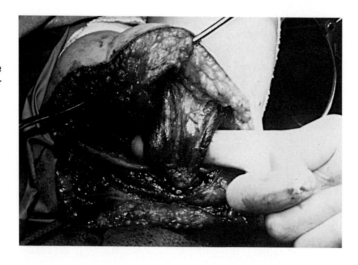

forearm supinated (Fig. 95–6). I have found this "finger test" to be most reliable in assuring that the transposition has been adequately mobilized.

■ REHABILITATION

For the first month after surgery, the patient is instructed in differential forearm, elbow, and wrist exercises to maintain joint mobilization without stressing the flexor pronator origin reattachment.[10] In this program, the elbow is taken through an active flexion-extension range of motion with the forearm held in full pronation and the wrist flexed. With the elbow flexed, the forearm can be taken through pronation and supination exercises and the wrist through a flexion and extension range. Shoulder mobilization should also be encouraged, of course. After approximately 3 weeks, the patient is instructed to begin combined forearm supination and elbow extension; wrist extension is added to this at 6 weeks. The goal is to have full active range of motion at approximately 6 weeks after surgery. The patient needs to be instructed that the performance of these exercises should be pain-free. Passive stretching should not be used, and the patient should use their protective splint when not exercising for the first 3 weeks. After that, the splint may be used on a more symptomatic basis. Once full range of motion is achieved, or when range of motion appears to have plateaued at a satisfactory range, gentle strengthening can begin. Typically, strengthening is started with a 1- to 2-lb lifting limit and gradually progresses over the next 6 weeks with weights that the patient can comfortably tolerate. If the elbow has a significant flexion contracture at 8 weeks, dynamic extension can be added.

Patients whose functional demands are relatively light often can return to restricted duty within a few weeks of surgery. Patients whose occupations include heavy bimanual activities are often unable to return to full unrestricted duty before 3 months postoperatively.

■ OUTCOMES

The reported results of submuscular transposition are generally good. Roughly 90% of patients are subjectively improved with regard to their presenting complaints.[12,14] Pain is most reliably improved, followed by sensibility; motor function is least predictably restored. Flexion contractures occur in a minority of patients and typically average 10° or less.

References

1. Adelaar RS, Foster WC, McDowell C: The treatment of the cubital tunnel syndrome. J Hand Surg, 1984; 9A:90–95.
2. Al-Qattan, Murray KA: The arcade of Struthers: an anatomical study. J Hand Surg, 1991; 16B: 311–314.
3. Amadio PC: Anatomical basis for a technique of ulnar nerve transposition. Surgical-Rad Anatomy, 1986; 8:155–161.

4. Amadio PC, Beckenbaugh RD: Entrapment of the ulnar nerve by the deep flexorpronator aponeurosis. J Hand Surg, 1986; 11A:83–87.
5. Broudy AS, Leffert RD, Smith RJ: Technical problems with ulnar nerve transposition at the elbow: findings and results of reoperation. J Hand Surg, 1978; 3:85–89.
6. Dellon AL: Musculotendinous variations about the medial humeral epicondyle. J Hand Surg, 1986; 11B:175–181.
7. Gabel GT, Amadio PC: Reoperation for failed decompression of the ulnar nerve in the region of the elbow. J Bone Joint Surg, 1990; 72A:213–219.
8. Inserra S, Spinner M: An anatomic factor significant in transposition of the ulnar nerve. J Hand Surg, 1986; 11A:80–82.
9. Janes PC, Mann RJ, Farnworth TK: Submuscular transposition of the ulnar nerve. Clin Orthop Rel Res, 1989; 238:225–232.
10. King PB, Aulicino PL: The postoperative rehabilitation of the Learmonth submuscular transposition of the ulnar nerve at the elbow. J Hand Therapy, 1990; 149–156.
11. Learmonth JR: A technique for transposition of the ulnar nerve. Surg Gynecol Obstet, 1942; 75:792–793.
12. Leffert RD: Anterior submuscular transposition of the ulnar nerves by the Learmonth technique. J Hand Surg, 1982; 7:147–155.
13. Mass DP, Silverberg B: Cubital tunnel syndrome: anterior transposition with epicondylar osteotomy. Orthopedics, 1986; 9:711–715.
14. Posner MA: Submuscular transposition for the ulnar nerve at the elbow. Bull Hosp Joint Dis Orthop Inst 1984; 44:406–423.
15. Rogers MR, Bergfield TG, Aulicino PL: The failed ulnar nerve transposition: etiology and treatment. Clin Orthop Rel Res 1991; 269:193–200.

Radial Tunnel Syndrome: Decompression by a Posterior Lateral Approach

■ HISTORY OF THE
TECHNIQUE

Radial tunnel syndrome is an entrapment, compressive neuropathy of the posterior interosseous branch of the radial nerve at the level of the radial neck. The posterior interosseous nerve (PIN) may be dynamically compressed by the conjoint tendon of origin of the wrist and finger extensors, compressing the nerve between the conjoint tendon and the underlying radial neck. The PIN also may be compressed by specific structures. From proximal to distal, the specific structures include fibrous bands which cross the radial nerve anteriorly and tether the nerve. These bands were initially described by Roles and Maudsley.[13] The second structure is a vascular leash, the fan of Henry, which includes small arteries and adjacent vena comitantes. The third anatomic structure that can compress the PIN is the fibrous edge of the extensor carpi radialis brevis. The next structure, and the most common anatomical structure to compress the PIN, is the fibrous proximal border of the superficial portion of the supinator, the arcade of Frohse. The fifth anatomic structure can be the fibrous edge of the distal portion of the superficial head of the supinator, as described by Sponseller and Engber.[15] The mnemonic FREAS, as recently sited by Gelberman and co-authors,[6] may allow one to remember those sites where the posterior interosseus nerve can be compressed throughout the radial tunnel: F (fibrous bands), R (recurrent radial vessels—the leash of Henry), E (extensor carpi radialis brevis), A (arcade of Frohse), and S (supinator—the distal, sometimes fibrous border).

At any level, the PIN also may be compressed by the presence of a ganglion[1] or lipoma.[11] The PIN can be compressed proximally by marked swelling of the elbow capsule due to rheumatoid synovitis as described by Millender and co-authors.[9] Radial tunnel syndrome may or may not be associated with lateral humeral epicondylitis.

Four operative approaches have been described for surgical management of radial tunnel syndrome. The first is the anterolateral approach. This approach begins in the arm four centimeters proximal to the anterior elbow crease. This incision leads to the interval between the brachialis and brachioradialis where the radial nerve is identified. At the level of the antecubital crease the incision is taken ulnarly and then distally along the radial border of the extensor mobile wad. After the radial nerve is located proximally, the nerve is followed to its division into the sensory and motor branches.

The second described approach is the posterior lateral approach as has been described by Hagert and co-authors.[7] The incision starts at a point just distal to the lateral humeral epicondyle and is taken 6 to 8 cm distally. The dissection plane is between the muscle bellies of the extensor carpi radialis brevis and the extensor digitorum communis. This approach is suggested for problems which exist in the more distal portion of the radial tunnel.

The third approach is the transbrachioradialis approach as described by Lister and co-authors.[8] A longitudinal 6-cm incision is made directly over the brachioradialis muscle in the region of the proximal portion of the radius. The fascia of the brachioradialis is opened longitudinally and dissection is then carried directly through the muscle fibers down to the posterior interosseous nerve. As pointed out by Lister, there are no specific landmarks in this procedure, one merely needs to proceed directly to the nerve. This incision has been fraught with the problems of postoperative keloid formation and Lister has subsequently suggested a transverse incision if possible.

The fourth approach is a more posterior approach also termed a posterior-lateral approach as described by Sanders.[14] The approach begins at the lateral humeral epicondyle and then extends distally to a point midway down the forearm on the mid posterior aspect of the forearm. The skin is elevated away from the underlying fascia and the fascia is incised longitudinally between the finger extensor muscles and the extensor carpi ulnaris muscle. Beneath the finger extensor muscles the superficial portion of the supinator can be visualized. The supinator may then be released from distal to proximal or from proximal to distal. The approach allows for visualization of all five potential compressing structures and visualization of the lateral humeral condyle, the conjoint tendon, fibroblastic proliferation related to a concomitant lateral epicondylitis, and the anconeus muscle. This approach allows one to address both radial tunnel syndrome and lateral humeral epicondylitis and also allows one to cover the area of the inflammation with an anconeus muscle rotation flap if so indicated.

The primary symptom of radial tunnel syndrome is aching pain at the dorsal aspect of the upper forearm. Radial tunnel syndrome can or cannot coexist with lateral humeral epicondylitis (tennis elbow). Radial tunnel syndrome may develop after lateral humeral epicondylitis has been operatively treated.

■ INDICATIONS AND CONTRAINDICATIONS

Lister and co-authors[8] lists three pathognomonic signs for radial tunnel syndrome. The first is tenderness to palpation about the area of the radial neck. This contrasts with lateral humeral epicondylitis where tenderness is present directly over the lateral epicondyle. The second sign is increased pain due to pressure on an actively extended long finger. Pressure on the long finger exerts stress on the ECRB and the edge of the ECRB can compress the radial nerve. The middle finger resistance test was initially described by Roles and Maudsley[13] but the specificity of this test has been questioned by Eversmann.[3] Personally, I have not found the middle finger extension test all that valuable because when the pain is elicited, the pain is reported anywhere from the mid forearm to the lateral humeral epicondyle. As well, tension on the ECRB may stimulate pain due to lateral humeral epicondylitis (tennis elbow). The third sign, as stated by Lister, is pain brought on by resisted supination of the forearm with the elbow fully extended.

Electromyography may help to establish the diagnosis of radial tunnel syndrome. Gelberman and co-authors[6] disagree with the need for electromyography stating that it will show no abnormalities. In my experience, 50 to 60% of patients who have clinically evident radial tunnel syndrome also have abnormal findings with the use of electromyographic evaluation.

As described by Morrey[10] and by Ritts and co-authors,[12] the use of 1 to 2 ml of plain Xylocaine placed near the arcade of Frohse may help to establish the diagnosis of radial tunnel syndrome by relieving the pain and by causing a temporary posterior interosseous paresis. The latter confirms that the posterior interosseous nerve was anesthetized. Morrey considers the relief of pain brought about by the use of Xylocaine as proof positive of an entrapped PIN, and as with Gelberman and co-authors,[6] Morrey does not believe that electromyographic studies are needed for further documentation of the diagnosis. Ritts and co-authors[12] consider the use of Xylocaine, when it does relieve symptoms, as a positive prognostic indicator for surgical release.

The injection of plain Xylocaine is done with a 1.5-inch, 25-gauge needle inserted at the upper third/middle third junction of the posterior forearm in the posterior midline. The location is approximately four finger breadths distal to the lateral humeral epicondyle. The tip of the needle is directed toward the anterior aspect of the radial neck, hence toward the arcade of Frohse. After the needle has been fully inserted, the Xylocaine is infiltrated near the PIN. No complications have been encountered using this injection technique and a temporary posterior interosseous paresis develops signifying that the PIN was blocked. The paresis resolves within 2 to 3 hours. The relief of pain brought about by the injection is extremely encouraging to the patient and is indicative of the pain relief that can be expected after surgical decompression.

When only a radial tunnel syndrome is present, the injection brings about a resolution of all pain. One also may separate radial tunnel syndrome from lateral humeral epicondylitis by doing differential blocks. If the above-mentioned block is ineffective, the patient may be asked to return in several days for a block directly over the lateral humeral epicondyle. If the injection of the Xylocaine directly over the lateral humeral epicondyle, as suggested by Eversmann,[3] relieves pain, then one may conclude that the cause of the pain is lateral epicondylitis and not radial tunnel syndrome.

Radial tunnel syndrome may be managed nonoperatively with the use of an orthosis, which keeps the wrist in extension. Stretching exercises for the structures about the elbow also are helpful. The conjoint tendon may be stretched by having the patient actively flex his wrist while the forearm is fully pronated and the elbow is fully extended. If these types of treatment prove to be ineffective, operative treatment should be considered.

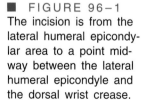

■ SURGICAL
TECHNIQUES

The patient is placed in the supine position with the upper extremity on an armboard or on a hand operating table. A pneumatic tourniquet is placed as high on the arm as possible. A general or plexus block anesthetic is provided. The procedure frequently takes too long for the use of an intravenous regional block anesthetic. Once the upper extremity is scrubbed and draped, the limb is elevated and exsanguinated with a Martin bandage or an Ace wrap.

The posterior-lateral approach extends from the lateral humeral epicondyle to a point midway between the lateral epicondyle and the dorsal wrist crease. The incision is a straight line on the mid-posterior surface of the forearm (Fig. 96–1). The incision needs to be extended to the mid forearm to release all of the superficial head of the supinator to release the potential fibrous band, which can be present at the distal border of the superficial head of the supinator.

The subcutaneous tissue is elevated away from the underlying posterior enveloping fascia of the forearm. Exposure is aided by the use of a pair of Gelpey retractors, which keep the subcutaneous and dermal tissues to the side.

Inspection of the enveloping fascia will reveal four underlying "envelopes" of muscle. The most anterior lying "envelope" contains the brachioradialis and the two radial wrist extensor muscles; the second "envelope" contains the extensor digitorum communis (EDC) and the extensor digiti minimi quinti (EDMQ); the third "envelope" contains the extensor carpi ulnaris (ECU); and the fourth envelope, which is noted only near the elbow, contains only the anconeus muscle.

The correct fascial incision is between the EDC/EDMQ and the ECU (Fig. 96–2). There is a septum between these two compartments and that septum is contiguous proximally with the radial collateral ligament of the elbow. Hence, one should stay just anterior to the septum to avoid injury to the radial collateral ligament.

■ FIGURE 96–1
The incision is from the lateral humeral epicondylar area to a point midway between the lateral humeral epicondyle and the dorsal wrist crease.

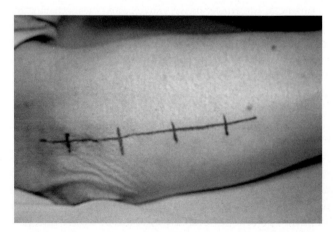

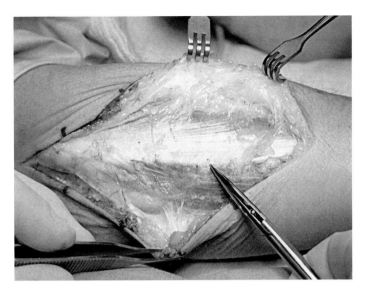

■ FIGURE 96-2
The underlying enveloping fascia of the forearm is visualized and an incision is made between the underlying finger extensor muscles and the extensor carpi ulnaris muscle.

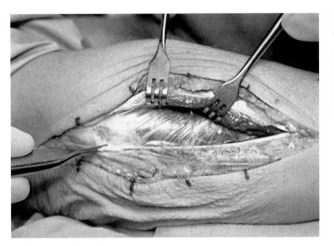

■ FIGURE 96-3
The supinator is found deep to the finger extensor muscles and the superficial portion of the supinator is slit longitudinally.

A helpful sign for the location of the correct interval between the EDC/EDMQ and the ECU is the location of small vessels exiting the fascia between these muscle groups. Caveat, small vessels also exit between the ECU and the anconeus, but this is only noted proximally near the elbow.

After the fascial incision has been established, the EDC/EDMQ fibers are followed posteriorly (dorsally), and the septum between the EDC/EDMQ and the ECU is noted. The septum may be followed proximally to the radial collateral ligament of the elbow. The underlying supinator can be visualized by elevating the EDC/EDMQ fibers anteriorly and one will then see the obliquely oriented, dense, fibromuscular fibers of the superficial head of the supinator (Fig. 96-3).

To decompress the posterior interosseous nerve, one may either locate the nerve proximally, at the level of the arcade of Frohse, or locate a branch of the posterior interosseous nerve distally as it exits from beneath the superficial head of the supinator as anatomically described by Fuss and Wurzl.[5] The identification of the PIN proximally is suggested because mobilizing the PIN distally has frequently caused a 6- to 12-week paresis of the finger extrinsic extensor muscles.

To locate the arcade of Frohse and the PIN, the incision that was started between the EDC/EDMQ and the ECU is continued proximally. One will be extending the incision into the conjoint tendon of origin of the wrist and finger extensors. The conjoint tendon may be released from the lateral humeral epicondyle. The conjoint tendon is then elevated anteriorly and one can visualize the underlying arcade of Frohse. The arcade of Frohse cannot be visualized without the previous incision and elevation of the conjoint tendon. The use of loupe magnification is suggested throughout the procedure and especially at any time when the PIN needs to be visualized.

Once the arcade of Frohse is noted, a leash of vessels are frequently seen passing over the PIN. The leash of vessels, the fan of Henry, should be cauterized with the use of a bipolar cautery. If there are any ligamentous tissues passing across the PIN, as described by Roles and Maudsley,[13] the structures should be divided. The arcade of Frohse can then be divided with a pair of scissors, such as Littler or Jamieson scissors. The PIN should be decompressed throughout its entire course beneath the superficial portion of the supinator. At the distal portion of the supinator a fibrous edge may exist, but more frequently than not the supinator becomes quite thin and has only muscle tissue distally rather than having fibrous tissue. At the exit site of the PIN from beneath the superficial portion of the supinator, branches of the PIN to the finger extensor muscles will be noted. Care must be taken not to injure these branches. If a fibrous edge does not exist, I do not attempt to decompress the PIN where it begins to arborize. The avoidance of the branches is done so as to prevent a postoperative paresis.

To decompress the PIN from distal to proximal, which is only done if the PIN cannot be visualized proximally, a leash of vessels at the distal aspect of the superficial head of the supinator are first located. The vessels may be elevated and beneath the vessels one will note the branches of the posterior interosseous nerve, those branches being the motor nerves to the finger extensors. The branches are followed to the posterior interosseous nerve. Care must be taken to preserve the branches. This is the most difficult and dangerous part of the procedure because mere retraction may injure the nerves, causing a postoperative finger extension palsy.

Once the PIN has been identified, the overlying supinator muscle is released from distal to proximal. The overlying conjoint tendon of origin of the wrist and finger extensors must be released in order to fully release the superficial portion of the supinator and the arcade of Frohse. Failure to release the conjoint tendon will result in inadequate visualization of all of the superficial head of the supinator and inadequate release of the arcade of Frohse. With adequate elevation and proximal release of the conjoint tendon, the arcade of Frohse may be easily visualized and the PIN may be fully released (Fig. 96–4). If any fibrous bands or vessels are traversing the PIN proximal to the arcade of Frohse, they should be fully released.

Once the PIN has been fully released, I place my index finger between the overlying conjoint tendon and the underlying PIN. The elbow is then extended, the forearm pronated, and the wrist flexed. If there is marked pressure on my finger, this indicates that the conjoint tendon needs to be recessed. The recession is carried out by making a transverse incision on the under surface of the conjoint tendon. In the central portion of the conjoint tendon one will notice a thickening of the fibrous tissue and this has been referred to by Sanders[14] as the central raphe. The central raphe should be incised transversely. The conjoint tendon is thereby lengthened. At the end of the procedure the fingers should be splinted in extension. If splinting is not done some patients may develop drooping, specifically of the long finger, since the central raphe appears to be most in line with the long finger and influences its extensor ability.

An additional advantage of the posterior approach is that degenerative fibroblastic tissue about the conjoint tendon and the radial head area may be excised. Myxoid, degenerative, fibroblastic proliferation is the abnormal finding noted at the time of operative management of lateral humeral epicondylitis (tennis elbow). If the degenerative, myxoid tissue is excised, a minimal lateral humeral epicondylectomy should also be performed, as suggested by Froimson,[4] to provide an area of raw bone to allow for healing of the tissues directly to the bone.

The void that is created by the excision of the myxoid, degenerative tissue may be covered with an anconeus muscle rotation flap. The anconeus can be located by elevating the proximal and posterior lying forearm fascia. The anconeus lies just posterior to the

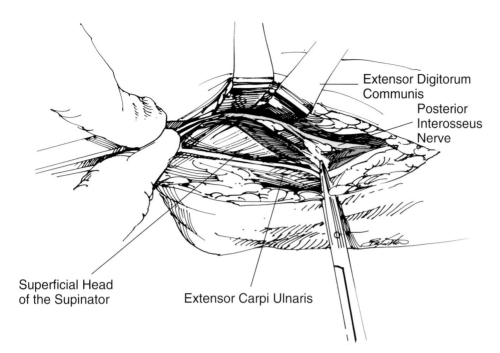

Extensor Digitorum Communis

Posterior Interosseus Nerve

Superficial Head of the Supinator

Extensor Carpi Ulnaris

■ FIGURE 96–4
After the superficial portion of the supinator has been completely decompressed, including transection of the arcade of Frohse, the underlying posterior interosseus nerve is fully visualized.

ECU. The anconeus is supplied by one neurovascular pedicle and after the anconeus has been mobilized from distal to proximal, it may be rotated on its neurovascular pedicle and utilized to cover the area of tissue void between the radial neck distally and the lateral epicondylectomy site proximally. The vascularized anconeus rotation flap provides a blood supply to the area. It should be attached to the radial neck and lateral epicondylectomy site with non-absorbable sutures or with the use of slowly absorbing PDS suture. The use of Vicryl (polyglycolic acid suture) is not recommended because it has resulted in the formation of numerous surgical granulomas.

Whether or not an anconeus muscle rotation flap or a lateral humeral epicondylectomy has been performed, the wound closure is essentially the same. The fascial interval between the EDC/EDMQ and the ECU is closed with a running 2-0 PDS suture. A hemovac drain is placed deeply and is brought out through the skin at a point distal to the distal end of the skin incision. Subcutaneous and dermal tissues are approximated with the use of absorbable 4-0 PDS undyed sutures with the knot buried. The skin is closed with a running, subcuticularly placed 2-0 Prolene suture. Skin tapes are also applied. Marcaine, without epinephrine, is infiltrated into the subdermal tissues along the skin incision area. Dressings are applied, and a long arm posterior splint is applied with the elbow at 90°, the forearm in neutral rotation, and the wrist and the finger metacarpophalangeal (MP) joints supported in slight extension.

One may ask, why use the posterior-lateral approach instead of the standard anterior approaches as suggested by Roles and Maudsley,[13] Lister and co-authors,[8] Cravens and Kline,[2] Eversmann,[3] and Hagert and co-authors?[7] The advantages of the posterior approach are two. The first is that the superficial radial nerve is not seen and is therefore not injured. The second advantage is that an unacceptable scar on the anterior surface of the elbow is avoided. Lister and co-authors[8] state that 2 of their 20 patients required steroid injections of the scar, and one required a revision of the scar when the brachioradialis splitting approach was used. The posterior approach provides a longitudinal incision on the dorsal aspect of the forearm and it heals quite nicely and is cosmetically acceptable (Fig. 96–5). The posterior-lateral approach also allows for the full release of all potentially compressing structures, allows for the performance of an elbow synovectomy and/or

■ TECHNICAL ALTERNATIVES

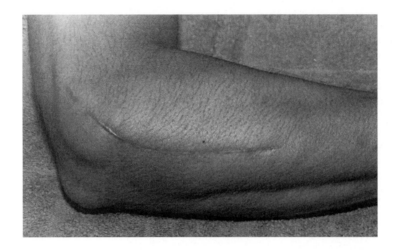

■ FIGURE 96–5
The posterior-lateral approach provides a scar that is fully cosmetically acceptable.

radial head excision, and allows for the performance of a lateral humeral epicondylectomy and a anconeus muscle rotation flap, if so needed.

The use of the anterior approach requires the visualization and mobilization of the superficial radial nerve. Use of this approach in my hands has resulted in a problem of persistent dysesthesias developing along the course of the superficial radial nerve.

The disadvantage of the posterior-lateral approach, in my experience, has been the occasional development of a finger drop palsy due to the irritation of the branches of the PIN that innervate the EDC and EDMQ. The irritation of the branches may be avoided by tracing the PIN from proximal to distal and stopping the dissection before the PIN arborizes.

An additional disadvantage of the posterior-lateral approach is the occasional weakness of the long finger due to the release of the conjoint tendon and its central raphe. This problem may be avoided by the use of a long arm splint, which immobilizes the finger MP joints in extension. If weakness of finger extension does develop, and specifically of the long finger, the problem has always resolved with the use of splinting and has always resolved within 4 to 6 weeks after surgery.

■ REHABILITATION

With the use of the posterior-lateral approach, whether or not a lateral epicondylectomy or anconeus muscle rotation flap has been performed, a long arm splint is used for 10 to 14 days after surgery. The position of the splint, as stated earlier, places the elbow at 90° of flexion, the forearm in neutral rotation, the wrist in slight extension and the finger MP joints in an extended position. The splint is used for 10 to 14 days. If drooping of the long finger is noted, the use of a short arm splint to maintain extension of the long finger is used for an additional 2 to 4 weeks.

The running subcuticularly placed 2-0 Prolene skin suture is removed at the first postoperative visit, usually after 10 days. The skin tapes are left in place until they fall off spontaneously. The skin tapes are kept in place to minimize widening of the scar.

Most patients do not require postoperative hand therapy. If, however, a patient has difficulty in attaining full grip strength, referral to a hand therapist is provided.

Most patients may begin activities of daily living after 10 to 14 days. Most patients require no further splinting after the initial 10 to 14 days. A return to work is usually possible 6 weeks after the operative procedure. Many workers are returned to part-time or to light duty first and then gradually progressed into a full schedule or into their full work load. Most patients that I have managed have not done heavy manual work but have done office-related work, such as filing and data entry.

■ OUTCOMES

From 1987 through mid 1994, I completed 55 posterior interosseous neuroplasties. Initially, the procedures were performed by an anterior approach. Dysesthesias along the course of the superficial radial nerve occurred for a transient period of time in eight of

17 patients. Also, a transient palsy of the finger extensors at the MP joints developed in two patients. In addition, I performed reoperations on two patients who had been initially operated on elsewhere via an anterior approach: one surgery was performed because dysesthesias developed along the course of the superficial radial nerve, and the other was performed because the patient did not have adequate decompression of the posterior interosseous nerve because it could not be located by the initial anterior approach.

Because of the complications with the anterior approach, the posterior-lateral approach was used. In 21 instances, the posterior interosseous nerve was explored from a distal to a proximal direction. Using this method, there were no cases of superficial radial nerve dysesthesias, but a postoperative palsy of the finger extensors at the MP joint level developed in seven patients. A permanent finger drop palsy of the ulnar three fingers developed in one of these patients. This individual was a man in his mid-60s with insulin-dependent diabetes mellitus.

Considering that the distal to proximal dissection of the PIN had a 33% incidence of a usually transient finger drop palsy, the preferred dissection now is from proximal to distal. Seventeen posterior-lateral, proximal to distal procedures have been completed, and there have been no patients with postoperative posterior interosseous nerve palsies or superficial radial nerve dysesthesias. One 50-year-old patient who received workers' compensation had ongoing pain and underwent a re-exploration. Despite the re-exploration, the patient continues to experience pain. Ritts and co-authors[12] have observed that not all patients who receive workers' compensation necessarily do well, even with an uncomplicated course. This certainly also has been my experience.

References

1. Bowen TL, Stone KH: Posterior interosseous nerve paralysis caused by ganglia at the elbow. J Bone Joint Surg, 1966; 48B:774–776.
2. Cravens G, Kline DG: Posterior interosseous nerve palsies. Neurosurgery, 1990; 27:397–402.
3. Eversmann WW Jr: Entrapment and Compression Neuropathies. In: Green DP (ed), Operative Hand Surgery, New York: Churchill Livingstone, 1993:1341–1385.
4. Froimson AI: Tenosynovitis and Tennis Elbow. In: Green DP (ed), Operative Hand Surgery, New York: Churchill Livingstone, 1993:1989–2006.
5. Fuss FK, Wurzl GH: Radial nerve entrapment at the elbow: surgical anatomy. J Hand Surg, 1991;16A:742–747.
6. Gelberman RH, Eaton R, Urbaniak JR: Peripheral nerve compression. J Bone Joint Surg, 1993; 75A:1854–1878.
7. Hagert CG, Lundborg G, Hansen T: Entrapment of the posterior interosseous nerve. Scand J Plast Reconstr Surg, 1977; 11:205–212.
8. Lister GD, Belsole RB, Kleinert HE: The radial tunnel syndrome. J Hand Surg, 1979; 4A: 52–59.
9. Millender LH, Nalebuff EA, Holdsworth DE: Posterior interosseous nerve syndrome secondary to rheumatoid synovitis. J Bone Joint Surgery, 1973; 55A:753–757.
10. Morrey BF: Reoperation for failed surgical treatment of refractory lateral epicondylitis. J Should Elbow Surg, 1992; 1:47–55.
11. Richmond DA: Lipoma causing a posterior interosseous nerve lesion. J Bone Joint Surgery, 1953; 35B:83.
12. Ritts GD, Wood MB, Linscheid RL: Radial tunnel syndrome. Clin Orthop Rel Res, 1987; 219: 201–205.
13. Roles NC, Maudsley RH: Radial tunnel syndrome. J Bone Joint Surgery, 1972; 54B:499–508.
14. Sanders WE: Radial tunnel syndrome: an investigation of compression neuropathy as a possible cause [letter]. J Bone Joint Surg, 1992; 74A:309–310.
15. Sponseller BD, Engber WD: Double-entrapment radial tunnel syndrome. J Hand Surg, 1983; 8A:420–423.

ROBERT M. SZABO

97

Median Nerve Release: Proximal Forearm

■ HISTORY OF THE
TECHNIQUE

In 1948, Parsonage and Turner first described paralysis of the flexor pollicis longus and the flexor digitorum profundus to the index finger. They called this condition "neuralgic amyotrophy" and attributed the pathology to an anterior horn cell lesion.[22] In 1952, Kiloh and Nevin reported isolated involvement of the anterior interosseous nerve in two cases.[16] Both cases were followed conservatively with only partial recovery after 1 year. They attributed the pathology to "isolated neuritis" rather than nerve compression. In 1965, Fearn and Goodfellow were first to propose mechanical compression as the cause of the lesion; they suggested that it be treated surgically.[5] Seyffarth first described pronator syndrome in 1951 when he reported on 17 patients treated nonoperatively.[24] Johnson and Spinner are credited with characterizing this syndrome based on observations in 103 operative decompressions.[12]

The most proximal site of median nerve entrapment in the cubital region is a supracondyloid process where the nerve is compressed as it passes underneath the ligament of Struthers.[2,4,25,30] At about the same level and slightly distal an accessory bicipital aponeurosis has been found to specifically cause anterior interosseous nerve palsy.[26] In the majority of reported cases, however, the compression in both anterior interosseous nerve palsy and pronator teres syndrome is caused by fibrous bands where the nerve passes between the two heads of the pronator teres.[12,18,20,38] If the deep head of the pronator is muscular, a fibrous arch usually develops where the two heads merge, whereas if the deep head is tendinous, it may act as a fibrous arch.[6] Other anatomic sites of compression include the flexor digitorum superficialis arch,[6] and fibromuscular bands in the distal forearm.[11] Several accessory and variant muscles have been noted as compressing structures including Gantzer's muscle (accessory head of the flexor pollicus longus), the palmaris profundus, and the flexor carpi radialis brevis.[28]

Traumatic etiologies include forearm fractures[7] and supracondylar fractures.[15,19,33] Pure anterior interosseous nerve palsy after supracondylar fracture is due to traction on the less mobile anterior interosseous nerve with sparing of the median nerve, which is more mobile in the proximal forearm.[27] Whether minimal repetitive trauma can cause proximal median nerve compression is unclear. Probably a preexisting anatomic abnormality must be present for symptoms to occur from strenuous activities or repetitive motion. I have operated on one adult spastic hemiplegic with a hypertrophied pronator teres muscle who got complete relief from his pronator syndrome. Direct trauma either from penetrating wounds or external compression can also produce a proximal median nerve compressive lesion. Pronator syndrome has also been attributed to a persistent median artery that passed completely through the proximal median nerve and then gave origin to a vascular leash to the flexor muscles that compressed the nerve.[14] Because of the topographic arrangement of the median nerve, it is possible to compress either the motor fibers or the sensory fibers within the pronator muscle and produce either an anterior interosseous motor palsy or a pronator teres sensory syndrome.

Clinical symptoms of pronator syndrome include forearm pain as well as paresthesias and hypesthesia in the cutaneous distribution of the median nerve (i.e., thumb, index, long and radial half of the ring finger). These sensory symptoms also may be present over the thenar eminence in the distribution of the palmar cutaneous nerve. Patients may experience weakness in the extremity. Patients' occupations frequently require repetitive use of their upper extremities.[3,9] Results of physical examination show pain on palpation of the median nerve in the proximal forearm. The pronator teres muscle can be tender, firm, or apparently enlarged.[13] There is no weakness of the median innervated intrinsic or extrinsic muscles. Percussion of the median nerve proximal may cause tingling and paresthesias, in contrast to carpal tunnel syndrome where this test is positive distally at the wrist. Paresthesias are increased with mild compression over the proximal muscle mass of the pronator teres. Severe muscle cramps and spasm perceived as "writer's cramp" are found in some cases.[13] Threshold testing with Semmes-Weinstein monofilaments may reveal decreased sensibility over the distribution of the median nerve including the thenar eminence.[31] Results of Phalen's wrist flexion test are negative. Specific provocative maneuvers that reproduce the pain and distal paresthesias are used to localize the site of compression. Resisted elbow flexion with the forearm in supination implicates compression by the bicipital aponeurosis. Resisted forearm pronation with the elbow in full extension suggests compression between the two heads of the pronator. Isolated proximal interphalangeal joint flexion of the middle finger producing paresthesias in the radial three digits suggests entrapment under the fibrous origin of the flexor digitorum superficialis (Table 97–1).[12,13] Palpation of the medial humeral condyle and distal diaphysis may reveal a bony prominence, which is a supracondyloid process. Before surgery, an anterior-posterior, lateral and oblique radiograph of the elbow should be obtained to rule out its presence.

The clinical symptoms of complete anterior interosseous nerve syndrome are loss of function of the FPL, flexor digitorum profundus index and sometimes long finger, and the pronator quadratus. Sensibility is unaffected. The incomplete syndrome can occur with either weakness or absence of FPL or FDP of the index finger with normal pronator quadratus function.[10] The thumb and index finger assume a classic position during pinch in this syndrome (Fig. 97–1). The index finger extends at the distal interphalangeal joint with compensatory increased flexion at the proximal interphalangeal joint. The thumb hyperextends at the interphalangeal joint and displays increased flexion of the metacarpophalangeal joint. Involvement of the pronator quadratus can be evaluated by testing the strength of resisted forced supination with the elbow maximally flexed. This eliminates the effect of the humeral head of the pronator teres, which is responsible for 75% of the rotational strength of this muscle.[7] The onset of symptoms is usually spontaneous, and electrophysiologic examination is valuable in making the diagnosis.

The most frequent cause of the entrapment is fibrous bands in the pronator teres muscle. The outcome after operation is better for complete lesions than for partial lesions that involve the thumb or index finger only.[38] Bilateral involvement should alert one to think about Parsonage-Turner syndrome or symmetrical polyneuropathy; however, at least one bilateral case has been attributed to anatomic nerve compressive lesions. Braun found on surgical exploration in each extremity of his patient with bilateral anterior interosseous nerve palsy enlarged communicating veins directly compressing the median nerve in the distal arms.[1] An anterior interosseous nerve palsy can occur as a complication of a closed both bone forearm fracture. Surgical exploration has been reported to show a bone spike from the proximal fragment perforating the median nerve.[7] Spinner reported four cases

TABLE 97–1 CLINICAL FEATURES OF COMPRESSION NEUROPATHY OF THE MEDIAN NERVE

	Carpal Tunnel Syndrome	Pronator Syndrome
Nerve Percussion	+ at wrist	+ proximal forearm
Nocturnal symptoms	+	−
Provocative tests	−	+
Wrist flexion	+	−

■ FIGURE 97–1
Characteristic pinch deformity demonstrated on the left with collapse of the thumb interphalangeal and the index distal interphalangeal joints into extension (with permission of Chidgey LK, Szabo RM. Anterior Interosseous Nerve Compression Syndrome. In: Szabo RM (ed), Nerve Compression Syndromes—Diagnosis and Treatment, Thorofare, NJ: Slack, 1989:153–162).

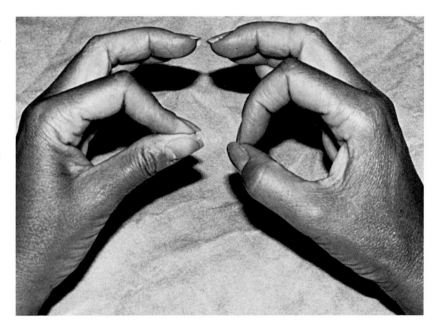

of anterior interosseous nerve palsy due to an accessory bicipital aponeurosis. Diagnosis in this case is characterized by the paresis or paralysis of muscles innervated by the anterior interosseous branch of the median nerve, the flexor pollicis longus, the flexor digitorum profundus, and the pronator quadratus, as well as the more proximal innervated muscles, the pronator teres and flexor carpi radialis. Sensibility remains intact and the site of the nerve percussion sign is found in the distal arm. The accessory aponeurosis can be visualized clinically in the distal third of the arm by resistance to elbow flexion with the forearm in supination.[26]

Of patients with a good clinical history and physical findings compatible with pronator syndrome, less than 50% can be confirmed by electrodiagnostic testing.[9] Nerve conduction velocity measurement of the median nerve in the proximal forearm is misleading because reduced velocity of conduction in the forearm has been noted in 20 to 32% of patients with carpal tunnel syndrome. Standard nerve conduction velocity tests measure the forearm segment in combination with the distal latency, and while this may not represent an accurate assessment of conduction in the proximal portion of the nerve, Pease and co-authors described a technique of direct evaluation of the forearm median nerve by the stimulation and recording of the forearm nerve action potential proximal to the wrist. They found that forearm median nerve conduction velocities in carpal tunnel syndrome patients are significantly slower than in normal subjects. Retrograde degeneration of the nerve axons may result from entrapment in the carpal tunnel.[23] Electrophysiologic findings, especially needle electromyography (EMG), may be more definitive than findings from clinical examination. The EMG diagnosis depends on seeing fibrillations, positive sharp waves, and reduced interference patterns in the FPL and pronator quadratus muscles. In one study, EMG and operative findings demonstrated that median nerve compression by the pronator teres produces denervation of this muscle as well as distal muscles. Electromyography cannot differentiate a median nerve lesion at the pronator teres from a more proximal lesion.[8]

The operative technique has evolved since Fearn and Goodfellow first described their approach to median nerve decompression via a longitudinal skin incision on the anterior forearm.[5] Johnson and Spinner recommend a volar zig-zag approach starting at the medial elbow crease progressing across the anterior forearm and back again medially.[12] They emphasize that a transverse incision will not provide sufficient visualization of the nerve and the associated areas of pathology. Nevertheless, Tsai recently reported on cadaver studies and clinical cases using a transverse incision in the proximal forearm, which he claims affords adequate exposure.[35] My preference is to use an extensile approach which can be extended proximally above the elbow and distally if needed.

■ INDICATIONS AND CONTRAINDICATIONS

In patients with symptoms of short duration, modification or termination of activities that provoke the syndrome should lead to its cessation. Steroid injections have little to offer in the conservative treatment of proximal median nerve compression since there is no "synovitis" causing compression along the course of the median nerve. Immobilization with a long arm removable splint can be offered with the elbow in 90° of flexion, the forearm in slight pronation and the wrist in slight flexion to relieve pressure and traction on the median nerve. Many patients will have satisfactory return of function and no recurrence of symptoms.

During the initial period of observation, baseline electrodiagnostic studies should be obtained, but not before 3 weeks have elapsed since the onset of the syndrome. Time is permitted for Wallerian degeneration to be detected electromyographically in the case of anterior interosseous nerve syndrome. If there is no sign of clinical improvement, or in anterior interosseous nerve palsy no electromyographic improvement in 2 to 3 months, surgical exploration is indicated.

■ SURGICAL TECHNIQUES

The surgical treatment of pronator teres syndrome and anterior interosseous nerve palsy is intimately related to the underlying anatomy. At the distal humerus both the median nerve and brachial artery pass through the antecubital fossa underneath a fibrous sheath, the bicipital aponeurosis, which takes origin from the biceps tendon and the fascia of the flexor-pronator mass. In this region, the median nerve separates from the brachial artery and continues most commonly between the deep (ulnar) and superficial (humeral) heads of the pronator teres, or it may pass posterior to both heads, or it may pierce the muscle's humeral head (Fig. 97–2). The main median nerve trunk and anterior interosseous nerve also can take different paths in relation to the pronator teres muscle.[18] The median nerve then enters the forearm deep to the fibrous arch of the flexor digitorum superficialis and emerges to a more superficial position in the distal third of the forearm. The pronator teres muscle receives one to four branches from the median nerve, and while these fibers separate from the bulk of the nerve proximal to the elbow joint, they share its perineural sheath. The fibers of the anterior interosseous nerve are posterior and the sensory fibers of the hand anterior at the level of the elbow. The fascicles of the anterior interosseous nerve are grouped separately from the remaining median nerve before the nerve divides into its main and anterior interosseous branches.[29] Other branches that originate from the median nerve before it passes through the pronator teres include branches to the palmaris longus, flexor carpi radialis, and flexor digitorum superficialis muscles, and rarely the flexor digitorum profundus muscle.[6] The fibrous arch of the pronator teres muscle (pronator arch) lies 3 to 7.5 cm below Hueter's line (a line through the tips of the humeral epicondyles). The fibrous arch of the flexor digitorum superficialis muscle (superficialis arch), which is always distal to the pronator arch, lies 6.5 cm below Hueter's line in its most proximal position.[6] Variations in the anatomy of the muscles and fibrous arches might cause compression of the median nerve in the forearm. The pronator teres always has a superficial head and usually a deep head; the flexor digitorum superficialis varies greatly in its site of origin and the median nerve might be crossed by two, one or no fibroaponeurotic arches.[4] Gantzer's muscle, an accessory head of flexor pollicis longus, is present in 45% of the cadavers.[4] The anterior interosseous nerve innervates the radial half of the flexor digitorum profundus, flexor pollicis longus, and the pronator quadratus. In the all-median hand, it can supply the entire profundi; occasionally, the ulnar nerve can innervate the long finger profundus. The median and ulnar nerves can be connected in the forearm in the form of a "Martin-Gruber" anastomosis 15% of the time.[34] In 50% of cases, this communicating branch from the median nerve originates from the anterior interosseous nerve. Median nerve fibers thus may supply some of the intrinsic hand muscles in 7.5% of limbs. The remaining median nerve courses distally to pass beneath the transverse carpal ligament. Five centimeters proximal to the proximal wrist crease, the

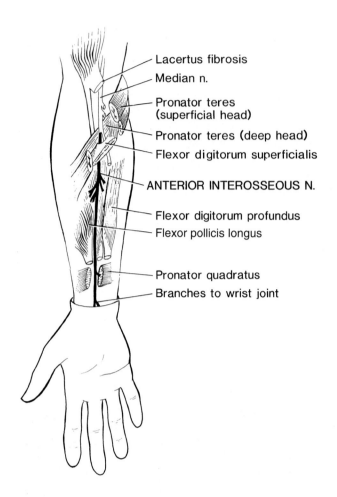

■ FIGURE 97–2
Anatomy of the anterior interosseous nerve (with permission of Chidgey LK, Szabo RM. Anterior Interosseous Nerve Compression Syndrome. In: Szabo RM (ed), Nerve Compression Syndromes—Diagnosis and Treatment, Thorofare, NJ: Slack, 1989:153–162).

Lacertus fibrosis
Median n.
Pronator teres (superficial head)
Pronator teres (deep head)
Flexor digitorum superficialis
ANTERIOR INTEROSSEOUS N.
Flexor digitorum profundus
Flexor pollicis longus
Pronator quadratus
Branches to wrist joint

palmar cutaneous branch originates and finally enters a short tunnel immediately medial to the flexor carpi radialis tendon before innervating the skin of the thenar eminence.[32] This area of sensibility is important in differentiating proximal median nerve compression from carpal tunnel syndrome.

The surgical approach and extent of median nerve exploration should be the same whether the diagnosis is anterior interosseous nerve palsy or pronator syndrome. The procedure is done under general or axillary block anesthesia. In most cases, the incision begins 5 cm proximal to the elbow flexion crease. However, if either a supracondyloid process or accessory bicipital aponeurosis has been identified, the incision should begin at least 10 cm proximal to the elbow crease. The incision curves distally just medial to the biceps tendon, zig-zags across the antecubital crease and gently curves back medially for 5 cm in the proximal forearm (Fig. 97–3). The medial antebrachial cutaneous nerve is identified and isolated with a small rubber drain as it courses next to the basilic vein. The median nerve is identified proximal to the elbow and isolated with a rubber drain. If a supracondylar process or accessory bicipital aponeurosis is diagnosed preoperatively, the median nerve is identified and isolated with a rubber drain in the most proximal portion of the incision and traced distally. The ligament of Struthers along with the supracondylar process are excised or if present the accessory bicipital aponeurosis is incised. The median nerve must be explored completely, as other proximal sites of compression can coexist.

The median nerve is dissected distally with a fine Jacobsen hemostat. The bicipital aponeurosis is incised and the nerve is followed to the proximal extent of the superficial (humeral) head of the pronator teres (Fig. 97–4). Retraction of the superficial head will assist in recognizing any variation of the nerve's course in relation to the two heads of the pronator. Tendinous or fibrous bands within the pronator are identified and incised.

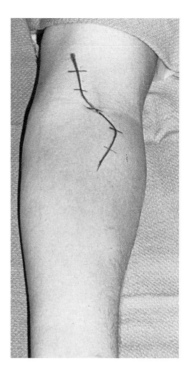

■ FIGURE 97–3
Incision used for exploration of the proximal median and anterior interosseous nerves.

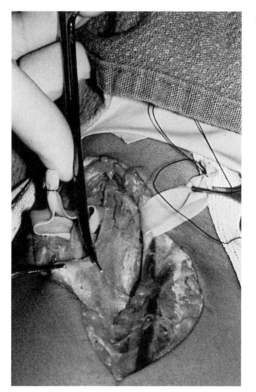

■ FIGURE 97–4
Exposure of the median nerve at the elbow. The median nerve is identified and tagged proximally. The bicipital aponeurosis is incised from proximal to distal further exposing the median nerve. Care is taken to identify and tag the medial antebrachial cutaneous nerve (forceps holding it tagged with a rubber drain).

If a median artery is found to penetrate the median nerve, the passage of the artery can be enlarged by interfascicular dissection. Ligation of this artery is avoided because it provides the dominant blood supply to the median nerve in 30% of cases and significantly contributes to the blood supply of the index and long fingers in select cases.[14] If, during exploration, a leash of muscular arterial branches from a median artery is found crossing

■ FIGURE 97–5
The median nerve courses between the superficial (SH.PRON.) and the deep (DH.PRON.) heads of the pronator teres muscle.

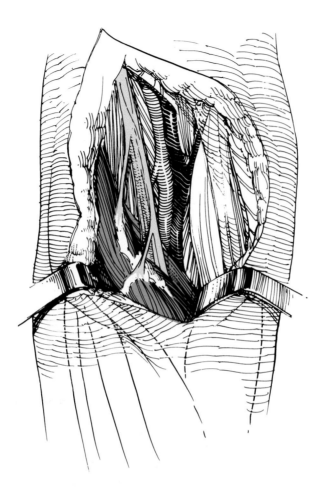

the nerve, these branches should be ligated. Most of the time the median nerve passes between the two heads of the pronator (Fig. 97–5). The anterior interosseous nerve can be visualized with retraction of the superficial head, but at times visualization is inadequate and the insertion of the superficial head is divided and tagged for later reattachment. If a variant is encountered such as the median and anterior interosseous nerves passing deep to both heads of the pronator, the deep (ulnar) head can be detached at its tendinous insertion on the radius and reflected proximal and ulnarly to fully expose the distal course of the nerves. If further exposure is needed, the radial origin of the superficialis can be released. Other anatomic variants are possible (Fig. 97–6).

Attention is next directed to the superficialis arcade. The anterior interosseous and median nerves pass deep to the superficialis arch distal to the pronator teres (Fig. 97–7). This arch is incised, as it may be a source of compression particularly if it is thickened. Careful dissection just distal to the arch is continued with attention to finding anatomic variations such as accessory muscles. Any site of compression is relieved.

The tourniquet is deflated and careful hemostasis is obtained with a bipolar cautery. The pronator teres is reattached if detachment was necessary. Care is taken not to shorten the muscle and tighten the attachment thereby creating a new compressive lesion. Epineurotomy or internal neurolysis is not necessary and may be harmful. Subcutaneous transposition of the median nerve is also not recommended. The subcutaneous layer is closed with 4-0 interrupted absorbable sutures and the skin edges with 5-0 nylon simple sutures.

Postoperatively, the extremity is placed in a bulky, plaster-reinforced, sterile, above-elbow dressing, maintaining the elbow at 90° of flexion, the forearm in 45° of pronation, and the wrist in slight flexion.

■ TECHNICAL
ALTERNATIVES

The most common pitfall is error in diagnosis. If one relies on an electrodiagnostic study that shows slowing of the median nerve in the proximal forearm in addition to signs of

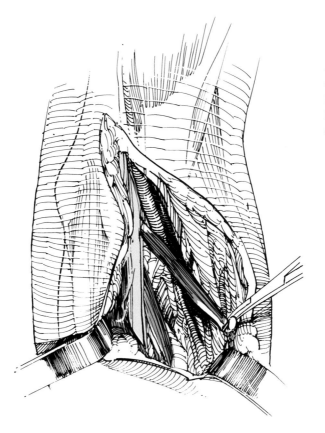

■ FIGURE 97–6
In this case, the median nerve passed superficial to the deep head and through the superficial head being compressed by a fibrous arch of this anatomic variant muscle.

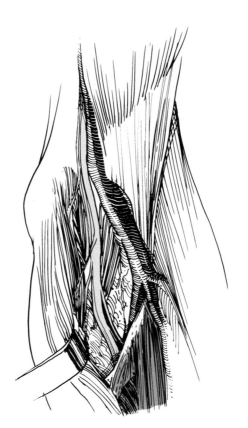

■ FIGURE 97–7
The median nerve accompanies the anterior interosseous nerve (AIN) underneath a tight arch of the flexor digitorum superficialis muscle (FDS).

distal compression in the carpal tunnel, usually the proximal finding is of no clinical significance. There is no substitute for a thorough clinical examination in the diagnosis of pronator syndrome. Sensory changes in the median nerve distribution may result from C6 (thumb) or C7 (fingers) radiculopathy. Patients with cervical spondylosis or arthritis are at greater risk for more distal nerve compression symptoms, the so-called "double-crush" syndrome.[21,37] Obtaining a history of neck pain with distal radiation is important in evaluating all extremity nerve compression lesions. Examination of the neck's range of motion, palpation of the cervical spine for tenderness, and radiographic examination is part of the work-up for differentiating proximal median nerve compression from other causes.

Carpal tunnel syndrome is the most important differential diagnosis relating to pronator syndrome. The history and presenting complaints are very similar, and frequently the diagnosis of pronator syndrome is made after a failed carpal tunnel release. Although electrodiagnostic studies can usually confirm median nerve compression at the wrist, this same compression can cause retrograde slowing of nerve conduction velocity in the proximal forearm. Careful use of provocative testing and absence of nocturnal symptoms will establish the diagnosis of proximal nerve compression.

Wood found that pronator teres syndrome may be found in patients with thoracic outlet syndrome as a double-crush phenomenon.[39] This phenomenon suggests that compression of a nerve at one site lessens the nerve's ability to withstand compression at a more distal site.[37] The pathophysiologic mechanism most likely relates to disturbances in axonal flow kinetics. Clinical studies confirm that less compression of the median nerve across the carpal tunnel is required to produce symptoms in the presence of more proximal root compression.[21] Isolated thoracic outlet syndrome (TOS) should not be confused with pronator syndrome. In TOS, the lower trunk is most commonly affected so symptoms are found in the ulnar innervated fingers. The Adson, costoclavicular, and hyperabduction maneuvers as well as the 3-minute elevation test are negative in pronator teres syndrome. If a history of heavy smoking is obtained or the patient is a female with history of breast carcinoma, a chest x-ray is probably warranted. Although rare, a Pancoast tumor often first presents with complaints of hand and forearm pain followed by weakness. Similarly, patients with axillary breast metastasis or radiation plexitis have first been diagnosed based on their strange upper extremity complaints.

Parsonage-Turner brachial neuritis, a peculiar entity of unknown etiology, is probably the most common differential diagnosis in anterior interosseous nerve palsy. First described in 1948,[22] it appears as pain around the shoulder and upper arm followed within a few hours to several days by atrophic paralysis.[36] In cases involving the anterior interosseous nerve, the pain also may be in the elbow and forearm. Pain may be bilateral in the shoulders but paralysis may appear only in one forearm. Frequently, a history may be obtained of recent surgery, a flu-like syndrome, or even a vaccination. Of 82 patients with a variety of nerve involvement, 23 incidents occurred 5 to 14 days after an operation: Recovery takes from 15 to 36 months, but recurrence is known to have occurred even after several years.[36] It is important to make this diagnosis because the treatment is observation whereas with anterior interosseus nerve compression, decompression is advised. Electrodiagnostic findings can be identical in these two conditions.

Isolated rupture of the flexor pollicus longus, or less commonly rupture of the flexor digitorum profundus to the index finger, also must be considered when establishing the diagnosis of anterior interosseous nerve palsy. These tendon ruptures occur secondary to attrition changes in diseases such as rheumatoid arthritis, osteoarthritis, gout, or scaphoid nonunion. Most commonly seen in rheumatoid arthritis, the FPL can rupture on an osteophyte from an eroded scaphoid.[17] Looking for a tenodesis effect on physical examination is very useful in differentiating tendon rupture from nerve palsy. Alternating wrist flexion and extension or squeezing the proximal forearm muscles will produce thumb and index distal interphalangeal joint flexion if the tendons are intact. The force may not reliably be transferred in severe rheumatoid arthritis or other conditions with wrist subluxation. Electromyography becomes particularly important in these cases.

There are few reported surgical complications for either pronator or anterior interosseous nerve syndromes.[9,13] The medial antebrachial cutaneous nerve is at risk during exposure. Proximally, one must anticipate the possibility of compression from a supracondylar process or accessory bicipital aponeurosis. The entire course of the nerve must be explored in the cubital region to inspect all possible sites of compression in every case. Scars from the incision can become hypertrophic or unsightly. Careful placement of the limb that crosses the elbow crease, closure without tension, the use of small sutures and prolonged use of steristrips after suture removal seems to produce the best cosmetic result.

If the function of the anterior interosseous nerve fails to return after decompression, appropriate tendon transfers are considered.

■ REHABILITATION

After 10 days, the sutures are removed and Steristrips applied to the wound. This is an incision that tends to spread, and careful early technique will improve the final cosmesis. Immobilization in a long arm fiberglass cast in the same position is continued for an additional 2 weeks. Then all immobilization is discontinued, and gentle elbow range of motion exercises are encouraged. Most patients do not require a supervised therapy program. Avoidance of any resistive activities is suggested for 6 to 8 weeks after surgery. Strength and symptoms gradually improve over 2 to 3 months. Full return of function can take longer than 6 months, particularly with anterior interosseous nerve palsy. Return to activities of daily living and work are dependent on the will and needs of the patient and the capacity to perform a specific task. Having said that, most patients with pronator syndrome are back to full function in 2 to 3 months. Patients with anterior interosseous nerve syndrome usually do not have full recovery by this time. Nevertheless, they have minimal disability in performing most tasks and are able to return to work.

■ OUTCOMES

In pronator syndrome, 50% of patients will respond to conservative therapy.[12] Surgery is successful in more than 85% of cases in most series.[9,12,13] Failure is generally attributed to misdiagnosis. In 32 cases followed for 3 to 88 months after surgery, Hartz and co-authors noted excellent or good results in 28 patients.[9] The most common lesions found in these patients were a taut bicipital aponeurosis or an intramuscular tendinous abnormality about the median nerve. The patients who faired poorly had less conspicuous lesions. Tsai reported 12 of 21 patients had excellent or good results using a transverse incision.[35]

In anterior interosseous nerve palsy, even though there are documented cases of return up to 18 months after the onset of this syndrome, expectant treatment has been less predictable than surgical intervention, and recovery is often incomplete.[16] Operative treatment results in a more rapid and predictable return of function.[10,28] If muscle is not reinnervated by 18 months, it becomes fibrotic and no longer functions.

References

1. Braun RM, Spinner RJ. Spontaneous bilateral median nerve compressions in the distal arm. J Hand Surg, 1991; 16A:244–247.
2. Crotti FM, Mangiagalli EP, Rampini P. Supracondyloid process and anomalous insertion of pronator teres as sources of median nerve neuralgia. J Neurosurg Sci, 1981; 25:41–44.
3. Danielsson LG. Iatrogenic pronator syndrome. Scand J Plast Reconstr Surg, 1980; 14:201–203.
4. Dellon AL, Mackinnon SE. Musculoaponeurotic variations along the course of the median nerve in the proximal forearm. J Hand Surg, 1987; 12B:359–363.
5. Fearn CBD, Goodfellow JW. Anterior interosseous nerve palsy. J Bone Joint Surg, 1965; 47B:91–93.
6. Fuss FK, Wurzl GH. Median nerve entrapment. Pronator teres syndrome. Surgical anatomy and correlation with symptom patterns. Surg Radiol Anat, 1990; 12:267–271.
7. Geissler WB, Fernandez DL, Graca R. Anterior interosseous nerve palsy complicating a forearm fracture in a child. J Hand Surg, 1990; 15A:44–47.
8. Gross PT, Jones HJ. Proximal median neuropathies: electromyographic and clinical correlation. Muscle Nerve, 1992; 15:390–395.
9. Hartz CR, Linscheid RL, Gramse RR, Daube JR. The pronator teres syndrome: Compressive neuropathy of the median nerve. J Bone Joint Surg, 1981; 63A:885–891.
10. Hill NA, Howard FM, Huffer BR. The incomplete anterior interosseous nerve syndrome. J Hand Surg, 1985; 10A:4–16.

11. Holtzman RNN, Mark MH, Patel MR. Median nerve neuralgia caused by a fibromuscular band in the distal forearm. J Hand Surg, 1986; 11A:894–895.
12. Johnson RK, Spinner M. Median Nerve Compression in the Forearm: The Pronator Tunnel Syndrome. In: Szabo RM (ed), Nerve Compression Syndromes—Diagnosis and Treatment, Thorofare, NJ: Slack, 1989:137–151.
13. Johnson RK, Spinner M, Shrewsbury MM. Median nerve entrapment syndrome in the proximal forearm. J Hand Surg, 1979; 4A:48–51.
14. Jones NF, Ming NL. Persistent median artery as a cause of pronator syndrome. J Hand Surg, 1988; 13A:728–732.
15. Karlsson J, Thorsteinsson T, Thorleifsson R, Arnason H. Entrapment of the median nerve and brachial artery after supracondylar fractures of the humerus in children. Arch Orthop Trauma Surg, 1986; 104:389–391.
16. Kiloh LG, Nevin S. Isolated neuritis of the anterior interosseous nerve. Br Med J, 1952; 1: 850–851.
17. Mannerfelt L, Norman O. Attrition ruptures of flexor tendons in rheumatoid arthritis caused by bony spurs in the carpal tunnel. A clinical and radiologic study. J Bone Joint Surg, 1969; 51B:270–277.
18. Megele R. Anterior interosseous nerve syndrome with atypical nerve course in relation to the pronator teres. Acta Neurochir (Wien), 1988; 91:144–146.
19. Moehring HD. Irreducible supracondylar fracture of the humerus complicated by anterior interosseous nerve palsy. Clin Orthop Rel Res, 1986; 206:228–232.
20. Nigst H, Dick W. Syndromes of compression of the median nerve in the proximal forearm (pronator teres syndrome: anterior interosseous nerve syndrome). Arch Orthop Trauma Surg, 1979; 93:307–312.
21. Osterman AL. The double crush syndrome. Orthop Clin North Am, 1988; 19:147–155.
22. Parsonage MJ, Turner JW. Neuralgic amyotrophy: the shoulder-girdle syndrome. Lancet, 1948; 1:973–978.
23. Pease WS, Lee HH, Johnson EW. Forearm median nerve conduction velocity in carpal tunnel syndrome. Electromyogr Clin Neurophysiol, 1990; 30:299–302.
24. Seyffarth H. Primary myoses in the m. pronator teres as cause of the n. medianus (the pronator syndrome). Acta Psychiatr Scand [Suppl], 1951; 74:251–254.
25. Smith RV, Fisher RG. Struthers ligament: a source of median nerve compression above the elbow. J Neurosurg, 1973; 38:778–779.
26. Spinner M. The anterior interosseous-nerve syndrome. With special attention to its variations. J Bone Joint Surg, 1970; 52A:84–94.
27. Spinner M, Schreiber SN. Anterior interosseous nerve paralysis as a complication of supracondylar fractures of the humerus in children. J Bone Joint Surg, 1969; 51A:1584–1590.
28. Spinner RJ, Carmichael SW, Spinner M. Partial median nerve entrapment in the distal arm because of an accessory bicipital aponeurosis. J Hand Surg, 1991; 16A:236–244.
29. Sunderland S. Nerves and Nerve Injuries, 2nd ed, Edinburgh: Churchill Livingstone, 1978: 655–690.
30. Suramyi L. Median nerve compression by Struthers ligament. J Neurol Neurosurg Psychiatry, 1983; 46:1047–1049.
31. Szabo RM, Gelberman RH. Peripheral nerve compression—Etiology, critical pressure threshold and clinical assessment. Orthopedics, 1984; 7:1461–1466.
32. Taleisnik J. The palmar cutaneous branch of the median nerve and the approach to the carpal tunnel. J Bone Joint Surg, 1973; 55A:1212–1217.
33. Thomas AP. Entrapment of the proximal fragment of supracondylar fractures. J Bone Joint Surg, 1990; 72B:321–322.
34. Thomson A. Third annual report on the Committee of Collective Investigation of the Anatomical Society of Great Britain and Ireland for the year 1891–1892. J Anat Physiol, 1893; 27:183.
35. Tsai T-M, Syed SA. A transverse skin incision approach for decompression of pronator teres syndrome. J Hand Surg, 1994; 19B:40–42.
36. Turner AJW, Parsonage MJ. Neuralgic amyotrophy (paralytic brachial neuritis) with special reference to prognosis. Lancet, 1957; 2:209–211.
37. Upton ARM, McComas AJ. The double crush in nerve-entrapment syndromes. Lancet, 1973; 2:359–362.
38. Werner CO. The anterior interosseous nerve syndrome. Int Orthop, 1989; 13:193–197.
39. Wood VE, Biondi J. Double-crush nerve compression in thoracic-outlet syndrome. J Bone Joint Surg, 1990; 72A:85–87.

PART

VII

Interpositional Nerve Grafting

98

Grafting of Digital Nerves

It is unclear when the first digital nerve graft was performed, but the first report of any nerve graft was by Philipeaux in 1870.[23] He bridged a gap of a hypoglossal nerve of a dog with an autologous lingual nerve. Albert is credited with the first nerve allograft in humans in 1878 and the first autograft in 1885, although he did not report the clinical outcome.[1]

In 1917, Mayo-Robinson reported the first successful nerve graft in humans when he used an allograft to span a 2.5-cm gap in a median nerve.[15] Bunnell reported success with digital nerve grafting as well as facial nerve grafting.[4,5] However, these reports of success were dampened by numerous reports of failure. Both Platt and Stopford reported universal failure in their series of nerve grafts published in 1920.[24,29] Thus, the prevailing opinion at the time was that nerve grafts had little role to play in the management of nerve injuries.[28]

World War II provided surgeons with a distressing number of nerve injuries. Woodhall and Beebe reported on 3415 peripheral nerve injuries in which nerve grafts were used on 0.9%.[38] Seddon reported on 1681 nerve injuries, of which 699 underwent some type of surgical repair and 59 underwent autogenous nerve grafting.[28] In 1963, Seddon reported a series of 109 nerve grafts with results comparable to direct suture repair in 70%.[27] His landmark data established that results of grafting are superior in distal nerve lesions, such as digital nerves, and superior in children.

The development of microneurosurgery in the 1960s, as well as the pioneering work of Millesi who introduced interfascicular grafting, enhanced interest in nerve grafting and led to increased clinical success. Millesi emphasized the importance of good microsurgical technique, including instrumentation, sutures, and magnification, in obtaining success with nerve grafts.[19] Both Millesi and Terzis showed experimentally that primary repair under tension was inferior to nerve grafting.[20,33]

Donor site morbidity in autologous nerve grafting has encouraged surgeons to explore alternate conduits to bridge nerve gaps. Both autologous vein grafts and polyglycolic tubes show promise, and are further discussed later in the chapter.[6,13,35]

Taylor reported the first successful vascularized nerve graft in 1976.[31] Both experimental and clinical work have yielded conflicting results, and, in general, vascularized nerve grafts have not been superior to conventional nerve grafts for digital nerve injuries, except in scarred and poorly vascularized tissue beds as shown by Rose.[17,25]

A gap in a nerve may be created in a variety of situations. This includes segmental loss secondary to injury, retraction, and loss of elasticity of nerves when direct repair is delayed, resection of a neuroma or glioma with delayed repair, and resection of a neuroma in continuity, or other nerve tumors. Nerve grafting of digital nerves is indicated whenever direct repair cannot be performed without undue tension. The obvious advantage of a single repair site for axons to traverse after direct repair is negated if the repair site is under tension. Gould advocates grafting of digital nerves when a gap exceeds 1 cm.[9]

The ten proper digital nerves do not have equal importance for hand function. Most surgeons believe that the critical nerves are the radial and ulnar digital nerve to the thumb, the radial digital nerve to the index and middle finger, and the ulnar digital nerve to the little finger. Reconstruction of the remaining nerves depends in part on the patient's occupation as well as the patient's desires.

Nerve grafting will decrease the risk of recurrence of painful neuromas after resection.

Nerve grafting also is recommended when direct repair places the repaired nerve in a dysvascular or scarred tissue bed. The additional length of a graft may allow placement of the nerve in an ideal tissue bed.

Although primary nerve grafting is rarely indicated, it is sometimes wise to perform nerve grafting during replantation surgery to prevent secondary operations, which may jeopardize vascular repairs.

Although some surgeons believe that nerve lacerations at or beyond the level of the distal interphalangeal joint will spontaneously regenerate, Wilgis has shown that grafting of these lesions is a useful procedure.[37]

Nerve grafting is contraindicated in the face of infection or when surrounding skin and soft tissue viability is questionable. The results of traditional nerve grafting in dysvascular and scarred tissue beds is poor.[3] However, this is now considered by some to be an indication for vascularized nerve grafting.[25]

■ SURGICAL TECHNIQUES

The decision to perform nerve grafting of a digital nerve is generally made after exposure and appropriate debridement of divided nerve ends, but it should be anticipated ahead of time. In preparation for any nerve repair or reconstruction, patients should receive informed consent regarding the possibility of nerve grafting, including the risk of permanent anesthesia in the cutaneous distribution of the donor nerve.

Surgery may be performed under general or regional anesthesia, although many surgeons prefer general anesthesia because any movement by the patient during microneurorrhaphy may jeopardize the result.

The neurovascular bundles to the fingers lie on the palmar side of the lumbrical muscles, nestled between the flexor tendons. In the palm the digital nerves lie deep to the common digital arteries, but, beyond the distal palmar crease, the nerves lie superficial to the arteries. The superficial palmar arch is at risk when exposing the digital nerves arising from the median nerve. The common digital nerves divide into proper digital nerves at the level of the palmar creases. The common digital arteries divide farther distally, approximately midway between the distal palmar crease and the margin of the web. Distal to the distal interphalangeal joint, the digital nerves divide into at least three and sometimes more terminal branches.

The three most important digital nerves, the radial digital nerve to the index finger and the two digital nerves to the thumb, are, ironically, the most vulnerable to injury as the remainder of the nerves lie deep to the palmar aponeurosis in the palm. When intact, the two digital nerves of the thumb may be palpated near the midline of the thumb at the level of the metacarpophalangeal crease. The radial nerve to the index finger may be palpated as it crosses the index metacarpal head 1 cm ulnar to the radial extent of the proximal palmar crease.

Initial dissection is performed under tourniquet control with $2.5\times$ to $4.5\times$ loupe magnification. A Bruner zigzag incision is used for wide exposure of lesions in the palm or proximal portion of the digit, but a midlateral incision is preferred for distal digital lesions. The initial laceration may dictate variations from these exposures.

Normal nerve is identified in an unscarred tissue bed both proximally and distally and dissection continues toward the zone of injury. The neuroma of the proximal stump and the glioma of the distal stump are resected sharply with a single-edged razor over a moistened wooden tongue depressor, or, alternatively, with a single stroke of a fresh scalpel blade or sharp serrated scissors. Trimming is continued as necessary until remaining nerve tissue appears normal under magnification, with bulging of fascicles from the cut end proximally and a normal appearing sheath distally.

Only after resection back to normal appearing unscarred nerve tissue can the decision regarding the need for a nerve graft be made definitively. If the nerve ends can be reapproximated without tension, direct suture is performed. A simple test for this is to see if nerve ends will remain opposed with a single 8-0 epineural suture. Flexing the interphalangeal joints to effect a direct repair is never tolerated, as this may lead to permanent joint contracture, or the regenerated axons may be disrupted when the finger is extended.

However, some flexion of the wrist or metacarpophalangeal (MP) joint for several weeks is permissible if it will obviate the need for grafting.

If grafting is necessary, the length of the graft is determined by measuring the gap created in the nerve when the wrist, MP and interphalangeal (IP) joints are held in extension, as described by Nunley.[22] Nerve grafts shrink 10% to 15%, so this additional length must be included.[28] Selecting a donor nerve from the ipsilateral arm or forearm simplifies the procedure and allows the surgery to be performed under regional anesthesia. Potential donors include the lateral antebrachial cutaneous nerve, the medial antebrachial cutaneous nerve, the terminal portion of the posterior interosseous nerve, the dorsal sensory branch of the ulnar nerve, digital nerves from noncritical sides of adjacent fingers, and, during replantation surgery, digital nerves from nonreplantable fingers.

In major reconstructive procedures in which multiple nerve grafts are needed, certain sensory nerves from the lower extremity may be used. Potential donors include the sural nerve, the lateral cutaneous nerve of the thigh, and the posterior cutaneous nerve of the thigh.

The lateral antebrachial cutaneous nerve is popular with some surgeons but may innervate portions of the thumb and should not be used if a digital nerve to the thumb is injured. It may be harvested with a transverse incision lateral to the biceps tendon, between the cephalic vein and the accessory cephalic vein; it lies deep to both. Up to 20 cm can be harvested using multiple small incisions.[16]

The terminal portion of the posterior interosseous nerve is preferred by some because there is no sensory deficit.[36] The posterior interosseous nerve is harvested through a longitudinal incision over the fourth dorsal wrist compartment, beginning distally at the level of Lister's tubercle and extending proximally 5 to 6 cm. The extensor retinaculum is partially divided over the fourth compartment and the extensor digitorum communis and extensor indicis proprius tendons are retracted. The nerve is located in the deep, radial aspect of the fourth compartment, lying proximally on the interosseous membrane, and distally on the periosteum of the radius, ulnar to Lister's tubercle.[36] The nerve is accompanied in the distal forearm by the posterior branch of the anterior interosseous artery and terminates in one or two major branches that supply the wrist capsule. It may be harvested from the level of the terminal motor branch in the forearm to the wrist capsule, supplying 5 to 10 cm of graft. The posterior interosseous nerve measures 1 to 5 mm in diameter.[36] Its diameter is well-suited for nerve grafting in the digit, but it is usually too small to graft digital nerves in the palm. Here, the lateral or medial antebrachial cutaneous nerve or sural nerve should be harvested.

Before suturing the graft, the tourniquet is deflated, and epineural bleeding is controlled with a bipolar microelectrocautery. The tourniquet may be reinflated if necessary. A colored plastic background is inserted. Although loupes are acceptable for nerve repair in the palm and proximal digit, most hand surgeons believe that higher magnification under a microscope allows more precise repairs.[10]

Excess epineural tissue at the ends of the graft and divided nerve is resected under the microscope to prevent it from interposing in the repair site. Either the proximal or the distal end of the graft is sutured in place. The graft is then placed in the bed, along the side of the end of the recipient nerve (Fig. 98–1). The required length is then accurately

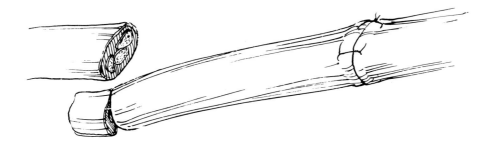

■ FIGURE 98–1
One end of the graft is sutured first, the graft is positioned in the bed, and the other end is then accurately trimmed.

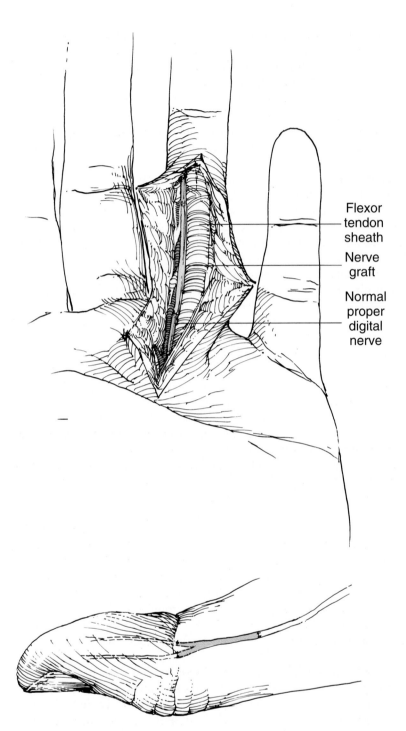

Flexor
tendon
sheath

Nerve
graft

Normal
proper
digital
nerve

estimated and the graft is sharply trimmed. The other end of the graft is then sutured into place (Fig. 98–2). Suturing is performed with 8–0 to 9–0 monofilament nylon on 75 to 130 μm taper-point needles. Epineural sutures are placed 180° apart and are tightened so that the epineurium approximates without bunching. Sutures may be placed at 90° intervals, if necessary, to prevent bulging of intraneural contents. Usually, two to four sutures are adequate.

In special cases where the reconstruction involves a bifurcation, the graft can be teased apart between fascicles. These surgically developed branches in the graft can then be repaired to the transected end of the injured nerve (Fig. 98–3).

The wound is closed, and a bulky, compressive dressing and splint are applied with the IP joints in full extension, the MP joints in 70° of flexion, and the wrist in slight flexion. Sutures are removed at ten days and gentle range of motion exercises are initiated, unless tension at surgery requires positioning of multiple joints in flexion. In that case, range of motion can commence approximately 1 week later.

There are five general methods available to overcome gaps in peripheral nerves: nerve mobilization, nerve transposition, joint immobilization, bone shortening, and bridging the gap with a nerve graft or other conduit. Not all of these are applicable to digital nerves injuries.

■ TECHNICAL ALTERNATIVES

Digital nerves may be mobilized in situ to provide several millimeters of additional length by dissecting along the epineurium and releasing soft tissues. When this is combined with joint positioning of the wrist and MP joints, gaps in digital nerves up to one cm can be overcome. Nerve rerouting and transposition, procedures useful for some nerve injuries, have no role in the treatment of digital nerve injuries. As previously mentioned, flexing the IP joints to overcome nerve gaps should never be tolerated. Bone shortening during replantations or revascularizations with associated fractures may prevent the need for nerve grafting. Most surgeons are reluctant to proceed with bone shortening if no fracture exists.

Much of the early experimentation in nerve grafting involved the use of xenografts and allografts.[26] The results of xenografts have been universally poor. The results of allografts also have been dismal in older clinical trials and have been scarcely used in modern times, although recent basic research holds some promise for their clinical use in the future.[12,18,34]

The morbidity of sacrificing normal sensory nerves to use as grafts continues to stimulate interest in alternative methods to bridge nerve gaps. Mackinnon and Dellon used tubes of bioabsorbable polyglycolic acid to bridge digital nerve gaps of 0.5 to 3.0 cm in 15 patients and reported results comparable to classic nerve grafting.[13] Walton used autogenous vein grafts to bridge digital nerve gaps of 1 to 3 cm.[35] In 13 acute reconstructions, 2 patients failed to regain two-point discrimination and the remaining 11 had a moving two-point discrimination of 8 mm or less. Only one of five delayed repairs had return of two-point discrimination. Chiu and Strauch reported an average static two-point discrimination of 11.1 mm and moving two-point discrimination of 6.5 mm following vein grafting of digital nerve gaps less than 3 cm.[6] Tang used reversed vein grafts to bridge gaps from 0.5 to 5.8 cm in digits undergoing simultaneous zone 2 flexor tendon surgery.[30] His reported results also were comparable to classic nerve graft techniques. Although these results appear promising, they await larger clinical trials and should still be considered investigational.

The risks that are unique to autologous nerve grafting techniques all involve donor site morbidity. This includes donor site anesthesia, painful neuromas, and unsightly scars. The use of synthetic conduits negates these risks and the use of vein conduits negates all but the potential of an unsightly scar.

When nerve repair or reconstruction is performed acutely, early postoperative rehabilitation is usually guided more by the associated bone and tendon injuries than by the nerve injury. However, since nerve grafting is almost always performed as a secondary procedure, associated injuries usually allow range of motion exercise to begin at the time of suture removal. Splinting is discontinued at the time of suture removal.

■ REHABILITATION

Nerve regeneration is followed by a Tinel's sign and advancement of 1 to 3 mm per day is anticipated after an initial delay of approximately 1 month. Pressure threshold testing using Semmes-Weinstein monofilaments and innervation density testing using static and dynamic two-point discrimination are useful in monitoring return of sensation. Dellon's moving two-point discrimination test allows an earlier assessment of discrimination than the static test. This is because it depends on quickly adapting fibers, which return sooner than the slowly adapting fibers needed for static discrimination. The clinician may find it useful to record both of these to compare with data in the literature because, unfortunately, many studies report only one or the other test.

Sensory re-education is begun early by hand therapists. Initially, patients lack protective

TABLE 98–1 STATIC TWO-POINT DISCRIMINATION FOR DIGITAL NERVE GRAFTS

Author	# of Grafts	Source	<6 mm	7–15 mm	>15 mm	No 2-PD	Ave. 2-PD
Young[41]	27	Sural	4	7	16	0	—
McFarlane[16]	13	LAC	0	6	5	2	16 mm
Greene[10]	15	D. Ulnar	4	6	2	3	9.5 mm
Tenny[32]	42	LAC	17	15	10	0	—
Nunley[22]	21	MAC	6	12	0	3	13.4 mm
Wilgis[37]	12	Sural/LAC	8	4	0	0	5.9 mm
Moneim[22]	3	MAC	2	1	0	0	—
Yamano[39]	8	LFC	0	8	0	0	10.5 mm
Hirasawa[11]	2	?	0	2	0	0	12.5 mm
Frykman[8]	24	?	1	5	3	15*	—
TOTAL	167		42 (25%)	66 (40%)	36 (22%)	23 (14%)	11.3 mm

LAC =   lateral antebrachial cutaneous nerve
D. Ulnar = dorsal sensory branch of ulnar nerve
MAC =   medial antebrachial cutaneous nerve
LFC =   lateral femoral cutaneous nerve
* 11 of these are in 2 patients with severe crush injuries

sensation and are taught to compensate for this by using both visual and cognitive awareness of hand position and use. Most patients experience dysesthesias during early nerve regeneration. These patients do well with desensitization techniques using graded stimuli.[2] When the patient develops the ability to identify the touch of the examiner's finger, localization training is begun followed by tactile gnosis training.[7]

■ OUTCOMES

There is no single test that adequately documents the return of functional sensibility. Different authors use a variety of tests to measure sensibility. This includes static and moving two-point discrimination, sharp versus dull discrimination, monofilament "threshold" testing, hot versus cold discrimination, vibration preception with tuning forks of 30 and 256 Hz, texture differentiation, and shape identification. Further confusion results from the fact that some authors anesthetize the opposite digital nerve to prevent "crossover" sensibility, while others do not.

Most authors have reported static two-point discrimination. The results of several modern studies using conventional nerve grafts (nonvascularized grafts) and microsurgical technique are listed in Table 98–1. An average two-point discrimination was calculated in studies, which included exact values for individual patients. From these data, one would predict that 25% of digital nerve grafts should obtain normal (less than 6 mm) two-point discrimination and that 86% of grafts should have some two-point discrimination.

The prognosis in children is excellent, and return of sensation is inversely related to age.[27] It must be recognized that adult patients with normal monofilament and two-point testing will not have normal sensibility. What is clear, however, is that useful and functional sensation should be anticipated with current microneural techniques.

References

1. Albert E: Einige Operationen an Nerven. Wien Med Presse, 1885; 26:1285.
2. Barber LM: Desensitization of the traumatized hand. In: Hunter JM, Schneider LH, Mackin EJ, Callahan AD (eds): Rehabilitation of the Hand, 2nd Ed, St Louis: C. V. Mosby, 1984: 493–502.
3. Beazley WC, Milek MA, Reiss BH: Results of nerve grafting in severe soft tissue injuries. Clin Orthop, 1984; 188:208–212.
4. Bunnell S: Surgery of nerves of the hand. Surg Gynecol Obstet, 1927; 44:145–152.

5. Bunnell S: Suture of facial nerve within temporal bone with report of first successful case. Surg Gynecol Obstet, 1927; 45:7–12.

6. Chiu D, Strauch B: A prospective clinical evaluation of autogenous vein grafts used as a nerve conduit for distal sensory nerve defects of 3 cm or less. Plast Reconstr Surg, 1990; 928–934.

7. Dellon AL, Curtis RM, Edgerton MT: Re-education of sensation in the hand following nerve injury. Plast Reconst Surg. 1974; 53:297–305.

8. Frykman GK, Cally D: Interfascicular nerve grafting. Orthop Clin North Am, 1988; 19:71–80.

9. Gould JS: Digital nerves. In: Gelberman RH (ed): Operative Nerve Repair and Reconstruction, Philadelphia: J. B. Lippincott, 1991:453–460.

10. Greene TL, Steichen JB: Digital nerve grafting using the dorsal sensory branch of the ulnar nerve. J Hand Surg, 1985; 10B:37–40.

11. Hirasawa Y, Katsumi Y, Tokioka T: Evaluation of sensibility after sensory reconstruction ot the thumb. J Bone Joint Surg, 1986; 67B:814–819.

12. Ishida O, Daves J, Tsai TM, Breidenbach WC, Firrell J: Regeneration following rejection of peirpheral nerve allografts of rats on withdrawal of cyclosporine. Plast Reconst Surg, 1993; 92:916–926.

13. Mackinnon SE, Dellon AL: Clinical nerve reconstruction with a bioabsorbable polyglycolic acid tube. Plast Reconstr Surg, 1990; 85:419–424.

14. MacKinnon SE, Hudson AR: Clinical application of peripheral nerve transplantation. Plast Reconst Surg, 1992; 90:695–699.

15. Mayo-Robinson AW: Nerve grafting as a means of restoring function in limbs paralysed by gunshot or other injuries. Br Med J, 1917; 1:117–118.

16. McFarlane R, Mayer J: Digital nerve grafts with the lateral antebrachial cutaneous nerve. J Hand Surg, 1976; 1:169–173.

17. Merle M, Dautel G: Vascularized nerve grafts. J Hand Surg, 1991; 16B:483–488.

18. Midha R, Mackinnon SE, Evans PJ, et al: Comparison of regeneration across nerve allografts with temporary or continuous cyclosporin A immunosuppression. J Neurosurg, 1993; 78: 90–100.

19. Millesi H, Meissl G, Berger A: Further experience with interfascicular grafting of the median, ulnar, and radial nerves. J Bone Joint Surg, 1976; 58A:209–218.

20. Millesi H, Meissl G, Berger A: The interfascicular nerve grafting of the median and ulnar nerves. J Bone Joint Surg, 1972; 54A:727–750.

21. Moneim MS: Interfascicular nerve grafting. Clin Orthop, 1982; 163:65–74.

22. Nunley JA, Ugino MR, Goldner RD, Regan N, Urbaniak JR: Use of the anterior branch of the medial antebrachial cutaneous nerve as a graft for the repair of defects of the digital nerve. J Bone Joint Surg, 1989; 71A:563–567.

23. Philipeaux JM, Vulpian A: Note sur les essais de greffe d'un troncon de nerf lingual entre les deux bouts de l'hypoglosse. Arch Physiol Norm Pathol, 1870; 3:618–620.

24. Platt H: On the results of bridging gaps in injured nerve trunks by autogenous fascial tubulization and autogenous nerve grafts. Br J Surg, 1920; 7:384–389.

25. Rose EH, Kowaslki TA, Norris MS: The reversed venous arterialized nerve graft in digital nerve reconstruction across scarred beds. Plast Reconstruc Surg, 1989; 83:593–602.

26. Sanders FK: The repair of large gaps in the peripheral nerves. Brain, 1942; 65:281–337.

27. Seddon HJ: Nerve grafting. J Bone Joint Surg, 1963; 45B:447–461.

28. Seddon HJ: The use of autogenous grafts for the repair of large gaps in peripheral nerves. Br J Surg, 1947; 35:151–167.

29. Stopford JSB: The treatment of large defects in peripheral nerve injuries. Lancet, 1920; 2: 1296–1297.

30. Tang JB, Gu YQ, Song YS: Repair of digital nerve defect with autogenous vein graft during flexor tendon surgery in zone 2. J Hand Surg, 1993; 18B:449–453.

31. Taylor GI, Ham F: The free vascularized nerve graft. Plast Reconstr Surg, 1976; 57:413–426.

32. Tenny JR, Lewis RC: Digital nerve-grafting for traumatic defects. Use of the lateral antebrachial cutaneous nerve. J Bone Joint Surg, 1984; 66A:1375–1379.

33. Terzis JK, Gaibisoff BA, Williams B. The nerve gap: Suture under tension versus graft. Plast Reconstr Surg, 1975; 56:166–170.

34. Trumble TE, Parvin D: Cell viability and migration in nerve isografts and allografts. J Reconst Microsurg, 1994; 10:27–34.

35. Walton RL, Brown RE, Matory WE, Borah GL, Dolph JL: Autogenous vein graft repair of

digital nerve defects in the finger: A retrospective clinical study. Plast Reconstr Surg, 1989; 84:944–952.

36. Waters PM, Schwartz JT: Posterior interosseous nerve: An anatomic study of potential nerve grafts. J Hand Surg, 1993; 18A:743–745.

37. Wilgis E, Maxwell G: Distal digital nerve grafts: Clinical and anatomical studies. J Hand Surg, 1979; 4:439–443.

38. Woodall B, Beebe WG: In: Peripheral Nerve Regeneration, A follow-up study of 3,656 World War II injuries. VA Medical Monograph, US Government Printing Office, Washington, D.C., 1956.

39. Yamano Y, Namba Y, Hino Y, et al: Digital nerve grafts in replanted digits. Hand, 1982; 14: 255–262.

40. Young L, Wray RC, Weeks PM: A randomized prospective comparison of fascicular and epineural digital nerve repairs. Plast Reconstr Surg, 1981; 68:89–92.

41. Young VL, Wray RC, Weeks PM: The results of nerve grafting in the wrist and hand. Ann Plast Surg, 1979; 5:212–215.

99

Median Nerve Grafting in the Forearm

Median nerve injuries in the forearm present as either low or high deficits. A low median nerve deficit is described as loss of thenar motor power and loss of sensation to the palm and volar aspect of the radial three and one half digits. A high median nerve deficit is similar to the low deficit plus the additional loss of the extrinsic flexor function of the pronator teres, flexor carpi radialis, flexor digitorum superficialis, index and long finger flexor digitorum profundus (FDP), flexor pollicus longus (FPL), and pronator quadratus. Injuries to isolated nerve branches such as the anterior interosseous nerve (AIN) present as loss of the FPL, FDP, and pronator quadratus function. High median nerve and AIN dysfunction usually results from trauma to the proximal third of the forearm. Low median nerve deficits result from trauma to the nerve in the mid and distal third of the forearm.

We discuss the repair of median nerve deficits in the forearm with consideration given to the historic perspective of nerve grafting in general, the specific indications for median nerve repair, and the surgical exposure necessary to perform that repair.

Nerve grafting was first described experimentally in 1810 by Phillipeaux. As early as 1885, Albert described the first nerve graft (a xenograft) used clinically to repair a nerve gap in humans. In 1928, Bunnell reported regeneration rates through autogenous grafts that equaled direct nerve repair rates. In 1927, he reported successful facial nerve repair by grafting, and in 1928 he reported successfully grafting a digital nerve defect.[3] Seddon described the technique of cable grafting in 1947.[17] Also, in 1947, the use of a vascularized nerve graft was introduced by Strange.[19]

Initially, free autogenous nerve grafting was associated with poor outcomes.[14,16] Millesi introduced grouped fascicular (funicular) repair of nerve gaps in 1972 and reported that the reliability of free nerve grafting could be improved if the nerve was separated into groups of fascicles and like-sized groups were reconnected with a tension-free repair.[11]

Nerve defects have been repaired with numerous materials. These include autogenous nonvascularized and vascularized autografts, allografts, and various conduits. Allografts and conduits are presently investigational tools and have as yet not proven to be reliable. The most commonly used donor material remains autogenous cable grafts harvested from the sural nerve, lateral femoral cutaneous nerve, dorsal antebrachial cutaneous nerve, lateral antebrachial cutaneous nerve, or superficial radial nerve. These nerve grafts have no inherent blood supply and are therefore vascularized by invasions of vessels from the surrounding soft tissue bed. The implication is that the viability of the nerve graft and its incorporation are intimately associated with an environment conducive to the formation of the adhesions necessary for vascular supply.

The role of free vascularized nerve grafts is still being defined. Recent reports state that vascularized grafts are indicated when a reconstruction is to be performed in a densely scarred area or the nerve gap is greater than 6 cm.[2] Whether immediately vascularized as free tissue transfer or vascularized by in-growth from adjacent tissue, Wallerian degeneration occurs within the nerve graft, and regeneration will dictate the final outcome.

Median nerve repair is indicated when wounds are clean, the skeleton stable, and there is adequate soft tissue coverage. This demands that, in open wounds, the zone of injury has been defined by removing all doubtfully viable tissue and the proximal and distal

■ HISTORY OF THE TECHNIQUE

■ INDICATIONS AND CONTRAINDICATIONS

775

extent of nerve injury has been determined. If these criteria can be met promptly after injury, reconstruction of the nerve should proceed straight away. This is especially true if a complex repair of other injured structures would preclude or inhibit later nerve repair. If wound stability is questionable, then nerve repair is delayed.

If the repair is delayed, then the possibility of nerve grafts should always be considered and discussed with the patient preoperatively. The potential need for grafts is not precluded by the mechanism of injury. Even the ends of a sharply lacerated nerve retract and, with time, will become densely scarred.

Graft reconstruction of an isolated AIN is seldom indicated for several reasons. Most injuries occur distal to the innervation of the FDP to the index and middle fingers and the FPL. A denervated pronator quadratus is not a significant impairment. Those injuries that denervate the FDP to the index and middle fingers and FPL can be readily reconstructed with tendon transfers. Index and middle FDP function is restored by side-to-side tenodesis with the ring and small finger FDP. FPL function can be reconstructed with transfer of the ring or the long finger flexor digitorum superficialis. The one possible indication for graft reconstruction of the AIN is when a complex injury of the forearm has resulted in a combined ulnar nerve and AIN deficit.

The length of any nerve deficit is defined by sharply resecting the nerve ends until internal architecture is identified and groups of fascicles protrude from the cut ends. The gap is measured, and one of three treatment options is chosen. First, if more than an 8-cm graft is required, then the benefits of reconstruction in an adult are questionable and the nerve repair may be abandoned.[3] Second, the nerve ends are mobilized and repaired under tension. Third, the gap is bridged with a graft.

Techniques for overcoming segmental defects in peripheral nerves, without interposition grafting, include in situ mobilization, transposition, joint positioning, and bone shortening. Only bone shortening renders a repair without some degree of tension-induced ischemia.

The tolerable length of nerve mobilization obtained by stripping mesoneurial attachments may be 45 times the nerve diameter or 8 to 12 cm along either end of a nerve in the forearm.[10] The exact amount of stretching that the human nerve will tolerate is not known, and experimental results are contradictory. Clark and co-authors have shown that stretching a rat sciatic nerve beyond 15% of original length markedly reduces blood flow within the nerve.[1] By inference, the human median nerve exposed over a length of 20 cm can accommodate gaps of no more than 3 cm in the average adult. Hentz examined nerve gaps in a primate model and concluded that single nerve repairs provided better results than cable grafts for gaps as large as 4 cm. The implication is that despite the tension with which the repairs were performed, one repair site is better than bridging 4-cm gaps with grafts using two repairs.

Zachary reported that the median nerve can be mobilized 3 to 4 cm with elbow flexion and 2 to 3 cm with wrist flexion.[22] Elbow flexion beyond 90° and wrist flexion beyond 40° should be avoided. The gains in nerve length obtained by joint positioning beyond these limits usually will fall short of any anticipated benefit. Releasing the lacertus fibrosis, pronator teres, and the origin of flexor digitorum superficialis will provide additional length.

Nerve grafting is indicated when end-to-end repairs cannot be performed. Age, timing, location, and length of nerve gaps should be considered before nerve grafts are performed. In a review of 132 median nerve reconstructions, Kallio and Vastamäaki presented consistently poor results associated with patients older than 54 years, an injury more than 56 cm proximal to the finger tips, a treatment delay of more than 24 months, and nerve gaps greater than 7 cm.[9] Millesi,[12] who reported predominantly satisfactory results with interfascicular cable grafts, suggests that nerve gaps greater than 2.5 cm should be grafted. He does not provide an upper limit to graft length but notes that the best results are in grafts less then 5 cm long.

As a rule, we believe that if a major peripheral nerve will not stay approximated with two 8–0 nylon sutures placed 180° apart in the epineurium, then interposition grafts should be considered. For smaller nerves, the same criteria are used with 9–0 nylon sutures.

The median nerve is composed of fibers from the fifth cervical through the first thoracic ventral spinal roots. The median nerve is formed from branches of the medial and lateral cords of the brachial plexus. In the forearm, the median nerve sequentially innervates the pronator teres, flexor digitorum superficialis, flexor carpi radialis, and palmaris longus. The AIN sequentially innervates the FDP, FPL, and pronator quadratus. In the hand, the median nerve sequentially innervates the flexor pollicis brevis, opponens pollicis, abductor pollicis brevis, the unipennate lumbricals (usually the index and middle), and the skin overlying the volar aspect of the thumb, index, long, and radial one half of the ring finger.

The median nerve enters the forearm posterior to the biciptal aponeurosis, medial to the brachial artery, and anterior to the brachialis muscle. It then courses deeper between the superficial (humeral) and deep (ulnar) heads of the pronator teres. As the nerve passes beneath the proximal edge of the pronator teres, the brachial artery branches into the radial and ulnar arteries. The radial artery remains lateral to the median nerve and continues its passage superficial to the tendon of the pronator teres and flexor digitorum superficialis muscle belly, respectively. The ulnar artery runs in a medial oblique direction passing beneath the median nerve and the humeroulnar origin of the flexor digitorum superficialis. Within 3 cm of its origin, the ulnar artery gives rise to the common interosseous artery. The median nerve traverses the origins of the pronator teres and dives beneath the fibrous arch from which the flexor digitorum superficialis originates. Just distal to this arch, the median nerve bifurcates into the larger median nerve trunk and the smaller AIN. The median nerve then travels between the flexor digitorum superficialis (FDS) and FDP. The nerve is bound to the under surface of FDS by the muscular investing fascia and sometimes travels within the substance of FDS. Distally, the median nerve emerges between the FDS and flexor carpi radialis 5 to 7 cm proximal to where the nerve enters the carpal tunnel.

The AIN arises from the dorsal surface of the median nerve, approximately 5 cm distal to the medial epicondyle and just as the median nerve passes beneath the origin to the FDS. The anterior interosseous artery (a branch from the common interosseous artery) then joins the AIN to travel between the FDS and profundus. At the midforearm level, the nerve passes between the profundus and the flexor pollicis longus to reach the interosseous membrane. The nerve follows the interosseous membrane to innervate the pronator quadratus from the dorsal surface of the muscle.

General anesthesia is used for most chronic cases because of the potential need to harvest nerve grafts from the lower extremities. Regional or general anesthesia is appropriate in the acute setting. The choice is usually dictated by the experience and acumen of the anesthetist. Gaul[4] advocates performing the initial exposure with a general anesthetic, dissecting the fascicles of the proximal and distal stumps, and waking the patient intraoperatively to determine the sensory fascicles proximally and the electrically active of fascicles distally. Mapping the proximal stump demands an excellent rapport among surgeon, anesthetist, and patient. Mapping the distal stump is futile after 1 week because of Wallerian degeneration. Gaul used the technique for both median and ulnar nerve injuries throughout the forearm with reported success. We find this technique to be helpful in the distal forearm but have been discouraged with attempts to identify fascicles that are predominantly sensory or motor in the proximal half of the forearm.

The patient is positioned on the operating table in the supine position with the shoulder abducted, the elbow extended, and the forearm held in supination. Hyperabduction of the shoulder and excessive traction on the brachial plexus is avoided. The injured extremity and one of the lower extremities is isolated in the operative field. The surgeon and assistant are positioned across from each other on either side of the forearm, and an operative microscope is positioned such that the anesthetist, the surgeons, and the nurse have adequate access to the patient. We bring the microscope either from the head of the bed or directly from the end of the hand table.

Dissection is conducted with a tourniquet inflated to 100 mm Hg above systolic blood pressure. Tourniquet duration is limited to 90 minutes and at least 10 minutes should pass before the tourniquet is reinflated. These parameters are based on two studies. Heppenstall and co-authors demonstrated that permanent changes will occur in nerves and muscles subjected to ischemia beyond 90 minutes. Newman used magnetic resonance spectroscopy to show that metabolic changes do not return to normal for at least 10 minutes after tourniquet deflation.[7,23]

Whether the trauma is acute or chronic, nerve injuries are best approached by identifying the nerve distal and proximal to the zone of injury and following the nerve into the area of trauma.

In Henry's text, two approaches to the volar forearm are described.[5] The first consists of an incision that crosses the antecubital fossa adjacent to the pronator teres until reaching the edge of the brachioradialis. The incision is then directed toward the radial styloid. This approach, often referred to as "Henry's" anterior approach to the forearm, was intended for exposure of the radius and is mentioned here to forewarn the reader that although the incision may provide access to the median nerve at the junction of the proximal and mid third of the forearm, the incision is inadequate for exposure of the median nerve elsewhere. In the distal one half to one third of the forearm, the incision is too radial for easy exposure and repair of the median nerve, does not provide access to the median nerve in the palm, and fails to provide access to the ulnar nerve in the case of a combined median and ulnar nerve injury. The second volar forearm incision described by Henry is credited to McConnell and is an excellent approach to the median and ulnar nerves in the forearm. The incision starts at the pisiform and goes straight to the medial epicondyle. The deeper dissection is between the muscle bellies of the FDS and the FDP. The median and ulnar nerve can be easily exposed in the distal three quarters of the forearm, but proximally the dissection is difficult. Millesi prefers this approach because this incision prevents placing surgical scars in the vicinity of the nerve repair and obviates any microvascular compromise that may result from scar contacture.[12] These concerns may be overlystated. With the exception of the elbow and the wrist, the median nerve in the forearm is covered by muscle, and the muscle acts as a barrier to contiguous scarring.

Littler proposed a lazy "S" incision, which incorporates the advantages of Henry's exposure of the proximal forearm and McConnell's exposure of the nerve in the distal forearm. The incision divides the forearm into a proximal, middle, and distal third. The proximal third incision runs from the medial epicondyle in a distal and radial direction parallel to the pronator teres. After reaching the radius, the middle third incision curves back toward the ulna, proximal to the wrist creases. In the distal third of the forearm, the incision is directed toward the palm.[18]

Roland, in the third edition of Green's *Operative Hand Surgery*, described an incision for use in the treatment of volar compartment syndromes that is easily adapted to extensile exposure of the median nerve throughout the forearm. In his presentation he stated that a broad exposure should meet the following five criteria: (1) damage to cutaneous nerves is avoided and as many longitudinal veins as possible are retained; (2) skin flaps are created to cover the median nerve at the wrist and the ulnar nerve at the elbow while awaiting secondary closure; (3) the median and ulnar nerves can be released as they pass through the the carpal tunnel and Guyon's canal, respectively; (4) the brachial artery may be explored; and (5) straight line incisions particularly across the wrist and elbow are avoided.[15]

Based on these criteria, Roland proposed the incision illustrated in Figure 99–1.

The incision described below is a modification of the above and provides exposure to the median nerve from above the elbow to the hand. The incision is divided into five parts (A to E) and differs from that described by Roland only in part B.

Part A: The palmar incision is similar to that proposed by Taleisnik for carpal tunnel release.[21] The incison begins at the intersection of two lines. The first line starts at the apex of the first web space and runs parallel to the proximal palmar crease. The second line runs parallel to the radial border of the ring finger. From this starting point the incision is carried longitudinally to the distal wrist crease.

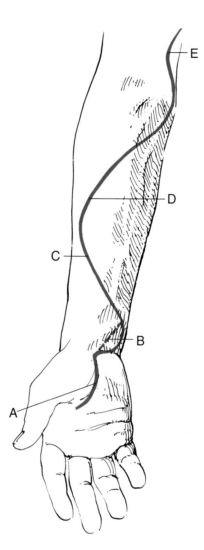

■ FIGURE 99-1
A utilitarian incision described by Roland (solid line) provides extensile exposure of the median and ulnar nerve in the forearm.[19] The dotted line at the wrist is our modification.

Part B: From the wrist, the incision is directed ulnarly at a 60° angle until reaching the radial border of the flexor carpi ulnaris. This is usually one to 2 cm proximal to the intersection of the flexor carpi ulnaris and the proximal wrist crease.

Roland advocated taking the incision transversely across the flexion crease to the ulnar boarder of the wrist and directing it upward to create a 5-cm wide flap. In our experience, using the incision described by Roland has been associated with dysesthesias along the base of the hypothenar eminence, perhaps resulting from injury to terminal cutaneous branches of the ulnar nerve. Since using the modification shown as a dotted line in Figure 99–1, there have been no problems with dysesthesias, nerve exposure, or wound closure.

Part C: From the radial border of the flexor carpi ulnaris, the incision is directed proximally and radially in a gentle curve to a point in line with the radius, halfway between the elbow flexion crease and the proximal wrist crease. It is in this region that the pronator teres passes beneath the brachioradialis to insert on the radius.

Part D: From the intersection of the pronator teres with the brachioradialis, the gentle curve turns ulnarly to run parallel to the pronator teres ending at a point just radial to the medial epicondyle of the elbow.

Part E: The final limb of the incision starts at the point just radial to the medial epicondyle and is directed along the medial midline of the arm. This last limb is necessary only when the median nerve must be identified in the arm.

For the sake of illustration, the forearm can be divided into proximal, middle, and distal thirds. The median nerve is exposed in the distal third of the forearm through parts B and C. Exposure into the hand is through part A. In the middle third of the forearm, the median nerve is exposed through parts C and D and occasionally part B. In the proximal third of the forearm, part D and the distal aspect of part E are used to approach the median nerve.

Proximally, there is no internervous plane between the biceps (musculocutaneous nerve) and brachialis muscles (musculocutaneous nerve). Distally, the internervous plane is between the pronator teres (median nerve) and the brachioradialis (radial nerve).

The superficial dissection divides the fascia in line with the skin incision (part D). At the elbow crease, the branches of the antecubital veins that cross between the basilic and cephalic venous systems are ligated. The bicipital aponeurosis is incised adjacent to the biceps tendon. At the level of the humeral epicondyles, the brachial artery and median nerve, the more medial structure, are identified immediately underneath the divided bicipital aponeurosis. Proceeding distally, the artery and nerve will sink into the depths of the antecubital fossa. As the superficial dissection passes radially the biceps tendon is identified and branches of the lateral antebrachial cutaneous nerve may be seen entering the forearm between the biceps and brachioradialis. These cutaneous branches are retracted radially. Distal to the biceps tendon, the superior edge of the pronator teres is encountered. The pronator is exposed from the medial epicondyle distally, where it passes beneath the medial edge of the brachioradialis (Fig. 99–2).

At this point in the dissection, it is helpful to envision the boundaries of the antecubital fossa. This is a triangular-shaped area defined by a proximally directed base, represented by a line connecting the humeral condyles; the walls consist of the pronator teres medially

■ FIGURE 99–2
The course of the median nerve as it traverses the antecubital fossa in the proximal third of the forearm.

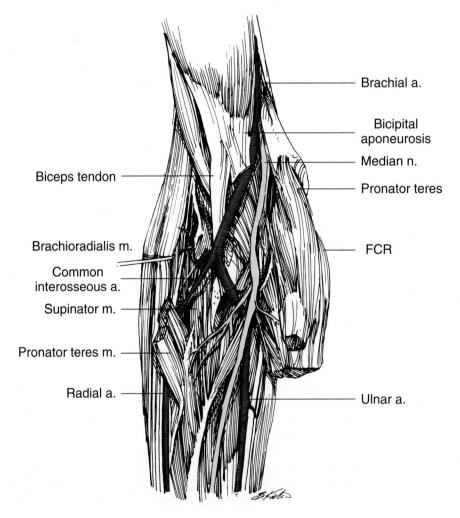

and the brachioradialis laterally; the floor is formed by the brachialis proximally and the supinator distally. The distal apex is just radial to a line dividing the forearm into medial and lateral halves. The brachial artery and the median nerve pass toward the midline as they travel through the antecubital fossa, heading for the apex.

The brachial artery divides into its radial and ulnar arteries within the antecubital fossa. The exact location of the arterial division is varied. In the majority of cases, the artery divides approximately 2 cm distal to the base of the triangle, close to where the biceps tendon dives toward its insertion onto the radius. A common variation is the division of the brachial artery at or above the base of the antecubital fossa, in which case the brachial artery will appear to be bifid. When this variant is encountered, distal dissection will reveal the smaller of the two arteries to be the radial artery and the larger to be the ulnar artery. The radial artery, no matter where it originates, enters the midforearm in the interval between pronator teres and the underbelly of the brachioradialis. The ulnar artery, in usual cases, passes beneath the median nerve just proximal to the apex of the antecubital fossa. If the ulnar artery has a high takeoff, it will enter the antecubital fossa more medial than usual, crossing beneath the median nerve at the base of the antecubital fossa rather than at the apex. The ulnar artery passes beneath the superior margin of the FDS and travels medially to lie along the radial side of the ulnar nerve in the midforearm.

The median nerve traverses the antecubital fossa medial to the brachial artery or in the case of the high brachial artery division medial to the radial artery. At the apex of the antecubital fossa, the radial artery and the median nerve part. The artery passes over the pronator teres as described above while the median nerve passes between the two heads of the pronator teres. The nerve is followed distally by developing the plane between the pronator teres and the flexor carpi radialis (Figs. 99-3A and 99-3B). The interval between these two muscles is identified distally, and the dissection proceeds cephalad, dividing the common raphe between the muscle bellies. The inferior margin of the pronator teres is retracted proximally, and the median nerve is identified passing beneath the arch of the FDS. The arch can be released with a subperiosteal dissection along the radial margin. This will expose the median nerve at the branch point for the AIN. If there is difficulty following or repairing the nerve under the pronator teres, then the tendon of the pronator teres' superficial head is divided (Fig. 99–3C). The tendon is cut in an oblique or stepcut fashion to facilitate later repair and retracted proximally. The median nerve is easily seen until it passes beneath the origin of the FDS. This method is particularly helpful if the nerve injury occurred within the muscle belly of the pronator teres. Full release of the radial origin of the superficialis permits further exposure; however, this is not necessary if the nerve is approached from "below" as explained in the dissection of the midforearm.

Injury to the branches of the median nerve in the proximal forearm can be avoided by keeping to the radial side of the median nerve as it passes through the antecubital fossa. All median nerve branches in the proximal forearm take off from the ulnar aspect of the nerve with the exception of the AIN, which arises from the under surface of the nerve in the vicinity of the FDS origin. By knowing this relationship, the AIN can be isolated by developing the interval between the brachial artery and subsequently the radial artery within the antecubital fossa. The median nerve is gently retracted by picking up the epineurium along its radial side. As the median nerve proceeds beneath the arch of the FDS, the AIN will be seen arising from the under surface of the median nerve. Further exposure requires elevation of the FDS origin on the radius.

Parts B and C of the incision illustrated in Figure 99–2 are used to expose the median nerve in the middle third of the forearm. The skin edges are elevated as fasciocutaneous flaps, raising the skin, subcutaneous fat, and forearm investing fascia as a single unit.

The flexor carpi radialis, palmaris longus, and FDP are identified, and the antebrachial fascia overlying the internervous plane between the flexor carpi ulnaris (ulnar nerve) and palmaris longus (median nerve) is incised. The common raphe between the flexor carpi radialis and the flexor carpi ulnaris muscle bellies is divided proximally. Lateral retraction of the palmaris longus and the flexor carpi radialis exposes the FDS and the ulnar artery and nerve. The interval between the ulnar neurovascular bundle and the FDS is easily

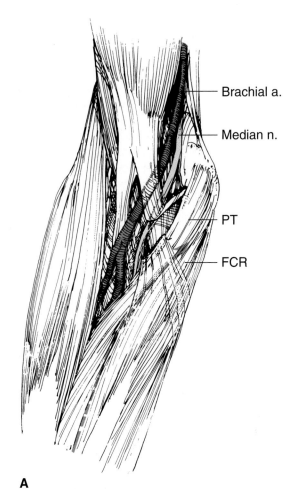

Brachial a.

Median n.

PT

FCR

A

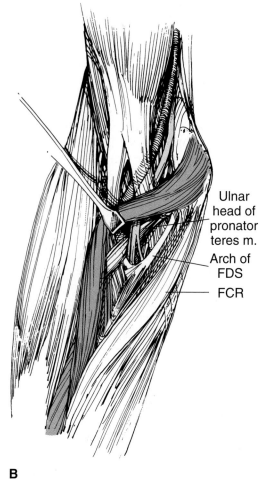

Ulnar head of pronator teres m.

Arch of FDS

FCR

B

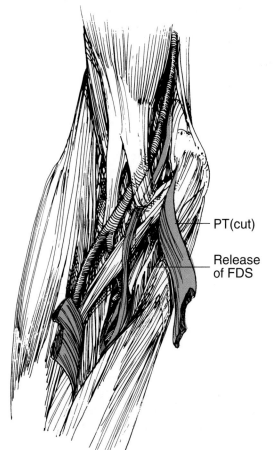

PT(cut)

Release of FDS

C

■ FIGURE 99–3

Exposure of the median nerve as it passes beneath the pronator teres. **A,** The interval between the pronator teres and the flexor carpi radialis is identified distally and dissected proximally. **B,** The inferior margin of the pronator teres is retracted cephalad and the median nerve is identified passing beneath the arch of the FDS. **C,** If there is difficulty following or repairing the nerve under the pronator teres the interval between the two heads of the pronator teres is developed and the tendon of the superficial head is divided. The tendon is retracted toward the pronator teres origin exposing the median nerve.

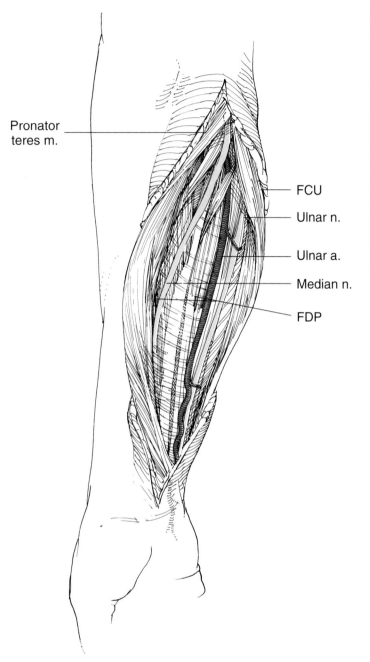

Pronator teres m.

FCU

Ulnar n.

Ulnar a.

Median n.

FDP

■ FIGURE 99–4
McConnell's exposure of the median nerve in the mid forearm. The fascia between the palmaris longus and flexor carpi ulnaris is incised. The palmaris longus and flexor carpi radialis are retracted radially. The interval between the flexor-digitorum superficialis is developed and the superficialis muscle belly is elevated by its ulnar border. The median nerve lies on the under belly of the FDS.

developed with blunt dissection. With the fingers and wrist flexed, the ulnar margin of the FDS is elevated and retracted radially. The median nerve will be seen running along the under belly of the muscle, held in place by the muscular investing fascia of the FDS (Fig. 99–4).

Once the median nerve is visualized, the investing fascia of the forearm is cut longitudinally, and the median nerve is followed proximally until joining the dissection of the proximal third of the forearm. The dissection will eventually be limited by the origin of the superficialis. In the proximal portion of this dissection, branches from the median nerve may be encountered that communicate with the ulnar nerve (a Martin-Gruber variation) and should be preserved. Nerve branches to the superficialis muscle also will be seen and should be preserved. In the cephalad extent of the dissection, the ulnar artery passes obliquely across the muscle belly of the FDP to join the ulnar nerve. If the artery is followed proximally, a number of muscular branches will be seen as well as a large branch, the common interosseous artery. All of these arterial branches pass deep to nerves including the vestigial median artery when present. With the branching of the median nerve and the brachial/ulnar artery, the dissection may become tedious. If indeed the dissection in this proximal extent becomes confusing, it is best to return to the antecubital fossa and follow the median nerve into the middle third of the forearm. This requires elevating the FDS from its radial origin until a two fingerbreadth opening communicates with the ulnar sided dissection. With this approach, the AIN must be identified as it takes off from the underside of the median nerve to run along the investing fascia of the FDP. The plane of dissection between the FDS and median nerve above, and the FDP and the AIN below, places the latter nerve at risk of traction injury during radial-sided dissections. This is especially true if one attempts to communicate with the ulnar FDS-FCU interval through minimal elevation of the FDS origin from the radius. The remaining course of the anterior interosseous artery can be followed from the radial side only if the pronator teres is divided. If the division is not desirable, then the nerve is marked with a vessel loop and approached from below through the FDS-FCU interval. The AIN is located between FDP and FPL in the midforearm. Distally, the nerve travels on the volar surface of the interosseous membrane. The innervation of the pronator teres, FDP to the index and middle fingers, and the FPL occur proximally, in close proximity to the pronator teres.

An alternative approach to the median nerve in the midforearm starts by incising the fascia over the flexor carpi radialis in the distal portion of the wound. As the flexor carpi radialis tendon is lifted up and retracted radialward, the median nerve will be seen passing from beneath the radial margin of the FDS. Care is taken to avoid dissecting on top of the nerve in the distal aspect of the wound. This prevents injury to the palmar cutaneous branch, which arises from the volar surface of the median nerve (Fig. 99–5). The median nerve is followed proximally by elevating the origin of the FDS from the radius. At the junction of the mid and distal third, the flexor carpi radialis needs to be retracted ulnarly to get to the origin of the FDS proximally. The radial artery is vulnerable in this region and should be mobilized by dividing muscular side branches along the ulnar side of the vessel. As one proceeds up the forearm, the interval between the flexor carpi radialis and brachioradialis is developed. The brachioradialis is retracted with care. The superficial radial nerve, found on the underbelly of the brachioradialis, is at risk for traction injuries or local crush from retractors. With these structures protected, the remainder of the origin of the superficialis is elevated from the radius, the humeral head of the pronator teres divided, and the median nerve followed into the proximal forearm.

A third approach to the median nerve in the midforearm is a combination of the previous two. The median nerve is identified radial to the flexor carpi radialis in the distal aspect of the midforearm and a colored vessel loop is passed around the nerve. Attention is directed to the FDS muscle and tendons, which are elevated from their ulnar margin, and the plane between the FDS and the FDP is followed distally. The median nerve, marked with the vessel loop, is identified and mobilized by incising the muscular investing fascia along the under belly of the FDS muscle. The exposure continues until encountering the point of injury or until the proximal and mid third exposures communicate.

Part B and the proximal portion of part C of Figure 99–1 are used to expose the median nerve in the distal forearm. If distal extension is necessary, part A of Figure 99–1 is used to expose the carpal tunnel. The forearm fascia is incised between the palmaris longus or, in the absence of a palmaris longus, the FCR and the FCU. Just proximal to the wrist creases, the nerve is identified as the most superficial structure about to enter the carpal tunnel. The nerve should be followed up the forearm along its ulnar side, thereby avoiding injury to the palmar cutaneous branch. At the junction between the mid and distal third of the forearm, the median nerve can be identified by two previously described approaches. The first develops the ulnar-sided plane between the FDS and the FDP and finds the nerve bound to the underbelly of the FDS. The second approach incises the forearm fascia over the FCR and radial artery. The FCR is retracted radially, and the median nerve is identified passing beneath the radial margin of the FDS. As explained in

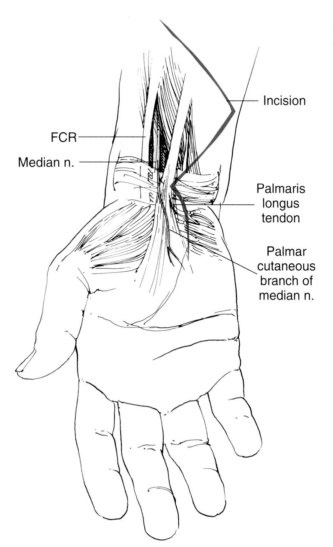

FCR

Median n.

Incision

Palmaris
longus
tendon

Palmar
cutaneous
branch of
median n.

■ FIGURE 99–5
The median nerve enters
the distal third of the forearm along the radial mar-
gin of the FDS. The pal-
mar cutaneous branch is
at risk of injury when dissecting in this region.

the dissection of the mid third of the median nerve, the palmar cutaneous branch is at risk with this exposure (Fig. 99–5).

Under loupe magnification, the nerve is identified and dissected from the surrounding scar tissue, working from normal to abnormal tissues. The proximal and distal nerve stumps are identified. The graft bed is evaluated. If the graft will cross a scarred bed, a different course through healthy, well-vascularized tissue is selected, even at the expense of needing a longer graft.

A dissecting microscope is used for the grafting procedure. All neuromatous tissue surrounding the nerve stumps is resected. Care is taken throughout the procedure to handle the nerve by manipulating either the neuromatous tip or the epineurium of the normal portion of the nerve. The extent of the neuroma is determined by gently running a jeweler's forceps along the nerve to identify areas of increased thickening and stiffness suggestive of scar tissue. The nerve is placed onto a moistened tongue depressor and cut with a razor blade. The end of the intact nerve is examined for healthy appearing tissue recognized by multiple shiny fascicles protruding several micrometers from the tip. Serial sectioning is performed until the cut surface has this appearance. This is more difficult distally, because Wallerian degeneration has occurred.

The orientations of the proximal and distal stumps are evaluated. Clues that aid in orienting these include the diameters of the fascicular groups, spatial relationships of the fascicular groups, and surface anatomy including vascular markings. Although Sunderland[20] described rapid changes of the internal fascicular topography, the grouped fascicular pattern remains constant over a much longer distance.[8]

The donor nerve graft selected is usually the sural nerve because it creates little morbidity, is easily harvested, and has enough length to provide multiple strands. The graft should be approximately 10% longer than the segmental defect being grafted.

Because the sural nerve is smaller caliber then the median nerve and about the same size as the AIN, graft repair presents the following possibilities: (1) *The graft and the nerve are the same size.* This is the typical situation for repair of the AIN in the proximal and mid third of the forearm. Coaptation of the nerve and the graft is accomplished with 10–0 nylon sutures passed through the epineurium 120° apart. (2) *The nerve is larger than the graft.* This is the typical setting for repair of the median nerve throughout the forearm. The topography of the median nerve in the proximal two thirds of the forearm is polyfascicular (more than five fascicles) with variable grouping. In the distal third of the forearm, the fascicles are usually bunched in easily definable groups.[22] If groups of fascicles are easily defined, then the graft repair should be from group to group. A 10–0 nylon is passed through the epineurium of the graft and sutured to the epineurium in the periphery of the group. No more than two sutures are used to secure the graft. Enough cables are used to completely cover both ends of the grouped fascicles. If groups of fascicles are not definable, the nerve should be covered with multiple grafts in roughly the same cross-sectional orientation at both the proximal and distal nerve ends. It is technically easiest to secure the deepest cables first rather than having to turn the nerve over after suturing the easier and more superficial portion of the defect.

Whether the graft repair is performed under tourniquet control is predicated on the length of ischemia time that the surgeon believes is appropriate. As stated earlier, we limit tourniquet time to 90 minutes.

Wounds are closed over suction drains and a compression dressing is applied. A plaster splint is applied with the elbow flexed 90°, the forearm in neutral pronation and supination, the wrist slightly dorsiflexed, and digits in a lumbrical-plus position. On the first postoperative day, the dressings about the fingers are removed, and active and passive range of motion exercises are begun. The wounds are usually dry enough to remove drains within 1 or 2 days, and the patient is discharged.

■ REHABILITATION

The splint is worn for 10 to 14 days, at which time the sutures are removed. A long-arm cast is worn for an additional 2 to 4 weeks for a total of 4 to 6 weeks of immobilization. Longer periods of immobilization are used for injuries near joints or if mandated by concomitant injuries.

Edema control and range of motion (active, active-assisted, and passive) are begun on the digits on the first postoperative day. At 4 to 6 weeks, scar massage, desensitization, and range of motion are started. A removable splint is often fabricated to maintain hand posture. The splint should be worn at night.

■ OUTCOMES

Following is a summary of the findings of Frykman and Gramyk, who reviewed the literature on nerve grafting.[3] They demonstrated that the results of nerve grafting were inversely related to age, graft length, and time lapse between injury and grafting. They noted that age was the best predictor and the level of injury had a significant impact on outcome. Also, for the motor recovery of the median nerve after grafting, the length of the graft had a significant impact on the outcome. For grafts less than 5 cm, 95% of the patients had return of useful motor function (powerful enough to resist gravity), and for grafts greater than 10 cm, only 66% of the patients had return of useful function.

Their inclusion criteria for their study were: (1) The results of each patient were described, allowing classification of motor and sensory recovery separately for mixed nerves; (2) Subgroups of age, time delay before grafting, and graft length were noted; (3) A minimum follow-up of 1 year after the nerve grafting procedure was reported; (4) The study was not performed before 1972 using the older methods of trunk grafting.

Using these criteria, they obtained 112 patients for motor loss evaluation and 116 patients for sensory loss evaluation. They used the Highet and Sanders' rating system with Mackinnon and Dellon's modification to grade motor and sensory results. For median nerve grafting, 81% of patients had useful motor recovery (i.e., M3 return in function of proximal and distal muscles such that all muscles have the ability to resist gravity). However, we add the caveat that 30% to 40% of patients with low median nerve injuries have adequate ulnar innervation to the thenar muscles to have functional opposition without any nerve grafting. Age was the best predictor of outcome, with 88% of the patients younger than 20 years of age obtaining useful motor function. This contrasts with only 64% of patients older than 40 years old obtaining useful motor function. Gap length had a marked effect on median nerve recovery after grafting. For gaps less than 5 cm, 95% obtained useful function, and for gaps greater than 10 cm, only 66% obtained useful motor function. A delay of greater than 6 months between injury and grafting was associated with 24% fewer patients obtaining useful function. For the location of the injury, they showed 50% useful recovery in high lesions, 92% recovery in middle lesions, and 81% recovery in low lesions.

Overall, 76% of patients obtained useful sensory recovery (i.e., static two-point discrimination of better than 15 to 20 mm). Again, age was the most significant prognostic factor: 98% of the patients younger than 20 years regained useful sensation, and 58% of patients older than 40 years regained useful sensation. Twenty-seven percent of patients younger than 20 years recovered normal (2 to 6 mm) static two-point discrimination, and no patients older than 40 years recovered normal two-point discrimination. Gap length was inversely proportional to outcome; however, 85% of grafts greater than 10 cm regained useful sensation. Greater than a 6-month delay between injury and grafting effected a 20% reduction in useful recovery. No patients with a high lesion obtained normal two-point discrimination; however, 30% of the patients with a low lesion obtained normal two-point discrimination.

References

1. Clark WB, Trumble TE, Swiontkowski MF: Nerve tension and blood flow in a rat model of immediate and delayed repairs. J Hand Surg, 1992; 17A:677–687.
2. Doi K, Tamaru K, Sakai K, Kuwata N, Kurafuji YSK: A comparison of vascularized and conventional sural nerve grafts. J Hand Surg Am, 1992; 17:670–676.
3. Frykman GK: Results of nerve grafting. In: Gelberman RH (ed): Operative nerve repair and reconstruction. Philadelphia: J. B. Lippincott, 1991:553–567.
4. Gaul JS: Electrical fascicular identification as an adjunct to nerve repair. J Hand Surg, 1983; 8A:289–296.
5. Henry KH: Extensile exposure, 2nd ed, Edinburgh and London: Churchill Livingstone, 1973: 90–111.
6. Hentz VR, Rosen JM, Xiao SJ, McGill KC, Abraham G: The nerve gap dilemma: A comparison of nerves repaired end to end under tension with nerve grafts in a primate model. J Hand Surg, 1993; 18A:417–425.
7. Heppenstall RB, Balderston R, Goodwin C: Pathophysiologic effects distal to a tourniquet in the dog. J Trauma, 1979; 19:234–238.
8. Jabaley ME, Wallace WH, Heckler HR: Internal topography of major nerves of the forearm and hand: A current review. J Hand Surg, 1980; 5:1–18.
9. Kallio PK, Vastamaki M: An analysis of the results of late reconstruction of 132 median nerves. J Hand Surg, 1993; 18B:97–105.
10. Lundborg G, Rydevik B: Effects of stretching the tibial nerve of the rabbit: A preliminary study of the interneural circulation and the barrier function of the perineurium. J Bone Joint Surg, 1973; 55B:390–401.
11. Millesi H, Meissl G, Berger A: The interfascicular nerve grafting of the median and ulnar nerves. J Bone Joint Surg, 1972; 54A:727–750.
12. Millesi H: Indications and techniques of nerve grafting. In: Gelberman RH (ed): Operative nerve repair and reconstruction. Philadelphia: J. B. Lippincott, 1991:525–543.
13. Newman RJ: Metabolic effects of tourniquet ischaemia studied by nuclear magnetic spectoscopy. J Bone Joint Surg, 1984; 66B:434–439.
14. Nicholson R, Seddon HJ: Nerve repair in civil practice: Results of treatment of median and ulnar nerve lesions. Br Med J, 1957; 11:1065–1071.

15. Roland SA. Fasciotomy: The treatment of compartment syndrome. In: Green DP (ed): Operative Hand Surgery, 3rd ed. New York: Churchill Livingstone, 1993:661–694.
16. Sakellarides H: A follow up study of 173 peripheral nerve injuries in the upper extremity in civilians. J Bone Joint Surg, 1962; 44A:140–148.
17. Seddon HJ: The use of autogenous grafts for the repair of large gaps in peripheral nerves. Br J Surg, 1947; 35:151–167.
18. Spinner M: Injuries to the major branches of peripheral nerves of the forearm. Philadelphia: W. B. Saunders, 1978:218.
19. Strange FG: An operation for nerve pedicle grafting: preliminary communication. Br J Surg, 1946; 34:423–425.
20. Sunderland S: The intraneural topography of the radial, median and ulnar nerve. Brain, 1945; 68:243–298.
21. Taleisnik J: The palmar cutaneous branch of the median nerve and the approach to the carpal tunnel. An anatomical study. J Bone Joint Surg, 1973; 55A:1212–1217.
22. Zachary RB: Results of nerve suture. In: Seddon HJ (ed): Peripheral Nerve Injuries. London: Her Majesty's Stationery Office, 1954:354–388.

DON A. COLEMAN
PAUL A. BINHAMMER

100

Ulnar Nerve Grafting in the Forearm

The first nerve grafts were probably performed by Philipeaux and Vulpian.[4] In 1863, they reported their failed results of optic nerve allografts between the hypoglossal and lingual nerves. The first clinical case using a zenograft was reported by Albert in 1878. The first report of a beneficial outcome was that by Mayo-Robson. In 1906, Sherren reported 16 cases of allografts with improvement in 6. However, it was not until the work of Millesi that nerve grafting became acceptable with the use of microsurgical technique and magnification.[14]

Millesi performed his surgery in a bloodless field with use of a pneumatic tourniquet. Using a dissecting microscope, normal fasciculi were identified proximal and distal to the nerve defect and dissected until the fascicles became fibrotic. The fasciculi were then transected individually with fine, sharp scissors. Sketches were then made of the fascicular pattern in the two stumps. For the ulnar nerve, four grafts from the sural nerve were usually adequate for reconstruction. One suture of 10-0 nylon was used in each graft end. The techniques that were developed and described by Millesi have changed little through the years. The technique for grafting the ulnar nerve that we describe is similar to the one he would have performed. We do add minimal modifications and technical clarifications.

■ HISTORY OF THE TECHNIQUE

Grafting for the ulnar nerve is indicated whenever there is a significant nerve gap and available graft material. Those patients whose injury is relatively recent and more distal in the extremity have the potential to regain not only sensation but motor function as well. Conversely, patients who have a long standing injury may not have return of motor function but only an improvement in their sensation.

The exact size of the gap that is significant and requires a graft is not known.[13] However, tension at the suture line in an end to end repair will compromise blood flow and affect the functional result. To close a small gap in the ulnar nerve, simple dissection and mobilization of the ulnar nerve proximal and distal to the site of injury may be all that is necessary. Nerve transposition or joint positioning may help decrease the gap even further. Anterior transposition of the ulnar nerve may provide 2 to 5 cm of excursion.[1,2] Transposition is more beneficial in proximal defects due to the branches to the flexor carpi ulnaris and flexor digitorum profundus more distally (Fig. 100-1). Elbow flexion, with or without transposition, may help decrease the gap. More distal gaps in the forearm may be decreased with wrist flexion. However, some surgeons prefer to repair or graft the nerve on maximal stretch so as to ensure that tension is eliminated during movement.[9] When the nerve ends cannot be approximated without undue tension, nerve grafting is indicated.

Contraindications or relative contraindications may be influenced by the age of the patient, the length of defect, the time since injury, the amount of graft material available, associated injuries, and condition of the recipient bed.

Children have a greater potential for regeneration than adults. Therefore, grafting in children should be a high priority. The results are less efficacious and less predictable in adults, and the operation is less readily recommended. However, the upper age limit at which the operation is contraindicated has not been clearly established.

The length of the defect has been shown to affect the functional results. The longer the gap, the worse the results. This also could be influenced by the amount of adequate graft

■ INDICATIONS AND CONTRAINDICATIONS

material available. Situations may arise where nerves such as the sural nerve, which has a high ratio of neural tissue to supporting structures, is not enough or not available. Associated injuries distal to the nerve injury site in the forearm may limit the potential for functional recovery making grafting not indicated. Also, recovery of the ulnar nerve may be of low priority if there is discontinuity more proximal (i.e., brachial plexus injury). The ulnar nerve may then serve as graft material, vascularized or nonvascularized, for reconstruction.

The condition of the recipient bed may influence the decision to perform grafting. A favorable vascular bed is preferable to allow revascularization of the nerve grafts. If the recipient bed is inadequate, the grafts may become fibrotic or necrotic. Free tissue transfer or rotational flaps may help restore an adequate vascular bed.

■ SURGICAL TECHNIQUES

Grafting of the ulnar nerve requires general anesthesia. This is because the nerve is large, requiring significant graft material from the sural nerve. Regional anesthesia is possible if the defect is known to be small and there is enough locally available donor material, but this is an unusual circumstance. General anesthesia also affords positioning of the patient.

The prone position is ideal for harvesting the sural nerve and accessing the ulnar nerve in the middle and distal aspects of the forearm. For these reasons, grafting at these levels is most easily done with the patient prone. For very proximal forearm or elbow grafting, the operation is best performed with the patient in the supine position. A sand bag placed under the hip along with knee flexion and internal hip rotation improves access to the sural nerve.

The path of the ulnar nerve can be outlined by first identifying the cubital tunnel proximally and the pisiform distally. A line joining these two points approximates the path of the ulnar nerve. Before proceeding with the operation, the surgeon should be knowledgeable of the ulnar nerve anatomy. Preservation of sensory and motor branches must be done. The sensory branches one must be aware of include the dorsal cutaneous branch, a branch off the nerve of Henle, and the palmar sensory branch. The latter two may supply sensation to the volar ulnar aspect of the distal forearm. The dorsal cutaneous branch leaves the ulnar nerve approximately 6 cm proximal to the head of the ulna passing deep to the flexor carpi ulnaris where it then pierces the forearm fascia to become subcutaneous approximately 5 cm from the pisiform. Sympathetic nerve supply to the ulnar artery typically originates 16 cm proximal to the ulnar styloid, then travels adjacent to the ulnar artery in 45% of extremities (nerve of Henle).[1,12] It then provides a branch that pierces the superficial fascia 6 cm proximal to the ulnar styloid to innervate the volar ulnar skin of the distal forearm.[1,12] A palmar sensory branch (atypical nerve of Henle) arises from the ulnar nerve 8 cm proximal to the ulnar styloid in 12% of extremities.[1,12]

The ulnar nerve supplies motor fascicles to the flexor carpi ulnaris and flexor digitorum very proximally in the forearm. The branches to the flexor carpi ulnaris can be dissected away from the ulnar nerve proximal to the cubital tunnel, retaining the flexor carpi ulnar innervation in proximal ulnar nerve injuries. The motor branch supplying the ulnar innervated intrinsic hand muscles can be dissected away from the ulnar nerve up to 9 cm proximal to the radial styloid.[3] This may be beneficial when accurate and feasible techniques are available for identifying motor and sensory fascicles.

The operation is performed in a bloodless field, using loupe magnification initially and then the operating microscope. The arm is first wrapped with an Esmarch bandage, and a tourniquet, having been placed about the arm, is inflated to 250 mm Hg. The Esmarch bandage is then removed, and the operation commences.

The skin can be incised through previous scars with longitudinal extension to provide access to normal tissue. If exposure is required across either the wrist or elbow, the incision should have a "Z" placed at this juncture. With the skin and subcutaneous tissue mobilized, the first structure to be encountered will be the flexor carpi ulnaris. It can be identified by its insertion into the pisiform. It is then best to approach the nerve by proceeding around the radial border of the flexor carpi ulnaris. The nerve has traveled from the cubital

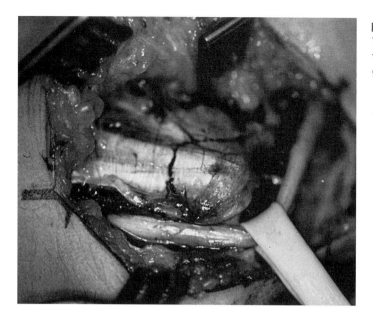

■ FIGURE 100-1
The ulnar nerve may be transposed anteriorly to gain length.

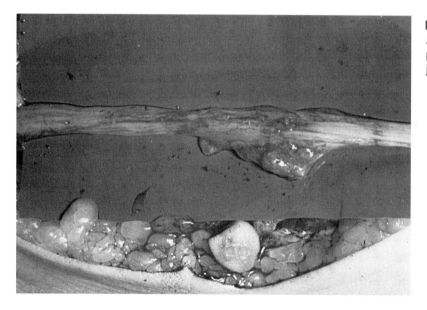

■ FIGURE 100-2
An ulnar nerve isolated proximal and distal to injury site.

tunnel and then deep to the two heads of the flexor carpi ulnaris. The ulnar artery and its venae commitantes are just radial to the nerve beginning in the proximal forearm and are located on, and somewhat adherent to, the flexor digitorum profundus.

The nerve is identified both proximally and distally to the zone of injury and is elevated for a short distance. If the nerve is in continuity, this may require only a small exposure (Fig. 100–2). A discontinuous nerve will require a larger exposure, and the identification of both ends is most easily achieved by dissecting in proximal and distal normal tissue. The area where the nerve is to be grafted requires a healthy vascular bed, lying on muscle rather than scar tissue.

Simultaneously, if possible, a common sural nerve graft is harvested. A tourniquet about the thigh is inflated after use of the Esmarch bandage. The sural nerve is identified between the lateral malleolus and the Achilles tendon where it travels with the short saphenous vein. A linear vertical (Fig. 100–3A) or multiple transverse (Fig. 100–3B) incisions are made extending proximally as the nerve is identified. An atraumatic technique is used as well as liberal irrigation of saline to prevent any desiccation. As the dissection proceeds,

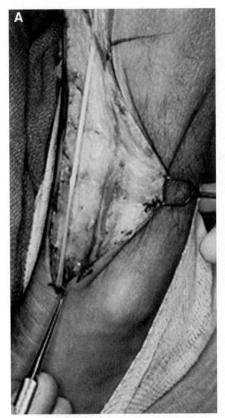

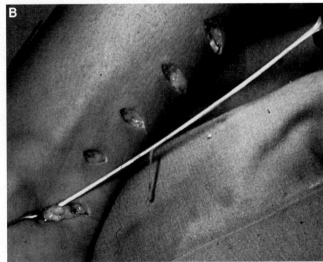

■ FIGURE 100–3
A, B, A linear incision or multiple transverse incisions for harvesting the sural nerve.

the distal incision is covered with saline gauze. Proximally, a contribution from the lateral sural nerve may be encountered in 75% of legs. The nerves, medial and lateral surals, can then be traced proximally to their origins from the posterior tibial and common peroneal. Once the nerve has been elevated throughout its length it is removed from the leg, wrapped in saline gauze, and passed to the team repairing the ulnar nerve. The leg tourniquet is deflated and hemostasis achieved using electrocautery. The skin incision is closed first with interrupted, subcuticular, 4-0, absorbable, long-lasting sutures, e.g. Vicryl or Dexon, and then a running intracuticular suture of similar material. The wound is dressed lightly and wrapped with an elasticized bandage.

The operating microscope is then positioned to view the forearm field. The proximal and distal ends of the nerve are transected using a new scalpel blade with a tongue blade acting as the cutting board. If there is a neuroma incontinuity with the clinical examination suggesting some intact fascicles, electrical intraoperative stimulation may help to identify intact motor fascicles. Careful dissection of the fascicles leading into the neuroma under high power also may help in identifying intact fascicles. This leaves intact fascicles within the neuroma and avoids a hazardous dissection through the neuroma.[10]

The appearance of the proximal and distal ends should be one of fascicles and not scar tissue. The ends of the nerve should be serially transected until this is achieved (Figs. 100-4A and 100-4B). The fascicular pattern is noted and drawn to compare the two ends. If possible, as in the hand and distal forearm, the motor and sensory fascicles are identified by their anatomic location. A decision is then made to match groups of fascicles proximally to specific groups distally. The distance between the nerve ends, lying in a vascular bed and free of tension, is measured: this is compared with the amount of nerve graft harvested and the number of strands of sural nerve anticipated to be used. It may be necessary at this stage to harvest more graft material.

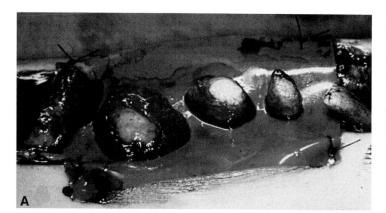

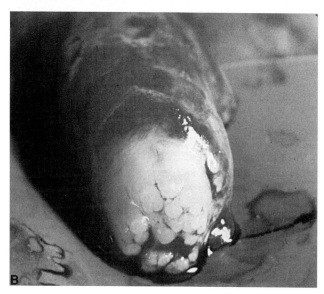

■ FIGURE 100–4
A, Multiple serial transections are made until fascicles are identified proximally and distally. **B,** Fascicles seen in cross section in a well prepared nerve. (Courtesy Graham Lister, MD.)

The proximal end of the sural nerve graft, which contains the largest fascicles and highest ratio of neural tissue to supporting tissue, is sutured to the proximal stump of the ulnar nerve. A 9-0 or 10-0 monofilament nonabsorbable suture is used, placing enough sutures to achieve coverage of the fascicles. The sural nerve is then stretched to its normal length and cut approximately 1 cm longer than the gap. The nerve graft is then sutured into place.

Rather than repeating the process of suturing the grafts first proximal then distal, which often requires readjusting the microscope, go proximal to distal with one graft, distal to proximal with the next graft, proximal to distal with the next graft, and so on until nerve grafting is complete (Fig. 100–5). Again, this will save time from having to adjust and, on occasion where there is a large defect, move the microscope as often.

The tourniquet is deflated, and meticulous hemostasis is achieved. It is essential to the revascularization of the graft that there be no hematoma formation. If there is any concern that a hematoma may form, a suction drain should be placed in such a manner that its removal will not injure the graft.

The skin incision is then closed in layered fashion. Subcutaneous tissues are approximated with absorbable interrupted sutures followed by either running absorbable subcutaneous or interrupted nonabsorbable sutures if increased skin tension occurs. The leg incision is closed in a similar manner with interrupted absorbable subcutaneous sutures and a running subcuticular suture. The arm is then splinted with the wrist in 30° of extension and the elbow in 90° of flexion. The dressing remains in place for 2 to 3 weeks. It is then removed, and the patient begins normal activities and proceeds with rehabilitation.

■ FIGURE 100–5
A completed grafting of
the ulnar nerve. (Cour-
tesy Douglas T. Hutchin-
son, MD.)

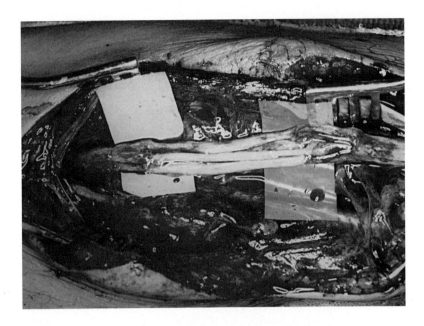

■ TECHNICAL
ALTERNATIVES

As mentioned, the ulnar nerve may be transposed or elevated to gain additional length from its proximal portion. Where there is a larger gap and limited amount of material, both these methods may be required to have enough material to graft all of the fascicles. The blood supply to the nerve should be preserved proximally and the ulnar artery and venue commitantes elevated with the nerve distally.

Nerves other than the sural are available for grafting but do not provide the same amount of neural material.[10]

Additional methods are available to identify the motor and sensory fascicles, other than the internal anatomy of the ulnar nerve. Rapid histochemical staining has been used and requires 1 hour.[8] Awake nerve stimulation involves waking the patient after identifying the proximal fascicles and stimulating the fascicles.[6] The patient is then able to localize the subjective sensation. The surgeon must then interpret this as motor or sensory and so identify the fascicles. In both cases, the proximal ends can be identified anatomically by dissecting out the fascicles if the lesions are distal enough. If a patient has an acute loss and can be grafted within days of the injury, it also is possible to stimulate the distal fascicles and identify the motor fascicles by muscle contraction.

The nerve gap has been treated by means other than autologous grafts. Absorbable tubes and freeze-thawed muscle grafts have been used.[2,10] The value of either of these insignificant gaps is certainly questionable at present.

■ REHABILITATION

During the postoperative immobilization period, the patient is encouraged to use the hand and to work on flexion and extension both actively and passively to keep the joints from becoming stiff and to decrease edema. After splint removal, gentle range of motion of the elbow and wrist is started. Certainly by 3 months, if not before, full motion of the extremity should be obtained. In the postoperative period, the patient should have frequent contact with a therapist, not only to prevent secondary contractures, but to possibly correct secondary contractures. Our preference to prevent secondary contractures is the "anti-claw" splint (Fig. 100–6). Activities that require grip, intraphalangeal joint extension, and thumb lateral pinch are encouraged to help with nerve retraining.

Sensory return after nerve repair is unpredictable. Sensory re-education may help maximize return. While the ulnar aspect of the hand and ulnar 1½ digits remain insensate, the patient should protect himself from extremes of heat and cold or sharp objects. Early return to sensation may be hyperesthetic and require desensitizing procedures. With further return, re-education using tuning forks and objects of various sizes, shapes, and textures, is useful.

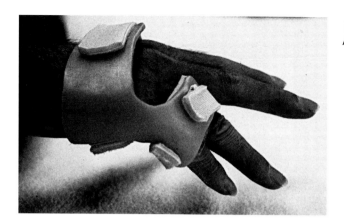

■ OUTCOMES

Millesi provided the best, early information on the results of ulnar nerve grafting in the forearm.[14] Adequate follow-up of more than 12 months was achieved in 18 of 32 patients. Motor function of M4 to M5 returned in 8 patients, M3 in 7 patients, and M2 in 3 patients. Two-point discrimination returned in 7 patients, and protective sensitivity returned in 11 patients. These results certainly suggest that grafting for ulnar nerve deficit is a worthwhile technique.

The results of grafting for ulnar nerve defects have been reviewed and summarized more recently by Frykman and Gramyk.[5] Only cases that met specific criteria and had a minimum of 1 year follow-up after grafting were included. Ulnar motor recovery overall was 63% M3 or better. Seventy-five percent of patients younger than 20 years of age achieved M3 or better, 66% of patients between 20 and 39 years of age achieved M3 or better, and approximately 50% of patients older than 40 years achieved M3 or better. A gap greater than 100 mm decreased the M4 and M5 results from 46% to 9%. Neither delay of grafting 6 months or more or the level of injury seemed to affect the motor return. Sensory return was described as useful in 87% of patients younger than 20 years and in 70% of those patients older than 20 years of age. Gaps greater than 100 mm achieved useful recovery 20% less than gaps 50 mm or less. A delay of 6 months or less between injury and grafting resulted in 87% useful sensory return compared with 71% with a delay from injuries to grafting greater than 6 months.

Kalomiri and co-authors also reviewed 85 patients with injuries involving only the ulnar nerve. Their results were better in younger patients and with shorter durations from injury to grafting.[7]

In summary, grafting for ulnar nerve defects in the forearm is a worthwhile procedure. Many factors may affect the outcome. From this review it appears that the ideal patient for such a procedure would be younger than 20 years of age, less than 6 months from injury to grafting, having a gap less than 50 mm, no associated injuries or fixed contractures, and an adequate recipient vascular bed.

References

1. Botte MJ, Cohen MS, Lavernia CJ, von Schroeder HP, Gellman H, Zinberg EM: The dorsal branch of the ulnar nerve: an anatomic study. J Hand Surg, 1990; 15A:603–607.
2. Calder JS, Norris RW: Repair of mixed peripheral nerves using muscle autografts: a preliminary communication. Br J Plast Surg, 1993; 46:557–564.
3. Chow JA, Van Beek AL, Bilos ZJ, Meyer DL, Johnson MD: Anatomical basis for repair of ulnar and median nerves in the distal part of the forearm by group fasicular suture and nerve grafting. J Bone Joint Surg, 1986; 68A:273–280.
4. Dellon ES, Dellon AL: The first nerve graft, Vulpian, and the nineteenth century neural regeneration controversy. J Hand Surg, 1993; 18A:369–372.
5. Frykman GK, Gramyk K: Results of Nerve Grafting. In: Operative Nerve Repair and Reconstruction, Philadelphia: J. B. Lippincott, 1991:553–567.

6. Gaul JS Jr: Electrical fascicle identification as an adjunct to nerve repair. Hand Clin, 1986; 4: 709–722.

7. Kalomiri DE, Soucacos PN, Beris AE: Nerve grafting in peripheral nerve microsurgery of the upper extremity. Microsurg, 1994; 15:506–511.

8. Kanaya F, Jevans AW: Rapid histochemical identification of the motor and sensory fascicles: preparation of the solutions. Plast Reconstruct Surg, 1992; 3:514–515.

9. Lister G: Reconstruction. In: The Hand: Diagnosis and Indications, 3rd Ed, Edinburgh: Churchill Livingstone, 1993:155–282.

10. Mackinnon SE, Dellon AL: Nerve Repair and Nerve Grafting. In: Surgery of the Peripheral Nerve, New York: Thieme, 1988:89–129.

11. Mackinnon SE, Glickman LT, Dagum A: A technique for the treatment of neuroma incontinuity. J Reconstruct Microsurg, 1992; 5:379–384.

12. McCabe SJ, Kleinert JM: The nerve of Henle. J Hand Surg, 1990; 15A:784–788.

13. Millesi H: The nerve gap: theory and clinical practice. Hand Clin, 1986; 4:651–664.

14. Millesi H, Meissl G, Berger A: The interfascicular nerve grafting of median and ulnar nerves. J Bone Joint Surg, 1972; 54A:727–750.

15. Vastamake M, Kallio PK, Solonen KA: The results of secondary microsurgical repair of ulnar nerve injury. J Hand Surg, 1993; 18B:325–326.

101

VINCENT R. HENTZ
BRETT J. SNYDER

Radial Nerve Grafting in the Arm

Although the radial nerve does not mediate the fine motor and sensory functions of the median and ulnar nerves, it plays a critical role in the positioning and strength of the hand. Radial nerve palsy produces significant disability not only from direct loss of extensor muscle groups, but from deterioration of functions mediated by the median and ulnar nerves, such as grip strength.[10]

Radial nerve injury is uncommon, accounting for approximately 10% of all upper extremity nerve injuries.[5] Fractures of the humerus are the most common cause of injury to the radial nerve.[5,7] Because most of these injuries are lesions in continuity, they do not require operative treatment.[4,12,14,19] In addition, because shortening of the humerus by 5 cm or less entails relatively few functional sequelae, this technique has frequently been used to overcome gaps and allow end-to-end approximation.

Historically, much of the literature on peripheral nerve injury and repair was compiled from wartime experience with a higher percentage of penetrating injuries.[14] Autogenous nerve grafting for defects of the radial nerve was attempted for World War I injuries. However, it was the opinion of British surgeons that autogenous nerve grafting was unlikely to yield functional results. The experience of World War II surgeons seems better, with Seddon reporting some useful results in over 100 patients with nerve grafts placed for defects in many peripheral nerves.[14] These early studies appeared to indicate that repair and, by inference, grafting of radial nerve injuries yield better results than for comparable median and ulnar nerve injuries.[18,19] Current techniques of nerve grafting owe much to the pioneering work of Millesi,[11] whose convincing arguments in favor of autogenous intrafascicular cable grafts inserted with the aid of magnification still guide our actions today. In fact, current techniques for grafting of radial nerve defects differ little from Millesi's[11] earlier work.

The radial nerve originates from the posterior cord of the brachial plexus just above the axilla. On entering the arm, the nerve immediately diverges from its neural fellow travelers and passes posteriorly and laterally in close approximation to the humerus. Appearing on the lateral aspect of the lower third of the upper arm, it is here well protected by a thick layer of muscles until its sensory branch becomes subcutaneously located in the distal forearm. This anatomic arrangement protects the radial nerve from many penetrating insults, but puts the nerve at special risk at the point where it is closely approximated to the humerus. In fact, fractures of the midshaft of the humerus are the single most frequent cause of radial nerve injuries. Because most of these fractures are closed injuries, their management requires some greater effort in surgical decision making than, for example, open injuries associated with loss of bone substance, or devastating avulsion injuries that might occur in association with injury from a rotating power take-off or large agricultural machinery.

As is true with any nerve injury, the principal factor determining whether direct repair or grafting is appropriate is the actual amount of nerve substance lost through injury or in debridement. Again, because of the anatomy of the radial nerve, only relatively minimal loss of nerve substance can be accommodated by surgical dissection or joint manipulation. In the upper arm, only about 2 to 3 cm can be gained by dissection and flexion of the

■ HISTORY OF THE TECHNIQUE

■ INDICATIONS AND CONTRAINDICATIONS

elbow. An additional 5 cm might be gained by humeral osteotomy and bone shortening. The other factor that plays an important role in deciding in favor of grafting a radial nerve defect that cannot be overcome to allow end-to-end repair is the near-perfect success rate of tendon transfers to substitute for absence of function of more distal, radially innervated muscles.

Few clinical circumstances associated with loss of nerve substance beg for immediate nerve grafting; resection of tumor associated with limb salvage operations comes to mind, but there are few other situations in which immediate grafting is the most appropriate course. Again, the anatomy of the nerve plays a role. Most injuries associated with loss of substance are high-energy injuries (e.g., high-velocity gunshot injuries, crush injuries). Because most patients presenting with radial nerve palsy do so after closed injuries, their management warrants some discussion.

Injuries associated with loss of radial nerve function may be separated into those requiring early exploration and those that allow closed treatment and observation. Radial nerve palsy, including cases associated with a penetrating injury, is not by itself an indication for exploration. Nerve exploration should be performed in cases where the clinical situation dictates early or immediate operation, including open injuries requiring debridement; vascular injuries, particularly those requiring vascular reconstruction; open fractures of the humerus and fractures requiring open reduction and stabilization; and instances in which the radial nerve was functioning before closed (or open) reduction of the humeral fracture but is not functioning postreduction.[1,2] Primary neurorrhaphy may be performed at initial exploration if the specific zone of injury can be determined and the resultant gap can be overcome by relatively simple maneuvers such as release of the intermuscular septum. Immediate nerve grafting for radial nerve injuries associated with humeral fractures seems relatively rarely called for, and, indeed, may be contraindicated. Otherwise, neurorrhaphy or nerve grafting should be delayed several weeks, at which time the extent of nerve injury will be better delineated.

The incidence of radial nerve palsy with humerus fractures has been estimated at 11%, with spontaneous recovery of nerve function in approximately 83% of these lesions. Studies using early exploration have found nerve transection in 12% of cases, whereas investigators favoring delayed exploration observed a 20% rate of nerve transection.[13,15] No differences in functional recovery were found in patients treated with early versus delayed exploration.[1,2] Therefore, the vast majority of radial nerve palsies that accompany closed humeral fractures will recover spontaneously, and observation is indicated except under the specific conditions detailed earlier.

Electrophysiologic studies should be considered in most cases of radial nerve palsy that lack convincing evidence of nerve recovery by 3 to 4 weeks after the injury. By this time, electrophysiologic studies can distinguish between a neurapraxic lesion that should recover spontaneously and relatively rapidly (weeks to a few months), and an injury associated with distal nerve degeneration. Unfortunately, a single electrical study cannot distinguish between any of the other grades of injury. Therefore, nerve recovery must be followed both by clinical examination, with careful observation for return of motor or sensory function in denervated areas, and serial electrical studies. An advancing Tinel sign is suggestive but not confirmatory of useful nerve regeneration. The same is true of electromyographic evidence of muscle reinnervation. A delay of several months beyond expected evidence of reinnervation of muscles closest to the presumed site of injury is an indication to proceed with exploration. While observing the course of nerve recovery, or lack thereof, the functional focus of this exercise should not be neglected. Hand therapy should be coordinated with a qualified therapist and concentrate on maintaining range of motion at the wrist and fingers. A custom static wrist extension splint should be fabricated and worn at all times except when performing range of motion exercises. Simple stabilization of the wrist will be very effective in enhancing hand function. Occasionally, a more complicated dynamic splint that both stabilizes the wrist and actively extends the digits may be necessary.

Delayed nerve exploration should be performed between 3 to 6 months after injury in the absence of clinical or electrophysiologic evidence for nerve recovery. Most studies have found significantly better results with nerve repair or grafting completed within 6 months of injury.[4,7] In cases of previously documented neurotmesis, secondary nerve reconstruction may be undertaken after allowing sufficient time for healing of adjacent bone and soft tissues. This will enable accurate assessment of the bed in which the nerve grafts will be placed, and avoidance of poorly vascularized or densely scarred areas. These factors must be judged on a case-by-case basis

General anesthesia is required because nerve grafts are likely to be needed. If the injury is associated with a humeral fracture, the surgeon should consider the option of positioning the patient in the prone position because extensive proximal dissection may be required. This position facilitates the surgical approach to the posterior aspect of the arm and the area of the spiral groove, the common site of radial nerve injury associated with fractures of the humerus. This position also facilitates harvesting of sural nerve grafts. In this case, induction of anesthesia and intubation is done while the patient is on the surgical gurney. After intubation, the patient can be turned prone onto the operating table with appropriate padding and elevation of the chest and abdomen to prevent restriction of ventilation. If the injury is presumed to be in the distal third of the arm, then a lateral decubitus position is indicated.

■ **SURGICAL TECHNIQUES**

The radial nerve is the terminal branch of the posterior cord of the brachial plexus, and contains elements from the C5 to C8 nerve roots. It provides motor branches to the triceps, brachioradialis, supinator, and the wrist, finger, and thumb extensors, and sensory innervation to the posterior and inferolateral arm, posterior forearm, and the dorsoradial wrist and hand. It enters the proximal arm behind the brachial artery and anterior to the subscapularis muscle, and the tendons of the latissimus dorsi and teres major.[20] It travels dorsolaterally with the profunda brachii artery between the medial and long head of the triceps around the posterior aspect of the humerus, separated from this bone by fibers of the medial head. The nerve pierces the lateral intermuscular septum approximately 10 cm above the lateral epicondyle, lying adjacent to but not within the spiral groove.[21] After entering the flexor compartment, the nerve proceeds within the intermuscular interval between the brachialis and the brachioradialis proximally and the extensor carpi radialis longus (ECRL) muscle distally.[20] It passes anterior to the tip of the lateral epicondyle as it enters the forearm, where it divides into superficial and deep terminal branches.

After formation of the main trunk in the axilla, the radial nerve gives off the posterior cutaneous nerve of the arm, and a branch to the long head of the triceps. The next branch, the ulnar collateral nerve, travels with the ulnar nerve distally in the arm while supplying the medial head. Leaving the nerve between the medial and lateral heads of the triceps are the posterior muscular branch, which innervates these muscles, and the common trunk of the inferior lateral cutaneous nerve of the arm and the posterior antebrachial cutaneous nerve. After piercing the lateral intermuscular septum, the main trunk gives off branches to the lateral portion of the brachialis (inconstant), the elbow joint, and the brachioradialis and ECRL muscle, whose branches arise 2 to 3 cm above the lateral epicondyle. The radial nerve divides into superficial and deep terminal branches anterior to the lateral epicondyle. The superficial branch terminates in the dorsal digital nerves, which provide sensation to the dorsal thumb and radial two and one-half fingers. A motor branch to the extensor carpi radialis brevis (ECRB) muscle arises from the superficial branch in more than 50% of subjects.[17] The deep terminal branch or posterior interosseous nerve (PIN) gives off branches to the ECRB and supinator muscles before piercing the latter muscle to emerge on the dorsal surface of the forearm. The PIN subsequently innervates the wrist, finger, and thumb extensors, in addition to providing sensory fibers to the wrist joint.[20]

Exposure of the radial nerve in the upper arm may be achieved by either a posterior or anterolateral approach, depending on the extent of exposure necessary, the pathologic process, and the need for exploration of associated structures.[15] Regardless of the approach, the patient should be placed in the lateral decubitus or prone position with a sterile tourniquet in place or available and the entire upper extremity draped free. The

■ FIGURE 101–1
The incision for an anterolateral exposure to the radial nerve is depicted. The proximal landmark is the interval between the deltoid and the lateral head of the triceps. The incision curves anteriorly toward the interval between the brachioradialis and biceps/brachialis.

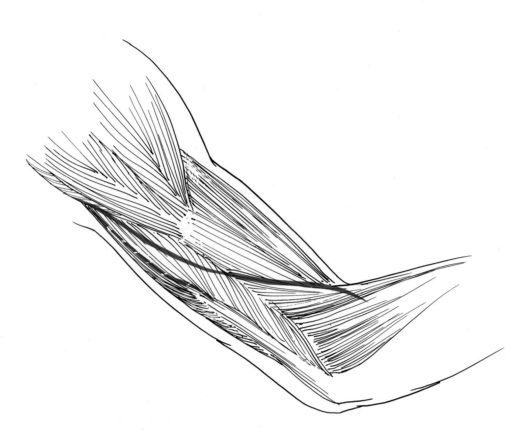

patient is not paralyzed until it is determined whether intraoperative nerve conduction studies will be required. The posterior approach may be used when the exploration will be limited to the upper arm; when further distal exposure may be necessary, the anterolateral approach is used. The more extensive anterolateral approach is illustrated (Fig. 101–1). The posterior approach is very similar to the upper portion of the anterolateral approach except for placement of the incision.

Bony landmarks for the posterior approach are the posterior border of the acromion and the tip of the olecranon. The incision is made along a line joining these landmarks, exposing the sulcus between the long and lateral heads of the triceps.[15] The fascia along the lateral border of the long head is incised in line with the skin incision, and the interval between the long and lateral heads developed with blunt dissection distally to the triceps tendon, which is incised sharply (Figs. 101-2 and 101-3). The superficial muscle bellies are then retracted to expose the radial nerve and profunda vessels in the superolateral aspect coursing obliquely across the medial head (Fig. 101–2). If the posterior aspect of the humeral shaft needs to be exposed, the medial head of the triceps may be incised sharply. Starting proximally, the radial nerve is gently retracted and the medial head is incised between the ulnar collateral nerve and a parallel branch to the lateral head.[8] Care must be taken to avoid damage to the main neurovascular bundle, which is located in the superomedial aspect of this exposure and comprises the median and ulnar nerves and brachial artery. The branch to the lateral head must also be identified and protected during this exposure. Elevation of the medial head allows visualization of the lateral intermuscular septum and the origins of the brachioradialis and ECRL. Division of this septum close to the humerus exposes the radial nerve. Adduction of the arm relaxes the nerve, allowing additional distal exposure. Proximally, further length may be gained by dividing the latissimus and teres major tendons, taking care to protect the radial and ulnar nerves lying anteriorly.[8] Experience has demonstrated the wisdom of beginning the actual dissection

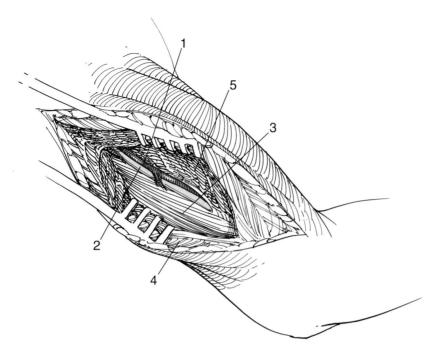

■ FIGURE 101–2
The fascia between the long and lateral heads of the triceps is incised to expose the radial nerve. The long and lateral heads are retracted, demonstrating the radial nerve covered in part by the medial head of the triceps. 1, profunda brachii artery; 2, radial nerve; 3, medial head of triceps; 4, long head of triceps; 5, lateral head of triceps.

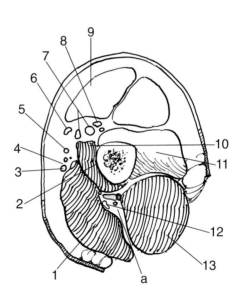

■ FIGURE 101–3
Cross-sectional anatomy of the middle upper arm (area of spiral groove). 1, long head of triceps; 2, medial head of triceps; 3, ulnar nerve; 4, medial cutaneous nerve of forearm; 5, basilic vein; 6, median nerve; 7, brachial artery with veni comitantes; 8, musculocutaneous nerve; 9, biceps; 10, coracobrachialis; 11, brachialis; 12, radial nerve with profunda brachii; 13, lateral head of triceps; a, surgical approach.

of the nerve in normal tissue proximal and distal to the site of injury, and then proceeding with dissection toward the zone of injury.

The anterolateral approach provides exposure of the radial nerve in the distal arm and may be easily extended when further exploration is required.[8] The incision may be started either anterior or posterior to the deltoid, depending on the type of exposure necessary. Anteriorly, the line of incision begins at the midportion of the deltoid and extends distally in the interval between the deltoid and the biceps. This may be extended proximally into the anteromedial approach to the shoulder.[3] If a more posterior approach is required, the incision may begin in the interval between the deltoid and the lateral head of the triceps, starting 8 cm below the posterior axillary crease (Fig. 101–1). Both incisions extend distally along the lateral border of the brachialis, curving anteriorly into the interval between the brachialis and brachioradialis (Figs. 101-4 and 101-5), and may be continued as for the anterolateral approach to the radial nerve in the forearm.[15]

The deep fascia is incised along the length of the incision and the biceps–brachialis retracted medially. The radial nerve may be exposed in the interval between the brachialis and brachioradialis (Figs. 101-5 and 101-6) just above the elbow, or in the lateral half of the brachialis after splitting this muscle longitudinally.[3,15] The nerve may be traced proximally to the lateral intermuscular septum, where further exposure may be obtained as in the posterior approach. Distally the nerve may be followed in the intermuscular interval into the forearm.

■ FIGURE 101–4
Distal extension of the anterolateral approach. The incision labeled "a" is the interval between the long and lateral head of the triceps, whereas fascial incision "b" is along the interval between the brachialis and brachioradialis.

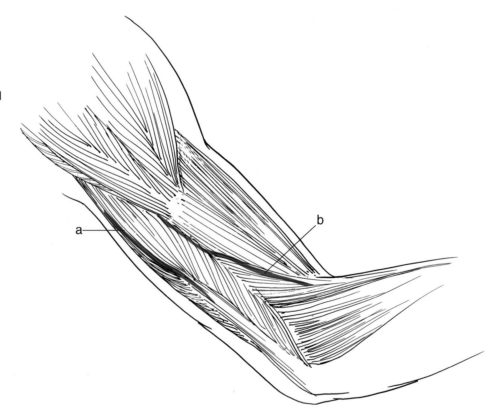

■ FIGURE 101–5
Cross-sectional anatomy of the distal upper arm. 1, brachialis; 2, radial nerve; 3, profunda brachii with veni comitantes; 4, brachioradialis; a, approach posterior to brachialis.

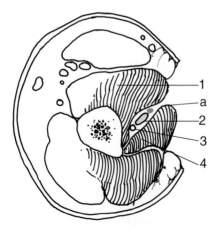

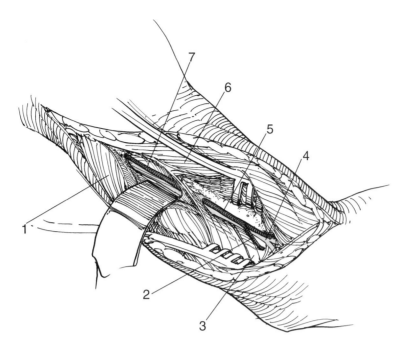

■ FIGURE 101–6
The radial nerve passes
through the intermuscular
septum to lie anterior to
it. 1, lateral head of triceps; 2, posterior de-
scending artery; 3, brachioradialis; 4, radial nerve;
5, anterior descending artery; 6, brachialis; 7, profunda brachii.

On identifying the site of nerve injury, careful dissection is performed to define the nature of the injury, its approximate extent, and the neural anatomy. The most critical issue becomes determining the extent of nerve injury, because only normal nerve must be grafted proximally and distally if recovery is to occur; if the nerve is in continuity one can use intraoperative electrophysiologic studies to assist in determining the nature of the neuroma-in-continuity. For example, if a large compound action potential (CAP) can be recorded from the distal nerve segment when stimulating the nerve proximal to the lesion, this indicates perhaps significant regeneration across the zone of injury. In this case, neurolysis may be indicated. If no signal can be recorded, or if signal averaging is necessary to document the presence of a distal CAP, then the damaged segment should be resected. The operating microscope is a useful adjunct in determining the level of distal and proximal resection. Proximal resection should commence just proximal to the grossly obvious neuroma. We prefer a #10 blade with as little slicing motion as possible. Several commercially available devices facilitate this step, but we have not used these. The surface of the nerve is observed for the presence of visible fascicular patterns and for the presence of abnormal-appearing vascular plexus. The cut end of the nerve is observed for the presence of bulging fascicle groups with minimal endoneurial or perifascicular thickening. However, if a significant stretch injury has occurred, the proximal nerve segment will never appear totally healthy, unless one is willing to resect far proximal to the neuroma. The distal segment is likewise examined, although its cut surface will lack bulging fascicle groups. After resection of the damaged segment, the length of the defect is then defined with the shoulder in abduction, the elbow in extension, and the wrist in slight extension. This allows mobilization of the limb without placing tension on the nerve graft. It makes little sense to go through the very major effort involved in grafting this nerve and then to flex the elbow to avoid an additional 2 cm of graft length.

The intraneural topography as described by Sunderland[19] should be applied when possible to optimize results from grafting the radial nerve. In the upper arm, the radial nerve has a polyfascicular architecture, with mixed motor and sensory bundles. Nevertheless, there is a rough distribution of motor fibers posteriorly and sensory fibers anteriorly (Fig. 101–7). Before branching from the main trunk, motor fascicles to the long and medial heads may be found posteromedially, and bundles to the lateral head, anterolaterally. Beyond the lateral intermuscular septum, fascicles to the brachioradialis, ECRL, and ECRB are located anterolaterally. Fascicles that will become the superficial sensory and the poste-

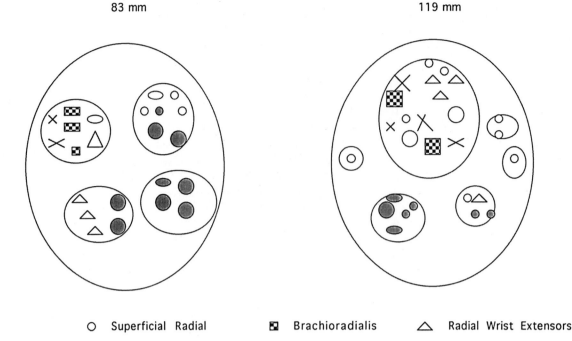

83 mm   119 mm

| ○ | Superficial Radial | ▣ | Brachioradialis | △ | Radial Wrist Extensors |
| ● | Posterior Interosseous | ✕ | Brachialis | | |

■ FIGURE 101–7

Topographic maps may be useful when a gap must be overcome by nerve grafts. On the left is the axon map of the radial nerve approximately 80 mm proximal to the humeral condyles, or at the level of the spiral groove. On the right is the radial nerve about 4 cm more proximal. Such maps may assist in aligning longer nerve grafts to maximize functional recovery by reducing the quantity of misdirected axons.

rior interosseous nerves (Fig. 101–7) are separated into the anterior and posterior portions of the nerve as high as 9 cm above its bifurcation.[9] Such proximal division of the radial nerve into motor and sensory components may account for historically better results obtained after repair of radial nerve injuries. Once topography has been determined, standard interfascicular nerve grafting techniques are used, as described in preceding chapters.

Several adjuncts in reconstruction are possible, including various histochemical techniques that permit the surgeon to differentiate primary motor and sensory fascicles in the proximal nerve stump. This is a potentially practical exercise in primary repair, where more normal distal stump anatomy is present. For the radial nerve with a large loss of substance, it may be difficult to identify the sensory component of the distal segment. However, the sensory fascicle(s) can be dissected from the primary motor fascicles far proximal in the nerve. We have used the sensory fascicle, so dissected, as a source of nerve graft. In addition, when the distal segment is considerably atrophied, it is advisable to avoid wasting precious distal motor endoneurial channels by identifying the sensory fascicle in the proximal stump and not covering this fascicle with a nerve graft cable.

Once grafting is completed, the wound is closed in layers using local or distant tissue as necessary to ensure adequate soft tissue coverage. The arm is splinted in the extended posture as described earlier to prevent scar adhesions around the graft in a flexed position.

■ TECHNICAL
ALTERNATIVES

The only practical technical alternatives involve simple sacrificing of radial nerve-innervated muscles and sensory territories and proceeding directly to muscle tendon transfers to restore wrist and digital extension. This approach may be considered when the interval between injury and operation is lengthy, or perhaps in the elderly. However, in general, the outcome of nerve reconstruction is favorable and the procedure worthwhile. Substitution for missing function by creative splinting has been mentioned.

Other adjuncts such as the use of vascularized nerve graft might be considered for very long defects (> 10 cm) or when the wound bed is vascularly compromised. Such steps hardly seem necessary in the enormous majority of cases of isolated radial nerve palsy because, as alluded to earlier, there exist so many successful alternatives, particularly reliable tendon transfers, to nerve reconstruction for this nerve.

The most common pitfall relates to failure to diagnose promptly a severe nerve injury associated with closed fracture of the humerus. There is no substitute for clinical experience in determining when to proceed with surgery. However, if the Tinel sign has advanced well beyond the typical motor point of proximal paralyzed muscles and no twitch can be appreciated, there is little reason to continue waiting. The most common technical pitfall relates to insufficient resection of damaged nerve. Compounding this error is insufficient proximal and distal exposure. Another potential error is failure to position the extremity with the shoulder abducted, elbow extended, and wrist extended when measuring and insetting nerve grafts. It may also be an error not to proceed to immediate tendon transfers when the length of the nerve gap exceeds 8 to 10 cm, for very proximal lesions, or in patients older than 40 years of age.

■ **REHABILITATION**

Postoperative care includes splinting of the upper extremity with the shoulder adducted, the elbow extended, and slight extension at the wrist. The extremity is elevated in the immediate postoperative period with frequent checks for vascular sufficiency. Immobilization is maintained for 10 to 14 days, at which time careful range of motion exercises are initiated. A static wrist extension splint is worn until adequate motor recovery has occurred. Nerve recovery is monitored clinically by physical examination. Because most injuries involve the middle and lower thirds of the upper arm, the brachioradialis is often the first muscle to regain function, usually within 4 to 6 months. Distal reinnervation as heralded by thumb extension generally takes another 7 to 9 months.[5] Tendon transfers should be considered if useful recovery of function has not been achieved by 9 months.

■ **OUTCOMES**

The poor results obtained with nerve grafting during the World Wars stifled its wide application. Millesi's results,[11] published in the early 1970s, rekindled interest in the technique, and interfascicular nerve grafting has become the procedure of choice for bridging nerve defects without tension. Frykman and Gramyk[7] compiled the published results for nerve grafting restricted to studies using microsurgical techniques and adhering to strict criteria for classification and follow-up. They found that "useful" motor recovery (> M3) occurred in 60% of grafts in the arm, 75% of those below the ECRL, and all grafts of the posterior interosseous nerve. This compares favorably with "useful" motor recovery in nerve grafts above the elbow in the median (50%) and ulnar (55%) nerves. Recovery of motor function displayed an inverse relationship with age, gap, delay to repair, and level of injury, with age being the best predictor. Results for sensory recovery in radial nerve grafts above the elbow were poor, with only 30% obtaining useful recovery. Delays of greater than 6 months did not have a significant effect on sensory recovery in the radial nerve.[6] Similar results with regard to motor and sensory recovery and factors affecting outcome have been found in recently published reviews for adults[16] and children.[1]

References

1. Barrios C, Pablos J: Surgical management of nerve of the upper extremity in children: A 15-year survey. J Pediatr Orthop, 1991; 11:641–645.
2. Bostman O, Bakalim G, Vainiopaa S, Wilppula E, Patiala H, Rokkanen P: Radial palsy in shaft fracture of the humerus. Acta Orthop Scand, 1986; 57:316–319.
3. Crenshaw AH: Surgical approaches. In: Crenshaw AH (ed): Campbell's Operative Orthopaedics, 7th Ed. St. Louis: CV Mosby, 1987:94–99.
4. Dellon AL, Mackinnon SE: Surgery of the Peripheral Nerve. New York: Thieme, 1988:121.

5. Dolene V: Radial nerve lesions and their treatment. Acta Neurochir, 1976; 34:235–243.

6. Fischer TR, McGeoch CM: Severe injuries of the radial nerve treated by sural nerve grafting. Injury, 1985; 16:411–414.

7. Frykman GD, Gramyk K: Results of nerve grafting. In: Gelberman RH (ed): Operative Nerve Repair and Reconstruction. Philadelphia: JB Lippincott, 1991:553–567.

8. Henry AK: Extensile Exposure, 2nd Ed. New York: Churchill Livingstone, 1970:15–40.

9. Jabaley ME, Wallace WH, Hecker FR: Internal topography of major nerves of the forearm and hand: A current view. J Hand Surg, 1980; 5:1–12.

10. Labosky DA, Waggy CA: Apparent weakness of the median and ulnar nerves in radial nerve palsy. J Hand Surg, 1986; 11A:528–533.

11. Millesi H: Indications and technique of nerve grafting. In: Gelberman RH (ed): Operative Nerve Repair and Reconstruction. Philadelphia: JB Lippincott, 1991:525–543.

12. Omer GE: Injury to nerves of the upper extremity. J Bone Joint Surg, 1974; 56A:1615–1624.

13. Pollock FH, Drake D, Bovill EG, Day L, Trafton PG: Treatment of radial neuropathy associated with fractures of the humerus. J Bone Joint Surg, 1981; 63A:239–243.

14. Seddon H: Surgical Disorders of the Peripheral Nerves, 2nd Ed. New York: Churchill Livingstone, 1975:303–307.

15. Siegel DB, Gelberman RH: Radial nerve: Applied anatomy and operative exposure. In: Gelberman RH (ed): Operative Nerve Repair and Reconstruction. Philadelphia: JB Lippincott, 1991:393–407.

16. Singh R, Mechelse K, Braakman R: Longterm results of transplantations to repair median, ulnar, and radial nerve lesions by a microsurgical interfascicular autogenous cable technique. Surg Neurol, 1992; 37:425–431.

17. Spinner M: Management of nerve compression lesions of the upper extremity. In: Omer GE, Spinner M (eds): Management of Peripheral Nerve Problems. Philadelphia: WB Saunders, 1980:569–587.

18. Steyers CM: Radial nerve results. In: Gelberman RH (ed): Operative Nerve Repair and Reconstruction. Philadelphia: JB Lippincott, 1991:409–412.

19. Sunderland S: Nerves and Nerve Injuries, 2nd Ed. New York: Churchill Livingstone, 1978: 838.

20. Warwick R, Williams PL (eds): Gray's Anatomy, 35th Ed (Br). Philadelphia: WB Saunders, 1973:1045–1048.

21. Whitson RO: Relation of the radial nerve to the shaft of the humerus. J Bone Joint Surg, 1954; 36A:85–88.

PART

VIII

Arthrodesis

102

Arthrodesis of the Distal Interphalangeal Joint with K-Wire Technique

Joint arthrodesis has been available as a reconstructive procedure for many years. Discussions on arthrodesis of the distal interphalangeal (DIP) joint often are combined with arthrodesis of other finger and hand joints. The goals of the surgery, painless and stable union in proper position, have remained unchanged with time. Reports in the literature reflect differences in bone preparation and fixation techniques.

Bunnell[5] stressed the importance of broad bony contact and fixation with two crossed Kirschner wires. Nemethi[14] believed that a single wire was adequate and prevented distraction at the arthrodesis site, which could occur with two wires. Robertson[16] was frustrated by the complication of nonunion and stressed the importance of proper bone preparation. He recommended the use of an oscillating power saw in preparing the bone ends because rongeurs or burrs did not provide flat and smooth bone ends. He believed that a single wire did not provide enough stability and two wires resulted in distraction. He, therefore, described wire-loop fixation, which provided compression at the arthrodesis site.

Moberg[12,13] added a new technique of bone grafting. While others suggested use of bone graft to stimulate healing, he used structural bone graft from the olecranon to transfix the arthrodesis site. Additional fixation was provided by K-wires. Potenza[15] modified this technique by using bone graft from the middle phalanx in arthrodesis of the DIP joint.

Carroll and Hill[7] described the cone in a cup technique of bone end preparation. They believed that this maximizes bone contact, yet allows adjustment in arthrodesis position in three planes before fixation. With the technique of squaring off the bone ends, the arthrodesis position is dictated by the angulation of the bone cuts and later cannot be adjusted.

Further developments centered on variations in fixation. Compression at the site of fixation increases stability.[19] Tension band wiring,[1] screw fixation,[17] plate fixation,[20] and external fixation[3] techniques have been described, all of which provide improved compression at the arthrodesis site. Unfortunately, most studies include other hand and finger joints in their results, making decisions on their use in the DIP joint difficult. Most frustrating is the lack of comparative study of the different methods.

■ HISTORY OF THE TECHNIQUE

The primary indication for DIP joint arthrodesis is pain or instability that is unresponsive to nonoperative treatment. Common causes include nonunion or malunion of intra-articular fractures, chronic collateral ligament or volar plate injuries, chronic flexor digitorum profundus avulsions, mallet finger deformity, or arthrosis. The DIP joint is a common site for hypertrophic degenerative arthrosis in the hand, which can cause restricted motion, prominent osteophytes (Heberden's nodes), and angular or rotational deformity. Often these changes occur without pain or functional compromise. Patients will frequently present with cosmetic concerns, but this is rarely an indication for surgical treatment. Pain or instability at the DIP joint that impairs the grasping or pinching activity of the finger warrants treatment.

Mucous cysts are ganglion cysts that often form about the DIP joint. They usually are

■ INDICATIONS AND CONTRAINDICATIONS

directly associated with an osteophyte from the distal phalanx, and if symptomatic can be simply excised with the osteophyte. Arthrodesis is indicated if the joint arthrosis is symptomatic as discussed previously or if there are symptomatic recurrent mucous cysts.

Nonoperative treatment options include nonsteroidal anti-inflammatory medications, activity modification, and splinting. These treatments often are helpful in degenerative arthrosis where pain will occur in the early stages but resolves with time.

Contraindications include active infection, inadequate bone, or significant loss of function in other fingers such that improved function of the operated finger would not be expected with an arthrodesis. Arthrodesis of an insensate or dysesthetic finger often results in poor function[12] and, therefore, should be considered a relative contraindication.

■ SURGICAL
TECHNIQUES

Adequate visualization is essential to minimize operative trauma and to identify important anatomic structures. This requires the use of a tourniquet. A finger tourniquet can be used comfortably with digital block or wrist block anesthesia. A distal forearm tourniquet also can be used, but intravenous sedation also may be required for tourniquet pain. I often use a wrist block and a distal forearm tourniquet. If the patient begins having tourniquet pain before the procedure is completed, I will then switch to a finger tourniquet. This minimizes the use of a finger tourniquet, which can cause digital nerve injury.[9,11] Alternatively, an axillary block or Bier block can be performed, which allows comfortable use of a proximal arm tourniquet. This is especially useful when multiple joints are to be treated, or if the arthrodesis is done in conjunction with other operative hand or wrist procedures.

A variety of incisions have been described to expose the DIP joint (Fig. 102–1). The incision must allow wide exposure of both sides of the joint while minimizing injury to the arterial and venous structures in the deep dermal layer. It also must avoid injury to the germinal nail matrix, which begins 1 mm distal to the insertion of the extensor tendon. Injury to the germinal matrix will result in nail growth abnormalities.

I prefer the Y incision because the longitudinal portion parallels the vasculature structures minimizing injury. Bipolar electrocautery is used for hemostasis of only actively bleeding vessels. Minimal injury to the dorsal veins is required to prevent problems with venous outflow, which would result in venous congestion and finger swelling. The incision is made sharply down to the extensor tendons. The soft tissues are sharply elevated off

■ FIGURE 102–1
Incisions for exposure of the DIP joint. **A,** Straight dorsal longitudinal incision with Y extension just distal to the level of the joint line. **B,** H-shaped incision. **C,** S-shaped incision. **D,** V-shaped incision with the apex at the lateral margin of the joint. **E,** Midlateral incision curved dorsally just proximal to nail fold. **F,** U-shaped incision based proximally.

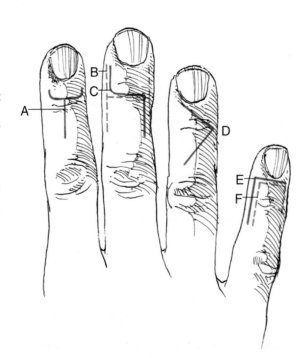

the tendon radially and ulnarly. Care is taken to avoid crushing the skin with forceps and to dissect carefully by spreading with scissors, which can injure the vascular structures. Distally, the skin is elevated to the level of the extensor tendon insertion. The extensor tendon is transversely transected 1 to 2 mm proximal to the joint. The tendon is retracted distally and elevated slightly (approximately 1 mm) from its insertion into the distal phalanx (Fig. 102–2). Care should be taken to make this dissection subperiosteal to avoid injury to the germinal matrix. The collateral ligaments are released from the middle phalanx. The joint is hyperflexed giving wide exposure to the joint. Marginal osteophytes are removed with a rongeur. The remaining cartilage and subchondral bone is removed from each bone end to allow opposing cancellous bone. The shape of the bone ends may vary. Each bone cut can be made at appropriate angles so that when opposed, the desired fusion angle is obtained (Fig. 102–3).[2,5,14,15] A small oscillating saw is recommended as it provides smooth bone ends for apposition.[16] Practically this is very difficult to perform in the DIP joint because of the small size of the bone ends. The other technique, which I favor, is to shape the distal end of the middle phalanx into a cone using a rongeur and the distal phalanx into a cup using a currette or small osteotome (Fig. 102–4).[7] With this shape, the arthrodesis

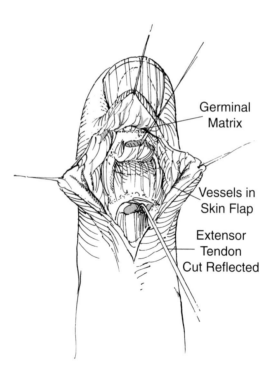

■ FIGURE 102–2
Dorsal Y exposure to the DIP joint. Full-thickness skin flaps are elevated with care taken to minimize injury to longitudinally oriented vessels. The extensor tendon is transected and reflected distally to expose the DIP joint.

Germinal Matrix

Vessels in Skin Flap

Extensor Tendon Cut Reflected

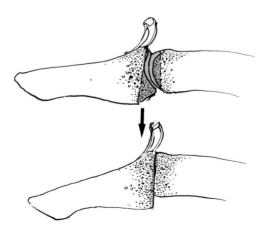

■ FIGURE 102–3
DIP joint arthrodesis. Straight angled cuts in bone ends.

■ FIGURE 102-4
DIP joint arthrodesis. Cup
in cone technique.

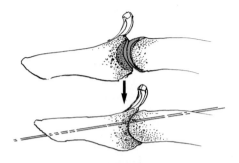

■ FIGURE 102-5
A and B, PA and lateral
radiographs using a longitudinal K-wire and an ad-
ditional oblique K-wire for
stability.

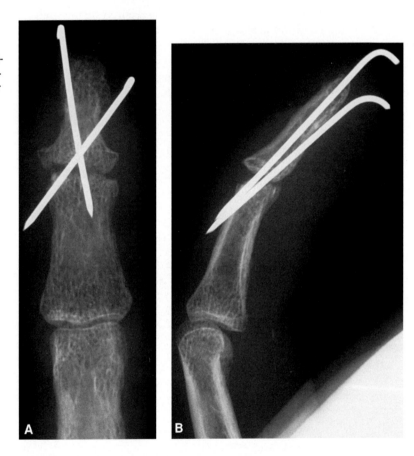

flexion angle can be adjusted before fixation and gives good cancellous bone contact. Portions of the resected cancellous bone can be used as bone graft.

The desired position for DIP arthrodesis is between 0° and 25° of flexion.[7] In general, more flexion is needed in the little finger and lesser amounts in the more radial fingers. This is because the ulnar fingers require more flexion for gripping while the radial fingers require a straighter position for tip-to-tip opposition to the thumb. It is important to correct any rotational deformity. The index finger may be slightly supinated to allow tip-to-tip opposition to the thumb. The little finger may be pronated slightly. Positioning is best adjusted to the patient's functional needs. This requires careful preoperative evaluation of the patient's specific activity needs.

Several methods of fixation have been described. I prefer fixation with one or two Kirshner wires. A 0.062- or 0.045-inch K-wire may be used depending on the size of the joint. The decision to use one or two wires is based on bone stability. If the bone is of good quality and length is well maintained, leaving good soft tissue tension, then a single longitudinal wire is used. If there is any instability after fixation, a second oblique wire is placed (Figs. 102-5A and 102-5B). Care must be taken to assure that the arthrodesis site is not distracted by the second wire. The wire can be cut beneath the skin, which decreases the chance of pin tract infection and allows the pin fixation to remain for a longer period of time. Alternatively, the wire can be bent and left external to the skin, which allows easier removal. The extensor tendon should be repaired to provide soft tissue coverage minimizing skin adhesion and avoiding swan neck deformity to the finger.[6]

The digit is immobilized with the metacarpophalangeal (MP) joint in flexion to prevent an extensor contracture and the proximal interphalangeal (PIP) joint in extension. If multiple fingers are operated, anterior-posterior plaster splints are used for immobilization. If just one or two fingers are operated, immobilization is achieved with an aluminum finger splint.

Technical alternatives involve the method of fixation. Although tension band technique provides better compression and stability, the additional dissection to place the tension wire risks injury to the germinal matrix. Also, the size of the bone makes this a technically difficult option compared with the PIP joint. However, tension band wiring can be combined with K-wire fixation to provide a stable construct for arthrodesis (Figs. 102-6A, 102-6B, 102-7A, and 102-7B). Screw fixation allows earlier motion without a splint; however, it is technically difficult to place because of the small bone size. Screw fixation becomes more difficult when greater flexion is needed in the arthrodesis. Also, screw fixation significantly increases the implant cost to the procedure. I will use screw fixation in a patient who desires minimal immobilization and does only light hand activity. The bone is too small to recommend plate fixation. Although I have no experience with external fixation, I would not recommend this because of potential pin tract infection, injury to the neurovascular structures, and bulkiness, which would interfere with adjacent finger function.

■ TECHNICAL ALTERNATIVES

Ten to fourteen days after surgery, the sutures are removed. The DIP joint is immobilized

■ REHABILITATION

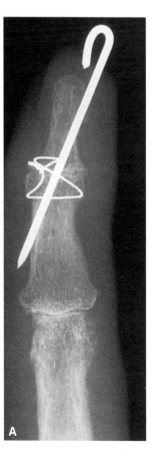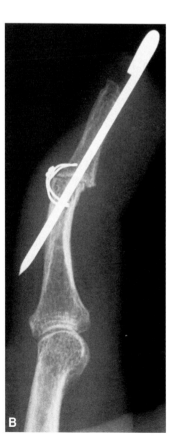

■ FIGURE 102–6
A and B, PA and lateral radiographs demonstrating the combined K-wire and tension band wire technique.

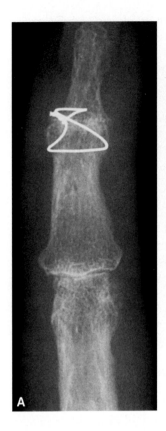
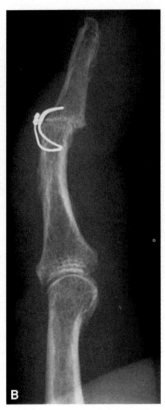

■ FIGURE 102–7
A and B, Postoperative PA and lateral radiographs with union of the arthrodesis. The tension wire can be retained if it is not problematic. The patient regained pain free use of the finger.

with an aluminum splint and aggressive motion of the MP and PIP joints begun. Maintaining motion of the MP and PIP joints is critical to maintaining overall finger mobility and therefore function.

The K-wire is generally removed approximately 6 to 8 weeks after surgery and splinting of the DIP joint continued with an aluminum splint until radiographic evidence of union is achieved (Fig. 102–6). Provided MP and PIP joint motion is maintained, the patient easily regains functional use of the finger.

■ OUTCOMES

With solid union, the patient can expect a painless joint with adequate stability to allow full hand activity without limitation.

Complications include pin tract infections, which usually respond well to pin removal and oral antibiotics. Nonunion or fibrous union is unusual being less than 10% in most reports. Repeat operation for these conditions is indicated if the finger remains painful. Malunion may result from inadequate fixation or bone preparation. Repeating the procedure is indicated if functional limitation exists. Wound dehiscence can be difficult to treat. Its occurrence can be minimized by attention to atraumatic operative technique and avoidance of tissue pressure or tension by fixation or splinting. If the dehiscence is mild, it may respond to local measures with soaking and dressing changes. If severe or if accompanied by infection, treatment may require tissue grafting or consideration of amputation.

References

1. Allende BT, Engelem JC: Tension band arthrodesis in the finger joints. J Hand Surg, 1980; 5: 269–271.
2. Beltran JE, Barjan R, Moreta D: A complication of distal interphalangeal joint arthrodesis. Hand, 1976; 8:36–38.
3. Braun RM, Rhoades CE: Dynamic compression for small bone arthrodesis. J Hand Surg, 1985; 10A:340–343.

4. Brockman R, Weiland AJ: Small joint arthrodesis. In: Green DP (ed): Operative Hand Surgery, New York: Churchill Livingstone, 1993:99–111.

5. Bunnell S: Joints. In: Boyes J (ed): Surgery of the Hand, 4th Ed, Philadelphia: J. B. Lippincott, 1948:320–324.

6. Burton RI, Margles SW, Lunseth PA: Small joint arthrodesis in the hand. J Hand Surg, 1986; 11A:678–682.

7. Carroll RE, Hill NA: Small joint arthrodesis in hand reconstruction. J Bone Joint Surg, 1969; 51A:19–12.

8. Culver JE, Fleegler EJ: Osteoarthritis of the distal interphalangeal joint. Hand Clinics, 1987; 3: 385–402.

9. Hixson FP, Shafiroff BB, Werner FW, Palmer AK: Digital tourniquets: A pressure study with clinical relevance. J Hand Surg, 1986; 11A:865–868.

10. Kilgore ES, Adams DR, Newmeyer WL: A preferred incision for dorsal finger exposure. Plast Reconstr Surg, 1971; 47:194–195.

11. Lubahn JD, Koeneman J, Kosar K: The digital tourniquet. How safe is it? J Hand Surg, 1985; 10A:664–669.

12. Moberg E: Arthrodesis of finger joints. Surg Clin North Am, 1960; 40:465–470.

13. Moberg E, Henrikson B: Technique for digital arthrodesis. A study of 150 cases. Acta Chir Scandinavica, 1959; 118:331–338.

14. Nemethi CE: Phalangeal fractures treated by open reduction and Kirshner wire fixation. Indust Med, 1954; 23:148.

15. Potenza AD: A technique for arthrodesis of finger joints. J Bone Joint Surg, 1973; 55A: 1534–1536.

16. Robertson DC: The fusion of interphalangeal joints. Can J Surg, 1964; 7:433–437.

17. Segmuller G: Surgical stabilization of the skeletal of the hand. Baltimore, Williams and Wilkins, 1977.

18. Swanson AB: Distal interphalangeal joint implant arthroplasty. In: Surgical Techniques for Flexible Implant Arthroplasty in the MP, PIP, DIP joints of the Hand, Grand Rapids: Orthopaedic and Reconstructive Surgeons, P.C., 1980:25.

19. Vanik RK, Weber RC, Matlouls HS, Sanger JR, Gingrass RP: The comparative strengths of internal fixation techniques. J Hand Surg, 1984; 9A:6–12.

20. Wright CS, McMurtry RY: AO arthrodesis in the hand. J Hand Surg, 1983; 8:932–935.

A. GEORGE DASS
MARK R. BELSKY

103

Arthrodesis of the Proximal Interphalangeal Joint with K-Wire Technique

■ HISTORY OF THE
TECHNIQUE

The term "arthrodesis" (artificial ankylosis) was coined by Eduard Albert of Vienna in 1882 in his treatment of an unstable ankle.[2] The first interphalangeal arthrodeses were probably spontaneous fusions that resulted from injury or infection. It is not clear from the literature who performed the first proximal interphalangeal (PIP) arthrodesis, but Emanuel Kaplan discussed the use of arthrodesis in the care of intrinsic deformities of the hand in 1937.[13,14]

There are several methods of surgical arthrodesis of the PIP joint that have been proven effective. The most popular techniques include the use of K-wires, tension band wiring, intraosseous wiring, Herbert and ASIF screw fixation, external compression devices, and miniplates.[1,4,6,8–10,17]

The use of two crossed K-wires for PIP joint arthrodesis is a popular technique and has been reported to be highly successful by Granovitz and Vainio,[9] Boyes,[3] Watson and Schaffer,[20] and Edwards et al.[7] A slight variation in the technique is well described by Carroll and Hill, who introduced the idea of one straight and one oblique wire.[5] Our preference is a modification using both a longitudinal and one or two oblique wires. In addition, there are several methods of bone preparation for PIP joint arthrodesis, including cup-and-cone, chevron, and tongue-and-groove techniques, each with its own theoretical advantages.[5,18,12] Often the bone quality limits the extent of reshaping that can be performed. Our preference is to maximize the bone contact surface with a shallow "ball and cup," comparable to a dome osteotomy in which all the stability is obtained with the internal fixation. Whatever method is chosen, it should be technically simple and reproducible, and have a high union rate and a low complication rate.

■ INDICATIONS AND
CONTRAINDICATIONS

The obvious total loss of motion that accompanies arthrodesis makes this technique a definitive choice in reconstruction. With the popularity of arthroplasty, there is often overlap of the surgical indications for these procedures. However, arthrodesis of the PIP joint in certain situations maximizes the function of the adjacent joints, gives complete relief of pain, and provides stability in a high percentage of cases.

The indications for PIP joint arthrodesis are to relieve pain, provide stability, correct deformity, and prevent progression of disease. If the patient has a painful articulation with loss of the cartilaginous surface of the joint but satisfactory soft tissue stability, then the choice is between arthroplasty and arthrodesis. Soft tissue stability includes the ligamentous support and the flexor and extensor tendon function. Arthrodesis is preferred in cases where deficient tendon function or collateral ligaments result in finger deformity. Occasionally there may be an angular or rotational deformity of the digit associated with PIP joint arthritis or instability. Arthrodesis facilitates correction of the alignment while providing joint stabilization.

Repositioning stiff joints for burn contractures, Dupuytren disease, or swan neck and boutonniere deformities secondary to rheumatoid arthritis and scleroderma (Fig. 103–1) is another indication. A limitation can be the quality of the overlying skin. It is not recommended that a skin graft be placed over the joint at the same time as arthrodesis. In this case, skeletal shortening or a staged procedure is recommended.

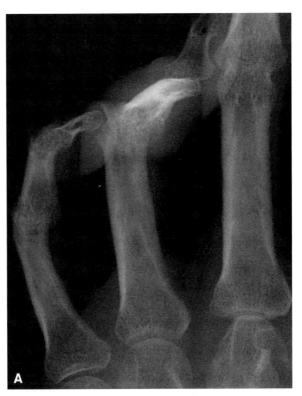

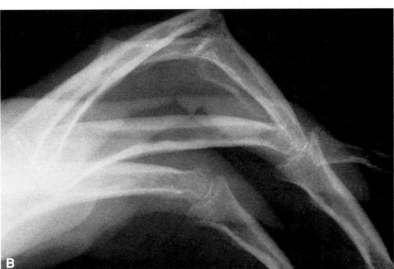

■ FIGURE 103–1
Posteroanterior **(A)** and lateral **(B)** radiographs of a boutonniere deformity of the ring finger in a patient with scleroderma.

Septic arthritis results in a joint that is often best treated by arthrodesis. The infection should be eradicated before arthrodesis with K-wires; active infection is a contraindication to using K-wires early in the treatment of an infected joint. Arthrodesis with K-wires is often done near the end stage of joint infection, with the final debridement. Additional bone graft should not be used unless the infection has been eradicated.

As with any bone operation, good soft tissue coverage is essential. Supple overlying skin provides for better excursion of the extensor apparatus through the lateral bands to the distal interphalangeal (DIP) joint. In addition, the wires are better protected, with better soft tissue coverage. The bone quality must be satisfactory to sustain the internal fixation necessary to support the arthrodesis. Ultimately, the internal fixation must keep the arthrodesis rigid or it will not heal in a reasonable time. Although this discussion is limited to the use of K-wires, it is most helpful to be familiar with several techniques to be prepared for certain individual variations in bone quality, the need to perform simultaneous procedures, and postoperative management. The final decision on the technique used in any individual patient is not made until the tissues are assessed during surgery.

Straub suggests that the PIP joints are best fused in the position of function.[19] Thus, the position varies from 25° in the index finger to 50° in the small finger. The position also depends on the status of the adjacent metacarpophalangeal and DIP joints. The priority for the ulnar border digits is that they must contribute to grasp functions yet still fit into the patient's pocket and into a glove.

■ SURGICAL TECHNIQUES

The procedure is performed under regional anesthesia with proximal arm tourniquet control. Loupe magnification is recommended to avoid injury to the adjacent delicate structures such as the dorsal cutaneous nerves. A 3- to 4-cm dorsal curvilinear incision is centered over the PIP joint. In patients with thin, delicate skin, the incision is made straight, with less flap elevation. Minimal dissection is performed between the skin and extensor mechanism. The incision is continued midline in the digit in a longitudinal fashion through the extensor tendon and dorsal capsule. This preserves integrity of the lateral band contribution to the terminal tendon.

Beginning on the dorsal edge of both collateral ligaments, the capsular–ligamentous complex is carefully scived from the head of the proximal phalanx. This continues until the joint can be opened like a "shotgun" (Fig. 103–2). It usually is not necessary to incise the ligaments from the middle phalanx; however, reflecting the ligaments distally to facilitate exposure is helpful. The volar plate is preserved unless the preoperative contracture is severe. Osteophytes are excised from both phalangeal surfaces to establish the anatomic joint lines, thereby aiding in the evaluation of the quality and quantity of bone for arthrodesis. At this point in the procedure, the techniques of bone preparation and internal fixation are decided.

■ FIGURE 103–2
The capsule and collateral ligaments are released from the head of the proximal phalanx until it can be opened like a "shotgun."

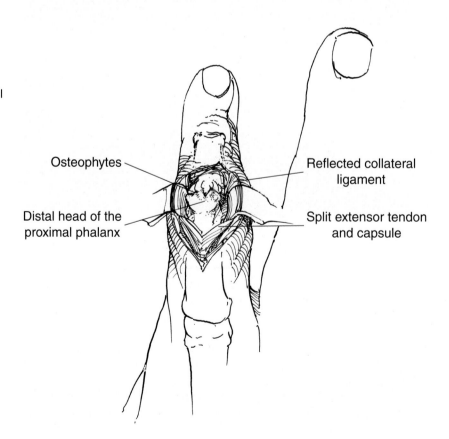

Osteophytes

Reflected collateral ligament

Distal head of the proximal phalanx

Split extensor tendon and capsule

Beginning with the proximal phalanx, the remaining articular cartilage and subchondral bone are excised. In osteoarthritis and in post-traumatic arthritis, the Midas Rex is used with a C-1 burr meticulously to remove the tissue down to the cancellous bone. Care is taken to preserve as much bone surface as possible. In patients with inflammatory arthritis, the bone is often soft enough to be removed with a sharp, delicate rongeur. Preparation of the proximal phalanx should extend volarly sufficiently to remove cartilage and subchondral bone. Attention is then directed to the middle phalanx. The remaining cartilage and subchondral bone is excised. The tendency is to create too deep a "cup"; a shallow concavity to match the convexity of the prepared head of the proximal phalanx is the goal. This modification of the Carroll and Hill technique[5] is an attempt to make the congruent cup and cone a bit more shallow; therefore, less bone shortening occurs (Fig. 103–3).

Every attempt is made to preserve the length of skeleton if the overlying soft tissues are adequate. However, in certain cases it is beneficial to shorten the skeleton to relieve tension on the soft tissues; a common example of this is in patients with psoriatic arthritis or scleroderma where a severe flexion contracture is often accompanied by thin dorsal soft tissues.[16]

Once the bone surfaces are prepared, appropriate flexion and alignment are set. Carefully align the digit. In the resting position, the fingers normally point toward the scaphoid. However, the nail plates are not all parallel and the digits do not all point to the same area on the scaphoid. The nail plates of the index and middle are slightly supinated, the index more than middle. The ring finger nail is often neutral and the small finger nail is slightly pronated. This should be assessed before surgery in both hands and set at this time in the procedure. The fingers rest in concert together and are best assessed by gently flexing and extending the wrist and observing the tenodesis on the digits.

The shallow "ball-and-socket" type surface preparation, analogous to a dome osteotomy, allows considerable freedom in setting position. The K-wires used are either 0.035" or 0.042" in diameter. The wires are introduced in an antegrade direction through the base of the middle phalanx. The intent is for the oblique wires to cross in the bone and not at the surface of the arthrodesis (Fig. 103–4A). The wires are drilled with a powered K-wire driver through the base and out the cortex of the middle phalanx. They are separated by 5 to 10 mm at the base of the middle phalanx. The third wire is centered longitudinally and driven dorsally out through the dorsal cortex of the middle phalanx. The angle of dorsal inclination should approximate the flexion angle at which the joint is to be set (Fig.

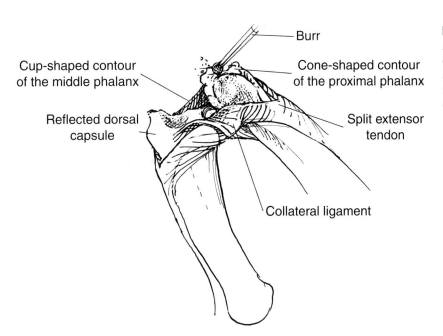

Burr

Cone-shaped contour
of the proximal phalanx

Cup-shaped contour
of the middle phalanx

Reflected dorsal
capsule

Split extensor
tendon

Collateral ligament

■ FIGURE 103–3
A burr is used to remove cartilage and a limited amount of subchondral bone to form a congruent cup and cone.

■ FIGURE 103–4
(A) The three-pin technique uses a central, longitudinal pin and two oblique pins that are 5 to 10 mm apart at the arthrodesis site. **(B)** The angle of dorsal inclination of the pin should approximate the arthrodesis angle.

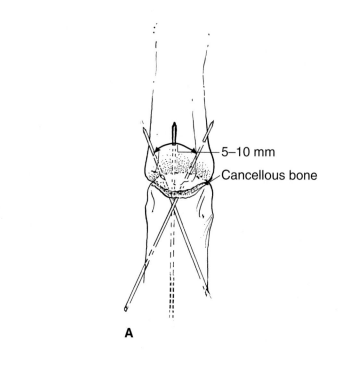

5–10 mm

Cancellous bone

A

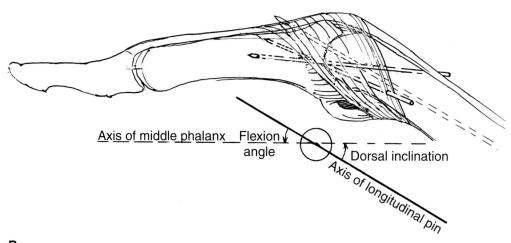

Axis of middle phalanx   Flexion angle

Dorsal inclination

Axis of longitudinal pin

B

103–4B). The drill is then placed distally to pull the wires further through the middle phalanx until the points are flush at the base.

The surgeon then holds the digit and compresses the two phalangeal surfaces with the proper alignment, while the assistant drills the previously placed wires in a retrograde fashion across the arthrodesis. Usually the longitudinal wire is drilled first and then the alignment is assessed. If satisfactory, the other wires are drilled.

The crossing wires' points are palpated under the skin as they pass through the cortex of the proximal phalanx. The longitudinal wire will pass down the canal of the proximal phalanx. Its length can be measured by placing another wire adjacent to it outside the skin. Depending on the individual patient, the wires are either cut off outside the skin or cut to rest just under the skin. The wires are left outside the skin under the following conditions: the soft tissues are thin; there are no other reasons that may delay healing; or no other procedures are being performed simultaneously. At least 3 mm of wire should remain outside the skin. Carefully check the skin tension, releasing it as necessary to avoid tenting. If the wires are cut under the skin, the points should be barely palpable to facilitate localization, without being long enough to cause pain. An end-biting wire cutter is very helpful in getting the wire cut short enough.

The collateral ligaments and capsule are repaired using 4-0 absorbable suture. The extensor is repaired separately. The extensor excursion must be preserved for the terminal tendon to function. It is preferable to bury the knots in the extensor so they are not palpable through the skin. The skin is closed with 5-0 nylon suture.

Tension band arthrodesis, intraosseous wiring, Herbert screw or ASIF screw fixation, compression arthrodesis, and miniplate fixation are all described methods for PIP arthrodesis.[1,4,6,8–10,17] All techniques provide more compression and rigid fixation of the arthrodesis than K-wires. Often additional splinting in the postoperative period is not required, and early motion of adjacent joints is facilitated. Each is a technically demanding procedure and carries with it other considerations.

■ **TECHNICAL ALTERNATIVES**

The tension band wire technique usually requires slightly more surgical exposure, especially of the middle phalanx. The idea is to leave the tension band wires permanently, but sometimes they become painful or break and require removal, usually necessitating another visit to the operating room and a small incision. Similar disadvantages are seen with the intraosseous wiring technique.

Herbert screw fixation can be a very effective technique for providing instant rigid fixation. However, it is quite unforgiving. If the initial screw placement is not perfect, the holes created often prevent reinsertion. Also, if bone stock is deficient or is of poor quality, Herbert screw fixation will fail. Finally, if the ends are not buried deep enough and the screw becomes painful, removal can be difficult by virtue of the bone ingrowth between the threads. Similar disadvantages are seen with the ASIF screw.

External compression arthrodesis, initially described by Charnley in 1953,[6] is best saved for those cases that have failed simpler means. In addition, it is used in primary arthrodesis for open, comminuted, intra-articular fracture dislocations and in septic arthritis of the PIP joint. The device is burdensome and can interfere with the remaining hand function. Pin tract infection can also be problematic.

Miniplate fixation, the most rigid of all techniques,[15] requires a large exposure and is technically demanding. The plate usually becomes painful, thus necessitating removal. The angle of arthrodesis may be difficult to control, and adjustments are fraught with loss of fixation. Poor soft tissue quality and coverage are contraindications to plate fixation.

Attention to certain details helps to avoid the pitfalls of K-wire fixation for arthrodesis. Bone surface contact must be ensured. Intraoperative radiographs may be helpful. Multiple passes of the K-wires through the bone and soft tissues should be avoided. Remember, the phalanx is in the dorsal two-thirds of the digit, and the wires never have to pass as volar as the midaxial line. This technique helps to protect the neurovascular bundles. As the wires pass through the skin, the digit should be held without stretching the skin. This maneuver will reduce skin tension at the pin sites. Any tension on the skin should be released by longitudinal incisions at the pin sites.

A hand dressing and volar splint are applied to immobilize adjacent digits and joints as well as adequately pad the ends of the wires. A solid cast is preferable. The dressing is changed and the sutures removed in 7 to 10 days, at the first postoperative visit. A radiograph is obtained to verify position of the arthrodesis and the wires. This film becomes the reference film for the radiographs to be obtained at 6 weeks. Depending on which digit is treated and individual patient considerations, the immobilization may vary. In some patients only a simple finger cast or splint is used. Other patients require a solid short arm cast extending out to the tip of the finger. The finger is protected for at least 6 weeks.

■ **REHABILITATION**

The dressings are changed during the biweekly office visits after surgery. The wire sites are examined for evidence of infection. Adjacent joints are gently passively moved to

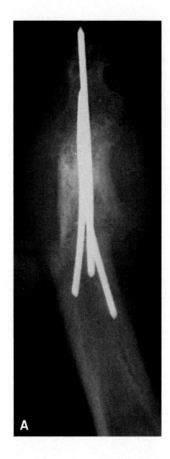
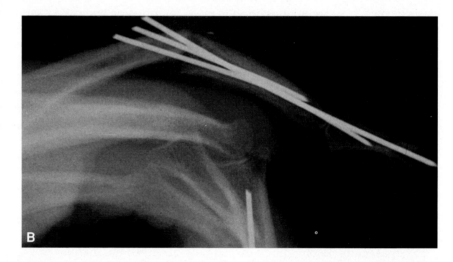

■ FIGURE 103–5

Posteroanterior **(A)** and lateral **(B)** radiographs after a PIP joint arthrodesis using a three-pin technique. In this case the pins were also placed across the DIP joint.

prevent stiffness. The most difficult joint to get moving is the DIP. By gently supporting the PIP joint, the DIP joint is passively and actively moved. With adequate healing of the arthrodesis confirmed radiographically, the wires are removed in the office at 6 to 8 weeks.

The care for the patient after arthrodesis, as suggested earlier, is individualized to a great degree. If the patient has diffuse osteoarthritis and only one finger is being treated, an isolated finger cast or splint is applied at the initial postoperative visit. The patient is educated about the importance of range of motion exercises of the adjacent fingers, wrist, elbow, and especially the shoulder. Too often, minor hand operations are accompanied by disabling stiffness in the proximal extremity. Each patient has his or her home exercise program to prevent stiffness. If necessary, the patient may be taught this program before surgery and visit a hand therapist after surgery.

Once solid arthrodesis is achieved, full hand function is restored (Fig. 103–5). No immobilization is used. Some patients require more extensive hand therapy if they are having difficulty with return of function or strength. An end point for therapy is full integration of the treated digit into hand function. Hand strength often continues to return over another 3 to 6 months.

■ OUTCOMES

The literature suggests that nonunion and delayed union are not very common.[1,4,5,8,9,18,20] Union rates have been reported to be 90% or better in most series, independent of fixation technique. Symptomatic nonunion is best treated by bone grafting and compression fixation. We have seen two patients in the last 13 years who had a nonunion and a delayed union. The nonunion was treated with bone grafting, and the delayed union eventually healed by 6 months.

Malunion is usually a result of technical error. Bone preparation techniques, including flat and chevron cuts, are difficult to make accurately, and rotational or angular malalignments may occur. Cup-and-cone preparations are much more forgiving and allow one to position the arthrodesis in three planes easily. If malunion becomes problematic, the fusion must be revised.

Infection is also uncommon. It occurs more often in situations where the quality of the soft tissue overlying the arthrodesis site is poor, as seen in trauma, burn, or scleroderma patients. According to Hill,[11] pin tract infections are more common when the pins are buried beneath the skin. If infection does occur, it usually resolves after pin removal, and debridement is not necessary.

The most common complication is loosening of a wire, which may require premature removal. If there are three wires well placed, loss of one does not necessarily become a problem. However, this patient would be treated with greater immobilization in the postoperative period to ensure healing.

References

 1. Allende BT, Engelem JC: Tension-band arthrodesis in the finger joints. J Hand Surg, 1980; 5: 269–271.
 2. Bick EM: In: Source Book of Orthopaedics. Baltimore: Williams & Wilkins, 1936.
 3. Boyes JH: In: Bunnell's Surgery of the Hand. Philadelphia: JB Lippincott, 1970:310.
 4. Buchler U, Aiken MA: Arthrodesis of the proximal interphalangeal joint by solid bone grafting and plate fixation in extensive injuries to the dorsal aspect of the finger. J Hand Surg [Am], 1988; 13:589–594.
 5. Carroll RE; Hill NA: Small joint arthrodesis in hand reconstruction. J Bone Joint Surg [Am], 1969; 51:1219–1221.
 6. Charnley J: In: Compression Arthrodesis. Edinburgh: Livingstone, 1953:172.
 7. Edwards GS, O'Brien ET, Heckman MM: Retrograde cross-pinning of transverse metacarpal and phalangeal fractures. Hand, 1982; 14:141–148.
 8. Faithfull DK, Herbert TJ: Small joint fusions of the hand using the Herbert bone screw. J Hand Surg [Br], 1984; 9:167–168.
 9. Granovitz S, Vainio K: Proximal interphalangeal joint arthrodesis in rheumatoid arthritis. Acta Orthop Scand, 1966; 37:301–309.
10. Heim U, Pfeiffer KM: In: Small Fragment Set Manual. Berlin: Springer-Verlag, 1982.
11. Hill NA: Small joint arthrodesis. In: Green DP (ed): Operative-Hand Surgery. New York: Churchill-Livingstone, 1988:121–134.
12. Hooper G: Techniques of interphalangeal arthrodesis: In: Bowers WH (ed): The Interphalangeal Joints. New York: Churchill-Livingstone, 1987:174–185.
13. Kaplan E: Extension deformities of the proximal interphalangeal joints of the fingers: Part I. J Bone Joint Surg, 1936; 18:781.
14. Kaplan E: Extension deformities of the proximal interphalangeal joints of the fingers: Part II. J Bone Joint Surg, 1937; 19:1144.
15. Kovach JC, Werner FW, Palmer AK, Greenkey S, Murphy DJ: Biomechanical analysis of internal fixation techniques for proximal interphalangeal joint arthrodesis. J Hand Surg [Am], 1986; 11:562–566.
16. Libscomb PR, Simons GW, Winkleman RK: Surgery for sclerodactylia of the hand: Experience with six cases. J Bone Joint Surg [Am], 1969; 51:1112–1117.
17. Lister GD: Intraosseous wiring of the digital skeleton. J Hand Surg, 1978; 3:427–435.
18. Omer EG: Evaluation and reconstruction of the forearm and hand after acute traumatic peripheral nerve injuries. J Bone Joint Surg [Am], 1968; 50:1454–1478.
19. Straub LR: The rheumatoid hand. Clin Orthop, 1959; 15:127–139.
20. Watson HK; Schaffer SR: Concave–convex arthrodesis in the joints of the hand. Plast Reconstr Surg, 1970; 46:368–371.

RICHARD A. RUFFIN

104

Tension-Band Arthrodesis of the Proximal Interphalangeal Joint

■ HISTORY OF THE TECHNIQUE

Tension-band arthrodesis of the hand has gained increasing popularity in the past decade. The AO group initially championed its use in patellar and olecrenon fractures, emphasizing the sound engineering principles necessary for a successful result.[9] Allende and Engelem first described the tension band technique in the English hand surgery literature.[1] Others, including Ijsseitein and co-workers,[4] Khuri,[6] Stern and Drury,[11] and Uhl and Schneider[12] have presented series describing techniques, results, and complications. The proximal interphalangeal (PIP) joint of the hand is ideally suited for arthrodesis by the tension-band technique. When properly performed in this joint, the dorsally placed wire absorbs the tension across the eccentrically loaded fusion site, converting distractive to compressive forces at the adjacent bone cortex.[6] My preferred technique does not differ significantly from the original description.

■ INDICATIONS AND CONTRAINDICATIONS

The primary indication for tension-band arthrodesis of the PIP joint is painful arthritis (osteoarthritis, rheumatoid arthritis and variants,[12] and post-traumatic arthritis[1,4]) (Fig. 104–1). In the small and ring fingers, arthroplasty is occasionally indicated when motion is desired, however arthrodesis remains more durable and complication-free. Severe spasticity with marked contracture causing hygiene problems[4] as well as Dupuytren's contracture also have been cited as indications. Salvage of the severely contracted or poorly controlled digit is a less common yet ideal situation for tension band arthrodesis.

Contraindications to arthrodesis include septic arthritis, osteomyelitis, soft tissue infection, and dorsal soft tissue defect. Intravenous antibiotics, debridement, and local flap coverage may be necessary before proceeding. The insensate and marginally perfused digit may best be served by amputation rather than arthrodesis. Bone loss, specifically lack of a sufficient volar buttress, is a contraindication.[1] An intercalary bone graft may allow successful fusion even with massive comminution and segmental loss.

■ SURGICAL TECHNIQUES

Regional or general anesthesia is preferred. In my experience, local or digital blocks have been insufficient. A gently curved dorsal longitudinal incision is centered over the joint undergoing arthrodesis. The skin edges are mobilized and sewn back. The extensor tendon is split longitudinally. The capsule and extensor are treated as separate layers. The capsule is dissected from the bone two thirds the way around the PIP joint, including proximal release of the collateral ligaments. Approximately 1.5 cm of the adjacent dorsal two thirds of the proximal and middle phalanges are exposed to facilitate drilling and pin placement.

A microsagital oscillating saw is used to cut the proximal phalanx at the desired angle of fusion; increasing from 20° to 50° in the index to the small fingers (Fig. 104–2). Remaining cartilage and subchondral bone are removed from the base of the middle phalanx with a small burr, rongeur, or curette, creating a flat surface perpendicular to the long axis of the middle phalanx. Two 0.045-inch wires (0.035-inch wire for smaller hands) are drilled retrograde from the midportion of the cut proximal phalanx surface, exiting dorsally 1 to 1.5 cm. from the osteotomy. A transverse drill hole (with a 0.035-inch wire) is placed dorsally 0.7 to 1 cm distal to the base of the middle phalanx to accommodate a 24-gauge wire (Fig. 104–3A). The cut surfaces are held snugly together by an assistant while the

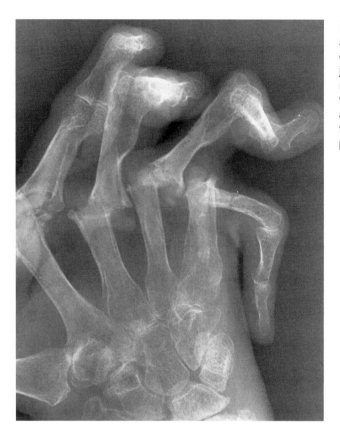

■ FIGURE 104-1
An oblique radiograph of eroded and subluxed PIP joints of the long and ring fingers in a patient who had MP joint arthroplasties for rheumatoid arthritis many years previously.

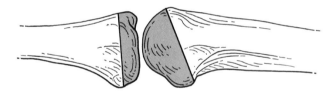

■ FIGURE 104-2
Shaded areas represent the desired osteotomy orientation with the angled cut of the proximal phalanx from 20° to 50°, increasing from the index to the small finger.

surgeon drills the 0.045-inch wires across the fusion site. Either distal intramedullary or volar cortex fixation is desirable. The 24-gauge wire is crossed over the dorsum of the bone in a figure-of-eight fashion, wrapped around the protruding proximal pins, and twist tightened on either aspect (Fig. 104–3B). An extra loop on the contralateral side may provide more uniform compression but adds more bulk.[6] Excessive wire length is cut off and the K-wires protruding proximally are bent and cut. They are then rotated against the side of the bone and gently tamped distally (Fig. 104–3C), Care should be taken that both the pin ends and wire twists are flush against the side of the bone (Fig. 104–4).

Radiographs or good quality fluoroscopic views confirm proper pin placement and length, as well as the angle of arthrodesis (Fig. 104–5). Adjustments in desired angle and rotation are very difficult after the initial attempt. Therefore, special care is necessary to avoid major technical errors. The pins are bent, cut short, and rotated flush to bone.

Closure is done in layers, suturing the capsule/periosteum and extensor separately with an interrupted absorbable suture and the skin with 5-0 or 6-0 monofilament suture. A bulky interdigital dressing and a dorsally placed padded aluminum splint are applied, with the metacarpophalangeal (MP) joint in 60° to 70° flexion, the PIP joint in the angle

■ FIGURE 104–3
A, 0.035- to 0.045-inch K-wires are used for intramedullary fixation with 24-gauge wire used for the tension band. **B,** The bone ends are approximated and the two K-wires advanced across the arthrodesis site. The 24-gauge wire is passed over the arthrodesis site in a figure-of-eight manner, with one end around the two K-wires. The 24-gauge wire is then twisted taut while maintaining gentle upward traction. **C,** Excessive wire length is cut off and the K-wires are bent proximally, rotated, and tamped distally.

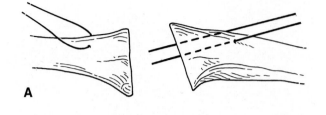

A

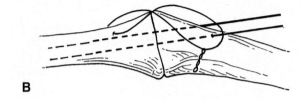

B

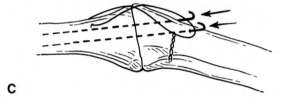

C

■ FIGURE 104–4
Completed arthrodesis with the proximal edges of the K-wires and residual 3 to 4 twists of tension band wire held flush against sides of bone.

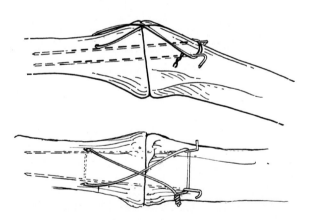

of fixation, and the distal interphalangeal (DIP) joint left free. Postoperative pain management may be aided by placing an intrathecal digital block.

■ TECHNICAL ALTERNATIVES

The method described above relies on readily available and relatively inexpensive equipment and hardware to achieve arthrodesis. Numerous other techniques have been used, including crossed K-wires, with or without an additional intramedullary wire,[5,8] the cup and cone method,[3] intraosseous wiring,[7] and plate and/or screw fixation.[13] Each has its proponents, with surgeon preference the major determinant of the technique chosen. Rigid fixation provided by tension band arthrodesis allows early active range of motion, preventing adjacent joint stiffness, with lower infection and pseudarthrosis rates.[1,4,6,12]

Certain pitfalls may lead to a less desirable result. First, the preparation of the fusion site must be meticulous, with precise proximal cuts and flush surfaces. Concave/convex reamers such as the Refine Fusion System (DePuy, Warsaw, IN) allow greater flexibility

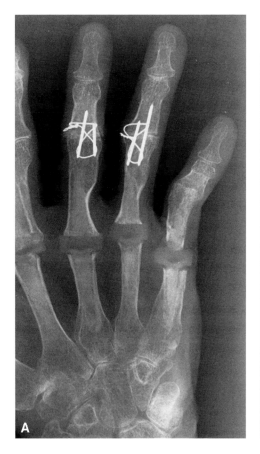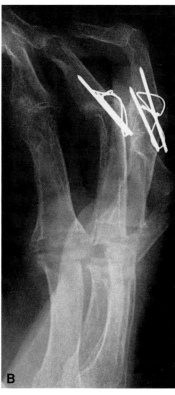

■ FIGURE 104–5
A and B, AP and lateral radiographs of successful arthrodeses using the tension band technique, as well as MP joint arthroplasty revision.

in angle adjustment and do not compromise pin and wire placement. Second, nonparallel placement of Kirschner wires may lower fusion rates. Uhl described a pin placement guide that has been developed to obviate this potential problem.[12] Third, excessive volar penetration of the pins causes postfusion pain, requiring pin removal and occasional tenolysis.[4,12]

Active range of motion of the DIP joint is encouraged immediately. The operative splint is removed between 1 and 2 weeks postoperatively. A supervised active range of motion program is initiated. A hand therapist is used if there is concern about compliance or patient confidence in an active range of motion program. A removable thermoplastic splint may be used for comfort during the rehabilitative phase. Fusion is usually evident radiographically between 6 and 8 weeks, but may take up to 6 months.[1] Resumption of normal work and activities of daily living are allowed unprotected after radiographic healing has occurred. Before this, use of a splint and modification of activities and work are recommended.

■ REHABILITATION

Successful arthrodesis is common with tension band arthrodesis. Other forms of rigid internal fixation also allow early range of motion and prevent stiffness of adjacent joints. Tension band principles have been shown by Kovach and co-workers[5] to be biomechanically superior to simple K-wire or intraosseous wire fixation. Tension band arthrodesis offers the additional advantages of less dissection and overall expense than plate and screw fixation.

Recent literature supports tension band arthrodesis as the preferred method of arthrodesis of the PIP joint. Allende and Engelem[1] popularized the tension band method with excellent results in a series of traumatized joints. Ijsselstein and co-workers,[4] also in a series consisting primarily of trauma cases, found tension band arthrodesis superior to

■ OUTCOMES

Kirschner wire fixation methods, with lower infection and rearthrodesis rates. Khuri[6] and subsequently Uhl and Schneider[12] found tension band arthrodesis to be an effective method for arthritic, paralytic, and post-traumatic conditions. In these above series, arthrodesis rates were greater than 90% and complications less than 10%. Although rheumatoid joints fuse readily with nearly all currently used techniques, use of tension band arthrodesis allows early protected range of motion, without compromise to the relatively osteoporotic bone.[6] Complications are few, and relate primarily to protruding hardware causing tendinitis or bursitis.[4,12] Difficult removal of the hardware has been cited as a disadvantage of the technique, with a formal operative procedure often needed.[4] Malunions can be avoided with attention to intraoperative detail and proper radiographs. Nonunion is caused by a number of factors, including massive bone loss, open injuries with infection, and poor technique.[1,4] Failure to mobilize the operated joint in a timely fashion (within 2 weeks) defeats the purpose and intent of the tension band and may contribute to delayed union or nonunion.

In summary, the tension band technique is an excellent choice for achieving arthrodesis of the PIP joint. Proper patient selection is important. Technical points to remember include wide dissection, precise boney cuts, parallel placement of K-wires, adequate tightening of the tension band wire, and recession of the cut wire edges.

Tension band arthrodesis has become my preferred method for stabilization of the arthritic and acutely traumatized PIP joint. I have not had the opportunity to assess the technique with congenital and paralytic conditions.

References

 1. Allende BT, Engelem JC: Tension band arthrodesis in the finger joints. J Hand Surg, 1980: 5: 269–271.
 2. Burton RI, Margles SW, Lunseth PA: Small joint arthrodesis of the hand. J Hand Surg, 1986; 11A:678–682.
 3. Carrol RE, Hill NA: Small joint arthrodesis in hand reconstruction. J Bone Joint Surg, 1969; 51A:1219–1221.
 4. Ijsselstein CB, van Egmond DB, Hovius SER, van der Meuien JC: Results of small joint arthrodesis: Comparison of firschner wire fixation with tension band wire technique. J Hand Surg, 1992: 17A:952–956.
 5. Kovach JC, Werner FW, Palmer AK, Groenkey S, Murphy DJ: Biomechanical analysis of internal fixation techniques for proximal interphalangeal arthrodesis. J Hand Surg, 1986: 11A: 562–566.
 6. Khuri SM: Tension band arthrodesis in the hand. J Hand Surg, 1986; 11A:41–45.
 7. Lister GD: Intraosseous wiring of the digital skeleton. J Hand Surg, 1978; 3:427–435.
 8. McGlynn JT, Smith RA, Bogumill GP: Arthrodesis of the small joint of the hand: A rapid and effective technique. Hand Surg, 1988; 13A:595–599.
 9. Muller ME, Allgower M, Schneider R, Willenegger H: Manual of Internal Fixation, Berlin: Springer-Verlag, 1979.
10. Segmuller G: Surgical Stabilization of the Skeleton of the Hand, Baltimore: Williams and Wilkins, 1977:42–59.
11. Stern PJ, Drury WJ: Tension-band arthrodesis of small joints. Contemp Orthop, 1984; 8:59–62.
12. Uhl RL, Schneider LH: Tension band arthrodesis of finger joints: A retrospective review of 76 consecutive cases. J Hand Surg, 1992; 17A:518–522.
13. Wright CS, McMurtry RY: AO arthrodesis in the hand. J Hand Surg 1983; 8:932–935.

105

Arthrodesis of the Thumb Metacarpophalangeal Joint with Tension Band Technique

Since the inception of the surgery of joints, arthrodesis has been used as a treatment. The technique of metacarpophalangeal (MP) joint arthrodesis has evolved from articular surface removal to various mitered shapes (i.e., Chevron osteotomy,[10] concave/convex technique,[2,15] tenon method,[8] and Moberg peg[9]). Methods of fixation have varied from simple pin fixation to multiple pin fixation, tension band wire,[1] screw fixation,[13] plate application,[16] and external fixation.[2,14]

Cup and cone arthrodesis was first discussed by Carroll and Hill[3] and then Watson and Shaffer[15] to increase the surface area of the bone for healing. This technique allows the surgeon to adjust the final angle of arthrodesis right up to the time of fixation. Recent modification of the technique includes use of curved saws and convex and concave reamers to shape the bone surface. This technique is readily applied to the MP joint of the thumb, using tension band wiring for fixation.

■ HISTORY OF THE TECHNIQUE

The foremost indications for MP joint arthrodesis are pain, deformity, and instability in the joint. Pain is usually caused by rheumatoid,[12] degenerative, traumatic,[5] or septic arthritis (Fig. 105–1). Deformity encompasses burn, paralytic,[6] and spastic etiologies.[4,7] Instability is most commonly due to chronic ulnar collateral ligament insufficiency, secondary to either trauma or chronic inflammatory disease. Arthrodesis also can be used as salvage for all previously failed procedures of the joint.

Arthrodesis is contraindicated if other joint motion sparing procedures have not been considered and used when indicated. These procedures would include soft tissue ligament reconstructions for ligament instability. Resurfacing procedures for arthritic joints using soft tissue, allograft, or manmade materials should be considered before fusion. Aggressive debridement coupled with intravenous antibiotics is required to alleviate infection before fusion for septic arthritis with joint destruction.

■ INDICATIONS AND CONTRAINDICATIONS

Regional or general anesthesia is administered. After preparation and exsanguination, a dorsal longitudinal skin incision is made (centered over the MP joint). Using a blunt scissors technique, the subcutaneous tissue and skin are elevated. Care is taken to identify and preserve small branches of the superficial radial nerve. Retraction of the skin is achieved by suturing it back to itself using 4-0 silk. The extensor hood is incised along the radial border of the extensor pollicis longus (EPL). The EPL is retracted ulnarly, and the extensor pollicis brevis (EPB) and capsular tissue are retracted radially (Fig. 105–2). The capsule and collateral ligaments are divided sharply from the metacarpal bone.

The metacarpal head is prepared using a fine Lempert rongeur. The head is rounded using the tip of the rongeur. The final shape of the head should be gently rounded, slightly larger in width transversely. This is done using the tip of the rongeur in fine small bites. A dental burr can be substituted for a rongeur when removing the articular surface. Care should be taken not to overheat the bone when using the burr. This can be achieved by using copious irrigation.

Attention then moves to the proximal phalanx. The periosteum is divided longitudinally

■ SURGICAL TECHNIQUES

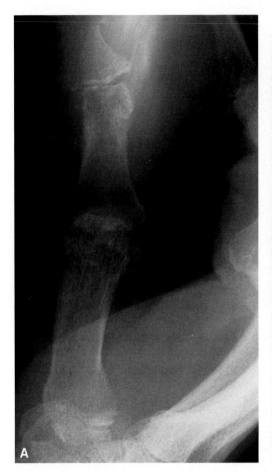
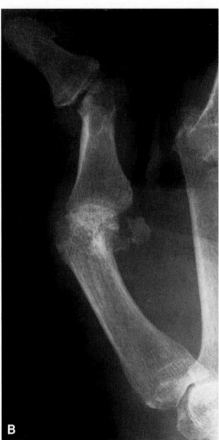

along the midline of the dorsum of the bone. The periosteum is elevated and retracted downward along the side of the phalanx to allow subsequent drilling and passing of the wire. The capsule is then released down the sides of the articular surface to gain exposure. The articular surface of the phalanx is curetted of any residual cartilage. If the bone is soft, gentle contouring of the phalanx is completed with the curette. If the bone is more dense, the dental burr may be appropriate. The resulting concavity of the phalanx should exactly match that of the metacarpal head, when positioned at 20° of flexion. A trial reduction to assess this congruency is performed. If the match is not satisfactory, recontouring of either surface should be completed.

Two parallel 0.045 Kirschner wires are drilled retrograde through the metacarpal head with the joint fully flexed to expose the prepared metacarpal bone surface. The joint is now reduced to an angle of approximately 20° to 25°.[3,11] The two K-wires are now driven distally into the proximal phalanx. The MP joint is passively moved to assure that the K-wires do not transfix the joint. If limited motion or crepitation is palpated, the offending pin or pins are backed out until the passive IP joint motion is free.

The position of the arthrodesis is generally confirmed at the time the fixation is placed. This can be done by fluoroscopy or plain films. At the base of the proximal phalanx a transverse hole is drilled dorsal to the K-wires. A 0.028 K-wire is used to drill the hole, then a 26-gauge wire is placed through the hole in a figure-of-eight fashion around the base of the K-wires on the dorsal surface of the metacarpal (Fig. 105–3). The 0.045 Kirschner wires are cut so that they extend approximately 1 mm beyond the width of the wire. They can be cut before or after the wire is tightened. This wire is tightened down using a wire twister or needle holder with the surgeon placing vertical tension on the wire when tightening it down. When the wire begins to lose its sheen, tightening is stopped. This

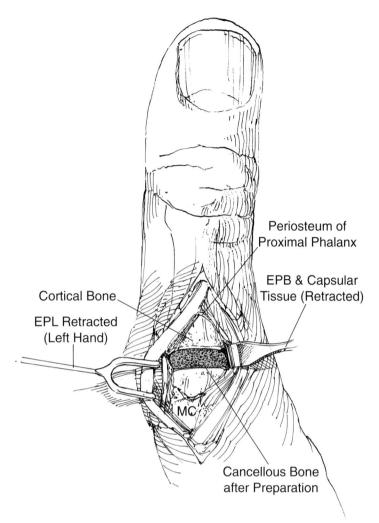

The dorsal approach to the MP joint of the thumb. The EPL is retracted ulnarly and the EPB radially. The metacarpal head is rounded down to cancellous bone.

Periosteum of
Proximal Phalanx

EPB & Capsular
Tissue (Retracted)

Cortical Bone

EPL Retracted
(Left Hand)

MC

Cancellous Bone
after Preparation

loss of sheen usually indicates impending wire breakage. The wire is cut to leave at least 2 twists, and the tip of the wire is bent down toward the surface of the bone to lay as flat as possible. The capsule is closed using 4-0 polydioxanone (PDS) on an RB-1 needle in a figure-of-eight buried knot technique. This is performed by inserting the initial pass of the needle on the undersurface of the tendon or capsule. The needle is passed twice to form two loops. A surgical knot is then tied; it should come to lie on the undersurface of the tendon or capsule. This is done to minimize irritation from the suture knots under the thin overlying soft tissue. The extensor hood is closed in a similar fashion. The skin is closed using 6-0 nylon. Dressings are placed and the patient is placed in a thumb spica splint.

Alternative techniques include the use of the lag-screw technique. The lag-screw technique is performed using a screw placed through the head of the metacarpal.[13] The screw is directed down the medullary canal of the proximal phalanx to achieve fixation. The arthrodesis angle can be difficult to achieve consistently with this technique.

Compression plating also has been used.[16] This technique usually involves placement of a dorsal contoured compression plate. Compression plating can be a very demanding procedure with increased dissection required for hardware placement. Hardware removal is generally desired as a consequence of its prominence.

The Moberg bone peg is a unique method of arthrodesis.[9] This technique involves using a cortical dowel to achieve fixation much the same as the lag-screw technique. However,

■ TECHNICAL
ALTERNATIVES

The prepared surfaces of the metacarpal head and proximal phalanx are approximated, parallel 0.045 K-wires are in place, and a figure-of-eight tension band of 26-gauge wire is twisted tight.

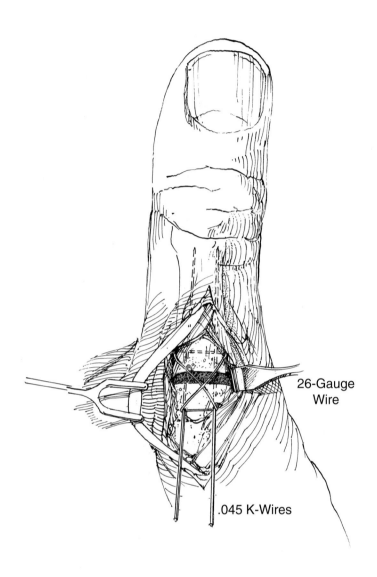

26-Gauge Wire

.045 K-Wires

it suffers the same disadvantages as the lag-screw technique and requires, in addition, a bone graft from a separate surgical site.

Technical pitfalls can be encountered during MP joint fusion. Primary emphasis should be placed on achieving good bony contact of the bone surfaces. The angle of the arthrodesis can be difficult to determine, and I recommend radiographic confirmation before wound closure. When osteoporotic bone is encountered, extra care should be taken when compression is applied at the arthrodesis site. Loss of fixation can occur by the wire cutting out through the bone.

Prominent hardware and suture material can be a problem after surgery. Areas of potential irritation should be palpated for excessive prominence during the operative procedure. If a prominence is encountered, the pins or suture material should be shortened.

■ REHABILITATION

Postoperatively, the patient returns for wound inspection and short arm thumb spica cast application after 3 to 5 days.

Active range of motion exercises for the thumb interphalangeal joint are initiated immediately after surgery.

The cast remains in place for 4 to 6 weeks or until radiographic evidence of healing has occurred.

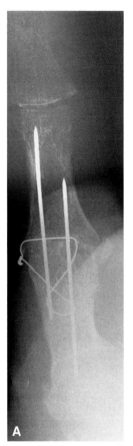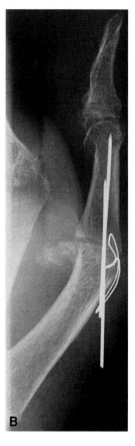

■ FIGURE 105–4
A and B, PA and lateral radiographs of the same patient 6 months after arthrodesis, showing healing of the bone. One of the pins is migrating out, requiring removal.

A short thumb spica splint is fabricated at approximately 4 to 6 weeks with the patient removing this splint to perform active range of motion exercises of the basal thumb joint. A hand therapist fabricates the splint and instructs the patient in the recommended range of motion exercises to be performed.

Patients are instructed not to lift more than 2 pounds for a period of 4 to 6 weeks. Patients may return to full activity after 8 weeks or when radiographic healing has been achieved.

■ OUTCOMES

Arthrodesis of the MP joint of the thumb has a high incidence of success using many techniques.[1–4,8,9,11,12,14–16] Tension band technique achieved 100% fusion rates in MP joints of the thumb.[1,5] Hagan and Hastings reported that 7 of 18 patients experienced complications. Superficial pin tract infections developed in four of the seven. The other three patients experienced prominent hardware difficulties, with two patients requiring hardware removal (Fig. 105–4).[5] Patients were evaluated by the Minnesota rate of manipulation test. Hagan and Hastings found 75% of the patients performed at or below average on the involved side.[5] In the same study, 69% performed poorly picking up small objects on the Jebson test.[5] Fourteen of 16 patients were employed before and after surgery. Return to work occurred at 42 to 154 days postoperatively, with an average of 96 days.[5] Postoperative patient satisfaction was regarded as high when compared with preoperative satisfaction.

The tension band wiring method of MP joint arthrodesis of the thumb offers simplicity of technique with significant biomechanical strength.

References

1. Allenda BT, Engelem JC: Tension band arthrodesis in the finger joints. J Hand Surg, 1980; 5: 269–271.

2. Brown RM, Rhoades CE: Dynamic compression for small bone arthrodesis. J Hand Surg, 1985; 10A:340–343.

3. Carroll RE, Hill NA: Small joint arthrodesis in hand reconstruction. J Bone Joint Surg, 1969; 51A:1219–1221.

4. Goldner LJ, Koman LA, Gilberman R, Levin S, Goldner RD: Arthrodesis of the metacarpophalangeal joint of the thumb in children and adults: Adjunctive treatment of thumb-in-hand deformity in cerebral palsy. Clin Orthop, 1990; 253:75–89.

5. Hagan HJ, Hastings H: Fusion of the thumb metacarpophalangeal joint to treat post-traumatic arthritis. J Hand Surg, 1988; 13A:750–752.

6. House JH: Reconstruction of the thumb in tetraplegia following spinal cord injury. Clin Orthop, 1985; 195:117–121.

7. Inglis AE, Cooper W, Bruton W: Surgical correction of thumb deformities in spastic paralysis. J Bone Joint Surg, 1970; 52A:253–258.

8. Lewis RC, Nordyke MD, Tenny JR: The tenon method of small joint arthrodesis in the hand. J Hand Surg, 1986; 11A:567–569.

9. Moberg E: Arthrodesis of finger joints. Surg Clin North Am, 1960; 40:465–470.

10. Omer GE: Evaluation and reconstruction of the forearm and hand after acute traumatic peripheral nerve injuries. J Bone Joint Surg, 1968; 50A:1454–1478.

11. Saldana MJ, Aulicide PL: The optimal position for arthrodesis of the metacarpophalangeal joint of the thumb; A clinical study. J Hand Surg, 1987; 12B:256–259.

12. Salgeback S, Eiken O, Haga T: Surgical treatment of the rheumatoid thumb: Special reference to the metacarpophalangeal joint. Scand J Plast Reconstr Surg, 1976; 10:153–156.

13. Segmuller G: Surgical Stabilization of the Skeleton of the Hand, Baltimore: Williams and Wilkins, 1977:42–59

14. Tupper JR: A compression arthrodesis device for small joints of the hand. Hand, 1972; 4:62–64.

15. Watson HK, Shaffer SR: Concave-convex arthrodesis in joints of the hand. Plast Reconstr Surg, 1970; 46:368–371.

16. Wright CS, McMurty RY: AO arthrodesis in the hand, J Hand Surg, 1983; 8:932–934.

106

WILLIAM B.
KLEINMAN

Scapho-Trapezio-Trapezoid Joint Arthrodesis

It has been more than 14 years since Watson and Hempton[34] first reported their speculative series of four patients with rotary subluxation of the scaphoid[2] treated by scapho-trapezio-trapezoid (STT) arthrodesis. It has been more than 12 years since my first publication describing the use of their procedure in the management of 12 patients treated for the same predegenerative problem.[20] Although Watson and Hempton reported good results in what they felt in 1980 was a "relatively untested" procedure, more recent articles from these authors and others[10,17,18,19,20,26,33] have supported the use of STT arthrodesis for chronic scapholunate (SL) dissociation with rotary subluxation of the scaphoid. The scaphoid can be reduced anatomically and prevented (by using the STT fusion technique) from recurrently collapsing into a mechanically more stable, but unphysiologic attitude, perpendicular to the longitudinal axis of the hand. The technique of reduction of a dissociated and malaligned scaphoid, and stabilizing its distal pole to the distal carpal row by STT arthrodesis, was first reported (without technical details) by Peterson and Lipscomb in 1967.[27] I have preferentially used the basic principles of the procedure popularized by Watson throughout my last 16 years of practice, representing a group of more than 80 patients.

Scapho-trapezio-trapezoid arthrodesis maintains scaphoid alignment the way an SL fusion would, but relies on a distal rather than a proximal scaphoid anchor. By anchoring the distal rather than proximal pole for stability, kinematic energy is allowed to dissipate *between* scaphoid and lunate, as is described in detail later in this chapter. In addition, an STT fusion is much easier technically to achieve than an SL fusion; the cancellous contact surface area is much greater at the STT joint, and the orientation of coapted surfaces is in a compression mode for the STT fusion, rather than in the shear or torque normally found at the SL joint. Although the concept of scaphoid stability through SL fusion may be logical, a plethora of authors have reported great frustration in attaining consistent bony unions.

Wrist kinematics consist of small aggregates of motion through the many articular surfaces within the carpus. With the hand–forearm unit held in neutral position, the carpal bones are maintained in positions relative to each other with stored-up potential energy; ligamentous "struts" and "guy-wires" holding the normal alignment of the carpus are located principally on the palmar surface (Fig. 106–1). If certain combinations of these retaining ligaments are injured or attenuated by disease, carpal relationships will collapse in a predictable manner into more mechanically stable, but less physiologic attitudes.[21] We call this result "carpal instability."

Scapholunate dissociation is a common example of this process, and is a consequence of severe hyperextension of the wrist under load. The hand–forearm unit is invariably in ulnar deviation at the time of impact-load, and the hand is forced into supination while the forearm is concomitantly pronated. Tension and torque develop within the intrinsic SL ligament, with enough load (and an appropriate time-action of injury) to cause failure of the ligamentous components that normally support the SL relationship (Fig. 106–2).[24,25] If the injury is severe and the scaphoid completely dissociated from the lunate, normal load transmitted through this bone creates a force-couple within the scaphoid; normal load transmitted through this bone results in scaphoid collapse from a physiologic 45° attitude to one more perpendicular to the plane of the palm (radioscaphoid angle > 60°).[2,13]

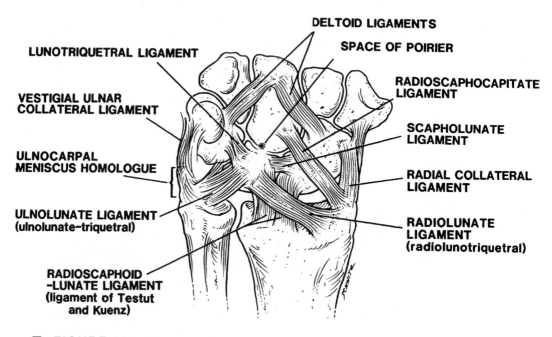

LUNOTRIQUETRAL LIGAMENT

VESTIGIAL ULNAR
COLLATERAL LIGAMENT

ULNOCARPAL
MENISCUS HOMOLOGUE

ULNOLUNATE LIGAMENT
(ulnolunate-triquetral)

RADIOSCAPHOID
-LUNATE LIGAMENT
(ligament of Testut
and Kuenz)

DELTOID LIGAMENTS

SPACE OF POIRIER

RADIOSCAPHOCAPITATE
LIGAMENT

SCAPHOLUNATE
LIGAMENT

RADIAL COLLATERAL
LIGAMENT

RADIOLUNATE
LIGAMENT
(radiolunotriquetral)

■ FIGURE 106–1

Schematic arrangement of the important extrinsic and intrinsic ligaments of the palmar aspect of the wrist. The mobile column (scaphoid) is suspended in a sling composed of radiocarpal extrinsic and deltoid intrinsic ligament. Similarly, the rotational column (triquetrum) is suspended between ulnocarpal and deltoid ligaments.

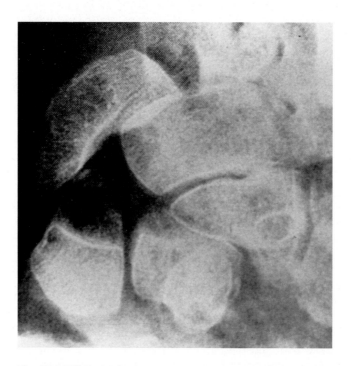

■ FIGURE 106–2

Laboratory studies by Mayfield and coworkers[24,25] demonstrate severe ulnar deviation, extension, and intercarpal supination of the hand on the forearm at the time of injury, leading to specific ligamentous failure (see text). This radiograph represents a grade II injury (progressive perilunar instability) leading to scapholunate dissociation and rotary subluxation of the scaphoid. (From Mayfield JK, Johnson RP, Kilcoyne RF: Carpal dislocations: Pathomechanics and progressive perilunar instability. J Hand Surg, 1980; 5:226; with permission.)

This posture is referred to as carpal instability-dissociative (CID), or SL dissociation with rotary scaphoid subluxation. Unleashed from the palmar-flexing influence of the scaphoid, the lunate will translate palmarly and rotate into an extended attitude, still coupled to the triquetrum (Fig. 106–3) assuming a position described as dorsal intercalated segment instability (DISI). This tendency for the lunate to extend is based on an intraosseous lunate force-couple, which results from load placed across nonaxisymmetric axes of flexion–extension at the radiolunate and lunatocapitate joints (Fig. 106–4). The internal scaphoid force-couple mechanism is responsible for the perpendicular attitude of the dissociated scaphoid (Fig. 106–5).[7,23] The mechanism of injury resulting in SL dissociation with rotary subluxation of the scaphoid ruptures the radial collateral ligament, the radioscaphocapi-

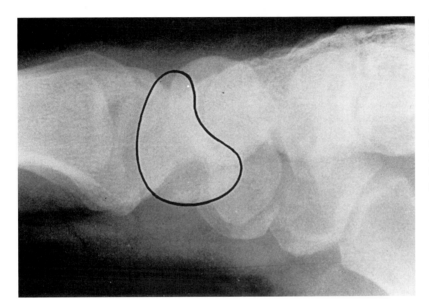

■ FIGURE 106–3
Dorsiflexion intercalated segment instability (DISI): without the palmar-flexing influence of the scaphoid on the lunate after scapholunate dissociation, the lunate slides palmarly on the radius and collapses (with the triquetrum) into a posture of extension.

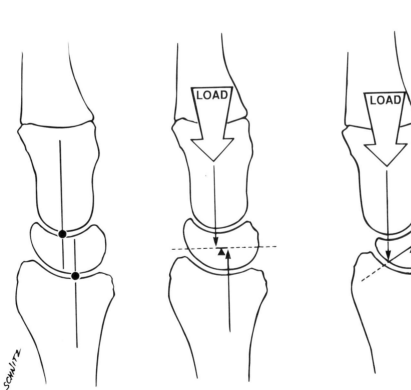

■ FIGURE 106–4
In the normal resting posture, the axes of rotation of the capitolunate and radiolunate joints are nonaxisymmetric. If separated from the palmar-flexing influence of the scaphoid, an internal mechanical force-couple precipitates lunate extension (DISI).

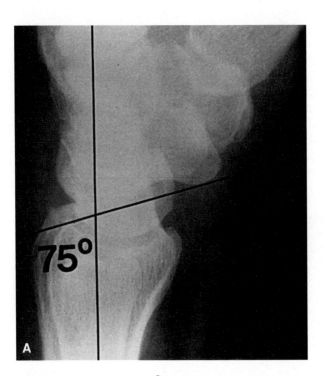

■ FIGURE 106–5
(A) "True" lateral projection of the wrist with longitudinal axes of the radius and third metacarpal collinear. In SL dissociation with rotary subluxation, the scaphoid collapses into a perpendicular attitude (relative to the plane of the palm), here shown to measure 75°. **(B)** Final resting posture is based on an intraosseous force-couple as load is transmitted from the hand to the forearm. (From Cooney WP, Linscheid RL, Dobyns JH, Wood MB: Scaphoid nonunion: Role of anterior interpositional bone grafts. J Hand Surg, 1988; 13A: 635–650; with permission.)

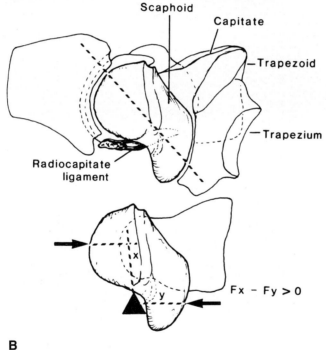

tate ligament, the interosseous SL ligament, and the radioscaphoid portion of the ligament of Testut. The mechanism is a combination of wrist extension, ulnar deviation, and intercarpal supination[24,25]; the long radiolunate ligament (radiolunatotriquetral ligament) is usually spared. Freed from the palmar-flexing influence of the scaphoid, the lunate may extend; but it will never translate ulnarward, unless the stabilizing long radiolunate ligament has been damaged. Even in an extended posture, the lunate maintains a stable relationship within the spherical lunate fossa of the radius. For this reason, arthritic changes rarely develop at this joint, even in very late untreated cases of SL advanced collapse (SLAC).[32] With separation of the scaphoid and lunate, and a potential rotational collapse of these two bones in different directions under load, the untreated wrist progressively undergoes proximal and radial migration of the capitate (intimately linked to the hamate and trapezoid), and results in the predictable pattern of arthritic changes observed in SLAC.[9,32] Normal compressional forces at hyaline cartilage surfaces become shear forces, and result in rapid cartilage destruction, synovitis, and arthritic change. In cases of untreated SL dissociation with rotary subluxation of the scaphoid, this deterioration initially occurs at the radial styloid–scaphoid interface; as the degree of degeneration progresses, it is seen at the elliptical (scaphoid) fossa of the radius; finally, with lateral capitate migration, it occurs at the capitolunate joint. As little as 5° of scaphoid subluxation will reduce the normal contact area of its proximal pole within the elliptical fossa of the radius by 44% (as the pole translates toward the dorsal lip of the radius). With 20° of subluxation, the contact area is reduced by 77%, with the proximal pole shifting radially toward the dorsal lip of the radial styloid.[6] These laboratory findings explain the progression of radioscaphoid arthritis in SLAC, from the tip of the radial styloid to the elliptical scaphoid fossa. They also emphasize the importance of operative anatomic reduction of the SL relationship in the prevention of progressive arthritis.

The goals of any reconstructive effort employed for this problem are: (1) to reduce pain and restore the patient's ability to pursue gainful employment and avocational activities; (2) to maintain a functional range of motion of the wrist, avoiding the need for total wrist arthrodesis; and (3) to prevent or retard the natural history of progressive arthritis inherent in surgically untreated SL dissociation with persistent rotary scaphoid subluxation. By anatomically reducing the scaphoid and anchoring its distal pole to the trapezium–trapezoid complex by fusion (with either autogenous iliac crest or radial bone graft), the proximal scaphoid pole can be more centrally maintained in the elliptical fossa of the radius, reducing the propensity for rapid degenerative change.[6]

The indications for surgery of this type combine clinical presentation with radiographic criteria. All patients relate some history of trauma, with resultant chronic pain. Every patient will have pain at the end-arcs of motion, with marked tenderness over the dorsal (and frequently palmar) SL joint. Pain at rest is usually not a complaint, but a general decreased range of wrist motion secondary to SL pain is usually observed. Profound weakness secondary to instability of the proximal row is present in each of these patients. Presence of a "click" or "clunk" using the provocative scaphoid stress test described by Watson (Fig. 106–6) may be inconsistent, but is pathognomonic of pathologic instability only when present on the injured wrist, absent on the normal side, and associated with either abnormal static or dynamic radiographic changes in the SL relationship. The scaphoid stress test should be performed with the patient's elbow on the examining table, the forearm in neutral rotation, and the fingers toward the ceiling. The hand is placed in ulnar deviation (scaphoid pulled into an extended position), and the examiner's ipsilateral thumb (e.g., patient's right wrist, examiner's right thumb) placed firmly under the tuberosity of the distal scaphoid; his medial four fingers support the patient's forearm. The examiner's opposite hand then passively moves the patient's hand from ulnar to radial deviation, while his thumb prevents the distal scaphoid from physiologically flexing (the normal mechanical action of the scaphoid as the wrist moves from ulnar to radial deviation). Forced passive radial deviation with a mechanical block to scaphoid flexion will transfer all load to the proximal portion of this bone. In the presence of an incompetent SL ligament, load transference in this manner will result in instability of the proximal scaphoid pole at the dorsal margin of the distal radius. A positive sign will either be a "click" or "clunk" relative to the examined opposite normal side; the symptom will be pain, also relative to normal side.

Radiographic criteria for patient selection should include an SL diastasis greater than 2 mm (the range among my own 80 studied patients was 3 to 10 mm). The ring-pole distance should be less than 7 mm,[17] and the radioscaphoid angle should be greater than 60° on a true lateral projection (Fig. 106–7). Candidates with even the earliest radiographic changes of arthrosis are never appropriate candidates for this operation.

■ INDICATIONS AND CONTRAINDICATIONS

■ **FIGURE 106–6**
The Watson maneuver.
Based on physiologic flexion of the scaphoid and
proximal carpal row in
passing from ulnar devia-
tion **(A)** to radial deviation **(B)**, the examiner's
thumb prevents scaphoid
flexion by upward pres-
sure under its distal pole,
forcing an unstable proximal pole dorsally, as the
hand is passively moved
into radial deviation. A
positive Watson maneu-
ver may cause severe
pain or "clunking" instability at the dorsal lip of the
radius.

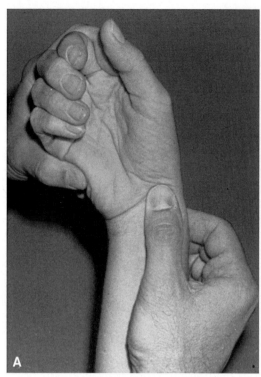
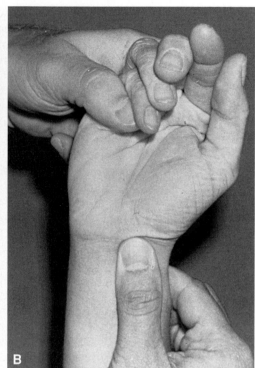

■ **FIGURE 106–7**
Criteria for static SL instability with rotary subluxation of the scaphoid. **(A)**
Scaphoid foreshortening
with SL diastasis; **(B)** a
flexed attitude of the
scaphoid greater than 60°
on true lateral projection.[8]

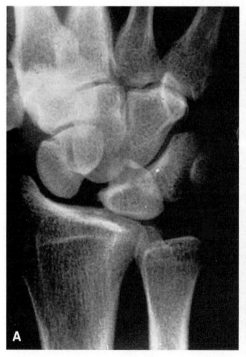
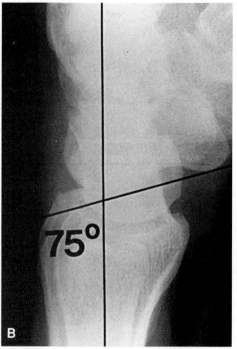

■ SURGICAL
TECHNIQUES

I use a general anesthetic when performing an STT arthrodesis, simply because I prefer the quality of autogenous cancellous iliac crest graft for the fusion. In addition, however, I have the anesthesiologist administer an axillary regional block, allowing the patient to be awakened after the bone graft has been harvested and the pelvic wound securely closed (bupivacaine can be injected around the graft donor site to afford patient comfort while the remainder of the surgery is performed under regional anesthesia alone).

The operation is accomplished through either a transverse or longitudinal skin incision 4 cm long and centered over the dorsal distal scaphoid. Because of the cosmetic advantages of any skin incision designed in Langher's lines, I prefer a transverse approach. A longitudinal incision is then made through the dorsal capsule, after mobilization and retraction of the radial artery; this capsular approach is designed between the first and second dorsal tendon compartments. The capsule is reflected off the underlying STT joint, exposing its articular surfaces. A hemostat should then be introduced under the palmar aspect of the distal neck of the malrotated scaphoid, along the radioscaphocapitate ligament. By gentle dorsal leverage the scaphoid can readily be derotated into its normal anatomic relationship with the adjacent carpus (Fig. 106–8). Reducing the scaphoid places its proximal pole securely within the elliptical fossa of the radius. Anatomic alignment can be judged by direct observation of the dorsal surfaces of the scaphoid and lunate, which will be coplanar if the reduction is anatomic. Orientation of the dorsal bony ridge of the scaphoid can also be used as an alignment landmark; ridge orientation should be about 25° to the transverse plane of the wrist. With increasing malrotation of the scaphoid, the ridge will become more perpendicular to the longitudinal axis of the hand. Bringing its orientation back to 25° helps the surgeon with the initial reduction. Regardless of the effectiveness of these technical tricks, however, radiographic confirmation of anatomic alignment must be obtained in the operating room after introduction of Kirschner wires (K-wires) to maintain the reduced posture. Because "normal" alignment is highly variable, patients who fit the clinical and radiographic criteria of SL dissociation with rotary subluxation of the scaphoid should have a preoperative posteroanterior and "true lateral" images taken of the contralateral normal wrist; this view provides the operating surgeon with a benchmark against which the patient's intraoperative alignment can be compared.

I prefer four percutaneous or subcutaneous K-wires to stabilize the STT relationship, and to support the reduced scaphoid to the capitate. No K-wires should cross the radiocarpal joint; no K-wire should penetrate the lunate. Two parallel wires anchor the scaphoid to the capitate; one wire holds the trapezium to the trapezoid; and one wire passes retrograde from the trapezium to the scaphoid. Care should be taken to avoid overcorrection of the scaphoid during the reduction maneuver. Levering it into an overly extended position will shift too much load onto the elliptical fossa of the radius. The ideal radioscaphoid

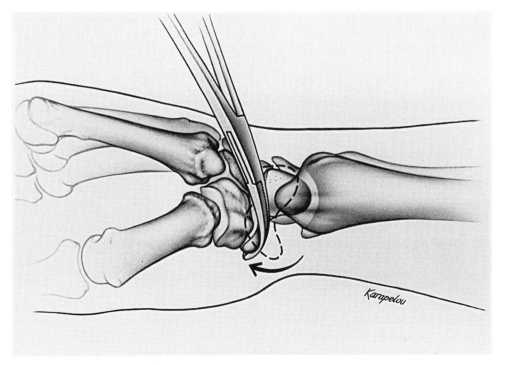

■ FIGURE 106–8 Gentle elevation of the perpendicular distal scaphoid pole is performed through a dorsoradial incision (transverse or longitudinal). Derotation is performed around the radioscaphocapitate ligament axis, followed by percutaneous K-wire internal fixation to the capitate and trapezium.

angle, as reported by Minamikawa et al,[26] ranges between 41 and 60°. I prefer reducing the scaphoid to a 45° posture, with anatomic (2-mm) closure of any preoperative SL diastasis. The final position must be confirmed by intraoperative radiographs.

After the STT joint has been effectively stabilized with K-wires, the dorsal two-thirds of cartilage and subchondral bone at each apposing joint surface are removed using a rongeur and curette. Use of power burring should be avoided because of its potential to cause thermal necrosis, even with continuous irrigation. The palmar third of the three-bone relationship should not be debrided; if left intact, carpal height is easily preserved, and an anatomic position of the reduced scaphoid can be ensured. Maintaining the palmar joint relationships also precludes palmar extrusion of cancellous bone graft as the graft is packed into the interstices of the three-bone mass. Autogenous bone graft can be harvested from either the iliac crest (which I prefer) or the distal metaphysis of the radius (through a separate transverse incision, if the initial incision was also transverse). During the packing process, no bone graft should be allowed to extrude into the scaphocapitate joint.

Once the three-bone fusion has been performed, the radial styloid should be removed at the radial origin of the radioscaphocapitate ligament, at an angle of 45° to the longitudinal axis of the radius. Approximately 7 mm should be removed, not violating the elliptical fossa. Performing a radial styloidectomy significantly decreases the propensity for styloid–scaphoid impingement; it does not, however, increase the postoperative range of wrist motion.

The capsule overlying the STT fusion mass should be closed with inverted 3-0 braided nylon, and the skin closed with subcuticular 4-0 absorbable suture material and Steri-Strips. Patients are immobilized in a long-arm, plaster-reinforced, thumb spica bulky compression dressing for 2 postoperative weeks, at which time the wound is checked.

■ TECHNICAL ALTERNATIVES

Efforts to restore normal alignment and to stabilize the relationship between the proximal pole of the scaphoid and scaphoid fossa of the radius after traumatic SL dissociation have, over the past 20 years, been predominantly based on three philosophic approaches (Table 106–1). In each, open reduction of the chronically malaligned scaphoid is performed through a dorsal or combined dorsal and palmar approach.[11] Regardless of the method

---

TABLE 106–1 ROTARY SUBLUXATION OF THE SCAPHOID: APPROACHES TO SURGICAL RECONSTRUCTION

Ligamentous reconstruction for scapho-lunate separation
Linscheid, et al, 1972[23]
Howard, et al, 1974[16]
Dobyns, et al, 1975[8]
Taleisnik, 1978[30]
Almquist, et al, 1991[1]
Augsberger, et al, 1992[3]
Lavernia, et al, 1992[22]

Scaphoid stabilization by ligamentodesis
Blatt, 1987,[4] 1992[5]

Scaphoid stabilization by limited (partial, intercarpal) wrist athrodesis
Howard, et al, 1974[16]
Watson, et al, 1980,[33] 1991[32]
Kleinman, et al, 1982,[20] 1987,[18] 1989,[17] 1990[19]
Essman, et al, 1990[11]
Hom and Ruby, 1991[14]
Pisano, et al, 1991[27]

selected, realignment of the carpus to preserve motion must be made *before* even the earliest signs of degenerative arthrosis at the radioscaphoid or midcarpal level. Reconstitution of ligament support by rebuilding the injured radioscapholunate ligament (Testut) or the intrinsic interosseous ligament has been proposed by many authors using either attached tendon[8,16,22,23] or free-tendon grafts,[31] after open anatomic reduction and temporary internal fixation of the scaphoid. Ligamentodesis or dorsal capsulodesis, using a proximally based portion of the dorsal wrist capsule, secured to the dorsal neck of the reduced scaphoid, has also been advocated as an option for long-term scaphoid stabilization.[4,5] A four-bone tendon weave using the distally attached extensor carpi radialis brevis has also been described.[1,3] Although the number of ligament reconstructive procedures from which to choose continues to grow, these approaches are complex, and highly unpredictable because of the viscoelastic properties of tendon substituted for ligament; they have not proven to be as reliable as partial carpal arthrodesis.[13,31,33]

As I mentioned earlier in this chapter, fusing the distal pole of the scaphoid to the trapezium and trapezoid has been clearly shown to be more reliable than efforts to fuse the proximal pole directly to the lunate.[14] Attaining a successful SL fusion is difficult: contact surfaces are small and physiologic compression is absent. The SL joint is normally in constant tension, generating only associated torque and shear with motion. An effort at SL arthrodesis becomes a rather poor choice for stabilization, with a high pseudarthrosis and failure rate. STT arthrodesis, as an alternative, can be performed with K-wires and bone graft alone, or with any type of fixation with which the surgeon feels comfortable. Shapiro staples and Herbert screws have both been described as effective, but I have found the compression screws to be very difficult to orient perfectly. After trying a variety of techniques for fixation, I find K-wires alone to be highly effective in providing the stability necessary to ensure fusion, while minimizing the risks of pseudarthrosis.

Traumatic SL dissociation eliminates the normal carpal shift influence of the proximal pole of the scaphoid on the lunate. Anatomic reduction of the scaphoid and stabilization of the distal pole by arthrodesis to the trapezium and trapezoid does not restore this shift influence; it has been permanently lost by destruction of the SL interosseous ligament. The scaphoid is unable to "pull" the lunate onto the spherical fossa of the radius in ulnar deviation (Fig. 106–9); it is also unable to influence extension of the remaining proximal row. Triquetrohamate mechanics, however, remain minimally affected.[18]

Because the distal scaphoid is now fixed to the distal carpal row and can no longer flex during radial deviation, and because the trapezium and trapezoid are unable physiologically to ride dorsally and proximally along the scaphoid neck, radial deviation after STT fusion is reduced to zero. Ulnar deviation, however, is only marginally compromised. Even without the carpal shift influence of the proximal scaphoid on the lunatotriquetral unit, the hamate can still engage the triquetrum along the medial column helicoidal joint in wrist extension and ulnar deviation, and actively extend the proximal carpal row. This influence of the hamate on proximal row extension has been observed consistently on postoperative videoradiograms and fluoroscopy in my own patient population. As expected, there is little observable change in the position of the lunate relative to the medial border of the radius. Postoperative absence of carpal shift influence is confirmed by a widening of SL diastasis in ulnar deviation, to the same observed preoperative "gap." Unless the SL relationship is surgically restored acutely at the time of initial trauma, and the interosseous ligament allowed to heal primarily, carpal shift influence of the scaphoid will be permanently lost. STT arthrodesis for chronic SL dissociation does not restore the influence of the proximal pole of the scaphoid on the lunate (Fig. 106–9); nevertheless, motion studies in my patient population of more than 80 cases show long-term postoperative ulnar deviation consistently greater than 25°.

Owing to minimally affected mechanics at the triquetrohamate joint, and the persistent loss of shift influence of the fusion mass on the lunatotriquetral unit, wrist motion takes place post-STT fusion through two planes: (1) midcarpal, dissipated through the SL joint; and (2) radiocarpal (Fig. 106–10). Through these two planes of motion, patients should be able to generate 60 to 75% of their normal flexion–extension arc. Although diminished, midcarpal mechanics still occur at both the lunatocapitate and triquetrohamate joints.

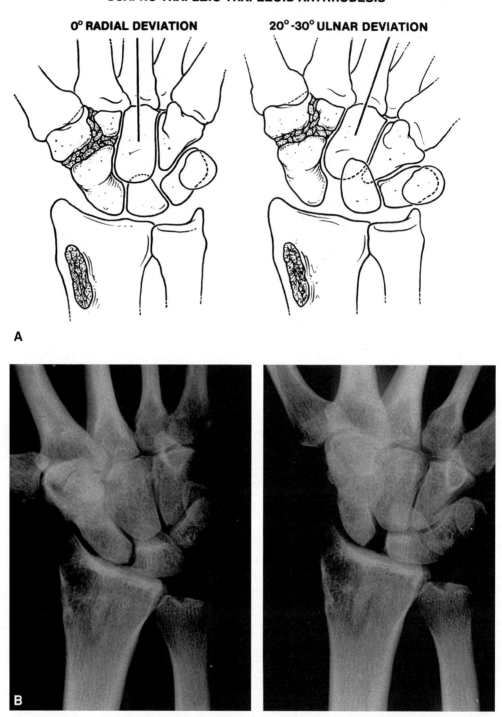

■ FIGURE 106–9

Schematic **(A)** and radiographic **(B)** depictions of significantly altered carpal mechanics following STT arthrodesis. Lost is the carpal shift influence of the scaphoid on the lunate. The lunate is no longer pulled radially in ulnar deviation; consequently, preoperative SL diastasis reappears in ulnar deviation. Although the fixed, postreduction scaphoid can no longer physiologically rotate, mechanics at the triquetrohamate joint are essentially normal. Flexion and extension of the remaining proximal row (lunate and triquetrum) still occur with radial and ulnar deviation.

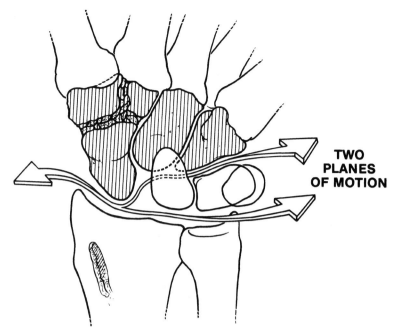

**TWO
PLANES
OF MOTION**

■ FIGURE 106-10
After STT arthrodesis,
kinematics at the trique-
trohamate joint remain essentially normal. Carpal
shift influence of the
scaphoid on the lunate is
lost, but the extending influence of the hamate on
the triquetrum in ulnar deviation is preserved. Wrist
motion occurs at both the
radiocarpal and intercar-
pal triquetrohamate and
capitolunate joints, com-
municating between the
separated scaphoid and
lunate.

NORMAL MECHANICS   **SCAPHO-TRAPEZIO-TRAPEZOID
ARTHRODESIS**

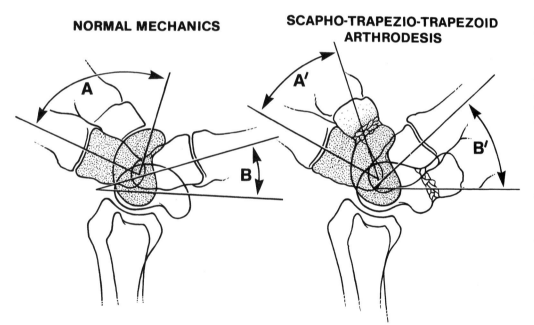

■ FIGURE 106-11
Videoradiographs demon-
strate that the angle be-
tween scaphoid and capi-
tate on lateral projection
changes greatly through
the normal extension–
flexion arc (compare angle
"A" in extension to angle
"B" in flexion). After STT
arthrodesis, this angle remains constant throughout
the extension–flexion arc
(angle A′ = angle B′),
clearly indicating that capitate movement is securely
linked to that of the STT fusion mass.

Plain radiographic, videoradiographic, and fluoroscopic studies of this large series of postoperative patients also demonstrate no motion between the scaphoid and capitate through the full postoperative flexion–extension arc (Fig. 106–11). The three-bone fusion mass behaves kinematically as a five-bone mass (scapho-trapezio-trapezoid-capito-hamate), through the short, strong intrinsic ligaments of the distal carpal row. After study-ing detailed postoperative videoradiographs of 12 patients, I concluded more than 12 years ago[20] that reduction of the malaligned scaphoid and arthrodesis of its distal pole to the trapezium and trapezoid would produce results identical to fusion of the scaphoid to the capitate alone. Postoperative kinematic behavior in each would be the same, as long as the anatomic relationships among the uninjured ligaments of the distal carpal row remained normal. That the behavior of the wrist after either STT arthrodesis or scaphocapitate arthrodesis should be mechanically similar has since been reported, first by Garcia-Elias et al, based on laboratory cadaver studies,[12] and more recently (from the Mayo Clinic biomechanics laboratory) by Horii et al.[15] These authors have shown that in cadaver studies comparing STT with scaphocapitate arthrodesis, transmission of load to the elliptical fossa of the radius, the spherical fossa of the radius, and the triangular fibrocartilage, under varying conditions, was essentially identical. In clinical trials involving 17 patients studied an average of 2 years, Pisano and colleagues found that the behavioral characteristics of scaphocapitate fusion closely parallel the results of STT fusion reported in the literature, including the ability of the scaphocapitate arthrodesis to "effectively preserve carpal relationships regained at the operation for rotary scaphoid subluxation."[28]

Certainly, a clear understanding of the consequences of permanent loss of carpal shift influence of the proximal pole of the scaphoid on the lunatotriquetral unit, and mechanical engagement of the triquetrum and hamate in ulnar deviation or extension, are critical in appreciating carpal kinematics after STT arthrodesis for chronic traumatic rotary subluxation of the scaphoid. But the surgeon performing this procedure (for the proper indications) should also understand that the single largest potential complication of the procedure is progressive arthrosis. In all cases reported in which progressive arthrosis was observed, each patient (in retrospective review) had an incompletely reduced SL relationship at the completion of surgery.[19]

It is clear that two of the fundamental principles the surgeon should observe to avoid major complications of this procedure are: (1) to make sure that no preoperative degenerative changes of early SLAC exist; and (2) to confirm radiographically anatomic scaphoid reduction before leaving the operating room.

■ REHABILITATION

The Indiana Hand Center is privileged to have associated with it the largest number of fully trained hand therapists anywhere in the United States. Through the close working relationship between surgeons and therapists at the Center, patients' postoperative function can be maximized. Each of the more than 80 patients reviewed for this chapter underwent extensive supervised rehabilitation, including active, active-assisted, and passive motion in three cardinal wrist motion planes; static and dynamic splinting as indicated; and strengthening exercises. After any major wrist reconstruction, small joint range of motion should begin immediately after surgery. Active and active-assisted motion of the medial four fingers should be encouraged, in addition to standard elevation and edema control. Contrary to the recommendations of Watson et al,[33,34] I have not found it necessary to immobilize the metacarpophalangeal (MP) joints of the index and middle fingers in the initial postoperative cast. Instead, my patients are maintained in a plaster-reinforced, long-arm, bulky compression dressing until postoperative swelling subsides; MP joints remain free for postoperative motion. A long-arm, cylinder plaster-of-Paris cast can be applied at 10 to 14 days, which should remain in place until the end of the sixth postoperative week. K-wires are removed and a short-arm, thumb spica cast (with the thumb interphalangeal joint free) replaces the long-arm cast until the STT fusion mass is clinically and radiographically healed (~ 10 weeks). Once the three-bone fusion mass is solid, aggressive rehabilitation of the wrist can begin.

Patients are encouraged to do no lifting with their operated hand until the fusion is healed. Usually 4 to 6 weeks of strengthening is required after cast removal to return the patient to any gainful employment that requires moderate lifting. Full rehabilitation of a patient who requires extraordinary strength for his or her routine job may require as much as 6 months of conditioning, and a rehabilitative program organized specifically to recreate their regular job activity.

■ OUTCOMES

Scapho-trapezio-trapezoid wrist arthrodesis has been well studied, and is an effective means of permanently stabilizing the reduced scaphoid in cases of traumatic SL dissociation. Wrist stability can be ensured, and chronic pain significantly improved. In those patients who have undergone the procedure before even the earliest radiographic signs of arthrosis, the need for total wrist arthrodesis can be obviated.

There are four *major* factors that directly affect the outcome of any large group of patients having undergone STT fusion for the indications discussed in this chapter. Two of these factors involve preoperative assessment of the surgical candidate; two involve technique.

First, I have found that even subtle changes of cartilage space narrowing, subchondral sclerosis, or radial styloid "beaking" are contraindications for this type of reconstruction. In the face of minor degenerative changes, even if the scaphoid is perfectly aligned during surgery, and if the fusion mass heals solidly, rapid degenerative changes will ensue; patients' potential to resume painless vocational and avocational activities will be poor. In the presence of preoperative degenerative changes, alternatives such as proximal row carpectomy, scaphoid excision and four-bone medial column fusion, or aggressive styloidectomy alone should be considered.

Patient outcome will also be severely compromised if the surgeon fails to appreciate before surgery the unusual case of injury to the long radiolunate ligament, with resultant preoperative medial translation of the lunate and triquetrum. Reduction of SL diastasis by simple operative scaphoid manipulation will not be successful. Failure to appreciate this severe problem before surgery invariably leads to a frustrating operative experience for the surgeon, and a poor outcome for the patient. Severe medial column pain is the usual outcome in these cases, precluding activities of gainful employment or avocational living. Salvage is usually by total wrist fusion.

The two major technical considerations that greatly compromise patient outcome are failure to reduce anatomically the malrotated scaphoid, and failure to perform a radial styloidectomy at the time of STT fusion. The first has been extensively dealt with earlier in this chapter. The incidence of progressive arthrosis in my large studied population was approximately 15%; each patient involved, retrospectively, had an imperfectly aligned scaphoid at the close of surgery. STT arthrodesis for chronic SL dissociation is not a panacea; however, it remains the most predictable means of preserving a relatively functional and painless wrist range of motion, with stability sufficient to allow patients to return to most of their preinjury activities. With or without the persistence of DISI, no progressive degenerative radiocarpal or midcarpal arthrosis has been observed in this large series over more than 15 years, as long as the normal anatomic posture of the pathologically rotated scaphoid can be restored.

Although chronic radial styloid–scaphoid impingement has not been a universal complication after STT arthrodesis, the rate of postoperative symptoms in the first 45 patients reported was only 5%[19] on early follow-up. This figure increased to 20% on reassessment of the initial group, 5 years later. I now agree with the recommendations of Rogers and Watson,[29] and routinely perform a radial styloidectomy when performing the three-bone STT fusion. Excision of 7 to 8 mm of styloid[30] allows the STT fusion mass to rotate through an arc of motion without impingement.

Chronic untreated traumatic instability of the SL relationship—either static or dynamic[19]—will result in SLAC, with its predictable patterns of arthritic change at the radiocarpal and midcarpal joints. From careful assessment of more than 80 patients undergoing STT arthrodesis for this problem over a 15-year period, it is clear that carpal mechanics are significantly altered by the operation, in spite of anatomic reduction of the malaligned scaphoid. Even in the presence of altered carpal mechanics, the pain of chronic scapholunate CID can be significantly reduced by the operation, while still preserving a functional arc of motion, averaging 50° of extension and 50% of flexion in this large series.

Patients incapacitated before surgery by wrist pain and weakness can frequently be returned to their preinjury gainful employment and avocational activities after the operation. The development of degenerative arthritis in this patient population on even longer-term follow-up remains to be determined.

References

1. Almquist EE, Bach AW, Sack JT, Fuhs SE, Newman DM: Four-bone ligament reconstruction for treatment of chronic complete scapholunate separation. J Hand Surg, 1991; 16A:322–327.
2. Armstrong GWD: Rotational subluxation of the scaphoid. Can J Surg, 1968; 11:306–314.
3. Augsberger S, Necking L, Horton J, Bach AW, Tencer AF: A comparison of scaphoid-trapezium-trapezoid fusion and four-bone tendon weave for scapholunate dissociation. J Hand Surg, 1992; 17A:360–369.

4. Blatt G: Capsulodesis in reconstructive hand surgery. Hand Clin, 1987; 3:81–102.
5. Blatt G, Ross N: Dorsal capsulodesis for rotary subluxation of the scaphoid—A review of long-term results. Presented at the 47th Annual Meeting of the American Society for Surgery of the Hand, Phoenix, Arizona, November 12, 1992.
6. Burgess RC: The effect of rotatory subluxation of the scaphoid on radioscaphoid contact. J Hand Surg, 1987; 12A:771–774.
7. Cooney WP, Linscheid RL, Dobyns JH, Wood MB: Scaphoid nonunion: Role of anterior interpositional bone grafts. J Hand Surg, 1988; 13A:635–650.
8. Dobyns JH, Linscheid RL, Chao EYS, et al: Traumatic instability of the wrist. In: AAOS Instructional Course Lecture. St. Louis: CV Mosby, 1975; 24:182–199.
9. Eaton RG, Akelman E, Eaton BH: Fascial implant arthroplasty for treatment of radioscaphoid degenerative disease. J Hand Surg , 1989; 14A:766–774.
10. Eckenrode JF, Louis DS, Greene TL: Scaphoid-trapezium-trapezoid fusion in the treatment of chronic scapholunate instability. J Hand Surg, 1986; 11A:497–502.
11. Essman JA, Reilly TJ, Forshew FC: Palmar approach for treatment of scapho-trapezio-trapezoid arthrodesis. J Hand Surg, 1990; 15A:672–674.
12. Garcia-Elias M, Cooney WP, An KN, Linscheid RL, Chao EYS: Wrist kinematics after limited intercarpal arthrodesis. J Hand Surg, 1989; 14A:791–799.
13. Glickel SL, Millender LH: Ligamentous reconstruction for chronic intercarpal instability. J Hand Surg, 1984; 9A:514–527.
14. Hom S, Ruby L: Attempted scapholunate arthrodesis for chronic scapholunate dissociation. J Hand Surg, 1991; 16A:334–339.
15. Horii E, Garcia-Elias M, An KN, et al: Effect on force transmission across the carpus in procedures used to treat Kienböck's disease. J Hand Surg, 1990; 15A:394–400.
16. Howard FM, Fahey T, Wojcik E: Rotary subluxation of the navicular. Clin Orthop, 1974; 104: 134-139.
17. Kleinman WB: Long-term study of chronic scapho-lunate instability treated by scapho-trapezio-trapezoid arthrodesis. J Hand Surg, 1989; 14A:429–445.
18. Kleinman WB: Management of chronic rotary subluxation of the scaphoid by scapho-trapezio-trapezoid arthrodesis. Hand Clin, 1987; 3:113–133.
19. Kleinman WB, Carroll C: Scapho-trapezio-trapezoid arthrodesis for treatment of chronic static and dynamic scapho-lunate instability: A 10 year perspective on pitfalls and complications. J Hand Surg, 1990; 15A:408–414.
20. Kleinman WB, Steichen JB, Strickland JW: Management of chronic rotary subluxation of the scaphoid by scapho-trapezio-trapezoid arthrodesis. J Hand Surg 1982; 7A:125–136.
21. Landsmeer JMF: Studies in the anatomy of articulation. Acta Morphol Neerl Scand 1961; 3: 87–321.
22. Lavernia C, Cohen M, Taleisnik J: Treatment of scapholunate dissociation by ligamentous repair and capsulodesis. J Hand Surg, 1992; 17A:354–359.
23. Linscheid RL, Dobyns JH, Beabout JW, Bryan RS: Traumatic instability of the wrist: Diagnosis, classification and pathomechanics. J Bone Joint Surg, 1972; 54A:1612-1632.
24. Mayfield JK, Johnson RP, Kilcoyne RF: Carpal injuries: An experimental approach, anatomy, kinematics and perilunate injuries. J Bone Joint Surg, 1975; 57A:725.
25. Mayfield JK, Johnson RP, Kilcoyne RF: Carpal dislocations: Pathomechanics and progressive perilunar instability. J Hand Surg 1980; 5:226–241.
26. Minamikawa Y, Peimer CA, Yamaguchi T, Medige J, Sherwin F: Ideal scaphoid angle for intercarpal arthrodesis. J Hand Surg, 1992; 17A:370–375.
27. Peterson HA, Lipscomb PR: Intercarpal arthrodesis. Arch Surg, 1967, 95:127–134.
28. Pisano S, Peimer C, Wheeler D, Sherwin F: Scaphocapitate intercarpal arthrodesis J Hand Surg, 1991; 16A:328–333.
29. Rogers WD, Watson HK: Degenerative arthritis at the triscaphe joint. J Hand Surg, 1990; 15A: 232–235.
30. Seigel DB, Gelberman RH: Radial styloidectomy: An anatomical study with special reference to radiocarpal intracapsular ligamentous morphology. J Hand Surg, 1991; 16A:40–44.
31. Taleisnik J: Wrists: Anatomy, function, and injury. In: AAOS Instructional Course Lecture. St. Louis: CV Mosby, 1978; 27:61–87.
32. Watson HK, Ballet FL: The SLAC wrist: Scapholunate advanced collapse pattern of degenerative arthritis. J Hand Surg, 1984; 9A:358–365.
33. Watson K, Belniak R, Garcia-Elias M: Treatment of scapholunate dissociation: Preferred treatment—STT fusion vs. other methods. Orthopedics, 1991; 14:365–370.
34. Watson HK, Hempton RF: Limited wrist arthrodesis: I. The triscaphoid joint. J Hand Surg 1980; 5:320–327.

MITCHELL B.
ROTMAN
TIMOTHY S. LOTH

107

Scaphocapitate Arthrodesis

Scaphocapitate (SC) arthrodesis was first described by Sutro in 1946 for the treatment of difficult scaphoid nonunions.[10] Local bone graft was used without any fixation. Union was usually obtained after 6 months of immobilization. Its use in the treatment of Kienböck disease and scapholunate (SL) instability was described 45 years later in a report by Pisano et al.[5] Fixation was achieved with either K-wires, a Herbert screw, or power-driven bone staples. Union was seen at 2.5 to 3 months.

The techniques that we present for SC arthrodesis are derived from techniques used for scaphocapitolunate arthrodesis,[6] taught to us by Paul R. Manske, M.D. The specific preferred technique presented in this chapter is a modification of techniques originally developed by the senior author (TSL). The concept of harvesting bone graft through the radial styloid osteotomy was contributed by MBR.

Scaphocapitate arthrodesis is most commonly indicated for the treatment of chronic, symptomatic incompetence of the SL joint (Fig. 107–1), resistant scaphoid nonunion with avascular necrosis or fragmentation of the proximal fragment that has failed previous bone grafting and internal fixation, and the treatment of stage IIIB (with collapse) Kienböck disease or stage IIIA (without collapse) after a failed leveling procedure (Fig. 107–2).[1] SC arthrodesis is contraindicated when degenerative changes involve joints other than the SC or radial styloid–scaphoid articulations.

We most commonly use axillary block anesthesia with a long-acting anesthetic, which helps in postoperative pain control. Under tourniquet control, an oblique dorsal skin incision is used that extends from the ulnar aspect of the distal radius and curves toward the distal pole of the scaphoid (Fig. 107–2). The wrist capsule is exposed in the interval between the third and fourth dorsal compartments. Only the distal half of the retinaculum between the two compartments needs to be released for exposure of the scaphocapitolunate articulation. Great care is taken to avoid injuring any terminal branches of the sensory radial nerve. A segment of the distal posterior interosseous nerve is easily found on the radial side of the fourth extensor compartment, and is excised.[3] The wrist capsule is then opened in an inverted T-fashion and the articular surfaces and carpal alignment of the scaphoid, capitate, lunate, and radius are inspected. Stripping of the dorsal ridge of the scaphoid is avoided to protect a significant portion of its blood supply. The articular cartilage and subchondral bone between the scaphoid and capitate is removed with rongeurs, curettes, and thin osteotomes. The use of larger osteotomes can cause cracks through the remaining articular surface and subchondral bone at critical joint surfaces proximal and distal to the intended site of fusion. Care should be taken to avoid straying into the capitolunate or SL joints. Power tools are avoided, preventing unnecessary necrosis from heat production. The architecture of the articular space is preserved by leaving a volar rim of cartilage and subchondral bone intact on both the capitate and scaphoid articular surfaces. K-wires 0.045″ in diameter are placed into the lunate and scaphoid proximal pole in a dorsal-to-volar direction and are used as "joysticks" to correct any malalignment. In Kienböck disease, we have removed the lunate only when it is sclerotic, fragmented, and lacks a cartilage envelope. We leave a volar shell with its ligamentous attachments; we have not replaced the lunate with any spacers. With scaphoid nonunions, we have not removed or replaced the fragmented proximal pole. Two 0.045″ K-wires are directed medially from the radial side of the scaphoid until they are seen at the SC interface and are pulled back flush with the scaphoid. A small, portable fluoroscopy unit has been very helpful for K-wire positioning.

■ HISTORY OF THE TECHNIQUE

■ INDICATIONS AND CONTRAINDICATIONS

■ SURGICAL TECHNIQUES

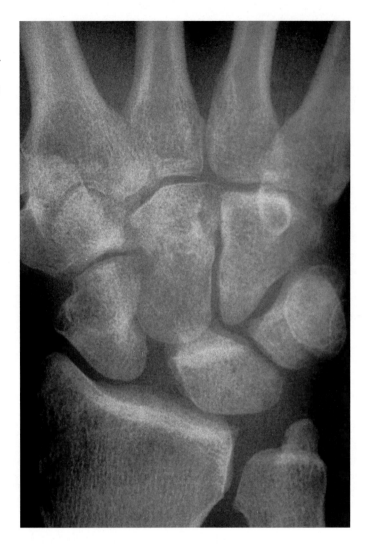

The radial styloid is then exposed between the first and second compartments. Osteotomes are used to perform a transverse radial styloidectomy, removing enough styloid to create an opening to introduce curettes to remove cancellous bone graft. A generous radial styloidectomy is done when there is radial styloid–scaphoid impingement or wear. Gelfoam (Upjohn, Kalamazoo, MI) is then placed into the distal radius and left there permanently. The cancellous bone graft is then packed into the area between the scaphoid and capitate, intercarpal relationships are reduced, and the K-wires are driven into or through the ulnar cortex of the capitate. The SL angle is corrected to approximately 45°; anywhere between 30 and 57° is acceptable.[2,5] If the scaphoid is fixed in a horizontal position, wrist extension is restricted more than wrist flexion, and ability to deviate radially is decreased. To hold an unstable SL joint, two more 0.045″ K-wires are driven across the SL and capitolunate joints, respectively, or both K-wires can be driven across the SL joint. We have been unsuccessful at closing a preexisting SL gap.

One to two power-driven 13 × 10 mm Shapiro staples[7] are placed after K-wire fixation (Figs. 107-3 and 107-4). The staples are placed in nonarticular portions of the capitate and scaphoid such that they do not impinge dorsally with passive range of motion of the wrist. All K-wires are cut beneath the skin. The wrist capsule and retinaculum are closed with 3-0 Ethibond and the skin is closed with 4-0 nylon. After surgery, the patients are immobilized in a sugar-tong splint with a thumb spica attachment, which is converted to a long-arm thumb spica cast. After 6 weeks, a short-arm thumb spica cast is applied. Wires are

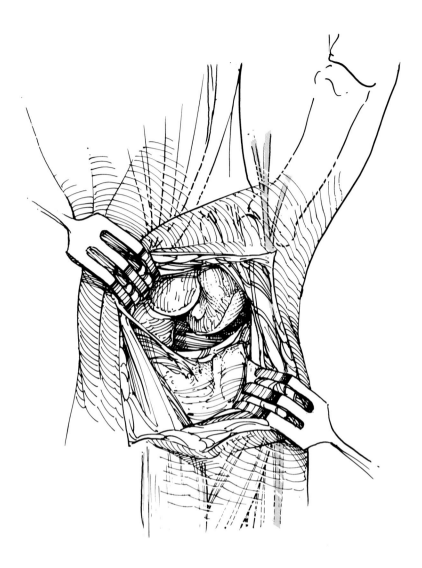

■ FIGURE 107–2
An oblique skin incision extends from the ulnar aspect of the distal radius and curves toward the distal pole of the scaphoid.

removed between 8 to 10 postoperative weeks if radiographs show early evidence of union (Fig. 107–5).

Instead of an oblique incision, a longitudinal incision can be used that extends 4 cm proximal and distal from Lister's tubercle, especially if the ulnar side of the wrist needs to be visualized. With the longitudinal exposure it is usually necessary to release the retinaculum between the third and fourth compartments entirely, which can be done in a step-cut fashion, allowing for easier closure. Bone graft can also be taken from the dorsal distal radius from deep to the second extensor compartment, or from the volar radius through a separate incision between the brachioradialis and radial artery, deep to the pronator quadratus.[9,12] K-wires alone or with a headless screw may also be used for fixation. When using staples, K-wires need to be driven across the arthrodesis site first to prevent a dorsal wedging effect from the staple. If K-wires are not cut deeply beneath the skin, skin necrosis can be a problem, necessitating early removal of the K-wires. We believe that K-wires left outside the skin are more prone to causing infection.

■ TECHNICAL ALTERNATIVES

Patients are placed into a thermoplastic thumb spica splint after pin removal. They are instructed in the techniques of scar massage and desensitization if necessary. Patients can remove the splint only for bathing until radiographic evidence of union is achieved. At that time, active and passive range of motion out of the splint is started, progressing to strengthening, which usually is started by 12 weeks. At that time the splint can be permanently removed. Most patients usually achieve unrestricted activities by 6 months.

■ REHABILITATION

The arthrodesis site with
K-wires, power staple,
and bone graft in place.

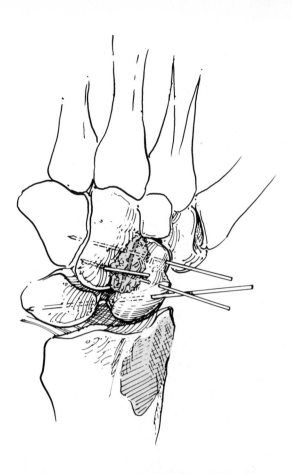

A postoperative radio-
graph showing the K-
wires and staple in place,
and the bone graft donor
site in the radial styloid.
Usually, two K-wires are
used to control the reduction of the scaphoid and
lunate.

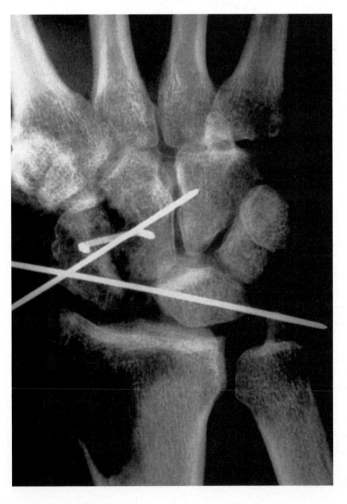

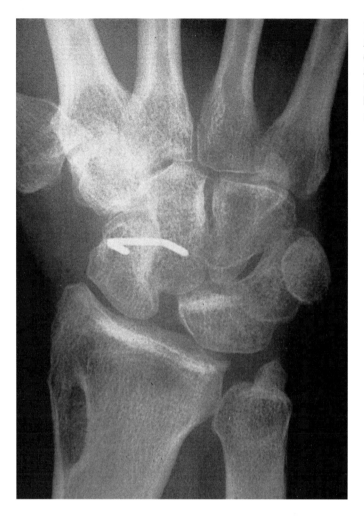

■ FIGURE 107–5
A scaphocapitate arthro-
desis site at 4 months
after surgery. The staple
is left in place and the
bone graft donor site is
repairing.

■ OUTCOMES

We have performed SC arthrodesis for SL instability since 1989, in nine patients. The patients' average age was 40 years (range, 19 to 58 years), and they included seven men and two women. Follow-up averaged 16 months (range, 5 to 25 months). Union was achieved in all patients by 12 weeks. Active range of motion averaged 47° of extension (range, 35 to 65°), 37° of flexion (range, 24 to 52°), 12° radial deviation (range, 5 to 16°), and 21° ulnar deviation (range, 15 to 30°). Grip strength averaged 74% of the opposite side. Pain was significantly reduced in 67% of the patients. Most patients were able to return to some kind of work by 6 months. Radiographic examination at last follow-up showed increased degenerative changes at the radiocarpal joints in two patients; one has required a complete wrist fusion.

A major concern about this procedure and all other intercarpal fusions is the lack of long-term follow-up studies. Short-term results have been promising with respect to pain relief, strength, stabilization of carpal architecture, and maintenance of a functional range of motion. The average follow-up from Pisano et al was 23.4 months; the maximum follow-up was 57 months.[5] Their study included patients with Kienböck's disease, who usually have stiff wrists before and after surgery, and thus their results were similar to ours except for slightly decreased range of motion. Over a third of their patients and all but one of our patients had pain with heavy use.

Viegas et al[11] and Short et al[8] have shown in SC and scapho-trapezial-trapezoid fusions that most of the load is transmitted through the scaphoid fossa, implying that, in time, we may see more changes at the radioscaphoid fossa in these patients. Viegas and co-workers showed that with scaphocapitolunate (SCL) arthrodesis, the load distributed through the lunate and scaphoid fossae was more proportionate.[11] We have seen one patient 30 years after an SC fusion done for the treatment of a scaphoid nonunion who presented with intermittent wrist pain and degenerative changes at the radioscaphoid fossa. A recent report on SCL fusions has been promising.[6] Longer follow-up of SCL arthrodesis and comparisons of SC and SCL arthrodesis will be necessary to establish more clearly the role of SC arthrodesis in surgical reconstruction of the wrist.

References

1. Alexander AH, Lichtman DM: Kienböck's disease. In: Lichtman DM (ed): The Wrist and Its Disorders. Philadelphia: WB Saunders, 1988:329–343.
2. Ambrose L, Posner MA, Green SM, Stuchin S: The effects of scaphoid intercarpal stabilizations on wrist mechanics: An experimental study. J Hand Surg, 1992; 17A:429–437.
3. Dellon AL: Partial dorsal wrist denervation: Resection of the distal posterior interosseous nerve. J Hand Surg, 1985; 10A:527–533.
4. Minamikawa Y, Peimer CA, Yamaguchi T, Medige J, Sherwin FS: Ideal scaphoid angle for intercarpal arthrodesis. J Hand Surg, 1992; 17A:370–375.
5. Pisano SM, Peimer CA, Wheeler DR, Sherwin F: Scaphocapitate intercarpal arthrodesis. J Hand Surg, 1991; 16A:328–333.
6. Rotman MB, Manske PR, Pruitt DL, Szerzinski JRN: Scaphocapitolunate arthrodesis. J Hand Surg, 1993;18A:26–33.
7. Shapiro JS: Power staple fixation in hand and wrist surgery: New applications of an old fixation device. J Hand Surg, 1987; 12A:218–227.
8. Short WH, Werner FW, Fortino MD, Palmar AK: Distribution of pressures and forces on the wrist after simulated intercarpal fusion and Kienböck's disease. J Hand Surg, 1992; 17A: 443–449.
9. Steichen JB, Schreiber DR.: Radial bone graft with prolonged immobilization for scaphoid nonunions. Contemporary Orthopedics, 1986; 12:19–24.
10. Sutro CJ: Treatment of nonunion of the carpal navicular bone. Surgery, 1946; 20:536–540.
11. Viegas SF, Patterson RM, Peterson PD, Poque DJ, Jenkins DK, Sweo TD, Hokanson JA: Evaluation of the biomechanical efficacy of limited intercarpal fusions for the treatment of scapho-lunate dissociation. J Hand Surg, 1990; 15:120–128.
12. Watson HK: Limited wrist arthrodesis. Clin Orthop, 1990; 149:126–136.

DAVID L. NELSON,
PAUL R. MANSKE

108

Lunotriquetral Arthrodesis

There was little written on wrist biomechanics and its clinical applications before 1972. (See Taleisnik[38] for a review of the pre-1972 literature.)

In 1972, Linscheid and co-authors[19] were the first authors in the English literature to recognize the pivotal role of the lunate with respect to carpal motion and how lunate position could be used to identify pathology. The importance of the scapholunate ligament was recognized in this seminal work but the lunotriquetral ligament was not yet identified as an important structure. While dorsal intercalated segmental instability (DISI) was correctly attributed to scapholunate ligament rupture, palmar intercalated segmental instability [PISI, later changed to volar intercalated segmental instability (VISI)] was attributed to "traumatic or congenital laxity of the palmar radiocarpal ligament." More than a decade elapsed before lunotriquetral disruption was recognized as a specific carpal injury, and, interestingly, it was recognized by the same group.[30] Later work by Trumble and co-authors[42] indicated that VISI was due to disruption of the lunotriquetral ligament and the ulnar half of the volar arcuate ligament, and Horii and co-authors[16] found that VISI was due to disruption of the lunotriquetral ligament and the dorsal radiotriquetral and dorsal scaphotriquetral ligaments. Our understanding of the lunotriquetral joint has lagged behind that of the scapholunate joint, and we would agree with Green[13] who stated in 1993 that "there is still a paucity of clinically applicable information regarding ligamentous injuries and instabilities on the ulnar side of the carpus . . . . "

Lunotriquetral pathology and its treatment is still controversial at this time. There is no consensus even on the terminology, some preferring the term lunotriquetral and others preferring triquetrolunate for the ligament between the lunate and the triquetrum bones. The recommended treatment of lunotriquetral injuries include immobilization,[1,30,38,40] injection,[40] open reduction with internal fixation,[1] lunotriquetral ligament repair,[1,30,40] lunotriquetral ligament reconstruction with tendon grafts,[1,38] and limited intercarpal fusion.[1,22,25,27,38,40] Ulnar shortening may be useful[38] (Rayhack, personal communication), but its success has not yet been reported. The recommended fusions include combinations of the capitate-lunate-triquetrum-hamate bones or the lunate-triquetrum-hamate bones,[41] in addition to just the lunate-triquetral bones.[14,22,30,32,41,44] The most common approach to the symptomatic lunotriquetral tear is fusion, and the most commonly fused joint has been the lunotriquetral joint. We have had limited experience with soft tissue repairs, but the outcome has not been good. Taleisnik has experience with soft tissue repairs and characterizes the lunotriquetral fusion as "easier and more reliable"[38] than soft tissue procedures. We now prefer to treat symptomatic lunotriquetral injuries with fusion of the lunate and triquetral bones with a Herbert screw and a single parallel Kirschner wire, due to the procedure's reasonably predictable outcome and good clinical function.

The differential diagnosis of ulnar-sided wrist pain is long, and the discrimination among these is difficult. The workup of ulnar-sided wrist pain is beyond the scope of this article and the reader is referred to Bottke and co-authors,[3] Pin and co-authors,[29] and Brown and Lichtman.[4] The diagnosis is initially based on the history of ulnar-sided wrist pain that usually follows a traumatic injury to the hand, although there are cases of repetitive, heavy manual labor with recurrent high magnitude stresses.[23] Attritional tears from repetitive light activity is unlikely to lead to symptomatic wrist pain. Physical examination should include the entire wrist, including the radiocarpal, radioulnar, and ulnocarpal joints.

■ HISTORY OF THE TECHNIQUE

■ INDICATIONS AND CONTRAINDICATIONS

855

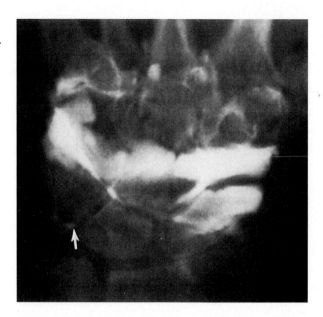

■ FIGURE 108–1
Patient with an lunotriquetral tear. Arthrogram of
the same wrist demon-
strating a lunotriquetral
defect (arrow).

The examination of the ulnar side of the wrist should include palpation of the triangular fibrocartilage complex (TFCC), the distal ulna, the distal radioulnar joint (DRUJ), and the extensor carpi ulnaris tendon, in addition to the lunotriquetral articulation. The most important finding in the physical examination for supporting a diagnosis of a lunotrique-tral tear is tenderness to direct pressure localized specifically to the lunotriquetral joint. The location of the lunate can easily be found by flexing and extending the wrist and palpating dorsally just distal to the radius, in the center of the wrist. (Radioulnar wrist motion may demonstrate the 90° out-of-plane flexion-extension of the lunate; lack of this motion may be a subtle indication of a scapholunate or lunotriquetral tear.) The location of the triquetrum can be found by radially and ulnarly deviating the wrist and palpating the dorsal translocation of the triquetrum on the helicoid surface of the triquetro-hamate joint (the triquetral lift test of Sennwald [personal communication]). The triquetrum will be found in line with the ulnar head, approximately 1 cm distal to it. The ballottement test of Reagan and co-authors[30] and the shear test of Kleinman[18] can be useful and should be performed. The plain radiographs are typically normal but are required to rule out other pathology, such as ulnar impaction, and to assess ulnar length.

The clinical diagnosis should be supported (note that we do not say "confirmed") in all patients by a videotaped arthrogram, with passage of contrast material through the lunotriquetral articulation (Fig. 108–1). A positive arthrogram, however, does not unequiv-ocally confirm the diagnosis, since asymptomatic lunotriquetral perforations (attritional lesions) as well as lunotriquetral tears (acute lesions) are not uncommon and may be merely coincidental. Viegas and co-authors dissected 393 wrists and found a 36% incidence of lunotriquetral tears.[43] Cantor and co-authors examined a series of 25 patients with unilateral ulnar-sided wrist pain (suspected lunotriquetral lesion) who underwent bilateral wrist arthrograms.[5] They found that 4 of 7 (59%) of the patients with a lunotriquetral perforation on the symptomatic side also had a similar lesion on the asymptomatic side. This study highlights the fact that the presence of a positive arthrogram is meaningful only if a defect is found in conjunction with tenderness localized to the lunotriquetral joint on physical examination. Before making a final diagnosis, an injection test (approxi-mately 0.25 to 0.5 ml lidocaine, with a steroid compound added, if desired) should be performed. The importance of this test cannot be overemphasized, and should be done before deciding to perform any limited carpal fusion. Patients who do not have significant temporary resolution of pain should have further evaluation. The injection also is useful to demonstrate to the patient the degree of pain relief that might be obtained with surgery. It is unlikely that the patient will achieve greater pain relief with surgery than they achieved with the lidocaine injection, and most patients will have some other pain in their wrists in addition to the lunotriquetral pain. The usefulness of this injection technique has been demonstrated so effectively in our practices that we often use it as soon as the presumptive diagnosis is made, not just as a final step before scheduling a procedure. Multiple injections can be very helpful in evaluating difficult wrist problems. One technique is to start at the joint(s) that is (are) suspected to be a source of pain but are less likely to be the main source of pain, and then progress to the joint suspected to be the most symptomatic.

Patients should initially be treated nonoperatively, with immobilization, nonsteroidal anti-inflammatory medication, steroid injection, or phonophoresis. Surgical treatment should be considered only after failure of conservative treatment, persistence of disabling pain, and a frank discussion of the likely outcomes of the procedure. We advise patients that complete pain relief in all activities is unlikely, that any limited carpal fusion may be the first stage of a complete wrist fusion, and that further surgery may be indicated if pain persists. Also, the long-term (more than 10 years) effect of the fusion is not known, although experience with congenital fusions of the lunotriquetral joint indicate that some optimism may be warranted.[32]

Magnetic resonance imaging (MRI) is not an adequate clinical diagnostic modality, even in most university settings, despite published reports (Yu[47] cites six in his review of MRI of the wrist) to the contrary and is not recommended.

Our experience with patients who have litigation pending, multiple complaints, or changing complaints at each visit would suggest that these factors are relative contraindications to the procedure. Worker's compensation patients present a particular challenge.

General or regional anesthesia can be used according to the surgeons' experience and preference. Bone graft can be obtained from the distal radius or the iliac crest. Our preferred approach is an ulnarly based, dorsal curving incision centered over the lunotriquetral joint (Fig. 108–2). The ulnar placement of the distal incision is particularly necessary to adequately visualize the lunotriquetral joint and place the Herbert screw. Loupe magnification makes avoiding injury to the dorsal branch of the ulnar nerve easier. The extensor retinaculum is opened longitudinally, distal to the ulna, through the fifth extensor compartment. The wrist capsule is opened longitudinally to expose the lunotriquetral joint. Radiographic confirmation that the correct joint has been entered is usually not necessary but should be performed if there is any doubt. The ulnar border of the triquetrum is exposed through a second retinacular and capsular incision at the ulnar side of the sixth extensor compartment for the placement of the Herbert screw. The cartilage and subchondral bone should be removed from the articular surfaces of the lunate and triquetrum with curettes, leaving a small rim of cartilage to help retain the bone graft within the arthrodesis site and to avoid damaging adjacent articular surfaces. Failure to adequately remove cartilage and subchondral bone will increase the incidence of nonunion. Cancellous bone graft obtained from the distal radius[21,36] is usually adequate, although patients older than 40 years may have poor bone stock at this location, and iliac crest graft may be necessary. As the bone graft is placed into the fusion site, care should be taken to keep the carpal bones in approximately their prefused position.

Two smooth K-wires are placed from the ulnar aspect of the triquetrum, across the arthrodesis site, into the lunate. Their position is checked radiographically. We have found the Fluoroscan or mini C-arm to be most helpful. The pin that is more centrally placed across the lunotriquetral joint is replaced with a Herbert screw placed free-hand using appropriate drills and taps. Alternatively, a Herbert-Whipple screw can be placed over the central K-wire wire before it is removed. The second K-wire is left in place, cut off beneath the skin, for 4 to 6 weeks to control potential rotational motion around the Herbert screw. The final position of the fixation device is documented by a plain radiograph.

Bupivacaine infiltration to the area will significantly decrease postoperative pain and pain medication requirements. One of the authors (DLN) adds morphine to the bupivacaine (approximately 5 mg of morphine to 20 to 30 ml of 0.5 or 0.75 mg/ml of bupivacaine),

■ SURGICAL TECHNIQUES

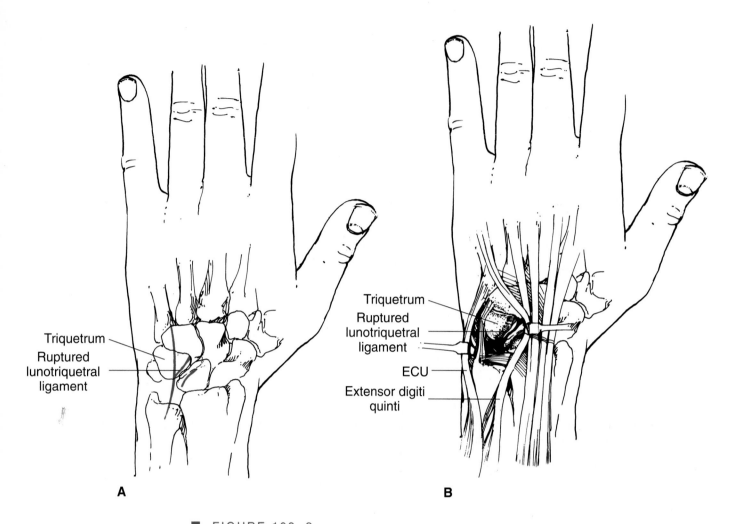

A

Triquetrum
Ruptured
lunotriquetral
ligament

B

Triquetrum
Ruptured
lunotriquetral
ligament
ECU
Extensor digiti
quinti

■ FIGURE 108–2
Surgical procedure. **A,** Preferred skin incision. **B,** Dissection between ECU and EDQ.

which decreases the postoperative pain over that provided by bupivacaine alone. The wrist capsule and extensor retinaculum are closed, followed by a subcuticular closure or simple interrupted skin closure.

A short arm cast should be worn for at least 6 weeks, and immobilization should not be discontinued until there is definite radiographic confirmation of union (Fig. 108–3). In our study,[23] all of our nonunions were initially judged to be "united" on the basis of PA and lateral radiographs of the wrist (Fig. 108–4). Upon review, these standard radiographs in all of our 22 cases, unions and nonunions alike, failed to adequately profile the lunotriquetral arthrodesis site. An unpublished retrospective study of 99 clinical radiographs has documented that PA and lateral radiographs routinely fail to profile the lunotriquetral joint (30% in the series), and rarely profile it as well as is required to assess union. Multiple spot radiographs with the wrist in varying degrees of rotation or tomography of the fusion site are essential to establish the presence of union. If required, fluoroscopic views should be obtained. The surgeon is cautioned not to discontinue immobilization on the basis of inadequate radiographs. The "unions" demonstrated on such films may not be proven false for several months or years, by which time repeat surgery (rather than further immobilization) will be required. If there is doubt about the status of union, some form of immobilization should be continued. The pin can be removed at 4 to 6 weeks.

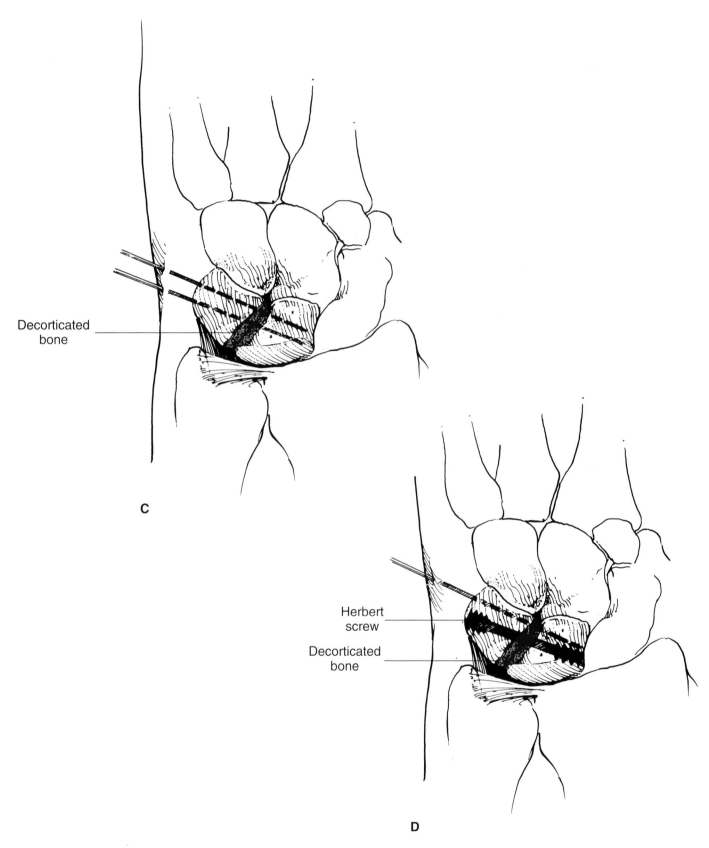

Decorticated
bone

C

Herbert
screw

Decorticated
bone

D

■ FIGURE 108–2
(continued) **C,** Two K-wires placed across the lunotriquetral joint. **D,** Herbert screw across the
lunotriquetral joint.

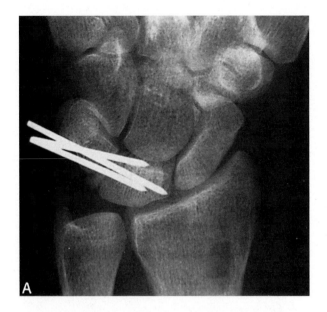
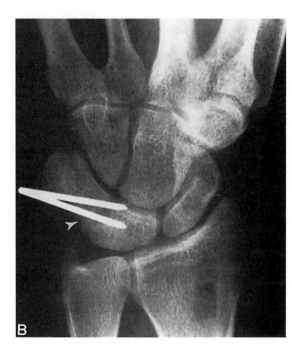
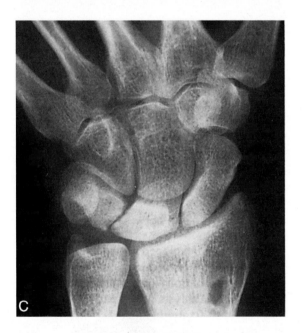

■ FIGURE 108-3

Sample case. **A,** Three K-wires transfix the lunotriquetral joint with graft material in the joint. **B,** One K wire has been removed approximately 2½ months after surgery. There appears to be graft incorporation (arrowhead). **C,** Twenty-two months after surgery, a definite lunotriquetral nonunion is evident.

■ TECHNICAL ALTERNATIVES

Although ligament repairs or reconstructions have been advocated,[1,30,40] there have not been any recent reports of these techniques. Linscheid no longer recommends the tendon interweaving technique but finds that a ligament repair with two sutures into the triquetrum works for small lunotriquetral lesions with adequate remaining lunotriquetral ligament. Larger lesions usually require fusion, and he prefers to use a Herbert screw (personal communication). Our experience with soft tissue procedures at the lunotriquetral joint is limited but not encouraging. Since the outcome of the fusion is fairly predictable and function is so good, fusion is preferred. Although we prefer a lunotriquetral arthrodesis, a fusion of the capitate-lunate-triquetrum-hamate bones may also be considered. Because

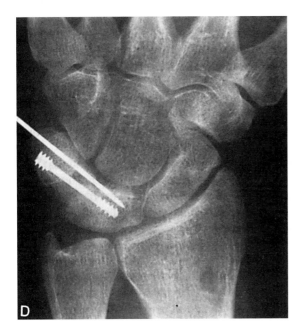 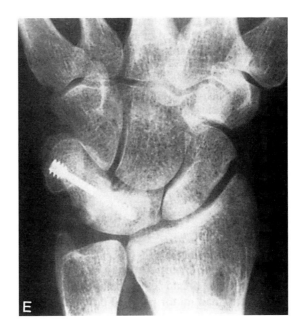

■ FIGURE 108-3

(continued) **D,** Twelve weeks after reoperation; a Herbert screw and K-wire transfix the lunotriquetral joint and the structure of the graft is smoothly blended with spongiosa of the lunate and triquetrum without adjacent lucencies. This appearance is strongly suggestive of solid union. **E,** Four months post second operation, the K-wire has been removed and solid lunotriquetral arthrodesis as evidenced by the bony bridging with medulary continuity.

this reduces the final range of motion by eliminating movement at the midcarpal joint, we use it only when there is associated pain or degenerative changes at the triquetrohamate joint (which is unusual), or as a salvage procedure if the lunotriquetral arthrodesis using the Herbert screw has failed.

Although there are no published papers on the use of ulnar shortening for this problem, the technique is being used with good results by some who have published work on lunotriquetral pathology (Rayhack, Linscheid, personal communications) and by the editor of this volume (Blair, personal communication). The indications for this procedure are an ulnar-positive wrist in association with the lunotriquetral tear. Since the arthrogram does not indicate the size of the lunotriquetral tear, Rayhack suggests examining the lunotriquetral joint at the time of surgery. If the tear is small, he only shortens the ulna, thereby unloading the lunotriquetral joint. If the tear is large, he fuses the lunotriquetral joint in addition to shortening the ulna. Linscheid has had the opportunity to re-arthrogram two patients with small lunotriquetral and TFC tears in combination with an ulnar-plus wrist who had been treated with ulnar shortening only. He found that the lunotriquetral and the TFC perforations had healed. We do not have any experience with ulnar shortening as the sole treatment for lunotriquetral pathology and therefore cannot recommend it, but the experience of other researchers in the field makes it seem promising.

The use of the cast immobilization is somewhat contrary to the concept of a compression screw, and might need further amplification. Shaw[33] demonstrated that the actual compressive forces of the Herbert screw are minimal. The value of the Herbert screw in this application is not due to its compression, but rather its stabilizing effect and its continuing presence. Percutaneous pins become irritated and erythematous at times, and subcutaneous pins become painful. Patients lose their patience with the pins, and at times with the surgeon. The surgeon, in turn, is tempted to remove the pins to keep peace with the patient. The radiograph, meanwhile, is not helpful, but is tantalizingly ambiguous. The value of the long-term presence of a completely intraosseous fixation device now becomes evident.

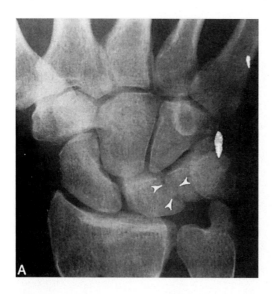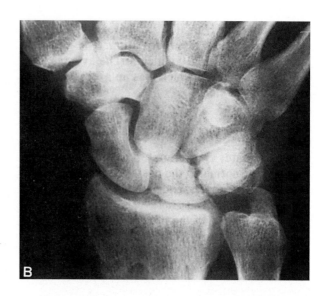

■ FIGURE 108–4

Proper profiling views are required. **A,** PA view of the wrist shows density in the midportion of the lunotriquetral joint suggesting a focal area of arthrodesis (between arrowheads). **B,** PA view of the same wrist the same day, with the lunotriquetral joint properly profiled, demonstrating a nonunion of the lunotriquetral joint.

■ REHABILITATION

Rehabilitation is initiated with preoperative counselling and starts on postoperative day one with finger, elbow, and shoulder range of motion. The cast must not restrict metacarpophalangeal joint motion. Once the cast is removed, we recommend further splint immobilization. The splint can be removed for gentle active, and later active assisted or passive, range of motion. However, initially it serves as a useful reminder to the patient to avoid forceful use of the hand for a further month or so. Four months after surgery the patients in most cases can resume aggressive physical activities or heavy lifting.

It is important to advise patients preoperatively that they will not have full range of motion after the procedure; in fact, full motion may not be desirable, since it may foster degenerative joint disease in adjacent joints. We stress that functional, painless motion is the goal, not full motion.[24,25] The time spent discussing these expected outcomes pays dividends in the long run, and needs to be discussed at the time that the decision is made to proceed with surgery, and should be repeated at each follow-up visit.

■ OUTCOMES

Taleisnik and co-authors[39] reported in 1982 the first case in the English literature of a patient with an lunotriquetral dissociation and a VISI deformity. He noted two prior reports of lunotriquetral injuries in the non-English literature. The outcomes were not reported. The first review of lunotriquetral injuries was a series of seven patients by Reagan and co-authors in 1984.[30] Fusion of the lunotriquetral joint resulted in two good, one fair, and four poor results, with an overall unsatisfactory rate of 72%. No mention was made of the rate of nonunion beyond describing its occurrence as "occasional." Several other authors have reported series suggesting that lunotriquetral fusion produces somewhat discouraging results.[14,17,19,22,34,41] Keck and Hastings[17] reported a series of 42 patients treated with K-wires and cancellous bone graft from the distal radius, with a 48% complication rate and a 29% nonunion rate. Smith and Rayhack[34] reported a series of 22 patients, treated with figure-of-eight compression wire and bone graft from the distal radius, with 2 nonunions and 3 questionable unions at an average follow-up of 5 months. They were disappointed with the ability of the procedure to provide the patients with pain relief. Two patients required re-operation for wire removal. Maitin and co-authors[22] reported 4 nonunions in 18 patients treated with lunotriquetral fusion for a nonunion rate of 22%; 2 of 3 failed to fuse who had Herbert screw fixation. The highest fusion rate reported was by Pin and co-authors,[28] who treated 11 chronic lunotriquetral tears with a 4.0 mm AO cortical screw; bone graft from the distal radius was used only if deemed necessary to maintain external carpal dimensions. There were no nonunions, but 27% had persistent pain. Only standard radiographic views (PA and lateral), which are a poor predictor of nonunions,[23] were used to analyze the fusion site in all of these series, and the true incidence of nonunion is unknown. None of these series analyzed their failures or made suggestions for treatment of these difficult problems. Nelson and co-authors[23] reported the results of 22 patients treated with lunotriquetral arthrodesis and internal fixation by various methods and analyzed the failures. While the overall fusion rate was only 68%, analysis on the basis of fixation showed that a Herbert screw supplemented with a K-wire yielded a 91% union rate and was superior to fixation with K-wires alone (60% union rate). Analysis on the basis of length of immobilization showed that immobilization longer than 6 weeks (86% union rate) was superior to immobilization less than 6 weeks (42% union rate). Importantly, the combined use of a Herbert screw supplemented with a K-wire and immobilization longer than 6 weeks had a 100% union rate, even when performed for nonunion after a prior attempted fusion. Pain was improved in all patients and all patients who previously were working returned to work. The results of this study and the study by Pin and co-authors[28] show that fusion can reliably be achieved, if adequate internal fixation and immobilization are used.

In our series of 22 patients,[23] the operative procedure was extremely successful in terms of range of motion, grip strength, and return to work. Range of motion averaged 107° (51° flexion to 56° extension). Grip strength, at an average 23 months follow-up, was 70% of the uninvolved wrist, with a trend toward further improvement. All but one patient had significant relief of pain compared to their preoperative condition, and all patients who were employed had returned to work. We continue to use this technique in our practices with good results.

References

1. Alexander CE, Lichtman DM: Ulnar carpal instabilities. Orth Clin North Am, 1984; 15: 307–320.
2. Botte MJ, Gelberman RH: Modified technique for Herbert screw insertion in fractures of the scaphoid. J Hand Surg, 1987; 12A:149–150.
3. Bottke CA, Louis DS, Braunstein EM: Diagnosis and treatment of obscure ulnar-sided wrist pain. Orthopedics, 1989; 12:1075–1079.
4. Brown DE, Lichtman DM: The evaluation of chronic wrist pain. Orth Clin North Am, 1984; 15:183–192.
5. Cantor RM, Stern PJ, Wyrick JD, Micheals SE: The relevance of ligament tears or perforations in the diagnosis of wrist pain: An arthrographic study. J Hand Surg, 1994; 19A:945–953.
6. Czitrom AA, Dobyns JH, Linscheid RL: Ulnar variance in carpal instability. J Hand Surg, 1987; 12A:206–208.
7. Dobyns JH, Linscheid RL, Chao EYS, Weber ER, Swanson GE: Traumatic instability of the wrist. In: American Academy of Orthopedic Surgeons, Instructional Course Lectures, Vol 24, St Louis: C. V. Mosby, 1975:182–199.
8. Fisk GF: Carpal instability and the fractured scaphoid. Ann R Coll Surg Engl, 1970; 46:63–76.
9. Frykman EB, Ekenstam FA, Wadin K: Triscaphoid arthrodesis and its complications. J Hand Surg, 1988; 13A:844–849.
10. Gilford WW, Bolton RH, Lambrinudi C: The mechanism of the wrist joint with special reference to fractures of the scaphoid. Guy Hosp Rep, 1943; 92:52–59.
11. Gilula LA: Carpal injuries: Analytic approach and case exercises. Radiology, 1979; 133: 503–517.
12. Goldner JL: Treatment of carpal instability without joint fusion-Current assessment. J Hand Surg, 1982; 7A:325–326.
13. Green DP: Carpal dislocations and instabilities. In: Green DP (ed): Operative Hand Surgery, New York: Churchill Livingstone, 1988:875–938.
14. Gross SC, Watson HK, Strickland JW, Palmer AK, Brenner LH: Triquetral-lunate arthritis secondary to synostosis. J Hand Surg, 1989; 14A:95–102.

15. Herbert TJ, Fisher WE: Management of the fractured scaphoid using a new bone screw. J Bone Joint Surg, 1984; 66B:114–123.
16. Horii E, Garcia-Elias M, An KN, Bishop AT, Cooney WP, Linscheid RL, Chao EYS: A kinematic study of luno-triquetral dissociations. J Hand Surg, 1991; 16A:355–362.
17. Keck CA, Hastings H: Lunotriquetral arthrodesis as treatment for lunotriquetral instability. ASSH Annual Meeting, 1989.
18. Kleinman WB: Am Soc Surg Hand Corr Newsl 1985:51.
19. Linscheid RL, Dobyns JH, Beabout JW, Bryan RS: Traumatic instability of the wrist: Diagnosis, classification, and pathomechanics. J Bone Joint Surg, 1972; 54A:1612–1632.
20. Linscheid RL, Dobyns JH, Beckenbaugh RD, Cooney WP, Wood MB: Instability patterns of the wrist. J Hand Surg, 1983; 8A:682–686.
21. MacCollum MS: Cancellous bone grafts from the distal radius for use in hand surgery. Plast Reconstr Surg, 1975; 55:477–478.
22. Maitin EC, Bora FW, Osterman AL: Lunato-triquetral instability: A cause of chronic wrist pain. J Hand Surg, 1988; 13A:309.
23. Nelson DL, Manske PR, Pruitt DL, Gilula LA, Martin RA: Lunotriquetral Arthrodesis. J Hand Surg, 1993; 18A:1113–1120.
24. Nelson DL, Kahn AS, Manske PR: Functional wrist range of motion in activities of daily living. J Hand Surg (submitted).
25. Nelson DL, Mitchell MA, Groszweski PG, Pennick SL, Manske PR: Wrist range of motion in activities of daily living. J Hand Surg (submitted).
26. Palmer AK, Dobyns JH, Linscheid RL: Management of post-traumatic instability of the wrist secondary to ligament rupture. J Hand Surg, 1978; 3A:507–532.
27. Palmer AK: The distal radioulnar joint. In: Lichtman DL (ed): The wrist and its disorders, Philadelphia: W. B. Saunders Company, 1988:220–231.
28. Pin PG, Young VL, Gilula LA, Weeks PM: Management of chronic lunotriquetral ligament tears. J Hand Surg, 1989; 14A:77–83.
29. Pin PG, Young VL, Gilula LA, Weeks PM: Wrist pain: A systematic approach to diagnosis. Plast Reconstr Surg, 1990; 85:42–46.
30. Reagan DS, Linscheid RL, Dobyns JH: Lunotriquetral sprains. J Hand Surg, 1984; 9A:502–514.
31. Sebald JR, Dobyns JH, Linscheid RL: The natural history of collapse deformities of the wrist. Clin Orthop, 1974; 104:140–148.
32. Sennwald G: The wrist: Anatomical and pathophysiological approach to diagnosis and treatment, Berlin: Springer-Verlag, 1987:206.
33. Shaw JA: A biomechanical comparison of scaphoid screws. J Hand Surg, 1987; 12A:347–353.
34. Smith AA, Rayhack JM: Luno-triquetral compression wire arthrodesis. ASSH Residents' and Fellows' Annual Meeting, 1989.
35. Stark HH, Rickard TA, Zemel NP, Ashworth CR: Treatment of ununited fractures of the scaphoid by iliac bone grafts and Kirschner-wire fixation. J Bone Joint Surg, 1988; 70A: 982–991.
36. Steichen JB, Schreiber DR: Radial bone graft with prolonged immobilization for scaphoid nonunions. Contemp Orthop, 1986;12:19–24.
37. Taleisnik J: Wrist: Anatomy, function, and injury. In: American Academy of Orthopedic Surgeons, Instructional Course Lectures, Vol 27. St Louis: C. V. Mosby, 1978:61–87.
38. Taleisnik J: The Wrist. New York: Churchill Livingstone, 1985: 281-291.
39. Taleisnik J, Malerich M, Prietto M: Palmar carpal instability secondary to dislocation of scaphoid and lunate: Report of case and review of the literature. J Hand Surg, 1982; 7A: 606–612.
40. Taleisnik J: Carpal instability. J Bone Joint Surg, 1988; 70A:1262–1268.
41. Trumble T, Bour CJ, Smith RJ, Edwards GS: Intercarpal arthrodesis for static and dynamic volar intercalated segment instability. J Hand Surg, 1988; 13A:384–390.
42. Trumble T, Bour CJ, Smith RJ, Glisson RR: Kinematics of the ulnar carpus related to the volar intercalated segment instability pattern. J Hand Surg, 1990; 15A:384–92.
43. Viegas SF, Patterson RM, Hokanson JA, Davis J: Wrist anatomy: Incidence, distribution, and correlation of anatomic variations, tears, and arthrosis. J Hand Surg, 1993; 18A:463–475.
44. Watson HK, Goodman ML, Johnson TR: Limited wrist arthrodesis. Part II: Intercarpal and radiocarpal combinations. J Hand Surg, 1981; 6:223–233.
45. Yu JS: MRI techniques and practical applications: MRI of the wrist. Orthopedics, 1994; 17: 1041–1048.

109

Four-Corner Arthrodesis

Over the last 50 years, there have been many articles and textbook chapters outlining the indications and technique for complete wrist arthrodesis.[3,4] This operation remains a very useful procedure for both post-traumatic and rheumatoid arthritis affecting the radiocarpal joint. More recently, limited intercarpal fusions have been performed for certain conditions affecting the wrist joint.[10,13] The obvious advantage of the intercarpal fusion technique is the preservation of some motion at the radiocarpal joint (specifically, the radiolunate joint). The procedure of scaphoid excision and capitate-lunate-triquetrum-hamate (CLTH) fusion has been worked out over the last 15 years, but the indications and various techniques are less widely known and accepted than complete wrist fusion. I did my hand fellowship at New York Orthopaedic Hospital in 1976. Dr. Robert E. Carroll ran a very busy service, and we performed many complete wrist fusions for both post-traumatic and systemic conditions. I did not perform a scaphoid excision and CLTH fusion during my fellowship. In the Division of Hand Surgery at Allegheny General Hospital in Pittsburgh, we now perform as many CLTH fusions as we perform complete wrist fusions. There is no doubt in my mind that the preservation of a painless limited arc of radiocarpal motion (approximately 65 to 70°) is functionally superior to a complete wrist fusion.[1]

H. Kirk Watson[13-15] has greatly contributed to our understanding of the indications and surgical technique for scaphoid excision and CLTH fusion. Through some very fine laboratory studies, others have helped us understand the biomechanical implications of this procedure and the anticipated results.[5,6,8]

The general indication for scaphoid excision and CLTH fusion is scapholunate advanced collapse (SLAC) wrist with degenerative arthritis at the radioscaphoid joint and the lunato capitate joint (Fig. 109–1). The common causes for SLAC wrist are nonunion of the scaphoid and chronic scapholunate dissociation. In both of these disorders, the normal congruous motion between the scaphoid and distal radius is disturbed. With time, the joint incongruity causes cartilage degeneration between the scaphoid and radius. The process may take years, and, remarkably, the radiolunate joint most often does not degenerate (Fig. 109–2) despite the fact that the lunate is often dorsiflexed relative to the radius. As the condition worsens, arthritis spreads distally through the lunatocapitate joint, and range of motion decreases and pain increases. Once there is radiographically apparent arthritis (plane radiographs or tomograms), it is too late to repair the scaphoid nonunion or reconstruct the scapholunate ligament. At this point, scaphoid excision and CLTH fusion is indicated because other procedures that attempt to preserve the scaphoid will fail. The only other choice at this point would be complete wrist fusion. (I do not consider total wrist arthroplasty an option in a patient younger than 60 years of age who must use his or her hand or wrist for any kind of work.) As stated earlier, the arthritic process proceeds from the radioscaphoid joint to the lunato capitate joint in SLAC wrist (Fig. 109–1).

The absolute contraindication for scaphoid excision and CLTH fusion is the presence of arthritis at the radiolunate joint. It is best to evaluate the radiocarpal and intercarpal joints by tomography if there is any doubt about the location or degree of the arthritic process. SLAC wrist, whether caused by scaphoid nonunion or scapholunate dissociation, is the result of trauma. Scaphoid excision and CLTH fusion is not performed in rheumatoid arthritis or other systemic arthritic conditions where progressive arthritis will occur at the radiolunate articulation.

■ HISTORY OF THE TECHNIQUE

■ INDICATIONS AND CONTRAINDICATIONS

■ FIGURE 109–1
Post-traumatic arthritis
with arthritic changes at
the radioscaphoid joint
and lunatocapitate
joint—the typical pattern
seen in SLAC wrist.

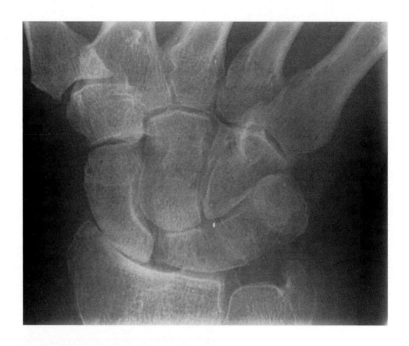

■ FIGURE 109–2
A lateral tomogram show-
ing the dorsiflexed posi-
tion of the lunate, but
preservation of the radiolunate joint.

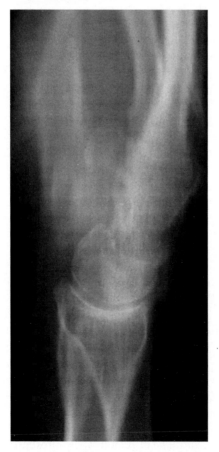

■ SURGICAL
TECHNIQUES

Scaphoid excision and CLTH fusion is performed through a dorsal incision that allows
exposure of the entire radiocarpal and intercarpal joints. The procedure takes between 60
and 90 minutes and can be performed under general or regional anesthesia. I perform
most of these procedures under axillary block using Nesacaine (Astra Pharmaceutical
Products, Westboro, MA). I most frequently use a longitudinal incision that is centered

over the radiocarpal joint for ease of exposure. Extensive subcutaneous dissection should be avoided after making the skin incision. The extensor retinaculum is incised between the third and fourth compartments. The extensor digitorum communis is retracted to the ulnar side. The retinaculum is sharply dissected from Lister's tubercle. The extensor pollicis longus is removed from the third compartment and retracted with the wrist extensors to the radial side. The wrist capsule is now totally exposed. A longitudinal incision is made in the midline of the capsule. The capsule and the extrinsic dorsal radiocarpal ligaments are dissected from the radius and the carpus. This results in two rectangular capsular flaps—one based radially and one based ulnarly. Extensive exposure is needed on the radial side for excision of the scaphoid. After exposure is complete, the scaphoid is removed. The scapholunate ligament is incised completely and the proximal pole grasped with a bone-holding forceps. Dissection is then carried down to and around the distal pole of the scaphoid. The attachments to the transverse carpal ligament and the scaphotrapezial ligaments are very thick, and sharp dissection is required to remove the distal pole. If difficulty is encountered with the exposure of the distal pole of the scaphoid, the scaphoid should be transected at its waist. The distal pole can then be removed with a rongeur. If the radial styloid is elongated because of the arthritic process, a styloidectomy can be performed before scaphoid removal. Radial styloidectomy aids in exposure and allows easy removal of the scaphoid. The excised scaphoid is morselized to be used as bone graft for the CLTH fusion.

After removal of the scaphoid, the cartilage and subchondral bone are removed from the lunatocapitate, the lunatotriquetrum, and the triquetrohamate joints. The bone can be removed with a rongeur in most cases. Occasionally, a high-speed burr is helpful if the subchondral bone is very dense and thick. The rounded surfaces of the proximal capitate and the distal lunate should be shaped so they fit snugly against one another when reduced. At this point, it is imperative that the lunate be placed in a neutral position relative to the radius. The natural tendency is to place the lunate in excessive dorsiflexion relative to the radius. The lunate can still fuse to the capitate in the dorsiflexed position, but postoperative wrist dorsiflexion will be severely limited. Malpositioning of the lunate is the most common technical problem I have seen with this procedure. Once the bones have been shaped and the proper reduction is possible, retrograde placement of the transfixion pins is performed. Two pins are driven through the capitate, one through the hamate, and one through the triquetrum. I use double-ended 0.045" stainless steel K-wires. The wires are pulled out flush to the fusion surfaces. Bone graft is then placed in the fusion site. The bones are reduced at this point, with the surgeon again being very aware of lunate position. Once the fusion site has been reduced, the K-wires are driven proximally across the fusion site and into the lunate and triquetrum (Figs. 109-3 and 109-4). The pins must be driven into the subchondral bone of the lunate proximally to gain adequate purchase. The fusion site should be checked at this point. The surface of the capitate and hamate should be flush with the lunate and triquetrum. Small gaps can be filled with the bone graft. If the scaphoid is an inadequate source of graft, cancellous bone from the distal radius may be used to supplement the graft. Iliac crest bone graft is not normally required for this procedure.

An intraoperative radiograph is taken to ensure proper reduction and pin placement. If the pins are across the radiocarpal joint, they need to be backed out. I cut the pins off below the skin at this point, but this is a personal preference. Many surgeons leave the pins exposed for easy removal in the office. The capsule is closed over the fusion site with absorbable suture once the fusion is adequately fixed. A hemovac drain is placed in the subcutaneous tissue over the capsule and brought out through a separate stab hole proximally. The skin is closed with interrupted nylon sutures. A bulky, well padded hand dressing using Adaptic on the wound with fluffs, ABD pads, and a webril and plaster splint is applied. Most often, we let the tourniquet down after the dressing is applied.

When the surgeon is confronted with the difficult problem of SLAC wrist, there are alternatives to simple scaphoid excision and CLTH fusion. Early in the development of SLAC wrist, the proximal capitate may not be degenerate, and the arthritis then is confined

■ TECHNICAL ALTERNATIVES

■ FIGURE 109–3
(A) The surfaces to be fused have been decorticated, and the pins are in position to be driven proximally. The scaphoid has been excised. C, capitate; H, hamate; T, triquetrum; L, lunate; R, radius; U, ulna; 1–4, K-wires. **(B)** The pins have been driven into place across the fusion sites. 1–4, K-wires.

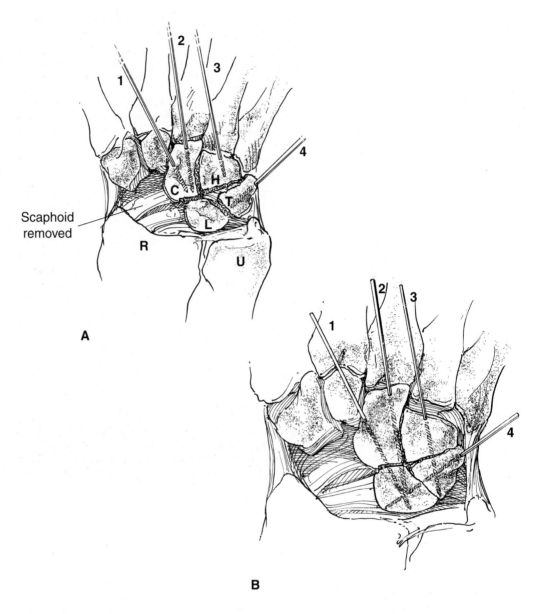

to the radioscaphoid articulation. At this stage, proximal row carpectomy (PRC) can be performed with the anticipation of good pain relief and a range of motion similar to that provided by scaphoid excision and fusion, but probably with less endurance.[2,7] The choice between PRC and CLTH fusion in this situation must be made by the individual surgeon based on the literature and his or her personal experience.[7] Some recommend fusion in all situations, whereas others see a place for PRC when the lunatocapitate and radiolunate joints are preserved. Once the capitate has degenerated, PRC is no longer a reasonable option. Some surgeons might recommend complete wrist fusion for the reliability of pain relief in severe SLAC wrist. Obviously, this sacrifices all wrist range of motion and certainly is not as functional as a pain-free CLTH fusion. After excising the scaphoid and performing a CLTH fusion, silicone implants have been used as spacers for the scaphoid. I have never routinely used silicone scaphoids, and at this point I believe they are contraindicated because of the possibility of particulate synovitis, and because they add very little to the final functional result.[11]

The success of scaphoid excision and CLTH fusion depends on obtaining a solid fusion with the lunate in proper position (neutral). It is imperative that the raw bone surface of the capitate coapts the raw bone surface of the lunate and that these surfaces are securely

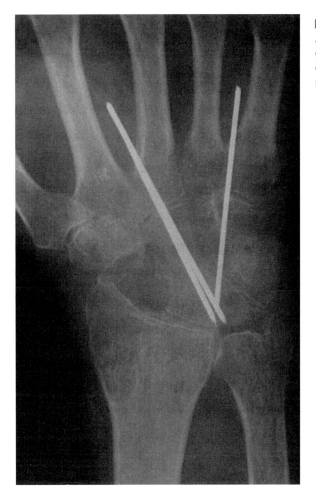

■ FIGURE 109–4
A posteroanterior radiograph showing scaphoid excision and pin placement.

internally fixed. Pin fixation can be supplemented with staples if the surgeon wishes. I find no advantage in using staples instead of pins.

Cast immobilization is necessary after this procedure for approximately 8 weeks. As the swelling decreases, occasionally a buried pin will irritate the skin, requiring removal. I have not had a problem with deep infection secondary to pin tract problems, although this is certainly a possibility, particularly if the pins protrude from the skin. Once radiographic healing has occurred, the pins can be removed under local anesthesia. At this point, range of motion and strengthening exercises are started. The patient sees a therapist approximately once a week for 6 weeks, and is given a home exercise program. Most of the patients are quite stiff after immobilization, and it takes 9 to 12 months to regain the desired flexion, extension, and strength. As long as the fusion has healed, this period of rehabilitation is not particularly painful, and patients quickly return to activities of daily living.

■ REHABILITATION

There are two objective parameters by which the success or failure of this procedure can be judged: the achievement of a solid fusion and the degree of long-term active range of motion. A solid fusion should eliminate most of the pain, and the long-term range of motion provided by the preserved radiocarpal joint should be adequate for most activities of daily living and even most work activities (Fig. 109–5). In most reported clinical series, CLTH fusions are combined with other intercarpal fusions, making it difficult to extract meaningful data. When two series of Watson's[13,14] and a series of Smith's[12] are combined,

■ OUTCOMES

■ FIGURE 109–5
An intercarpal fusion 1
year after surgery. This
patient had a total flex-
ion–extension arc of mo-
tion of 70°.

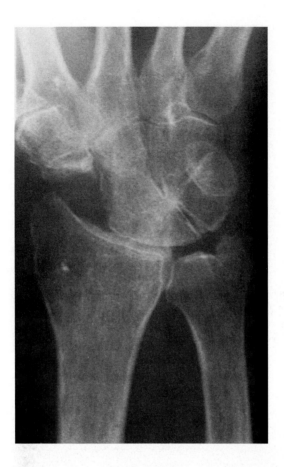

there were 4 nonunions in 41 patients (10%) who had a CLTH fusion with scaphoid excision. Three of these nonunions were successfully salvaged by repeat bone grafting. In other small series, the nonunion rate also appears to be about 10%. Most patients with nonunions will have persistent pain.

A number of laboratory studies have been performed to determine the effect of various intercarpal fusions on wrist motion. Meyerdierks et al[8] concluded that 67% of the flexion–extension arc and 76% of the ulnar deviation–radial deviation arc should be preserved after fusion of the proximal to the distal carpal row. This study was performed by simulating fusions in cadaver specimens. Likewise, Douglas et al[5] found that 64% of the flexion–extension arc and 71% of the ulnar–radial deviation arc remained after simulated intercarpal fusion between the proximal and distal rows. Assuming that the total arc of active wrist motion is 133°,[9] the theoretical range of motion remaining after fusion of the proximal to the distal row should be almost 90°.

In the clinical setting, scaphoid excision and CLTH fusion does not result in a 90° arc of flexion–extension. In combined clinical series, the flexion–extension arc of patients undergoing this operation is approximately 70°.[12,13] Postoperative radial deviation averaged 12°, and ulnar deviation 26°. This range of motion is certainly adequate for routine activities and most jobs, as determined by Brumfield and Shampoux.[1] If we compare these numbers to Palmer and colleagues'[9] determination that the average wrist moves actively through an arc of 130°, then we see that given the proper technique and adequate postoperative rehabilitation, the surgeon can expect approximately 50% of the normal flexion–extension arc of wrist motion. Before surgery, I explain to my patients that, if successful, this procedure will afford good pain relief, will allow approximately 50% of normal wrist motion, and will allow them to do most jobs without pain. They may be somewhat limited in more vigorous activities, including sports requiring extremes of wrist motion. Once the fusion has healed and the initial postoperative stiffness has abated, most patients are happy with the procedure. There is no evidence at this time of an increased incidence of degenerative changes at the radiocarpal joint.

References

1. Brumfield RH, Shampoux JA: A Biomechanical study of normal functional wrist motion. Clin Orthop, 1984; 187:23–25.
2. Buterbaugh GA, Imbriglia JE, Hagberg WC: The surgical management of SLAC wrist: Proximal row carpectomy vs. scaphoid excision with four-bone fusion. (In press).
3. Campbell CJ, Keokarn T: Total and subtotal arthrodesis of the wrist. J Bone Joint Surg, 1964; 46A:1520–1533.
4. Dick HM: Wrist and intercarpal arthrodesis. In: Green DP (ed): Operative Hand Surgery. New York: Churchill-Livingstone, 1982:127–139.
5. Douglas DP, Pimer CA, Koniuch MP: Motion of the wrist after simulated limited intercarpal arthrodesis. J Bone Joint Surg, 1987; 69A:1413–1418.
6. Gellman J, Kauffman D, Lenihan M, Botte M, Sarmiento A: An in-vitro analysis of wrist motion: The effect of limited intercarpal arthrodesis in the contributions of the radiocarpal and midcarpal joints. J Hand Surg, 1988; 13A:378–382.
7. Imbriglia J, Broudy A, Hagberg W, McKeirnan D: Proximal row carpectomy: A clinical evaluation. J Hand Surg, 1990; 15A:426–430.
8. Meyerdierks EM, Mosher JP, Werner FW: Limited wrist arthrodesis: A laboratory study. J Hand Surg, 1987; 12A:526–529.
9. Palmer AK, Werner FW, Murphy B, Glisson R: Functional wrist motion: A biomechanical study. J Hand Surg, 1985; 10A:39–46.
10. Peterson HA, Lipscond PR: Intercarpal arthrodesis. Arch Surg, 1967; 95:127–134.
11. Smith RH, Atkinson RE, Jupiter JB: Silicone synovitis of the wrist. J Hand Surg, 1985; 10A: 47–60.
12. Trumble T, Bour CJ, Smith RJ, Edwards F: Intercarpal arthrodesis for static and dynamic volar intercalated segment instability. J Hand Surg, 1988; 13A:384–390.
13. Watson HK: Limited wrist arthrodesis. Clin Orthop, 1980; 149:126–136.
14. Watson HK, Goodman ML, Johnson TR: Limited wrist arthrodesis: Part 2. Intercarpal and radiocarpal combinations. J Hand Surg, 1981; 6:223–233.
15. Watson HK, Ballet FL: SLAC wrist: Scapholunate advanced collapse pattern of degenerative arthritis. J Hand Surg, 1984; 9A:358–365.

JEFFREY J. TIEDEMAN

110

Radioscaphoid Arthrodesis

■ HISTORY OF THE
TECHNIQUE

Degenerative arthritis of the wrist usually develops in specific sequential patterns.[12,13] The first area of involvement typically is the radioscaphoid joint. Despite this prevalence, there are few reports in the literature of isolated radioscaphoid arthrodesis. The procedure was first described in a series of 13 patients by Schwartz in 1967.[10] Cambell and Keokarn used an inlay bone graft to achieve subtotal wrist arthrodesis while preserving unaffected joints.[3] The concept of limited wrist arthrodesis did not gain in popularity, however, until the report by Watson et al in 1981.[11] Of the 28 arthrodeses performed in that study, only 3 were confined to the radioscaphoid joint. It is evident that radioscaphoid arthrodesis is an uncommon operation with narrow indications.

The primary advantage of limited carpal arthrodesis is the preservation of some wrist motion.[7,9] Although a complete wrist fusion usually provides predictable pain relief, the resultant restriction of motion is considered unacceptable by many patients. In addition, the wrist can be a difficult joint to fuse and the operation is associated with a high rate of complications, including pseudarthrosis, infection, neuroma, and fracture.[4] Radioscaphoid arthrodesis is technically less demanding and may be an alternative to total wrist fusion in certain patients. Another potential advantage of radioscaphoid arthrodesis is the opportunity to convert a limited carpal arthrodesis to a total wrist arthrodesis if the first operation fails to provide adequate clinical response.

■ INDICATIONS AND
CONTRAINDICATIONS

The primary indication for radioscaphoid arthrodesis is degenerative or post-traumatic arthritis limited to that joint in a patient with wrist pain refractory to conservative management (Fig. 110–1). This procedure has also been used to stabilize a flail wrist in radial nerve palsy and to correct wrist deformity associated with cerebral palsy.[10] Contraindications to this operation include arthritis in other articulations in the wrist. Specifically, these would include the scaphocapitate, capitolunate, or radiolunate joints. Also, widening of the scapholunate interval secondary to attenuation or rupture of the scapholunate interosseous ligament is a contraindication.

■ SURGICAL
TECHNIQUES

The operation is preferably performed under a general anesthetic. A pneumatic tourniquet is placed on the upper arm over abundant soft roll padding. The tourniquet is inflated after exsanguinating the limb with an elastic bandage. A 6- to 8-cm longitudinal skin incision is made on the dorsum of the wrist, centered over Lister's tubercle. Dissection is performed down to the extensor retinaculum, and medial and lateral subcutaneous flaps are developed and held retracted with retention sutures of 4-0 nylon. Meticulous hemostasis is required to prevent postoperative hematoma formation. Abundant dorsal veins present in this region are either protected, cauterized, or ligated, based on their position and caliber. The third dorsal compartment is identified just ulnar to Lister's tubercle. The retinaculum overlying this compartment is longitudinally divided, exposing the extensor pollicis longus (EPL) tendon. The EPL is then retracted radially with a vessel loop. Access to the radiocarpal joint is gained through the base of the third compartment. While preserving the dorsal wrist capsule, the fourth dorsal compartment is subperiosteally elevated from the distal radius and retracted. Similarly, subperiosteal dissection is also performed radially under the second compartment. With the dorsal capsule exposed, an "H"-shaped capsular incision is made with the transverse limbs of the incision centered over the radiocarpal and midcarpal joints (Fig. 110–2). The capsular flaps are subperiosteally elevated from the underlying carpus and held retracted with retention sutures. The articular sur-

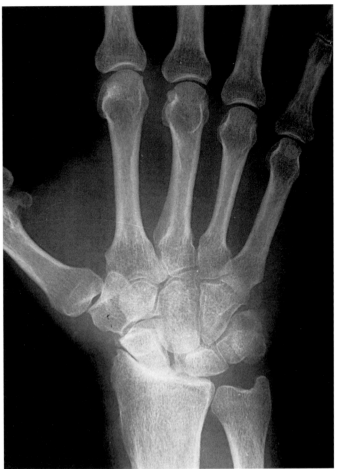

■ FIGURE 110–1
Posteroanterior radio-
graph of the wrist show-
ing severe degenerative
arthritis confined to the
radioscaphoid joint.

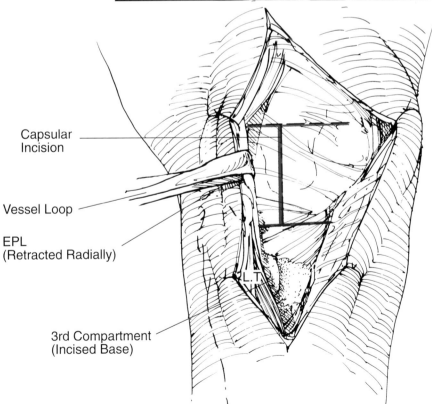

■ FIGURE 110–2
"H"-shaped dorsal capsu-
lar incision used to ex-
pose the radiocarpal and
midcarpal joints. EPL, extensor pollicis longus; LT,
Lister's tubercle.

Capsular
Incision

Vessel Loop

EPL
(Retracted Radially)

L.T.

3rd Compartment
(Incised Base)

■ FIGURE 110–3
Exposure of the capitate, scaphoid, lunate, and distal radius articular surfaces after capsular subperiosteal elevation. C, capitate; H, hamate; L, lunate.

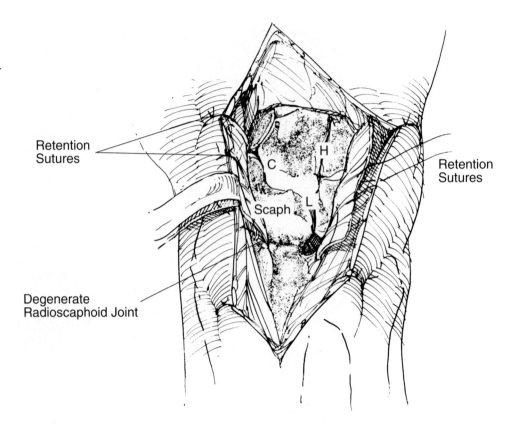

Retention Sutures

Retention Sutures

Scaph

Degenerate Radioscaphoid Joint

faces of the scaphoid, lunate, capitate, and distal radius are closely inspected (Fig. 110–3). A radioscaphoid arthrodesis is completed only if degenerative changes are confined to that joint. If degenerative changes are evident in the radiolunate joint or proximal capitate, alternative surgical techniques are indicated. Once arthritic involvement of only the radioscaphoid joint has been confirmed, all remaining articular cartilage on the proximal scaphoid and the scaphoid fossa of the radius is removed with a curette. Care is taken to avoid the articular surfaces of the lunate and radial lunate fossa. To prepare the bone surfaces adequately, debridement should be continued until subchondral cancellous bone is evident. This may be difficult if areas of dense, sclerotic, eburnated bone are present. Repetitively drilling these regions with a small, 0.028″ K-wire to promote vascular ingrowth may be helpful. The scaphoid is then then held in a reduced position. A temporary 0.062″ K-wire can be placed into the dorsum of the scaphoid to aid this manipulative reduction. Good bony contact between the scaphoid and radius is achieved through digital pressure on the dorsal K-wire. When properly reduced, the scaphoid should be aligned so that its proximal articular surface is concentric with the scaphoid fossa of the radius. The radioscaphoid joint is percutaneously pinned, preferably with three 0.062″ K-wires directed through the radial styloid into the scaphoid (Figs. 110-4 and 110-5). The pins should not penetrate beyond the confines of the scaphoid. Typically, this can be ascertained through direct inspection of the midcarpal joint. The arthrodesis site is augmented with corticocancellous bone graft obtained either from the ipsilateral distal radius or from an iliac crest. If radial bone graft is used, the distal metaphysis between the second and third dorsal compartments is the preferred harvest site. The bone graft is firmly packed into any remaining areas of bone deficit in the radioscaphoid joint.

Closure is initiated first by reapproximating the capsular flaps with multiple 3-0 absorbable sutures placed in a figure-of-eight fashion. The EPL tendon is returned to its normal anatomic location and the extensor retinaculum is closed with 3-0 absorbable suture in an interrupted or running fashion. Skin closure is accomplished with a combination of several evenly spaced horizontal mattress stitches and then a running stitch of 5-0 nylon. The K-wires are bent over and cut superficial to the level of the skin. The wound edges

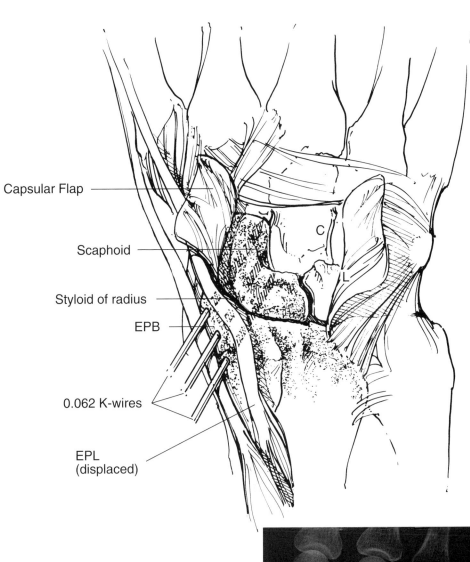

Capsular Flap

Scaphoid

Styloid of radius

EPB

0.062 K-wires

EPL
(displaced)

C

L

FIGURE 110–4
Stabilization of the radioscaphoid joint with three 0.062″ K-wires, directed through the styloid into the scaphoid. C, capitate; L, lunate; EPB, extensor pollicis brevis; EPL, extensor pollicis longus.

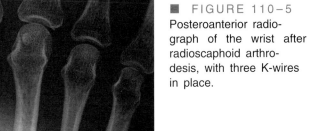

FIGURE 110–5
Posteroanterior radiograph of the wrist after radioscaphoid arthrodesis, with three K-wires in place.

are infiltrated with several milliliters of 0.5% bupivacaine without epinephrine for postoperative pain relief. A sterile dressing is applied, followed by volar and dorsal splints to keep the wrist immobilized in a neutral position. Sutures are removed in the clinic in 10 to 14 days, and a short-arm thumb spica cast is placed with a window over the pins to facilitate pin care and alleviate pressure from the cast on the pins.

■ TECHNICAL ALTERNATIVES

There are several technical alternatives to the described technique. The approach to the radioscaphoid joint could also be accomplished through the fourth dorsal compartment rather than the third. The advantages of the approach through the third compartment, however, include closer proximity to the radioscaphoid joint and the avoidance of direct manipulation of the common extensor tendons. This technique appears to facilitate postoperative rehabilitation and diminish the risk of postoperative tendon adhesion.

There are also different alternatives available to stabilize the radioscaphoid joint after the bone surfaces have been adequately prepared. Although using K-wires is technically simple, there are occasional problems associated with their use. These problems include pin tract infection, migration, breakage, or loosening with loss of fixation. Another option is to stabilize the joint with one or two screws, such as AO cancellous bone screws or Herbert screws. If properly countersunk, these screws seldom require removal. Wider dissection or an additional incision near the radial styloid is required to place these screws, however. Alternatively, some authors have achieved a satisfactory fusion without the use of hardware, by drilling a cylindrical cavity in the region of the radioscaphoid joint and packing the cavity with autogenous bone graft.[10]

There are also several procedural alternatives to the described technique of radioscaphoid arthrodesis. The operative indications for these procedures usually are different, however, precluding any fair comparison. Bach et al have reported that a proximal row fusion (radioscapholunate arthrodesis) has a high probability of providing good functional results.[1] Several patients in their series had degenerative changes in the radiolunate joint secondary to Kienböck disease, thus necessitating inclusion of that joint in the fusion. Some authors would prefer a proximal row carpectomy under those circumstances, provided the proximal capitate and radial lunate fossa are free of degenerative changes.[5] Alternatively, if there are degenerative changes in the proximal capitate and radioscaphoid joint, but the radiolunate joint is spared, then scaphoid excision and "four-corner fusion" would be an appropriate choice.[12] For pancarpal arthritis, a total wrist arthrodesis may be the only option. Last, if degenerative changes are confined to the distal pole of the scaphoid and radial styloid region, no fusion at all may be necessary and the patient might be best treated with a limited radial styloidectomy, taking care to preserve the volar carpal ligaments. Ultimately, the radiocarpal and midcarpal joints should be closely inspected at the time of surgery, and the appropriate procedure performed based on those findings.

Pitfalls associated with radioscaphoid arthrodesis are common to all limited radiocarpal and intercarpal arthrodeses. Possible complications include nonunion or malunion of the arthrodesis site, and pin tract-related problems such as infection or migration. The risk of nonunion is minimized by adequate preparation of the bone surfaces and complete packing of the fusion site with a sufficient quantity of bone graft. Immobilization should be continued until solid radiographic union is evident. If a nonunion does develop, some authors have achieved a successful outcome through reoperation and bone grafting.[1,12] Malunion of the fusion could further limit the resultant wrist motion. This is avoided by ensuring concentric reduction of the scaphoid in the scaphoid fossa of the radius. Over-reduction of the scaphoid, so that the bone is too horizontal, reduces the scapholunate angle and results in diminished radial deviation. Over-reduction can be prevented by obtaining preoperative, true lateral comparative radiographs. Intraoperative spot films can then be used to confirm pin placement and scaphoid orientation. Last, meticulous daily pin care can usually prevent subsequent pin-related problems. If a pin tract infection occurs, most are superficial and respond to a short course of oral antibiotics. A lack of clinical response or involvement of deeper structures requires a more aggressive approach, with formal debridement and possible pin removal.

Cast immobilization generally is continued for 8 postoperative weeks. At that point the pins are removed in the clinic. Hand therapy is then initiated. A volar orthoplast splint is fabricated and worn full-time, except for exercises, for an additional month. Exercises consist of gentle active range of motion three times a day. If adequate bony union is evident (Fig. 110–6), the patient is then weaned from the splint and released to normal activities, typically around 4 months after surgery.

■ REHABILITATION

There are few reports in the literature concerning radioscaphoid arthrodesis. Consequently, little data exist regarding expected surgical outcome. Schwartz achieved good results in 12 of 13 patients in his series, which included 5 patients with post-traumatic arthritis.[10] Of the three patients in Watson's series who were treated with radioscaphoid fusions, two went on to nonunion. One was successfully regrafted and the other subsequently underwent silicone scaphoid replacement. The two patients with solid fusions were pleased with their results and subjectively had less pain.[11] In our experience, radioscaphoid arthrodesis has been a successful and predictable operation with high patient satisfaction.

■ OUTCOMES

Radioscaphoid arthrodesis does restrict wrist motion, however. In fact, Meyerdierks et al found experimentally in a cadaveric study that fusions that cross the radiocarpal row lost 55% of wrist flexion and extension, and 45% of ulnar and radial deviation.[6] Their study, however, did not take into account the associated soft tissue involvement that occurs with wrist arthritis, so the percentage of motion lost with radioscaphoid fusion may be greater in the clinical setting. Reported rates of wrist motion after radioscaphoid arthrodesis have varied from a total arc of 28 to 52° (average 35°) of flexion and extension, and 20 to 40° (average 25°) of radial and ulnar deviation. This is consistent with our

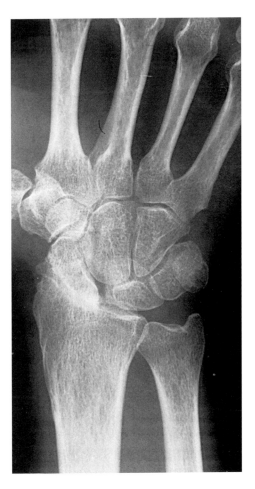

■ FIGURE 110–6
Posteroanterior radiograph 6 months after radioscaphoid arthrodesis, with solid bony union evident.

clinical experience. This restricted motion that results after radioscaphoid arthrodesis is not necessarily functionally detrimental. Several studies have shown that the optimum range for functional motion of the wrist to accomplish most activities is 10° of flexion, 30° of extension, 10° of radial deviation, and 15° of ulnar deviation.[2,8] An attempt should be made, therefore, to fuse the radioscaphoid joint in a position that will keep its retained motion in the functional range.[8] In conclusion, radioscaphoid arthrodesis is a technically straightforward operation ideal for patients with arthritis limited to that joint and pain refractory to conservative management. Although wrist motion is significantly restricted after this operation, the motion retained typically allows the patient to remain quite functional.

References

1. Bach AW, Almquist EE, Newman DM: Proximal row fusion as a solution for radiocarpal arthritis. J Hand Surg, 1991; 16:424–431.
2. Brumfield RH, Campoux JA: A biomechanical study of normal functional wrist motion. Clin Orthop, 1984; 187:23–25.
3. Cambell CJ, Keokarn T: Total and subtotal arthrodesis of the wrist. Inlay technique. J Bone Joint Surg, 1964; 46A:1520–1533.
4. Clendenin MB, Green DP: Arthrodesis of the wrist. J Hand Surg, 1981; 6A:253–257.
5. Imbriglia JE, Broudy AS, Hagberg WC, McKernan D: Proximal row carpectomy: Clinical evaluation. J Hand Surg, 1990; 15A:426–430.
6. Meyerdierks EM, Mosher JF, Werner FW: Limited wrist arthrodesis: A laboratory study. J Hand Surg, 1987; 12A:526–529.
7. Minami A, Ogino T, Minami M: Limited wrist fusion. J Hand Surg, 1988; 13A:660–667.
8. Palmer AK, Werner FW, Murphy D, Glisson R: Functional wrist motion: A biomechanical study. J Hand Surg, 1985; 10A:39–46.
9. Rozing PM, Kauer JMG: Partial arthrodesis of the wrist. Acta Orthop Scand, 1984; 55:66–68.
10. Schwartz S: Localized fusion at the wrist joint. J Bone Joint Surg, 1967; 49A:1591–1596.
11. Watson HK, Goodman ML, Johnson TR: Limited wrist arthrodesis: Part II. Intercarpal and radiocarpal combinations. J Hand Surg, 1981; 6A:223–233.
12. Watson HK, Ballet FL: The SLAC wrist: Scapholunate advanced collapse pattern of degenerative arthritis. J Hand Surg, 1984; 9A:358–365.
13. Watson HK, Ryu J: Evolution of arthritis of the wrist. Clin Orthop, 1986; 202:57–67.

111

Radiolunate Arthrodesis

The goal of partial arthrodesis of the wrist is to retain the maximum amount of mobility compatible with a painless, strong, and stable wrist. Several investigators have attempted to determine the potential loss of motion resulting from limited carpal arthrodeses through internal fixation of groups of different carpal bones performed in cadaver specimens.[1,9,10,19,24,25] These studies have little clinical significance, because the location and extent of an arthrodesis should be based on pathologic findings, and be designed to maximize residual mobility within a functional, pain-free range, regardless of the theoretical advantage of one type of partial arthrodesis over another. Furthermore, there are "in vivo" examples of the effects of surgically performed arthrodeses, because these procedures mimic congenital synostosis, or spontaneously occurring fusions, seen for example in rheumatoid arthritis, where the residual range of motion is entirely compatible with excellent function.

In general, partial arthrodeses were initially performed for isolated degenerative or post-traumatic changes, or instability.[2–4,8,11,12,13,14,15,17,18,21,27,30,32–34] Radiolunate fusions were also first proposed for degenerative changes, usually postfracture, occurring strictly between the lunate facet of the distal radius and the lunate.[34] Spontaneous radiolunate fusions in wrists with rheumatoid arthritis provided a naturally occurring model for the application of this technique to other carpal and radiocarpal problems.[5,6,28]

■ HISTORY OF THE TECHNIQUE

The disorders that are effectively treated by radiolunate arthrodesis fall into three general categories.

Post-traumatic degenerative changes limited to the radiolunate joint are seen after unreduced or malunited die-punch fractures of the distal radius.

The use of radiolunate fusions for the treatment of ulnar translation in wrists with rheumatoid arthritis was prompted by the observation that such wrists, after spontaneous radiolunate fusions, remain aligned, stable, pain-free, and functional.[5,6,28] The use of this procedure in nonrheumatoid wrists, and for carpal instabilities other than ulnar translations, has been exceptional.[17,22] Indeed, for traumatic ulnar translations, soft tissue repairs have been used in preference to partial fusions.[20,22] Stabilization of the lunate to the radius through a localized arthrodesis for these nonrheumatoid patients, however, would seem to be a logical extension of the excellent experience with rheumatoid wrists (Fig. 111–1).

Radiolunate arthrodeses may also be used for other forms of carpal instability in which the lunate, as the carpal keystone, is out of alignment and tilting into dynamic or static forms of volar intercalated segmental instability (VISI) or dorsal intercalated segmental instability (DISI). The same rationale behind the use of radiolunate fusions to stabilize the laterally displaced carpus seen in ulnar translation may thus be applied to correct the abnormal dorsopalmar displacement seen in these other forms of carpal instability. A more normal radiocarpal relationship is restored through stabilization of the lunate, the carpal keystone, to the radius, in neutral alignment (Fig. 111–2).[7] In my experience, the loss of motion after radiolunate arthrodesis is less than anticipated based on cadaver studies (Fig. 111–1C, D).

Other than for insufficient bone stock, as may be encountered in wrists with rheumatoid arthritis, the only potential contraindications are degenerative changes between scaphoid and radius, in which case extension of the fusion to include the scaphoid is preferable, and scapholunate dissociation coexisting with static VISI or DISI deformities, a more complex type of dissociative carpal instability. In these wrists, the unstable scaphoid rotates

■ INDICATIONS AND CONTRAINDICATIONS

■ FIGURE 111–1
Traumatic ulnar transla-
tion. **(A)** Initial posteroanterior radiograph shows
ulnar displacement of the
entire carpus. **(B)** Appearance after reduction and
radiolunate arthrodesis.

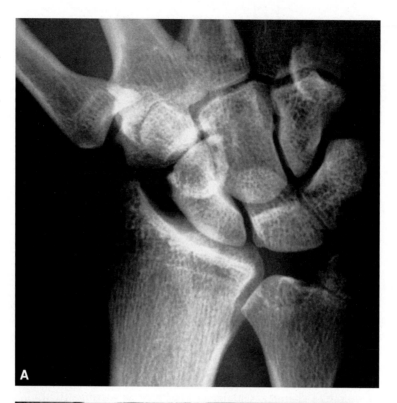

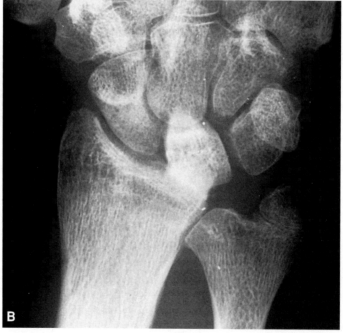

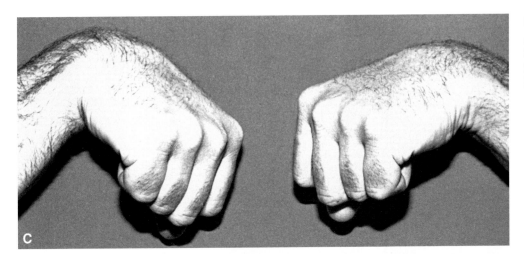

(continued) **(C)** Range of flexion (involved wrist is to the reader's right). **(D)** Range of extension.

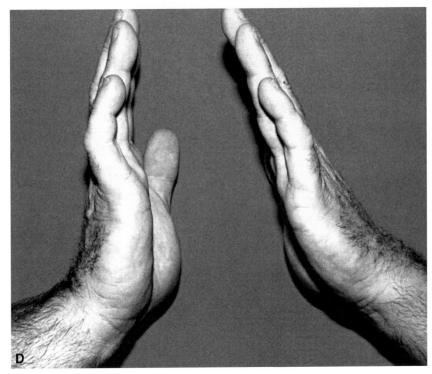

into palmar flexion, allowing the capitate to drift radial to the fixed lunate, into the scapholunate gap. This has not been a problem in patients with ulnar translation, both rheumatoid and post-traumatic, who may also present with widening of the scapholunate space (ulnar translation type II).[29] In these wrists, the scaphoid remains stable, and is joined by the lunate in restoring a glenoid cavity for the head of the capitate, after the lunate is reduced and fused to the radius.

This procedure is performed under general or regional anesthesia. The radiocarpal joint is approached using a dorsal, longitudinal incision, placed immediately ulnar to the palpable prominence of Lister's tubercle. The incision extends from the projection of the head of the capitate distally, in a proximal and slightly ulnar direction, for an average of 8 cm. Both skin flaps are elevated from the dorsal retinaculum, and carry with them the cutaneous branches of the radial and ulnar nerves. The radiocarpal joint is exposed through the fourth dorsal wrist compartment because this allows a more direct approach to the radiolunate joint, particularly when the carpus has translated ulnarly. Routinely, the dorsal

■ SURGICAL TECHNIQUES

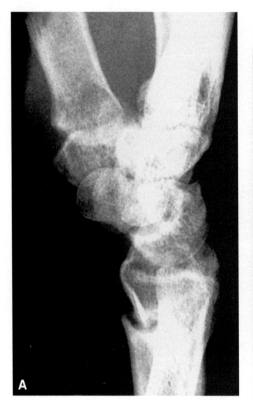

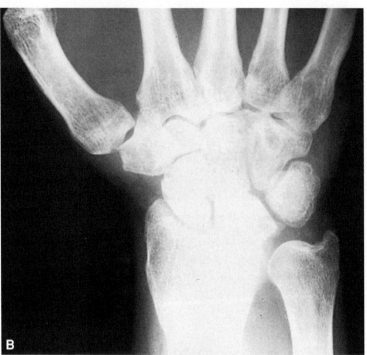

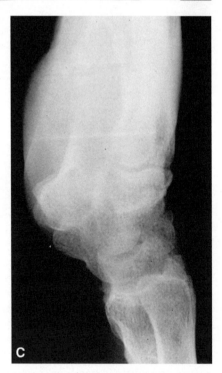

■ FIGURE 111-2

Traumatic static VISI deformity. **(A)** Initial lateral radiograph shows a minimally displaced fracture of the distal radius and a static VISI deformity. **(B)** Appearance after reduction and radiolunate arthrodesis. The fracture of the radius is well healed. **(C)** Postoperative lateral projection demonstrates a satisfactory radiolunocapitate alignment.

interosseous neurovascular bundle is coagulated and divided. It is found just proximal to the distal radioulnar joint, lying on the interosseous membrane deep to the extensor tendons about to enter the fourth dorsal wrist compartment. The dorsal retinaculum is divided and the extensor tendons are retracted to expose the retrotendinous layer, which is incised transversely, together with the radiocarpal capsule. Proximally, a narrow capsular remnant is left attached to the dorsal rim of the radius, for later repair.

The articular surfaces of the radius and lunate are identified and are excised until healthy cancellous bone is exposed (Fig. 111–3A). Next, the distal radius is exposed subperiosteally, between the tendons of the extensors carpi radialis brevis and longus. A cortical window is elevated at the level of the base of the radial styloid to obtain a sufficient amount of cancellous bone, preferably as a large single block (Fig. 111–3B). Two parallel Kirschner wires proportionate in size to the dimensions of the wrist and the lunate (usually 0.045 to 0.062") are then inserted obliquely, eventually to engage the lunate and the lunate facet of the radius. This may be done distally to proximally along the triquetrum and lunate (Fig. 111–3C), or proximally to distally through the radius. In either case, the wires are advanced until their tips are visible at the level of the the fusion surfaces of radius or lunate. If at all possible, avoid traversing the midcarpal joint. Because of the area of weakness created in the distal radius by removing the bone graft, the Kirschner wires should pass through the radial cortices that are preserved, usually proximal to the graft donor site. As for all types of limited arthrodesis, compression of the surfaces to be fused is avoided, because the outside dimension and shape of the fused radiolunate unit must remain unchanged from normal, so as not to interfere with the function of neighboring joints.[33,34] This is particularly important here because the normal width of the joint space between radius and scaphoid must also remain unchanged for this remaining segment of the radiocarpal joint to continue to function unimpeded. The lunate alignment is carefully determined, to correct ulnar translation, or abnormal rotation into VISI or DISI. It is advantageous at this point to advance the most peripheral of the Kirschner wires across the radiolunate space to secure the alignment of the lunate.

When inserting the bone graft, bone chips may be inadvertently spilled between radius and scaphoid, or radius and ulnar head. To avoid this, a small, narrow osteotome is placed with the flat of the blade closing off the ulnar side of the radiolunate cavity. Next to this, a large cancellous bone piece cut out of the single cancellous bone block previously obtained is packed against the osteotome. Additional bone chips are inserted from laterally against the medial single bony block (Fig. 111–3D). Another single cancellous piece is finally used to wall off the radioscaphoid space from the fusion. A cortical graft may be slotted to cover the dorsal radiolunate area for further support. The remaining Kirschner wire is then advanced. Closure is performed in layers. I prefer to use absorbable suture material for the capsular, retinacular, and subcutaneous layers. Immediate immobilization after surgery is provided in a long-arm thumb spica cast, changed to below-elbow immobilization at 4 postoperative weeks. The total immobilization time has ranged from 7 to 10 weeks in my experience.

■ TECHNICAL ALTERNATIVES

In my opinion, there are no satisfactory alternatives to radiolunate arthrodesis for the treatment of post-traumatic changes localized to the radiolunate joint. When the degenerative process extends to the radioscaphoid joint, then a radioscapholunate arthrodesis is the procedure of choice.

As for the other conditions for which radiolunate fusions may be used, a review of the literature reveals that different surgical procedures have been proposed to correct ulnar translation and static or dynamic VISI and DISI instabilities. Rayhack and colleagues evaluated seven patients with ulnar translation treated by ligamentous repair. Three of the seven required subsequent wrist arthrodesis and were considered treatment failures. Four of the remaining five patients had recurrent ulnar translation.[22] Mulier et al[20] reported an isolated instance of a successful ligamentous repair for a recent ulnar translation.

Triquetrolunate dissociations that result in a static VISI have been most commonly treated by triquetrolunate arthrodesis.[14,18,23,31] The two cases reported by Regan et al[23] experienced relief of pain. Both, however, showed no change in their VISI alignment. In

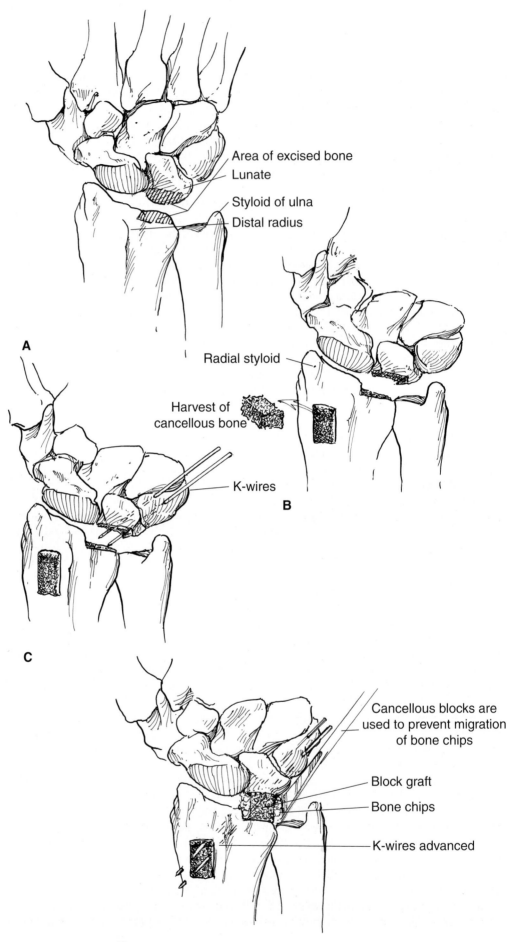

■ FIGURE 111-3

Surgical technique. **(A)** Extent of excision of articular surfaces of lunate and radius. **(B)** Cancellous bone block and bone chips are obtained from the distal radius. **(C)** K-wires are advanced proximally to distally or, as depicted here, distally to proximally, until the tips are visible at the surface to be fused. One wire may be advanced through the lunate to maintain its reduction. **(D)** Cancellous bone is packed between the radius and lunate. A cancellous block is used medially to "wall off" the fusion site and prevent displacement of bony chips into the distal radioulnar joint. A similar bony block is used laterally, to keep bone chips from spilling into the radioscaphoid joint. Avoid collapse or compression of the radioscaphoid space.

Area of excised bone
Lunate
Styloid of ulna
Distal radius

A

Radial styloid

Harvest of cancellous bone

K-wires

B

C

Cancellous blocks are used to prevent migration of bone chips

Block graft
Bone chips
K-wires advanced

D

some of the remaining studies, it was difficult to differentiate the results of those patients with fixed VISI deformities from those without.[14,18,31] I believe that lunotriquetral stabilization by ligamentodesis or arthrodesis is the procedure of choice for lunotriquetral dissociations without VISI. However, this procedure alone is insufficient to correct a static VISI deformity.

As for the dynamic VISI/DISI deformities, usually manifested as a painful, catch-up "clunk" produced by subluxation at the midcarpal level during ulnar–radial deviation, these have been treated in various manners, including ligamentous reconstructions and partial arthrodesis, with no single treatment having been uniformly successful.[16,31]

Radiolunate arthrodesis is an accepted procedure for stabilization of ulnar translation in rheumatoid wrists.[5,6,26,28] Its application to ulnar translation and other forms of carpal instability in nonrheumatoid patients has been less popular, but should be considered.[7,22]

Once plaster immobilization and pin fixation are discontinued, patients are placed in a removable splint and instructed in active range of motion exercises for the wrist. Throughout the period of immobilization, active full range of motion of the fingers and shoulder, and the elbow when free (including pronation–supination), is encouraged. The wrist splint is then worn at all times for 1 to 3 weeks, except during exercises.

Exercises designed to increase grip strength are prescribed as soon as the fusion appears radiographically solid. Progressive activities are allowed as long as they remain pain-free.

■ REHABILITATION

A major problem in evaluating radiolunate arthrodeses is the relatively small number of patients amenable to treatment using this technique. Our experience with post-traumatic ulnar translation shows that patient satisfaction is excellent, without clinical or radiographic recurrence and with few complications.[7] Patient satisfaction correlates with the relief of pain and restoration of stability. There is no correlation, however, between the postoperative range of motion and the degree of patient satisfaction. Clinical alignment, and the "catch-up midcarpal clunk" typical of dynamic instabilities, are routinely corrected, and the correction is maintained.

■ OUTCOMES

The postoperative range of motion compared to the uninvolved wrist averages, in my experience, 75% of dorsiflexion, 65% of palmar flexion, 65% of radial deviation, and 75% of ulnar deviation. This postoperative range is remarkably similar to the preoperative range of motion of the injured wrist, already self-limited by the patient, owing to pain or to post-traumatic ankylosis. The only exception has been a moderate postoperative loss of ulnar deviation compared to that existing before surgery. Grip strength also improves after surgery.

In spite of the lengthy postoperative follow-up of over 10 years in some of my patients, I have remained concerned that radiolunate fusions may still result in degenerative changes at the lunocapitate level, particularly when this procedure is used in patients with scapholunate instability, because the capitate may displace into a scapholunate gap, resulting in excessive, abnormal loads between the head of the capitate and the fixed lunate. I am also concerned that ulnocarpal impingement may result, as was seen in one of my cases. However, this particular complication may be prevented by adequate preservation of carpal height, and if the complication occurs, it may be corrected by ulnar shortening or by one of the several resection arthroplasties of the distal ulna.

The final range of motion that was obtained in our patients was greater than that anticipated based on cadaver studies reported in the literature[19] (Fig. 111–1C, D).

Complications include nonunion, distal radioulnar joint dysfunction due to penetration of the distal radioulnar joint by bone chips, and in one patient in my experience, symptoms of ulnar nerve entrapment at the level of the canal of Guyon. These complications are minimized by careful attention to technique.

References

1. Ambrose L, Posner MA, Green SM, Stuchin S: The effects of scaphoid intercarpal stabilizations on wrist mechanics: An experimental study. J Hand Surg, 1992; 17A:429–437.

2. Bertheusen K: Partial carpal arthrodesis as treatment of local degenerative changes in the wrist joint. Acta Orthop Scand, 1981; 52:629–631.
3. Campbell CH, Keokarn T: Total and subtotal arthrodesis of the wrist: Inlay technique. J Bone Joint Surg, 1964; 46A:1520–1533.
4. Carstam N, Eiken O, Andren L: Osteoarthritis of the trapezio-scaphoid joint. Acta Orthop Scand, 1968; 39:354–358.
5. Chamay A, Della Santa D, Vilaseca A: Radiolunate arthrodesis: Factor of stability for the rheumatoid wrist. Ann Chir Main, 1983; 2:5–17.
6. Chamay A, Della Santa D: Radiolunate arthrodesis in rheumatoid wrist. Ann Chir Main, 1991; 10:197–206.
7. Colello-Abraham K, Taleisnik J: Radiolunate arthrodesis. Presented at the 13th Annual Meeting of the American Society of Hand Therapists, 1990, Toronto, Canada.
8. Crosby EB, Linscheid RL, Dobyns JH: Scapho-trapezial Trapezoid arthrodesis. J Hand Surg, 1978; 3:223–234.
9. Douglas DP, Peimer CA, Koniuch MP: Motion of the wrist after simulated limited intercarpal arthrodeses: An experimental study. J Bone Joint Surg, 1987; 69A:1413–1418.
10. Gellman H, Kauffman D, Lenihan M, Botte MJ, Sarmiento A: An in vitro analysis of wrist motion: The effect of limited intercarpal arthrodesis and the contributions of the radiocarpal and midcarpal joints. J Hand Surg, 1988; 13A:390–395.
11. Gordon LH, King D: Partial wrist arthrodesis for old ununited fractures of the carpal navicular. Am J Surg, 1961; 102:460–464.
12. Graner O, Lopes, EI, Costa Carvalho B, Atlas S: Arthrodesis of the carpal bones in the treatment of Kienböck's disease, painful ununited fractures of the navicular and lunate bones with avascular necrosis, and old fracture-dislocations of carpal bones. J Bone Joint Surg, 1966; 48A:767–774.
13. Helfet AJ: A new operation for ununited fracture of the scaphoid. J Bone Joint Surg, 1952; 34B:329.
14. Keck CA, Hastings A: Lunotriquetral arthrodesis as treatment for lunotriquetral Instability. Presented at the 44th Annual Meeting of the American Society for Surgery of the Hand, Seattle, Washington, 1989.
15. Kleinman WB, Steichen JB, Strickland JW: Management of chronic rotary subluxation of the scaphoid by scaphotrapezio-trapezoid arthrodesis. J Hand Surg, 1982; 7:125–136.
16. Lichtman DM, Noble WH, Alexander CE: Dynamic triquetrolunate instability: Case report. J Hand Surg, 1984; 9A:185–187.
17. Linscheid RL, Dobyns JH: Radiolunate arthrodesis. J Hand Surg, 1985; 10A:821–829.
18. Maitin EC, Bora FW, Osterman AL: Lunato-triquetral instability: A cause of chronic wrist pain. J Hand Surg, 1988; 13A:309.
19. Mayerdierks EM, Mosher JF, Werner FW: Limited wrist arthrodesis: A laboratory study. J Hand Surg, 1987; 12A:526–529.
20. Mulier T, Reynders P, Broos P, Fabry G: Posttraumatic ulnar translation of the carpus: A case report. Acta Orthop Scand, 1992; 63:102–103.
21. Peterson HA, Lipscomb PR: Intercarpal arthrodesis. Arch Surg, 1967; 95:127–134.
22. Rayhack JM, Linscheid RL, Dobyns JH, Smith JH: Posttraumatic ulnar translation of the carpus. J Hand Surg, 1987; 12A:180–189.
23. Regan DS, Linscheid RL, Dobyns JH: Lunotriquetral sprains. J Hand Surg, 1984; 9A:502–514.
24. Rongières M, Mansat M, Devallet P, Bonnevialle P, Railhac JJ: An experimental study of partial intercarpal arthrodesis. Ann Chir Main, 1987; 6:269–275.
25. Rozing PM, Kauer JMG: Partial arthrodesis of the wrist: An investigation in cadavers. Acta Orthop Scand, 1985; 55:66–68.
26. Stanley JK, Boot DA: Radio-lunate arthrodesis. J Hand Surg, 1989; 14B:283–287.
27. Sutro CJ: Treatment of nonunion of the carpal navicular bone. Surgery, 1946; 20:536–540.
28. Taleisnik J: Subtotal arthrodesis of the wrist joint. Clin Orthop, 1984; 187:81–88.
29. Taleisnik J: The Wrist. New York: Churchill-Livingstone, 1985.
30. Thornton L: Old dislocation of os magnum: Open reduction and stabilization. South Med J, 1924; 17:430–434.
31. Trumble T, Bour CJ, Smith RJ, Edwards GS: Intercarpal arthrodesis for static and dynamic volar intercalated segment instability. J Hand Surg, 1988; 13A:384–390.
32. Uematsu A: Intercarpal fusion for treatment of carpal instability: A preliminary report. Clin Orthop, 1979; 144:159–165.
33. Watson HK, Hempton RF: Limited wrist arthrodesis: Part I. The triscaphoid joint. J Hand Surg, 1980; 5:320–327.
34. Watson HK, Goodman ML, Johnson TR: Limited arthrodesis: Part II. Intercarpal and radiocarpal considerations. J Hand Surg, 1981; 6:223–233.

112

EDWARD DIAO
JAYARAM S.
HARIHARAN

Wrist Arthrodesis with an Intramedullary Rod

Wrist arthrodesis has been an integral part of upper extremity surgery since it was first reported by Ely[6] in 1910. Traditionally, wrist arthrodesis was performed with the use of a large, autogenous, corticocancellous bone graft to bridge the entire carpus from the distal radius to the bases of the second and third metacarpals. These early techniques relied on the use of external cast immobilization to maintain wrist position until solid fusion was achieved, and usually used iliac grafts to provide both stability and a stimulus for bony fusion. The technique of Haddad and Riordan[8] used a radial exposure and a rectangular iliac graft. The Carroll and Dick[1,5] technique incorporated a dorsal approach, with an iliac graft shaped as a rabbit-ear with two prongs distally that were designed for insertion into the medullary cavities of the second and third metacarpals.

In the 1960s and 1970s, use of intramedullary pin fixation to augment wrist arthrodesis procedures became popular. In 1965, Clayton,[2,3] in his report of surgical treatment of the wrist in rheumatoid arthritis, described the use of a buried Steinmann pin extending from the radius into the third metacarpal, inserted retrograde, 3/32" in diameter, to maintain alignment and stability after placement of a dorsal corticocancellous autogenous bone graft from either the iliac bone, or a sliding radial graft. Plaster immobilization was recommended until solid union, from 8 to 11 weeks. In 1971, Mannerfelt and Malmsten[9] described a technique for arthrodesis of the wrist in rheumatoid arthritis that incorporated a Rush rod introduced into the shaft of the third metacarpal and driven in a retrograde manner into the medullary canal of the radius, with supplemental fixation provided by a staple. In 1973, Millender and Nalebuff[10] described a simplified technique of rheumatoid wrist arthrodesis incorporating a Steinmann pin placed from the medullary space of the radius through the carpus into either the second or third web space of the hand. The authors noted the following advantages: (1) decreased operating time, (2) the ease with which other concomitant procedures can be performed, and (3) short recuperation time, allowing immediate mobilization of adjacent joints (e.g., the use of the extremity in platform crutch ambulation). These authors believed that bone graft from the resected distal ulna in conjunction with the prepared surfaces of the radiocarpal and intercarpal joints was sufficient for satisfactory arthrodesis without the need for distant autogenous bone grafts. Millender and Nalebuff[10] noted that the use of the Steinmann pin dictated a neutral position of the wrist at the time of fusion. They noted that one of the virtues of the Mannerfelt and Malmsten method, because of the flexibility of the Rush rod, was that the wrist could be fused in different degrees of flexion or extension.

The method of Millender and Nalebuff has enjoyed great popularity, particularly for rheumatoid patients. In addition to its relative simplicity, the likelihood of pseudarthrosis or loss of position of the wrist is significantly reduced, compared to other methods.[4] Some other, more recent modifications have made it possible to use their techniques and provide for alternative positions of the wrist at arthrodesis. Viegas and co-authors[13] described a study evaluating grip strength and wrist position in 25 healthy subjects. They found that grip strength was maximal when the wrist was in slight extension and in slight ulnar deviation. This correlates with information generated by Palmer and co-authors[12] Based on these findings, these authors modified the Steinmann pin arthrodesis technique by introducing the Steinmann pin through a stab wound in the first web space of the hand, then drilling along the base of the second metacarpal, through the carpus, and into the medullary canal of the radius.

Feldon and co-authors[7] described a modification of the Millender and Nalebuff technique. Instead of using a large, single Steinmann pin, two relatively thin Steinmann pins (3/32″–7/64″ in diameter) are inserted through the second and third web spaces between the metacarpal bones across the carpus, and into the medullary canal of the radius. The result of the "stacked-pin" effect in the radius was that rotational stability as well as anteroposterior and lateral stability was provided, without the need for supplementary staple or K-wire fixation. Moreover, the pins are thin enough to be bent after insertion into the radius, allowing for adjustment of the wrist arthrodesis position from strictly neutral.

■ INDICATIONS AND CONTRAINDICATIONS

The primary indication for wrist arthrodesis with intramedullary rod technique is rheumatoid arthritis (Figs. 112-1–112-4). The intramedullary rod technique in rheumatoid arthritis affords speed and simplicity over other techniques, while maintaining control of overall wrist position. In the osteopenic bone routinely encountered in rheumatoid arthritis surgery, intramedullary fixation can be superior to fixation using plates and screws. This technique of wrist arthrodesis can easily be performed in conjunction with other procedures, such as metacarpophalangeal (MP) joint arthroplasty with Silastic implants, extensor tendon repair or reconstruction, and distal ulna resection.

The indications for arthrodesis in rheumatoid arthritis are deformity, instability, or pain (Figs. 112-1–112-4). These factors, when present alone or in combination to a degree that significantly interferes with wrist, hand, and upper extremity function, are appropriate indications for arthrodesis. Other indications for wrist arthrodesis with intramedullary rod fixation include other connective tissue disorders, such as systemic lupus erythematosus and psoriatic arthritis. Post-traumatic or degenerative arthritis were the most common categories for patients treated with wrist fusion using the intramedullary rod technique in the series by Viegas and co-authors,[13] and also in a recent presentation by O'Donovan

■ FIGURE 112–1
Preoperative photograph of the arthritic left hand and wrist. Note the flexed position of the ring metacarpophalangeal joint due to extensor tendon rupture.

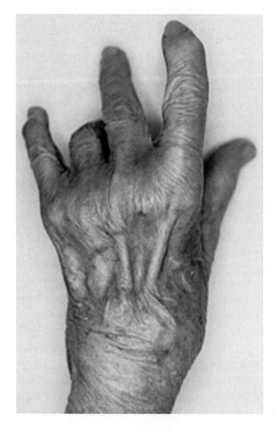

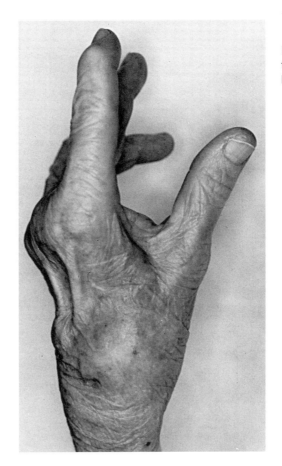

■ FIGURE 112–2
Preoperative lateral photograph of the arthritic left hand and wrist.

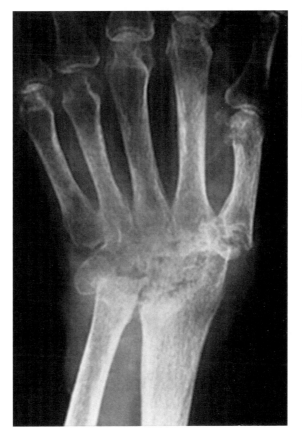

■ FIGURE 112–3
Preoperative posteroanterior radiograph of the arthritic left wrist. Note complete destruction of the carpal bones and severe wrist arthritis.

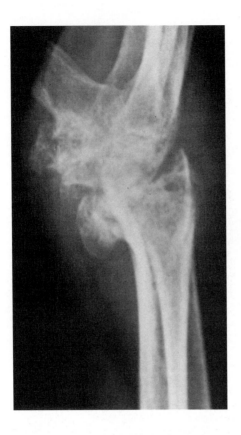

■ FIGURE 112–4
Preoperative lateral radiograph of the arthritic left wrist. Note severe arthritis and volar translation of the carpus.

and co-authors[11]. Arthrodesis of the wrist is the treatment of choice for significant post-traumatic or degenerative arthritis, particularly in patients who desire one procedure with a high likelihood of long-term success, as well as in patients who require wrist stability, pain relief, and strength for heavy use. Arthrodesis is most appropriate when lesser procedures, such as synovectomy, Darrach distal ulna resection alone, limited intercarpal arthrodesis, radioscapholunate arthrodesis, limited carpectomy, or proximal row carpectomy have been eliminated as alternative procedures.

The third general category in which wrist arthrodesis with intramedullary rod fixation is indicated is patients with paralytic disorders with resultant wrist flexion deformity. Patients with cerebral vascular accidents, brain injury, or cerebral palsy in certain circumstances require wrist fusion to correct wrist deformity and pain. This may or may not be augmented with muscle balancing procedures to release tightened muscle tendon units. In paralytic cases, wrist arthrodesis is also indicated when wrist motors can then be made available for tendon transfers to enhance overall function of the extremity.

Wrist arthrodesis should be considered, with either intramedullary rod fixation or plate fixation, in situations of previous failed arthroplasty of the radiocarpal joint. For failed total wrist arthroplasty, there may be significant bone defects that will require large bone grafts, and if remaining bone stock is reasonable, plate fixation may be superior to intramedullary fixation in holding the wrist and bone graft rigidly to prevent nonunion formation. In acute trauma with significant bone loss or reconstruction after segmental tumor resection, similar needs for large bone grafts may make plate fixation wrist arthrodesis techniques superior to those that rely on intramedullary fixation. These instances are relative contraindications to the technique described in this chapter. There are other, more general contraindications to wrist arthrodesis of any kind. When the patient is skeletally immature and the epiphyseal plate of the distal radius is open, wrist arthrodesis will result in extremity shortening. In situations where alternatives to wrist arthrodesis are feasible and the demands for that upper extremity are low (i.e., in the nondominant hand of the older patient with sedentary life demands), lesser procedures that retain some wrist motion may be desirable. Paralytic patients who require wrist motion for grasp and transfer functions are contraindicated for wrist arthrodesis. In instances with sensory loss in the hand through neurologic primary diseases or neurologic injury, arthrodesis should be avoided.

Regional axillary block or general anesthesia are appropriate for performing satisfactory wrist arthrodesis. A pneumatic tourniquet should be used at the forearm or upper arm level.

If a longitudinal incision is used, it should be based generally over the dorsal midline of the wrist over Lister's tubercle. If the transverse incision is used, it is placed along Langer's lines between the radial and ulnar styloids dorsally. The radiocarpal joint should be palpated as a guide. We prefer a dorsal longitudinal incision that is placed in the midline over the dorsum of the wrist (see Fig. 112–8). Care should be taken to preserve the dorsal veins and maintain a thick skin flap. Skin flaps and subcutaneous tissues are dissected from the extensor retinaculum. Dorsal branches of radial and ulnar nerves should be preserved. The extensor retinaculum is opened through a longitudinal incision in the sixth dorsal compartment. The contents of the dorsal compartments are then placed around a Penrose drain for retraction.

Reflection of the extensor retinaculum is performed through a longitudinal incision (Fig. 112–5) in the sixth dorsal compartment, with transverse incisions above and below the flaps to reflect it radially. Enough extensor retinaculum is preserved to allow later dorsal transposition of the retinaculum to protect the extensor tendons from the underlying bony surfaces. In the floor of the fourth dorsal compartment is the terminal branch of the posterior interosseous nerve, which is resected to partially denervate the wrist to decrease joint pain. A longitudinal incision is made in the wrist capsule, and flaps elevated to expose the radiocarpal and intercarpal joints. Using techniques of traction and flexion of the wrist over a bolster, the radiocarpal and intercarpal synovectomies are performed (Fig. 112–5). The radial collateral ligaments should be released from the radial styloid. The abductor pollicis longus and extensor pollicis brevis tendons in the first extensor compartment should be preserved. A complete synovectomy is performed with rongeurs and curettes. Periarticular erosions, if present, are curetted. After synovectomy, cartilage from the radio-

■ SURGICAL TECHNIQUES

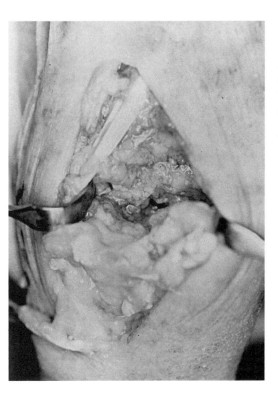

■ FIGURE 112–5
Intraoperative view of the dorsum of the flexed left wrist after dissection of the joint capsule. Note severe arthritic changes in the distal radius and the carpal bones.

carpal and intercarpal joints is removed completely with a rongeur and curettes (Fig. 112–5). A power burr is used to remove residual cartilage, and if there is some sclerotic bone, this should be prepared with a burr. A drilled K-wire (0.32″) can be used to create multiple drill holes in sclerotic bone to promote repair and, subsequently, arthrodesis. The carpometacarpal joints do not need to be resected.

Next, the distal radioulnar joint is exposed through an extension of the capsular incision. The ulna is exposed subperiosteally and resected minimally with an oscillating power saw. In most patients with rheumatoid arthritis, the distal ulna requires resection. In some patients with post-traumatic arthritis, however, especially if they remain in ulnar-negative variance, the ulna may not require resection. If ulnar resection is required, the triangular fibrocartilage complex should be carefully preserved. These soft tissues will be important to use in the reconstruction at the end of the procedure to prevent painful subluxation of the distal ulna, and possible digital extensor tendon rupture as a consequence.

After preparation of the bony surfaces, the fusion site is supplemented with bone grafts harvested from the distal ulnar resection. In post-traumatic and degenerative arthritis, supplemental iliac crest cancellous bone graft may be required.

Pin placement is performed in a variety of techniques. We prefer the Feldon dual-rod modification of the Millender-Nalebuff technique.

Millender-Nalebuff Technique[10]   The intramedullary canal of the radius is entered with a pointed awl, and the largest Steinmann pin that the medullary canal will accommodate is selected. This Steinmann pin is then drilled retrograde through the carpus via the dorsal wrist wound to exit either between the second and third or between the third and fourth metacarpals, depending on the alignment that is optimal in the given patient. Care should be exercised to have the pin exit through the dorsal portion of the interspace. The pin is

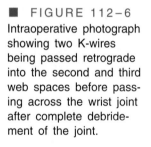

■ FIGURE 112–6
Intraoperative photograph showing two K-wires being passed retrograde into the second and third web spaces before passing across the wrist joint after complete debridement of the joint.

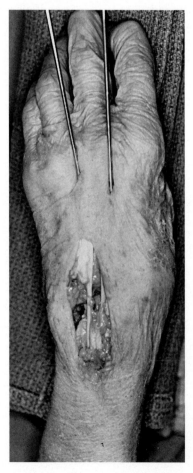

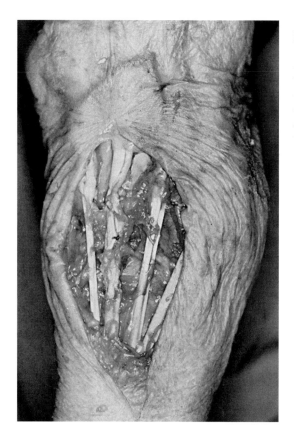

■ FIGURE 112–7
Intraoperative photograph
after wrist arthrodesis,
volar transposition of the
extensor retinaculum, and
extensor tendon recon-
struction by tendon
transfer.

advanced until its tip emerges between the web spaces, as described earlier. The drill is then placed on the exposed distal tip of the Steinmann pin and the pin further advanced until the proximal end is flush with the wrist arthrodesis site. The wrist is then aligned and the Steinmann pin tapped in a retrograde fashion into the intramedullary space of the radius. The pin should be countersunk into the intermetacarpal space using a bone tamp. This fixation can be supplemented by staples to span the radiocarpal joint. However, staples can also migrate and be a source of dorsal soft tissue irritation.

Millender-Nalebuff Technique With Concomitant MP Arthroplasty[10]   In situations in which simultaneous MP arthroplasty that includes the third metacarpal will be performed, the Steinmann pin can be driven right through the third metacarpal shaft. For these cases, exposure of the metacarpals followed by metacarpal head resection can be performed first, followed by the wrist arthrodesis procedure. In this way, retrograde introduction of the Steinmann pin through the distal metacarpal is facilitated without damage to extensor tendons or other structures. The Steinmann pin is countersunk so as not to interfere with MP arthroplasty placement subsequently.

Viegas and Co-workers' Technique[13]   A large Steinmann pin is introduced through a stab wound in the first web space of the hand. The pin is placed on the drill or hand chuck for positioning. The Steinmann pin may then be passed alongside the base of the second metacarpal. It is drilled through the metacarpal, through the carpus, and into the medullary canal of the radius until a satisfactory length has been placed in the intramedullary canal, or until the ulnar border of the radius is contacted. The wrist in this manner can be placed in 0° to 25° of extension and 0° to 25° of ulnar deviation. A large curette or bone tamp and mallet can be used to advance the pin and bury it below the skin.

Feldon Dual-Rod Technique[7,11]   Instead of using a single, large Steinmann pin, two smaller Steinmann pins are inserted through the second and third web spaces dorsally between the metacarpal bones, across the carpus, and into the medullary canal of the radius (Fig. 112–6). Because of their smaller size (3/32"–7/64" in diameter), the pins can be directly drilled through the dorsal aspect of the second and third web spaces and retrograde across the carpus into the radius. After insertion of the pins, the attitude of the wrist can be adjusted by manipulation with subsequent bending of the pins to allow some wrist extension and ulnar deviation if desired. The pins can be cut short beneath the skin (Fig. 112–7) to lie in the web spaces, and removed electively at 6 to 12 postoperative months. No other supplemental internal fixation is required with this technique.

At the end of the procedure, if the distal radioulnar joint has been treated with resection, the triangular fibrocartilage complex and radioulnar ligamentous complex should be sutured to the dorsal and ulnar aspect of the ulna, either to ligaments, capsule, or periosteum, with nonabsorbable suture. The floor of the sixth dorsal compartment can also be used to stabilize the distal ulna. The dorsal capsule should be approximated to cover the arthrodesis site. Extensor retinaculum that has been preserved should be transposed volarly (Fig. 112–7) to provide added protection for the digital extensor tendons. A nonabsorbable suture should be used to close this portion of the wound. The tourniquet should be released before skin closure, and hemostasis obtained. A negative-pressure suction drain should be placed through a separate stab wound and removed in 24 to 48 hours. Skin closure should be performed with 3-0 Dexon deep sutures, followed by 4-0 nylon (Fig. 112–8) or skin staples to close the skin. Sterile wraps and soft bandages are applied, followed by a bulky dressing. External immobilization is provided through a short arm cast or dorsal/volar splints. If a concomitant procedure has been performed, such as distal ulna resection or ligamentous reconstruction, the distal radioulnar joint needs protection. In such an event, a long arm cast with the forearm supinated is desirable for 2 to 3 weeks. At 2 weeks, dressings can be removed, and a custom thermoplastic volar splint used to protect the operative site until evidence of fusion is obtained radiographically. Usually, 4 to 6 weeks of immobilization in a cast or splint are sufficient.

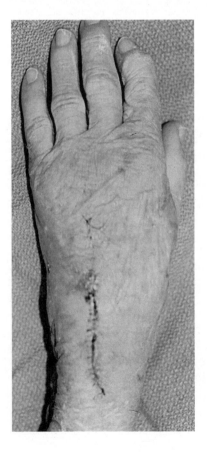

■ FIGURE 112–8
Postoperative photograph showing dorsal longitudinal incision.

Pins are not removed unless they cause pain or have migrated. If pin removal is required before fusion has occurred, supplementary external immobilization will be necessary.

In general, the major technical alternative to intramedullary rod fixation in wrist arthrodesis is the use of dorsal plates. Plate immobilization may offer sufficient rigidity to render postoperative immobilization optional. The plate techniques are most applicable in post-traumatic and osteoarthritic situations, as opposed to patients with rheumatoid arthritis.

Only limited numbers of patients with rheumatoid arthritis are candidates for partial wrist arthrodesis. Wrist arthroplasties with Silastic wrist implants or metal and plastic wrist arthroplasties have not enjoyed the durability of wrist arthrodesis, and have relatively limited indications.

Severe S-shaped, zig-zag, or oblique skin incisions should be avoided in the rheumatoid patient because of increased risk of vascular compromise and skin slough. This is particularly true in patients with atrophic skin or those who are on systemic steroid medications. An alternative with some cosmetic advantages is the transverse dorsal incision.

In terms of exposing the wrist joint, the extensor retinaculum can be incised through any dorsal compartment, as long as the tendons are preserved and retracted, and the extensor retinaculum transposed volarly at the end of the procedure.

The major pitfall of arthrodesis surgery is failure to achieve arthrodesis. A review by Clendenin and Green[4] in 1981 analyzed and compared results in 33 patients with three different types of wrist arthrodesis: two techniques of noninstrumented bone grafting versus the Millender-Nalebuff[10] technique. As opposed to a pseudarthrosis rate of 20% to 28.5% in the noninstrumented techniques, only 1 of 12 cases using the Nalebuff technique (8.3%) resulted in pseudarthrosis.

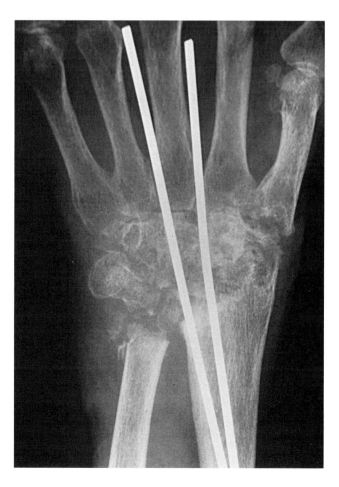

■ FIGURE 112–9
Postoperative posteroanterior radiograph showing dual intramedullary rod technique for wrist arthrodesis, combined with distal ulnar resection.

Occult median nerve injury as a result of arthrodesis preparation or malposition of the carpal bones is a potentially serious complication. Careful volar palpation of the arthrodesis site and thorough scrutiny of radiographs from a portable fluoroscopy unit or C-arm should be a standard part of the procedure to assess positioning of the intramedullary rod or rods, and to assess the overall alignment of the wrist and carpal bones.

Dorsal skin complications can arise through injudicious handling of compromised soft tissue, or hematoma formation. Careful hemostasis plus the use of a drain are important to avoid these types of complications. Pin complications can occur early if Steinmann pins are left prominent. Assessment of pin position clinically by palpation and radiographically should be performed before the end of the procedure.

■ REHABILITATION

The main goals are to provide enough supplemental fixation to ensure bony union, and to prevent stiffness in adjacent joints. Clearly, if extensor tendon reconstructions, MP arthroplasties, or other procedures are performed in the hand and digits, the appropriate rehabilitation for these procedures is warranted. In general, the postoperative dressing and immobilization can be kept in place for up to a month without significant problems. Alternatively, dressings can be removed at 1 to 2 weeks, followed by fabrication of a custom thermoplastic orthosis. This is the technique we prefer. Elbow flexion and extension exercises, pronation and supination if there has not been concomitant distal radioulnar joint surgery, and digital motion if there are no contraindications, are encouraged.

■ OUTCOMES

The techniques described here should result in a reliable, predictable wrist arthrodesis for most patients (Figs. 112–9 and 112–10). In Millender and Nalebuff's original description,[10] 70 arthrodeses were performed in 60 patients, and fusion was successful in all but 2 patients. Their patients with pins placed in the intermetacarpal interspaces were immobilized 4 to 5 months in a long or short arm cast. However, in those patients with supplemental staple or intramedullary pin fixation into the fifth metacarpal, immobiliza-

■ FIGURE 112–10
Postoperative lateral radiograph after wrist arthrodesis, showing the dual-rod system in place. Note the correction of volar translation of the carpus that was visible in Figure 112–4.

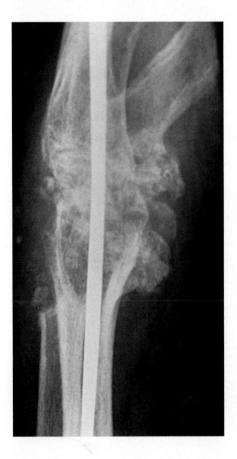

tion time was decreased to somewhere between 2 and 6 weeks. In their series, one patient had a deep wound infection that was cured by debridement and antibiotics. Two patients with pseudarthrosis had premature removal of the Steinmann pin, resulting in painless, stable wrists with 10° to 15° of motion. Twelve patients had distal migration of the pin associated with pain, necessitating pin removal. In cases where pin removal was required before bony fusion had consolidated, the wrists were then immobilized in plaster casts. The authors noted that after introduction of pin countersinking and the addition of staples, there have been no difficulties with pin migration. Skin slough occurred in three of the patients.

In Viegas and co-authors'[13] series of 10 patients, all did well. There were two complications among the 10 patients, one with a superficial infection treated with incision and drainage, the other with a prominent Steinmann pin that required early removal.

O'Donovan and co-authors[11] reported on 33 wrists and 31 patients with an average follow-up of 4 years. All 33 wrists fused by radiographic and clinical examination within 16 weeks. All the rheumatoid patients had excellent pain relief, had subjective increases in grip strength, and were pleased with the cosmetic appearance of their wrists. The nonrheumatoid patients all had relief of wrist pain, and 11 of 12 patients followed for longer than 2 years had documented increases in their grip strength.

In our experience, the intramedullary rod techniques are ideally suited for the rheumatoid patient, for selected patients with post-traumatic or degenerative arthritis, and for paralytic patients. We favor the dual-rod fixation over the single Steinmann pin fixation because of the added rotational stability, the ability to adjust the angle of the wrist more easily, and the ability to avoid use of supplemental staples or K-wires.

References

1. Carroll RE, Dick HM: Arthrodesis of the wrist for rheumatoid arthritis. J Bone Joint Surg, 1971; 53A:1365–1369.
2. Clayton ML: Surgical treatment at the wrist in rheumatoid arthritis. J Bone Joint Surg, 1965; 47A:741–750.
3. Clayton ML, Ferlic DC: Arthrodesis of the arthritic wrist. Clin Orthop, 1984; 187:89–93.
4. Clendenin MB, Green DP: Arthrodesis of the wrist: Complications and their management. J Hand Surg, 1981; 6:253–257.
5. Dick HM: Wrist arthrodesis. In: Green DP (ed): Operative Hand Surgery. New York: Churchill-Livingstone, 1982:155–166.
6. Ely LW: Study of the joint tuberculosis. Surg Gynecol Obstet, 1910; 10:561–572.
7. Feldon P, Millender LH, Nalebuff EA: Rheumatoid arthritis of the hand and wrist. In: Green DP (ed): Operative Hand Surgery. New York: Churchill-Livingstone, 1982:1587–1690.
8. Haddad RJ Jr, Riordan DC: Arthrodesis of the wrist. J Bone Joint Surg, 1967; 49A:950–954.
9. Mannerfelt L, Malmsten M: Arthrodesis of the wrist in rheumatoid arthritis. Scand J Plast Reconstr Surg, 1971; 5:124–130.
10. Millender LH, Nalebuff EA: Arthrodesis of the rheumatoid wrist. J Bone Joint Surg, 1973; 55A:1026–1034.
11. O'Donovan T, Feldon P, Belsky MR: Dual rod internal fixation for wrist fusion. Annual Meeting of the American Society for Surgery of the Hand. Toronto, Ontario, Canada. September, 1990.
12. Palmer AK, Werner FK, Murphy D: Functional wrist motion: A biomechanical study. J Hand Surg, 1985; 10A:39–46.
13. Viegas SF, Rimoldi R, Patterson R: Modified technique of intramedullary fixation for wrist arthrodesis. J Hand Surg, 1989; 14A:618–623.

ARNOLD-PETER C.
WEISS

113

Wrist Arthrodesis with Plate Fixation

■ HISTORY OF THE
TECHNIQUE

Wrist arthrodesis has been used since the early 1900s as a salvage technique for patients with severe degenerative arthritis of the carpus, massive infection, or tumor destruction of bone.[5] Many techniques for accomplishing wrist fusion have been described, with a natural evolution to methods involving more rigid internal fixation.[2-4,6,7,11,12,15] The use of iliac crest bone graft augmentation of the fusion site has always been a prerequisite for this type of procedure, but with newer and more rigid fixation techniques, this requirement has come into question.[1]

The development of rigid internal fixation plates for the treatment of fractures has led to the use of these plates in obtaining rigid fixation from the metacarpal, across the carpus, to the distal radius.[10,16] This type of fixation allows immediate postoperative rehabilitation with little immobilization and a very high predictable fusion rate. Recently, plate fixation has been used in wrist fusions with bone graft augmentation using local bone only, with excellent results.[9,14]

■ INDICATIONS AND
CONTRAINDICATIONS

The classic indications for the use of a plate in wrist arthrodesis have comprised those conditions, other than rheumatoid arthritis, that involve significant post-traumatic degenerative carpal joint destruction (Fig. 113–1), massive infection with loss of bone substance, or tumor destruction of bone. The use of a plate in wrist arthrodesis in these patients is highly advantageous because of the immediate postoperative rigidity provided by the plate in situations where intrinsic stability to the wrist is lost. Absolute indications for the use of plate fixation in wrist arthrodesis are those conditions with significant carpal or distal radius bone loss requiring postoperative maintenance of carpal height and rigidity. Relative indications for this procedure are conditions involving degenerative joint changes in the carpus from post-traumatic causes that have not undergone significant carpal collapse, but for which early rehabilitation exercises are deemed advantageous.

Relative contraindications to this procedure include those patients with rheumatoid arthritis because simpler techniques with less absolute rigidity provide a highly predictable fusion rate.[3,4,11]

■ SURGICAL
TECHNIQUES

This operation is done with the patient undergoing either general or axillary block anesthesia. A bloodless field, which is essential when performing a total wrist arthrodesis, is accomplished by a pneumatic tourniquet. A straight longitudinal incision of approximately 10 to 12 cm in length is made over the dorsal aspect of the wrist, centered over Lister's tubercle. It is extended distally to the proximal aspect of the third metacarpal shaft. The entire dissection is done using a scalpel. The plane between the subcutaneous tissue and extensor retinaculum is developed in both a radial and ulnar direction, avoiding injury to the sensory branch of the radial nerve. The retinaculum of the third compartment is incised beginning at Lister's tubercle and extending distally and proximally. The entire extensor pollicis longus tendon is then removed from its compartment and transposed radially, taking care to use dissecting scissors to release the muscle belly entirely from any proximal constriction (Fig. 113–2).[8] The floor of the third compartment is incised between the second and fourth compartments from the dorsal radius proximally to the dorsal carpal capsule distally. This longitudinal incision is carried out over the dorsal

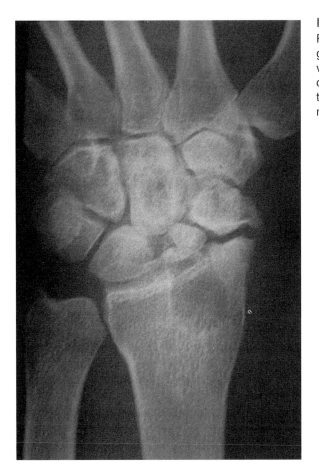

■ FIGURE 113-1
Posteroanterior radio-
graph of a wrist with ad-
vanced degenerative
changes. Arthrodesis with
the plate fixation tech-
nique is indicated.

aspect of the third metacarpal. Capsular flaps are elevated off the carpus, maintaining as much thickness as possible, in both a radial and ulnar direction. The vestigial sensory component of the posterior interosseous nerve can be transected in the floor of the fourth compartment, for denervation of the carpus, should this be desired. An osteotome is used to remove Lister's tubercle, to provide a flat surface along the dorsal radius. The dorsal one-quarter of the carpus itself, including, at least, the scaphoid, lunate, capitate, and third carpometacarpal joint, is removed using an osteotome. Sequential thin osteotomes and rongeurs of small and large size are then used to denude the articular surfaces of both the radiocarpal, intercarpal, and third carpometacarpal joints of cartilage and the immediate subchondral bone (Fig. 113–3). Preparation of these structures should be done to appropriate cancellous bone. The volar-most portion of the carpal articular surfaces may be left intact to maintain appropriate intercarpal spacing, which aids in avoiding any change in relative carpal alignment during the plate placement procedure.

Local bone graft is obtained from the distal radius using a large curette, with the entry site in the region proximal to the denuded Lister's tubercle (Fig. 113–4). A 1-cm width of intact cancellous bone should be maintained between the bone graft donor site and the radiocarpal joint so that secondary problems are not encountered while obtaining the fusion. In general, sufficient amounts of bone graft can be obtained from the distal radius site. A 3.5-mm dynamic compression plate of an appropriate length (usually, a 10-hole plate) or a wrist fusion plate (2.7 mm–3.5 mm) is then chosen to span the third metacarpal–carpal–radius region. In the region of the capitate, a normal volar dip in the contour of the carpus occurs, and the dynamic compression plate is contoured appropriately with a volar convex dip. This technique allows the plate to maintain constant contact with all the osseous structures included in the wrist fusion. An essential minimum plate length

■ FIGURE 113–2
The extensor pollicis longus tendon is transposed
and the capsule is in-
cised distally between the
second and fourth com-
partments (dotted line).

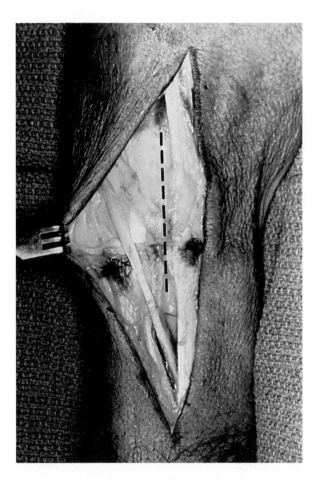

should accommodate screws to secure six cortices of bone in the proximal metacarpal and six cortices of bone in the distal radius. The intervening holes can be used to place one or two cancellous screws through selected carpal bones, most commonly the capitate, for further fixation of the carpus itself. After the plate has been contoured and positioned to ensure appropriate length and fit, the distal-most holes are drilled and tapped in the metacarpal to align the plate optimally. The plate should be placed so that at least three bicortical screws are present in the third metacarpal. However, the plate should be placed as far proximal as possible when accomplishing this goal; distal positioning of the plate can cause postoperative impingement between the plate edge and overlying extensor tendons, and should be avoided. For the same reason, the plate should always be affixed distally first because there is far more leeway in axial plate alignment over the distal radius than over the metacarpal shaft.

With the plate firmly affixed to the metacarpal distally, local bone graft is packed into all joint surfaces to be fused (previously prepared by removal of cartilage and hard sub-chondral bone). The third carpometacarpal joint should always be fused. In general, suffi-cient local bone graft is available from the distal radius and Lister's tubercle to accomplish this task. After packing the bone graft, the plate is fixed along the distal radius with at least three bicortical screws (Fig. 113–5). The wrist usually is fused in 10 to 15° of extension, which should have been previously contoured into the plate. In heavy laborers and those requiring significant power grip, some ulnar deviation of the wrist may be desired and can be accomplished with slight ulnar deviation of the plate in the coronal plane combined with contouring of the plate so that it remains flush to the radial shaft, avoiding any proximal impingement between the plate and forearm musculature. The distal radioulnar joint is not treated by surgical excision or modification unless it was symptomatic before surgery. Intraoperative radiographs are taken to check plate placement and screw length

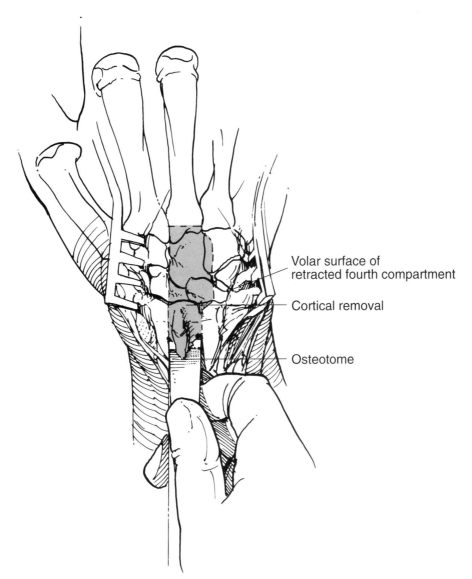

Volar surface of
retracted fourth compartment

Cortical removal

Osteotome

■ FIGURE 113–3
Resection of the dorsal
one-quarter of the carpal
bones and third metacar-
pal before removal of the
cartilage.

(Fig. 113–6). A medium suction drain is usually placed in the wound and the capsule is closed over the plate using 3-0 absorbable sutures to provide a buffer between the plate and the extensor tendons. The extensor pollicis longus is transposed above the retinaculum, preventing any impingement between this tendon and the plate itself. The skin is then reapproximated and closed using 5-0 nylon interrupted sutures in a horizontal mattress fashion.

A well padded, bulky short-arm dressing with a volar plaster splint is applied in the operating room. The splint allows for full active and passive range of motion in the digits and elbow, which is begun immediately on the night of surgery. Strict elevation for several days is important to limit secondary edema.

Although excellent fusion rates have been obtained with the use of local bone graft only combined with plate fixation, additional autogenous cancellous bone graft can be obtained from the iliac crest and used for augmentation. This technique imparts an increased morbidity for the patient but can be useful when there is insufficient distal radius bone graft. Several alternative techniques of fixation have been described using intermedullary rods, staples, and K-wires to provide appropriate fixation. Because postoperative fixation in

**■ TECHNICAL
ALTERNATIVES**

■ FIGURE 113–4
Local cancellous bone
graft is obtained with a
curette through a cortical
window in the dorsal dis-
tal radius, where Lister's
tubercle was previously
removed by an osteo-
tome. A 1-cm bridge of
cancellous bone at the
distal radius should not
be violated by the cu-
rette.

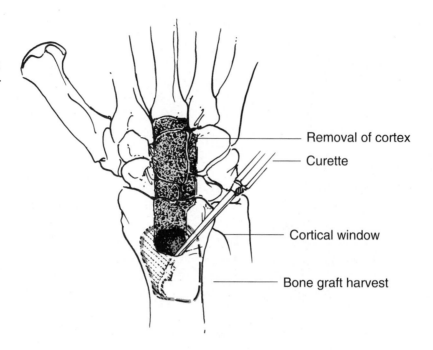

Removal of cortex

Curette

Cortical window

Bone graft harvest

■ FIGURE 113–5
The dorsal plate in appropriate alignment with cancellous packing of the
carpus using local graft
only. The plate is tita-
nium and specifically de-
signed for wrist fusion.

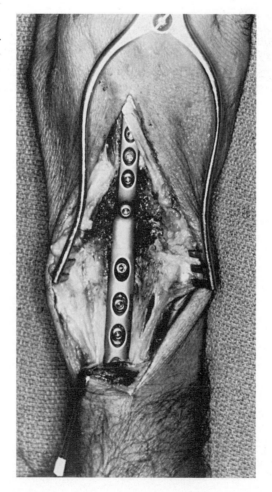

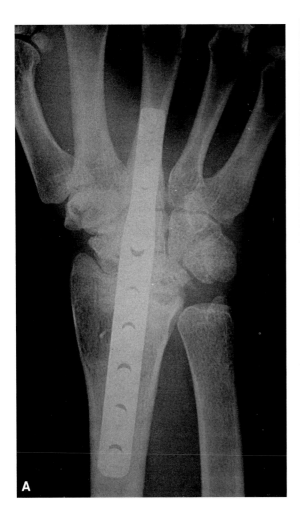 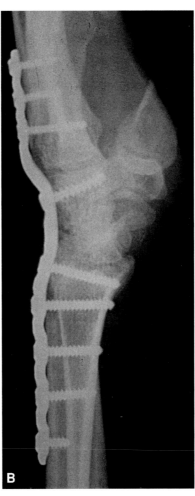

■ FIGURE 113–6
Posteroanterior **(A)** and
lateral **(B)** postoperative
radiographs demonstrat-
ing appropriate plate
alignment and contact,
and screw placement and
length.

any of these techniques is less than that obtained with the plate technique, augmentation with autogenous iliac crest bone graft should be done in all patients (with the exception of those with rheumatoid arthritis) to improve the fusion rate. Because no alternative technique provides the rigid fixation that can be obtained with the plate technique, some care must be taken in the postoperative management of these patients to avoid excessive motion in the fusion sites.

Pitfalls involving the use of this technique usually can be avoided by a sequential approach to exposure and plate placement. With transposition of the extensor pollicis longus tendon, one must ensure that no "pulley-type" tethering is present proximally after transposition of the muscle itself. Postoperative closure under the extensor pollicis longus tendon should be done with care to avoid any impingement between this muscle–tendon unit and the plate itself. Thick retinacular and capsular flaps should be maintained throughout the procedure because they aid significantly in reconstruction of the soft tissue buffer over the plate after fixation. The plate should always be placed distally first and should be checked for appropriate length and contour before any screw fixation. Complete contouring of the plate should be accomplished before any screw fixation. The plate should always be placed as proximal on the third metacarpal as possible, yet still providing six cortical screw interfaces, thereby avoiding any impingement problems between the distal plate and the extensor tendons dorsally. Always fuse the third carpometacarpal joint. If some degree of postoperative ulnar deviation is required for the patient, this can be accomplished by plate contouring over the distal radius with angulation of the plate as previously detailed, or, alternatively, by transfixing the plate to the second metacarpal shaft instead of the third metacarpal shaft to accomplish ulnar deviation of the wrist. A

1-cm region of subchondral and metaphyseal bone should not be violated during bone graft harvesting to ensure appropriate fusion and bone-to-bone contact.

■ REHABILITATION

Little formal hand rehabilitation is required for these patients after fusion with the exception of instruction in active and passive range of motion exercises for the digits and elbow during the immediate postoperative period. In general, patients can make a full fist within 4 to 5 postoperative days. A molded plastic splint is used for approximately 4 to 5 weeks for protection, when some consolidation of the fusion mass is noted on radiographs. The patient should be instructed in maintaining range of motion of the shoulder and elbow because these can commonly undergo secondary stiffness if not addressed in the postoperative period.

Complete consolidation of the wrist fusion generally occurs at 10 weeks, when full-use activities of the hand are encouraged, including manual labor work activities. Patients frequently note a "learning curve" for 4 to 6 months after surgery in how to use the fused wrist most effectively in accomplishing activities of daily living. Perineal care and use of the hand in tight spaces are frequently cited as items that are difficult to perform efficiently.[14]

■ OUTCOMES

Patients who undergo wrist arthrodesis using plate fixation with local bone graft only demonstrate an extremely high fusion rate, excellent postoperative range of motion of the fingers, and an improvement of grip strength over their preoperative status. The fusion rate is between 98 and 100% using rigid plate fixation with bone graft augmentation.[9,13] A limited prospective study of 18 patients demonstrated final total active motion (index through small fingers) of 259° and in the thumb of 127°; grip strength improved from 27 pounds before surgery to 42 pounds after surgery (contralateral normal grip strength averaged 81 pounds) in this series.[13] Postoperative infection or delayed wound healing is extremely rare. Plate removal is occasionally required because of extensor tendinitis in approximately 12% of patients fused with standard dynamic compression plates.[9] The use of local bone graft eliminates the morbidity associated with an iliac crest grafting procedure.

After a 3- to 6-month learning curve in the use of their fused wrist, patients usually can perform all activities of daily living as long as their elbow and shoulder have normal range of motion. Patients have noted some difficulty in the use of the fused hand in personal hygiene, but have demonstrated little difficulty in adjusting with the other hand. The greatest advantage of this technique is the opportunity for immediate postoperative rehabilitation with little risk of fixation failure. The plate fixation technique provides a very predictable fusion rate and a pain-free, stable wrist for the patient over the long term.

References

1. Abbott LC, Saunders JBDM, Bost FC: Arthrodesis of the wrist with the use of grafts of cancellous bone. J Bone Joint Surg, 1942; 24A:883–898.
2. Campbell CJ, Keokarn T: Total and subtotal arthrodesis of the wrist. J Bone Joint Surg, 1964; 46A:1520–1533.
3. Carroll RE, Dick HM: Arthrodesis of the wrist for rheumatoid arthritis. J Bone Joint Surg, 1971; 53A:1365–1369.
4. Clayton ML, Ferlic DC: Arthrodesis of the arthritic wrist. Clin Orthop, 1984; 187:89–93.
5. Ely LW: Study of the joint tuberculosis. Surg Gynecol Obstet, 1910; 10:561–572.
6. Evans D: Wedge arthrodesis of the wrist. J Bone Joint Surg [Br], 1955; 37A:126–134.
7. Haddad RJ, Riordan DC: Arthrodesis of the wrist: A surgical technique. J Bone Joint Surg, 1967; 49A:950–954.
8. Hastings II H, Leibovic SJ: Dorsal approach to the distal radius through the third dorsal compartment. J Hand Surg (in press).
9. Hastings H II, Weiss APC, Strickland JW: Wrist fusion: Indication, technique, functional consequences for the hand and wrist. Orthopade, 1993; 22:86–91.
10. Larsson SE: Compression arthrodesis of the wrist: A consecutive series of 23 cases. Clin Orthop, 1974; 99:146–153.

11. Millender LH, Nalebuff EA: Arthrodesis of the rheumatoid wrist: An evaluation of sixty patients and a description of a different surgical technique. J Bone Joint Surg, 1973; 55A: 1026–1034.
12. Rayan GM: Wrist arthrodesis. J Hand Surg, 1986; 11A:356–364.
13. Weiss APC, Hastings H II: Wrist arthrodesis for post-traumatic conditions: A study of plate and local bone graft application. J Hand Surg, 1995; 20A:50–56.
14. Wiedeman GP, Quenzer D, Strickland JW, Hastings J, Steichen JB, Kleinman WB: Arthrodesis for post-traumatic arthritis of the wrist: Reliability and function. J Hand Surg, 1988; 13A: 305–306.
15. Wood MB: Wrist arthrodesis using dorsal radial bone graft. J Hand Surg, 1987; 12A:28–212.
16. Wright CS, McMurtry RY: AO arthrodesis in the hand. J Hand Surg, 1983; 8:932–935.

PART

IX

Arthroplasty

MICHAEL E. JABALEY
ALAN E. FREELAND

114

Capsulectomy of the Proximal Interphalangeal Joint

"The PIP joint is the epicenter of the hand"

Raymond M. Curtis (1913–1994)

Even in the formative years of the specialty of hand surgery, there was an awareness of joint stiffness and its surgical correction. Curtis[2] classified the causes of proximal interphalangeal (PIP) joint stiffness in flexion and extension in 1954 and described their surgical treatment. His approach was based on careful analysis of the injury to identify the offending structures and on excision of the collateral ligaments or volar plate, coupled with appropriate freeing of tendons and surrounding structures from scar. A better understanding of anatomy has allowed subsequent refinements in technique.

Watson[12] described division of the proximal check-rein ligaments, thus releasing the flexion contracture while retaining the functional integrity of the volar plate. Diao and Eaton[5] reinforced the concept of complete excision of the collateral ligaments through bilateral midaxial incisions.

This chapter will address surgical capsulectomy of the PIP joint, but not contractures due to deficits or scarring of skin or subcutaneous tissue. The role of tendon and tendon sheath involvement will be mentioned only briefly. Remarks will be limited to those structures in and about the PIP joint that more purely ankylose the joint and limit its range of motion: the capsule, the collateral ligament complex, the volar plate and retrocondylar recess, and the articular surfaces of the phalanges themselves.[10] The surgical procedures described herein are largely those of the late Raymond M. Curtis.[1,3,11]

The ideal patient for surgical correction of PIP joint stiffness is a motivated person with normal bony architecture and contracture of specific, identifiable structures, either ligaments or volar plate, but without primary scarring of these structures. Such patients make up the minority of candidates for surgery, and the importance and involvement of other structures and injuries must be carefully weighed in decision-making.

Curtis[3] separated PIP joint stiffness into two categories: those stiff in flexion (flexion contractures) and those stiff in extension (extension contractures). He enumerated the causes and treatment of each (Table 1). This classification is still valid and is quite useful in assessing severity, treatment, and outcome. Each structure, in its turn, should be inspected and examined. The surgeon should consider those structures that must be addressed during surgery and be prepared to deal with each.

Surgery is preferably deferred until the remodeling stage of wound healing has been reached, usually 4 to 6 months from the injury or most recent surgery. Scar maturity can be clinically monitored by serially recording the specific range of active and passive motion in the joint and noting the time at which improvement plateaus.

Capsulectomy for extension contracture is indicated when the range of active flexion is poor and prehension is weak. If other joints are normal, 60° of active motion at the PIP joint is considered adequate. Flexed joints may result from contracture of skin and subcutaneous tissue, the flexor tendons and their sheath, or the volar plate and collateral ligaments. Passive extension will usually be the same regardless of metacarpophalangeal (MP) joint position if the primary problem is the volar plate. This may not be the case in flexor tendon adhesion. Joint pain is an ominous symptom, which portends arthrosis. A true lateral

■ HISTORY OF THE TECHNIQUE

■ INDICATIONS AND CONTRAINDICATIONS

909

TABLE 114–1

Structures Limiting PIP Joint Flexion	*Structures Limiting PIP Joint Extension*
1. dorsal skin	1. volar skin
2. extensor mechanism	2. superficial fascia
3. interosseous muscle/tendon	3. tendon sheath
4. retinacular ligament	4. flexor tendons
5. collateral ligaments	5. volar plate
6. volar plate	6. retinacular ligaments
7. bone block/exostosis	7. accessory collateral ligaments
8. flexor tendon/sheath	8. proper collateral ligaments
	9. bone block or exostosis

radiograph is essential in all cases to detect joint narrowing, arthrosis, subluxation, or postfracture deformities.

Surgery should be deferred in the recently injured or operated patient who is still improving with nonoperative therapy. It may be contraindicated in the noncompliant patient. Relative contraindications include inadequate flexor or extensor tendon function and inadequate soft tissue cover. The PIP joint that is severely flexed and subluxated presents special problems of surgical exposure and may, in the absence of severe pain, be best treated by no surgery or by either arthrodesis or a resection arthroplasty and implant.

■ SURGICAL TECHNIQUES

The anesthetic of choice is 0.5% intravenous lidocaine block and sedation,[9] although a digital block can be used if a single joint is being treated. A well-padded upper arm tourniquet and pressure of 100 mm above systolic blood pressure will allow 75 to 90 minutes of operating time. Before tourniquet deflation, digital blocks with 0.25% bipivicaine are performed, permitting intraoperative assessment of motion.

Antibiotics and methylprednisolone are administered preoperatively, and ibuprofen is given for 10 to 14 days postoperatively to minimize swelling and pain during the vital postoperative therapy.

For the joint that is stiffened in extension, a dorsal curvilinear incision is centered over the PIP joint and extends from the distal portion of the middle phalanx to the midportion of the proximal phalanx. Dissection is performed in the areolar subcutaneous plane, exposing the extensor mechanism down to Cleland's ligament on either side. This ligament can be divided if necessary, to allow further exposure of the neuromuscular bundle and the other volar structures.

At issue currently is the management of the transverse retinacular ligament (TRL). It must be incised to gain access to the deeper joint structures (Fig. 114–1). In the Curtis capsulectomy, that structure was considered important for joint stability, and he recommended either retracting it or incising and repairing it.[4] Eaton incises it or, if scarred, excises it and does not repair it and reports no postoperative instability.[5] If unscarred, one may manage the TRL in either fashion. The question of the role of the TRL in joint stability cannot be answered at this time.

To obtain PIP joint flexion, it is important to excise the entire proper collateral ligament on each side. This can be done by sharply shaving it off its tubercle of origin on the proximal phalanx and cutting it flush at its insertion into the base of the middle phalanx. A portion or all of the accessory collateral ligament should be removed as necessary to permit free passive flexion of the joint. A thin, curved elevator should next be passed beneath the central slip of the extensor tendon and beneath the lateral bands to assure that these structures will glide satisfactorily and permit the joint to go into flexion. The

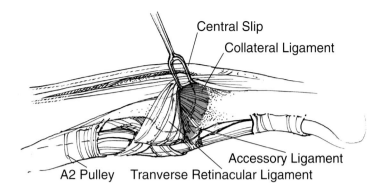

Central Slip

Collateral Ligament

Accessory Ligament

A2 Pulley   Tranverse Retinacular Ligament

■ FIGURE 114-1

For a dorsal capsulectomy a longitudinal skin incision permits exposure of the central and lateral bands, and the transverse retinacular ligaments (TRL). To the extent possible, the TRL is retracted proximally and dorsally, permitting complete excision of the collateral ligaments as well as a portion or all of the accessory collateral ligaments.

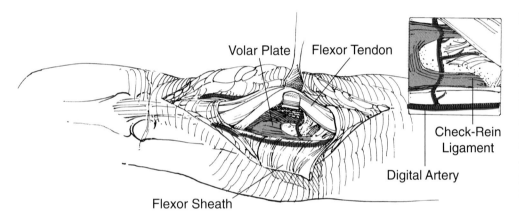

Volar Plate | Flexor Tendon

Check-Rein
Ligament

Digital Artery

Flexor Sheath

■ FIGURE 114-2

For a volar capsulectomy a Bruner skin incision allows exposure of the flexor tendon sheath. The sheath is opened by releasing cruciate and the A3 pulleys; the flexor tendons are then retracted. The inset shows the transverse arterial branch between the radial and ulnar digital arteries.

same elevator should be used to separate adhesions and assess the articular surfaces and the retrocondylar recess (beneath the head of the proximal phalanx). Removal of osteophytes or offending fragments of bone can be accomplished by small osteotome and rongeur. Appropriate intrinsic releases should be performed when necessary. At this point, the joint should go easily into passive flexion. If it does not, each structure must be reexamined for causes of residual tightness. Active flexion can be easily tested in the awake patient. During general anesthesia, one should make a palmar incision proximal to the A_1 pulley and apply traction to the flexor tendons to evaluate joint flexion.

The joint that is stiff in flexion is approached through a volar zigzag incision or a longitudinal incision with Z-plasty closure, extending from the distal interphalangeal (DIP) joint to the MP joint crease. The apex of the zig zag is ulnar in the index, long, and ring fingers and radial in the small finger. The A_3 pulley is either excised or divided in a step-wise fashion. The flexor tendons are retracted, taking care not to injure the vincula to the superficialis tendon (Fig. 114–2). Tendolysis is performed when necessary.

The check-rein ligaments are next incised proximally and transversely, taking care to protect the transverse branches of the digital artery crossing immediately beneath them. The volar plate is elevated in a proximal-to-distal direction to relieve the contracture.

If the joint does not passively extend after division of the check-rein ligaments, one should incise along both sides of the volar plate and either incise or excise a portion of the accessory collateral ligaments to gain extension (Fig. 114–3). The proper collateral ligaments are neither visualized nor incised in this procedure. Exposure can be especially

■ FIGURE 114–3
To release the PIP joint, the check-rein ligaments are incised, the volar plate is elevated, and, if needed, a portion of the accessory collateral ligament is excised.

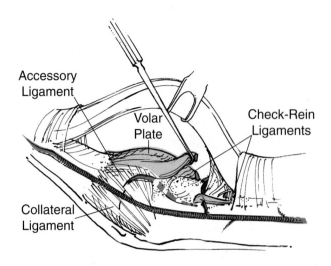

Accessory Ligament

Volar Plate

Check-Rein Ligaments

Collateral Ligament

difficult if the contracture is severe or if there is subluxation of the joint (see Indications and Contraindications section).

In the severely flexed PIP joint, the other surrounding soft tissues may also be contracted. A temporary Kirschner wire is used to maintain alignment in the extended position for 5 to 6 days. It is important to check the joint position with the tourniquet deflated to be sure that circulation to the finger is adequate. If necessary, the K-wire should be removed and the joint repositioned in more flexion.

After either procedure, a bulky dressing and plaster splint are applied with the MP joints and the PIP joints comfortably flexed. Hand elevation is continued for 48 hours before beginning therapy. Sutures are removed in 10 to 14 days.

■ TECHNICAL ALTERNATIVES

The best alternative to surgery is an aggressive therapy program.[6,13] Many patients with joint stiffness can be improved substantially by the use of physical modalities, dynamic splinting, passive stretching, and active use of the hand in a supervised setting. Surgery should be reserved for those cases where such a program fails to produce adequate joint motion. Before surgery, one should evaluate pain very carefully and be sure that its cause is not an arthrosis or painful arthritis. The painful joint is doomed to failure because the patient will avoid motion, and restiffening will invariably occur.

An alternative to the dorsal incision is the bilateral midaxial incisions recommended by Eaton.[5] This approach avoids a dorsal skin scar but is less versatile than the dorsal incision. In either approach, wound closure is performed with a single layer with interrupted or running skin sutures.

The surgeon should be particularly careful when approaching the joint that is subluxated in flexion. The surgical release of such joints, however difficult, can usually be accomplished, but it is at the price of considerable operative trauma. Such trauma is cumulative, resulting in pain and swelling postoperatively, with the final result substantially reduced. In addition, the extensor mechanism of such a joint is usually stretched and will be incapable of extending an otherwise moveable joint, again compromising the final result.

A particularly subtle problem in patients who have had previous flexor tendon surgery is the loss of two or more pulleys and contracture due to intact flexor tendons bowstringing across the volar surface of the PIP joint. This results in a space between the tendons and the volar plate that fills with scar and inexorably produces flexion of the PIP joint, resistant to therapy or surgery.

Complications following surgical procedures about the PIP joint are mercifully rare, but mediocre results are not. Infection is seen occasionally but may be more common when Kirschner wires are used. Skin loss from previous scarring and aggressive surgical dissection is a major problem. Joint swelling and pain from over-aggressive surgery is the most common cause of poor results. A complacent or noncompliant patient who will not or cannot follow the postoperative routine will invariably negate otherwise excellent surgery.

It is prudent to recognize, in advance, those joints which can only be straightened by heroic surgery. The long-term improvement rarely justifies this approach and alternative procedures such as arthrodesis or arthroplasty should be considered.

The postoperative treatment is based on an understanding of the wound-healing process.[6] The PIP joint must be managed progressively through the phases of inflammation, fibroplasia, and scar remodeling. The compressive dressing is removed after 48 to 72 hours. Once the inflammation of surgery begins to subside and before collagen appears, the patient should begin motion (oral nonsteroidal anti-inflammatory drugs are helpful). This consists of passively flexing and extending the PIP joint a few times every 30 minutes while awake and allowing active motion. One progresses to dynamic splinting, both in flexion and extension. The objective is to move the joint through the range of motion that was achieved at surgery, recognizing that this will be difficult to completely accomplish because of the limitations of pain and swelling. Various compressive mechanisms, such as a pneumatic sleeve, elastic wraps, and active and passive flexion of the digit can be helpful in speeding the resolution of edema. Further therapy is guided by the patient's response during the period of fibroplasia. Care should be taken not to further inflame the joint by overwork in the early postoperative period.

■ REHABILITATION

It is important to continue therapy during the period of fibroplasia (4 to 6 weeks) and to measure and record the patient's progress frequently. Splinting can be adjusted if the joint tends too much either toward flexion or extension.

After 6 weeks, swelling and pain should be substantially less, and the patient should move progressively through light activity to further activities of daily living. Lastly, from 3 to 6 months, strengthening exercises are added.

The final outcome depends on careful patient selection, precise and gentle surgery, and diligent postoperative therapy. The therapy program is critical and may be supervised either by the surgeon or a trained hand therapist. The patient must understand the procedure that has been performed and must ultimately perform the exercises that will determine the degree of obtainable improvement.

■ OUTCOMES

The degree of improvement varies with etiology.[7,8,11] Burns, crush injuries, and PIP joint fractures gain less motion after capsulectomy than do nerve injuries and distant trauma.[7,11] Joints stiff in extension fare better than those with flexion contractures. Harrison found that 72% of 30 joint studies gained over 20° of motion and 36% gained over 40° after capsulectomy.[8] The average gain for extension contractures was 55°, but for flexion contractures the gain was only 24°. Sprague noted that patients retained only 40% of the motion gained at operation and this figure decreased as more complex surgery was required.[11] Weeks and co-authors[13] found that 87% of an unselected group of patients with joint stiffness gained 30° to 40° *without surgery*, emphasizing the value of hand therapy.

The very best reported results for extension contractures are those of Curtis.[4] The average gain in flexion of 125 joints in 100 patients undergoing capsulectomy was 50°, a testament to both his surgical skill and postoperative management.

The normal PIP joint can move easily from 0° to 110°. An excellent surgical result is one that achieves 70° to 80° of painless motion in the functional range (i.e., lacking no more than 15° or 20° of extension and 15° or 20° of flexion).

Trauma to the PIP joint often leaves residual stiffness and incomplete motion. An appreciation of joint mechanics and selective surgical removal or release of specific anatomic structures, as described for both extension and flexion contractness, can lessen these deformities and improve overall function.

References

1. Bowers WH: Injuries and complications of injuries to the capsular structures of the interphalangeal joints. In: Bowers WH (ed): The Hand and Upper Limb, Volume I—The Interphalangeal Joints. Edinburgh: Churchill Livingstone, 1987:56–76.

2. Curtis RM: Capsulectomy of the interphalangeal joints of the fingers. J Bone Joint Surg, 1954; 36A:1219–1232.

3. Curtis RM: Stiff finger joints. In: Grabb WC and Smith JW (eds): Plastic Surgery, 3rd Ed, Boston: Little Brown & Co., 1979:598–603.

4. Curtis RM: The interphalangeal joints. In: Tubiana R (ed): The Hand, Vol. II, Philadelphia: WB Saunders Company, 1985:1054–1064.

5. Diao E, Eaton RG: Total collateral ligament excision for contractures of the proximal interphalangeal joint. Hand Surg, 1993; 18A:395–402.

6. Gorman RJ: Metacarpal and proximal interphalangeal joint capsulectomy. In: Clark GL, Wilgis EFS, Aiello B, Eckhaus D, Eddington LV (eds): Hand Rehabilitation: A Practical Guide, New York: Churchill Livingstone, 1993:287–296.

7. Gould JS, Nicholson BG: Capsulectomy of the metacarpophalangeal and proximal interphalangeal joints. J Hand Surg, 1979; 4:482–486.

8. Harrison DH: The stiff proximal interphalangeal joint. Hand, 1977; 9:102–108.

9. Jabaley ME: Electrical nerve stimulation in the awake patient. Bulletin of the Hospital for Joint Diseases Orthopaedic Institute, 1984; 44:248–259.

10. Kuczynski K: Less-known aspects of the proximal interphalangeal joints of the human hand. Hand, 1975; 7:31–33.

11. Sprague BL: Proximal interphalangeal joint contractures and their treatment. J Trauma, 1976; 16:259–265.

12. Watson HK, Light TR, Johnson TR: Checkrein resection for flexion contracture of the middle joint. J Hand Surg, 1979; 4:67–71.

13. Weeks P, Wray RC Jr, Kuxhaus M: The results of nonoperative management of stiff joints in the hand. Plas Reconstr Surg, 1978; 61:58–63.

115

Volar Plate Arthroplasty of the Proximal Interphalangeal Joint

It has long been recognized that fracture–dislocations of the proximal interphalangeal (PIP) joint carry the potential for producing major finger disabilities. The earliest published methods of treatment involved traction techniques,[11,16] which addressed the problems of reduction but left accurate articular restoration somewhat to chance. There are no published long-term results of these early traction techniques.

Open reduction has likewise been advocated,[6,8,14,17] attempting to restore, by direct manipulation, the comminuted volar articular surface of the middle phalanx. Results of these open procedures depend largely on the size of the fragments and the degree of comminution.

Agee, in 1978, introduced an ingenious force-couple device requiring percutaneous insertion of K-wires and having a dynamic reduction moment.[1] In theory, this force-couple, when constructed in perfect alignment, should maintain reduction and permit immediate motion. Even so, it also fails to ensure anatomic restoration of comminuted and depressed articular fragments.

In 1967, advancement of the volar plate to resurface a defect representing 50% of the articular surface of an acute fracture–dislocation of the middle phalanx was successfully accomplished.[3] This technique also serves to maintain a stable reduction of the middle phalanx. Results of 10 years' experience with this technique were published in 1980.[4] Since that time, the indications for the volar plate advancement arthroplasty have gradually expanded to include even osteoarthritic PIP joints.

The rationale for the volar plate advancement arthroplasty is easily explained. Comminuted and irreducible dorsal fracture dislocations of the middle phalanx create two problems. The first is mechanical, due to disruption of the arcuate contour of the volar lip of the middle phalanx as well as the volar plate insertion to the middle phalanx.[2] The second is articular, because there is a major disruption or impaction of the volar articular surface of the middle phalanx. Volar plate advancement specifically corrects each of these problems. The most significant feature of this advancement–arthroplasty is the resurfacing of the severely damaged articular surface with a vascularized fibrocartilage pedicle.

■ HISTORY OF THE TECHNIQUE

Volar plate arthroplasty is particularly well suited for acute and chronic fracture dislocations involving more than 40% of the articular surface of the middle phalanx (Fig. 115–1). Likewise, it is effective for acute or chronic intra-articular fractures of the middle phalanx that are not subluxed but have a depressed or impacted central segment (Fig. 115–2). Last, the resurfacing provided by volar plate advancement can be used for patients with traumatic or degenerative arthritis, provided that the middle phalangeal condyle remains intact as a concentric arc in the lateral radiograph.

This same advancement principle may also be applied to other intra-articular acute or reconstruction problems. One variation involves resurfacing a single proximal condyle by advancing the appropriate half of the volar plate. Another modification is advancement of the volar plate for a fracture dislocation of the distal phalanx of the thumb.

Volar plate arthroplasty is contraindicated for fracture dislocations in which lateral angulation is greater than 20° across the fracture site or for a fracture dislocation with an accompanying fracture through the metaphysis of the middle phalanx. In this combination,

■ INDICATIONS AND CONTRAINDICATIONS

■ FIGURE 115–1
Radiograph of an acute fracture–dislocation of the PIP joint with disruption of more than 40% of the middle phalanx volar articular surface.

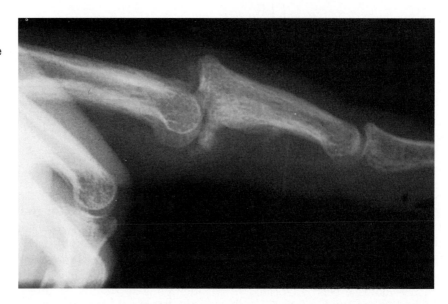

■ FIGURE 115–2
Radiograph of an impacted intra-articular fracture of the middle phalanx. Note the central subchondral fragments embedded within the metaphysis. Figure 115–4 shows an intraoperative view of these articular surfaces.

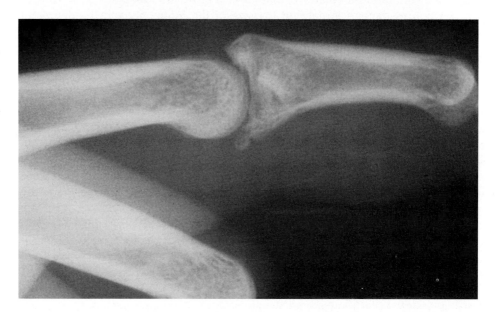

one would primarily reduce and fix the metaphyseal fracture, performing a volar plate arthroplasty once healing had occurred and solid bone stock had been restored. Extensive damage or fibrosis of the extensor mechanism accompanying the fracture–dislocation is also a contraindication, as are fracture–dislocations with an accompanying displaced fracture of the proximal phalangeal condyle. In patients with degenerative arthritis, loss of the concentric arc contour of the condyle of the proximal phalanx would be a contraindication to the volar plate arthroplasty.

A relative contraindication to this arthroplasty would be a situation in which the surgeon has a limited knowledge of PIP joint anatomy and minimal experience with the specific details of this technically demanding procedure.

■ SURGICAL TECHNIQUES

The incision is a volar "V" incision centered on the PIP flexion crease.[3,7] The flexor sheath between the A2 and A4 pulleys is resected. The neurovascular bundles should be mobilized at least 1.5 cm proximal and distal to the PIP joint. Both flexor tendons are retracted by passing a soft rubber drain between the volar plate and the superficialis tendon, permitting the volar plate and volar portions of the collateral ligament to be clearly

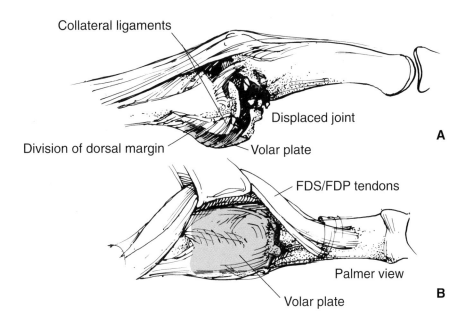

Collateral ligaments

Division of dorsal margin

Displaced joint

Volar plate

A

FDS/FDP tendons

Palmer view

Volar plate

B

■ FIGURE 115–3
(A) Schema of the anatomic disruption that oc-
curs with displacement.
Joint exposure is
achieved by dividing the
longitudinal collateral ligament insertion into the
dorsal margin of the
plate. FDS, flexor dig-
itorum superficialis; FDP,
flexor digitorum profun-
dus. **(B)** The ligament incision is continuous with
the transverse disruption
of the distal insertion.

visualized. The longitudinal insertion of the collateral ligament into the dorsal margin of the volar plate is incised along the radial and ulnar margins (Fig. 115–3A). The incision is connected distally by a transverse incision across the volar periosteum of the middle phalanx, if it is not already disrupted, or to the insertion of the flexor digitorum superficialis tendon in late, healed cases. The entire width of the volar plate or the volar periosteum must be incised to create a rectangular, proximally based fibrocartilaginous flap, hinged on the proximal check ligaments (Fig. 115–3B). In acute injuries, the attached fragments of the middle phalanx articular cartilage and subcondylar bone are conservatively debrided.

The collateral ligaments are incised at the joint line, permitting the joint to be maximally hyperextended to expose fully the condyles of the proximal phalanx and the base of the middle phalanx. The exposure is similar to that of opening a shotgun to load it. With this exposure, the condyles and the disrupted middle phalanx articular surface are aligned in a single plane (Fig. 115–4). The full width of each collateral ligament, from volar to dorsal, must be incised to accomplish this maneuver. All of the collateral ligament attaching to the proximal condyle is then completely excised. The distal collateral ligament is also excised except for a 3-mm tag (Fig. 115–4, arrow), which will subsequently serve as a lateral mooring to suture the margins of the advanced volar plate.

In the hyperextended "shotgun" position, the damage can be accurately evaluated. The disrupted volar one half or two thirds of the articular surface of the middle phalanx is conservatively debrided to accommodate the 3-mm thickness of the volar plate as it is advanced to replace the disrupted articular surface. Even impacted fragments can be retained as long as no portion encroaches on the space being created for the advanced volar plate.

When an angular deformity is present, due to an asymmetric impaction of the articular cartilage, additional debridement of the less impacted (more normal) facet must be done to realign the middle phalanx. This trough or volar depression should be created perpendicular to the long axis of the middle phalanx to restore alignment across the joint. It is not possible to correct angular deformities much greater than 20°. In such situations, the aligning maneuver as described can be done, and the volar plate arthroplasty performed, in the expectation of doing a corrective osteotomy across the base of the middle phalanx 6 to 10 months later, when volar plate motion has begun to plateau and when the local tissue reaction has returned to normal.

With the collateral ligaments removed, the joint should reduce easily and achieve full

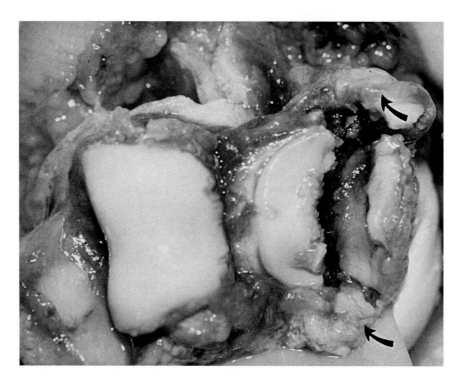

■ FIGURE 115–4
The "shotgun" exposure, obtained through hyperextension of the joint. Only the dorsal capsule remains in continuity, like the binding of an open book. The volar plate lies to the left. The central articular fragment is deeply depressed. This displacement can be predicted by careful evaluation of the preoperative radiograph (see Fig. 115–2). The dorsal condyle is scored by the intact dorsal edge of the middle phalanx. An arrow marks the distal tag of the ligament.

passive flexion. After prolonged subluxation, however, the dorsal capsule and extensor mechanism become inelastic and may restrain full flexion. Full passive flexion should be done gently to stretch rather than tear the dorsal capsule and central portion of the extensor mechanism. Excessive force can produce a dehiscence of this complex mechanism, leading to a mild boutonnière deformity and some loss of active extension after surgery.

In patients undergoing late reconstruction who have varying degrees of healing of the impacted volar articular surface, superficial debridement to a depth of 2 to 3 mm must be done to prepare a bed to accommodate the volar plate. The volar 50 to 60% of the middle phalanx surface should be prepared in this fashion. Cadaver studies have shown that the dorsal 30 to 40% of the middle phalanx surface bears little of the compressive forces across the PIP joint, and thus does not need the same perfect resurfacing as does the volar 60%.[12] As long as this segment is intact and in continuity with the dorsal cortex and extensor tendon insertion, volar plate advancement can be performed.

Using a double-ended, 3-0 monofilament nonabsorbable suture, a lateral trap or spiral (baseball) suture is placed along the lateral margins of the volar plate. The two free ends should emerge from each distal corner of the plate. A Keith needle is then drilled from each dorsolateral corner of the previously prepared depression in the middle phalanx (Fig. 115–5), with the needle directed to emerge on the mid-dorsum of the middle phalanx. The distal interphalangeal (DIP) joint should be flexed 15 to 20° as the needle penetrates the extensor tendon, to prevent tethering of the DIP in full extension.

The middle phalanx is then reduced and flexed 70 to 80° as traction is applied on the volar plate fixation sutures, which now emerge on the dorsum of the middle phalanx. They are tied down over a button. The first knot is a surgeon's knot to stabilize this tension while the volar plate is visualized to verify full advancement into the joint. When satisfied that the plate is fully advanced, the final ties are completed (Fig. 115–6). At this point, a

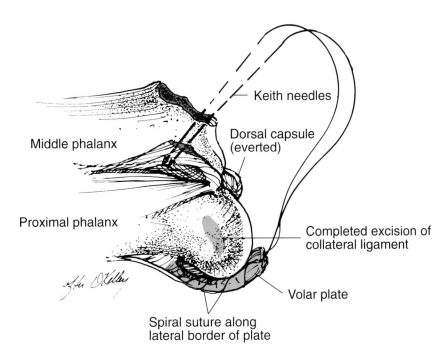

■ FIGURE 115–5
Schema of the suture placement. The Keith needles are drilled as dorsally and laterally as possible in the prepared depression.

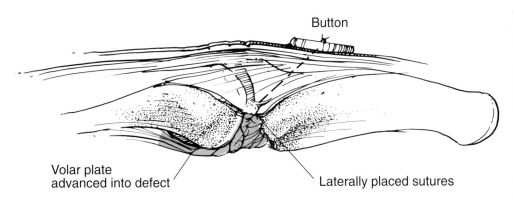

■ FIGURE 115–6
Advancement of the volar plate into the defect. The plate is stretched around the concentric curve of the condyle on which it will subsequently glide. A suture is placed to secure each lateral margin to the tag of distal ligament to stretch the plate laterally and to further secure the advancement.

lateral radiograph should be obtained to confirm complete and congruous reduction. With the PIP joint securely reduced, it should then be extended as far as possible. With the joint in maximum passive extension, the proximal check ligaments, both radial and ulnar, are fractionally lengthened by teasing the tight fibers gently until the PIP joint is fully extended (Fig. 115–7).

To maintain reduction in optimal extension during the 3 weeks of immobilization, a Kirschner wire is passed across the PIP joint in 15 to 20° of flexion. The volar plate is further secured as well as stretched laterally by suturing each lateral margin to the tag of collateral ligament preserved at the base of the middle phalanx. This suture also serves as a back-up in the event that the pull-out suture ruptures. After skin closure, a well padded cast is applied, incorporating an adjacent digit. The distal joint is left free.

Many alternate techniques for reducing PIP dislocation and restoring the comminuted articular surface have been proposed. Nonoperative treatment of PIP fracture–dislocations is an alternative to surgical treatment and has numerous advocates. It is important in evaluating results of such treatment, however, to distinguish between fractures that involve more from those that involve less than 40% of the articular surface of the middle phalanx. Fractures involving less than 40% are usually stable and congruous once reduced,

■ TECHNICAL ALTERNATIVES

■ FIGURE 115-7
(A) The joint is extended with gentle teasing of the check ligaments until full extension is achieved. **(B)** Fractional incisions in the cord-like check ligaments produce lengthening without loss of continuity.

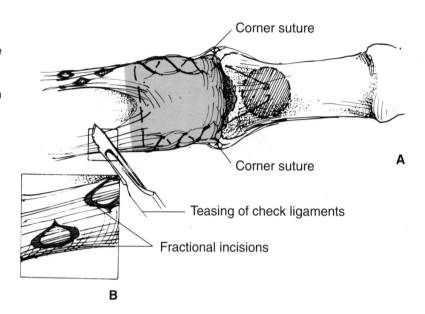

Corner suture

Corner suture

A

Teasing of check ligaments

Fractional incisions

B

and have a good to excellent prognosis. Fractures involving more than 40 to 50% of the articular surface have lost, in addition, a significant portion of the collateral ligament insertion on the middle phalanx, and are therefore less stable as well as having articular irregularities. Extension block splinting is an excellent nonoperative technique for maintaining reduction while permitting sufficient motion to permit cartilage healing[9] via the continuous motion principle. It is less effective, however, for fractures involving more than 40% of the articular surface, even if a fairly congruous reduction can be maintained.

Open reduction has been suggested in the past and continues to be proposed, using some of the many highly sophisticated internal fixation techniques not previously available.[5,15] Complex dynamic traction devices have also been proposed.[13] Although reduction may be accomplished, anatomic restoration to a truly congruous articular surface is extremely difficult to achieve. Radiographic alignment does not accurately reflect the true condition of the articular surface; open reduction has significant limitations because many small fragments are impossible to replace. Furthermore, with open reduction most of the collateral ligament is left in place, making complete visualization and restoration of the damaged surfaces very difficult. Retaining damaged ligaments also permits fibrosis and restriction of the ultimate range of motion.

In patients with chronic fracture dislocations or osteoarthritis, alternate treatment would include PIP arthrodesis or silicone PIP arthroplasty. Arthrodesis provides stability and complete relief of pain at the cost of all movement through this central articulation. Silicone implant arthroplasty usually provides pain relief and moderate motion, but does not ensure lateral joint stability.[10] It is usually reserved for low-stress hands. The volar plate arthroplasty provides freedom from pain, excellent stability, and at least a functional range of motion.

In the surgical technique of volar plate arthroplasty, there are several technical omissions that must be avoided.

Incomplete exposure of both articular surfaces is one potential problem. The "shotgun" maneuver fully exposes both proximal and distal articular surfaces. With such exposure, the bed into which the volar plate is advanced can be most effectively prepared and drill holes more accurately placed. To achieve this exposure, both collateral ligaments must be divided and ultimately excised.

Failure to excise completely the collateral ligaments can also be a problem. Once the "shotgun" exposure has been achieved by sectioning both ligaments and hyperextending the joint, the proximal portion of the ligament must be completely excised. All but a 2-

to 3-mm slip of the distal insertion is also excised. This serves as a mooring for an anchoring suture for the fully advanced volar plate. Retained portions of the damaged collateral ligaments appear to produce an intense fibrous reaction that serves to inhibit final range of motion. Postoperative instability has not occurred because new ligaments apparently develop and are palpable within 4 to 6 weeks.

Failure to obtain a reduction and complete passive flexion of the middle phalanx can prevent eventual recovery of full active flexion. Once the collateral ligaments are excised, the joint must be gently reduced and fully flexed. The dorsal capsule and extensor mechanism may become taut or shortened as a result of protracted dorsal dislocation. If these structures are not stretched to full length, it is difficult to obtain full postoperative flexion despite an apparent congruous reduction.

Failure to achieve full passive extension after volar plate advancement can prevent eventual, full active extension. A complete fractional lengthening or teasing of the proximal check ligaments of the volar plate is easily accomplished once the plate has been fully advanced and sutured. These tough cords are teased as the PIP joint is gently extended to neutral.

The cast and Kirschner wire are both removed at 3 weeks and an extension block splint in 20° of flexion is applied. Full active flexion within this range is encouraged. At 4 weeks, all daytime splinting is discontinued and a full active range of motion begun. Use of a static dorsal night splint in maximum passive extension is very helpful in preventing overnight finger flexion, which may contribute to a late loss of PIP extension.

By 5 weeks, if any extension lag remains, a dynamic outrigger extension splint should be applied. A schedule of 10 minutes progressing to 20 minutes of dynamic extension, three times daily, will improve extension rapidly. Excessive force or prolonged splinting, which may produce PIP swelling, should be avoided. A short course of systemic prednisone may be given if swelling persists much beyond 6 weeks. Full activity is encouraged at 6 weeks. A range of motion exercise program, however, should continue until motion is essentially normal, with improvement expected to continue up to at least 1 year after surgery.

■ REHABILITATION

The initial description of this procedure, with a 10-year follow-up, reported an average postoperative range of motion of 95° in patients undergoing surgery within 6 weeks of injury, and a 78° range in patients operated on 6 months to 2 years after injury.[4] In the earliest cases, it was noted that in patients whose collateral ligaments were not completely excised, the final range of motion was less than when complete excision was done. In the author's experience, the long-term results of this procedure remain as initially reported.

The fibrocartilaginous surface provided by the volar plate appears to wear quite well over time. Not infrequently, the defect in the volar base of the middle phalanx fills in with what appears radiographically to be trabecular and cortical bone with almost complete restoration of the outline of the base of the middle phalanx. The initial patient to undergo volar plate arthroplasty has been evaluated 20 years after surgery. He has maintained a 105° range of PIP motion and has no pain. Radiographs show a congruous but somewhat narrow joint space. One must indeed wonder if the same articular longevity is possible for patients having less-than-perfect resurfacing after open or distraction reduction of displaced intra-articular fractures.

Complications are quite rare. However, a full 110° range of motion is rarely achieved. When motion is restricted, it is more likely to be extension that is lost. Recurrent dorsal subluxation of the joint is quite rare in my experience, possibly owing to careful attention to regaining full passive flexion–extension at the time of surgery and the postoperative use of a longitudinal K-wire. When dorsal subluxation does occur, it can be corrected by closed reduction and pin fixation in a reduced 20° flexed position for an additional 2 weeks. Mobilization using an extension block splint for 3 to 4 weeks longer is likewise recommended.

Angular deformities may occur in patients who have more than 15° preoperative angula-

■ OUTCOMES

tion. In the rare occasion when this does occur, a corrective osteotomy through the metaphysis of the middle phalanx should be considered. Corrective osteotomy is not usually necessary unless the persisting angulation exceeds 15°. Intraoperative correction of angular deformities is discussed under Surgical Techniques. Rarely can preoperative angular deformities exceeding 20° be completely corrected.

The volar plate advancement arthroplasty in the author's experience has proved a most valuable procedure over the past 25 years. Although technically demanding, it is a procedure that with thoughtful and critical experience yields progressively more satisfactory results. The patient, however, often requires more than a year to reach final PIP joint active motion, and unless late evaluation is carried out, the surgeon may not appreciate the ultimate effect of his or her labors. It is absolutely essential that in performing the first few volar plate arthroplasties, the surgeon follow the described technique to the last detail, because it represents the culmination of the author's highly critical trial-and-error evaluation over 25 years. Undoubtedly, improvements are possible, but the present technique should not be varied until a solid clinical experience with this time-proven technique has been achieved.

References

1. Agee JM: Unstable fracture dislocations of the proximal interphalangeal joint: Treatment with a force couple splint. Clin Orthop, 1987; 214:101–112.
2. Bowers WH, Wolf JW, Nehil JL, Bittinger S: The proximal interphalangeal joint volar plate: I. An anatomical and biomechanical study. J Hand Surg, 1980; 5:79–88.
3. Eaton RG: Joint Injuries of the Hand. Springfield, IL: Charles C Thomas, 1971.
4. Eaton RG, Malerich MW: Volar plate arthroplasty of the proximal interphalangeal joint: A review of 10 years' experience. J Hand Surg, 1980; 5:260–268.
5. Hastings H II, Carrol C IV: Treatment of closed articular fractures of the metacarpophalangeal and proximal interphalangeal joints. Hand Clin, 1988; 4:503–527.
6. Lee MLH: Intra-articular and peri-articular fractures of phalanges. J Bone Joint Surg, 1963; 45B:103–107.
7. Littler JW: The extremities. In: Cooper P (ed): The Craft of Surgery. Boston: Little, Brown, & Co., 1965.
8. McCue FC, Honner R, Johnson MC, Gieck JH: Athletic injuries of the proximal interphalangeal joint requiring surgical treatment. J Bone Joint Surg, 1970; 52A:937–956.
9. McElfresh EC, Dobyns JH, O'Brien ET: Management of fracture–dislocation of the proximal interphalangeal joints by extension-block splinting. J Bone Joint Surg, 1972; 54A:1705–1711.
10. Pelligrini VD, Burton RI: Osteoarthritis of the proximal interphalangeal joint of the hand: Arthroplasty or fusion? J Hand Surg, 1990; 15A:194–209.
11. Robertson RC, Cawley JJ, Faris AM: Treatment of fracture–dislocation of the interphalangeal joints of the hand. J Bone Joint Surg, 1946; 28:68–70.
12. Scarangella SF, Klein MJ, Eaton RG: Analysis of proximal interphalangeal joint wear patterns with aging using a human cadaver model. New York Society for Surgery of the Hand Residence Program, June, 1992.
13. Schenck RR: Dynamic traction and early passive movement for fractures of the proximal interphalangeal joint. J Hand Surg, 1986; 11A:850–858.
14. Stark HH: Use of internal fixation for closed fractures of the phalanges and metacarpals. J Bone Joint Surg, 1966; 46A:1365.
15. Stern PJ, Roman RJ, Kiefhaber TR, McDonough JJ: Pilon fractures of the proximal interphalangeal joint. J Hand Surg, 1991; 16A:844–850.
16. Wantabe K, Wataya S, Saito T: Skeletal traction in old fracture dislocations of the interphalangeal joint of the fingers. J Bone Joint Surg, 1964; 46A:214.
17. Wilson JN, Rowland SA: Fracture–dislocation of the proximal interphalangeal joint of the finger. J Bone Joint Surg, 1966; 48A:493–502.

LEONARD S. BODELL
MARC E. GOTTLIEB

116

Dorsal Capsulectomy of the Metacarpophalangeal Joint

Metacarpophalangeal (MP) joint dorsal capsulectomy is a surgical procedure used to treat patients with disabling contractures.[1,7,11,15] The causes of joint, and in particular, MP stiffness and contractures are numerous. Almost any form of direct trauma resulting in structural pathology in and about the joint or indirect trauma resulting in an inflammatory response can be causative.[11] Systemic conditions, such as diabetes, Dupuytren disease, multiple trauma, infections, underlying arthritis, substance abuse, seizure disorders, or use of immune-altering drugs add to a specific patient's risk or predisposition to development of MP joint contracture. Because limitation of range of motion can pose a major impairment to hand function,[12] efforts to understand its evolution, methods of prevention, and treatment options are essential to treating patients with these hand problems.

An understanding of MP joint anatomy is necessary for performing this operation. The MP joints of the fingers are best viewed as two-axis joints, with their centers lying in the metacarpal head.[3] This concept, when applied to a metacarpal head that is wider volarly than dorsally, explains the observed normal biomechanics as well as the typical extension contracture that is seen after trauma.[2,3,20] In the normal state, the MP joint is capable of abduction–adduction while in extension, but only a small amount of rotation occurs in the flexed position.[3] The thick, more dorsal, quadrangle-shaped portion of the collateral ligament, which stretches from the subcapital depression on the metacarpal head to the lateral tubercle of the proximal phalangeal base, becomes increasingly taut as the MP joint is flexed to 70°. The volar portion, sometimes called the accessory portion of the collateral ligament, or, as described by Flatt and Fischer, the metacarpal glenoid ligament, is typically taut in extension and hyperextension and lax in the flexed position of the MP joint.[9]

The joint contact surfaces are larger in flexion and, conversely, the intracapsular space available for fluid or synovial inflammation is greatest in extension. In addition, the volar plate, consisting of many crisscross collagen fibers, is highly compressible and uncommonly associated with fibrosis.[19]

Trauma, immobilization, and some systemic conditions can result in dynamic changes that effectively increase fluid within the capsule, collateral ligaments, and joints.[9] Alteration of the viscoelastic properties, development of adhesions about the synovial folds, and proliferations of fibrofatty tissue all force the MP joint into the position best able to accommodate these changes, and that is extension! Long-term capsular and collateral ligament thickening and contracture become fixed and may extend to involve the dorsal tendon and hood mechanisms, with development of tendon adhesions. Arthrofibrosis and ultimately cartilage atrophy with surface irregularities can result in a painful, deformed, and arthritic joint for which only a salvage fusion or arthroplasty procedure may prove helpful.[7,8,11,16]

As Curtis has pointed out, there are a number of anatomic factors specific to the MP joint that may limit flexion.[7] These can include: 1) scarring, contracture, or inadequacy of dorsal skin in patients with burns over the dorsum of the hand, particularly where the hand has been immobilized in a position of MP extension; 2) dorsal tendon and extensor hood adhesions, which can be the result of underlying bony injury or soft tissue responses to trauma, such as the deposition of edema fluid with subsequent fibrosis; 3) thickening and contracture of the dorsal capsule and the main portion of the collateral ligaments,

■ HISTORY OF THE
TECHNIQUE

usually a result of the accumulation of edema fluid resulting in soft tissue fibrosis; and 4) bony deformity, which can be the result of malunion of intra-articular or extra-articular fractures of the metacarpals. An example would include transverse fractures healing with an apex dorsal deformity. Additional factors include intra-articular bony blocks associated with osteophyte formation and intra-articular calcifications associated with chronic disease states.

Dr. R. M. Curtis is given credit for popularizing the surgical approach and treatment program for the management of MP extension contractions. Although his name is intimately attached to the procedure at the proximal interphalangeal (PIP) joint, it is equally appropriate to credit him for soft tissue procedures for contractures at the MP joint. Dr. Curtis described using individual linear incisions over the MP joints, splitting the extensor tendons longitudinally, retracting and reflecting them to either the radial or ulnar side as necessary, incising or resecting the dorsal capsule, and then removing only that portion of the dorsal aspect of the collateral ligament necessary to gain release of the joint. He made a particular point to maintain the volar attachment so as to maintain joint stability and normal gliding flexion of the joint. His work is in part based on some earlier clinical work done by Bunnell, Doherty, and Curtis that was published in *Plastic and Reconstructive Surgery* in 1948.[5] One year earlier, Dr. S. B. Fowler published in the *Journal of Bone and Joint Surgery* his concepts of joint mobilization.[10] There have been few articles on this procedure since Dr. Curtis' publication. Kirk Watson has described in brief his technique modifications, and Buch published a report on use of a transverse incision and preservation of the tendons.[4,18] Tsuge[17] in his atlas has described a technique that basically is that of Curtis'. This, in our opinion, reflects the general high level of success of this procedure based on the concepts and understanding of the anatomy, proper patient selection, and good postoperative therapy.

■ INDICATIONS AND CONTRAINDICATIONS

Dorsal capsulectomy should be reserved for patients with functional disability resulting from extension contracture of the MP joint in one or more fingers. The operation is rarely indicated for an isolated index finger contracture when 30° or more of flexion is present. Patients with index finger and middle finger flexion to less than 30° and ring finger and little finger flexion to less than 50° are candidates for this procedure. The presence of skin involvement that would require grafts and flaps, neurovascular status, hand dominance, presence of other deformities, and dysfunction in other joints must be considered as well. The patient's motivation, present work status, and life goals round out the issues that must be considered before proceeding with surgery.

Although we could find no review indicating that arthritic changes are a contraindication to this type of surgery, our experience suggests that dorsal capsulectomies on MP joints with changes greater than Larson type III[13] result in poor outcomes without improvement in range of motion. The presence of diabetes, Dupuytren diathesis, scleroderma, systemic lupus erythematosus, psoriatic arthritis, and other conditions (Fig. 116–1) requires an understanding of the altered or exaggerated responses possible when performing surgical procedures (including the increased risk of reflex sympathetic dystrophy), and represent modifications for the indications to surgery.

Dorsal capsulectomy with or without release of the collateral ligaments as an isolated procedure cannot effectively improve range of motion in the face of fixed bony deformities, either intra-articular or extra-articular. Therefore, it is essential that the nature of these deformities be assessed and that they be treated in conjunction with the soft tissue procedure. As an example, it may be necessary to perform a corrective metacarpal osteotomy, fixing the osteotomy site with rigid fixation techniques, then performing the dorsal capsulectomy and collateral ligament release at the same time. If this cannot be effectively accomplished at one surgical procedure, then it would be better, in our opinion, to perform the corrective bony surgery first and do the soft tissue releases at a second stage.

Consideration of indications for this operation should include comments about prevention, which is certainly the best treatment we can offer a patient. In principle, therefore, if a contracture in the early stages after trauma is showing evidence of progressive improvement and is responding to conservative treatment, operations should be delayed.

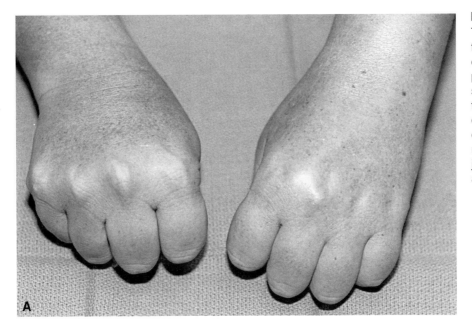

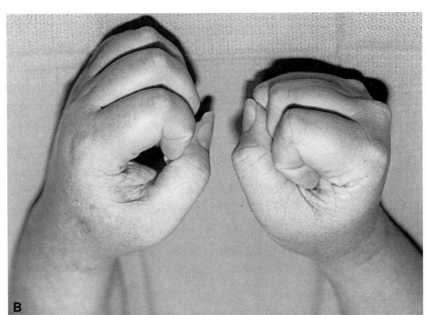

■ FIGURE 116–1
This patient had a Colles fracture treated with an external fixator. She experienced post-traumatic swelling of the dorsum of the hand **(A)**, and initial difficulty in performing digit flexion activities **(B)**, resulting in limited MP joint flexion many months after the fracture healed.

However, it is probably counterproductive to continue therapy in a patient with a fixed contracture that is failing to demonstrate improvement much beyond 8 weeks.

This procedure is most often performed on an outpatient basis. If indicated from the medical history, appropriate medical preoperative clearance and testing should be performed. Dorsal capsulectomy can effectively be done under either Bier block or axillary block, although both the patient and the anesthesiologist often prefer general anesthetic over regional blocks. The one limitation to the Bier block is that the anesthesia is lost relatively rapidly once the tourniquet comes down, necessitating either local supplementation or not releasing the tourniquet until after final dressing application. We prefer not to let the tourniquet down before closure, but this is a personal preference. We find that when the tourniquet is let down, there frequently are edematous changes within the tissues that make closure and reconstruction difficult. One way to avoid this is to complete all of the reconstruction, let the tourniquet down, and establish hemostasis; essentially all

■ SURGICAL
TECHNIQUES

that is then left to do is close the skin. We avoid local anesthesia as a primary method, especially if multiple digits are to be operated on, and find that even with a forearm tourniquet, our patients do not tolerate the tourniquet times necessary to perform some of the more extensive operative procedures.

The choice of incision depends on the number of MP joints being released and the quality of the dorsal skin. If only one digit is involved, we prefer a dorsal longitudinal incision centered over the MP joint. It affords good exposure to the dorsal tendon and can be lengthened or altered to permit local flap closure if necessary. When operating on two adjacent digits, a single longitudinal incision placed between the metacarpals will often suffice, but only in milder forms where there is good skin quality. In more severe contractures, or when performing surgery on three or four MP joints, our preference is a standard dorsal transverse incision located just proximal to the metacarpal heads. Through this approach, we can atraumatically elevate skin flaps proximally and distally, exposing the extensor tendons to perform tenolysis if needed. This approach provides adequate visualization of the dorsal capsule, collateral ligaments, lateral bands, and volar structures through the joint. The transverse incision allows visualization, as well, of the dorsal neurovascular structures, permitting their atraumatic retraction and protection. This approach is cosmetic and permits placement of skin grafts when necessary.

After incising the skin, there may be marked dermal fibrosis and difficulty identifying clean tissue planes. In cases of contracture secondary to nerve injury, or in association with systemic conditions such as reflex sympathetic dystrophy or steroid dependence, skin and subcutaneous tissue atrophy is not uncommon. In cases of burn contracture, the skin contracture, in contrast to the joint capsule and ligament, may be the limiting factor to motion, and an accurate preoperative plan to deal with the possibility of a large graft or flap coverage should be devised. As the deeper layers are approached, longitudinally directed veins are typically encountered in the interosseous gutters. The terminal branches of the dorsal nerves should be looked for and protected, particularly on the radial side of the index finger and ulnar side of the little finger. At this point, the dorsal tendons are clearly in view. Rarely will these tendons be subluxed into the ulnar gutter. We prefer initially to elevate the sagittal bands from the underlying joint capsule and retract them distally (Fig. 116–2). Using a small Cottle or Freer elevator, we gently lyse any adhesions at this stage and assess the excursion of the extensor tendons. In milder cases, a transverse dorsal capsulotomy can be performed where the capsule reflects off the dorsal distal metacarpal. The incision should extend across the metacarpal head to the origins of the thick quadrangular portion of the collateral ligaments. In many cases, full 90° of motion can be obtained. Using a short-handled small Smilie-type beaver blade (#9082) often facilitates the dorsal capsulotomy through this limited exposure. Care should be taken to be certain that the resulting motion is flexion and gliding, and not hinging like a book. An intraoperative fluoroscope can save time and assist in assessment if there is any uncertainty.

When the capsule is thickened or associated with surface irregularities and inflammation, we believe capsulectomy should be performed using an alternative method. When operating on joints with severe or long-standing contracture, sufficient exposure often requires incision of the sagittal bands. We have found this uniformly to be the situation if active and passive range of motion is less than 20° of flexion and the condition is present for more than 6 months. On exposing the joint by retracting the dorsal tendon, the tightness of the capsule and collateral ligament is usually apparent. Dorsal capsulotomy is performed as previously described. We have performed a complete dorsal capsulectomy, when leaving the capsule would leave a tissue flap that could interpose into the joint. We also believe a capsule that is markedly thickened, fibrotic, and associated with synovial reaction requires excision. Again, at this point, flexion of the joint should be attempted. If flexion is incomplete, we place a probe in the volar recess and release any adhesions about the volar plate. Flexion is attempted once again, but most often in the moderate to severe cases the collateral ligaments have thickened and shortened and cannot clear the wider volar area of the metacarpal head. A stepwise release of both the ulnar and radial collateral ligament is performed at their origin on the metacarpal neck until gliding flexion through a full range of motion can easily be obtained. It is important to make certain that normal gliding-type flexion and extension occurs, and that this motion can be reproduced

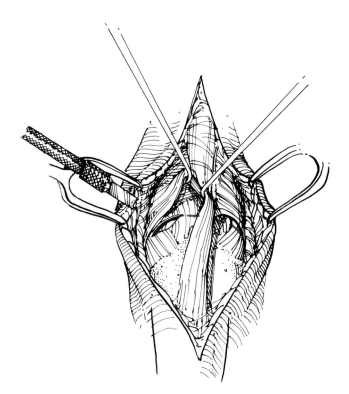

A dorsal view demonstrating a limited longitudinal exposure that allows performance of a capsulotomy and release of the collateral ligaments.

when the dorsal apparatus is repositioned. It is rarely necessary to lengthen the tendon in our experience. When indicated, we perform a stepcut proximal to the sagittal bands and repair the tendon with 3-0 or 4-0 nonabsorbable suture. The sagittal bands must be repaired to the tendon, and for this we use an absorbable monocryl suture, size 3-0 or 4-0, depending on the size of the hand and tissue quality. We have not noticed any untoward reactions with the use of absorbable suture in this operation.

Before skin closure, motion and joint balance are reassessed and documented. The tourniquet can be released electively at this time and hemostasis confirmed and secured with cautery. Closure is performed with 4-0 or 5-0 absorbable suture for the subcutaneous layer and 5-0 nylon on skin. During the course of the procedure, and on closure, the wounds are copiously irrigated with an antibiotic solution. On closure, we usually use one or two small polyethylene tubes (#7522). For dressing, we use a #40 fine-mesh gauze wrapped over a thin layer of sheet cotton which is first soaked in antibiotic irrigation solution (a dressing the senior author learned from Dr. James Dobyns). The moist cotton acts as a wick, drawing out excess blood. The remainder of the dressing includes Kerlex fluffs to increase the relative anterior–posterior diameter of the hand. The MP joints are placed in 70° of flexion, and outer rolls of Kerlex, soft roll, and plaster strips to maintain position are followed by bias stockinette to complete the dressing. The patient is advised to keep the hand at heart level and every few hours flex the fingers into the soft palmar part of the dressing. If skin grafts are used and there are other soft tissue concerns, dressings can remain in place up to 10 days. Typically, the patient is reevaluated at approximately 48 hours and therapy initiated.

Tsuge[17] has presented a technique that is essentially that described by Dr. Ray Curtis.[7] Curtis' technique for the MP joint release is a modification of his somewhat better known arthroplasty technique for PIP joint contractures.[6] His method uses longitudinal incisions for each digit and then does a tendon-splitting incision followed by a capsulectomy and sectioning of the "cord-like" portion of the collateral ligament, which is excised only near the tubercle of the metacarpal head. This is obviously an excellent technique that has been used for many years. Its limitations are that four incisions are used instead of one and it

■ TECHNICAL ALTERNATIVES

■ FIGURE 116-3
A lateral view showing instrument placement for
lysis of adhesions in the
volar pouch.

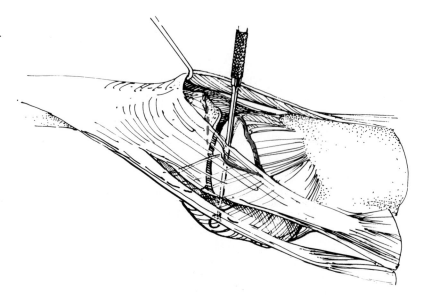

■ FIGURE 116-3
A lateral view showing instrument placement for lysis of adhesions in the volar pouch.

is inflexible relative to skin grafting. The transverse incision for this particular procedure, in our opinion, affords greater flexibility and is a better choice when more complex surgical reconstruction such as skin grafting or flaps are required. We prefer incising the sagittal band when a greater degree of exposure is necessary, rather than splitting the tendon. There are fewer postoperative adhesions, and cutting the ulnar side facilitates centralization in cases in which the dorsal tendon has a tendency to sublux ulnarward in flexion (Fig. 116-3). One of the potential complications with tendon splitting is alluded to by Curtis when he suggests that finger flexion should be initiated early but not to such an extent that the repaired tendon splits open over the metacarpal head.[7] In addition, fascial grafts, synovial or dermal tissue for capsule reconstruction, lengthening of collateral ligaments, or reefing of the sagittal bands can be performed as additional procedures.

Technically, it is important to release all tight structures. We have not found step-cut lengthening or grafting to lengthen the collateral ligaments necessary. It is important to be conservative when releasing the collateral ligaments and only release the amount necessary to restore joint motion while preserving stability. It is important to incise as much of the thick or main portion of the collateral ligament as necessary to gain full motion, but the ligament attachment distally should be preserved to help ensure maintenance of proper joint mechanics.[7] Limited resection of the redundant thick component of the collateral ligament should be done close to the metacarpal recess. Preservation of the continuity of the metacarpoglenoidal (accessory) portion of the collateral ligament is important to the stability of the MP joint and thus the success of this operation.

The therapist must be familiar with the extent of the surgery. A program that is too aggressive could cause tendon rupture, splitting of the extensor tendon if a tendon-splitting incision was used,[7] and joint synovial reaction with effusion and wound healing problems. Insufficient therapy or inappropriate splints might facilitate recurrence of deformity.

■ REHABILITATION

After capsulotomy or capsulectomy and partial collateral ligament release, splinting in 70 to 90° flexion and active assistive range of motion can be initiated at the first dressing change. A home program of 5 minutes of exercise every 2 hours while awake is recommended for cooperative patients. If tendon lengthening was required, only passive motion into extension is permitted for 4 weeks. Where minimal soft tissue work was performed, active range of motion is allowed at 1 to 2 weeks (wound permitting), and night splints maintaining MP flexion are provided. These splints should be worn for at least 6 weeks and weaned away slowly over several months. Dynamic splints with flexor slings can be provided in highly motivated and cooperative patients in whom extensor tendon repair or lengthening was not required. In more complex situations, free active motion is not initially permitted and usually is started at 4 weeks. Before that, therapy, including active assistive or passive range of motion, is performed in the attempt to minimize a postoperative inflammatory reaction and facilitate formation of a nonadherent and lengthened capsule and collateral ligaments. In the unlikely event an extension lag develops in a patient, the use of alternating flexion- and extension-assist dynamic splinting can overcome this problem. Similarly, in situations where there has been a tendon lengthening or tenolysis, the combined use of both flexor and extensor slings may be needed.

With proper indications and rehabilitation, the outcomes from this operation can be excellent. Excluding burn patients and other patients with fixed hyperextension deformity that require skin grafts or flap coverage,[4] motion to near 90° of flexion can be anticipated over 90% of the time, with an average increase in range of motion greater than 60°. When skin grafts or flaps are required, the relative improvement may be more dramatic, but the results are less predictable, and depend a great deal on the limits imposed on therapy by the surgery and other associated tissue problems. Because of this, when a distant flap is needed, a free flap that would permit early motion is preferred to a traditional abdominal flap.[4] If used appropriately and carefully, we believe dorsal capsulotomy or capsulectomy with selective release of the collateral ligaments can be of great benefit and a valuable procedure in the surgeon's armamentarium for the treatment of extension contractures of the MP joint level.

■ OUTCOMES

References

1. Akeson WH, Amirl D, Abel MF, Garfin SR, Woosl Y: Effects of immobilization on joints. Clin Orthop, 1987; 219:28–37.
2. Berme N, Paul JP, Purues WK: A biomechanical analysis of the metacarpophalangeal joint. J Biomech, 1977; 10:409–412.
3. Brand PW, Hollister A: Clinical Mechanics of the Hand, 2nd Ed. St. Louis: Mosby Yearbook, 1993:35–59.
4. Buch VI: Clinical and functional assessment of the hand after metacarpophalangeal capsulotomy. Plast Reconstr Surg, 1974; 53:452–457.
5. Bunnell S, Doherty EW, Curtis RM: Ischemic contracture, local, in hand. Plast & Reconstruct Surg, 1948; 3:424–433.
6. Curtis RM: Capsulectomy of the interphalangeal joints of the fingers. J Bone Joint Surg, 1954; 36A:1219–1232.
7. Curtis RM: Stiff finger joints. In: Grabb WC, Smith JW (eds): Plastic Surgery, 3rd Ed. Boston: Little, Brown, & Co., 1979:598–603.
8. Field PL, Hueston JT: Articular cartilage loss in long-standing immobilization of interphalangeal joints. Br J Plast Surg, 1970; 23:186–191.
9. Flatt AE, Fischer GW: Restraints of the metacarpophalangeal joints: A force analysis. Surg Forum, 1968; 19:459–460.
10. Fowler SB: Mobilization of metacarpophalangeal joints. Arthroplasty and capsulotomy. J Bone Joint Surg, 1947; 29:193–202.
11. Hettinga DL: I. Normal joint structures and their reaction to injury. JOSPT, 1979; 1:16–22.
12. Hume MC, Gellman H, McKellop H, Brumfield RH: Functional range of motion of the joints of the hand. J Hand Surg, 1990; 15A:240–243.
13. Larsen A, Dale K, Eek M, et al: Radiographic evaluation of rheumatoid arthritis by standard reference forms. J Hand Surg, 1983; 8:667–669.
14. Laseter AF: Management of the stiff hand: A practical approach. Orthop Clin North Am, 1983; 14:749–765.
15. Radin EL, Paul IL: A consolidated concept of joint lubrication. J Bone Joint Surg, 1972; 54A:607–616.
16. Randall T, Portney L, Harris BA: Effects of joint mobilization of joint stiffness and active motion of the metacarpal-phalangeal joint. JOSPT, 1992; 16(1):30–36.
17. Tsuge K: Comprehensive atlas of hand surgery. Chicago: Year Book Medical Publishers, 1989.
18. Watson HK, Dhillon HS: Stiff joints. In: Green DP (ed): Operative Hand Surgery, 3rd Ed. New York: Churchill Livingstone, 1993:549–562.
19. Watson HK, Light TR, Johnson TR: Checkrein resection for flexion contracture of the middle joint. J Hand Surg, 1979; 4:67–71.
20. Youm Y, Gillespie TE, Flatt AE, Sprague BL: Kinematics investigation of normal MCP joint. J Biomech, 1978; 11:109–118.

LEWIS H. MILLENDER
ANDREW L. TERRONO

117

Silicone Arthroplasty of the Proximal Interphalangeal Joint

■ HISTORY OF THE TECHNIQUE

The proximal interphalangeal (PIP) joint silicone rubber arthroplasty was originally used in 1966[8–11] in conjunction with the silicone prostheses for the metacarpophalangeal (MP) joint in rheumatoid arthritis. Initially the prosthesis was used primarily in the patient with rheumatoid or degenerative arthritis; however, over the years the indications have changed. Now the procedure is used most commonly in patients with degenerative arthritis, and certain cases of traumatic arthritis.[1,2]

The purpose of this chapter is to describe the volar approach for PIP joint silicone arthroplasty. The indications, contraindications, and alternatives as well as rehabilitation and outcomes are discussed.

■ INDICATIONS AND CONTRAINDICATIONS

The procedure is primarily used in patients who have persistent PIP joint pain that has been refractory to several months of intensive nonoperative therapy, including nonsteroidal anti-inflammatory drugs, occasional cortisone injections, temporary splinting, and activity modification. Carefully prescribed hand therapy focuses on modifying activities of daily living, and not on increasing range of motion. It usually becomes evident when surgical intervention is indicated because the patient will complain of persistent, severe pain associated with activities, and even night pain.

The reason for using caution and restraint before recommending PIP arthroplasty is related to several factors. Prolonged nonoperative therapy often is effective in eliminating pain in these patients. Also, many of these patients are older, and if their pain is tolerable they function well in spite of deformity and limited motion. The postoperative motion will vary in any individual case and it is difficult to predict the result. Therefore, if motion is greater than 70° or the patient can touch his or her palm, we would recommend PIP arthroplasty cautiously.

The best candidate for PIP joint arthroplasty is the patient with a painful PIP joint secondary to degenerative or post-traumatic arthritis in one of the ulnar three digits and who has near full extension and 30 to 40° of flexion. When there is good bone stock, minimal deformity, and preserved extensor and flexor mechanisms, the prognosis for eliminating pain and improving motion is good (Fig. 117–1).

We caution against PIP arthroplasty in painless degenerative arthritis, especially if there is good MP and distal interphalangeal (DIP) joint motion. However, there are occasional patients with a single long, ring, or small finger that is stiff in an extended position who are candidates for the procedure when apprised that the amount of flexion is unpredictable.

The indications for PIP arthroplasty in traumatic arthritis are similar to those described above, but there are other considerations. The best patient for the procedure is the patient who has sustained a comminuted intra-articular PIP joint fracture that is stiff in extension. In these cases, the bone stock usually is preserved and the soft tissues are not injured. The prognosis for restoring a favorable range of motion (ROM) is good.[3,7] We have also been successful in restoring motion after low-velocity gunshot wounds to the PIP joint that did not cause severe bone loss or massive injury to the extensor or flexor mechanisms.

There are several advantages to the volar approach. If one is planning to perform a volar plate arthroplasty and at the time of surgery it is determined that there is too much joint destruction, it is then appropriate to convert the procedure to a silicone prosthesis

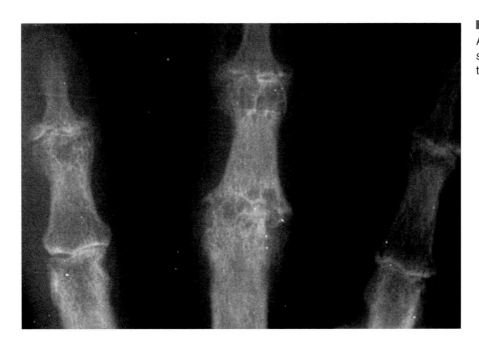

■ FIGURE 117-1

A preoperative radiograph showing PIP joint post-traumatic arthritis.

using the same approach. Alternatively, if there is a significant swan-neck deformity with traumatic arthritis from an old volar plate injury, this approach allows one to repair the volar plate. Also, when one believes that flexor tendon adhesions are an additional issue, this approach allows easy access to the tendons.

Proximal interphalangeal joint arthroplasty is usually unsuccessful in patients with severe rheumatoid involvement.[1,2] In addition, combining PIP joint arthroplasty with MP joint arthroplasty either as a combined procedure or in two stages usually is not successful. Most times, we recommend PIP joint fusions combined with MP joint arthroplasty for combined involvement. However, in the unusual case of an isolated painful digit with little deformity, preserved bone stock, and functional extensor and flexor mechanisms, PIP arthroplasty is appropriate. In most cases patients with PIP joint involvement in rheumatoid arthritis have complex problems with boutonniere, swan-neck, or lateral deformity associated with bone loss and soft tissue involvement, and flexible silicone implant arthroplasty is not appropriate.

Contraindications for PIP joint arthroplasty include patients who have had PIP joint infections or who have had previous failed attempts at flexor or extensor tenolysis. This arthroplasty usually fails secondarily to recurrent scarring. Massive bone loss, severe deformity, and repeated surgery including initial extensive open reduction are certainly relative contraindications for the procedure, and arthrodesis should be considered.

One should be very cautions recommending PIP arthroplasty in digits with significant fixed flexion contractures in the range of 50° or more. In these cases, one must remove excessive bone to insert the prosthesis, and it often requires extensive reconstruction of the extensor mechanism, which requires prolonged splinting. Results after these procedures generally are not good, and the patient is left with a stiff finger in extension that is more disabling than the previous flexion contracture. In these situations when surgery is indicated, it is preferable to consider arthrodesis in a more functional position.

Classically, PIP arthrodesis is recommended for the index digit because flexion is not as crucial, strong pinch is necessary, and lateral deviation after PIP arthroplasty is reported.[5,11] Although we subscribe to these recommendations, we would not absolutely exclude the procedure in the index PIP joint.

The volar approach for PIP joint arthroplasty is our preferred approach. Once one is familiar with the approach, it is simple and provides excellent exposure without interfering

■ SURGICAL
TECHNIQUES

■ FIGURE 117–2
The neurovascular structures are mobilized and protected. The flexor tendon sheath is opened from the A2 to A4 pulley. The flexor tendons are retracted. FDP, flexor digitorum profundus; FDS, flexor digitorum superficialis.

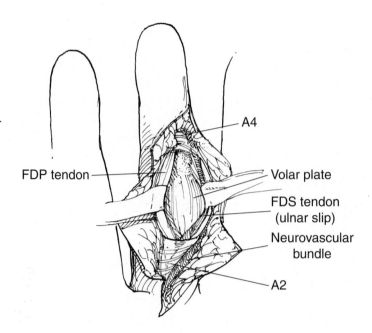

A4

FDP tendon

Volar plate

FDS tendon (ulnar slip)

Neurovascular bundle

A2

with the extensor tendons. Almost any anesthesia that is appropriate for the patient is suitable for the procedure. This includes intravenous sedation with a metacarpal-level digital block, intravenous regional anesthesia, axillary block, or general anesthesia. However, we prefer axillary block or general anesthesia. Usually this is an outpatient procedure, and tourniquet control is used.

A generous volar zigzag incision is used extending 5 to 6 cm, centered over the PIP joint. Skin retraction sutures are used for flap retraction. The neurovascular structures are mobilized and protected. A 2- to 3-cm flap of volar pulley, including a small portion of A2 and A4, is raised (Fig. 117–2). This exposes the volar plate, which is detached from its membranous proximal origin and the accessory collateral ligaments, but left widely attached to the base of the middle phalanx for later reconstruction. Penrose drains can be passed around each flexor tendon to retract them to either side of the joint. The collateral ligaments are detached from the base of the proximal phalanx to allow complete hyperextension of the joint and excellent exposure of the proximal phalanx. A #15 blade is inserted parallel to the phalanx and into the sulcus between the collateral ligament and the phalanx. By using careful, short strokes, the ligament can be detached and preserved. After the ligaments are completely detached the joint can be hyperextended and carefully dislocated. This must be a gentle, controlled dislocation to prevent stretching the neurovascular structures and traumatizing the soft tissues. The flexor tendons are guided to either side of the joint (Fig. 117–3).

With the joint dislocated, bone reconstruction can be carried out. Depending on the preference of the surgeon, a rongeur or oscillating saw is used to osteotomize the proximal phalangeal condyles. Sometimes the rongeur is safer because of the small size of the joint, and the saw can injure the soft tissues. Next, the middle phalanx is prepared. This can be the most difficult part of the procedure, depending on the amount of deformity of the base of the middle phalanx. When there are erosions with large lateral ridges on the sides, they must be removed. To remove these ridges, the assistant lifts the base and supports the phalanx while the surgeon carefully releases the collateral ligament from the ridges only. Care is taken not to detach completely the entire ligament from the middle phalanx. Then a sharp rongeur is used to osteotomize the ridge, thereby preparing a flat surface on which to seat the prosthesis.

The medullary canals of the proximal and middle phalanx are prepared to accept the stem of the prosthesis. An awl is used to perforate the subchondral bone. Then power reamers and square hand reamers are used to ream and fashion the canal. The surgeon

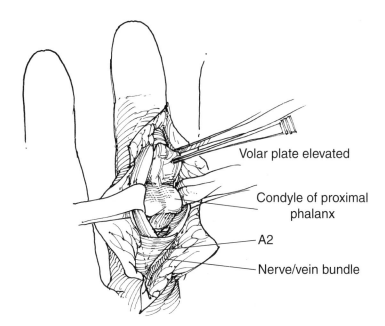

■ FIGURE 117–3
The joint is slowly hyper-extended as the flexor tendons are guided to the side of the joint.

Volar plate elevated

Condyle of proximal phalanx

A2

Nerve/vein bundle

should hold the phalanx with one hand and ream with the other hand to prevent accidental perforation of the cortex, which is easily done in the narrow middle phalanx. Trial insertion and testing of the prosthesis is then begun. Rarely does one use a size larger than a #2 Swanson prosthesis; often a size #1 is adequate. The prosthesis is inserted with the slot in the hinge facing volar. The prosthesis should rest on the proximal and middle phalanx without a tendency to rotate or to buckle. If the hinge of the prosthesis is not flush with the bony surfaces, additional reaming is carried out or a smaller prosthesis is chosen. Also, if the prosthesis buckles or tends to rotate, one must shorten the bones, look for additional causes for the rotation, or insert a smaller trial. The fit is adequate when the digit can be carried through a full ROM without buckling, rotation, or tendency to dislocate.

The flexor tendon must be assessed if preoperative full active flexion was not present. A trigger-finger incision can be used to access the flexor tendons in the palm. Through this incision, traction can be applied to the tendons to ensure full flexion. Alternatively, if local or intravenous regional anesthesia has been used, the tourniquet can be deflated and active flexion checked.

Two or three drill holes are then made in the base of the proximal phalanx. The prosthesis is inserted using the "no touch" technique. The volar plate and accessory collateral ligament are then sutured to the proximal phalanx using the previously drilled holes (Fig. 117–4). The flexor sheath can be used to reinforce the volar plate by placing it deep to the tendons, but it is usually placed in its anatomic position. The tourniquet is deflated and meticulous homeostasis is obtained because a postoperative hematoma or excessive swelling can jeopardize the early exercise program. A bulky homeostatic dressing is applied with a volar splint holding the digits in extension. A radiograph will demonstrate a good joint space without residual osteophytes or prosthetic buckling (Fig. 117–5).

When nonoperative treatment of the painful PIP joint has failed, arthrodesis must be considered instead of PIP arthroplasty. Arthrodesis is best suited for the isolated index finger PIP joint with good DIP and MP joint motion. Joints with previous infection or severe scarring of the flexor or extensor mechanism are also best treated with arthrodesis.

The dorsal approach is an alternative to the volar approach. It was the original approach, and does have some specific indications. Its primary indication would be in situations where there is a significant PIP flexion contracture that must be corrected, or where tenolysis or reconstruction of the extensor mechanism is needed. In this approach the extensor mechanism must be carefully handled, reattached, and then protected during the rehabilitation phase.

■ TECHNICAL ALTERNATIVES

■ FIGURE 117–4
The joint is reduced with
the implant in place. The
volar plate is reattached
through previously drilled
holes in the proximal phalanx. FDP, flexor dig-
itorum profundus; FDS,
flexor digitorum superfi-
cialis.

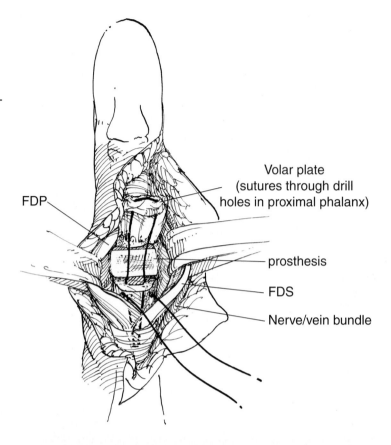

■ FIGURE 117–4
The joint is reduced with
the implant in place. The
volar plate is reattached
through previously drilled
holes in the proximal phalanx. FDP, flexor dig-
itorum profundus; FDS,
flexor digitorum superfi-
cialis.

Volar plate
(sutures through drill
holes in proximal phalanx)

FDP

prosthesis

FDS

Nerve/vein bundle

■ FIGURE 117–5
A postoperative radio-
graph of a Silastic PIP
arthroplasty.

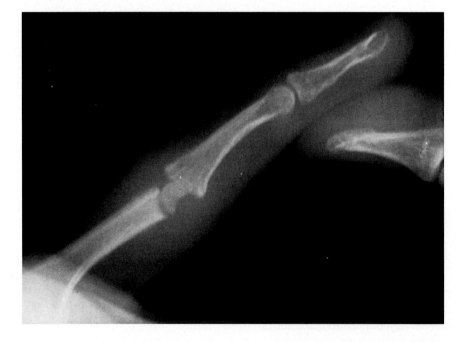

Another alternative in very selected cases is the volar plate arthroplasty as described by Eaton.[11] If the post-traumatic arthritis is localized to the volar articular surface of the middle phalanx, this may be possible.

An adequate incision must be used to allow exposure with adequate retraction and protection of the neurovascular structures. The soft tissues must be kept moist and handled with care. The collateral ligaments must be completely released proximally and a controlled dislocation performed to prevent fracture or soft tissue injury. Proper bone cuts will allow the joint to function properly with good alignment, stability, and motion.

After 3 to 5 days, the dressing is changed and supervised hand therapy started. Extension block splinting with the operated PIP joint flexed approximately 20° is begun. Splinting includes both the involved and one adjacent digit. Active flexion and extension may be started without worrying about tendon repair or reconstruction. The digits are splinted in extension between exercise periods. This is continued for 4 to 6 postoperative weeks. Strapping to the adjacent digit to protect the collateral ligaments is continued for 3 months.

■ REHABILITATION

Flexible silicone arthroplasty is an excellent procedure for relieving pain while restoring functional motion in the ulnar digits of patients with post-traumatic or degenerative arthritis in the PIP joints. Complications are rare in patients without rheumatoid arthritis. However, the types of complications vary, and include infection, fracture, dislocation, bone resorption, instability, stiffness, and recurrent deformity.[11]

■ OUTCOMES

Our results are similar to those reported in the literature, with excellent pain relief, good motion, and stability without fracture, dislocation, or infection. In our series of PIP joint arthroplasties in patients with post-traumatic arthritis, the average active ROM was 48° without deterioration or pain, with an average follow-up of 7 years.[3] A review of the literature shows the average ROM to be 45 to 60°,[4,6,11] with approximately 70% of patients getting greater than 40°.[11]

The incidence of infection and dislocation in a large series is approximately 0.4%.[10] The implant fracture rate is about 6%,[4,11] with an overall revision rate of 10%.[11] Reports of bone resorption vary from 1.2[11] to 35%[5] and may vary with the length of follow-up and the person evaluating the radiographs. In our long-term follow-up, this has not been a significant clinical problem.

At this time, we would recommend the flexible silicone arthroplasty for the PIP joint in ulnar digits of patients with post-traumatic and degenerative arthritis. The volar approach can be used in most patients; it is simple and allows early rehabilitation. Further study to discover the optimal arthroplasty is warranted.

References

 1. Dryer RF, Blair WF, Shurr DG, Buckwalter JA: Proximal interphalangeal joint arthroplasty. Clin Orthop, 1983; 185:187–194.
 2. Eaton RG, Malerich MM: Volar plate arthroplasty of the proximal interphalangeal joint: a review of ten years experience. J Hand Surg, 1980; 5:260–268.
 3. Ferenz CC, Millender LH: Silicone rubber arthroplasty for post traumatic proximal interphalangeal arthritis: A long term follow-up. Orthop Trans, 1989; 13:516–517.
 4. Green SM, Posner NA, Garay A: Silicone rubber arthroplasty of the proximal interphalangeal joint: Dorsal and lateral approaches. Surgical Arthroplasty, 1991; 2:130–139.
 5. Pellegrini VD, Burton RI: Osteoarthritis of the proximal interphalangeal joint of the hand: Arthroplasty or fusion?. J Hand Surg, 1990; 15A:194–209.
 6. Schneider LH: Proximal interphalangeal joint arthroplasty: The volar approach. Surgical Arthroplasty, 1991; 2:139–147.
 7. Strickland JW, Dustman JA, Selzer L, et al: Posttraumatic arthritis of the proximal interphalangeal joint. Orthop Rev, 1982; 11:75–83.
 8. Swanson AB: Flexible implant arthroplasty for arthritic finger joints. J Bone Joint Surg, 1972; 54A:435–455.
 9. Swanson AB: Implant resection arthroplasty of the proximal interphalangeal joint. Orthop Clin North Am, 1973; 4:1007–1029.
10. Swanson AB, Matev IB, Waller T: The proximal interphalangeal joint in arthritic disabilities and experiences in the use of the silicone rubber implant arthroplasty. J Bone Joint Surg, 1968; 50A:634.
11. Swanson AB, Maupin BK, Gajjar NV, Swanson GD: Flexible implant arthroplasty in the proximal interphalangeal joint of the hand. J Hand Surg, 1985; 10A:796–805.

EDWARD A.
NALEBUFF

118

Silicone Arthroplasty of the Metacarpophalangeal Joint

■ HISTORY OF THE TECHNIQUE

The current management of deformities of the metacarpophalangeal (MP) joints in rheumatoid arthritis includes, at different stages, synovectomy, intrinsic releases, extensor tendon relocations, and arthroplasties. In the late 1950s and early 1960s, Riordan and Fowler,[12] Fowler,[3] and Vainio and others[2,15] described techniques to correct the severe deformities of the MP joints in rheumatoid arthritis. They resected the MP joints and interposed soft tissues between the metacarpal and proximal phalanx. Kirschner wires were used to hold the fingers temporarily in alignment. Using these techniques, it was possible greatly to improve digital alignment while obtaining moderate motion at the resected joint. However, the results were unpredictable and recurrent deformities were common.[2,15]

In the mid-1960s, Swanson[13] devised a flexible hinge implant that was designed as a spacer to improve the reliability of the resection arthroplasty. The implant was not thought to be a "joint" but rather an internal splint that would maintain alignment and stimulate a capsular response (encapsulation). These implants were simple in design and made from a silicone material that withstood millions of cyclic bendings in the laboratory. It was thought that the material was "nonreactive," and would be well tolerated by the body. Field trials in centers around the world were started, and the early results of this new technique were very promising in achieving realignment of the digits while maintaining motion. With experience, it was apparent that strict attention to detail was needed with this operation, which was refined by Swanson and others.[5,6,14] When the procedure was introduced, it was thought that the simple hinge design was just a first step in the development a prosthesis for the MP joint. Other designs have come and gone, but this flexible hinge with modification to "toughen" the rubber to be more tear-resistant has stood the test of time. Twenty-five years after the introduction of this prosthesis, its use in arthroplasty is still the most accepted and performed technique to treat the severely involved MP joint in rheumatoid arthritis.

■ INDICATIONS AND CONTRAINDICATIONS

The indications for silicone arthroplasty are to relieve pain, correct deformity, and improve function.[6,9] As a result of synovitis, the supporting structures of the MP joint are stretched. Ulnar deviation of the fingers, volar subluxation of the proximal phalanx, and the development of fixed flexion deformities of the MP joint are common (Fig. 118–1A). Each of these indications can be treated by implant arthroplasty. Pain at the MP joint level is not frequently associated with ulnar deviation, but is common with fixed flexion deformities or volar dislocations. As the patient attempts extension, pain is increased, and the need for surgery becomes more apparent. Patients can continue to function fairly well with ulnar deviation of the fingers; they compensate for this deformity by radially deviating the wrist. In addition to the cosmetic deformity, these patients often have considerable weakness in grasping and holding on to objects because of the lack of radial collateral ligament support in the MP joints.[4] When you support the fingers in less ulnar deviation, the patient has a definite feeling of increased strength in holding on to large objects. When fixed flexion deformities are present, patients often cannot hold on to objects such as a glass without using two hands. In the typical patient, there is often an element of each of these problems. MP arthroplasty can improve the patient's function, as well as relieving pain and improving appearance. In my early years with MP arthroplasty, I would wait

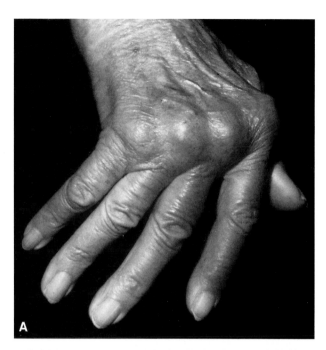

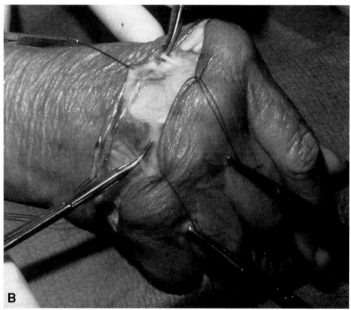

■ FIGURE 118-1
Surgical technique of MP arthroplasty. **(A)** Preoperative appearance with moderate ulnar drift of digits. **(B)** Transverse skin incision with preservation of superficial nerves.

until the deformity became severe before advising surgery. With increased confidence in the arthroplasty, I now prefer to do the surgery in less deformed hands to obtain the best results.[10] If the joints are subluxed instead of dislocated, it allows the surgeon to resect less bone. The supporting structures, including the capsule and collateral ligaments, are in better condition.

Under these conditions, excellent functional results are more likely. I do not talk patients into this surgery, but do advise them that the best results can be obtained when less bone needs to be resected and the supporting soft tissues can be repaired. I ordinarily do not recommend surgery at the first consultation. It is important to get to know the patient and appreciate how they function over a period of a few months' observation. At this point in the treatment cycle, our hand therapist can help the patient with ways to improve his or her function in activities of daily living.

■ FIGURE 118-1
(continued) **(C)** Resection of metacarpal head and creation of adequate space for prostheses. **(D)** Preparation of medullary canals to provide supinating force to index finger.

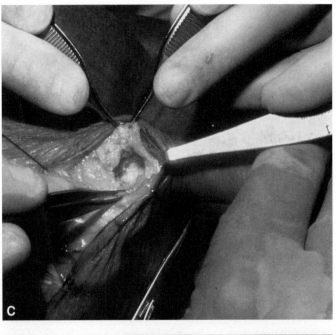

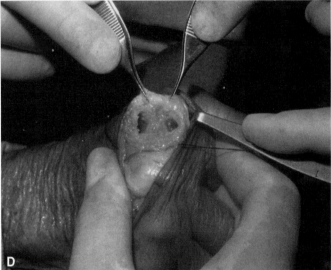

There are definite contraindications to MP arthroplasty;[10,13,14] these include a deformed or painful wrist. The ability to grasp is reduced with wrist pain, and radially deviated metacarpals secondary to wrist disease will lead to recurrent ulnar deviation of the fingers after arthroplasty. The absence of active digital flexion because of flexor tendon ruptures is a strong contraindication to MP arthroplasty. The presence of extensor tendon function does not rule out MP arthroplasties. In this situation, I stage the reconstruction with the MP arthroplasties as the first stage and restoration of extensor tendon activity at a second operative procedure. I believe that MP arthroplasty should not be performed with arthritis mutilans.[8] In these patients, an "egg cup" deformity develops at the MP level, and they maintain significant motion without the implant. The presence of an implant does not stop the bone destruction characteristic of this condition. Bone loss in these patients can be halted only by fusions, and I recommend this approach at the interphalangeal level to preserve digital length.[8]

In some patients with juvenile rheumatoid arthritis onset, there is an underdevelopment of the intramedullary canals, which makes it impossible to insert even the smallest implant.

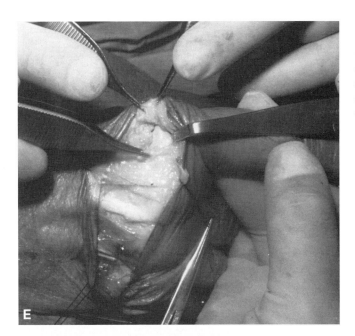

(continued) **(E)** Prosthesis in place. Note abundant capsular tissue for closure. **(F)** Capsular closure with realignment of digit.

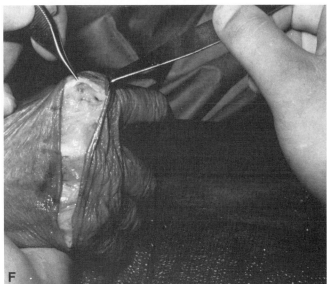

In these patients a resection arthroplasty may be needed to realign the digits. For me, a previous infection of the MP joint is another contraindication to implant surgery.

The surgical procedure is technique-intensive. There are no shortcuts! Careful attention to detail is important, both during the operation and after surgery, to obtain optimum results. I prefer axillary block anesthesia. It is the safest of the anesthesia choices and can provide a number of hours of postoperative pain relief. My second choice is general anesthesia, although the presence of cervical spine changes is a contraindication to this method. I avoid the intravenous regional anesthesia technique because the patients often do not tolerate the 2-hour surgical time that is often required. The skin incision can either be a single transverse cut just proximal to the MP joints or an individual longitudinal incision when the surgery is confined to single digits, or when it is done in combination with proximal interphalangeal (PIP) joint surgery. In these patients, the skin is quite thin, and care is therefore needed to avoid damage to the underlying veins and superficial nerves (Fig. 118–1B). The skin is retracted both proximally and distally to facilitate wide

■ SURGICAL
TECHNIQUES

■ FIGURE 118–1
(continued) **(G,H)** Postoperative extension and flexion at 5 weeks.

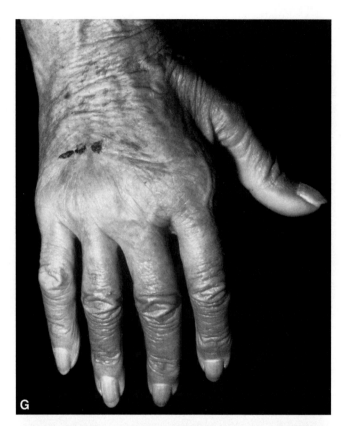

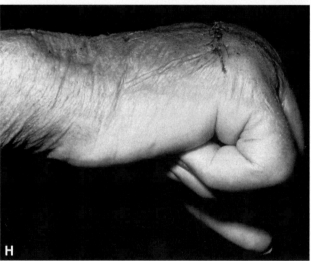

exposure. I use 3-0 silk traction stitches to avoid compromising the skin margins with forceps. The extensor mechanism of the digits is next exposed by blunt dissection.

It is common to note ulnar translocation of the tendons with stretching of the radial sagittal fibers. The tendons must be dissected away from the underlying joint capsules. This requires a division of the sagittal fibers along the lateral margins of the tendon. I prefer to release the shortened fibers on the ulnar side of the tendons. For the index and small fingers, it is possible to expose the joint capsule by splitting between the extensor digitorum communis and the extensor indicis proprius or extensor digitorum minimi. It is usually necessary to divide the junctura between the index and long fingers and to separate the conjoint tendon going to the ring and small fingers. I start my surgery on the index finger and proceed in sequence to the small finger. My assistant retracts the soft tissues to expose the ulnar intrinsic, which is released. This facilitates retraction of the extensor tendon mechanism from the joint capsule.

In most cases, I divide the ulnar intrinsic to help correct ulnar deviation of the finger and to weaken the extensor force to the PIP joint when there is an associated swan-neck deformity. The division of the intrinsic does reduce the patient's ability to spread the fingers in a normal fashion after the arthroplasty. With less ulnar deviation, I may not completely divide the ulnar intrinsic. I make the final decision in this regard after resecting the metacarpal head. Swanson believes that the ulnar intrinsic to the index finger acts as a supinating force. For this reason, he avoids dividing this particular intrinsic in most cases. With the intrinsic divided, I next carefully separate the extensor tendon from the underlying joint capsule. The capsule often has a dorsal rent with protruding synovium. To preserve capsular tissues, the next incision is made longitudinally, directly through the capsular rent, and carried onto the base of the proximal phalanx. With the MP joint in flexion, attention is directed to the collateral ligaments. They are dissected off the metacarpal head while maintaining their attachment to the base of the proximal phalanx. With a scalpel, I next make a transverse incision in the periosteum across the dorsum of the metacarpal neck. The periosteum is stripped proximally. This provides tissue for subsequent capsular closure. Using an oscillating saw, the metacarpal head is divided perpendicular to the shaft. The amount of bone to be removed varies depending on the shape of the base of the proximal phalanx. If the base is sloped, it will have to be cut square to the shaft of the phalanx. Thus, less bone will need to be resected from the metacarpal to provide sufficient space for the implant (Fig. 118–1C). In early cases with less subluxation, I divide the metacarpal head just at the level of the insertion of the collateral ligaments. After removal of the metacarpal head, the medullary canal is opened. To do this, I use a pointed awl. The canal is prepared with various-sized hand reamers. The Swanson reamers shaped like the prosthesis are very helpful with soft bone.

In some cases, it is necessary to use power burrs to prepare the metacarpal shaft. Attention is next addressed to the base of the proximal phalanx. The assistant brings the base of the phalanx into the wound with the digit flexed. It may be necessary to release the soft tissues along the volar aspect of the phalanx to make this possible. Care is taken to avoid injury to the flexor tendons. The base of the phalanx is cut to provide a flat surface. An awl is used to perforate the canal. A small, straight hemostat is a good instrument to sound the canal and to avoid perforation. The Swanson reamers are used to shape the opening in a rectangular fashion. The rectangular opening in the index and long fingers should not be parallel to the volar surface of the proximal phalanx, which would be a neutral position. Making the opening more volar radialward and dorsal on the ulnar side provides a supinating force to the finger when the implant is inserted (Fig. 118–1D). The rectangular shaping is important because it controls rotation of the prosthesis. I next determine if sufficient space has been achieved to insert a prosthesis without buckling (Fig. 118–1E). A 1-cm space is ideal. If the space achieved falls short of this, there is difficulty inserting the prosthesis and motion is restricted. Additional space can be produced by: 1) Cutting more bone from the metacarpal or the base of the phalanx; 2) releasing and resecting the ulnar capsule and intrinsic tendon; and 3) releasing or excising the volar plate. The initial incision in the volar plate is longitudinal. The flexor tendons are visualized and a portion of the volar plate is excised. This releases the tight volar structure and makes it possible to bring the base of the proximal phalanx dorsal to the metacarpal.

Once the canals have been prepared with sufficient space, I concentrate on the prosthesis insertion and repair of the soft tissues. I use a 000 absorbable suture woven into the radial collateral ligament at the base of the proximal phalanx. In most cases, I am able to suture the capsular issues to the previously prepared periosteal sleeve. The reattachment of the radial collateral ligament realigns the digit.

A second suture is used to provide a transverse closure of the capsule at the base of the phalanx. Additional stitches are added to obtain coverage of the prosthesis. Because the original capsular cut is longitudinal and midline, minimal capsular tissue is lost and the prosthesis usually can be covered (Fig. 118–1F). Other experienced surgeons do not believe that this is necessary, but when accomplished, it protects against prosthetic dislocation and allows the fingers to be splinted in a flexed position, without the fear of implant dislocation.

If the radial sagittal fibers are very lax and the extensor tendon is ulnarly displaced even after implant insertion, several 4-0 absorbable sutures can be used to reinforce the radial support to the tendon. This is accomplished with horizontal mattress stitches, which shorten the radial sagittal fibers, bringing the extensor tendon into a centralized position. Once all implants are in place, I repair the previously divided tendon junctura. At the conclusion of the procedure, the fingers should align in a normal fashion without ulnar deviation. Passive MP joint flexion of 70 to 80° should be possible without disrupting the capsular sutures. I infiltrate the operative area with 0.5% bupivacaine before closure to reduce postoperative pain.

The skin edges are closed with fine 5-0 nylon stitches. If the tourniquet time exceeds 2 hours, it is wise to let down the tourniquet before bandaging. In most cases, with careful attention to small blood vessels throughout the procedure, it is possible to close the skin with the tourniquet still inflated. Multiple drains can facilitate drainage, but a loose closure accomplishes the same result. A well adapted dressing with fluffs and Kerlex is applied. The wrist is supported with a plaster splint that extends beyond the MP level but allows PIP joint motion. The fingers are held in neutral or slight radial deviation.

The position of the fingers is influenced by the preoperative status.[10] If the major problem was ulnar deviation or subluxation without fixed flexion, I will put the fingers in a functional position with the MP joints flexed, with the fingers pointing to the base of the thumb. The intact capsular closure makes this feasible without fear of implant dislocation. If the preoperative posture of the fingers was in severe MP joint flexion with weak or absent extension, I splint the digits in extension. To protect against ulnar deviation, I often use paper tape to each digit, supporting the finger in a radially deviated alignment. The hand is elevated the first night to minimize swelling.

■ TECHNICAL ALTERNATIVES

Patients with significant MP ulnar deviation without subluxation or dislocation can be treated by techniques other than arthroplasty. Blair and colleagues[11] have reported their results with crossed intrinsic transfer. In this procedure, the ulnar intrinsic is released and then transferred to the lateral band or radial collateral ligament of the adjacent finger. It has been shown that correction of ulnar deviation has held up for 5 years with this technique. Another soft tissue alternative for ulnar deviation is to release the ulnar intrinsic and relocate the extensor tendon directly over the MP joint. To minimize recurrent subluxation of the tendon, a tenodesis of the tendon to the capsular tissues or bone just distal to the MP joint is carried out. I have had success with this approach in early cases of lupus with ulnar deviation and subluxed tendons. Without the tenodesis, tendon subluxation occurs with recurrent deformity. I indicated in the section on Surgical Techniques that I release the extensor tendon along its ulnar border, leaving the radial sagittal fibers intact. Other surgeons approach the joint through the stretched radial sagittal fibers, and then shorten them after the implant is in place.[1,2] I also indicated that I suture the radial capsule and collateral ligament to the periosteal sleeve prepared before dividing the bone.

Swanson routinely repairs the capsule of the index and middle fingers to the metacarpal. He prepares two small holes in the metacarpal with a 1-mm drill,[14] ensuring a strong reattachment of the radial soft tissues. He does not believe this is required for the ring and small digits.

There are pitfalls in performing an MP arthroplasty with a silicone implant. You must provide enough space for the implant to be inserted without buckling of the stems. If enough space is not provided, MP joint extension will be limited and implant fracture is more likely. In some patients with prolonged volar dislocations, the proximal end of the proximal phalanx becomes flattened, and it appears that the dorsal surface of the phalanx is the proximal end. Perforation of the phalanx through the dorsal surface for insertion of the distal stem can occur unless the surgeon recognizes that the articular surface of the phalanx has been deformed. If this complication occurs, it is possible with care gradually to reopen the phalanx to insert the distal stem into the phalanx properly. In reaming the proximal phalanx, it is also possible to perforate the volar cortex. If this occurs, the distal stem will enter the flexor tendon sheath. The use of blunt reamers aimed slightly dorsally will minimize this pitfall. You must be careful not to excise too much bone; otherwise, the prosthesis will not fit flush against the bone surfaces. The shaping of the opening in the proximal phalanx is important. It should be rectangular to reduce the tendency for the prosthesis to rotate out of ideal position. It is important not to handle the prosthesis with the surgical glove, because talc on the glove will adhere to the prosthesis and can lead to a particulate synovitis.

I think it is very important to change the entire dressing on the first postoperative day. The dressing can be blood soaked and constrictive. This dressing change often reduces pain and the need for narcotics.

■ REHABILITATION

Most patients are comfortable enough to leave the hospital on the first or second day after surgery. I reexamine and redress the hand at about 10 days. I teach patients how to splint the fingers in proper alignment with paper tape. They are instructed in an exercise program specifically designed around their preoperative deformity and condition of the soft tissues at surgery. Dynamic splinting is helpful for patients with an extensor lag, but is not routinely used in my practice. I prefer custom splints with low profiles that are fitted to the patient. The continuous passive motion machine can be considered in selected patients with excellent soft tissue closure. This technique can be initiated after 1 week, and significantly increases the postoperative range of motion. Splinting of the PIP joint to concentrate motion at the MP level is also helpful.

■ OUTCOMES

The results of MP arthroplasty are as varied as the patients undergoing the procedure.[1,10,16] You can expect between 30 and 80° of motion in the MP joint (Fig. 118–1G,H). This wide range of flexion is influenced by many factors, including the type of arthritis, the condition of adjacent joints, the controlling tendons, and the tissue elasticity of the patient. Patients with psoriatic arthritis achieve much less motion than patients with lupus. If there is normal PIP joint motion, the patients tend to get less MP joint motion than patients with stiff PIP joints. In this latter group of patients, all motion is concentrated at the MP level and the range of MP joint motion may be great, but the overall gripping ability is less than in patients with full PIP joint motion with less mobile but aligned MP arthroplasties. The strength and condition of the flexor and extensor tendons have a profound effect on the ultimate range of motion and functional result. Ruptures of the extensor tendons should not be repaired before correction of MP joint subluxation or dislocation. I do the arthroplasties in two stages, with realignment of the digits with implant insertion followed by dynamic splinting to maintain extension until the extensor tendons can be repaired or substituted by tendon transfer. Flexor tendon function should be restored before performing MP arthroplasties.

I consider it a contraindication to MP arthroplasty if flexor tendon function is not achieved. Repair of the radial collateral ligaments helps to keep the fingers aligned. The condition of the wrist influences the ultimate finger alignment. With carpal collapse, there may be metacarpal radial deviation, which tends to cause recurrent ulnar deviation of the fingers. For this reason I advise correction of wrist position and relief of wrist pain before MP arthroplasty (Fig. 118–2). This can be accomplished by wrist fusion in advanced cases or by transfer of the extensor carpi radialis longus to the extensor carpi ulnaris in some cases with good passive motion.

There are complications associated with MP arthroplasties, including recurrent ulnar deviation, implant fractures, and infections.[7] Postoperative splinting, keeping the fingers radially deviated, helps to reduce recurrent ulnar deviation. Most patients do have 5° of recurrent ulnar deviation. Implant fractures occur in 10 to 20% of cases.[14] Usually this is a radiographic diagnosis, because the encapsulation of the implant tends to maintain a functional joint even with a fracture of the implant. The use of tear-resistant silicone

■ FIGURE 118–2
Patient with multiple
areas of hand and wrist
involvement. **(A)** Preoperative clinical appearance
of hand. **(B)** Preoperative
radiograph shows wrist,
MP, and PIP deformities.

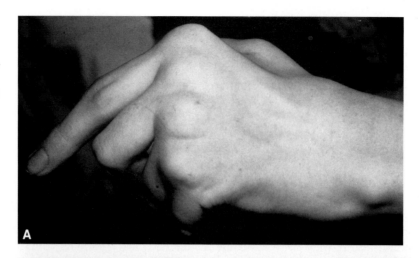

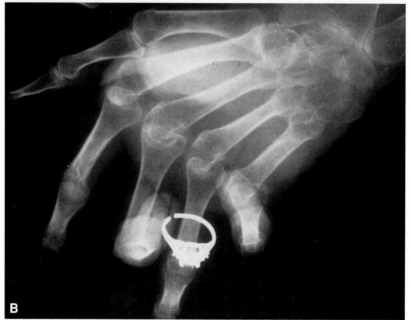

prostheses has reduced the incidence of implant fracture, but not eliminated it. Titanium grommets can be used to protect the stems of the implant against the bone edges. However, the insertion and fitting of the grommets adds to the complexity of the procedure. I tend to limit their use to cases with previous implant fracture or when the resected bone edges are particularly sharp. Infections around the implants are rare. In a series of 2000 implants, Millender and I[7] had only 12 joints become infected. Removal of the implant with a short period of antibiotic coverage controls the problem. I do not attempt to reinsert an implant after the infection of the MP joint has been brought under control. By removing the implant, the operation is converted to a "resection" arthroplasty. The range of motion is reduced, but pain is eliminated and digital alignment can be maintained by splinting for 6 weeks. In general, patients are pleased with the results of MP arthroplasties.

In my practice it is uncommon for patients with bilateral hand deformities not to request MP arthroplasties in the second hand. To me, this is the best test of patient satisfaction with the operation. The MP replacement arthroplasty has been reliable in reaching its goals of improved function, correction of deformity, and relief of pain. Attention to detail in the selection of patients as well as following the technical steps needed to insert the prosthesis goes a long way toward achieving the goals of arthroplasty.

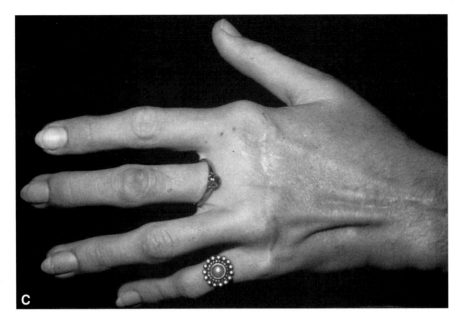

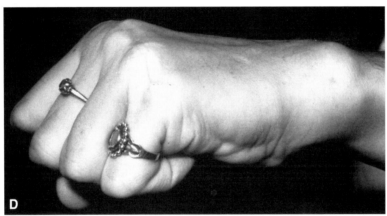

■ FIGURE 118–2 *(continued)* **(C,D)** Postoperative function after staged procedures. Stage 1 **(C)**, wrist fusion and correction of boutonniere deformity of the middle finger. Stage 2 **(D)**, MP arthroplasties with prostheses.

References

1. Blair WF, Shurr DG, Buckwalter JA: Metacarpophalangeal implant arthroplasty with a Silastic spacer. J Bone Joint Surg, 1984; 66A:365–370.
2. Flatt AE: The Care of the Rheumatoid Hand. St. Louis: CV Mosby.
3. Fowler SB: Arthroplasty of the metacarpophalangeal joint in rheumatoid arthritis. J Bone Joint Surg, 1962; 44A:1037–1038.
4. Madden JW, De Vore G, Arem AJ: A rational postoperative management program for metacarpophalangeal implant arthroplasty. J Hand Surg, 1977; 2:358–366.
5. Mannerfelt LG, Anderson K: Silastic arthroplasty of the metacarpophalangeal joint in rheumatoid arthritis. J Bone Joint Surg, 1975; 57A:484–489.
6. Nalebuff EA, Millender LH: Metacarpophalangeal joint arthroplasty utilizing the silicone rubber prosthesis. Orthop Clin North Am, 1973; 4:349–371.
7. Nalebuff EA, Millender LH: Analysis of infections after silicone rubber prosthesis in the hand. J Bone Joint Surg, 1975; 57A:825–829.
8. Nalebuff EA, Garrett J: Opera-glass hand in rheumatoid arthritis. J Hand Surg, 1976; 1: 210–220.
9. Nalebuff EA, Millender LH, Feldon P: Rheumatoid arthritis. In: Green DP (ed): Operative Hand Surgery. New York: Churchill Livingstone, 1982:1161–1262.
10. Nalebuff EA: Factors influencing the results of implant surgery in the rheumatoid hand, J Hand Surg, 1990; 15B:395–403.
11. Oster LH, Blair WF, Steyers CM, et al: Crossed intrinsic transfer. J Hand Surg, 1989; 14A: 963–971.

12. Riordan D, Fowler SB: Surgical treatment of rheumatoid deformities of the hand. J Bone Joint Surg, 1958; 40A:1431–1432.

13. Swanson AB: Silicone rubber implants for replacement of arthritic or destroyed joints in the hand. Surg Clin North Am, 1968; 48:1113–1127.

14. Swanson AB: Flexible Implant Resection Arthroplasty in the Hand and Extremities. St. Louis: CV Mosby, 1973.

15. Vainio K, Reiman I, Pulkki T: Results of arthroplasty of the metacarpophalangeal joints in rheumatoid arthritis. Reconstr Surg Traumatol, 1967; 9:1–7.

16. Vahvanen V, Viljalkka T: Silicone rubber implant arthroplasty of the metacarpophalangeal joint in rheumatoid arthritis: A follow-up study of 32 patients. J Hand Surg, 1986; 11A: 333–339.

119

Ligament Reconstruction of the Thumb Carpometacarpal Joint

Just as painful instabilities of major joints (shoulder, elbow, wrist, knee, and ankle) have been increasingly acknowledged over recent decades as clinical entities needing treatment, so too has painful instability of the prearthritic thumb carpometacarpal (CMC) joint, although only recently. This is probably because the arthritic CMC joint has drawn so much attention in the literature that painful instability of the joint before the onset of arthritis has been relatively ignored.

Littler and Eaton first performed ligament reconstruction of this joint in 1967.[2] They developed their procedure with the goal of preserving motion and restoring stability in painful CMC joints because previous techniques for CMC pain had been the more radical trapeziometacarpal arthrodesis and trapezium excision.[1] Although these latter procedures were appropriate for treatment of CMC arthritis, Littler and Eaton wanted to save the joint and preserve motion in nonarthritic patients.

■ HISTORY OF THE TECHNIQUE

The most difficult aspect of properly treating painful CMC instability is making an accurate diagnosis. When there is a clear history of trauma, pain on palpation, or obvious painful instability of the joint, the diagnosis is straightforward. Often, however, the diagnosis is quite difficult to establish. The joint may be no more unstable than the contralateral thumb. The pain may be of insidious onset, may radiate from the mid-forearm to the thumb tip, or may be perceived in the first web or metacarpophalangeal (MP) region. Painful CMC instability has been misdiagnosed as de Quervain tenosynovitis, occult scaphoid fracture, MP joint sprain, and carpal tunnel syndrome.[5] An intra-articular injection of anesthetic or a period of immobilization may be necessary to establish the diagnosis.

Once the diagnosis has been made, the primary indication for ligament reconstruction is persistently disabling pain refractory to conservative treatment. Usual conservative methods include nonsteroidal anti-inflammatory medication, rest, immobilization, and change of hobby or job (if feasible). Intra-articular steroid injections are rarely helpful. An infrequent indication for ligament reconstruction is to stabilize the CMC joint after Bennett fracture when the volar fracture fragment is small or comminuted and when usual methods have failed.[5]

This procedure is contraindicated when the CMC or scaphotrapeziotrapezoid joints, or both, are arthritic, when the CMC joint is not unstable, or when the diagnosis is in question.[2–4]

■ INDICATIONS AND CONTRAINDICATIONS

In brief, the procedure stabilizes the CMC joint with a harvested slip of the flexor carpi radialis (FCR), which is routed through a gouge hole in the base of the first metacarpal, passed under the abductor pollicis longus (APB) and around the FCR, and finally secured over the radial side of the joint.

Ligament reconstruction of the CMC joint can be readily performed under regional anesthesia and pneumatic tourniquet control. The arm is abducted on an arm board, and the surgeon should sit on the "axillary" side. With the forearm supinated, a skin incision is drawn from the level of the first metacarpal neck proximally along the border of the glabrous and nonglabrous skin to the wrist crease. The incision then gently curves ulnarly along the wrist crease to the ulnar edge of the FCR. Two 2-cm transverse incisions are

■ SURGICAL TECHNIQUES

drawn at equal intervals over the FCR, with the most proximal one 8 cm proximal to the wrist crease. If not palpable now, the FCR can be identified later and the FCR incision drawn at that time. The hand and arm are wrapped with an Esmarch tourniquet and the pneumatic upper arm tourniquet is then inflated.

The incision is made as drawn in the palm and carefully deepened through the subcutaneous tissue to the thenar fascia. Branches of the radial nerve course parallel to or cross the distal two-thirds of the incision. These branches are mobilized and retracted, if possible. If not, they are divided as close to their skin insertions as possible to try to reduce the chance of neuroma formation. Neuroma or adhesion formation of the nerve stumps can lead to a sensitive symptomatic scar or even reflex sympathetic dystrophy. Therefore, meticulously delicate technique is called for here. Proximally, the superficial branch of the radial artery and its companion branches cross the wrist crease radial to the FCR. If possible, the superficial branch of the radial artery is skeletonized and preserved while the other structures are cauterized and divided. The palmar cutaneous branch of the median nerve may be encountered. If so, it, too, must be carefully protected to avoid neuroma formation.

The thenar fascia is incised near its insertion on the first metacarpal and the thenar muscles are sharply elevated off the bone *extraperiosteally*. This dissection is continued proximally. The muscle fibers are sharply dissected off the CMC joint capsule, the trapezium, and the distal scaphoid. The muscle is dissected deeply enough to allow exposure of the proximal-volar aspect of the first metacarpal and the ridge of the trapezium, deep to which is the FCR.

Occasionally, the attachment of the abductor pollicis longus (APL) is on the radial or dorsoradial aspect of the CMC joint. Also, it is common that a slip of the APL inserts on the APB. It will be necessary to release the APL slip that inserts on the APB to gain adequate exposure, and helpful but not essential to repair the same slip when closing. The major attachment of the APL to the first metacarpal, however, must be securely reattached during closure if it is released during the exposure.

The CMC joint must be inspected to verify that there is no arthritic change. First, look at the capsule of the CMC joint. Very often it is thinned or torn. A tear will need to be repaired later. Make an incision in the joint capsule parallel to the articular margin. If the joint surface is healthy, close the capsule (and repair the tear, if present) with reabsorbable 4-0 suture. If the joint has degenerative changes, the surgeon should be prepared to perform an alternative reconstructive procedure. (This should have been fully explained to the patient before surgery.) A small (1-cm) incision should also be made in the scaphotrapezial joint to verify that it, also, is free of degenerative change. The arthrotomy should be closed with 4-0 reabsorbable suture.

Expose a small area on the dorsal cortex of the proximal end of the first metacarpal by retracting the extensor pollicis brevis (EPB) and any radial nerve branches (Fig. 119–1). Make a small (1-cm) "X"-shaped incision through the periosteum in the dorsal midline and expose the cortex just distal to the proximal edge of the first metacarpal. Using increasingly larger gouges, create a channel 6 to 8 mm distal to the joint margin, perpendicular to the plane of the thumb nail and parallel to the articular surface, through the first metacarpal, out the volar cortex. Do not enter the joint. The channel must be large enough to permit the harvested FCR tendon slip to slide through. A drill may be used, but it is easy to "wind-up" soft tissue structures, so extreme care is needed here. Pass a 4-0 stainless steel suture through the first metacarpal, cut off the needle, and tag it with a hemostat. The steel suture will be used later for passage of the tendon slip through the metacarpal. Place damp sponges in the wound after irrigation, and direct attention to the volar forearm.

The "new" ligament will be harvested from the FCR tendon (Fig. 119–2). Make a short transverse incision 8 to 10 cm proximal to the wrist crease over the FCR tendon, expose the tendon, and lift it superficially with a small curved scissors or hemostat. Incise tendon longitudinally 40 to 50% from its ulnar margin and divide this ulnar slip transversely. Pulling up on the slip with a hemostat, separate it from the rest of the intact tendon. If tension is held on the slip, it should easily and cleanly separate from the body of the

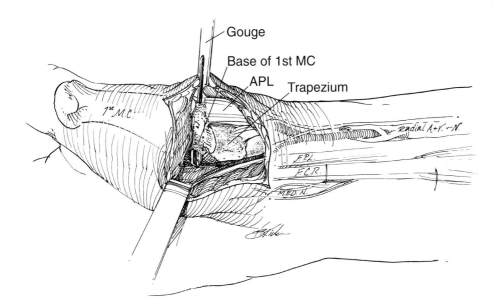

FIGURE 119–1
A gouge tract is created in the proximal aspect of the first metacarpal. The tract is oriented perpendicular to the plane of the nail, from the dorsal midline through the volar cortex, parallel to, and 6 to 8 mm distal to, the joint surface. APL, abductor pollicis longus; FCR, flexor carpi radialis; FPL, flexor pollicis longus; MC, metacarpal; MED N, median nerve; Radial A, V, N, radial artery, vein, nerve.

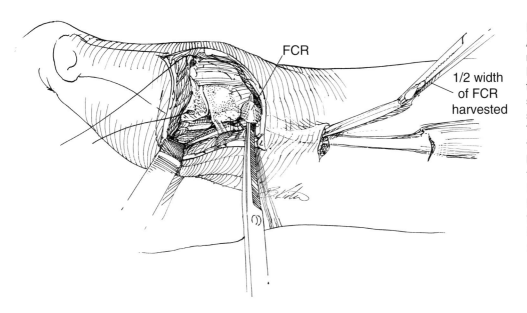

FIGURE 119–2
A slip of the flexor carpi radialis (FCR) is created. It is a strip 40 to 50% the width of the tendon, split away from the ulnar side of the intact tendon. The slip is harvested from proximal to distal, beginning 10 cm proximal to the wrist crease, and is passed beneath skin bridges to a point 5 mm from the distal end of the FCR tunnel under the ridge of the trapezium.

tendon. Use a scalpel, scissors, or both as needed to facilitate this. Flex the wrist to reach more tendon distally. Keep the tendon moist with a damp sponge. Estimate the length of tendon already split, make another incision more distally, and identify the tendon. Place a small tendon passer in this new wound, advance it retrograde through the tendon sheath out the proximal wound, grab the tip of the tendon slip, and pull the slip beneath the skin bridge out this newest incision. Repeat the process to bring the tendon slip into the palmar wound by passing the tendon passer up the FCR sheath from the palmar wound. Incise the FCR tunnel (the attachment of the transverse carpal ligament) so that only the last 5 mm of the tunnel remains intact. With scissors, lyse those fibers from the FCR still attached to the slip. Pass the tendon slip through the metacarpal channel with the steel wire. If tugging on the slip after it has been passed dorsally deviates the intact FCR volarly, tack down the slip where it leaves the FCR canal on the volar side.

At this point in the procedure, the slip should be tensioned to secure the metacarpal against the trapezium. Often it is easier to first pass the slip around the APB (first dorsoulnar, then deep and palmar) and hold it with a clamp at its tip. With one hand, seat the metacarpal into the CMC joint, and with the other hand pull on the new ligament, setting tension. The metacarpal should not be secured too tightly because CMC motion must be preserved. Test stability by applying radioulnar stress to the base of the metacarpal. When satisfied with the tension, suture the new ligament dorsally with 3-0 nonreabsorbable suture. Usually, there is inadequate periosteum to which to sew. By suturing to the edge of the dorsal capsule, which is usually substantial, secure fixation for the new ligament can be obtained. After the suture is tied, immediately test the stability. Be prepared to tighten or loosen it if the tension is unsatisfactory. Be fussy! This is the most critical step in the procedure. Add an additional suture or two for security.

Pass the slip obliquely-proximally, deep to the FCR tendon, then distally over the CMC joint. Suturing the slip to itself as it courses around the FCR, at any point of change in direction, and at several points around the CMC joint will enhance stability of the CMC joint volarly, dorsally, and radially (Fig. 119–3). Before closing, test motion and stability of the CMC joint. If it is too tight or too loose, adjust tension by replacing sutures. Resect and discard any extra tendon slip. (I have found the stability to be quite sufficient and I do not use a K-wire for fixation, in contrast to the originally published description.[2])

If it was noted that the MP joint hyperextended during power pinch at the time of preoperative physical examination, it is appropriate to perform either a tenotomy of the EPB, or a volar tenodesis of the MP joint. Although a tenodesis is better theoretically, it delays the postoperative recovery significantly, and sometimes will stretch out over time. The EPB tenotomy, at the level of the CMC joint, is easily performed and is helpful. Care must be taken not to injure the radial sensory branch.

If the first metacarpal is noted to lie in relative adduction and the APL to be relatively lax, the APL should be reefed/advanced to place the first metacarpal in more abduction. This will also potentiate the benefit of the EPB tenotomy.

After irrigating the wounds and confirming hemostasis, replace and tack down the thenar muscles, and close the thenar fascia with 4-0 reabsorbable sutures. If a slip of the APL had been divided, repair it. The palmar and forearm wounds are closed in routine fashion. Apply a bulky soft dressing (including the thumb as far as the interphalangeal [IP] joint) and dorsal and volar splints (as a thumb spica). Limited thumb MP flexion–extension and full finger motion should be permitted by the splints. The hand is elevated for the first day or two if there is significant swelling or pain, and thereafter as needed. Narcotic analgesics are routinely prescribed.

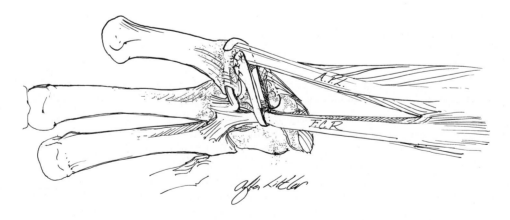

■ FIGURE 119–3

The harvested slip of the flexor carpi radialis (FCR) is passed through the metacarpal from volar to dorsal, under the abductor pollicis longus (APL), around the FCR, and back over the radial side of the joint. It is first sutured dorsally under appropriate tension and then secured as needed to prevent its migration. Thus, it reinforces the dorsal and radial aspects of the joint, as well as setting tension on the reconstructed volar trapeziometacarpal ligament.

This operative procedure is a unique treatment for a very specific problem. There is essentially no other comparable procedure or technique in the literature to treat CMC instability other than arthrodesis. The main pitfall in this technique is to make the ligament too tight or too loose. Experience with stability testing of many thumb CMC joints is the best preparation for the surgeon to know how to set the tension "just right." A second pitfall is that the FCR slip can be harvested too thick or too thin: The former would create difficulty in passing it through the first metacarpal, and the latter place it at risk to rupture. The harvested slip should be 40% of the original FCR tendon.

■ TECHNICAL ALTERNATIVES

At 2 postoperative weeks, if the patient is comfortable and the reconstruction was felt to be solid, a hand-mounted thumb spica orthosis allowing full IP and limited MP motion is applied, and therapy is begun. The splint is removed for hygiene and limited flexion–extension three times per day. If the pain is significant or any doubt about the stability exists, a small fiberglass thumb spica cast is applied until 4 postoperative weeks, and only MP and IP exercises are done.

At 4 weeks, a progressive motion (including flexion–extension and circumduction) and strengthening program is started. The orthosis is weaned gradually over 3 months according to pain and the demands of the patient's lifestyle. Sports and work in the splint are permitted as soon as the patient is comfortable, with the exception of high-stress contact sports or work. These exceptions must be evaluated on an individual basis.

■ REHABILITATION

Results of this surgical procedure[2–4] show that the procedure is reliable, durable, and predictable with a follow-up of up to 13 years. This author's results[5] confirm those of Littler and Eaton. Patients should expect to be able to return to all, or nearly all, previous activities and regain strength. Half of the patients will lose some palmar abduction and may not be able to place the hand fully on a flat surface. Postoperative soreness often lingers for 3 to 6 months, and patients frequently do not achieve their full recovery until 12 months after surgery. Complications are infrequent, although sensitivity around the wound from adhesions to the radial nerve or the palmar cutaneous branch of the median nerve does occur. The results also show that the procedure does not work for patients with arthritic CMC joints, and is in fact contraindicated for this group.

■ OUTCOMES

References

1. Eaton RG, Littler JW: A study of the basal joint of the thumb, treatment of its disabilities by fusion. J Bone Joint Surg, 1969; 52A:661–668.
2. Eaton RG, Littler JW: Ligament reconstruction for the painful thumb carpometacarpal joint. J Bone Joint Surg, 1973; 55A:1655–1666.
3. Eaton RG, Lane LB, Littler JW, Keyser JJ: Ligament reconstruction for the painful thumb carpometacarpal joint: A long term assessment. J Hand Surg, 1984; 9A:692–699.
4. Lane LB, Eaton RG: Ligament reconstruction for the painful "prearthritic" thumb carpometacarpal joint. Clin Orthop, 1987; 220:52–57.
5. Lane LB, Scarangella SF: Ligament reconstruction of the painful, unstable, non-arthritic thumb carpometacarpal joint [Abstract]. Orthop Trans, 1994; 17–353.

MATTHEW M.
TOMAINO
RICHARD I. BURTON

120

Ligament Reconstruction with Tendon Interposition Arthroplasty for the Thumb Carpometacarpal Joint

■ HISTORY OF THE TECHNIQUE

The carpometacarpal (CMC) joint of the thumb is frequently afflicted with osteoarthritis, especially in postmenopausal women.[4,15,16] Although reciprocal concave surfaces on the base of the thumb metacarpal and the distal articular surface of the trapezium afford this joint exceptional mobility, stability during functional activity is predicated almost completely on ligamentous restraint.[5,13] The primary contact area during functional activities involving flexion–adduction of the thumb, such as lateral key pinch and grip, involves the palmar surfaces of the trapezium and metacarpal.[17] Analysis of postmortem specimens has demonstrated a close correlation between degeneration of the metacarpal attachment of the stabilizing palmar oblique ligament and the severity of disease on the adjacent cartilage surfaces.[13,14] The presence of more advanced eburnation in the palmar contact region of surgically harvested osteoarthritic trapeziometacarpal joints supports the role of instability and shear in the pathogenesis of basal joint arthritis.[14]

The rationale for ligament reconstruction with tendon interposition (LRTI) arthroplasty centers around three fundamental principles: trapezium excision to remove painful arthritic joint surfaces, palmar oblique ligament reconstruction to restore thumb metacarpal stability and prevent axial shortening, and fascial interposition to reduce the likelihood of impingement between neighboring bony surfaces.[2,4,19] The impetus for its development was the senior author's observation in the late 1970s that instability and weakness complicated the long-term use of silicone implant arthroplasty.[16] Although the cannulated Eaton prosthesis allowed stabilization with a slip of the abductor pollicis longus,[8] improved stability resulted in greater cold flow deformation and particulate synovitis.[16]

Based on favorable results after ligament reconstruction of the unstable basal joint without arthritis using one-half the width of the flexor carpi radialis (FCR) tendon, as described by Eaton and Littler,[7] in 1980 the senior author began combining trapezium excision, as first recommended by Gervis,[9] with fascial interposition as described by Froimson,[11] in an attempt to rectify the long-term problems of instability and particulate synovitis. The FCR tendon was rerouted through the base of the thumb metacarpal after removal of its arthritic articular surface to create a sling for stability and suspension, and its excess length was then interposed into the space remaining after trapezium excision.[2,4]

Since its original description in 1983[2] and the first reports of results in 1986,[4] the procedure has been modified to facilitate its performance and to eliminate potential complications. Originally, the extent of trapezium excision depended on the severity of web space contracture and the presence of pantrapezial arthritis. Complete excision was preferentially used in cases of more severe web space contracture and when arthritis involved the scaphotrapezial joint. Similarly, only one-half the width of the FCR tendon was used for ligament reconstruction and tendon interposition. The procedure has evolved over time to include routine excision of the entire trapezium because this provides broader exposure of the FCR tendon and facilitates its use in ligament reconstruction. In addition, removal of the entire trapezium minimizes the likelihood of bony impingement between the thumb metacarpal and trapezial remnant as well as the risk that unrecognized scaphotrapezial arthritis could result in persistent postoperative pain. In younger patients in whom arthrodesis remains a useful salvage in the event that ligament reconstruction were to attenuate with time, hemitrapeziectomy is performed to preserve bone stock. The entire width of the FCR tendon is now routinely used because this not only facilitates its harvest more proximally in the forearm, but provides a bulkier piece of tissue for both ligament reconstruction and interposition into the arthroplasty space. These modifications have been employed over the last 6 years; the procedure as it is currently performed by the senior author is described herein.[19]

The patient with a painful basal joint in which cartilage wear, eburnation, and joint space narrowing are secondary to osteoarthritis or post-traumatic arthritis is a candidate for the LRTI arthroplasty. Physical examination should reveal tenderness along the thumb CMC joint, and the traditional crank-and-grind test performed with axial compression, flexion–extension, and circumduction characteristically incites crepitance and pain. Preliminary nonoperative modes of treatment include anti-inflammatory medications, intraarticular steroid injection, and splint immobilization followed by thenar muscle strengthening exercises, but symptomatic relief is frequently short-lived. Radiographic examination consisting of posteroanterior (PA) stress views as described by Eaton and Littler,[7] a lateral, and a pronated AP view should demonstrate CMC joint narrowing and sclerosis as well as subluxation, depending on the degree of ligament incompetence (Fig. 120–1). The triad of intractable pain, progressive functional disability, and radiographic evidence of CMC joint arthritis is indication for surgery.[1,3,4,19]

In light of potentially weakened osteoporotic metacarpal bone and degenerative changes in the FCR tendon in the patient with rheumatoid disease, we have not routinely recommended this procedure for rheumatoid arthritis, but prefer using silicone implant arthroplasty instead because, in these cases, low demand diminishes the potential for instability and particulate synovitis. In select cases, however, the LRTI arthroplasty has restored useful function in the rheumatoid patient. Concern about patient compliance with postoperative hand therapy constitutes a second relative contraindication to the use of the LRTI arthroplasty because a lengthy period is required before objective strength improvements plateau.[19]

■ INDICATIONS AND CONTRAINDICATIONS

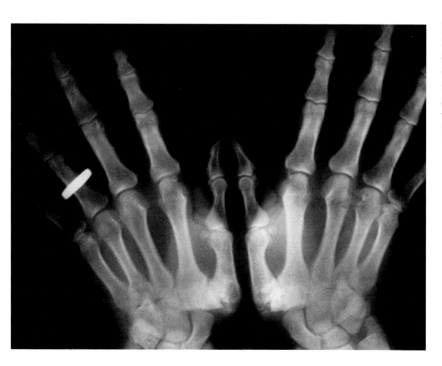

■ FIGURE 120–1
Preoperative posteroanterior stress radiograph demonstrates bilateral CMC joint subluxation and pantrapezial arthritis with osteophyte and loose body formation.

■ FIGURE 120–2
A modified Wagner "triradiate" incision is used to expose the basal joint. The thumb CMC joint level is marked by the dashed line. The dorsal end of the incision facilitates exposure of the radial artery, as marked.

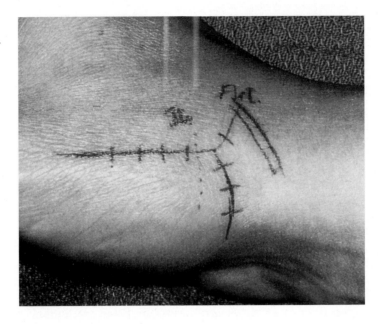

In preparation for basal joint reconstruction, it is critical to evaluate the patient's hand for signs or symptoms of carpal tunnel syndrome,[3,10] de Quervain disease, metacarpophalangeal (MP) joint instability, and scaphotrapezial arthritis, for the following reasons. Swelling after basal joint arthroplasty may exacerbate coexistent mild carpal tunnel syndrome. Pain secondary to de Quervain tenosynovitis may compromise compliance with postoperative hand therapy. Unaddressed longitudinal collapse deformity and scaphotrapezial disease may result in arthroplasty instability, recurrent web space contracture, and incomplete pain relief after surgery. Accordingly, preoperative electrodiagnostic tests may be warranted, and if carpal tunnel syndrome is confirmed, transverse carpal ligament release should accompany the arthroplasty procedure. Similarly, the first extensor compartment should be released if tenosynovitis exists. Last, because exposure of the basal joint involves mobilization of the radial artery, patency of both radial and ulnar arteries must be verified by the Allen test before surgery.

■ SURGICAL TECHNIQUES

The procedure is performed under regional anesthesia (axillary block) and tourniquet control to ensure lengthy pain relief and a hemostatic field. Prophylactic antibiotics, usually a first-generation cephalosporin, are routinely administered before inflation of the tourniquet and are continued intravenously for 48 hours after surgery.

The basal joint is exposed using a modified Wagner "triradiate" incision with a longitudinal limb along the thumb metacarpal, a limb extending around the volar palmar aspect at the base of the thenar cone, and a shorter dorsal limb to facilitate safe exposure and mobilization of the radial artery (Fig. 120–2). Great care is taken to identify and protect the dorsal sensory branches of the radial nerve in the process of dividing subcutaneous tissue. The radial artery is easily identified in the fat pad just proximal to the base of the thumb metacarpal, lying directly over the scaphotrapezial joint. The artery is carefully mobilized proximally and protected, dividing and coagulating multiple articular branches in the process. Broad exposure of the capsule overlying the basal joint is obtained before longitudinally incising it and dissecting it off the surface of the trapezium. Its radial and ulnar edges are tagged with 4-0 nonabsorbable suture to facilitate exposure of the underlying trapezium as well as capsular closure (capsuloplasty) at the conclusion of the procedure.

With traction placed on the thumb, the thumb CMC, scaphotrapezial, and scaphotrapezoidal joints are inspected. If scaphotrapezoidal disease exists, debridement with a rongeur or fascial interposition using local capsular tissue are options to prevent subsequent pain

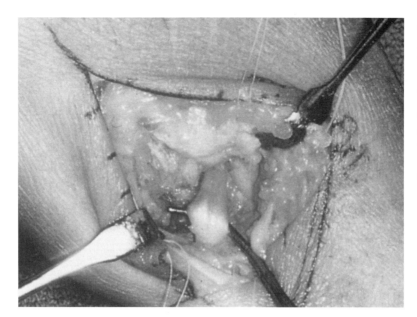

■ FIGURE 120–3
After trapezium excision, the FCR tendon is visualized at the base of the arthroplasty space, passing obliquely with respect to the longitudinal access of the thumb metacarpal to its insertion on the base of the index metacarpal.

secondary to unaddressed arthritis at this joint. The articular surface and subchondral bone are removed from the base of the thumb metacarpal with a power sagittal saw so as to leave intact the abductor pollicis longus insertion. Longitudinal traction placed on the thumb tip facilitates this initial cut. Next, a saw cut is made in the trapezium to a depth of three-fourths of its full thickness parallel to the course of the FCR tendon, which passes obliquely, relative to the longitudinal axis of the thumb metacarpal, to its insertion on the base of the index metacarpal. A sharp osteotome is placed in the space created by the saw, carefully twisting it to complete infraction of the trapezium without damaging the underlying FCR tendon (Fig. 120–3). A rongeur is used to remove the bone, including osteophytes, from the medial base of the thumb metacarpal and the radial margin of the trapezoid. In addition, free ossicles that may be embedded in the capsule itself should be excised. These measures ensure the absence of impingement between the thumb metacarpal base and the trapezoid when the thumb is brought into abduction and extension. Any defects made in the deep capsule in the process of excising the trapezium are repaired with 4-0 nonabsorbable suture. This same suture material is then placed in the deep capsule at the distal margin of the scaphoid and left long to be used later for stabilization of the interposition material.

Next, an oblique hole is made in the dorsal cortex of the thumb metacarpal in the plane of the nail approximately 1 cm distal to its squared-off base and extending through the intramedullary canal (Fig. 120–4). Gouges of increasing size are used to make and enlarge the initial hole, and a series of curettes facilitates selective removal of bone from the distal margin of the hole to prevent narrowing of the bony bridge between the hole and the metacarpal base.

The entire FCR tendon is harvested from its musculotendinous junction to its insertion on the volar base of the index metacarpal. Use of the entire width of the tendon allows harvest using only one proximal transverse incision (Fig. 120–5). After dividing subcutaneous tissue, the wrist is flexed to facilitate exposure of the more distal tendon to allow release of overlying fascia and tendinous adhesions. After dividing the tendon at the musculotendinous junction, it is delivered into the distal wound by placing a curved clamp beneath the FCR tendon, as shown in Figure 120–3, and gently pulling. The tendon must be freed to its insertion on the base of the index metacarpal so that it accurately simulates the vector of the original palmar oblique ligament after its passage through the hole in the thumb metacarpal base. The tendon is easily passed through this hole by first placing a 28 gauge monofilament wire through the hole dorsally and out the base and tying it

■ FIGURE 120-4
A hole is made in the dorsal cortex of the thumb metacarpal 1 cm distal to its base in the plane of the nail and exiting out the intramedullary canal. The FCR tendon is visualized in the depths of the wound.

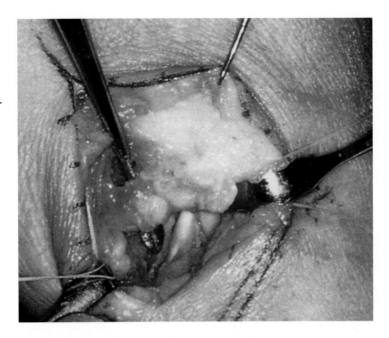

■ FIGURE 120-5
The FCR tendon is harvested through a transverse incision at the palpable musculotendinous junction. A second, more distal incision can be made if fascial bands and tendinous adhesions necessitate improved exposure.

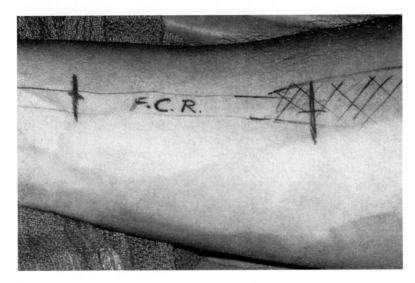

around the tendon near its distal end. Irrigation of the tendon facilitates its passage through the intramedullary canal and out the dorsal hole (Fig. 120–6).

With the thumb metacarpal base positioned at the same level as the base of the index metacarpal, the path of the tendon sling should be perpendicular to the index metacarpal's long axis. The thumb metacarpal is then stabilized in the abducted fist projection (the metacarpal base should be abducted and extended), effectively restoring the first web space, and a single oblique 0.045″ K-wire is advanced through the radial cortex of the metacarpal shaft ulnarly into the trapezoid or scaphotrapezoidal interval. The FCR tendon is then held under snug tension and sutured to the periosteum, where it exits the bone hole dorsally. This tension will be appropriate because the thumb metacarpal has already been accurately positioned and stabilized by the K-wire. It is then folded across the base of the thumb metacarpal and sutured to itself. At this point, the ligament reconstruction component of this arthroplasty has been completed and the residual length of the FCR tendon is fashioned into an "anchovy" by using a Keith needle over which the tendon length can be folded on itself like an accordion (Fig. 120–7). The four corners of the anchovy

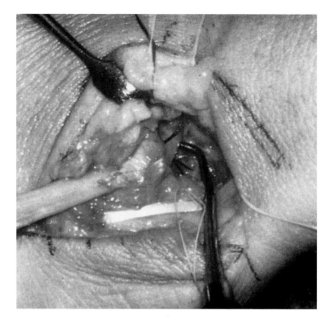

■ FIGURE 120–6
The FCR tendon is mobilized to its insertion on the base of the index metacarpal and delivered through the base of the thumb metacarpal out the dorsal hole. The hand probe demonstrates that the vector of the ligament reconstruction is perpendicular to the axis of the thumb metacarpal.

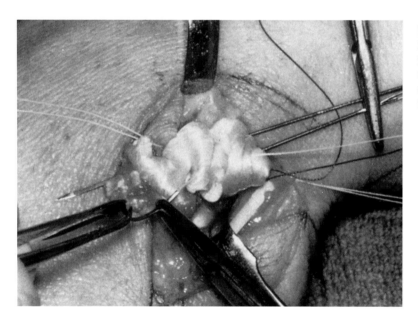

■ FIGURE 120–7
Residual length of FCR tendon is folded on itself over Keith needles and sutured at its corners to form the "anchovy."

are then sutured together using 4-0 nonabsorbable material and a second Keith needle is placed through this interposition mass parallel to the first. The previously placed suture in the volar capsule is then used, threading both limbs through the two Keith needles so that the anchovy can be recessed into the arthroplasty space and secured with the tying of this suture. The dorsal capsule is carefully repaired in a two-layered closure over the interposition material; the surface of this material and the superficial portion of the reconstructed ligament can be incorporated into the repair if necessary.

If the MP joint has not been stabilized, the extensor pollicis brevis tendon is divided and tenodesed to the metacarpal shaft to remove its hyperextension deforming force from the proximal phalanx. Residual length of this tendon distal to the site of tenodesis is placed in the hole in the dorsal cortex. If longitudinal collapse deformity at the MP joint is present, we prefer to address it after trapezium excision and FCR tendon harvest so that the manipulation required to perform the LRTI arthroplasty up to this point does not disrupt a previously stabilized MP joint.

Failure to address an unstable MP joint will result in potential collapse of the thumb with longitudinal pinch. The hyperextension of the MP joint imposes thumb metacarpal adduction, and increases stresses on the ligament reconstruction. If there is more than 30° of hyperextension instability to passive stress, we recommend arthrodesis in 10° of flexion. Although volar capsulodesis[6] is an alternative, we elect arthrodesis in light of its predictability, durability, and the minimal disability accompanying fusion of this joint. If hyperextension instability is less than 30°, temporary stabilization with a K-wire is used for a period of 4 weeks.

K-wires are cut short outside the skin and coated with collodion, and incisions are closed with 5-0 nonabsorbable monofilament suture, being careful not to incorporate superficial sensory branches of the radial nerve. The patient is placed in a short-arm thumb spica dressing with external plaster cast immobilization after the procedure, and hospital discharge typically occurs on postoperative day 2.

■ TECHNICAL ALTERNATIVES

A number of variations to the LRTI technique detailed herein have been described,[12,18,20] but each appropriately prioritizes ligament reconstruction. Thompson's suspensionplasty uses the abductor pollicis longus tendon,[18] and evolved originally as a salvage procedure for revision of failed silicone implant arthroplasty. Indeed, it serves as a useful bail-out should the FCR tendon be damaged during the LRTI procedure or found to be incompetent. We believe that the FCR tendon is the most suitable donor, however, because of the proximity of its insertion to the base of the thumb metacarpal, an intact vascular supply based on injection studies, and close simulation of the vector of the native palmar oblique ligament.[2,4] In our initial description[2] of the LRTI arthroplasty, we used only one-half the width of the FCR tendon, and advocated complete trapezium excision only when degenerative disease involved both CMC and scaphotrapezial joints. We have noted no weakness in wrist flexion related to use of the full width of the FCR tendon, which provides a stronger ligament and bulkier interposition material. Compared to hemitrapeziectomy, complete trapezium excision both maximizes web space correction and facilitates FCR exposure, and has not been predictive of poor subjective outcome or associated with weaker or radiographically less stable thumbs.[19]

As suggested during description of surgical technique, a number of potential pitfalls exist that may compromise the postoperative result. These range from failure to diagnose fully and surgically address carpal tunnel syndrome, de Quervain disease, and concomitant scaphotrapezoidal arthritis, which may compromise postoperative pain relief and compliance with therapy; to failure to address longitudinal collapse deformity at the MP joint, which can compromise arthroplasty stability and web space correction. In addition, inadequate attention to surgical detail may result in injury to the radial artery or sensory branches of the radial nerve, damage to the FCR tendon, fracture of the bony bridge on the dorsal thumb metacarpal base, impingement between osteophytes on the medial aspect of the thumb metacarpal and the radial aspect of the trapezoid during lateral pinch, and interposition material instability and herniation secondary to insufficient capsuloplasty.

■ REHABILITATION

At 4 weeks, the original plaster dressing, K-wire, and sutures are removed. If the MP joint has been fused, we maintain those K-wires until the fusion site is nontender or there is radiographic evidence of union. The patient is then placed in an isoprene thumb spica splint extending from the interphalangeal (IP) joint level of the thumb to the junction of the proximal and middle third of the forearm. The patient removes this splint four times a day for a limited exercise program consisting of active motion exercises at the MP joint (if not stabilized) and IP joints, and isometric thenar abduction strengthening. At 2 months after surgery, active mobilization of the basal joint is begun, consisting of flexion–adduction exercises. Weaning from the splint begins at this time; splinting is discontinued when thenar strength has improved to a level that allows pain-free pinch and grip as would be required to perform activities of daily living, typically around 3 months. Resistive lateral pinch and grip strengthening are begun at 3 months, with gradual resumption of unrestricted activity as return of strength allows, typically by 4 to 6 postoperative months. The first postoperative radiographs are usually obtained at approximately 3 months unless earlier examination of a fused MP joint has been required.

The LRTI arthroplasty has been most effective in providing pain relief and restoring effective pinch and grip strength. Patients have been very satisfied with the performance of their thumbs, including activities like opening jar tops and using keys. Objective grip and pinch strengths have routinely improved compared to preoperative values, and thumb mobility, stability, and web space restoration have been well maintained over time. Longitudinal analysis of strength measurements from our original cohort of patients[4] at intermediate and long-term follow-up intervals has shown that grip and tip pinch strengths steadily improve for as long as 6 years before plateauing, and improvements over preoperative values of between 65 and 95% can be expected.[19] Although key pinch strength may improve more slowly than grip strength, lateral pinch has been well tolerated and effective.

Few complications have arisen. One patient required reoperation because the interposition material herniated through a defect in the volar capsule; hence, attention to the repair of these defects is mandatory. Symptoms consistent with reflex sympathetic dystrophy in only a few patients have been transient, as have complaints of pulling in the volar aspect of the forearm referable to FCR tendon harvest. Although objective strength gains have been lower when this procedure has been performed as revision arthroplasty for failed silicone implants, subjective results have been favorable, and there has been no correlation with deterioration in radiographic appearance.

Our experience with the LRTI arthroplasty has demonstrated convincingly that thumbs continue to improve for as long as 6 years after surgery, underscoring the protracted time necessary to achieve maximum strength recovery after the procedure.[19] Documentation of such durable long-term performance after the LRTI arthroplasty contrasts markedly with the experiences of prosthetic trapezium replacement and trapezium excision with fascial interposition, for which stability and strength appear to decline as time progresses (Fig. 120–8).[2,11]

■ OUTCOMES

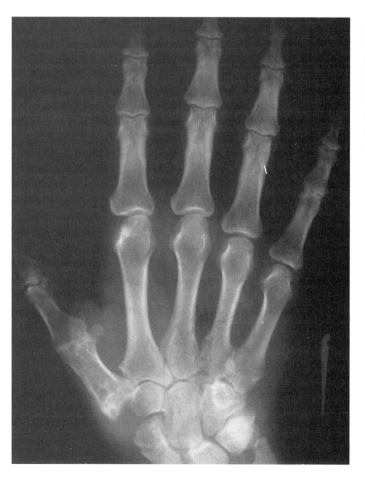

■ FIGURE 120–8
Nine-year follow-up stress radiograph after LRTI arthroplasty and MP joint arthrodesis demonstrating maintenance of arthroplasty height and absence of metacarpal subluxation.

In summary, outcome after the LRTI arthroplasty is characterized by excellent pain relief and significant improvement in strength. These observations imply persistent integrity of the palmar oblique ligament reconstruction as an effective suspensionplasty of the metacarpal, and underscore the importance of duplicating normal anatomy in providing a stable, functional, and durable thumb reconstruction.

References

1. Burton RI: Basal joint arthrosis of the thumb. Orthop Clin North Am, 1973; 4:331–348.
2. Burton RI: The arthritic hand. In: Evarts CM (ed): Surgery of the Musculoskeletal System. New York: Churchill-Livingstone, 1983:670–681.
3. Burton RI: The arthritic hand. In: Evarts CM (ed): Surgery of the Musculoskeletal System, 2nd Ed. New York: Churchill-Livingstone, 1990:1134–1143.
4. Burton RI, Pellegrini VD Jr: Surgical management of basal joint arthritis of the thumb: Part II. Ligament reconstruction with tendon interposition arthroplasty. J Hand Surg, 1986; 11A: 324–332.
5. Cooney WP, Lucca MP, Chao EYS, Linscheid RC: The kinesiology of the thumb trapeziometacarpal joint. J Bone Joint Surg, 1981; 63A:1371–1380.
6. Eaton RG, Floyd WE: Thumb metacarpophalangeal capsulodesis: An adjunct procedure to basal joint arthroplasty for collapse deformity of the first ray. J Hand Surg, 1988; 13A: 461–465.
7. Eaton RG, Littler JW: Ligament reconstruction for the painful thumb carpometacarpal joint. J Bone Joint Surg, 1973; 55A:1655–1666.
8. Eaton RG: Replacement of the trapezium for arthritis of basal articulations. J Bone Joint Surg, 1979; 61A:76-82.
9. Gervis WH: Excision of the trapezium for osteoarthritis of the trapeziometacarpal joint. J Bone Joint Surg, 1949; 31B:537–539.
10. Florack TM, Miller RJ, Pellegrini VD Jr, Burton RI, Dunn MG: The prevalence of carpal tunnel syndrome in patients with basal joint arthritis of the thumb. J Hand Surg, 1992; 17A: 624–630.
11. Froimson AJ: Tendon arthroplasty of the trapeziometacarpal joint. Clin Orthrop, 1987; 70: 191–199.
12. Kleinman WB, Eckenrode JF: Tendon suspension sling arthroplasty for thumb trapeziometacarpal arthritis. J Hand Surg, 1991; 16A:983–991.
13. Pellegrini VD Jr: Osteoarthritis of the trapeziometacarpal joint: The pathophysiology of articular cartilage degeneration. I. Anatomy and pathology of the aging joint. J Hand Surg, 1991; 16A:967–974.
14. Pellegrini VD Jr: Osteoarthritis of the trapeziometacarpal joint: The pathophysiology of articular cartilage degeneration. II. Articular wear patterns in the osteoarthritic joint. J Hand Surg, 1991; 16A:975–982.
15. Pellegrini VD Jr: Osteoarthritis at the base of the thumb. Orthop Clin North Am, 1992; 23: 83–102.
16. Pellegrini VD Jr, Burton RI: Surgical management of basal joint arthritis of the thumb: Part I. Long-term results of silicone implant arthroplasty. J Hand Surg, 1986; 11A:309–324.
17. Pellegrini VD Jr, Olcott C, Hollenberg G: Contact patterns in the trapeziometacarpal joint: The role of the palmar beak ligament. J Hand Surg, 1993; 18A:238–244.
18. Thompson JS: Complications and salvage of trapeziometacarpal arthroplasties. AAOS Instructional Course Lectures, 1989; 38:3–13.
19. Tomaino MM, Pellegrini VD Jr, Burton RI: Arthroplasty of the thumb basal joint: Long-term follow-up of ligament reconstruction with tendon interposition. J Bone Joint Surg, 1995; 77A: 346–355.
20. Uriburu IJF, Olazabal AE, Ciaffi M: Trapeziometacarpal osteoarthritis: Surgical technique and results of "stabilized resection–arthroplasty." J Hand Surg, 1992; 17A:598–604.

DAVID M. LICHTMAN
GREGORY G. DEGNAN

121

Proximal Row Carpectomy

T. T. Stamm of Guy's Hospital in London first reported on proximal row carpectomy in 1944.[11] Stamm, however, credits Lambrinudi with suggesting the idea that excision of the proximal row for scaphoid nonunion would convert an unstable link joint system into a simple hinge joint. Stack first reported on proximal row excision in this country for treatment of transcaphoid perilunate dislocations in 1948.[10]

Since its initial description, proximal row carpectomy has had an undeservedly poor reputation. Almost every report in the literature makes mention of this poor reputation, and yet there is no large series that substantiates this. Every reasonably large series of proximal row carpectomies has shown favorable long-term results when the procedure is used to treat post-traumatic disorders limited to the proximal row.[1,3,5,7,8] As a result, proximal row carpectomy has been gaining popularity in recent years as a salvage for these difficult problems.

Often, with long-standing post-traumatic disorders of the lunate or scaphoid, collapse and degeneration of both bones will occur. Proximal row carpectomy may be well suited for this situation. These disorders include long-standing scaphoid nonunions, rotary subluxation of the scaphoid with radioscaphoid arthritis, stage IV osteonecrosis of the lunate, and severe perilunate dislocations and fracture dislocations.[1,3–5,8] Less common indications include severe flexion deformities related to arthrogryposis, septic arthritis, and Volkman ischemic contracture.[12] Omer and Capen also describe its use in spastic paralysis.[9] In our experience, calcium pyrophosphate deposition disease has also been an indication for this procedure. In advanced cases the wrist ligaments are stiffened by crystal deposition and lose their elasticity. This predisposes them to rupture and can cause a scapholunate dissociation with eventual chronic degenerative changes. Crystal deposition in articular cartilage also hastens joint degeneration. These changes respond well to proximal row carpectomy.

The one absolute contraindication to proximal row carpectomy, as performed by us, is significant degeneration of the articular surface of the capitate or lunate fossa of the radius.[1,3,8] Relative contraindications include rheumatoid arthritis and the patient who cannot be trusted to perform an aggressive postoperative regimen.[2] It is also contraindicated in the patient who would prefer a totally stable and pain-free wrist to one that retains partial mobility. For this patient, we would recommend limited intercarpal or total wrist arthrodesis.

Proximal row carpectomy can be carried out under regional anesthesia. Because bone graft is not necessary and operative times are routinely less than 2 hours, axillary block or interscalene block is adequate. More commonly, however, we use a general anesthetic so that a bone graft may be harvested if intraoperative conditions (severe degeneration of the capitate or lunate fossa) dictate a change from proximal row carpectomy to intercarpal arthrodesis or wrist arthrodesis.

After routine skin preparation and sterile draping, the external landmarks of the wrist are identified and outlined with the marking pen. The radial styloid, the proximal pole of the scaphoid, base of the third metacarpal, and Lister's tubercle are outlined. A straight dorsal longitudinal incision is used, extending from the base of the third metacarpal to a point 2 to 3 cm proximal and just ulnar to Lister's tubercle. The dissection is carried down to the extensor retinaculum in line with the skin incision using double-sharp curved dissection scissors. After defining the level of the retinaculum, radial and ulnar flaps are

■ HISTORY OF THE
TECHNIQUE

■ INDICATIONS AND
CONTRAINDICATIONS

■ SURGICAL
TECHNIQUES

developed in this plane to ensure thick subcutaneous flaps containing the superficial nerves and vessels. These flaps are developed in one of two ways. While maintaining straight dorsal retraction with heavy skin hooks, the plane is developed using a spread-and-snip technique with the scissors, or using an inverted #15 blade to "feather" or "paint" the subcutaneous tissues off the retinaculum. As the radial flap is developed, care should be taken to identify and protect the superficial sensory branch of the radial nerve. Similarly, the dorsal sensory branch of the ulnar nerve is identified and protected in the ulnar flap.

The distal one-half to one-third of the extensor retinaculum is divided between the third and fourth compartments. The tendons of the second, third, and fourth compartments are mobilized and the extensor pollicis longus is subluxed out of the groove at Lister's tubercle. The tendons of the second and third compartments are retracted radially and the tendons of the fourth compartment retracted ulnarly, exposing the dorsal wrist capsule.

The level of the radiocarpal joint is identified using a Bunnell probe while flexing and extending the wrist. The wrist capsule is incised transversely over the proximal row, ensuring that a sufficient cuff of tissue remains proximally along the dorsal rim of the radius to allow subsequent repair. The incision is "T"ed centrally and distally to the level of the middle one-third of the capitate (Fig. 121–1). The dorsal capsule is separated from

■ FIGURE 121–1
To expose the proximal row, a transverse capsular incision is "T"ed centrally to the body of the capitate and the capsule is dissected free from the proximal carpal bones. Proximally the capsule and periosteum are also "T"ed to allow subperiosteal dissection of a radial flap. This provides the exposure for radial styloidectomy. EPL, extensor pollicis longus; MC, metacarpal.

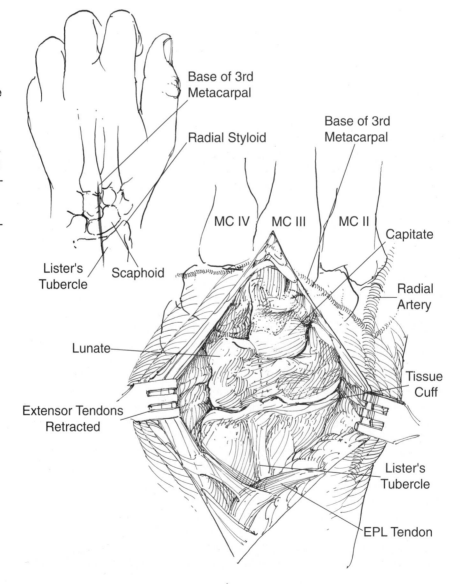

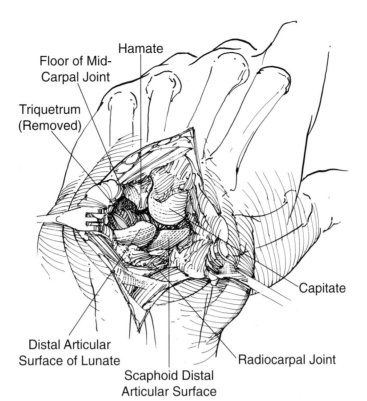

Hamate

Floor of Mid-
Carpal Joint

Triquetrum
(Removed)

Distal Articular
Surface of Lunate

Scaphoid Distal
Articular Surface

Capitate

Radiocarpal Joint

■ FIGURE 121–2
The wrist is then flexed
to visualize the articular
surface of the capitate
and the lunate fossa. Significant degenerative
change would result in
selection of an alternate
procedure.

the bones of the proximal row using sharp dissection with a knife blade. When developing the dorsal flap distal to the scaphoid, care is taken not to injure the radial artery, which overlies the scaphotrapezotrapezoid joint. This is done by identifying the vascular bundle first with blunt dissection and retracting it gently to the radial side with a small Myerding retractor.

Before excising the proximal row, the articular surfaces of the lunatocapitate and radiolunate joints are visualized. This is facilitated by manual distraction of the wrist combined with forced flexion (Fig. 121–2). If either of these surfaces show significant wear or degenerative changes, an alternative procedure is performed. Mild wear is not considered a contraindication to proximal row excision because it has been demonstrated that it does not adversely affect the clinical outcome, and significant progression of the degenerative arthritis does not occur.[1,4] The bones are removed in ulnar to radial sequence, with the triquetrum being excised first (Fig. 121–2). It should be noted that the pisiform is a sesamoid bone palmar to the wrist, and is not excised with the remainder of the proximal row. Excision of these bones can be challenging, and it is easier to remove them in a piecemeal fashion. The osteotome is used to split the bone and then to strip the soft tissues while the fragments are stabilized with rongeurs (Fig. 121–3). The rongeurs are also used to reduce the size of the fragments, facilitating removal. The distal pole of the scaphoid is by far the most difficult portion to remove, and we occasionally use a 0.062″ K-wire as a "joystick" to manipulate the bone.

There are two key points to remember when excising the proximal row. First, it is essential to avoid damage to the articular surfaces of the lunate fossa and the capitate. Second, it is crucial to preserve the volar capsule and ligaments. In particular, as previously noted by Green,[3] preservation of the radioscaphocapitate ligament is of critical importance. This ligament is largely responsible for the stability of the capitate in the lunate fossa.

After the proximal row is removed, the capitate is positioned in the lunate fossa and the wrist is placed in neutral and then radial deviation to check for impingement of the

■ FIGURE 121–3
An osteotome is used to split the lunate after previous triquetral excision. The osteotome is then used to lever the fragments and dissect soft tissue free from the bone. This technique significantly facilitates removal of these bones. C, capitate; H, hamate; SC, scaphoid; TR, triquetrum; TZ, trapezoid.

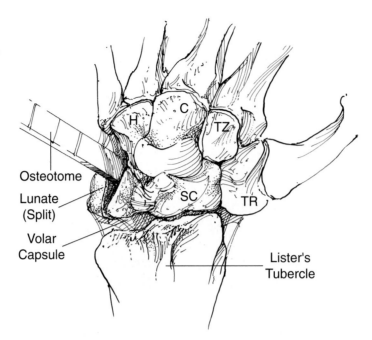

Osteotome

Lunate (Split)

Volar Capsule

Lister's Tubercle

radial styloid on the trapezium. If impingement is present, radial styloidectomy is performed. An index finger on the styloid tip can detect impingement when the wrist is radially deviated.

To perform styloidectomy, the proximal capsule and dorsal periosteum are "T"ed centrally and proximally. The radial flap is then developed subperiosteally using a #15 blade and a periosteal elevator. This dissection is carried out around the styloid to the volar aspect of the radius. During this subperiosteal dissection it is easy to enter the first dorsal compartment, and care is taken not to damage the abductor tendons. Approximately 1 to 1.5 cm of articular surface is excised using a sharp osteotome. It may be helpful to place a K-wire into the styloid in line with the proposed cut and check the position with the image intensifier.

At this point the wound is copiously irrigated, the tourniquet is released, and hemostasis is obtained. We check routinely for injury to the deep branch of the radial artery in the region of the proximal trapezium. After 10 minutes, the tourniquet is reinflated before closure. The capitate is seated in the lunate fossa, the wrist is placed in neutral, and the dorsal capsule is closed with interrupted 3-0 Vicryl sutures. There is often some capsular redundancy and the distal flaps are advanced proximally to aid in stabilizing the capitate. After capsular closure the stability of the capitate is assessed. If translation does not seem excessive, closure is continued. If, however, translation does seem excessive, crossed K-wires are placed across the radiocarpal joint into the capitate, avoiding the articular portion of the capitate in the lunate fossa (Fig. 121–4). The K-wires are placed in such a fashion that the capitate is not actually in contact with the radius to avoid pressure across these articular surfaces.

The extensor retinaculum is reapproximated with 5-0 nylon with specific care taken to avoid making the repair too tight. A Z-plasty closure of the retinaculum is used if the closure is tight. Stenosing tenosynovitis can be a troublesome complication if this is overlooked. The skin is approximated with 4-0 nylon using horizontal mattress sutures, and a bulky sterile dressing is applied out to the fingertips. A splint is then placed with the wrist in neutral position.

Perioperative antibiotics are administered for 24 hours, and the hand is elevated above the level of the heart. Oral pain medication is administered liberally, but the administration of parenteral pain medication is always preceded by examination by skilled personnel to ensure that neurovascular compromise is not occurring.

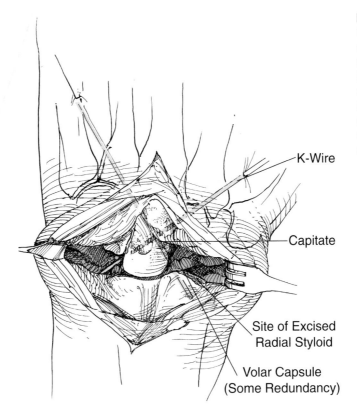

■ FIGURE 121–4
Crossed K-wires can be used to stabilize the capitate in the lunate fossa. Note that the wires do not penetrate the articular surface. Usually the capsule is closed before K-wire placement to better assess stability.

K-Wire

Capitate

Site of Excised
Radial Styloid

Volar Capsule
(Some Redundancy)

Proximal row carpectomy is commonly performed through a transverse dorsal incision along the line from the ulnar styloid to the radial styloid.[3–5] Although this is certainly an acceptable technique, we believe the straight dorsal longitudinal incision is more versatile. If the articular surface of either the capitate or lunate fossa is degenerative, this incision provides excellent exposure for limited intercarpal fusion or wrist arthrodesis.

Exposure of the proximal row is sometimes performed through two capsular incisions, one on either side of the fourth compartment. We believe, however, that this makes it more difficult to visualize the position of the capitate on the radius after excision of the proximal row.

There are several serious potential errors that adversely affect the outcome of this procedure. First, care must be taken to ensure that the capsular flaps are removed from bone and kept thick to allow for solid repair. If insufficient capsule remains proximally, the distal flap must be repaired through drill holes in the distal radius. During excision of the proximal row, the volar capsule, particularly the radioscaphocapitate ligament, must be protected to preserve subsequent stability of the capitate.[3] This occasionally requires that a cortical shell of distal scaphoid be left behind where it is intimate with the palmar capsular ligaments. This shell of bone, although radiographically visible, does not adversely affect the clinical outcome in any way. During excision of the proximal row the surgeon must be careful not to damage the articular surfaces of the capitate and lunate fossa. Perhaps the two most common pitfalls are failure to recognize significant degenerative changes, which should preclude this procedure, and failure to recognize impingement of the trapezium on the radial styloid.[3,8]

■ TECHNICAL ALTERNATIVES

After surgery, the patient is placed in a bulky compressive dressing for 10 to 12 days. At that time the sutures are removed and a well molded short-arm cast is applied. At 4 postoperative weeks the cast—and pins, if present—are removed. A well molded, removable volar splint is applied and a nonresistive exercise program is begun to mobilize the wrist. Strengthening exercises are begun at 6 to 8 postoperative weeks. Maximum strength

■ REHABILITATION

and motion may not be achieved for 6 to 12 months. Occasionally patients will complain of inability to flex or extend their fingers in the early postoperative period. This may be the result of the relative lengthening of the tendons and the alteration in Blick's curve. The patient and the therapist are made aware that this is transient and will resolve with therapy.

■ OUTCOMES

In almost all reported series, patients have experienced a subjective sense of weakness in the operated wrist.[1,3,5,8] Objective measurements, however, have revealed grip strengths that are routinely between 60 and 90% of normal.[1,3–5,8] Most major series report an average of 44° of extension, 45° of flexion, 30° of ulnar deviation, and 5° of radial deviation at the wrist.[3–5,8] The final range of motion and maximum strength may not be achieved for up to 1 year. Almost all patients note a significant improvement in pain, and most patients are able to return to their normal preoperative avocations and occupations regardless of the type of work.[1,3–5,8] In general, all series report excellent overall patient satisfaction with the procedure and its outcome. On the basis of these published outcomes and our own experience, we recommend proximal row carpectomy when appropriately indicated for the treatment of wrist pain or deformity.[6]

References

1. Crabbe WA: Excision of the proximal row of the carpus. J Bone Joint Surg, 1964; 46B:708–711.
2. Ferlic DC, Mack LC, Mills MF: Proximal row carpectomy: Review of rheumatoid and nonrheumatoid wrists. J Hand Surg, 1991; 16A:420–424.
3. Green DP: Proximal row carpectomy. Hand Clin, 1987; 3:163–168.
4. Inglis AE: Proximal row carpectomy for diseases of the proximal row. J Bone Joint Surg, 1977; 59A:460–463.
5. Jorgenson EC: Proximal-row carpectomy: An end result study of twenty-two cases. J Bone Joint Surg, 1969; 51A:1104–1111.
6. Mack GR, Lichtman DM: Proximal row carpectomy. In: Lichtman DM (ed): The Wrist and Its Disorders. Philadelphia: WB Saunders, 1988:320–322.
7. Mclaughlin HL, Babb OD: Carpectomy. Surg Clin North Am, 1951; 31:451–461.
8. Neviaser RJ: Proximal row carpectomy for post traumatic disorders of the carpus. J Hand Surg, 1983; 8:301–305.
9. Omer EG, Capen DA: Proximal row carpectomy with muscle transfers for spastic paralysis. J Hand Surg, 1976; 1:197–204.
10. Stack JK: End results of excision of the carpal bones. Arch Surg, 1948; 57:245–252.
11. Stamm TT: Excision of the proximal row of the carpus. Proc R Soc Med, 1944; 38:74–75.
12. White JW, Stubbins SG: Carpectomy for intractable flexion deformities of the wrist. J Bone Joint Surg, 1944; 26:131–138.

122

ROBERT H.
BRUMFIELD

Shelf Arthroplasty of the Radiocarpal Joint

Wrist involvement in patients who have rheumatoid arthritis often produces pain, loss of motion, weakness, and impaired function. This is the result of progressive synovitis, which produces alteration of wrist ligaments, destruction of wrist joints, and loss of stability.

Early efforts to halt the progression of synovitis with modalities, splints, and various types of medications may prevent or delay the progression of wrist deformities. Once significant intra-articular changes have developed, arthrodeses and arthroplasties are usually recommended. However, patients prefer to retain at least some wrist motion.

Upper extremity function, positioning the hand in space to perform activities of daily living, requires a stable, pain-free wrist. An electrogoniometric study[3] done in our pathokinesiology laboratory found that 35° of extension and 10° of flexion were necessary in the wrist to perform routine activities of daily living. Other studies[7] found similar requirements in range of motion. Thus, we became interested in the concept of arthroplasties. Murphy probably was the first to write about wrist arthroplasty.[8] However, this operation was thought to be of limited value because of instability and loss of motion, resulting in loss of function. The subsequent reports of Lipscomb,[7] Linscheid,[6] Straub and Ranawat,[10] and Albright and Chase[1] encouraged us to start performing arthroplasties at Rancho Los Amigos Hospital in 1970. We perform the procedure as described by Albright and Chase with slight modifications.

■ HISTORY OF THE TECHNIQUE

The indication for this operation is primarily wrist pain unresponsive to conservative care in a patient with rheumatoid arthritis. Clinical findings during physical examination would typically include mild palmar subluxation of the carpus and increased pain with motion. Radiographic findings would confirm palmar subluxation and show minimal joint space narrowing and bone destruction.

Contraindications to palmar shelf arthroplasty include sepsis, nonfunctioning wrist extensors, severe instability, and advanced bone destruction on radiographs.

■ INDICATIONS AND CONTRAINDICATIONS

The procedure is done under general anesthesia, using standard upper extremity preparations and draping, and is done with tourniquet control. Prophylactic antibiotics are recommended.

The skin incision is almost straight, with an oblique orientation. If it is too "S" shaped, it can cause skin necrosis with subsequent delayed healing, dehiscence, or infection. The skin flaps are carefully mobilized, along with subcutaneous fat, from the underlying retinaculum. The longitudinal veins are preserved because disruption can lead to venous stasis, swelling, and decreased arterial supply, with its complications.

The dorsal retinaculum is detached (as suggested by Clayton)[4] from the ulnar side of the wrist. Each successive dorsal compartment is opened and tenosynovectomies are performed. The retinaculum is left attached on the radial side for transfer under the extensor tendons, thus lessening the chance of postoperative extensor tendon rupture.

The distal ulna is resected if indicated to treat instability, pain, or arthritic changes in the distal radioulnar joint (DRUJ). Less than three quarters of an inch should be removed because removing more can cause instability of the distal ulna (Fig. 122–1).

■ SURGICAL TECHNIQUES

■ FIGURE 122–1
Diagram of the resected distal radius; resection of the distal ulna is indicated only for pain or instability.

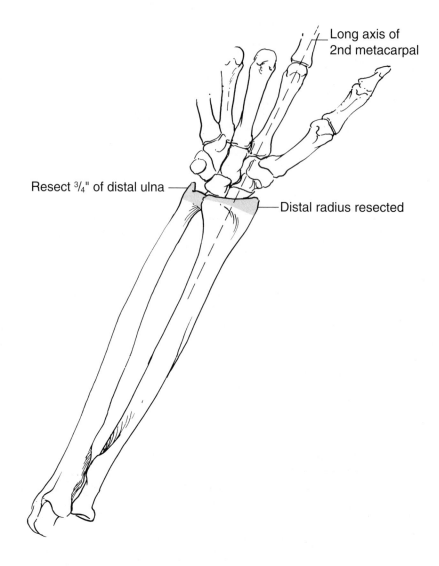

Long axis of 2nd metacarpal

Resect ³/₄" of distal ulna

Distal radius resected

The dorsal wrist capsule is opened in an "H"-shaped (or similar) fashion. Synovectomies of the radiocarpal, radioulnar, and ulnocarpal joints are then done.

The distal radius is shortened to correct the flexion deformity and prepared to receive the proximal carpal row. Either a palmar shelf or a crescent-shaped distal radius is created (Fig. 122–2). The carpus is then reduced on the radius, passive motion is checked, and further bone resection is done as necessary to correct the flexion deformity. The proximal carpal bones are not osteotomized (partially or completely) unless absolutely necessary for relocation of the wrist or correction of the flexion deformity, because this one factor increases the chance of spontaneous fusion. The wrist is immobilized in the desired position (neutral with slight ulnar deviation) with one or two crossed Steinmann pins or with a Rush nail.

The capsule is closed with interrupted absorbable sutures. The dorsal retinaculum is sutured under the extensor tendons as protection against rupture (bone erosion or recurrent synovitis). Ruptured finger extensors are reconstructed using tendon transfers or interpositional grafts, or a combination of techniques. Skin closure is with interrupted sutures. A forearm splint with a compression dressing is applied and changed 5 to 7 days after surgery.

■ TECHNICAL
ALTERNATIVES

Alternatives to this technique include interposition arthroplasties, and limited and total wrist arthrodeses.

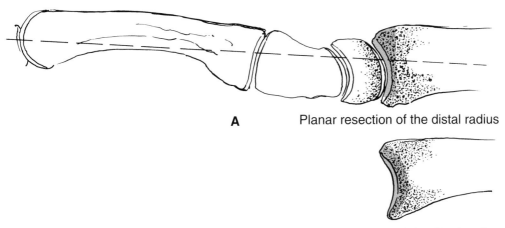

A Planar resection of the distal radius

B Or a crescentic resection of the distal radius

■ FIGURE 122–2
Diagram from a lateral perspective of the resected distal radius. The palmar shelf can be fashioned from straight osteotomy cuts **(A)** or a concentric resection **(B)** to receive the carpal bones.

The potential technical problems with this operation are many: skin necrosis with infections (superficial and deep), radiocarpal and DRUJ instability, spontaneous fusion, and recurrence of synovitis.

■ REHABILITATION

A short arm cast is applied at the first dressing change. It is used until 5 to 6 postoperative weeks, when the pins are removed. A short arm splint is then applied and the patient is instructed on active range of motion exercises. At 9 weeks, the splint is used at night only, until 3 postoperative months. The rehabilitation is supervised by a hand therapist, who emphasizes wrist extensor strength, edema control, and return to light activities of daily living. The patient is closely observed to detect any signs of early reflex sympathetic dystrophy. Full activities of daily living are not permitted until 3 postoperative months.

■ OUTCOMES

In 1979,[2] we reported on 93 procedures on 95 patients. These patients, who had rheumatoid arthritis for an average of 14 years before surgery, were followed for a minimum of 12 months and an average of 26 months. Adjacent joints were involved in all patients. Five patients (six operations) were lost to follow-up from 2 to 8 postoperative months, providing acceptable follow-up of 87 procedures in 70 patients.

Postoperative relief of pain was obtained in 72 of the 87 wrists (83%). Seventy-one of the 87 wrists (91%) were stable after surgery. An arthrodesis was done on one of the unstable arthroplasties, and the others were satisfactorily treated with orthoses. Loss of wrist motion occurred in all cases, averaging a 40° loss (55%), from a preoperative average range of 73° to a postoperative average range of 33°, which was equally distributed in extension and flexion. Spontaneous fusion occurred in 14 of 87 wrists (16%). Other complications included recurrence of synovitis in 7 of 87 wrists (8%), postoperative infection in 7 of 87 cases (8%), and carpal tunnel syndrome in 1 of 87 (which required surgical decompression with poor results).

In 1989,[5] we reported on 63 of these procedures in 49 of the original patients. The length of follow-up averaged 83 months (minimum, 12 months for the wrists that fused and 24 months for those that did not). Before surgery, all wrists were painful, with 96% being moderately or severely so. Carpal subluxation was present in 79% of the wrists. After surgery, pain recurred in 84% of the wrists, but it was less severe (mild in 48%, moderate in 35%, and severe in 2%). Sixty-eight percent of the wrists fused spontaneously and were no longer painful. Of the 20 wrists (32%) that did not fuse, 70% were mildly or moderately painful.

In patients who have rheumatoid arthritis, we found that palmar shelf arthroplasty provides early, encouraging results. Longer-term results are associated with a high rate of delayed spontaneous fusion and an unacceptably high rate of recurrent pain, although the pain was less severe. Currently, I recommend this procedure very infrequently.

References

1. Albright JA, Chase RA: Palmar shelf arthroplasty of the wrist in rheumatoid arthritis. J Bone Joint Surg, 1970; 52A:896–906.
2. Brumfield RH, Conaty JP, Mays JD: Surgery of the wrist in rheumatoid arthritis. Clin Orthop, 1979; 142:159–163.
3. Brumfield RH, Champoux JA: A biomechanical study of normal functional wrist motion. Clin Orthop, 1984; 187:23–25.
4. Clayton ML: Surgical treatment at the wrist in rheumatoid arthritis. A review of thirty-seven patients. J Bone Joint Surg, 1965; 47A:741–750.
5. Gellman H, Rankin G, Brumfield R, Chandler D, Williams B: Palmar shelf arthroplasty in the rheumatoid wrist. J Bone Joint Surg, 1989; 71A:223–227.
6. Linscheid RL: Surgery for rheumatoid arthritis: Timing and techniques: the upper extremity. J Bone Joint Surg, 1968; 50A:605–613.
7. Lipscomb PR: Surgery for rheumatoid arthritis: Timing and techniques: Summary. J Bone Joint Surg, 1968; 50A:614–617.
8. Murphy JB: Arthroplasty. Ann Surg, 1913; 57:593–647.
9. Palmar AK, Werner FW, Murphy D, Glisson R: Functional wrist motion: A biomechanical study. J Hand Surg, 1985; 10A:39–46.
10. Straub LR, Ranawat CS: The wrist in rheumatoid arthritis: Surgical treatment and results. J Bone Joint Surg, 1969; 51A:1–10.

MICHEL Y. BENOIT,
JOHN F. FATTI

123

Wrist Arthroplasty with a Silastic Implant

The development of the silicone wrist prosthesis began in the early 1960s with the pioneering work of Alfred B. Swanson, M.D. The successful experience gained in flexible intramedullary stemmed hinged implants for the fingers led to the development of the flexible silicone prosthesis for the radiocarpal joint in 1967.[15,16] The prosthesis is a silicone rubber spacer that has a thickened central barrel section serving as a hinge and intramedullary stems, which are placed into the third metacarpal and the distal radius. Since its introduction, some modifications have been made to the prosthesis. The initial silicone prosthesis was reinforced with Dacron. In 1974, another version of the Swanson wrist implant was introduced using a more durable high-performance silicone elastomer.[17] More recently, in 1982, titanium grommets were added to the silicone implant to decrease the amount of prosthetic wear at the bone–silicone interface.

The surgical technique was described by Swanson at the time of the introduction of the prosthesis in 1967.[16] Except for the abandonment of the use of the silicone cap replacing the ulnar head, the technique itself has not significantly changed since its inception. Therefore, in the subsequent section of this chapter, the surgical technique reflects the Swanson technique. The distal ulna is now simply resected. Finally, some modifications to this technique that we have used are described in the technical alternatives section.

The principle indication for wrist arthroplasty is the relief of arthritic pain where some motion is an important functional factor (especially in polyarticular disease involving the upper extremity). However, in light of the recent reports on long-term follow-up of patients with silicone prostheses,[3,7–9] we believe that the indications should be limited to patients with inflammatory arthritis, whose arthritis is under control, who have low demands on their wrist, have a well-aligned wrist with good bone stock, have intact wrist extensor tendons, and do not need their upper extremity for ambulatory support (Fig. 123–1). Posttraumatic arthritis, Kienbock's disease, osteoarthritis, wrist instability leading to arthritic changes, and similar conditions in an otherwise healthy patient should be considered as relative contraindications. Patients with a history of wrist infection would probably be better served with wrist arthrodesis. Ideally, ipsilateral elbow and shoulder pain or deformity should be treated before wrist implant arthroplasty so that the hand and wrist can be adequately positioned in space.

General or regional anesthetic can be used for this procedure. In all cases, proper positioning of the patient is mandatory. This requires attention to the limited range of motion of other joints because of the patients' frequent polyarticular involvement. Perioperative intravenous antibiotics should be used. The use of a well-padded upper arm tourniquet is recommended when performing this procedure. Inflating the tourniquet to approximately 100 to 125 mm Hg above systolic blood pressure is usually sufficient.

Although the anatomy of the wrist can be quite distorted in patients with advanced inflammatory arthritis, the dorsal aspect of the distal radius and the shaft of the third metacarpal are the standard landmarks. A longitudinal dorsal midline incision centered over the radiocarpal joint should follow the long axis of the radius and third metacarpal. In rheumatoid patients, one should be extremely careful with the delicate skin, which can

■ HISTORY OF THE TECHNIQUE

■ INDICATIONS AND CONTRAINDICATIONS

■ SURGICAL TECHNIQUES

971

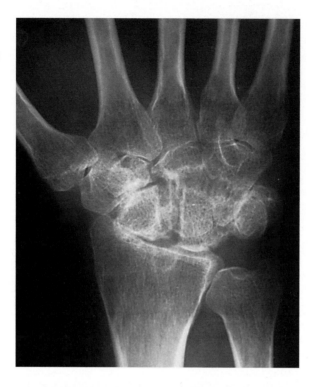

be easily torn with simple traction. Therefore, extension of the incision may be appropriate
to decrease skin tension. Skin and subcutaneous tissue are elevated, revealing the extensor
retinaculum. The retinaculum itself is incised longitudinally over the center of the fourth
compartment. If a tenosynovectomy is necessary, the retinaculum is elevated radially
and ulnarly to open the other extensor tendon compartments. With the extensor tendons
unroofed and retracted, a wrist capsulotomy is performed. A U-type incision that is distally
based is made in the capsule. The transverse branch of the U is made at the radiocarpal
joint. This capsular flap is carefully preserved for later resuturing.

Because of the distortion of the carpal anatomy caused by the disease, proper identification of the different carpal bones is mandatory, as is protection of the structures volar to
these carpal bones. The lunate and proximal portions of the scaphoid, capitate, and triquetrum are resected to provide a distal flat surface. The distal radius is then cut perpendicular
to its long axis, just proximal to the articular surface, using an oscillating saw. The resection
of bone should result in a 1.5-cm gap between these two parallel flat surfaces of bone (Fig.
123–2). The capitate and base of the third metacarpal are then reamed with broaches,
curettes, and power tools. A K-wire can be used initially to find the medullary canal of
the third metacarpal through the capitate and an intraoperative radiograph can be obtained
if there is any incertitude regarding this important technical aspect of this procedure. The
prosthesis size testing is carried out distally because the size of the prosthesis is usually
determined by the diameter of the third metacarpal reaming. The distal fit into the third
metacarpal is deemed satisfactory if the barrel (hinge) of the trial prosthesis fits flush
against the carpal bones with the distal stem all the way into the third metacarpal. The
radius is then reamed and tailored to accept the proper size prosthesis based on the size
previously determined distally. To judge if the proper size prosthesis has been selected,
the hinge of the trial implant should rest on the cortical margin of the distal radius (especially radially and ulnarly) to prevent settling (Fig. 123–3). Soft tissue contracture or
marked bone deformity may cause difficulty in insertion of the proper size trial. In this
case, further bone resection should be done, preferably from the radius. Proper bone
preparation and prosthetic choice should allow 60° of passive motion without buckling
or impingement of the implant. Finally, less than 2 cm of distal ulna is resected to obtain
a smooth bony surface that will not impinge upon the distal radius and remaining carpal

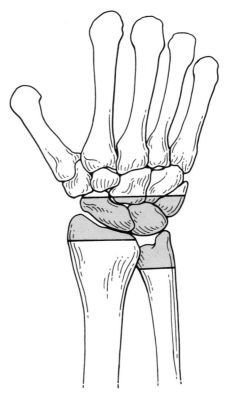

FIGURE 123–2
A diagram of the bone resection necessary to obtain 2 parallel surfaces approximately 1 to 1.5 cm apart.

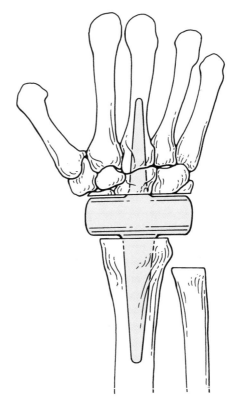

FIGURE 123–3
A diagram of a prosthetic implant.

■ FIGURE 123–4
The intraoperative ap-
pearance of the implant
with the wrist in a neutral
position.

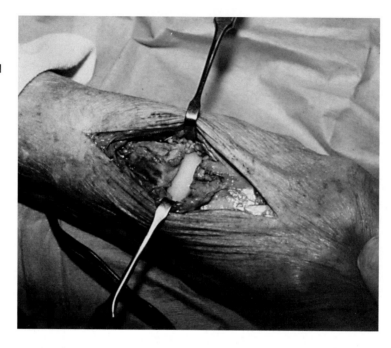

bones. The bony surface in contact with the prosthesis should be smoothed to decrease the chance of prosthetic damage. The final prosthesis can then be inserted (Figs. 123–4 and 123–5).

The wound closure is preceded by thorough irrigation. The wrist capsule is carefully closed to enhance structural support of the implant. The transverse capsulotomy is repaired through holes made in the distal radius with the wrist in mild dorsiflexion. For this purpose, three or four stitches of absorbable material are usually passed through the dorsal cortex of the radius before the final insertion of the prosthesis. The two longitudinal branches of the distally based U capsulotomy are closed with absorbable suture material using figure-of-eight stitches. A 2-0 or larger size suture should be used for this step. The capsule is closed over a suction drain and brought out through a separate small skin incision. The extensor retinaculum is then closed using a 4-0 absorbable suture after being divided transversely and placing the distal half deep to the extensor tendons to reinforce the wrist capsular closure. The proximal portion is placed superficial to the extensor tendons to prevent tendon bowstringing. If necessary, a transfer of the extensor carpi radialis longus to the extensor carpi ulnaris is performed.[10] The need for this tendon transfer is indicated if preoperatively the patient has a radially deviated wrist that cannot be actively ulnarly deviated to a neutral position. Wrist balance, including residual radial deviation, also is assessed intraoperatively after the prosthesis has been placed. With careful handling of the skin, the wound is closed using interrupted vertical mattress sutures of 4–0 nonabsorbable material.

A bulky dressing is applied to the hand and forearm. The dressing should leave the fingers free for movement. A well-padded short arm plaster splint with the wrist in neutral position is then applied to the hand and forearm. Pressure points, which could cause trauma to the fragile skin, are avoided. Finger motion is started on the day of the operation by instructing the patient during the postoperative check. The drain is removed on the first day after surgery, and the patient is discharged. At 5 to 7 days after surgery, the splint is changed to a short arm cast, keeping the wrist in neutral position. The stitches are left in place for approximately 14 days to allow healing of the skin of patients, who often are receiving corticosteroid medication.

■ TECHNICAL
ALTERNATIVES

As mentioned earlier, this surgical technique represents the original description by Swanson. There are a few modifications to the technique that we occasionally have found

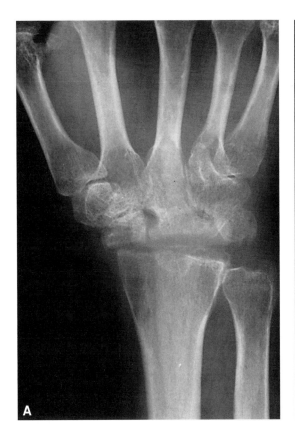
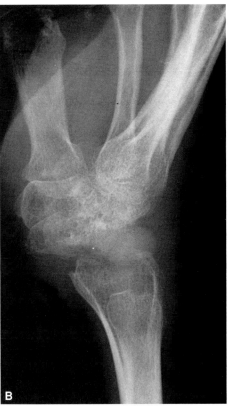

■ FIGURE 123–5
A and B, Immediate postoperative PA and lateral radiographs of a well-positioned implant.

useful. An alternative approach to the extensor retinaculum can be used if a tenosynovectomy needs to be performed. The second, third, fifth, and sixth compartments all could be opened if necessary. Conversely, if the extensor tenosynovium is in good condition, a technique that allows exposure of the wrist without entering the fourth compartment can be used. In this case, the extensor retinaculum is incised over the third extensor compartment at the distal radius level and over the wrist extensors more distally. An incision is carefully made over the ulnar side of Lister's tubercle, which can be easily palpated. The third compartment is then opened with scissors proximally and distally. Distally, the opening of the extensor retinaculum follows the course of the extensor pollicis longus until it crosses the second compartment. The extensor pollicis longus, now unroofed, is allowed to sublux radially. The deeper incision distally follows the ulnar side of the wrist extensors. The floor of the third and second compartment, which is the dorsal wrist capsule, can be incised longitudinally. A subperiosteal dissection of the distal radius proximally and carpal bones distally then exposes the wrist joint without entering any of the extensor tendon compartments other than the third. This technique minimizes postoperative pain during finger motion exercises. Closure of the wrist joint is done in a fashion as previously described but leaving the extensor pollicis longus superficial to the extensor retinaculum. Lister's tubercle should be removed if there are any sharp bone edges present.

   Another alternative technique includes the use of grommets with the silicone prosthesis.[17] Our experience is limited with their use, but, technically, the procedure is similar to what has been described except for a slightly larger opening in the medullary canals to accommodate the grommets. Proximally, the grommet is placed on the palmar aspect of the prosthesis, whereas the distal grommet is placed on the dorsal portion of the prosthesis. The grommets partially cover the stem and hinge of the prosthesis.

Transfer of the extensor carpi radialis longus to the extensor carpi ulnaris remains a rarely performed procedure.[10] If necessary, the extensor carpi radialis longus is divided from its insertion at the base of the second metacarpal. The tendon is then rerouted superficially over the common extensor tendon of the fingers. The tendon is then sutured to the extensor carpi ulnaris. The tension to be placed on the extensor carpi radialis longus is estimated with the wrist in neutral position. Finally, extensor tendon repair or extensor tendon transfer for ruptured rheumatoid tendons should be done as indicated.

■ REHABILITATION

A short arm cast is worn for a total of 6 weeks. The importance of this period of immobilization has been stressed by many authors who believe that limited postoperative wrist motion decreases the incidence of breakage of the prosthesis. After the initial 6 weeks of immobilization, the wrist is placed in a removable orthoplast splint. At that time, a hand therapist supervises range of motion and strengthening exercises. The goal is to regain a functional range of motion of 20° to 30° of both flexion and extension, as well as 10° of radial and ulnar deviation. The wrist splint is usually weaned over a period of 3 to 4 weeks as the therapy reaches its goal. At this point, unrestricted activity is allowed.

■ OUTCOMES

In 1973, Swanson reported the first series of patients who had a silicone wrist arthroplasty. He reported excellent results in 15 patients.[17] Since that time, there have been numerous other authors who have reported the benefit of this wrist implant in the treatment of their patients.[2,9,11] In early follow-up, patients regained pinch and grip strength and were satisfied with the range of motion and pain relief. Subjective satisfaction of the patients approached almost 100% (Fig. 123–6).

However, recent reports based on long-term follow-up have shown that patients' satisfaction, objective measurements, and radiographic evaluation all deteriorate in time.[1,5,7,12,13] In one study, more than 50% of the patients were having moderate or severe pain, and 41% were having mild pain at an average of 5.8 years of follow-up.[8] By that time, 41% of the patients required additional surgery for their wrists. Worse results were

■ FIGURE 123–6
A 6-month postoperative PA radiograph.

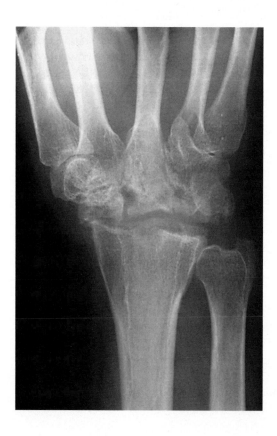

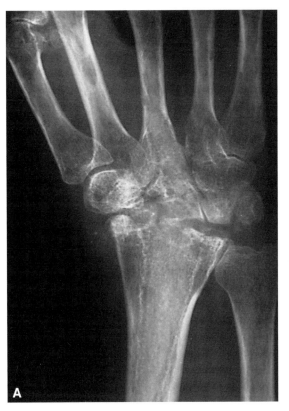
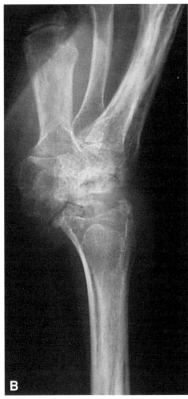

■ FIGURE 123-7
A and B, Five-year post-operative radiographs. Note the subsidence of the prosthesis into the radius and carpus, ulnar deviation of the wrist, and bone resorption.

noted in noninflammatory arthritis or uncontrolled systemic rheumatoid arthritis. More specifically, 36% of the wrist prosthesis fractured, the majority of which required a revision. Another study demonstrated a prosthesis fracture rate of 65%.[7] Similarly, the wrist alignment deteriorated in 44% of the cases (Fig. 123-7). Finally, approximately 25% of the prostheses caused silicone synovitis, which has a destructive effect on the bone. This complication is related to the wear debris from the prosthesis. Other complications, including dislocation of the prosthesis, infection, fracture of the distal radius or third metacarpal, reflex sympathetic dystrophy, and carpal tunnel syndrome, have been documented. Overall, after an average of almost 6 years of follow-up, the evaluation of the Swanson wrist arthroplasty resulted in only 26% of the patients having good or excellent results. These results have extremely narrowed the indications for implantation of this prosthesis. It is our opinion that rheumatoid patients with good bone stock and exceedingly low demand on their wrists are the rare candidates for this procedure. Other wrist reconstructive procedures such as wrist synovectomy and distal ulnar resection, radiocarpal arthrodesis, and total wrist arthrodesis are considered to be more durable procedures.[4,6,14,18]

References

1. Atkinson RE, Smith RJ: Silicone synovitis following silicone implant arthroplasty. Hand Clinics, 1986; 2:291-299.
2. Beckenbaugh RD: Implant arthroplasty in the rheumatoid hand and wrist: Current state of the art in the United States. J Hand Surg, 1983; 8:675-678.
3. Brase D, Millender L: Failure of silicone wrist arthroplasty in rheumatoid arthritis. J Hand Surg, 1986; 11:175-183.
4. Carrol RE, Dick HM: Arthrodesis of the wrist for rheumatoid arthritis. J Bone Joint Surg, 1971; 53A:1365-1369.
5. Carter PR, Benton LJ, Dysert PA: Silicone rubber carpal implants: A study of the incidence of late osseous complications. J Hand Surg, 1986; 11A:639-644.
6. Clayton ML: Surgical treatment of the wrist in rheumatoid arthritis: A review of thirty-seven cases. J Bone Joint Surg, 1965; 47A:741-750.

7. Comstock CP, Louis DS, Eckenrode JF: Silicone wrist implant: Long-term follow-up study. J Hand Surg, 1988; 13A:201–205.

8. Fatti JF, Palmer AK, Greenky S, Mosher JF: Long-term results of Swanson interpositional wrist arthroplasty: Part II. J Hand Surg, 1991; 16A:432–437.

9. Fatti JF, Palmer AK, Mosher JF: The long-term results of Swanson silicone rubber interpositional wrist arthroplasty. J Hand Surg, 1986; 11A:166–175.

10. Ferlic DC, Clayton ML: Tendon transfer for radial rotation in the rheumatoid wrist. J Bone Joint Surg, 1973; 55:880-881.

11. Goodman MJ, Millender LH, Nalebuff EA, Philips CA: Arthroplasty of the rheumatoid wrist with silicone rubber: an early evaluation. J Hand Surg, 1980; 5:114–121.

12. Gordon M, Bullough PG: Synovial and osseous inflammation in failed silicone rubber prostheses. A report of six cases. J Bone Joint Surg, 1982; 64A:574–580.

13. Peimer CA, Medige J, Eckert BS, Wright JR, Howard CS: Reactive synovitis after silicone arthroplasty. J Hand Surg, 1986; 11A:624–638.

14. Straub LR, Ranawat CS. The wrist in rheumatoid arthritis. Surgical treatment and results. J Bone Joint Surg, 1969; 51A:1–20.

15. Swanson AB: Flexible implant arthroplasty for arthritic disabilities of the radiocarpal joint. Orthop Clin North Am, 1973; 4:383–394.

16. Swanson AB: Flexible implant resection arthroplasty in the hand and extremities, St. Louis: Mosby, 1973:254–264.

17. Swanson AB, Swanson GD, Maupin BK: Flexible implant arthroplasty of the radiocarpal joint: Surgical technique and long-term study. Clin Orthop, 1984; 187:94–106.

18. Taleisnik J: Rheumatoid arthritis of the wrist. Hand Clinics, 1989; 5:257–278.

MARY LYNN BROWN,
ROBERT
BECKENBAUGH

124

Wrist Arthroplasty with the Biaxial Prosthesis

The goals of arthroplasty in the surgical management of wrist arthritis are to preserve functional range of motion and to provide wrist stability while relieving pain. Total wrist arthroplasty can achieve these goals.

There have been many options described for treatment of rheumatoid arthritis of the wrist. Synovectomy of the wrist is a viable option when there is limited articular destruction and early deformity. Although the disease process continues, synovectomy can relieve pain and improve function. Other possibilities include limited wrist fusions and wrist arthrodesis. Arthrodesis of the wrist is popular for treatment of rheumatoid arthritis. The procedure provides a stable pain free wrist that is functional if other upper extremity joints are not severely involved in the disease process. However, eliminating wrist motion in patients with severe shoulder and elbow disease may prevent or severely hinder activities such as eating and personal hygiene.

Swanson[6] introduced the first wrist joint replacement in the late 1960s. Silastic prostheses were initially used quite extensively. Success in metal and polyethylene cemented hip prosthesis stimulated the development of fixed fulcrum wrist implants by Meuli and Volz in the early 1970s.[4,7] Although initial results were promising, the longevity of these and other prostheses have not approached those achieved with total hip arthroplasty. Problems with these designs included unacceptable loosening rates and prosthetic migration into the carpal canal.[1,3] Therefore, from 1978 through 1982 the biaxial total wrist was developed to provide improved anatomic function and better fixation. The implant is ellipsoidal with convex-concave articulating surfaces oriented in the planes of wrist motion. The stems are porous coated to enhance fixation.

The primary indication for use of the biaxial prosthesis is multiple upper extremity joint involvement and the need for motion in patients with rheumatoid arthritis. Pain and significant deformity also are typically present in these patients (Fig. 124–1).

Total wrist arthroplasty may be relatively contraindicated in patients with post-traumatic or degenerative arthritis of the wrist. These patients typically do not have other upper extremity joint involvement and the lack of wrist motion after an arthrodesis is well tolerated. In addition, total wrist arthroplasty in this group of patients will loosen and even ultimately fail with highly stressful activities such as heavy repetitive labor or high impact sports.[1] Therefore, if the patient insists on the maintenance of motion, they must be carefully selected and be aware of the functional limitations and possibility of complications. A second relative contraindication is marked osteoporosis or absence of adequate bone stock for fixation.

Previous surgical procedures, including previous prosthetic insertion, also are not necessarily contraindications to arthroplasty. Provided that the extensor retinaculum is intact, total wrist arthroplasty can be accomplished after synovectomy or distal ulna resection. In the case of a previous arthroplasty or arthrodesis, the complication rate is higher, and a custom prosthesis may be needed, but revision can be achieved in the patient who requires motion. Also, excessive bone loss does not preclude arthroplasty. Fixation is improved with retention of a portion of the distal carpal row but the distal component can be inserted directly into the metacarpals.[2]

■ HISTORY OF THE TECHNIQUE

■ INDICATIONS AND CONTRAINDICATIONS

■ FIGURE 124–1
A and B, Preoperative radiographs in a 44-year-old man.

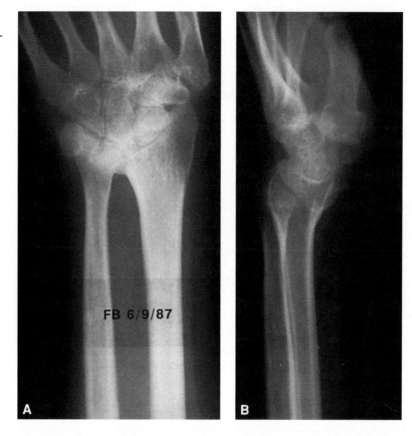

FB 6/9/87

A   B

Two absolute contraindications to total wrist arthroplasty are absence of the radial wrist extensors or the extensor retinaculum. Deficiency of the retinaculum allows the wrist and finger extensors to sublux also, resulting in wrist deformity after total wrist arthroplasty. If the radial wrist extensors or retinaculum cannot be adequately repaired, then arthroplasty must be abandoned.

Finally, a relative contraindication to total wrist arthroplasty is a previous history of sepsis. Guidelines such as those developed for total hip and knee arthroplasty patients with a history of sepsis should be followed before consideration of wrist arthroplasty.

■ SURGICAL
TECHNIQUES

The technique for the biaxial prosthesis begins with careful preoperative planning. This includes the use of templates that allow determination of the appropriate prosthesis (the largest possible) and the amount of bone to be resected.

The choice of anesthesia is made in consultation with the anesthesiologist. A general anesthetic is usually preferred. If there is a pre-existing medical problem or cervical disease in a rheumatoid patient, then a regional (i.e., axillary block) anesthetic may be preferred.

The patient is placed in a supine position with the arm on a table, using a pneumatic tourniquet. A longitudinal incision is made over the dorsum of the wrist, in line with and starting at the midportion of the third metacarpal. Subcutaneous flaps are elevated radially and ulnarly from the underlying extensor retinaculum. The retinaculum is divided over the fourth dorsal compartment and tenosynovectomy is performed as needed. The third dorsal compartment is opened and the extensor pollicis longus tendon is retracted radially. Using subperiosteal dissection, the second and first compartments are elevated off the distal radius. In particular, the extensor pollicis brevis and abductor pollicis longus tendons are identified and protected as they course over the radial styloid during resection of the distal radius. Tenosynovectomies are performed as needed.

Dissection is extended subperiosteally to the ulnar side of the wrist through the initial incision. The distal radioulnar joint is exposed by taking down the dorsal ligaments and

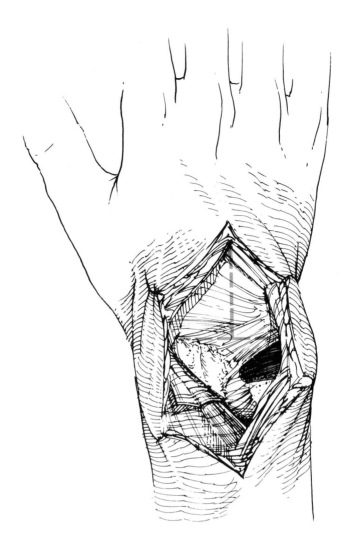

preserving radial soft tissue attachments for closure. The distal ulna is exposed subperiosteally, leaving the fifth and sixth dorsal compartments intact. Approximately two centimeters of distal ulna is resected with a sagittal saw.

A T-shaped incision is made in the wrist capsule with the base of the incision along the
radiocarpal joint, extending the T onto the base of the third metacarpal (Fig. 124–2). The
flaps are elevated so that the carpus is exposed. The distal end of the radius is resected
perpendicular to the long axis of the radius. The amount of bone that is removed is variable
but, in general, the least amount that will provide a perpendicular surface is resected. The
carpus is resected through the neck of the capitate using a slightly concave osteotomy
(Figs. 124-3A and 124-3B). An approximately 2.5-cm wide space should be left for the
prosthesis. The volar capsule should be preserved if possible. Any remaining carpus that
is subluxed volar to the radius must be excised.

The periosteum is carefully elevated off of the base of the third metacarpal to allow two
small Hohman retractors to be placed around the third metacarpal. The wrist is flexed
volarly and a sharp pointed awl or 3.0-mm Steinmann pin is passed down the capitate
into the third metacarpal shaft. After identifying the endpoint of the metacarpal head, the
medullary canal can be opened with awls, presized reamers, and power burrs to accept
the prosthesis. A side cutting awl or burr can be used to enlarge the base of the capitate
and to prepare the hole in the base of the trapezoid for the radial stud of the prosthesis. The
appropriate metacarpal rasp (as measured with the templates preoperatively) is impacted
down the third metacarpal medullary canal.

■ FIGURE 124-3
A and B, Bone resection
for biaxial total wrist
arthroplasty.

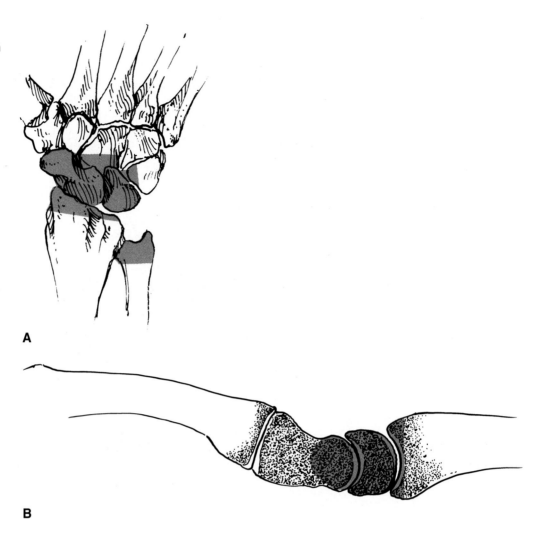

A

B

Similarly, an awl is passed down the center of the medullary canal of the radius. Any hard cortical bone at the distal surface of the radius is removed with a rongeur. Appropriately sized rasps are progressively impacted with a mallet. A trial reduction is performed. The largest sized prosthesis possible should be used and tension adjusted such that the wrist can be distracted 1 to 2 mm (normal fit). If the proper prosthesis has been selected, the only additional bone resection needed is to increase the size of the trapezoidal stud opening since the porous coated stem is 1 mm larger in diameter than the trial prosthesis. Radiographs are checked to assure proper placement. If the fit is too tight and the wrist cannot be distracted, more bone can be resected from the radius until normal tension is obtained. If the fit is loose (greater than 1 to 2 mm of distraction), and a larger prosthesis is not appropriate, longer immobilization is needed.

After an adequate trial reduction, the final prosthesis is selected and cement prepared. The distal component is almost always cemented. However, with the exception of extensive osteoporosis or previous implants, cement is not usually used proximally. The use of cement with the proximal prosthesis is believed to increase the likelihood of stress shielding and subsequent loosening.

The distal component is inserted first after placing a small piece of cancellous bone down the third metacarpal as a plug. A 12-ml syringe with an expanded tip is used to fill the medullary canal. After seating the distal component, excess cement is trimmed and the proximal component is inserted. The components are reduced and immobilized while the cement sets. Radiographs should be rechecked. After the cement is solid, both passive range of motion and tension are tested. If there is any evidence of impingement (especially on the ulnar aspect), the involved bone is excised.

Wound closure progresses in a layered fashion. The dorsal capsular flaps are closed over a suction drain to the capsular remnants or drill holes in the radius. While holding the ulna volarly, the distal radioulnar ligaments are repaired with a 2–0 or 1–0 nonabsorbable suture. The extensor retinaculum is anatomically repaired. The skin and subcutaneous tissues are closed over a second suction drain and a long arm plaster splint is applied.

The placement of the arm postoperatively and the length of immobilization are important aspects of the postoperative period. The elbow is placed in 90° of flexion and the forearm is supinated. The wrist is placed in neutral radial and ulnar deviation. Ten degrees of wrist extension is preferred if flexion and extension are equivalent during gentle passive motion after prosthesis insertion. If soft tissue tension limits palmar flexion, then the wrist should be splinted in slight palmar flexion; if wrist extension is limited, the wrist should splinted in slight extension.

■ REHABILITATION

The drains are removed at 36 to 48 hours. The dressings are changed after 4 days, and a long arm splint is reapplied. At 2 weeks, sutures are removed, and the patient is placed in a short arm cast. The length of immobilization depends on the fit determined during surgery.

Normal fit—short arm casting for two more weeks followed by a resting splint in 10° to 20° of dorsiflexion.

Loose fit—Short arm casting for 6 additional weeks followed by splinting.

Tight fit—Splinting is begun unless fit loosens, then casting.

After the splint is applied, the patient is instructed in gentle active range of motion and isometric strengthening. Weaning of the splint is begun 2 weeks later and in most patients it is discontinued 12 weeks postoperatively. The goals of therapy are limited in respect to both wrist flexion-extension and radioulnar deviation. Range of motion beyond 40° of either dorsiflexion or palmar flexion and 10° of radial or ulnar deviation can result in prosthetic imbalance, subluxation, and loosening.[5]

■ OUTCOMES

The results of biaxial total wrist arthroplasty were reviewed in 68 wrists of patients who underwent surgery between January 1983 and July 1987.[2] The patients were followed for an average of 41 months (24 to 77 months). Postoperative measurements were obtained on 56 wrists (Table 124–1). Nineteen patients had previous surgery in the same wrist or hand and eight of these patients had one or more failed arthoplasties of various designs.Range of motion averaged dorsiflexion 34.8°, palmar flexion 27.9°, radial deviation 8.6°, and ulnar deviation 17.6°. Improvements in range of motion were seen in all planes with the exception of a 9.5° decrease in palmar flexion postoperatively. With regard to subjective measurements, 85% of patients were satisfied with surgery at the time of last follow-up and 86% remained pain-free (Fig. 124–4).

The total complication rate in this series was 28%, which included a rate of 62% in patients with previous surgeries such as arthroplasties or arthrodesis. The most common complication, which also has been seen with other prostheses, is loosening. Twelve patients have demonstrated evidence of radiographic loosening, with an additional 11 patients showing partial lucent lines. Three patients experienced late dislocation of the prosthesis. One patient had an intraoperative distal radius fracture, which resulted in a nonunion and one patient had a late postoperative infection at 51 months.

More recently, the biaxial design total wrist arthroplasty was used to salvage 13 failed arthroplasties of various designs.[5] After an average 31.3 month follow-up period, two wrists had undergone further revision for loosening and one wrist was fused. Two other arthroplasties were loose. In the 10 patients with revision prostheses in place, 8 reported no pain, 1 had mild pain, and 1 had moderate pain. Range of motion averaged 35.5° dorsiflexion, 18.5° palmar flexion, 5.5° radial deviation, and 15.0° ulnar deviation.

Based on the present prostheses available, total wrist arthroplasty can offer the rheumatoid patient a potential period of excellent wrist function and pain relief with an anticipated

■ FIGURE 124–4
A and B, Postoperative radiographs with a biaxial prosthesis in place.

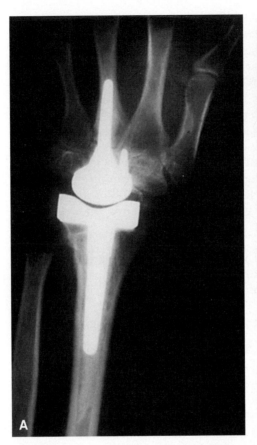
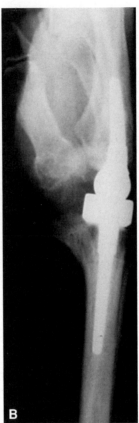

TABLE 124–1   POST-OPERATIVE ROM

Dorsiflexion	34.8°	+5.1°
Palmar Flexion	27.9°	−9.5°
Radial Deviation	8.6°	+3.8°
Ulna Deviation	17.6°	+0.8°

chance of requiring revision following primary surgery. Patients who require wrist motion and who have had previous failed arthroplasties show a higher complication rate, but can still be considered candidates for this procedure. Although problems with loosening persist, pain relief, good motion, and stability can be achieved today.

References

1. Beckenbaugh RD, Brown ML: Preliminary experience with biaxial total wrist arthroplasty. Orthop Trans, 1990; 4:678.
2. Brown ML, Beckenbaugh RD: Experience with a new design of total wrist arthroplasty. American Society for Surgery of the Hand. Toronto, Ontario, September 1990.
3. Cooney WP, Beckenbaugh RD, Linscheid RL: Total wrist arthroplasty. Problems with implant failures. Clin Orthop, 1984; 187:121-128.
4. Meuli HC: Arthroplasty of the wrist. Clin Orthop 1980; 149:118-125.
5. Rettig ME, Beckenbaugh RD: Revision total wrist arthroplasty. J Hand Surg, 1993; 18A: 798–804.
6. Swanson AB: Flexible implant arthroplasties for arthritic disabilities of the radial-carpal joint: A silicone rubber intramedullary stemmed flexible implant for the wrist joint. Orthop Clin North Am 1973; 4:383–394.
7. Volz RG: The development of a total wrist arthroplasty. Clin Orthop 1976; 116–209.

125

Hemiresection Arthroplasty of the Distal Radioulnar Joint

The hemiresection interposition technique (HIT) for arthroplasty of the distal radioulnar joint (DRUJ) was first described by Bowers in 1985.[2] A similar procedure, termed the "matched resection" technique, was described a year later by Watson and co-authors.[15] The purpose of both of these procedures is the reconstruction of a painful DRUJ by resecting the articular portion of the ulnar head while maintaining the integrity of the ulnar styloid–carpus axis. The integrity of this axis is maintained by preserving the triangular fibrocartilage complex (TFCC) connections between the radius, ulnar styloid, and ulnar carpus. Through these retained attachments the ulna is stabilized.

The Darrach-type excisional arthroplasty of the distal ulna has been unpredictable in its maintenance of distal ulna stability.[1,10,11,14] The philosophy of the HIT procedure is based on an analysis of Darrach procedures with good or excellent results. Dingman found that patients with good or excellent results had very little bone removed or had substantial regenerated bone extending distally into the region previously occupied by the styloid.[6] These patients had, in effect, reconstituted an ulnar styloid axis, resulting in improved stability and strength.

The initial reports of the HIT procedure were made up largely of patients with rheumatoid arthritis. The procedure has been useful in patients before the late stages of their rheumatoid disease, before the TFCC has been destroyed and is not reconstructible. Patients in later disease stages usually demonstrate radiocarpal translocation in addition to DRUJ involvement. Later-stage wrists are better treated with a radiolunate arthrodesis combined with either a Darrach procedure or a Sauve-Kapandji procedure.[4,12] In addition to rheumatoid arthritis, HIT has also been successful in treating osteoarthritis of the DRUJ.

Ulnocarpal impingement syndrome, where the DRUJ cartilage is still intact, may be treated by alternative procedures. The Feldon wafer resection is useful if the positive ulnar variance is less than 2 mm.[7] A formal shortening osteotomy in the diaphyseal region of the ulna may be used for positive ulnar variance of a greater magnitude.[5] However, neither of these procedures will give adequate pain relief if the cartilage surface of the ulnar head or the sigmoid notch of the radius is disrupted. In this situation HIT may be combined with an ulna shortening procedure. It is critical to combine HIT with some method of shortening the ulnar styloid axis; otherwise, stylocarpal impingement will continue.

For patients with painful instability of the DRUJ, hemiresection arthroplasty will not restore stability. However, it may substitute a less painful instability. If the articular cartilage is intact, reconstruction of the ligamentous structures should be considered before HIT.

Post-traumatic contracture combined with incompetent articular surfaces of the DRUJ may be improved with capsular release combined with HIT. If the articular surfaces are competent, a capsular release alone may be sufficient.

A contraindication to HIT is an incompetent or nonreconstructible TFCC. The stability of the ulnocarpal axis depends on the biomechanical characteristics of this anatomic structure. Experience has demonstrated that most patients with a nonreconstructible TFCC have advanced rheumatoid arthritis.[2]

■ HISTORY OF THE TECHNIQUE

■ INDICATIONS AND CONTRAINDICATIONS

■ SURGICAL
TECHNIQUES

This description of the hemiresection arthroplasty closely follows that of Bowers.[2] The operation may be done either under regional block or general anesthesia. The procedure is started with the forearm extended out on a hand table in the fully pronated position. A dorsal-ulnar incision is begun three finger-breadths proximal to the ulnar styloid, extending along the ulnar shaft (Fig. 125–1). The incision curves radially at the ulnar head, extending to the mid-carpus dorsally. The incision is then directed back in an ulnar-distal direction for several centimeters to create a flap, which should incorporate the dorsal sensory branches of the ulnar nerve. Mobilization of the flaps should incorporate the entire subcutaneous tissue down to the extensor retinaculum to protect these sensory branches. The distal ulnar shaft can then be identified between the tendons of the extensor carpi ulnaris (ECU) and the extensor digiti minimi (EDM). The muscle of the extensor indicis proprius can also be identified as it originates from the ulnar shaft just under the EDM. The capsule of the DRUJ overlying the ulnar head is evident just proximal to the extensor retinaculum. ECU stability should be evaluated at this time (preoperative assessment is also critical). If the ECU tendon is stable within the groove just radial to the ulnar styloid, then later reconstruction of the ECU sheath will not be needed. It is important to determine the stability of the ECU tendon at this stage, because if the first extensor retinacular flap will be needed for ECU stabilization, then this flap length needs to be made as long as possible. The first extensor retinacular flap is outlined in the proximal and ulnar half of the extensor retinaculum, basing the flap radially (Fig. 125–2). The ulnar incision of this retinacular flap needs to be carried around the ulnar border as far as possible to gain

■ FIGURE 125–1
Incision, highlighting the dorsal sensory branch of the ulnar nerve, which must be protected.

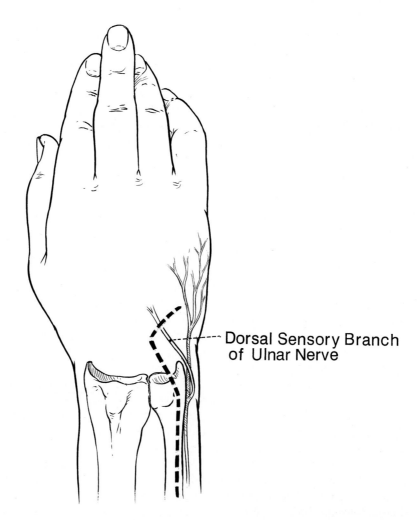

Dorsal Sensory Branch
of Ulnar Nerve

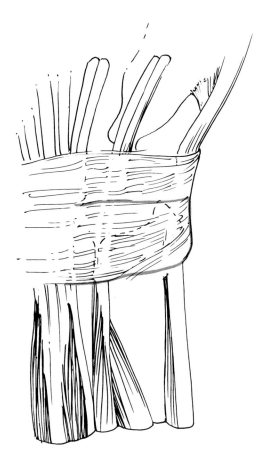

■ FIGURE 125–2
The first extensor retinacular flap is based radially
and encompasses the
proximal half to two
thirds of the retinaculum.

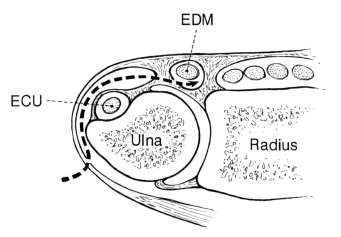

EDM

ECU

Ulna   Radius

■ FIGURE 125–3
The retinaculum flap is
reflected superficial to the
ECU subsheath–joint cap-
sule; flap reflection is
stopped before entering
the EDC compartment.

length if this flap is to be used for ECU sheath reconstruction. It is important to reflect
this flap superficial to the deeper ECU subsheath and joint capsule (Fig. 125–3). The reflection of this flap is carried radially through the EDM compartment, stopping before entering
the extensor digitorum communis (EDC) compartment. The EDM is retracted radially to
expose fully the underlying joint capsule, TFCC, and dorsal margin of the sigmoid notch
of the radius. The DRUJ capsule is detached from the radius, leaving a 1-mm cuff for later
repair (Fig. 125–4). The capsular flap is mobilized from the margin of the TFCC and
reflected ulnarly. Care is taken to preserve the integrity of the ECU subsheath by reflecting
it from the ulnar groove subperiosteally (Fig. 125–5). In most nonrheumatoid cases, this
subsheath elevation can be accomplished, and later retinacular reconstruction for ECU

■ FIGURE 125–4
The DRUJ capsule is detached from the radius, leaving a 1-mm cuff for later repair.

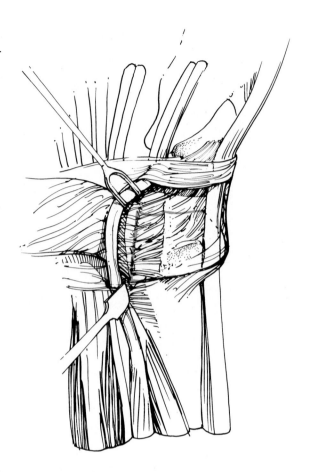

■ FIGURE 125–5
The plane of dissection for reflecting the capsular flap and elevating the ECU subsheath is subperiosteal.

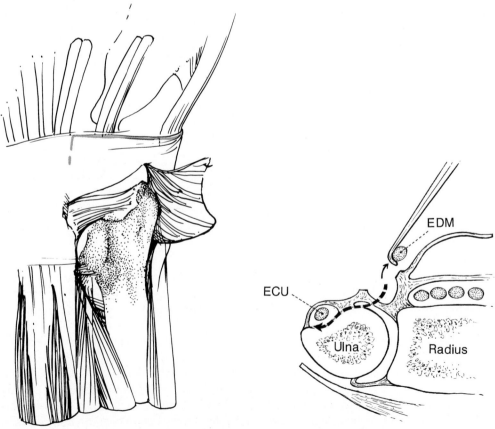

stabilization is not needed. When the capsule is repaired the ECU subsheath can be laid back into its groove, where it will heal satisfactorily, restoring ECU stability. For better exposure of the sigmoid notch and the undersurface of the TFCC, the forearm may be brought to neutral rotation. A small lamina spreader placed between the distal shafts of the radius and ulna may help expose the sigmoid notch. A small right-angle retractor may be used to retract the dorsal radioulnar ligament distally and dorsally to expose the central portion of the TFCC. Central defects of the TFCC are inconsequential. However, integrity of the dorsal and palmer radioulnar ligaments is critical. If these are detached from the ulnar styloid, reconstruction of this structure must be carried out before proceeding with the procedure. In rheumatoid patients, synovectomy may be needed to expose fully the joint surfaces and the TFCC. Further exposure of the TFCC may be accomplished by reflecting the distal ulnar half of the extensor retinaculum in an ulnar direction, opposite to the first flap (Fig. 125–6). The distal retinaculum is divided along the septum between the EDM compartment and the EDC compartment. Reflection is then carried over the ECU tendon around the ulnar side of the styloid. If the ECU tendon is unstable and later retinacular reconstruction of the sheath is required, the tendon can be mobilized all the way out to its insertion on the fifth metacarpal for better mobilization. For inspection of the ulnocarpal joint, an incision may be made in line with the fibers between the radiotriquetral ligament and the distal margin of the TFCC. The dorsal portion of the TFCC blends with this dorsal ligamentous complex, and the interval must be established sharply. The lunate and triquetral surfaces, as well as the distal surface of the TFCC, may be inspected through this incision. Routine inspection of the ulnocarpal joint and the distal portion of the TFCC

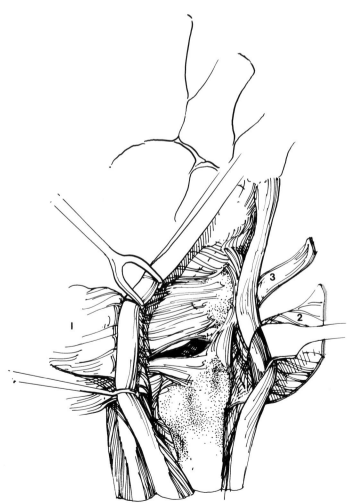

■ FIGURE 125–6
The distal retinacular flap is reflected opposite to the first flap. This flap is developed only if further exposure of the TFCC or radiocarpal joint, or both, is needed. The radiocarpal joint is accessed through an incision between the radiotriquetral ligament and the distal margin of the TFCC.

The articular portion of the ulnar head is removed first with an oblique cut using an osteotome. The remaining palmar and dorsal portions of the head are removed with a rongeur.

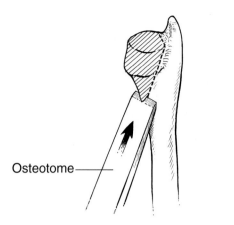
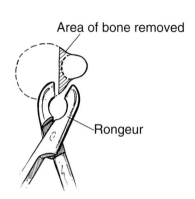

Osteotome

Area of bone removed

Rongeur

is not needed unless a pathologic process is suspected. In rheumatoid patients, opening this area for synovectomy may be warranted. After a synovectomy of the DRUJ is complete, the articular surface and underlying bone of the ulnar head is removed by first making an oblique cut with an osteotome and then removing the remainder of the bone with a rongeur (Fig. 125–7). Osteophytes may be present along the margin of the sigmoid notch. These should be removed. The radius should be rotated to expose the palmar and dorsal aspects of the ulna, and the distal ulna tapered to resemble a long, slender cone. The potential for stylocarpal impingement should now be assessed. The forearm should be taken through a full range of motion with the radius and ulna shafts compressed together while simultaneously ulnarly deviating the wrist. If there is any question that the ulnar styloid will impinge the ulnar carpus, then the ulna should be shortened. This can be carried out by detaching the ulnar styloid through the metaphyseal area of the ulna and resecting an appropriate amount of metaphysis. The ulnar styloid then can be reattached to the remaining ulna with a compression interosseous wire loop (24- to 26-gauge). If stylocarpal impingement is equivocal, instead of ulna shortening, the space between the radius and ulna can be filled with an interposition "anchovy." Enough tendon material to approximate the amount of bone resected can be harvested from the palmaris longus, ECU, or flexor carpi ulnaris. This tendon substance is rolled into a ball and sutured to the dorsal and volar capsules. Tendon interposition alone has been found adequate only in borderline cases of stylocarpal impingement (0 variant ±1 mm).

For closure, the reflected dorsal capsule is folded into the resection site as interposition material and to cover the exposed cancellous bone at the resection site (Fig. 125–8). The dorsal capsule is sutured to the volar capsule. I use a braided 4-0 nonabsorbable suture material and either interrupted simple or mattress stitches for all capsular and retinacular repairs. If a tendon "anchovy" is interposed in the joint, the dorsal capsule is repaired back to the dorsal margin of the sigmoid notch to maintain the tendon material in place. If the distal retinacular flap was elevated, it can either be repaired back over the ECU and EDM or brought under the ECU and reattached to the dorsal margin of the sigmoid notch to augment a deficient TFCC. If stabilization of the ECU is needed, the first retinacular flap is passed under and around the ECU tendon. The flap is sewn back in a more distal position to create a sling for the ECU tendon. If the ECU tendon was left intact in its subsheath, the extensor retinacular flap is repaired back to its former insertion site. The skin is closed with interrupted 4-0 nylon sutures.

■ TECHNICAL
ALTERNATIVES

Hemiresection arthroplasty will fail if the procedure is carried out in a patient with an incompetent TFCC that is not reconstructible. Assessment must be carried out both before and during surgery. If the TFCC is incompetent intraoperatively, then reconstruction can be carried out. In advanced rheumatoid arthritis there may not be sufficient tissue for reconstruction, and alternative procedures should be carried out. This may involve a radiolunate fusion combined with a Darrach or Sauve-Kapandji procedure. Most traumatic

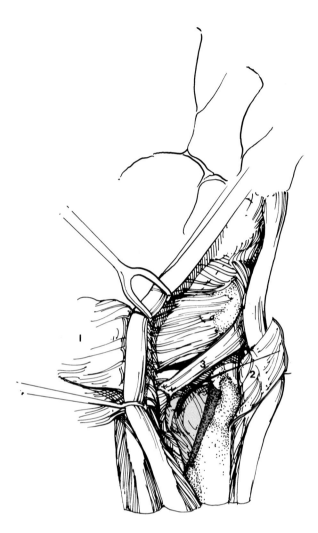

■ FIGURE 125–8
The dorsal capsular flap
(2) is interposed in the resection site and sutured
to the volar capsule. If a
tendon "anchovy" is
used, the dorsal capsular
flap is sutured back to
the dorsal margin of the
sigmoid notch. The distal
retinacular flap (3) may
be passed under the
EDU tendon and used to
augment a deficient
TFCC. The proximal reti-
nacular flap (1) may be
passed under the EDM
and then under and
around the ECU tendon
to create a sling if the
ECU tendon is unstable.

disruptions of the TFCC can be reconstructed. In the presence of degenerative changes in the DRUJ, technical modifications may be necessary (Fig. 125–9).

The two most common technical pitfalls involve inadequate bone resection and persistent stylocarpal impingement. Persistent osteophytes may be one cause of inadequate bone excision. Assessing the adequacy of ulnar head resection in only one plane is another cause. The forearm must be rotated through a full range of motion to ensure adequate bone from the volar and dorsal aspects of the ulnar head has been resected. The contour of the remaining ulnar shaft and styloid should approximate a long, slender cone.

Assessment of possible stylocarpal impingement should begin before surgery. The normal articular ulnar head provides a stable seat around which the radius rotates and translates during forearm rotation. Ulnar head resection allows the two shafts to come closer together, especially in a power grip. The maximum migration of the radius toward the ulna is no more than 0.75 cm.[3] This figure has been determined by measuring the distance between the radial styloid and the ulnar styloid with and without a power grip. If a preoperative posteroanterior radiograph of the wrist in neutral forearm rotation and ulnar wrist deviation shows that this amount of narrowing will bring the styloid within 2 mm of the ulnar carpus, then stylocarpal impingement can be expected and ulna shortening should be done. My preferred method of ulna shortening during an HIT procedure is through the distal metaphysis, but, as an alternative, a formal ulnar diaphyseal shortening osteotomy with plate fixation can be carried out. If the likelihood of impingement is assessed to be borderline, I consider tendon arterposition instead of shortening.

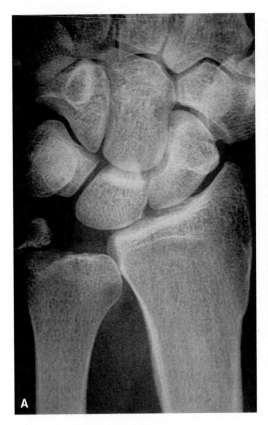
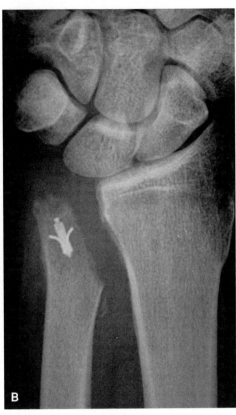

■ FIGURE 125-9

(A) Distal radioulnar joint instability with early arthrosis (more evident intraoperatively) after TFCC avulsion and ulnar styloid nonunion. Even though there is an ulnar negative variance, intraoperative assessment showed that styloid shortening was required to avoid impingement. **(B)** To accomplish ulnar axis shortening, the ulnar styloid fragment was excised and the TFCC reattached to the ulna using a suture anchor. Despite the successful use of a suture anchor in this case, I would recommend reattachment through drill holes in the ulna cortex because the anchor may easily cut out through the cancellous bone.

■ REHABILITATION

If no ulnar shortening is done, a short arm bulky dressing incorporating a short arm plaster splint is used. Finger motion is encouraged with a small amount of forearm rotation allowed. At 2 weeks, the sutures are removed and a short arm thermoplast wrist splint applied. Forearm rotation is encouraged and the patient can resume most activities of daily living and light work with the splint. At 4 postoperative weeks, the thermoplast splint is used only for heavy activities, and full wrist and forearm motion is encouraged. Heavy lifting is not recommended until after 3 months. If an ulnar shortening has been accomplished through the metaphyseal region, the initial dressing incorporates a sugar-tong splint. At 2 weeks, the sutures are removed and a sugar-tong thermoplast splint is placed for an additional 4 weeks. Six weeks after surgery, forearm motion is begun with an intermittent wrist support splint being used for the next several weeks when doing lifting or repetitive activities. Heavy lifting is not allowed for at least 3 months. If an osteotomy in the diaphyseal region has been carried out, a thermoplast forearm splint is needed until union is evident. Activity restrictions must be coordinated with the diaphyseal osteotomy healing.

■ OUTCOMES

Bowers reported on 38 cases in 1985, 27 of which were rheumatoid.[2] In 1986, Watson and colleagues reported on 44 cases, 34 of which were rheumatoid.[15] Other authors have added to these numbers, bringing the total number of patients reported in the literature to 152.[8,9,13] The diagnoses have been 42% rheumatoid, 29% instability, 21% ulnocarpal impingement, 5% primary osteoarthritis, and 3% a variety of other traumatic problems. After hemiresection arthroplasty, 76% of patients were pain free and 24% had mild pain, but described this mild pain as better than their preoperative pain. No patient had a poor result. In the hemiresection arthroplasty patients with postoperative mild pain, the pain was secondary to persistent stylocarpal impingement in 2% and was corrected by a secondary shortening osteotomy. These patients were later classified as pain free. Of those patients who did not demonstrate preoperative instability, none reported postoperative distal ulnar instability. Of those patients who had preoperative instability, the hemiresection arthroplasty replaced painful instability with less painful instability. The major demonstrable advantage over a Darrach-type total resection arthroplasty is the lack of distal ulnar instability. Up to 7% of patients after Darrach resection demonstrate painful distal ulnar instability, and they consider themselves worse than they were before surgery.[1] I have also had problems with instability of the distal ulna stump after the Sauve-Kapandji procedure, especially in young manual laborers. In my hands, the HIT is most useful in the young patient with post-traumatic arthrosis of the DRUJ and in rheumatoid patients with relatively early DRUJ involvement.

References

1. Bieber EJ, Lindscheid RL, Dobyns JH, Beckenbaugh RD: Failed distal ulnar resections. J Hand Surg, 1988; 13A:193–200.
2. Bowers WH: Distal radioulnar joint arthroplasty: The hemiresection–interposition technique. J Hand Surg, 1985; 10A:169–178.
3. Bowers WH: Distal radioulnar joint arthroplasty. Clin Orthop, 1992; 275:104–109.
4. Chamay A, Santa DD: Radiolunate arthrodesis in rheumatoid wrist (21 cases). Ann Chir Main, 1991; 10:197–206.
5. Chun S, Palmer AK: The ulnar impaction syndrome: Follow-up of ulnar shortening osteotomy. J Hand Surg, 1993; 18A:46–53.
6. Dingman PV: Resection of the distal end of the ulna (Darrach operation): An end-result study of twenty-four cases. J Bone Joint Surg, 1952; 34A:893–900.
7. Feldon P, Terrono AL, Belsky MR: Wafer distal ulna resection for triangular fibrocartilage tears and/or ulna impaction syndrome. J Hand Surg, 1992; 17A:731–737.
8. Fernandez DL: Radial osteotomy and Bowers arthroplasty for malunited fractures of the distal end of the radius. J Bone Joint Surg, 1988; 70A:1538–1551.
9. Imbriglia JE, Matthews D: The treatment of chronic traumatic subluxation of the distal ulna by hemiresection interposition arthroplasty. Hand Clin North Am, 1991; 7:329–334.
10. Kessler I, Hecht O: Present application of the Darrach procedure. Clin Orthop, 1970; 72: 254–260.
11. Leslie BM, Carlson G, Ruby LK: Results of extensor carpi ulnaris tenodesis in the rheumatoid wrist undergoing a distal ulnar excision. J Hand Surg, 1990; 15A:547–551.
12. Linscheid RL, Dobyns JH: Radiolunate arthrodesis. J Hand Surg, 1985; 10A:821–829.
13. Minami A, Ogind T, Minami M: Treatment of distal radioulnar disorders. J Hand Surg, 1987; 12A:189–196.
14. Newmeyer WL, Green DP: Rupture of extensor tendons following resection of the distal ulna. J Bone Joint Surg, 1982; 64A:178–182.
15. Watson AK, Ryu J, Burgess RC: Matched distal ulnar resection. J Hand Surg, 1986; 11A: 812–817.

PART
X

Skeletal Reconstruction

TERI S. FORMANEK
BARRY P. SIMMONS

126

Phalangeal Derotational Osteotomy

Malrotation of the digits may occur in conjunction with traumatic, congenital, and developmental disorders. Malrotation can also occur at various levels within the phalanges. Traumatic disorders result in combinations of angulatory and rotational deformity. The clinical deformity is magnified when the site of malrotation is more proximal in the digit. Significant malrotation may cause functional impairment because of the overlap of adjacent digits, the inability simultaneously to close all digits comfortably, and the inhibition of opposition. As little as 10° of rotation may result in significant functional deformity and may also be cosmetically unacceptable. Rotational deformities in children do not spontaneously correct with growth, and therefore will need surgical correction to achieve realignment.

Very few techniques for performing phalangeal derotation osteotomy have been described in the literature. Most textbooks mention the need for this operation but offer no technical suggestions. The techniques that follow are a result of the authors' experience with the treatment of phalangeal fractures and rotational deformities. They have been refined over time by incorporation of ideas from the literature.

Many authors have recommended that phalangeal malrotation be corrected through metacarpal osteotomy.[4,7,8] They object to phalangeal osteotomy, citing difficulties with angular deformity, internal fixation of small bone fragments, delayed union, and tendon rupture or adherence. However, the amount of rotational correction obtainable through a metacarpal osteotomy is limited to between 15 to 20° owing to the soft tissue constraints on the metacarpal.[2] Likewise, a large rotational correction through the metacarpal may lead to altered kinematics at the metacarpophalangeal (MP) joint during flexion. The change in mechanics results from the change produced in the axial alignment of the MP joint relative to the axis of finger flexion and extension. The force vectors of the flexor tendons and the extensor apparatus across the MP joint remain the same after metacarpal rotation osteotomy. The change in the MP joint axial alignment relative to the unchanged tendon forces results in the MP joint moving through an altered arc of rotation, with constraint from the collateral ligament increasing through the flexion arc. Cadaveric studies confirm that basal metacarpal osteotomies may correct phalangeal malrotation only over a limited range of flexion.[6] There clearly remain indications for correction of rotational deformities of the fingers by phalangeal derotation osteotomy. Certainly, larger magnitudes of malrotation (>25°) will necessitate correction at the phalangeal level. Congenital or developmental rotational deformities of the phalanges should be corrected at the site of rotation. Rotational deformities associated with phalangeal angulation should also be corrected at the phalangeal level to address most effectively both deformities.

There are no absolute contraindications to derotation osteotomy at the phalangeal level. Unstable soft tissues at the site of rotation is a relative contraindication to correction at the phalangeal level. The risk of compromise to the dorsal and flexor apparatuses or adjacent growth plates must be considered when contemplating phalangeal osteotomy. Significant digital stiffness may limit the need for corrective osteotomy because overlap will not occur owing to limited flexion. Certainly, soft tissue equilibrium should be present

■ HISTORY OF THE TECHNIQUE

■ INDICATIONS AND CONTRAINDICATIONS

before performing derotation osteotomy. This implies that maximum active range of motion should be obtained before performing the operation.

The technique for phalangeal derotation osteotomy requires meticulous attention to detail for optimal results. Soft tissue handling must minimize the insult to the tendinous structures. In general, osteotomy is best performed at the metaphyseal level where cancellous surfaces allow for rapid and consistent union. However, if AO plating is planned or open physes are present, then diaphyseal level osteotomies must be used. Adequate internal fixation must ensure that correction of the deformity is maintained until union. Fixation must not interfere with the dorsal apparatus function while allowing for early mobilization to prevent tendon adhesion. Both metaphyseal and diaphyseal techniques are important, and both are described.

Metaphyseal Osteotomy Technique   Regional or general anesthesia is preferred, enabling tourniquet control for a bloodless field. Midaxial incisions are used to minimize insult to the tendinous structures (Fig. 126–1). Superficially, the common neurovascular bundle is identified and carried volarly. The dorsal branch of the proper digital nerve is elevated dorsally with the other subcutaneous tissues. Occasionally, it may be necessary to sacrifice this branch. The interval between the dorsal apparatus and flexor apparatus is developed. At the proximal phalangeal level, the lateral bands are gently retracted dorsally to allow exposure. At the middle phalangeal level, the oblique retinacular ligament is likewise lifted dorsally. After longitudinal incision of the periosteum, a subperiosteal dissection is carried out to expose the phalanx at the level of planned osteotomy. Under fluoroscopic guidance, 0.045″ K-wires are placed through the periarticular metaphyseal bone from both ulnar and radial aspects. The wires should be positioned just short of the planned osteotomy and such that they will cross at this site (Fig. 126–2). An elevator or similar instrument is placed in the subperiosteal position to prevent soft tissue injury. A micro-oscillating

■ FIGURE 126–1
The midaxial approach allows careful protection of dorsal and volar neurovascular structures.

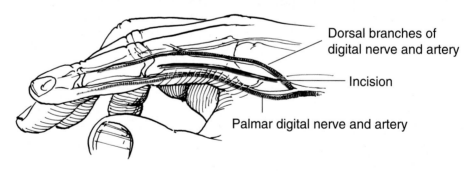

Dorsal branches of
digital nerve and artery

Incision

Palmar digital nerve and artery

■ FIGURE 126–2
Subperiosteal exposure and preplacement of fixation wires are done before the osteotomy. Note circumferential soft tissue protection at the osteotomy site.

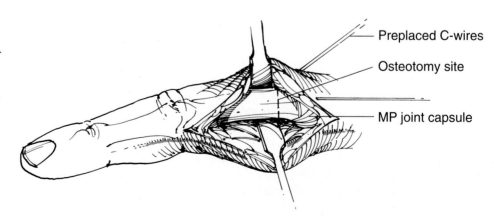

Preplaced C-wires

Osteotomy site

MP joint capsule

saw is used to make a transverse osteotomy, carefully protecting the soft tissues. The digit is rotated to the corrected position, securing the osteotomy by advancement of the preplaced wires. The correct rotation is frequently difficult to judge. The alignment is assessed while observing the tenodesis effect on the digits during passive wrist flexion and extension. Alignment is also judged by viewing the nail alignment axially. Visual access to the opposite hand is helpful in determining the "normal" alignment. The C-wires are advanced through the diaphyseal bone until the tips are in a subcutaneous position at the periarticular level (Fig. 126–3). The C-wires are cut short and bent to 90° at the diaphyseal level. They should remain protruding through the skin. The periosteum and dorsal apparatus are allowed to fall back into position and the skin is closed with 5-0 nylon suture. Xerofoam gauze is place around the protruding pins and a sterile hand dressing is used. The fingers should be immobilized in the safe position with a dorsal plaster splint.

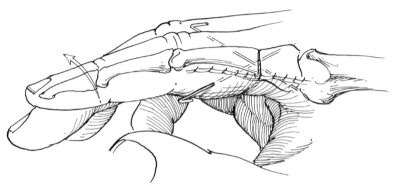

■ FIGURE 126–3
The osteotomy is completed, the phalanx derotated, and the wires are advanced.

Completed osteotomy and pinning after derotation

Diaphyseal Technique This technique is indicated in the presence of open physes in a child. The anesthetic and approach techniques are those used for the metaphyseal osteotomy. The diaphysis is exposed using a subperiosteal dissection (Fig. 126–4). A micro-oscillating saw is used to complete a transverse, mid-diaphyseal osteotomy (Fig. 126–4).

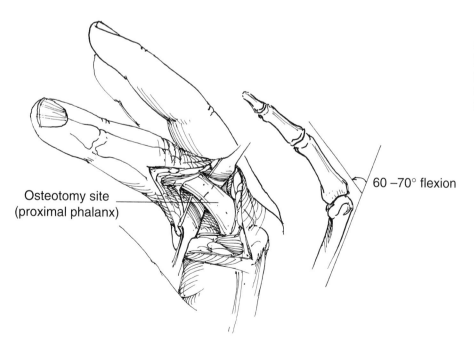

■ FIGURE 126–4
Subperiosteal dissection is completed at the diaphyseal level. The tissues are protected circumferentially.

Osteotomy site
(proximal phalanx)

60 –70° flexion

■ FIGURE 126-5
■ FIGURE 126-5
The longitudinal wires
pass through the MP
joint, across the osteot-
omy site, and through the
derotated distal fragment.
Note MP joint flexion at
60 to 70°.

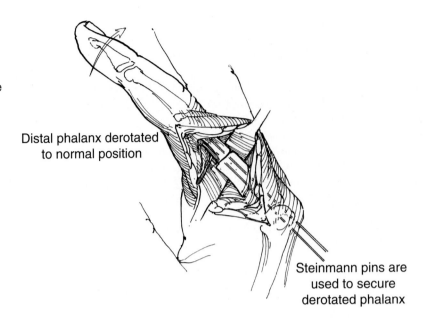

Distal phalanx derotated
to normal position

Steinmann pins are
used to secure
derotated phalanx

■ FIGURE 126-6
The advanced wires re-
mained across the MP
joint, leaving the proximal
interphalangeal (PIP) joint
free.

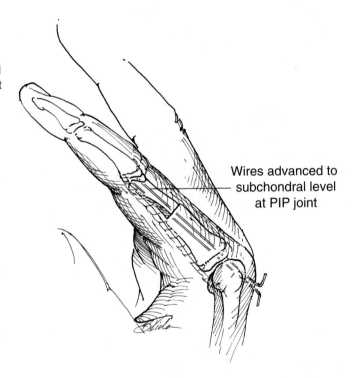

Wires advanced to
subchondral level
at PIP joint

With the MP joints flexed 60 to 70°, two 0.028″ or 0.035″ C-wires are driven centrally across the MP joint, physis, and osteotomy site in a longitudinal fashion. The C-wires are advanced to the subchondral bone distal to the osteotomy, with care taken to avoid penetration of the adjacent joint (Fig. 126–5). The C-wires are cut short and bent to a 90° angle, leaving them protruding from the skin (Fig. 126–6). The skin is closed with interrupted 5-0 chromic sutures and xerofoam gauze is placed around protruding pins. The hand should be placed in the safe position in a cast extending to the fingertips at the time of surgery.

■ TECHNICAL
ALTERNATIVES

Other techniques have been used and are mentioned for sake of completeness. Froimson[1] recommends a dorsal midline extensor tendon-splitting incision. This technique may be advantageous for osteotomizing the proximal metaphysis of the proximal phalanx. A single axial or oblique C-wire for fixation is acceptable if combined with postoperative taping of the finger to an adjacent digit. Pichora[6] recommends a step-cut osteotomy to correct rotatory deformity. This is particularly applicable in those cases necessitating tenolysis or capsulotomy. This technique requires a dorsal approach to expose a significant portion of the phalanx. A longitudinal cut is made in the dorsal cortex through the diaphyseal region. The width of the longitudinal cut determines the amount of rotational correction. He recommends beginning with a narrow osteotomy and gradually increasing the width until the correct amount of rotation is obtained. The distal transverse cut must point in the direction of correction or the longitudinal gap will open, not close, during the correction. Hence, the proximal transverse cut must exit opposite the direction of deformity. This type of osteotomy requires rigid internal fixation with interosseous wires or screws to enable immediate rehabilitation of the involved tendon and adjacent joints. The remainder of the operative technique is otherwise similar.

Internal fixation of osteotomies with various miniplates is acceptable. This technique is particularly applicable in the patient requiring extensor tenolysis. Miniplate fixation requires exacting technique to ensure that correction is adequate. Nunley and Kloen[5] have shown by cadaveric studies that application of miniplates to proximal phalanges significantly limits the active proximal interphalangeal (PIP) joint flexion. Extensor lag may also develop after this technique. These complications can be minimized through use of the miniblade plate. This plate is applied laterally, gives excellent fixation, and allows early motion while minimizing the limitation on PIP joint flexion. A subsequent operation to remove the plate is usually necessary. Therefore, the potential complications compared to the benefits of plate fixation must be considered before using these fixation devices. These techniques have been outlined in other sources.[3]

Tendon adherence is minimized by careful soft tissue handling and early mobilization. The difficulty of working with small bone fragments is avoided if wires and screws are predrilled or prepositioned before osteotomy. Placement of the osteotomy in the metaphyseal area also provides larger bone surfaces with which to work.

REHABILITATION

The hand should be immobilized initially in a hand dressing for antiedema and comfort. Between a week and 10 days after surgery, the sutures are removed and a therapy program should be instituted. This should consist of a supervised home program of active and active-assisted range of motion of the involved digit. A protective hand-based orthosis that is removable is necessary to protect the osteotomy site. The addition of other static and dynamic splints may be necessary depending on the progress made in regaining both active and passive motion of the digit. With rigid internal fixation using AO plates, the ability to begin a more aggressive rehabilitation program is possible.

For children treated with the open physeal technique, the osteotomy is allowed to heal for 3 to 4 weeks, at which time the pins are removed and a similar rehabilitation program is begun. The problem of residual stiffness is much less of a concern with the pediatric population. This allows for immobilization of the osteotomy site for a longer period of time before instituting a rehabilitation program.

OUTCOMES

Rotatory deformities at the phalangeal level can significantly impair hand function. The excellent results of correction of rotational deformities by metacarpal derotational osteotomy must be considered when correction of digital malrotation is contemplated. Despite this, phalangeal derotation osteotomy remains an important technique in the hand surgeon's armamentarium. Although clinical results for these techniques are gratifying, there is no published documentation of the objective results. Strict attention to soft tissue handling and a supervised rehabilitation program are essential to satisfactory outcomes. Radiographic evidence of union occurs after clinical union, but should be evident in all patients by 8 weeks.[6] Maintenance of preoperative range of motion is expected. Nonunion at the osteotomy site is rare, and full correction of the deformity can be achieved in essentially all patients.

References

1. Froimson AI: Osteotomy for digital deformity. J Hand Surg, 1981; 6:585–589.
2. Gross MS, Gelberman RH: Metacarpal rotational osteotomy. J Hand Surg, 1985; 10A:105–108.
3. Heim U, Pfeiffer KM: Small Fragment Manual. Berlin: Springer-Verlag, 1982.
4. Manktelow RT, Mahoney JL: Step osteotomy: A precise rotation osteotomy to correct scissoring deformities of the fingers. Plast Reconstr Surg, 1981; 68:571–576.
5. Nunley JA, Kloen P: Biomechanical and functional testing of plate fixation devices for proximal phalangeal fractures. J Hand Surg, 1991; 16A:991–998.
6. Pichora DR, Meyer R, Masear VR: Rotational step-cut osteotomy for treatment of metacarpal and phalangeal malunion. J Hand Surg, 1991; 16A:551–555.
7. Pieron AP: Correction of rotational malunion of a phalanx by metacarpal osteotomy. J Bone Joint Surg, 1972; 54A:516–519.
8. Weckesser EC: Rotational osteotomy of the metacarpal for overlapping fingers. J Bone Joint Surg, 1965; 47A:751–756.

127

Angulatory Osteotomy of Phalanges

Angulatory osteotomies of phalanges are needed for two problems—congenital deformities such as delta phalanges, and malunions. The method of performing the osteotomy, the choice of fixation types, and postoperative rehabilitation depends on the nature of the underlying cause.

Little mention of corrective osteotomies in the hand occurred until Bunnell's first edition of *Surgery of the Hand*, in 1944.[2] His method of corrective osteotomy included autologous matchstick grafts from the olecranon, fitted in a mortise-and-tenon fashion, using a special anvil to achieve the osteotomy with hand tools.[2] The first edition of Campbell's *Operative Orthopaedics* from 1939 makes no mention of osteotomy for phalangeal angulation.[3]

Most commonly, angulatory deformities must be corrected by performing an osteotomy at the level of the deformity. If the deformity is at the level of a joint, then an osteotomy just proximal or distal to the joint will realign the transverse axis of the joint and the digit. On the other hand, an osteotomy of the phalanx can be complicated by joint adhesions. Rigid internal fixation allows early joint motion, but sometimes the soft tissue cover is inadequate to allow the use of plates and screws. Use of the miniblade plate fixation can be immensely helpful in avoiding extensor adhesions.

As has been noted during closed reduction and percutaneous pinning of hand fractures, the degree of difficulty in surgeries of this type is often underestimated, because the bone is more dorsal than commonly expected by the occasional hand surgeon. When plans for digital osteotomy include the use of less rigid fixation, such as K-wires, the actual joint surfaces are more distal than one might expect based on a cursory surface examination. Because correction of angulatory malunion usually requires more precise alignment, open surgical techniques are mandated rather than percutaneous methods.

Digits with crossover deformities are ideal for corrective osteotomies of the phalanges, unless the angular deformity is very minimal. If hand function is obviously compromised because of the angular deformity, then corrective osteotomy is indicated. It is not the radiographic appearance of the digit that determines whether correction is needed. Progressive deformity in a growing child is an excellent indication. This can occur with delta phalanges or bracket epiphyses.[4,5,8,10,12,13] Gross deformities should be corrected, but mild deformities with good joint motion are best left alone.

Physical examination determines whether the deformity in an individual finger is a problem of malrotation, angulation in the sagittal plane, angulation in the frontal plane, or a combination of these. Also, assessment must be made as to how much the problem affects function, and secondarily as to cosmesis. A 5 or 10° angulation of a phalanx is often a minimal cosmetic deformity, and is certainly not a functional disability. One should do nothing rather than perform an osteotomy under these circumstances.

Very mild deformities should not be corrected (Fig. 127–1). Ill-advised surgery can be associated with serious compromise of otherwise good hand function. Active infection or inadequate soft tissue cover are contraindications to osteotomies. Chronic osteomyelitis, persisting nonunions, and tendon and joint adhesions can compromise the best-planned surgeries and make a fairly good hand worse. Patients who will not or cannot comply with a vigorous rehabilitation regimen should be advised to avoid corrective osteotomy.

■ HISTORY OF THE TECHNIQUE

■ INDICATIONS AND CONTRAINDICATIONS

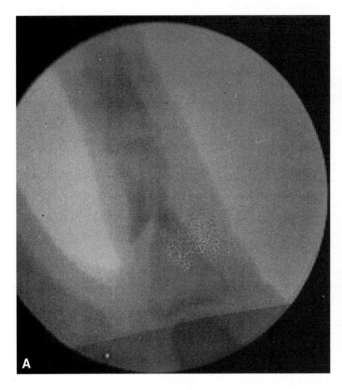
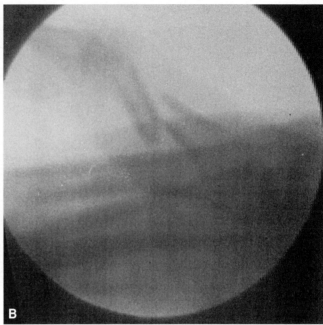

■ FIGURE 127–1

(A) Radiograph of an apparent malunion 5 weeks after a proximal phalangeal fracture of the small finger in a 32-year-old man. **(B)** A lateral radiograph of an apparent malunion in the same finger.

■ SURGICAL
TECHNIQUES

This operation can be done under axillary block or general anesthesia. Surgical incisions must be placed carefully. If a preexisting laceration or incision is present, it should be incorporated in the operative planning to avoid skin slough. If no incision or laceration is present, extensile approaches are suitable. Straight longitudinal dorsal or midlateral approaches work well. Despite the "one wound" concept by which dorsal finger incisions must curve to avoid wound contracture, a straight dorsal longitudinal incision may be used along most of the entire length of the finger without significant risk of extension contracture. A sharply angled curvilinear incision can result in skin necrosis. This problem can cause exposed tendon, which can desiccate and slough.

Radial or ulnar midlateral incisions are well suited approaches for these osteotomies, but the occasional hypertrophic or sensitive scar should be avoided by meticulous search for the dorsal sensory branches of the digital nerves. The radial border of the thumb or little finger is a wiser choice than the ulnar side, just as one would use the ulnar border of the index, middle, or ring finger. If the approach results in a dorsal sensory neuroma, it is on the side of that particular finger that experiences less contact in use patterns of the hand.

If the extensor expansion has not had previous surgery or laceration, the exposure is accomplished by releasing both transverse retinacular ligaments and raising the extensor mechanism mesially (toward the midline) with a moistened Penrose drain. Central longitudinal incisions through the extensor expansion can also be used. Intraosseous or tension band wiring provides good fixation, especially when supplemented with a K-wire. The fixation is not as rigid as a miniplate, but it can serve the purpose.

The quality of the soft tissues often influences the choice of fixation. If there is poor soft tissue coverage, one should use small or mini external fixators, or rigid internal fixation with miniplates and screws, to allow early motion. For example, if there is tendon adhesion related to prior injury or surgery, one must determine whether very rigid fixation can be

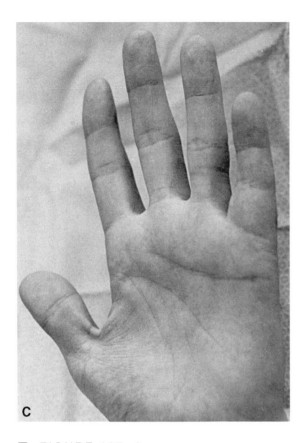

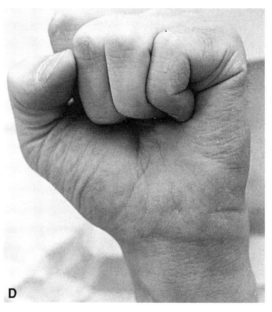

■ FIGURE 127–1
(continued)
(C) Full extension after about 18 days of hand therapy. **(D)** Full flexion of the same hand. Although radiographs suggest malunion, clinically there is no functional deficit or cosmetic deformity.

applied, to allow early range of motion. This is preferable to the alternative, which is to do staged procedures with either tenolysis and capsulotomy first, then osteotomy second, or osteotomy and realignment first, and tenolysis and capsulotomy second.

The type of correction depends on the problem. If a recent fracture results in a malunion, takedown at that site and osteosynthesis are indicated, using standard principles. The approach to a healed fracture with combined rotatory and angular malunion is often best accomplished by making the osteotomy transversely at the level of the original fracture.

Realignment should fully correct the malunion (Fig. 127–2A). It can be accomplished with a variety of techniques, including opening wedges (Fig. 127–2B), closing wedges (Fig. 127–2C), dome-shaped wedges (Fig. 127–2D), reversed wedges (Fig. 127–2F), or reversed partial wedges (Fig. 127–2E). Radiographs of the digit are used in planning. With prior templating of the radiographs, the desired result is more likely than with the "eyeball" method—in which one "guesstimates" the amount of angulatory correction, and then makes approximate cuts accordingly.

When planning the osteotomy, paper or plastic templates are very helpful. Anatomic landmarks also can be used at time of surgery. For instance, during the operation, alignment can be restored by using the anatomic contours of the original cortex. This verifies that correction has been achieved. It is also important to preshape the bone grafts and fixation devices to fit the resulting contours.

A closing wedge (Fig. 127–2C) can relatively lengthen the extensor expansion, which can result in a lack of proper tension on the extensor surface. The flexors overpower the extensors, a palmar-flexed phalanx results, and a mallet deformity or a boutonniere

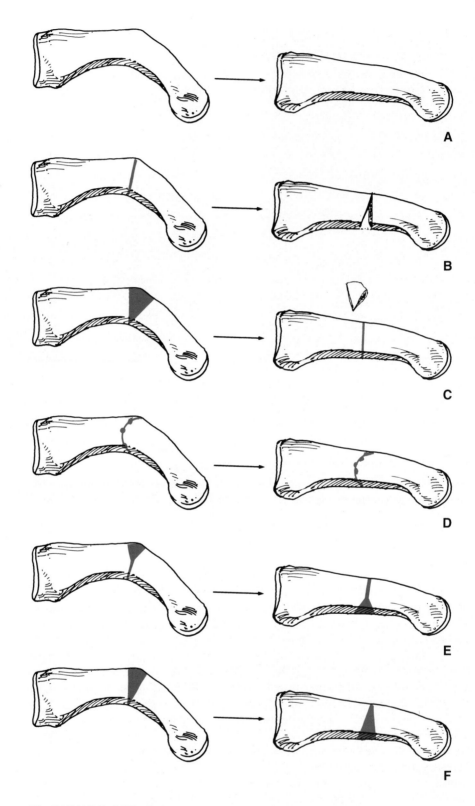

■ FIGURE 127–2
(A–F) Alternative osteotomies to achieve correction of an angulatory malunion.

deformity can occur. For this reason, an opening wedge (Fig. 127–2B) should be considered. Yet, with this opening wedge osteotomy, delayed union may occur because of the interposed graft. Opening wedges may also leave a gap at the osteotomy site on the opened side of the bone. Opening wedge osteotomies may be best suited for small corrective angles, because new bone can form more readily across the gap.

Another option is the more difficult dome-shaped osteotomy (Fig. 127–2D). Although it can be accomplished without special equipment, using multiple K-wire holes and small osteotomes, dome-shaped saw blades can help. Dome osteotomies allow better bone-to-bone apposition without excessive shortening, and allow minor corrections to be adjusted at the time of surgery. This is our procedure of choice when it can be used.

A well chosen alternative is a reversed total or partial wedge osteotomy. If a wedge is chosen, a "V"- or "Y"-shaped cut is made (Fig. 127–2E,F). The angular deformity to be corrected is measured. The reversed wedge (total or partial) is moved from the convex cortex to the concave side. The angle of either wedge should be one half of the total planned correction; hence, when removed from one side and moved to the other, the correction will be complete. A minitemplate helps, so that the correct size and angle of the half wedge is transected. Then, a "V" or a "Y" (based on half the degree of correction needed) is cut from the remainder. This wedge is then reversed and inserted on the opposite side. It can be held with the hardware that had been chosen in advance. This is our procedure of choice for osteotomies for delta phalanges.

If the patient is a young child, because the nonunion rate is lower in children, simple K-wire fixation can be used. It is less time consuming, more forgiving, and well suited to the needs. Nonetheless, K-wires are not rigid fixation, and they are more prone to fatigue fracture or loosening than are plates and screws. Yet, because the hole diameter is smaller for pins, the strength of the remaining bone is better after osteosynthesis with pins than with plates and screws. The decision must be made between cutting the ends of the pins short and burying them near the bone surface, below the skin, or leaving them percutaneous, penetrating the skin and subcutaneous tissue.[6] Removal in the office setting is much easier if the pins are not buried.

Intraosseous wiring of the phalanges is also an acceptable method of fixation (Fig. 127–3). Although the construct is not as rigid as plates and screws, it certainly can suffice. Tension-band wiring is an alternate form of wiring that serves the purpose well, also.[1]

To accomplish rigid fixation, the technique of choice is the use of miniplates and screws. Midlateral placement allows the tendons to glide better over the plate and osteotomy site.[9] Wherever possible, periosteal closure over the plate and screw heads probably allows better gliding. If a midlateral incision is used, one may excise the portion of the extensor hood on the side of the hardware. This can give good results, because tendon adhesions limit function severely in this situation. It is wisest to achieve provisional reduction and fixation with K-wires, then obtain radiographs in the operating room before rigid fixation, rather than completing the procedure without provisional reduction and planning, then obtaining radiographs documenting bad position of the fragments.[9]

Staples can be used for osteosynthesis.[7] Staples achieve compression at the fracture site if they are modified before use, by bending the prongs apart slightly. A number of suitable implants allow one a good choice, based on local wound factors, particular experience with each of the devices, host factors such as age and ability to comply with the rehabilitation regimen, and mechanical factors of the operative construct.

If tenolysis and capsulotomies are contemplated, obtaining rigid fixation is mandatory. A decision must be made whether to perform staged procedures such as osteotomy at one sitting, followed by subsequent tenolysis and capsulotomy; or the opposite, which is even less likely to yield a good result. One would prefer to perform all together: tenolysis, capsulotomy, and correction of angulatory deformity. Ideally, motion exercises should begin within 24 hours of surgery to limit adhesions. Because of the necessity for early motion, rigid internal fixation is a prerequisite.

Fine nonabsorbable sutures for skin closure prevent the intense inflammatory response occasionally seen with absorbable suture material. Interrupted sutures maintain good approximation during flexion and extension of the finger. Interrupted sutures are prefera-

■ FIGURE 127-3

(A) A lateral radiograph of a malunion of the proximal phalanx of the long finger 8 weeks after fracture. Incomplete flexion was present because of tendon adhesions and incomplete extension because of relative lengthening of the dorsal apparatus. **(B)** Posteroanterior radiograph of the same finger. **(C)** A lateral radiograph after osteotomy and union. Intraosseous wiring was used (a supplemental K-wire has been removed) to obtain union along with simultaneous tenolysis and capsulotomy. **(D)** Postoperative posteroanterior radiograph of the same finger. The total active range of motion was 220°.

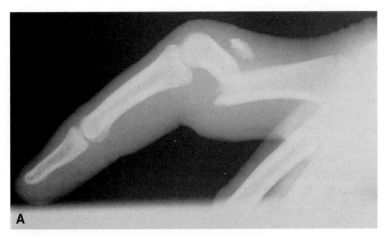

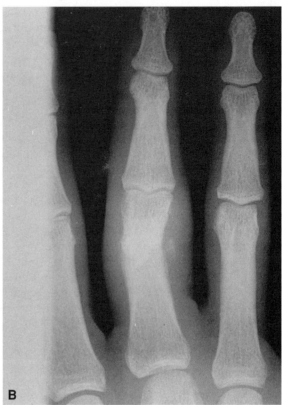

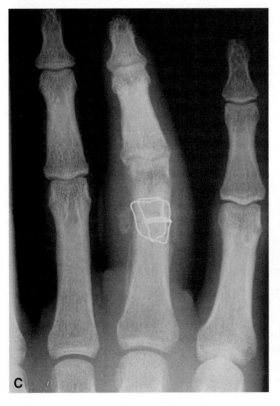

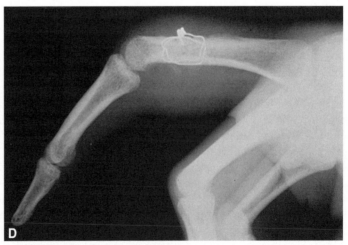

ble to running sutures because they allow movement without the suture line becoming too loose or too taut. Running sutures cause ischemic dorsal skin during finger flexion if they are too tight, and they are too loose during extension if they are just right with full finger flexion.

Delta Phalanges   Delta phalanges are a special case. If a delta phalanx is present, it has the potential of worsening with growth. If it is progressive, osteotomy with a wedge removal and reversal to the opposite side of the correction is often wisest (Fig. 127–4). This wedge should be half the desired degree of angular correction, such that when it is reversed, the correction will be achieved. This reversed wedge interrupts the C-shaped epiphysis (true physis) and thereby interrupts the cause of the progressive nature of the deformity. An excellent way to cut this delta phalanx is to use a bone-cutting forceps. This helps avoid the problem caused by shortening the bone as a result of removal of bone by the width of the saw cut. This maintains maximum length of the digit. Good correction and arrest of the progressive deformity can be accomplished with this technique (Fig. 127–5).

Consideration must be given to the position and alignment of the normal hand when performing the osteotomy. It has commonly been said that all fingers point to the scaphoid tuberosity. All flexed fingers do not normally point directly to the scaphoid tuberosity, and perhaps not even to the scaphoid. Even so, some normal digits are curved somewhat. Some individuals have straighter digits than others.

Prior planning improves technical performance. To attempt repeated adjustments of the osteosynthesis is fraught with hazards. The fragments are prone to fracture, loss of correction, and implant loosening, especially if the hardware fails to hold the fragments well after repeated attempts.

It always seems that an inordinate amount of time is spent awaiting the arrival of the radiography equipment and personnel. The use of small, mobile, portable fluoroscopy equipment, with or without hard-copy image capabilities, can avoid this. One may call

■ TECHNICAL
ALTERNATIVES

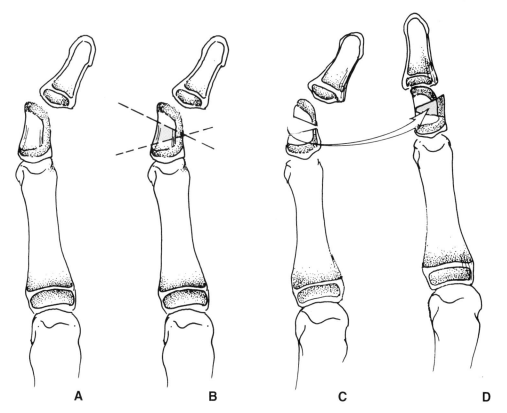

■ FIGURE 127–4
(A) Preoperative diagram of a delta phalanx. **(B)** Orientation of the planned wedge cuts. **(C)** The wedge is cut and reversed. **(D)** After the reverse wedge is inserted, it is fixed with a small longitudinal K-wire.

A   B   C   D

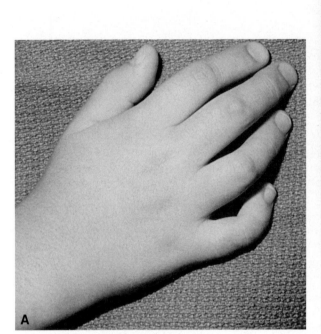
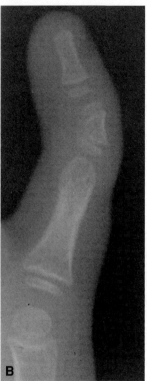
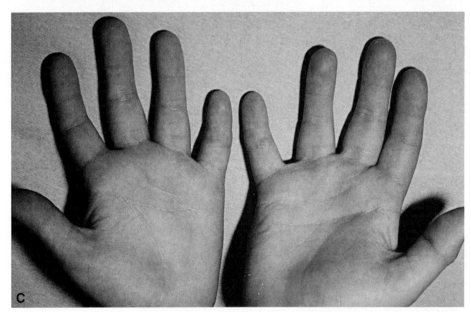

■ FIGURE 127–5
(A) The hand of a 7-year-old boy with clinodactyly of the small finger. **(B)** Radiographs confirm a delta phalanx with a "U"-shaped physis in the middle phalanx. Correction was planned using the techniques outlined by Dr. Richard J. Smith. **(C)** Postoperative view with the fingers in extension.

for the radiography team while simultaneously exposing the osteotomy site. It is far better to note malposition of the osteotomy in the operating room than it is to discover that the position is unacceptable after the patient has already left the operating room. This problem is much easier to correct in the operating room than after departure. One may wish to delay closure until the permanent radiographs return for inspection. One often accepts an imperfect position if the skin has been closed and the splints and dressings have been

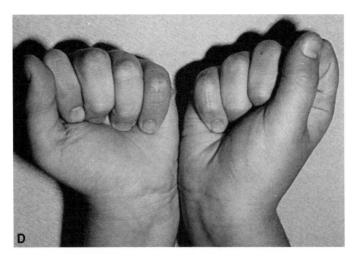

■ FIGURE 127-5 *(continued)* **(D)** A postoperative view with the fingers flexed. **(E)** Postoperative posteroanterior and lateral radiographs demonstrating incorporation of the reversed wedge.

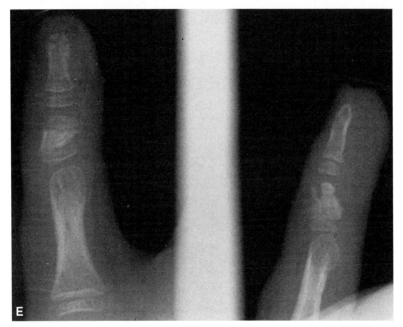

applied; the psychological mind-set is different after the wound is closed. Closure of wounds before final radiographic inspection should be done only when one is committed to reopen if the position is unacceptable.

The use of biodegradable pins has been recommended for fixation of fractures and osteotomies. Reports of intense inflammatory response in the area of absorbable pins is a cause for caution in phalangeal osteotomies. It is obvious that a large biodegradable pin can degrade only if it is absorbed by means of an inflammatory response. This response can mimic severe inflammatory responses after use of absorbable sutures.

Rehabilitation after surgery is easiest with rigid internal fixation, and should begin as soon as possible without risking loss of position and alignment. This time span is generally within the first week or less for very rigid fixation, as with screws or screw–plate combinations. If osteosynthesis is very rigid and if tenolysis and capsulotomy were combined, then hand therapy can begin within the first 24 hours. Formal hand therapy given by occupational therapists is not always used, because highly motivated patients can often begin on their own with suitable direction by the surgeon, and formal hand therapy can then be used only if the patient is unable to regain good to excellent active motion quickly over the first 8 to 12 weeks. With crossed K-wires and other inherently less stable forms of fixation, one must delay early motion, but preferably motion exercises should begin

■ REHABILITATION

within 2 weeks of K-wire fixation. If formal hand therapy is required, the therapist can monitor progressive increases in motion. Regardless of whether formal hand therapy is required, the surgeon will know when the patient has maximized return of motion (reached a plateau in improvement). Clinical assessment of tenderness at the osteotomy site is the best index of the rate of union of the osteotomy; radiographic assessment is done infrequently to assess completion of remodeling. It is more difficult to base decisions on radiographic assessment of time to union than on clinical assessment of union (lack of tenderness, and no motion at osteotomy site). Phalangeal osteotomies often heal quickly, within 5 to 6 weeks, unless delayed union occurs. Most patients after single osteotomy will return to activities of daily living within 10 to 14 days. Return to work status depends on occupation—laboring occupations may require 4 months before return to full duties, whereas desk duties may allow return to work within 2 weeks. Enough time must be allowed each day for appropriate exercises, with or without supervised hand therapy.

■ OUTCOMES

Osteotomies for phalangeal deformities are seldom indicated. These operations were much more frequent during the time of Bunnell's early career, in the 1940s. The few phalangeal osteotomies that most hand surgeons do leave very few patients for statistical analyses of data. Most phalangeal fractures can be managed nonoperatively, and usually do not result in malunion. Other causes of angular deformity are rare. Severe multiple hand trauma probably results in most malunions.

Lucas and Pfeiffer[9] reported on results of corrections of phalangeal and metacarpal malunions using AO techniques. Only 36 osteotomies were recorded in the AO Documentation Center, of which 23 were rated as very good, 8 as good, and 5 as poor. This yielded an overall satisfactory result rate of 86%.

Most recently, Sanders and Frederick[11] reported on their results of treatment of 10 metacarpal and phalangeal malunions at an average of 30 months' follow-up. All patients had healed osteotomies with correct alignment. Their preference was for plates and screws whenever possible, because the rehabilitation was made easier in their opinion. They had no postoperative tendon adhesions, nonunions, or delayed unions.

When this operation is indicated on the basis of functional loss rather than radiographic appearances, and performed using careful and well planned osteotomies, it can play a valuable role in reconstruction of the hand.

References

1. Allende BT: Tension band arthrodesis in the finger joints. J Hand Surg, 1980; 5:169–171.
2. Bunnell Sterling: Surgery of the Hand. Philadelphia: JB Lippincott, 1944:185–192.
3. Campbell WC: Operative Orthopaedics, Illustrated. St. Louis: CV Mosby, 1939.
4. Carstam N, Theander G: Surgical treatment of clinodactyly caused by longitudinally bracketed diaphysis. Scand J Plast Reconstr Surg, 1975; 9:199–202.
5. Flatt AE: Crooked fingers. In: Flatt AE (ed): The Care of Congenital Hand Anomalies. St. Louis: CV Mosby, 1977:146–163.
6. Halpern FP, Trebal MJ, Hodge W: Contamination and infection rate of percutaneous Kirschner wires in foot surgery. J Am Podiatr Med Assoc, 1990; 80:433–437.
7. Krackow KA, Mecherikunnel P: Influence of bone staple design on interfragmentary compression. Orthopedics, 1992; 14:751–755.
8. Light TR: The longitudinal epiphyseal bracket: Implications for surgical correction. J Pediatr Orthop, 1981; 1:299–305.
9. Lucas GL, Pfeiffer CM: Osteotomy of the metacarpals and phalanges stabilized by AO plates and screws. Ann Chir Main, 1989; 8:30–38.
10. Peimer CA: Combined reduction osteotomy for triphalangeal thumb. J Hand Surg, 1985; 10A: 376–381.
11. Sanders RA, Frederick HA: Metacarpal and phalangeal osteotomy with miniplate fixation. Orthopaedic Review, 1991; 20:449–456.
12. Smith RJ: Osteotomy for correction of "delta phalanx" deformity. Clin Orthop, 1977; 123: 91–94.
13. Wood VE, Flatt AE: Congenital triangular bones in the hand. J Hand Surg, 1977; 2:179–193.

A. GEORGE DASS
MARK R. BELSKY

128

Derotation Osteotomy of the Metacarpals

Corrective osteotomy for metacarpal rotational malunion has been described by a number of authors.[2–6,8–11,13] Weckesser in 1965 described this type of osteotomy through the metacarpal base with K-wire fixation across the osteotomy site into the adjacent metacarpal in eight patients for both phalangeal and metacarpal rotational malunion.[13] No postoperative immobilization was used because of the fixation and rapid union through cancellous metaphyseal bone. In the 1970s, Butler[3] described a similar osteotomy using a K-wire and small staple for fixation, whereas Pieron[10] used plate and screw fixation. A step-cut osteotomy has been advocated by Manktelow and Mahoney,[8] and more recently by Pichora and colleagues.[9] This is a technically demanding procedure, requiring removal of a longitudinal strip of dorsal cortex, controlled fracture of the volar cortex, and fixation with interosseous wires.

Despite improved knowledge about and treatment of metacarpal fractures, limited patient compliance, loss of reductions, and complex cases may result in rotational malunion of the metacarpal or metacarpals. Derotation osteotomy continues to be an important operation for this clinical problem.

Most metacarpal fractures can be treated by closed techniques.[1] The interosseous muscles, fascia, and the deep intermetacarpal ligaments prevent significant fracture displacement. However, rotational malalignment of the digits may occur with oblique and spiral metacarpal shaft fractures (Fig. 128–1). The distal fragment rotates and migrates proximally, thus shortening the metacarpal. This rotational malalignment may result in deformity, digital pain, or weakness in grip. This deformity may be overlooked if the fingers are examined in extension only. By passively extending the wrist, the fingers are brought into flexion by the tenodesis effect. This maneuver facilitates visual assessment of the rotational malalignment.

Many patients can tolerate mild rotational deformities of the digits. Derotational osteotomy of a metacarpal is indicated for rotational malalignment that produces irritation of the fingers when crossed, digital pain when gripping objects, or weakness of grip. A secondary indication for derotational osteotomy is to improve cosmesis. Phalangeal rotatory malunion may also be corrected via metacarpal osteotomy.[10] Because of the intimate relationship of the flexor and extensor mechanisms, postoperative scarring may occur, resulting in stiffness if the osteotomy is done at the phalangeal level.[8] However, if a large rotatory deformity exists, full derotation may be possible only if the osteotomy is made at the phalangeal level.[6]

Metacarpal shortening, as an isolated deformity, is not clinically significant and is not an indication for surgery. Contraindications include fracture nonunion, infection, or any other systemic conditions that preclude surgery.

The procedure is done under regional anesthesia using axillary or Bier block. The limb is prepared, draped, and exsanguinated in a standard manner. Loupe magnification is recommended. A 4-cm longitudinal incision, centered over the proximal metaphyseal–diaphyseal junction, is made over the ulnar or radial border of the involved metacarpal (Fig. 128–1). If multiple metacarpals are involved, the incision is made between the metacarpals.

■ HISTORY OF THE TECHNIQUE

■ INDICATIONS AND CONTRAINDICATIONS

■ SURGICAL TECHNIQUES

Spiral fracture of a metacarpal that resulted in a clinical rotational deformity.

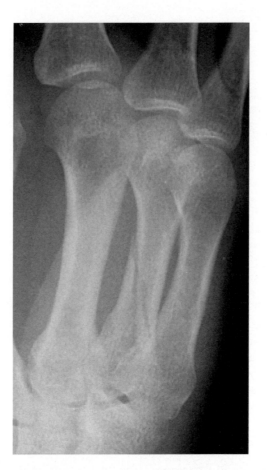

The incision is carried down between the extensor tendons. In this manner, adhesions to the extensor tendons are minimized. The interosseous muscles of the involved metacarpal are reflected in an extraperiosteal fashion. Dissection is limited to the extent of plate fixation. Small baby Homan or Bennett retractors are placed on either side of the metacarpal. The transverse osteotomy site is then marked with a pen at the proximal metaphyseal–diaphyseal junction and the dorsal cortex is scored longitudinally with the electrocautery. The periosteum is incised and stripped circumferentially at the osteotomy site. The transverse osteotomy is made with a narrow oscillating saw with a thin kerf to minimize bone shortening, debris, and damage to the soft tissues (Fig. 128–2). Saline irrigation is used as a coolant to minimize bone necrosis.

To determine the degree of correction needed, the diameter of the metacarpal is measured at the osteotomy site. By calculating the circumference of the metacarpal and dividing into 360°, the correction is obtained in degrees per millimeter of rotation. For example and simplicity, a given diameter of 11.5 mm yields:

$$
\begin{aligned}
\text{Circumference} \ &= \text{pi} \times \text{Diameter} \\
&= 3.14 \times 11.5 \text{ mm} \\
&\sim 36 \text{ mm}
\end{aligned}
$$

$$
\text{Correction} = \frac{360°}{\text{Circumference}} = \frac{360°}{36 \text{ mm}} = 10°/\text{mm}
$$

Therefore, for every 1 mm of derotation, 10° of correction is obtained. Gross and Gelberman determined from their cadaveric study the potential digital correction after derotational metacarpal osteotomy.[6] Phalangeal rotation was 70% of metacarpal rotation owing to the viscoelastic nature of the soft tissues at the metacarpophalangeal joint. Therefore, in the example, for every 1 mm of derotation at the osteotomy site, 7° of phalangeal

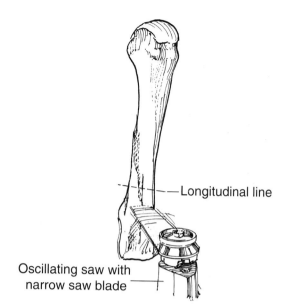

Longitudinal line

Oscillating saw with
narrow saw blade

■ FIGURE 128–2
A longitudinal straight line
is made on the bone with
electrocautery. A trans-
verse osteotomy is com-
pleted using a narrow
saw blade with a thin
kerf.

correction is obtained. This calculation is an estimate and should be used in collaboration with the clinical assessment of correction. The important message is that a small amount of derotation at the metacarpal results in a relatively large amount of phalangeal correction.

The desired derotation is performed (Fig. 128–3A) and a ¼ tubular plate or 2.0-mm minifragment plate (Synthes, Paoli, PA) is selected for fixation. These plates have a lower profile than the 2.7-mm dynamic compression plate, yet some compression is still achieved. A four- or five-hole plate is used to secure a minimum of four cortices proximal and four cortices distal to the osteotomy. The plate is contoured to the dorsoulnar or dorsoradial cortex and secured to the proximal fragment using 2.0-mm cortical screws. The metacarpal bone is triangular in cross-section and affords better fixation on its dorsoulnar or dorsora-dial cortex. In addition, the plate should not be placed directly beneath the extensor tendon because it may interfere with tendon excursion. The derotation is checked again and main-tained with a Verbrugge clamp, holding the plate to the distal fragment. The first hole on the distal side is eccentrically drilled away from the osteotomy. As this screw is tightened, it moves from its eccentric position to the center of the screw hole. This movement of the screw and bone toward the fracture results in axial compression and closes the osteotomy site. The last screw is then placed in the unloaded or neutral position (Fig. 128–3B). Postop-erative radiographs are obtained to confirm satisfactory position of the plate and screws (Fig. 128–4).

The wound is thoroughly irrigated, removing any bony debris. The periosteum is closed with 3-0 absorbable suture. The skin is closed with 5-0 nylon suture. After surgery, the patient is splinted, immobilizing the wrist in 20° of extension and the metacarpophalangeal (MP) joints in 70° of flexion. The interphalangeal (IP) joints are left free.

If the osteotomy is made more proximally at the metacarpal base, which precludes the use of a straight plate for proximal fixation, a 2.0 or 2.7 T or L plate may be used.[2] When either of these plates are secured, the transverse arms of the plate should be secured to the proximal fragment before the straight portion to the distal fragment.[7] If the straight portion of the plate is secured first, rotation of the underlying bone may result as the screws in the transverse portion pull the distal fragment to the plate.

Methods other than plate fixation have been previously mentioned.[3,4,8–11,13] Although K-wire fixation is technically easier, rigid internal fixation is not achieved. Longer postop-erative immobilization is needed to ensure union. However, K-wires are easier to remove and no immobilization is needed after hardware removal. A period of protected mobiliza-

■ TECHNICAL
ALTERNATIVES

■ FIGURE 128–3
(A) Derotation of the metacarpal using a measure of dorsal scoring separation. **(B)** Fixation using a ¼ tubular or 2.0-mm minifragment plate under compression.

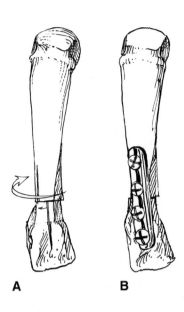

A   B

■ FIGURE 128–4
Posteroanterior **(A)** and oblique **(B)** radiographs after derotation osteotomy. Note that the plate is applied to the dorsoradial cortex of the metacarpal.

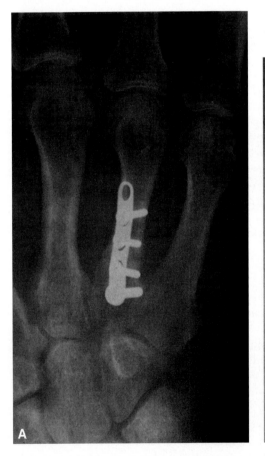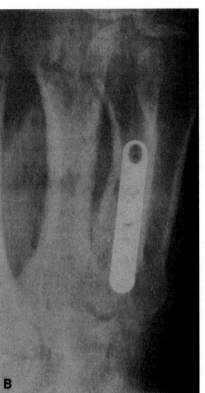

tion is needed after plate and screw removal because the bone may refracture owing to localized osteoporosis (stress shielding) occurring beneath the plate.

Staple fixation has problems similar to those with K-wire fixation. In addition, compression at the osteotomy site may be minimal with staple fixation. Maintaining the correct rotational alignment during staple impaction is also difficult, and provisional fixation with K-wires may be needed.

The precise step-cut osteotomy advocated by Manktelow and Mahoney[8] and Pichora and co-authors[9] is technically demanding, requiring a larger dissection. Larger cancellous surfaces at the osteotomy site promote bony union. However, a larger osteotomy may produce more scarring, resulting in greater stiffness. In addition, if dorsal or volar comminution occurs at the time of controlled longitudinal fracture, more rigid internal fixation may be required than that provided by interosseous wires.

The surgical technique outlined here is straightforward, but the following technical points are important. Limit periosteal stripping to the osteotomy site, but go circumferentially to obtain full correction. This may reduce nonunion rates. The osteotomy must be made perpendicular to the metacarpal shaft, otherwise an angular deformity may result. At times, this may be desirable, but biplane osteotomy is difficult to control. Do not divide the deep intermetacarpal ligament in an attempt to gain more correction. Instability of the first ray and loss of the transverse metacarpal arch will occur.[6] Check rotational alignment before final screw placement. If screws have to be removed and placed again, fixation may be compromised.

■ REHABILITATION

The patient returns 3 days after surgery for dressing change and wound check. A well padded, nonremovable short arm splint or cast is applied again with the wrist in 20° extension. The MP and IP joints are left free. Active and passive motion of the MP and IP joints is stressed to limit extensor and flexor scarring and joint stiffness. Early postoperative mobilization can be initiated because of the rigid internal fixation. Sutures are removed at 2 weeks. A removable volar wrist splint is used for another 2 weeks. Thermoplastic splints may be used, but are unnecessary for this short period of immobilization. Most patients are able to do the postoperative exercises themselves. Formal hand therapy supervised by a therapist is instituted if range of motion is not progressing. Goals of therapy include full IP motion by the first week and full MP motion by 4 weeks. Strengthening exercises using putty and light weights and wrist range of motion exercises are then started. Postoperative radiographs usually show union by 8 weeks. Patients are allowed to resume full, unrestricted activities by 8 to 10 weeks, once they have achieved full motion and strength.

Plates usually are not removed after bony union occurs. These lower-profile plates cause less irritation when placed on the dorsoulnar or dorsoradial cortices of the metacarpals. If hardware irritation does occur, the plates may be removed no earlier than 6 months after osteotomy. Protected mobilization is advised for 4 weeks after plate removal.

■ OUTCOMES

The reported rates of union are virtually 100%, regardless of the technique.[8–11,13] One report of delayed union with diaphyseal osteotomy and plate fixation required additional bone grafting to achieve union.[2] Malunion has been reported by Stern and colleagues[12] after metacarpal derotational osteotomy. This complication can be avoided by careful preoperative planning and surgical technique.

The two largest series, totaling 33 osteotomies, were reported using the step-cut technique.[8,9] Both series showed 100% union by 8 weeks using early range of motion in the postoperative period. Patient satisfaction was reported as good in all cases. However, postoperative stiffness did occur in several patients. In fact, stiffness, defined as total active motion less than 190°, was the most common complication after metacarpal plating in Sterns and co-authors' series.[12] Stiffness was related to the extent of soft tissue dissection and plate interference with tendon gliding. Infection has not been reported after derotational osteotomy of the metacarpals.

The technique described for derotational osteotomy of the metacarpals is simple and precise. Rigid internal fixation allows early postoperative mobilization. Patient satisfaction can be maximized and complications reduced if meticulous surgical technique is implemented.

References

1. Belsky MR, Eaton RG: Displaced fractures of the ring and little finger metacarpals. Orthop Trans, 1982; 6:349–350.
2. Breen TF: Metacarpal rotational osteotomy for metacarpal and phalangeal fracture rotatory malunions. Techn Orthop, 1991; 6(2):19–22.
3. Butler B: Complications of treatment of injuries to the hand. In: Epps CH (ed): Complications in Orthopaedic Surgery. Philadelphia: JB Lippincott, 1978:428–429.
4. Clinkscales GS: Complications in the management of fractures in hand injuries. South Med J, 1970; 63:704–707.
5. Freeland AE, Jabaley ME, Hughs J: Stable Fixation of the Hand and Wrist. New York: Springer-Verlag, 1986.
6. Gross MS, Gelberman RH: Metacarpal rotational osteotomy. J Hand Surg, 1985; 10A:105–108.
7. Hastings H: Unstable metacarpal and phalangeal fracture treatment with screws and plates. Clin Orthop, 1987; 214:37–52.
8. Manktelow RH, Mahoney JL: Step osteotomy: A precise rotation osteotomy to correct scissoring deformities of the fingers. Plast Reconstr Surg, 1981; 68:571–576.
9. Pichora DR, Meyer R, Masear VR: Rotational step-cut osteotomy for treatment of metacarpal and phalangeal nonunion. J Hand Surg, 1991; 16A:551–555.
10. Pieron AP: Correction of rotational malunion of a phalanx by metacarpal osteotomy. J Bone Joint Surg, 1972; 54B:516–519.
11. Seitz WH, Froimson AI: Management of malunited fractures of the metacarpal and phalangeal shafts. Hand Clin, 1988; 4:529–536.
12. Stern PJ, Weiser MJ, Reilly DG: Complications of plate fixation in the hand skeleton. Clin Orthop, 1987; 214:59–65.
13. Weckesser EC: Rotational osteotomy of the metacarpal for overlapping fingers. J Bone Joint Surg, 1965; 47B:751–756.

129

Angular Osteotomy of Metacarpals

Metacarpal fractures, although extremely common and usually not difficult to treat, are not universally free of complications. Complications include malunion, nonunion, tendon adhesions, infection, and limitation of adjacent joint motion. These complications do not necessarily exist in isolation, and combinations of the listed complications are frequently seen.[1,2] Malunion per se can create significant problems when angular deformity upsets muscle balance, thereby weakening pinch and grip. Pain due to localized pressure in the palm, fatigue with repeated gripping, and a sense of aching in the hand are common complaints of patients who present with a metacarpal malunion.

There is a logical solution to the metacarpal malunion problem—namely, osteotomy, just as would be done in the femur, tibia, or any other long bone. Although the sequelae of malunion of metacarpals and phalanges have been known for decades, there has been a reluctance to perform osteotomy in the small bones of the hand for fear of creating additional complications such as joint stiffness or nonunion. The long-prevalent attitude regarding small bone osteotomy is perhaps best summed up by Milford, who said in several editions of *Campbell's Operative Orthopaedics*, "not every malunited fracture should be treated . . . Ill-advised treatment usually fails to improve function and sometimes makes it worse. Unless the deformity is gross it should usually be accepted . . . . For treatment by osteotomy may lead not only to nonunion but also to difficulty in reestablishing satisfactory joint motion."[9] It is certainly true that not every malunited fracture should be treated, but concern for further complications seems to account for the paucity of accounts of metacarpal osteotomy in the literature before the current era. The development of small plates and screws by the AO group and the success of rigid fixation in other long bones as taught and promulgated by the practitioners of the AO method has been important in obviating many of the concerns about small bone fixation.[5] Use of plates and screws in the hand has been a natural evolution from their use in larger bones. Development of plate and screw or wiring constructs in the hand is an important consideration that has allowed successful metacarpal osteotomy in recent years.

Rotary malunion is perhaps a greater problem than angular malunion, and accounts for most of the literature on the subject of metacarpal osteotomy.[4,8,10] Actually, rotary and angular deformity may exist in the same digit, so that it is difficult to separate the two problems for discussion purposes. Pieron in 1972 provided the first report of stabilizing a metacarpal osteotomy with plate and screws, and, in the following year, Heim and co-authors included 21 cases of osteotomy in a large series of hand fractures treated with AO methods of osteosynthesis.[5,11] Thus, osteotomy of the metacarpals in general and stabilization with plates and screws in particular has been part of our armamentarium for the past two decades, with isolated examples having been performed before that.

The indication for performance of a corrective osteotomy in a metacarpal is a metacarpal malunion that causes significant pain, impairment of hand function, or, rarely, cosmetic deformity. How much angular deformity can be tolerated is quite variable from patient to patient on account of handedness, age, occupation, and suppleness of adjacent joints and from metacarpal to metacarpal. The thumb metacarpal, for example, can tolerate considerable angular malunion owing to the wide excursion of the carpometacarpal (CMC)

■ HISTORY OF THE TECHNIQUE

■ INDICATIONS AND CONTRAINDICATIONS

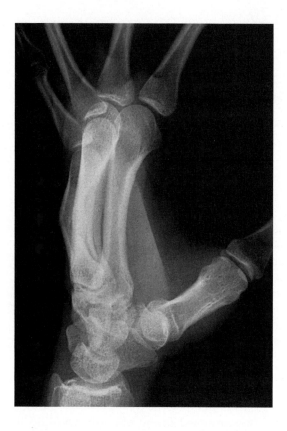

and the metacarpophalangeal (MP) joints. Similarly, the fifth metacarpal can often tolerate 70° of angular malunion in flexion, although 40° of deformity is a more usual figure for symptomatic malunion (Fig. 129–1).[6] Virtually all angular metacarpal malunions create flexion deformities, incidentally. When the metacarpal head is depressed, compensatory hyperextension at the MP joint occurs and secondary contracture of the collateral ligaments in a shortened position can occur. In the fifth metacarpal, a palmarly displaced metacarpal head can be compensated for by the 30° of motion at the CMC joint, thus avoiding undue pressure over the metacarpal head in the palm. This is true to a considerably lesser extent for the ring finger, but compensation at the index and middle finger rays is essentially nil because of the limited motion of their respective CMC joints. Thus, in the second and third ray, flexion deformity at the metacarpal neck will cause the metacarpal to remain fixed in the palm and create pain with grasp. Volar angulation in the diaphysis is even less well tolerated and should be corrected when the angulation reaches 20 to 25°. Patients are much more likely to complain of shaft angulation than metacarpal neck angulation, and osteotomy is more likely done in this region of the metacarpal for the lesser angular deformities. As mentioned, angulation and rotation may exist in the same bone, and correction must be planned to address both problems as well as accompanying soft tissue lesions such as tendon adherence or joint contracture.

Contraindications are few but include all the concerns for any surgical procedure, such as anesthetic risks, systemic illness, potential noncompliance with a postoperative rehabilitation regimen, and unrealistic expectations for the outcome of the procedure. Specific contraindications include infection, unremediable tendon loss or adherence, and severe stiffness of adjacent joints.

■ SURGICAL
TECHNIQUES

The surgical procedure begins with preoperative planning of the amount of correction to be achieved. This can be done most easily by tracing the configuration of the malunited metacarpal on either tracing paper or clear radiographic film and then drawing the osteotomy and the wedge of bone to be excised to restore proper alignment. In cases of bone loss with angulation, a cortical bone peg can be used to restore length and correct angulation at the same time, but in most instances palmar angulation is corrected by a dorsal closing wedge osteotomy, which can be simply, but precisely, planned out by the paper "cut-out" method.

Metacarpal osteotomy can be easily performed on an ambulatory basis under axillary block anesthesia, thus decreasing hospital costs and risks to the patient from general anesthesia. After the block is administered, a pneumatic tourniquet is placed about the upper arm and routine orthopaedic skin preparation is carried out. The tourniquet is then inflated after the limb has been exsanguinated with an elastic bandage. Surface anatomic features are easily noted, with the apex of the deformity visible and palpable along the metacarpal axis. A longitudinal incision is made centered over the apex of the deformity and extended approximately 2 cm distally and proximally from the apex of the deformity. Sensory nerve branches should be identified and protected. The extensor tendon is retracted and the interosseous fascia and periosteum over the metacarpal incised longitudinally along the dorsoulnar or dorsoradial margin, and then gently stripped with a dental elevator on each side of the metacarpal to expose the site of intended osteotomy. A longitudinal orientation line is drawn on the bone with a scalpel or cautery and the proximal osteotomy cut marked on the bone. A four- or five-hole plate is selected depending on the location of the osteotomy, and the proximal or distal half of the plate affixed to the metacarpal shaft in the routine manner using the appropriate drill, tap, and screws (Fig. 129–2). The screws need not be fully tightened and, indeed, the screw closest the osteotomy site can be removed and the farther one loosened to allow the plate to swing out of the way while the osteotomy is performed with a small drill and osteotome or a thin-bladed reciprocating saw (Fig. 129–3). The distance between the two dorsal osteotomy sites has been predetermined by the preoperative planning tracing. Once the osteotomy cuts have been completed, with care taken to preserve the palmar periosteum and perhaps even some cortical bone, the wedge of bone is removed and the bone ends approximated (Fig. 129–4). Observation of the previously marked orientation line is important at this point. When a satisfactory position has been achieved, and this can be checked by provisional

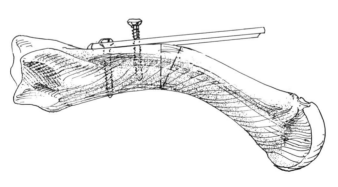

■ FIGURE 129–2
The appropriately sized plate is attached through screw holes proximal to the intended osteotomy site.

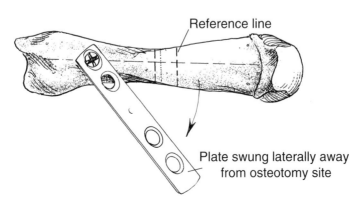

Reference line

Plate swung laterally away from osteotomy site

■ FIGURE 129–3
The plate is rotated out of the way before osteotomizing the metacarpal, and a reference line is made on the metacarpal.

■ FIGURE 129–4
The osteotomy cuts are completed and the dorsal wedge of bone is removed, preserving the palmar periosteum.

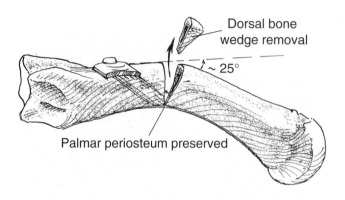

Dorsal bone wedge removal

~ 25°

Palmar periosteum preserved

■ FIGURE 129–5
The bone is reduced and the plate is applied through additional screw holes.

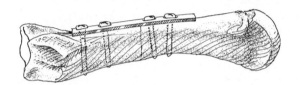

stabilization with a small K-wire and an intraoperative radiograph, the mobile segment of the metacarpal is stabilized to the plate in a similar manner with properly drilled, measured, and tapped screws (Fig. 129–5). Usually the 2.7 dynamic compression plate (DCP) with the 3.5-mm cortical screws or the ⅓semitubular plate with 3.5-mm screws are used for stabilization of metacarpal osteotomies, but in smaller bones ¼semitubular plates and 2.7-mm screws may be appropriate. If the ¼semitubular plate is used instead of the DCP, some compression at the osteotomy site can still be achieved by eccentrically drilling the third and fourth drill holes away from the osteotomy line. Tightening of the screws should be done in the 1, 3, 2, 4 sequence. For metacarpal neck or metacarpal base osteotomy, a "T"- or "L"-shaped plate may be preferable. If such plates are used, the side arms should be applied first to prevent rotatory deformity when the screws in the straight portion of the plate are tightened. Four cortices of screw purchase on each side of the osteotomy site is adequate. If correction is satisfactory as judged by intraoperative radiographs, the periosteum/fascial flap is loosely closed over the plate with 4-0 absorbable suture and the skin closed over a miniflap drain using 4-0 or 5-0 interrupted sutures. Gauze squares and a padded palmar or ulnar gutter splint complete the dressing.

■ TECHNICAL ALTERNATIVES

Accurate realignment of the metacarpal and secure internal fixation with plates and screws will avoid most of the pitfalls of this operation in terms of delayed union or nonunion and postoperative impairment in joint motion. Tendon adherence and scar formation about the plate can be minimized by covering the plate with periosteum and using early finger motion to restore tendon gliding before adhesions are irreversibly formed. Alternative forms of bony stabilization such as K-wires, interosseous wiring techniques, or tension-band wiring have been employed, but these forms of stabilization are not as reliable for angular osteotomy fixation as dorsally applied plates and screws.[12] Obviously, some form of protection of the hand and avoidance of unprotected stresses must be emphasized to the patient to prevent disruption at the osteotomy site or even plate breakage. Infection in this type of elective hand surgery should be nearly nil, and, in the author's opinion, there is no need to use prophylactic antibiotics.

As described, early range of motion exercises supervised either by the surgeon or the hand therapist are critical. Use of continuous passive motion (CPM) machines is an attractive luxury but not essential to success if the patient is cooperative and the therapist (surgeon or hand therapist) is diligent. Scar massage is helpful in preventing tendon adherence, and occasionally other modalities such as heat or ultrasound may be used to soften

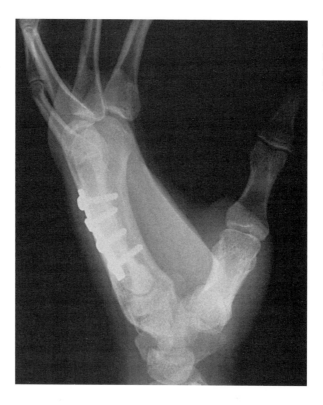

A postoperative lateral radiograph showing a well applied plate and corrected malunion.

tissues and encourage free and painless joint motion. Occasionally elastic-loop type splints may be used to foster flexion of the involved digit.

The patient is instructed to remove the drain the following day and leave the splint and dressing in place until seen on the tenth postoperative day for suture removal. If postoperative joint stiffness is anticipated, earlier motion may be achieved with the use of a CPM machine, but this is seldom necessary. After the sutures are removed and a postoperative radiograph is obtained and found satisfactory (Fig. 129–6), active motion of the hand is begun and practiced several times daily. At other times the hand is supported with a removable splint or elastic bandage. Hand therapy is a useful adjunct but usually not essential, but if the patient is not making steady progress in regaining motion, the services of a therapist must be enlisted. As healing progresses, the splint may be discarded and support provided by buddy taping to adjacent digits as range of motion exercises are performed. Supervised strengthening exercises should be started when union of the osteotomy site seems assured. Patients may return to light occupations within 1 to 2 weeks, but manual workers will need longer time off work (up to 8 weeks).

Plate removal is occasionally necessary, and the patient who is having difficulty regaining motion may be improved by hardware removal and extensor tenolysis. In my experience, no special protection seems necessary after plate and screw removal in the metacarpals.

■ REHABILITATION

In the properly selected patient who is operated on following AO principles, a satisfactory outcome can be anticipated. Operative correction should be offered to those patients who have symptomatic angular deformities of the metacarpals with the expectation of significant benefit. Previous attitudes of pessimism regarding small bone osteotomy are worthy of note, but should not persist in the current era of stable bone fixation, which allows early joint motion. Several recent articles have attested to the value of metacarpal and phalangeal osteotomy, the most extensive being that of the author and K. M. Pfeiffer, who reported the AO experience in 1989.[7] This study, as do several others, includes many examples of rotatory osteotomy or combined rotatory and angular correction, but 23 of

■ OUTCOMES

the 36 cases reported are of pure angular deformity. For the entire series, 100% of the osteotomy sites united, and in 86% there was no or minimal joint stiffness. I have personally done nearly 50 metacarpal and phalangeal osteotomies with equally good results. The most recent article on the subject (1991) indicates exceptionally good results when similar guidelines for patient selection and surgical procedures were carried out.[10] Thus, I am confident in agreeing that, "when deformity impairs function or is cosmetically unacceptable, surgical correction is indicated."[3]

References

1. Bouchon Y, Merle M, Foucher G, Michon J: Malunions of the metacarpals and phalanges: Results of surgical treatment. Rev Chir Orthop, 1982; 62:549–555.
2. Clinkscales GS: Complications in the management of fractures in hand injuries. South Med J, 1970; 63:704–707.
3. Froimson AI: Osteotomy for digital deformity. J Hand Surg, 1981; 6:585–589.
4. Gross MH, Gelberman RH: Metacarpal rotational osteotomy. J Hand Surg, 1985; 10A: 105–108.
5. Heim U, Pfeiffer KM, Mueli HC: Resultate von AO Osteosynthesen des Handskelettes. Handchirurgie, 1973; 5:71–78.
6. Hunter JH, Cowen NJ: Fifth metacarpal fractures in a compensation clinic population. J Bone Joint Surg, 1970; 53A:1159–1165.
7. Lucas GL, Pfeiffer KM: Osteotomy of the metacarpals and phalanges stabilized by AO plates and screws. Ann Chir Main, 1989; 8:30–38.
8. Manktelow RT, Mahoney JL: Step osteotomy: A precise rotation osteotomy to correct scissoring deformities of the finger. J Plast Reconstr Surg, 1981; 68:571–576.
9. Milford L: In: Campbell's Operative Orthopaedics, 7th Ed. St. Louis: CV Mosby, 1987:200.
10. Pichora DR, Meyer R, Masear VR: Rotational step-cut osteotomy for treatment of metacarpal and phalangeal nonunion. J Hand Surg, 1991; 16A:551–555.
11. Pieron AP: Correction of rotational malunion of a phalanx by metacarpal osteotomy. J Bone Joint Surg, 1972; 54B:516–519.
12. Vanik RK, Weber RC, Matloub HS, Sanger JR, Gingrass RP: The comparative strengths of internal fixation techniques. J Hand Surg, 1984; 9A:216–221.

130

Bone Grafting for Metacarpal Diaphyseal Defects

Metacarpal shaft defects often result from complex hand trauma associated with extensive soft tissue injury and wound contamination.[4,7,12] Bone grafting is only one component of the reconstruction necessary to restore hand function. Traditionally, a grafting procedure was delayed for several weeks or months after injury until soft tissue healing was well advanced.[4,12] Littler reported the first large series of metacarpal bone grafting in 1947.[9] Many of his patients had large or multiple bony defects and some also had chronic osteomyelitis. More recently, Peimer and co-authors demonstrated the benefits of temporary skeletal fixation using K-wires or external fixation to maintain skeletal length until definitive bone reconstruction was performed.[12] Although this approach remains an appropriate alternative, Freeland and co-authors showed that improved techniques in skeletal fixation and soft tissue reconstruction provide an effective means to achieve earlier skeletal restoration.[7]

Primary or delayed primary bone grafting offers distinct advantages in the care of these complex injuries.[7,14] The bone graft is placed in a vascularized, unscarred bed, allowing skeletal length and alignment to be reestablished more easily. Early bone grafting with stable fixation provides the foundation for repair of other structures and allows an accelerated rehabilitation program that will optimize the functional result. However, early definitive reconstruction of a multistructural injury requires meticulous wound debridement complemented by full-thickness soft tissue coverage at the time of bone grafting.

Although traumatic bone loss presents an obvious indication for metacarpal bone grafting, debridement of a chronic infection or resection of a tumor can create substantial defects. Early bone grafting of these defects provides the same advantages that exist for traumatic bone loss. However, the graft bed must be properly prepared to accept the graft because residual infection or tumor may prevent graft healing and cause recurrence of the destructive process.

Factors integral to the success of bone grafting, regardless of the clinical problem, are the quality of the graft and the stability of bone fixation.[14] By virtue of its abundant vascular supply, the hand can provide an excellent bed for a bone graft despite significant trauma. Bone from amputated parts may be suitable for reconstruction of the metacarpal when early wound closure can be achieved.[7,9] Under most circumstances, an autogenous corticocancellous bone graft obtained form the iliac crest is most appropriate. The cancellous portion is united and remodeled more reliably than cortical bone, whereas the cortical portion offers greater strength and can be incorporated into the fixation to enhance stability. Bone grafts without adequate fixation require prolonged external immobilization. This causes joint stiffness and tendon adhesions, which compromise the goals of early reconstruction. In adults, stabilization of a corticocancellous bone graft is best achieved by rigid internal fixation. In children, sufficient metacarpal may not be available for rigid fixation without endangering the physis. Less stable internal fixation combined with cast immobilization can be used successfully in children because rapid bone union occurs and allows early removal of the cast and initiation of rehabilitation (Fig. 130–1).

A common indication for grafting metacarpals is open fractures with loss of diaphyseal bone resulting from gunshot wounds, explosions, and industrial accidents.[4,7,9,12] Provided

■ HISTORY OF THE TECHNIQUE

■ INDICATIONS AND CONTRAINDICATIONS

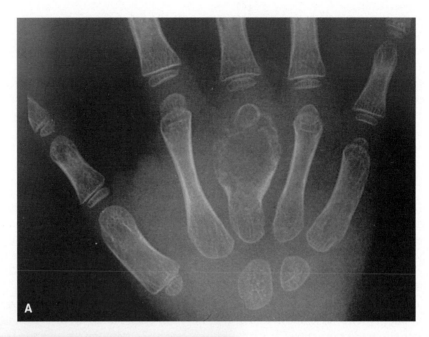

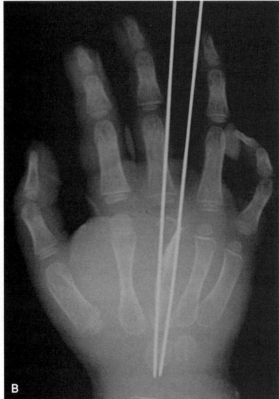

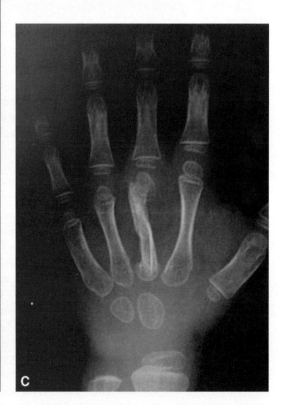

■ FIGURE 130–1

(A) Giant cell tumor of bone in the third metacarpal of a child. There is advanced bone destruction with metacarpal deformity. **(B)** Intraoperative radiograph shows a corticocancellous bone graft fixed by K-wires in the metacarpal defect after tumor resection. An attempt was made to spare the distal physis. Graft was taken from the iliac crest. **(C)** Result 6 months after surgery. The graft healed and the child regained full motion in the finger. However, some growth disturbance occurred.

wound debridement creates a clean bed, bone grafting should proceed in conjunction with soft tissue repair and wound coverage. A gunshot wound or severe crush injury may cause severe comminution with devitalized or poorly vascularized fragments. Thus, a substantial deficit that is not apparent on the initial radiograph may be created by wound debridement.

Although chronic osteomyelitis can be treated effectively by debridement and antibiotic therapy without complete loss of bone integrity, a more extensive debridement is occasionally required to eradicate the infection.[9,11] In this circumstance, bone grafting should be delayed to minimize the risk of recurrent infection. Alignment and space for future grafting can be maintained by temporary skeletal fixation and perhaps antibiotic-impregnated cement, making delayed reconstruction easier.[5]

Benign tumors of the metacarpal can present initially with advanced bone destruction. The more common benign tumors include enchondroma, giant cell tumor of bone, and aneurysmal bone cyst.[6] Primary bone grafting is indicated when complete tumor resection can be accomplished. Curettage, with or without bone grafting, is usually sufficient treatment for enchondromas.[2,8] The treatment of other tumors can require removal of substantial diaphyseal bone with loss of skeletal continuity.[1] These defects require structural restoration with large bone grafts (Fig. 130–1).

In the traumatized hand, wound debridement must be repeated until all contaminated and devitalized tissues are removed before reconstruction. Full-thickness soft tissue coverage of the bone graft and placement of internal fixation materials should be accomplished at the time of the grafting procedure. In most cases, split-thickness or full-thickness skin grafts will not provide adequate coverage. However, they may be used to complement other techniques, such as small skin defects over intrinsic muscle or intact paratenon away from the bone graft site. Requirements of local or distant flap coverage should be considered during preoperative planning. Delayed skeletal reconstruction is indicated when a question of residual contamination, infection, or tumor exists.

Although early restoration provides the potential for an optimal result, delayed and staged procedures offer lower risks of major complications in some complex hand problems.[4,9,12] During preoperative planning, it should be clear that reconstruction can be performed with minimal risk to surrounding uninjured structures.

■ SURGICAL TECHNIQUES

General anesthesia provides the option to obtain bone graft and flap coverage from distant sites. Regional anesthesia is appropriate in adults when bone graft is obtained locally or allograft is used. A dorsal longitudinal incision over the metacarpal or a longitudinal extension of a traumatic wound is preferable to minimize damage to veins on the dorsum of the hand. Dividing the juncturae tendinae, with later repair, may facilitate exposure. The thumb metacarpal is approached through an incision along the dorsoradial edge of the metacarpal. The radial sensory nerve branches are carefully identified and protected. The extensor pollicis brevis tendon is retracted, the periosteum is incised dorsally, and the thenar muscles are elevated subperiosteally. For the finger metacarpals, the periosteum is incised in the midline between the origins of the interosseous muscles, and subperiosteal elevation is gently performed. A T extension made in the periosteum proximally at the metacarpal base will provide greater exposure of the metacarpal and reduce muscle damage. A similar extension can be made distally, just proximal to the metacarpophalangeal joint capsule. For an intramedullary benign tumor or localized infection, a bone window is made over the involved area, with care taken to avoid a circumferential fracture. After curettage of a tumor, cancellous bone graft can be packed into the defect. Special care should be exercised during subperiosteal dissection on the palmar surface to avoid further damage to traumatized interosseous muscles and potentially exposed flexor tendons and neurovascular structures.

Preoperative radiographic assessment of the metacarpal and its defect or deformity is essential to reestablish normal skeletal length and contour. Even when temporary fixation has been used to maintain alignment, some degree of deformity is usually present. The metacarpals contribute to the longitudinal arch of the hand through the slight dorsal convexity of their shafts. In addition, the distal transverse arch and breadth of the hand are formed by the metacarpal heads. Therefore, restoring the natural alignment of the metacarpal shafts is important for normal hand contour. A corticocancellous graft slightly larger than the defect is harvested from the iliac crest. A unicortical or bicortical graft is appropriate, whereas a tricortical graft is too bulky and unnecessary. If more than one metacarpal requires grafting, a single graft spanning multiple defects is often simpler and justified in traumatic wounds. The graft is fashioned to the appropriate length and width. The iliac crest has a slight convexity which can be used to approximate the convexity of the metacarpal shaft. Protruding dowels of cancellous bone can be left extending from the graft ends. These can be inserted into the medullary canal of the metacarpal to add stability and increase contact area for bone union. Occasionally a step cut in the bone ends can be used to achieve greater surface contact. Bone contact is essential and may require further removal of the metacarpal to obtain appropriate fit. Devitalized or poorly vascularized cortical bone in the metacarpal diaphysis delays healing and should be removed in favor of bridging the defect with corticocancellous graft. This encourages graft union by providing contact with the metacarpal metaphyseal cancellous bone.

Stable internal fixation of the graft is an important goal. No one method of fixation is appropriate for all cases. A combination of techniques may be required, with each end of the graft fixed in a different manner. A dorsal plate provides the most secure fixation, but requires substantial remaining metacarpal for screw placement (Fig. 130–2A). To obtain additional screw fixation in the proximal or distal end of the metacarpal, a T- or L-plate can be used instead of a straight plate (Fig. 130–2B). Interfragmentary screws between graft and metacarpal are effective if a step-cut fit is possible (Fig. 130–2C). K-wires placed obliquely or crossed is often the easiest fixation to perform. However, stability is difficult to achieve with K-wires alone. Interosseous wiring techniques using a dorsal tension band or wire loops can add significant stability to the bone construct (Fig. 130–2B,C). Penetration of the metacarpophalangeal joint and extensor mechanism with wires should be avoided if possible to allow free joint mobility and tendon gliding. Stability is assessed under direct vision while the involved digits are manipulated. Additional fixation is attempted if stability has not been obtained.

During closure, the interosseous muscles are allowed to seek their own position, whereas thenar muscles are reapproximated to their origins without excessive tension. Reconstruction of extensor tendon injuries can be initiated or completed during this same operative session. However, the principles of tendon reconstruction must be followed. Depending on the extent of tendon injury, primary repairs, tendon transfers, or secondary reconstruction using intercalary grafts or temporary Silastic rods can be performed. Prominent hardware that impinges on overlying extensor tendons must be corrected to avoid attrition ruptures.

Primary skin closure or full-thickness flap coverage must completely cover the bone graft and hardware. In the traumatized hand, avoid primary closure with excessive tension that will cause skin necrosis. If a local flap from the dorsum of the hand is not possible, a regional pedicle flap such as the reverse radial artery forearm flap or posterior interosseous artery flap can be considered. Regional flaps offer an advantage over distant pedicle flaps that require the hand to be placed in positions that compromise rehabilitation. Free tissue transfers are reserved for the most difficult problems.

A suction drain and prophylactic antibiotics are used for 48 hours. A bulky gauze dressing supported by a plaster splint is applied. Provided that no protection of a soft tissue injury or repair is necessary, and skeletal fixation is stable, the metacarpophalangeal joints are allowed free motion, but protected by a dorsal extension of the splint.

■ TECHNICAL ALTERNATIVES

Alternative techniques are indicated when reconstructive requirements are complex or compromised by wound condition. External fixation may be the only means to achieve fixation when bone loss is extensive.[5,11,12] An external device can provide stabilization of combined bone and joint injuries without immobilizing uninjured joints, and it can allow access for wound care.

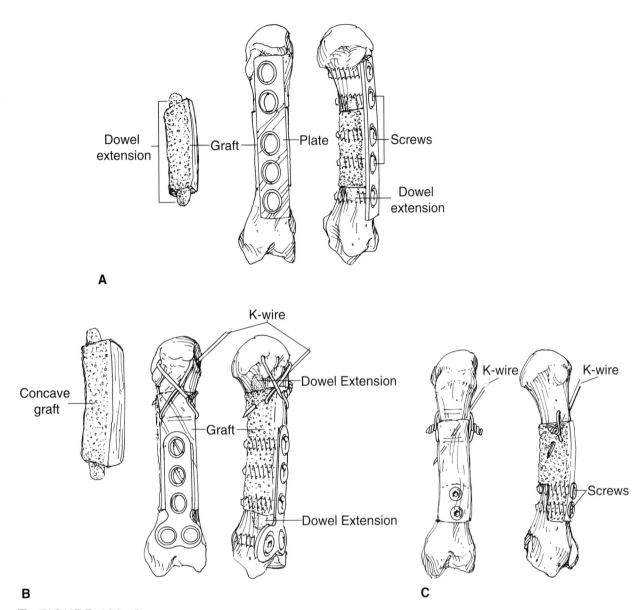

A

B   **C**

■ FIGURE 130–2
Several methods are available to fix a corticocancellous graft in a metacarpal defect. The methods chosen depend primarily on the amount of metacarpal bone remaining at each end. **(A)** A
dorsal 2.7-mm ¼ tubular plate is spanning the defect. Stable fixation is obtained with screws
engaging each metacarpal end and additional screws in the graft. Interfragmentary screw fixation through the plate will add stability. **(B)** A 2.7-mm T-plate is applied to the proximal graft
junction. The distal end is fixed with tension band wiring and an oblique K-wire. **(C)** A step-cut
fit with interfragmentary screws provides proximal fixation. Distal fixation is obtained with an interosseous wire loop and an oblique K-wire.

Although most surgeons prefer autogenous bone graft for hand reconstruction, allograft
has been used successfully.[2,16] Osteocutaneous flaps have been used to reconstruct both
bone and soft tissue defects simultaneously.[3,10,13,15] They can be raised as a pedicle or
transferred as a free vascularized flap. Although these procedures are technically more
demanding, a one-stage reconstruction has definite advantages over multiple, staged procedures.

The surgeon must avoid the pitfall of embarking on a difficult bone grafting procedure
that requires extensive soft tissue dissection, only to find that it is impossible to achieve
adequate bone fixation and wound coverage. Despite a satisfactory radiographic appear-

ance, long-term cast immobilization and secondary wound healing will severely compromise the functional result.

■ REHABILITATION

The rehabilitation program depends on the stability of bone fixation and the status of the soft tissue injuries. Provided bone fixation is secure, rehabilitation should begin in the immediate postoperative period and include passive and active range of motion of all joints to minimize joint stiffness and tendon adhesion. All too commonly, functional outcome is compromised by a failure to appreciate the importance of a well planned therapy program.

■ OUTCOMES

Bone grafting of metacarpal defects results in a high union rate owing to the excellent vascularity of the hand.[7,9,12] In Littler's series, 53 of 56 metacarpal grafts in 44 patients united by 3 months.[9] He concluded that bone grafting was a worthwhile procedure for relieving pain at the fracture site and for restoring the architecture, strength, and function of the hand. Although severe open wounds with large bone defects have been reconstructed by technically successful operations, hand function is usually compromised in these complex injuries.[4,7] Functional outcome depends primarily on associated hand injuries and the ability to initiate early rehabilitation.[7,12] Using techniques of early bone and soft tissue reconstruction, Freeland and co-authors demonstrated that more rapid and better functional recovery occurred than was reported in previous series using staged procedures. Twenty of 21 bone grafts united, and most patients recovered function within 2 to 3 months.[7] Several case reports have described one-stage reconstructions of severe wounds with bone and joint loss using composite tissue transfers.[3,10,13,15]

The treatment of enchondromas in the hand by curettage is highly successful.[2,8] However, the importance of filling the defect with bone graft is unclear. Hasselgren and co-authors reported that curettage without bone grafting was safe and effective.[8] Allograft bone has been used successfully, but the incorporation of graft is prolonged compared to autogenous graft.[2] More aggressive tumors, such as giant cell tumors of bone, require more extensive resection and grafting. The results have been good if the tumor does not recur.[1] Bone grafts have been used for defects caused by osteomyelitis primarily to restore gross structural alignment and stability.[5,9] Their use in smaller defects without bony instability is probably unnecessary and risky. Complications and poor results after bone grafting procedures for all clinical problems result from failing to obtain a clean, disease-free graft bed and not achieving stable bone fixation with complete soft tissue coverage.

References

1. Averill RM, Smith RJ, Campbell CJ: Giant-cell tumors of the hand. J Hand Surg, 1980; 5: 39–50.
2. Bauer RD, Lewis MM, Posner MA: Treatment of enchondromas of the hand with allograft bone. J Hand Surg, 1988; 13A:908–916.
3. Chacha B, Soin K, Tan KC: One stage reconstruction of intercalated defect of the thumb using the osteocutaneous radial forearm flap. J Hand Surg, 1987; 12A:86–92.
4. Chait LA, Cort A, Braun S: Metacarpal reconstruction in compound contaminated injuries of the hand. Hand, 1981; 13:152–157.
5. Cziffer E, Farkas J, Turch nyi B: Management of potentially infected complex hand injuries. J Hand Surg, 1991; 16A:832–834.
6. Dahlin DC, Unni KK: Bone Tumors: General Aspects and Data of 8,542 Cases, 4th Ed. Springfield, IL: Charles C Thomas, 1986.
7. Freeland AE, Jabaley ME, Burkhalter WE, Chaves AMV: Delayed primary bone grafting in the hand and wrist after traumatic bone loss. J Hand Surg, 1984; 9A:22–28.
8. Hasselgren G, Forssblad P, Törnvall A: Bone grafting unnecessary in the treatment of enchondromas in the hand. J Hand Surg, 1991; 16A:139–142.
9. Littler JW: Metacarpal reconstruction. J Bone Joint Surg, 1947; 29:723–737.
10. Matev I: The osteocutaneous pedicle forearm flap. J Hand Surg, 1985; 10B:179–181.
11. O'Brien ET: Fractures of the metacarpals and phalanges. In: Green DP (ed): Operative Hand Surgery, Vol. 1. New York: Churchill-Livingstone, 1988:709–733.

12. Peimer CA, Smith RJ, Leffert RD: Distraction–fixation in the primary treatment of metacarpal bone loss. J Hand Surg, 1981; 6:111–124.
13. Reinisch JF, Winters R, Puckett CL: The use of the osteocutaneous groin flap in gunshot wounds of the hand. J Hand Surg, 1984; 9A:12–17.
14. Segmüller G: Indications for stable internal fixation in hand injuries. In: Chapman MW (ed): Operative Orthopaedics, Vol. 2. Philadelphia: JB Lippincott, 1988:1219–1233.
15. Swartz WM: Immediate reconstruction of the wrist and dorsum of the hand with a free osteocutaneous groin flap. J Hand Surg, 1984; 9A:18–21.
16. Upton J, Glowacki J: Hand reconstruction with allograft demineralized bone: Twenty-six implants in twelve patients. J Hand Surg, 1992; 17A:704–713.

RICHARD L. UHL
RAYMOND J. KOBUS

131

Metacarpal Lengthening by Distraction Osteosynthesis

■ HISTORY OF THE TECHNIQUE

Lengthening the metacarpal bones of the hand has been done as a one-step distraction procedure with bone graft, or by daily distraction with an external fixator and secondary bone grafting once the desired length has been achieved.[2-6,8-11,14,17] Attempts at metacarpal lengthening with single daily distractions have not resulted in consistent regenerative bone formation. Ilizarov found that by preserving the periosteal sleeve around the cut bone and by lengthening the bone gradually, regenerative bone forms predictably.[7,12] Instead of a single daily lengthening, a smaller amount of distraction, several times a day, results in more consistent regenerative bone formation, even in adults.[13,15,16]

■ INDICATIONS AND CONTRAINDICATIONS

The technique of distraction osteosynthesis is useful in cases of congenital shortening of the metacarpals (Fig. 131–1) and in cases of traumatic loss of the end of the thumb (Fig. 131–2). In adults, this method is usually better suited to reconstruction after trauma rather than to correct congenital deformities. Although lengthening may improve the appearance of the hand, the functional improvement should always be the prime consideration. Lengthening for cosmetic reasons alone is discouraged.

In cases of lengthening for congenital shortening, the part to be lengthened should have adequate function (tendons, joints, and sensation all near normal). Lengthening of a traumatically amputated part should be performed carefully if there is a question of skin stability at the tip. If there is evidence of decreased vascular supply or skin breakdown during lengthening, a break in the daily distraction will let the skin and the vessels "catch up" with the bony distraction.

This procedure requires good patient (or parental) compliance and cooperation. The results will be unpredictable if the patient is unable or unwilling to cooperate. Lengthening is painful, and usually requires narcotic analgesia for control of the pain. The patient must understand and agree to the commitment required, because once started there is little alternative to completion.

■ SURGICAL TECHNIQUES

A linear distraction device with half-pins is best suited for lengthening of the metacarpals. Preoperative planning, including device position and location of the bone cut, is essential. The apparatus must be small enough to fit the bone to be lengthened, yet sturdy enough so that the pins will not deform as the lengthening progresses.

An open technique should be used so that the extensor tendons may be exposed and isolated. Under regional or general anesthesia, an incision is made on the dorsum of the hand, in line with the bone to be lengthened. The extensor tendons are identified and retracted. The periosteum of the metacarpal is incised longitudinally and carefully elevated away from the bone. Care must be taken not to damage the periosteum, because this is essential for the formation of the regenerative bone.[7,12,13,15] At no time should any transverse cuts be made in the periosteum because this will delay regenerative bone formation (G. A. Ilizarov, personal communication). If possible, the distraction device should be situated so that the bony cut will be in the metaphyseal region; lengthenings through the diaphyseal region exhibit less regenerative bone formation.[7,15] In some cases this requires crossing the carpometacarpal joint, which does not present a problem in those joints where there is minimal motion (such as the second or third metacarpal).

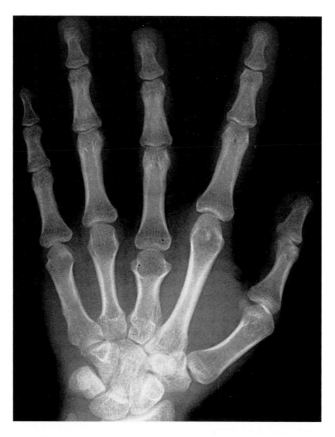

■ FIGURE 131–1
Posteroanterior radiograph of a 16-year-old girl with congenital brachymetacarpia. The patient has difficulty using the hand because of the proximal position of the third metacarpophalangeal joint.

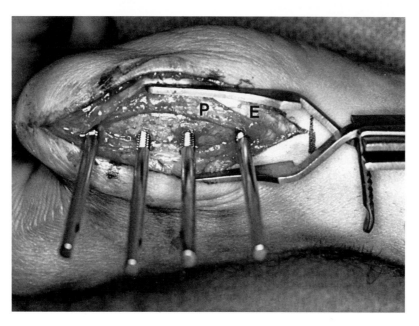

■ FIGURE 131–2
The fixator pins are inserted before cutting the bone. The extensor tendon (E) and the periosteum (P) must be protected throughout the corticotomy.

There are several advantages to inserting the fixator pins before corticotomy (Fig. 131–2). Pin placement in the intact bone helps to ensure accurate alignment after the bone is cut. The pins are easier to insert and the fixator can be applied to ensure a proper fit. Pin insertion after the cut may increase motion at the corticotomy site and damage the periosteum.

Pin sites should be predrilled and the pins inserted by hand. Self-drilling pins inserted with power may lead to bone necrosis. Once the pins have been inserted, the bone is cut

■ FIGURE 131–3
(A) After the bone is cut, the fixator is attached and distracted slightly to ensure that the cut is complete. **(B)** The bone ends are then compressed and left compressed for 5 days.

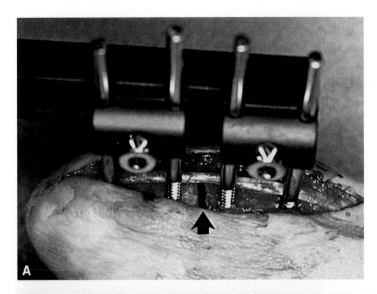

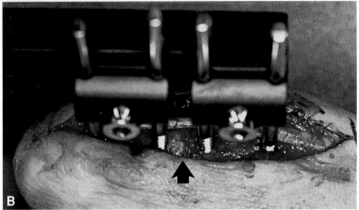

using a hand-sharpened osteotome. Modification of the osteotome by rounding one corner provides a blunt edge and serves as an additional means of protecting the periosteum. An oscillating saw should not be used because this may damage the periosteum, create a larger bone gap, and burn the ends of the bone, making the formation of adequate regenerative bone less predictable. After the bone has been cut, the lengthening device is attached to the pins and distracted very slightly to ensure that the cut is complete (Fig. 131–3A). The corticotomy is then compressed and left compressed for the first 5 postoperative days (Fig. 131–3B). Intraoperative radiographs should be taken to ensure proper device application.

The periosteum is closed with absorbable suture, the skin is closed with nylon suture, and a compressive bandage applied. After surgery, the patient is encouraged to open and close the hand to maintain motion of the joints. Patients may spend the first postoperative night in the hospital, although postoperative pain, before lengthening, is usually minimal.

The patient returns to the office on the fifth postoperative day, and distraction is usually started. If the periosteum was accidentally damaged during the surgical procedure, approximately 10 days should be allowed before lengthening. In these cases, this additional delay leads to more reliable consolidation (G. A. Ilizarov, personal communication).

Patients (or parents in the case of a child) are taught by the physician how to advance the lengthening device. They are told both the direction and the amount to turn the apparatus, and must demonstrate understanding of this before leaving the office. We call the patients 2 days later to make sure they are progressing without any problems, and bring them back to the office if there is any question that the lengthening is not being done properly. Patients are also taught pin care. We start cleaning the pins with hydrogen peroxide and normal saline at the first office visit. Patients continue pin care three times daily at home. If, during the treatment, the pin sites become erythematous or begin to drain, we place the patients on a 5- to 7-day course of oral antibiotics.

Once lengthening has begun, both the distance per adjustment (the rate) and the number of adjustments per day (the rhythm) are important. Greater distances per adjustment with the same number of adjustments per day will give slower consolidation, whereas more frequent adjustments with a smaller distance per adjustment will give faster consolidation.[7,12] A distraction rate of 0.25 mm, four times a day (for an overall daily lengthening of 1 mm) is the rate and rhythm usually used for extremity lengthening, but this can be too much for the small bones of the hand. On the other hand, rates slower than 0.5 mm/ day, especially in children, lead to premature consolidation.

The distraction should proceed until the desired overall length has been achieved. Radiographs are taken on a weekly basis to monitor the degree of lengthening and overall alignment (Fig. 131–4A). Most patients have moderate to significant discomfort throughout the lengthening and usually require narcotic analgesia for pain relief. If the patient is unable to tolerate continued lengthening on a daily basis, it may be necessary to wait 1 to 2 days without any distraction, and then resume the distraction at the previous level until the desired length is achieved.

Once the final length has been attained, the device must remain in place while the regenerative bone matures. Radiographs should be taken every 2 to 3 weeks to monitor

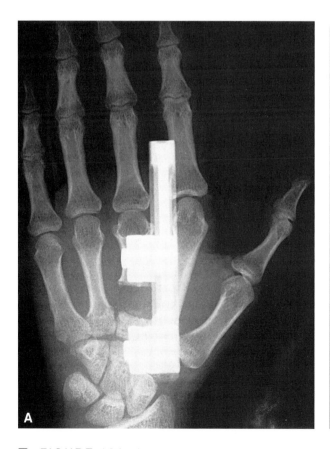 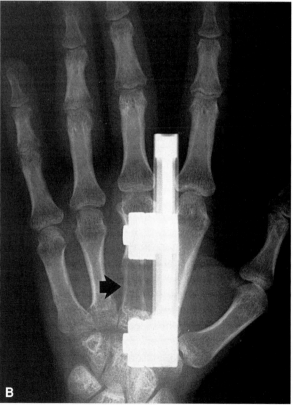

■ FIGURE 131–4
(A) The patient presented in Figure 131–1, after 2 weeks of distraction. There is minimal regenerative bone at this point. Excessive regenerative bone indicates a distraction rate that is too slow, and may lead to premature consolidation. **(B)** The final length is achieved, and there is abundant regenerative bone. A "neocortex" (arrow) is beginning to form.

■ FIGURE 131–4
(continued)
(C) After device removal. Note that the most proximal pin was placed in the capitate to allow a metaphyseal corticotomy.

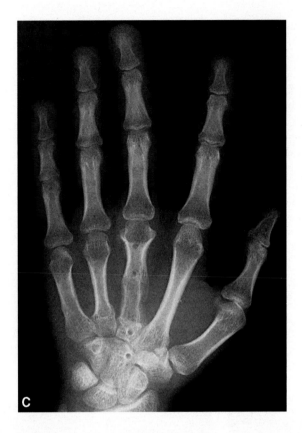

regenerative bone formation (Fig. 131–4B). When the radiographs indicate the formation of a new cortex within the regenerative bone, the device may be removed. Usually, this takes two to three times as long as it took to achieve the desired length (Fig. 131–4C).

■ TECHNICAL ALTERNATIVES

The technique illustrated is useful when lengthening of more than 1 cm is required. For lengths less than 1 cm, a one-step lengthening, with interposition graft (iliac crest or toe phalanx) and pinning, may be preferable.[6] Acute lengthening greater than 1 cm is limited by the neurovascular and musculotendinous structures.

The method of distraction osteogenesis has many potential pitfalls. Most can be avoided by careful preoperative planning (e.g., the fixator and pins do not fit the length of bone available), by careful operative technique (e.g., pins inserted into joints, damage to the periosteum or tendons, incomplete bone cut), and by meticulous postoperative care (e.g., prevention of angulation when distracting, development of contractures). At no time should a large, one-stage distraction be performed because this will damage the periosteum.[7] Gradual distraction with several lengthenings per day is best suited for regenerative bone formation. Single daily lengthenings have not been shown to produce consistent regenerative bone formation.[15] Once regenerative bone has formed, the fixator must be left in place until that bone has sufficient strength to allow removal.

■ REHABILITATION

All patients go to hand therapy throughout the treatment period. Active range of motion exercises should be continued throughout the distraction and consolidation period. This is important not only to maintain motion, but to aid in maturation of the regenerative bone.[1] Often during lengthening a muscle imbalance will occur, and either a flexion or extension contracture will develop. In our experience, the type of contracture that develops is somewhat unpredictable, emphasizing the need for careful follow-up and monitoring by both the physician and therapist. Once a contracture begins, aggressive splinting should be instituted to correct the condition. Often, holding distraction for several days will allow the muscle imbalance to improve.

With careful patient selection and meticulous attention to the many details, the procedure can be most rewarding. The total time in the external fixator will be 3 to 5 days for each millimeter of length desired. Most patients will develop stiffness during lengthening, and all have pain. Streaks of early bone formation are usually seen at the distraction site by the third or fourth week of lengthening. We have had one case of early consolidation (in a child) and one case of delayed bone formation (in an adult). Should the regenerative bone not form within an acceptable time, a second-stage bone grafting can be performed. All of our pin tract problems have been adequately managed with local care and oral antibiotics; however, it may sometimes be necessary to replace or remove an infected pin if these measures do not control the problem.

■ OUTCOMES

References

1. Aronson J, Good B, Stewart C, Harrison B, Harp J: Preliminary studies of mineralization during distraction osteogenesis. Clin Orthop, 1990; 250:43–49.
2. Cobb TK, Stocks GW, May WF, Strauss MR, Lewis RC: Thumb reconstruction by metacarpal lengthening after traumatic loss at the level of the interphalangeal joint. Orthop Rev, 1990; 19:47–51.
3. Cowan NJ: Surgical management of the hypoplastic hand. In: Cowan NJ (ed): Practical Surgery of the Hand. Chicago: Yearbook Medical, 1979:173–205.
4. Cowan NJ, Loftus JM: Distraction augmentation manoplasty: Technique for lengthening digits or entire hands. Orthop Rev, 1978; 7:45–53.
5. Flatt AE: The care of congenital hand anomalies. St. Louis: CV Mosby, 1977:123–125.
6. Fultz CW, Lester DK, Hunter JM: Single stage lengthening by intercalary bone graft in patients with congenital hand deformities. J Hand Surg, 1986; 11B:40–46.
7. Ilizarov GA: Epiphysealysis and corticotomy lengthening (abstract). Second Annual International Conference on Ilizarov Techniques for Management of Difficult Skeletal Problems, New York, New York, December 1988.
8. Kessler I, Baruch A, Hecht O: Experience with distraction lengthening of digital rays in congenital anomalies. J Hand Surg, 1977; 2:394–401.
9. Kessler I, Hecht O, Baruch A: Distraction lengthening of digital rays in the management of the injured hand. J Bone Joint Surg, 1979; 61A:83–87.
10. Matev IB: Thumb reconstruction after amputation of the metacarpophalangeal joint by bone lengthening. J Bone Joint Surg, 1970; 52A:957–965.
11. Matev IB: Thumb reconstruction in children through metacarpal lengthening. Plast Reconstr Surg, 1979; 64:665–669.
12. Paley D: Current techniques of limb lengthening. J Pediatr Orthop, 1988; 8:73-92.
13. Paley D, Catagni M, Argnani F, Villa A, Benedetti G, Cattaneo R: Ilizarov treatment of tibial non-unions with bone loss. Clin Orthop, 1989; 241:146–165.
14. Paneva-Holevich E, Yankov EA: Distraction method for lengthening of the finger metacarpals: A preliminary report. J Hand Surg, 1980; 5:160–167.
15. Schwartsman V, McMurray MR, Martin SN: The Ilizarov method: The basics. Contemporary Orthopaedics, 1989; 19:628–638.
16. Seitz WH Jr, Froimson AI: Callotasis lengthening in the upper extremity: Indications, techniques, and pitfalls. J Hand Surg, 1991; 16A:560–563.
17. Smith RJ, Brushart TM: Allograft bone for metacarpal reconstruction. J Hand Surg, 1985; 10A:325–334.

132

Transposition of the Index Ray

■ HISTORY OF THE
TECHNIQUE

Prehension after traumatic amputation of the middle finger is compromised, particularly three point or chuck pinch. The index finger, in an attempt to make better contact with the thumb and ring finger, tends to deviate in an ulnar direction (Figs. 132-1A to 132-1C). The degree of deviation depends on the length of the amputation stump; the shorter the stump, the greater the scissoring. Frequently, the stump protrudes during grasp, and patients find this annoying because the stump tends to be traumatized. Small objects may also fall from grasp, and the aesthetic appearance of the hand is distorted by the space left by the missing finger.

Sterling Bunnell is credited with performing the first ray transposition in 1931,[5] but it was not until World War II that the procedure became more widely used. During the war years, regional hand centers were established by the United States Army to treat hand injuries, and Bunnell, who served as the civilian consultant, helped introduce the procedure for the treatment of severe gunshot and shrapnel injuries.[5] However, it was the dedication and ingenuity of the military surgeons at the centers who developed the protocol to make it an effective procedure.[2,4,13] The technical aspects of the procedure as originally described remain valid today, although improvements have been made in the placement of the surgical incisions and the type of osteotomy used to transpose the second metacarpal. Regarding the surgical incisions, they are placed on the sides of the proximal segments of the fingers rather than in the depths of the web spaces to avoid scarring of the newly formed web. This technique was reported by the author in 1979,[11] and its importance was later emphsisized in an article by Plasschaert and Hage[10] in 1988. Regarding the osteotomy, it is performed in a fashion that will maximize the surface area of bone-to-bone contact to hasten healing. This is best achieved by step-cut rather than straight osteotomies through the cancelleous metaphyseal portions of the bases of the second and third metacarpals. A cortical-cancellous strut removed from the amputated portion of the third metacarpal and inserted into the medullary portion of the base of the third metacarpal and cancellous chips packed around the osteotomy also will aid healing.

■ INDICATIONS AND
CONTRAINDICATIONS

Transposition of the second or index ray with its extrinsic tendons, intrinsic muscles, and neurovascular bundles is an effective procedure to restore function and improve the aesthetic appearance of the hand after loss of the middle finger. It also can be used in conjunction with surgical ablation of a middle finger that has been rendered useless by trauma, involved with tumor, or is congenitally hypoplastic.[7,11]

Several factors must be taken into consideration when contemplating an index ray transposition. Ideally, the finger should have normal mobility and sensibility. While a mild impairment in mobility or sensibility is not a contraindication to the procedure, a finger with limited mobility and absence of protective sensibility is a contraindication. The index finger must be free of any chronic soft tissue or bone infection and its circulation intact. In cases where there is extensive scarring in the palm and the patency of the arterial arch or common digital arteries is suspect, a preoperative arteriogram should be obtained. A potential disadvantage of the procedure is that it narrows the breadth of the palm, which decreases grip strength. However, this has not been a significant problem, particularly when the stump of the middle finger is painful preoperatively. Removing the stump

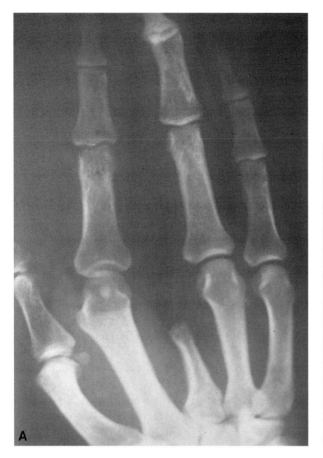
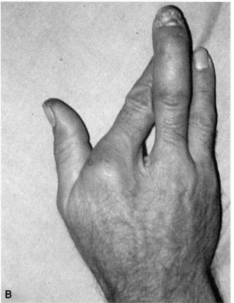
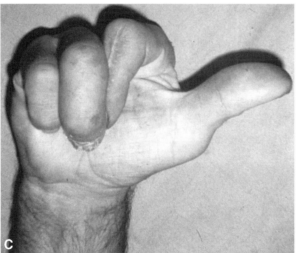

■ FIGURE 132–1

A, A 65-year-old retired construction worker sustained a traumatic amputation of his right middle finger 10 years earlier. Primary care at that time consisted of debridement; the head of the third metacarpal was removed to obtain skin closure. **B and C,** Several months after the injury, the patient noted ulnar deviation of the index finger, scissoring of the finger with flexion, and impaired use with motions of the ring finger.

eliminates the pain, which was the primary reason for their weakened grasp. These specific patients often report an increase in grip strength after surgery.

The operation is performed under tourniquet control using regional block anesthesia, with general anesthesia generally reserved for children. The skin incisions are carefully planned to avoid later scar contractures in the new web between the transposed index finger and the ring finger as well as in the palm. Avoiding a scar contracture in the new web is accomplished by not making incisions in the second and third webs. Rather, curved incisions are made on the ulnar sides of the proximal segments of the index and middle fingers, 1.5 cm distal to their respective webs (Figs. 132-2A and 132-2B). If there is scarring on the ulnar side of the proximal segment of the middle finger, the curved incision is made on its radial side, with a corresponding incision on the radial side of the ring finger. When the middle finger has been traumatically amputated through its base, leaving little or no stump, these incisions cannot be used, and the only option is to make straight incisions through the second and third web spaces. Dorsally, the incisions are carried proximally in a V-shaped configuration to converge at the base of the third metacarpal. They also converge volarly, but this occurs in the thenar crease. Rather than making straight incisions in the palm, they are zig-zagged at the metacarpophalangeal (MP) flexion crease and at the distal palmar crease to avoid later scar contractures at these sites. Skin flaps are mobilized, and the palmar fascia in the operative area is excised and the neurovascular bundles identified. The radial and ulnar arteries to the middle finger are ligated and divided as they arise from their common digital arteries. The radial and ulnar digital nerves also are divided, but at a much more proximal level to avoid later tender neuromata. This is accomplished by mobilizing each digital nerve by interfascicular dissection of its respective common digital nerve into the proximal palm before it is divided. The ulnar digital nerve to the index finger and the radial digital nerve to the ring finger are carefully

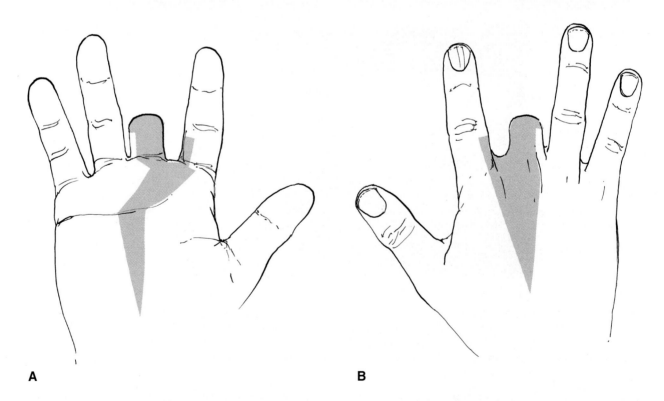

A

B

■ FIGURE 132–2
A and B, Skin incisions for transposition of the index ray. A-A', B-B', and C-C' come together after excision of the shaded portions of the skin.

protected during this dissection. Longitudinal traction is applied to both flexor tendons to the middle finger with the wrist in flexion, and the tendons are divided, allowing their ends to retract proximally into the carpal tunnel. In post-traumatic amputations, the cut ends of the flexor tendons are usually scarred in the distal palm, where they must be released before being divided more proximally. The deep transverse metacarpal ligaments on both sides of the palmar plate are sectioned as close to the plate as possible, which leaves sufficient tissue to facilitate later closure. The transverse head of the adductor pollicis is detached subperiosteally from the volar surface of the third metacarpal, and care is taken to protect the motor branch of the ulnar nerve, which courses between the transverse and oblique heads of the muscle.

Dorsally, the interconnections (juncturae tendinum) between the extensor digitorum communis tendon to the middle finger and the adjacent extensor tendons are divided. The extensor tendon itself is then sectioned as far proximal as possible. The fascia over the interosseous muscles to either side of the third metacarpal is released. Using blunt and sharp dissection, the second dorsal interosseous, which will be removed with the middle ray, is separated from the first volar interosseous, which is saved. Similarly, the third dorsal interosseous on the ulnar side of the metacarpal is separated from the second volar interosseous, which also is saved. The second and third metacarpals are then osteotomized at their bases where the bones flare. Each osteotomy is carried out in a step-cut fashion with the higher step on the ulnar side of the bone. This facilitates shifting the second metacarpal onto the base of the third (Fig. 132–3A). A power sagittal saw with a narrow blade is used when making the osteotomies to avoid inadvertently fracturing either bone. Cancellous bone chips from the head of the third metacarpal are frequently added to the osteotomy site. An intramedullary cortical-cancellous strut also can be inserted across the osteotomy site.

The transposed index ray is stabilized both to the base of the third metacarpal and to the fourth and fifth metacarpal using Kirschner wires. At least two wires (0.045 to 0.062)

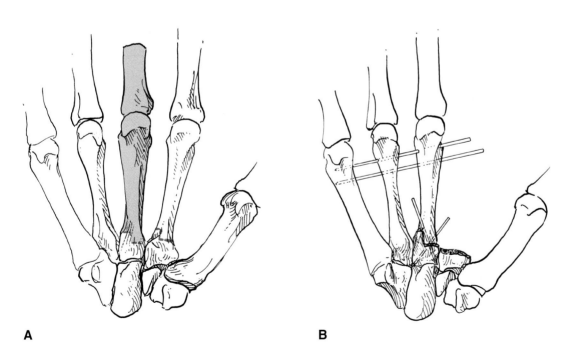

A   **B**

■ FIGURE 132–3
A and B, A diagram of the step-cut osteotomies through the bases of the second and third metacarpals. The osteotomies are carried out at the same level in each bone. After the index ray is transposed, the higher step at the base of its metacarpal is usually removed, leveling the base.

are used to stabilize the second metacarpal into the adjacent metacarpals. These wires are inserted transversely, while the wires used to stabilize the osteotomy site (0.035 to 0.045) are inserted obliquely and are usually crossed (Fig. 132–3B). A cortical screw can be substituted for the wires at the osetotomy site, but a plate should be avoided.[12] Care must be taken to insure that the second metacarpal is properly positioned. The head of the metacarpal should be slightly dorsal to the heads of the fourth and fifth metacarpals to maintain the normal curvature of the transverse metacarpal arch. More importantly, the index finger must not be malrotated. This is assessed by passively flexing and extending it. The finger should neither cross the adjacent middle finger nor diverge from it. After the index ray is positioned and rigidly stabilized, the deep transverse metacarpal ligament is repaired and the transverse head of the adductor pollicis is reattached to the periosteal tissues on the radial side of the fourth metacarpal. Monofilament (4-0) nylon is generally used for both repairs. The tourniquet is released, bleeding points cauterized or ligated, and the skin incisions closed. The skin flap that was elevated from the ulnar side of the proximal segment of the middle finger will inset into the defect on the ulnar side of the index finger. A volar plaster splint is applied, immobilizing the wrist in slight extension and the MP joints of all fingers in flexion to avoid later extension contractures. After the normal postoperative swelling has subsided, usually within 2 weeks, a more comfortable splint is fabricated by a hand therapist using a lightweight but rigid thermoplastic material. The splint immobilizes the wrist and the MP joint of the transposed ray. The splint is removed for periodic active range of motion exercises, but it is worn at all other times until the osteotomy has healed, as demonstrated by radiographs. Bone healing generally occurs in 8 to

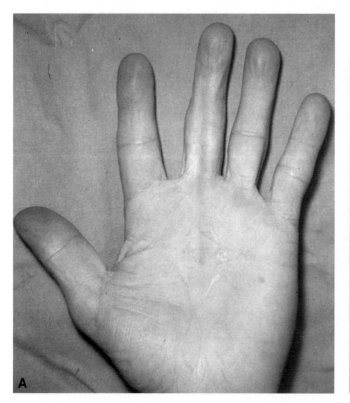
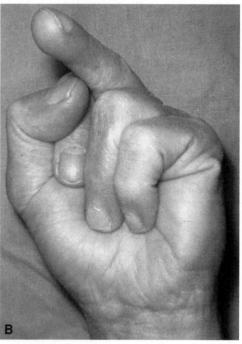

■ FIGURE 132–4

A and B, A 35-year-old carpenter sustained a power saw injury to the volar aspect of his dominant right middle finger almost 2 years earlier. He had two unsuccessful operations, including nerve grafts and a staged flexor tendon reconstruction. The finger was stiff with only a few degrees of passive mobility at either interphalangeal joint, the tendon graft was bowstrung, and the finger was anesthetic.

12 weeks. There is never any urgency about removing the Kirschner wires, which all were cut beneath the skin. They are removed only if they cause discomfort, and usually this is an office procedure.

Two other techniques for transposition of the index ray have been described, both involving excision of the entire third metacarpal. Bunnell[1] in 1944 and later Slocum[13] in 1959 recommended bringing the heads of the second and third metacarpals closer together by simply suturing the deep transverse metacarpal ligament between them. A Kirschner wire also was drilled transversely across both metacarpals to provide additional support. Since the carpometacarpal joint of the index finger is normally rigid, the finger always appeared angulated, and the new web space between it and the ring finger was wider than normal. This technique is not nearly as effective as transposing the index ray onto the base of the third metacarpal via osteotomies. Perhaps it is indicated in very rare clinical situations when postoperative immobilization cannot exceed 3 weeks.[6]

Peze and Iselin[9] modified the procedure by performing a wedge resection of the capitate after they excised the third metacarpal. By removing a distally based wedge from the capitate with its apex at the lunate-capitate articulation, they were able to close the interval between the second and fourth metacarpal, thereby bringing the index and ring fingers closer together. Although they claimed their technique reduced the risk of nonunion of

■ TECHNICAL ALTERNATIVES

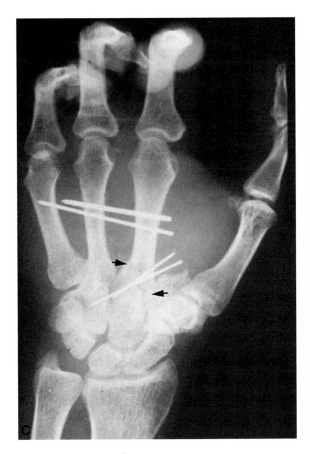

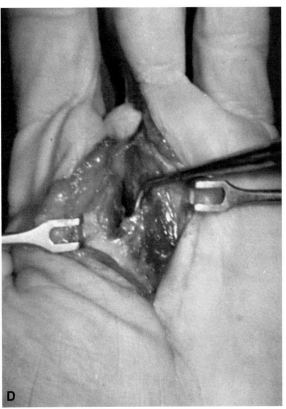

■ FIGURE 132–4
(continued)
C, Radiograph of the hand after the index ray transposition. The step-cut configuration of the osteotomy (arrows) is clearly seen. The step at the second metacarpal base had been leveled.
D, The transverse head of the adductor pollicis was reattached to the radial side of the fourth metacarpal.

the metacarpal osteotomy, it resulted in incongruity of the midcarpal joint, which has potential consequences for limiting wrist motion.

■ REHABILITATION

Rehabilitation after transposition of the index ray is as important as the operative procedure itself. Active range of motion exercises are encouraged immediately after surgery for all joints except the wrist and the MP joints. After 2 weeks, when the thermoplastic splint has been fabricated, periodic active exercises for these joints are begun. As bone healing progresses, active resistive exercises are instituted to restore strength to the extrinsic muscles in the forearm as well as to the intrinsic muscles in the hand. Strengthening the thumb intrinsics, particularly the adductor pollicis, is important because the transverse head of the muscle was detached before resection of the third metacarpal and reattached to the fourth metacarpal. Strengthening this muscle is accomplished by adducting the thumb against the resistance of a sponge inserted in the first web space. Initially, a soft sponge is used, but as strength improves the resistive exercises are increased by using denser sponges. Strengthening the thenar intrinsic muscles, which are primarily abductors of the thumb, is achieved by abducting the thumb against the resistance of a rubber band

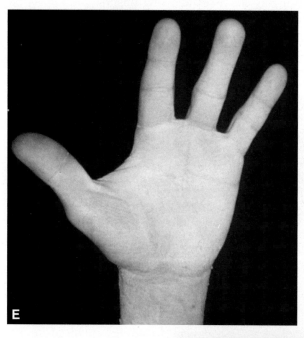
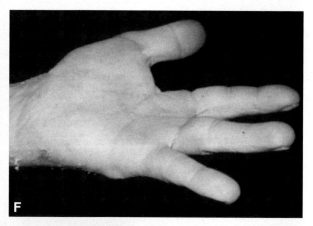
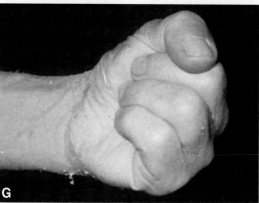

■ FIGURE 132–4

(continued)

E to G, Postoperative range of motion and appearance of the hand.

wrapped around it and the palm. Initially, the rubber band should provide sufficient strength to be effective without overpowering the weakened muscles. If the rubber bands are too strong, a muscle strain can result. As muscle strength improves, thicker or multiple rubber bands are used. The frequency of exercises is more important than their duration, and patients are instructed to exercise hourly, performing up to 10 repetitions of each exercise.

■ OUTCOMES

The functional results of index ray transpositions were evaluated by Colen and co-authors,[3] who measured grip and pinch strength as a percentage of the nonoperated side. In their group of 11 patients, grip strength averaged 74% and pinch strength 73%. Their results emphasize the importance of postoperative resistive exercises. Although some loss of grip strength is inevitable after any ray transposition, pinch strength will be less affected provided the patient exercises effectively. Index ray transpositions are effective reconstructive procedures that predictably improve prehension and aesthetics (Figs. 132-4A to 132-4G).

References

1. Bunnell S: Surgery of the Hand, Philadelphia: J. B. Lippincott, 1944:478.
2. Carroll RE: Transposition of the index finger to replace the middle finger. Clin Orthop, 1959; 15:27–34.
3. Colen L, Bunkis J, Gordon L, Walton R: Functional assessment of ray transfer for central digital loss. J Hand Surg, 1985; 10A:232–237.
4. Graham WC, Brown JB, Cannon C, Riordan DC: Transposition of the fingers in severe injuries of the hand. J Bone Joint Surg, 1947; 29:998–1004.
5. Hygroop GL: Transfer of a metacarpal, with or without its digit, for improving function of the crippled hand. Plast Reconstr Surg, 1949; 4:45–58.
6. Louis DS: Amputations. In: Green D (ed): Operative Hand Surgery, 3rd Ed, New York: Churchill Livingston, 1993:66–72.
7. Malek R: Digital transposition in children. Hand, 1975; 7:57–59.
8. Peacock EE: Metacarpal transfer following amputation of a central digit. Plast Reconstr Surg, 1962; 20:345–355.
9. Peze W, Iselin F: Cosmetic amputation of the long finger with carpal osteotomy. Ann Chir Main, 1984; 3:232–236.
10. Plasschaert MJJT, Hage JJ: A web saving skin incision for amputation of the third and fourth ray of the hand. J Hand Surg, 1988; 13B:340–341.
11. Posner MA: Ray transposition for central digital loss. J Hand Surg, 1979; 3:242–257.
12. Razemon JP: Technique of Digital Transposition. In: Tubiana R (ed): The Hand, Volume 3, Chapter 94, Philadelphia: W. B. Saunders, 1988:1065–1070.
13. Slocum DB: Amputations of the fingers of the hand. Clin Orthop, 1959; 15:35–39.

MARTIN A. POSNER

133

Transposition of the Small Ray

■ HISTORY OF THE
TECHNIQUE

Although amputation of the ring finger is not as common as amputation of the middle finger, many of the problems are the same after either injury. Small objects fall from grasp, especially when the stump of the ring finger is short, and the little finger scissors in a radial direction, disturbing the appearance of the hand. The only difference between loss of either central digit is that three-point chuck pinch is generally not compromised with loss of the ring finger. An effective operation to restore function and improve the aesthetic appearance of the hand in these patients is radial transposition of the small ray.[2,4,6] Technically, the operation involves either transposing the ray onto the base of the fourth metacarpal or simply allowing the small ray to shift radially on the hamate. The advantages and disadvantages for each technique will be discussed as well as a technique that involves an intracarpal osteotomy. The technique for transposition of the small ray after loss of both middle and ring fingers also will be discussed.

However, there is one slight but significant difference regarding the technique for performing the osteotomies. Although step-cut osteotomies also are used, they are performed at different levels in the fourth and fifth metacarpals—the osteotomy in the fourth metacarpal at a more distal level than that in the fifth, which effectively "lengthens" the little finger.[6]

■ INDICATIONS AND
CONTRAINDICATIONS

Transposition of the fifth ray, with its extrinsic tendons, intrinsic muscles, and neurovascular bundles, is an effective procedure to restore function and improve the aesthetic appearance of the hand after loss of the ring finger. It also can be used as a component of hand reconstruction after amputation of a ring finger that is profoundly impaired as a result of previous trauma, tumor, or congenital deformity. The small finger ray is indicated for transposition only when it has normal mobility and sensibility or in the presence of limited impairment. Mild deficits in mobility or sensibility are not necessarily a contraindication to the procedure. A finger with advanced loss in mobility or absence of protective sensation is contraindicated for transposition. The small finger must be free of any chronic soft tissue or bone infection, and circulation must be intact. Extensive scarring in the palm, about the base of the small finger, or occlusion of the arterial arch or common digital arteries also are contraindications to this procedure.

A potential disadvantage of the procedure is that it narrows the width of the palm, which decreases grip strength. However, this has not been a significant problem, particularly when the stump of the ring finger is painful before surgery. If pain interferes with peak grip activity, removing the ring finger amputation stump may result in an increase in postoperative grip strength.

■ SURGICAL
TECHNIQUES

The technique for transposition of the small ray after traumatic loss of the ring finger or when it is performed in conjunction with amputation of a diseased, damaged, or congenitally hypoplastic ring finger, is similar to the technique for transposition of the index ray. The skin incisions are designed to avoid contractures in the newly formed web between the middle and little fingers,[5,6] as well as in the palm (Figs. 133-1A and 133-1B). Curved incisions are made on the ulnar sides of the proximal segments of the ring and middle fingers or, if there are scars in either area, on the radial sides of the proximal segments

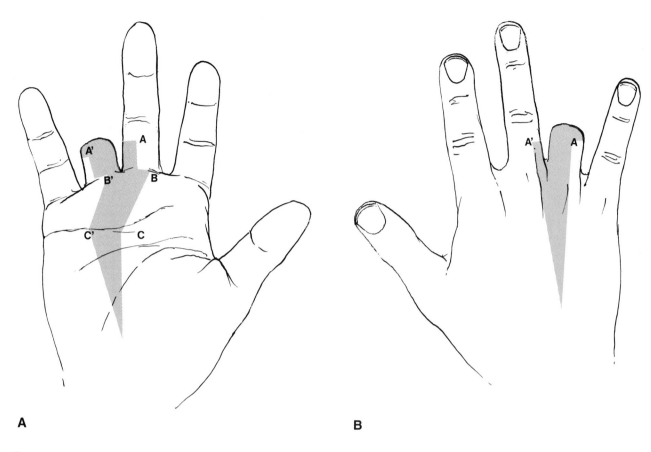

A

B

■ FIGURE 133–1
A and B, Skin incisions for transposition of the small ray.

of the ring and little fingers. Dorsally, the incisions are carried proximally to converge at the base of the fourth metacarpal and volarly in a zig-zag fashion, corresponding to the direction of the palmar creases, to converge in or slightly to the ulnar side of the thenar crease. The dissection in the palm involves excising the palmar fascia and then visualizing the common digital nerves and vessels to the ulnar three fingers. The radial and ulnar digital arteries to the ring finger are ligated and divided as they arise from their respective common digital arteries. The digital nerves to the ring finger are dissected proximally by interfascicular dissection of their respective common digital nerves and cut as far proximally as possible to avoid later tender neuromata. Longitudinal traction is applied to both flexor tendons with the wrist flexed and then divided proximally and allowed to retract into the carpal tunnel. Dorsally, the juncturae tendinum connections to the extensor digitorum communis tendon to the ring finger are released and the extensor tendon itself is divided proximally. The interossei muscles that will be sacrificed with the ring ray (second volar and fourth dorsal) are separated from the interosseous muscles that will be saved, the third dorsal interosseous to the middle finger and the third volar interosseous to the little finger.

Transposition of the small ray is commonly done either via osteotomies through the bases of the fourth and fifth metacarpals or by excising the entire fourth metacarpal and then shifting the fifth metacarpal radially on the hamate. The preferred technique is via metacarpal osteotomies because rotation and angulation of the transposed small ray can be better controlled. Osteotomies also provide a means to "lengthen" the little finger, which normally is considerably shorter than the middle finger (Figs. 133-2A and 133-2B). Lengthening the little finger up to 1.5 cm can be achieved by cutting the fourth metacarpal

■ FIGURE 133–2
A and B, A diagram of the osteotomies through the fourth and fifth metacarpals. The osteotomies are carried out at different levels, with the one in the fourth at a more distal level than the one in the fifth. This technique "lengthens" the little finger.

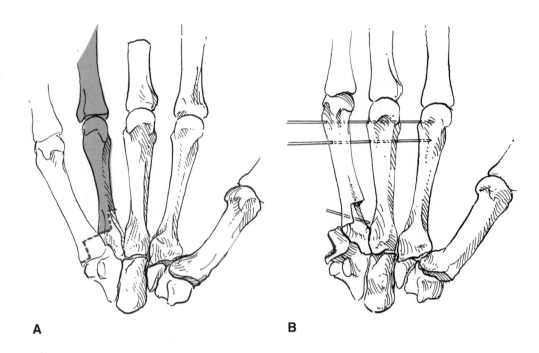

A   **B**

at a more distal level than the fifth. Step-cut osteotomies are used for each bone to maximize bone to bone contact, and the higher step of each osteotomy is on the radial side of the bone, which facilitates shifting the fifth metacarpal in a radial direction. By lengthening the small ray, the symmetry of the little finger to the remaining index and middle fingers is enhanced. The potential for malrotation is greater after transposition of the small ray than after transposition of the index ray, and this must be carefully checked at the time of surgery. Rigid fixation is obtained using Kirschner wires in a similar fashion as described for transposing the index ray. Although failure of the osteotomy to heal has not been a problem, the possibility exists because the fourth metacarpal is the narrowest of all the metacarpals and the level of the osteotomy tends to be in its diaphyseal portion. To promote healing, cancellous bone chips from the resected portion of the metacarpal should be added to the osteotomy site. They also can be inserted in an intramedullary fashion when the fifth metacarpal is shifted onto the fourth (Fig. 133–3A).

■ TECHNICAL
ALTERNATIVES

The other commonly used technique for transposing the small ray is based on the anatomy of the fourth metacarpal and the carpometacarpal joints of the ring and little fingers. The fourth metacarpal is the only one that has no tendon attachments at its base. Therefore, excising it will not affect wrist mobility. Because it is also the narrowest, the gap created by its removal will not be as large as the gap following excision of the third metacarpal. Regarding the anatomy of the carpometacarpal joints, the fourth and fifth metacarpals share a common articulation with the hamate. In contradistinction to the carpometacarpal joints of the index and middle fingers, which are normally rigid, the carpometacarpal joints of the ring and little fingers permit 15° to 30° of mobility. After the soft tissue dissection in the palm and dorsal aspect of the hand has been completed, the joint between the fourth metacarpal and hamate is identified and the dorsal ligaments divided. By flexing the metacarpal, the volar ligaments are visualized and they also are divided with care taken not to damage the ulnar nerve and artery, which lie immediately volar to them. The fourth metacarpal is removed, and the fifth metacarpal now has the potential to slide radially. Actually, the shift is minimal because strong ligaments continue to tether it to the hamate. Sectioning these ligaments has been suggested[4] as a method to more effectively shift the metacarpal closer to the third metacarpal. Kirschner wires are used to stabilize the fifth metacarpal in its new position. Although closing the gap is more suited for excision of the fourth metacarpal than the third, some angulation of the little finger is common.[7]

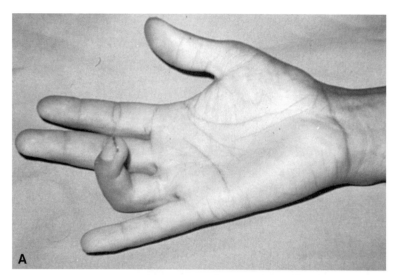

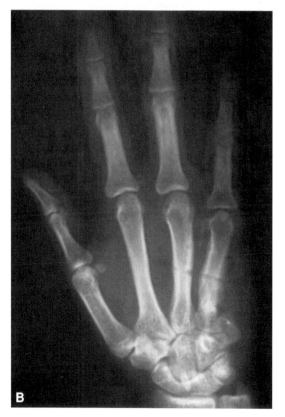

■ **FIGURE 133–3**
A, A 42-year-old mechanic with a fixed flexion contracture of his left ring finger following a crushing-lacerating injury to the digit 1 year earlier. In addition to being rigid, the finger also was anesthetic. **B,** Radiograph of the hand after healing of the metacarpal osteotomy and pin removal.

Le Viet proposed another technique that involves resection of the entire fourth ray, an osteotomy of the lateral part of the hamate, and a capitohamate arthrodesis.[3] He claimed that his procedure did not alter the course of the hypothenar muscles and also preserved the carpometacarpal joint of the small ray, two factors be considered important. However, calculating the angle of the cuneiform osteotomy is complicated, and there is a risk of the little finger being improperly positioned, which Le Viet acknowledged was a complication in many of his early cases.

In rare situations, both middle and ring fingers have been traumatically amputated or must be surgically ablated. While tip pinch between the thumb and index finger in these patients is relatively spared, grip strength is seriously impaired. The large gap between the remaining two fingers also interferes with effective three-point chuck pinch. Although

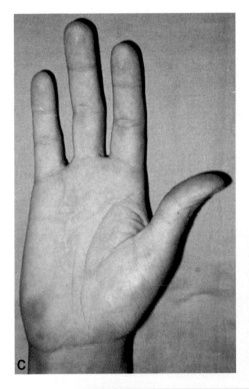

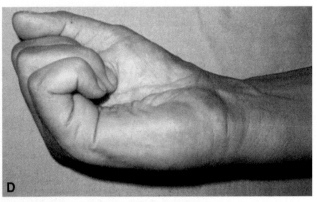

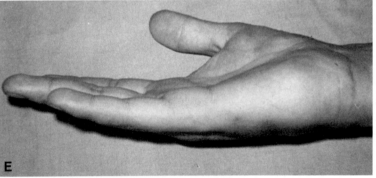

■ FIGURE 133–3

(continued)

C to E, Postoperative photographs of the hand. "Lengthening" the little finger when it was transposed improved the appearance of the hand.

it is impossible to restore normal prehension in these patients, some functional improvement can be achieved by transposition of the small ray, which also improves, even to a slight degree, the aesthetic appearance of the hand. Transposing the fifth metacarpal onto the base of the third metacarpal is technically feasible, but it may position the little finger too close to the index finger. Transposing the fifth metacarpal to the fourth metacarpal also may be unsatisfactory, because the little finger may remain too apart from the index finger. Often the best position for the transposed fifth metacarpal is the base of the fourth, but only after most of the third metacarpal is resected including the interossei muscles to the middle finger.

The principles regarding the skin incisions are the same as previously discussed for transposition of the small ray after loss of the ring finger. When both central fingers have been amputated, the soft tissue dissection is obviously more extensive. The common digital artery to the middle and ring fingers is ligated close to the transverse arterial arch and the common digital nerve is divided at the same level. The common digital arteries to the index and middle fingers, and to the ring and little fingers are preserved, but their branches to the middle and the ring fingers are ligated. The digital nerves accompanying these braches are mobilized proximally by interfascicular dissection of their respective common digital nerves and sectioned at the same level as was the previously divided common digital nerve to the middle and ring fingers. Unless contraindicated for reason of adequacy of tumor resection, the transverse head of the adductor pollicis is saved. It is removed subperiosteally from the third metacarpal and reattached to the fifth metacarpal after it is transposed. The second and third volar interossei on the second and fifth metacarpals respectively are also saved and separated from the interossei on the third and fourth metacarpal, which are excised with those bones. As when transposing the small ray after amputation of only the ring finger, the stepcut osteotomy through the base of its metacarpal is at a more proximal level than the osteotomy through the third or fourth metacarpal. The small ray is then shifted radially either onto the base of the fourth or third metacarpal depending on which bone provides the more optimum position for the little finger.

Rehabilitation after transposition of the small ray is similar to that after transposition of the index ray and also is as important as the operation itself. Active range of motion exercises are begun immediately postoperatively for all joints except the wrist and metacarpophalangeal joints. Two weeks postoperatively, a thermoplastic splint is fabricated and active exercises of these joints are added. As bone healing begins, active resistance exercises are begun for the extrinsic and intrinsic muscles of the hand. Strengthening the small finger intrinsic muscles, particularly the abductor digiti quinti, is important. Strengthening this muscle is accomplished by abducting the small finger against the resistance of a rubber band(s) wrapped around the fingers. The splint is discontinued at 8 to 12 weeks postoperatively, when radiographic evidence of bone healing is present.

■ REHABILITATION

Colen and co-authors[1] reported that grip and pinch strength were less affected after small ray transpositions than after index ray transpositions. Pinch strength was only minimally impaired (98%), which would be expected because the little finger is not involved in that activity. However, their finding that grip strength was only slightly affected and averaged 87% of the nonoperated hand has not been my experience. Generally, grip strength is more impaired following loss of a ring finger than a middle finger since the ulnar two fingers are important for power grip. While transposing the small ray following loss of a ring finger will improve overall prehension, it will not significantly improve grip strength.

■ OUTCOMES

References

1. Colen L, Bunkis J, Gordon L, Walton R: Fuctional assessment of ray transfer for central digital loss. J Hand Surg, 1985; 10A:232–237.
2. Hygroop GL: Transfer of a metacarpal, with or without its digit, for improving function of the crippled hand. Plast Reconstr Surg, 1949; 4:45–58.
3. Le Viet D: Transposition of the Fifth Digital Ray by Intracarpal Osteotomy. In: Tubiana R (ed): The Hand, Volume 3, Chapter 95, Philadelphia: W. B. Saunders, 1988:1071–1080.
4. Louis DS: Amputations. In: Green D (ed): Operative Hand Surgery, 3rd Ed, New York: Churchill Livingston, 1993:66–72.
5. Plasschaert MJJT, Hage JJ: A web saving skin incision for amputation of the third and fourth ray of the hand. J Hand Surg, 1988; 13B:340–341.
6. Posner MA: Ray transposition for central digital loss. J Hand Surg, 1979; 4:242–257.
7. Steichen JB, Idler RS: Results of central ray resection without bony transposition. J Hand Surg, 1980; 11A:466–474.

Bone Grafting for Scaphoid Nonunion

■ HISTORY OF THE TECHNIQUE

Five percent of fractures of the scaphoid fail to unite for a variety of reasons.[11,12] The sites of the nonunions are 70% in the waist of the bone, 20% through the proximal third, and 10% in the distal scaphoid tubercle.[12] Proximal-third scaphoid nonunions have the worst prognosis for healing because of a precarious blood supply[4] and a higher incidence of avascular necrosis.[2]

The currently recommended treatment of bone grafting a scaphoid nonunion is not a new concept. Adams and Leonard reported using a cortical bone peg in the scaphoid in 1928.[1] Six years later, Murray used a cortical bone peg driven across the nonunion site.[10] In 1936, Matti[9] described resecting the bone and detritus at the nonunion site of the scaphoid through a dorsal approach and filling the defect with cancellous bone. Russe,[12] in 1960, inserted a corticocancellous graft across the nonunion defect and packed the surrounding area with cancellous bone. This was done through a volar approach. The technique of bone grafting a scaphoid nonunion with corticocancellous graft through a volar approach is usually referred to as the Matti-Russe procedure.

■ INDICATIONS AND CONTRAINDICATIONS

If a scaphoid fracture fails to unite after 4 to 6 months, regardless of the treatment used, it is considered a nonunion. The patient usually complains of pain in the wrist that is aggravated by activity, stiffness of the wrist, and a weak grip.

Although a nonunion of the scaphoid can usually be seen on routine radiographs (posteroanterior, lateral, oblique, and radial deviation and ulnar deviation stress views), if there is any question as to the extent of healing of the bone, a computed tomography (CT) scan of the scaphoid in the sagittal and coronal planes is indicated. The CT scan will allow an accurate assessment of bony healing even if the hand and wrist are immobilized in the cast. If further information is needed, a CT reconstruction of the nonunited bone can be obtained. Although some individuals prefer to use tomography to evaluate scaphoid healing, I feel a sharper, crisper image of the bone is obtained from a CT scan. Slight motion of the extremity by the patient can cause blurring of the tomographic image, and this may result in a false radiographic interpretation.

Open reduction, bone grafting, and internal fixation of the scaphoid are ideally suited for nonunions of the waist (middle third) and in the proximal third of the bone. The rate of healing of proximal-third nonunions is less than for nonunions of the middle third of the bone.[5,14] Avascular necrosis of the proximal pole of the scaphoid is not a contraindication to this operation. A small, fragmented, sclerotic proximal pole of the scaphoid is a contraindication to doing a bone graft, and some other reconstructive procedure should be considered.[11,16]

Scaphoid nonunions with significant resorption of the palmar side of the bone, extension of the proximal segment, and a secondary dorsal intercalated segment instability deformity of the carpus should be treated by an anterior wedge graft to correct the dorsal angulation of the scaphoid. This technique is discussed in another chapter.

■ SURGICAL TECHNIQUES

The operation is done under general anesthesia. The entire upper extremity and iliac crest are thoroughly cleaned with povidone–iodine or some other antiseptic solution.

The palmar radial side of the wrist is opened through a longitudinal incision in the

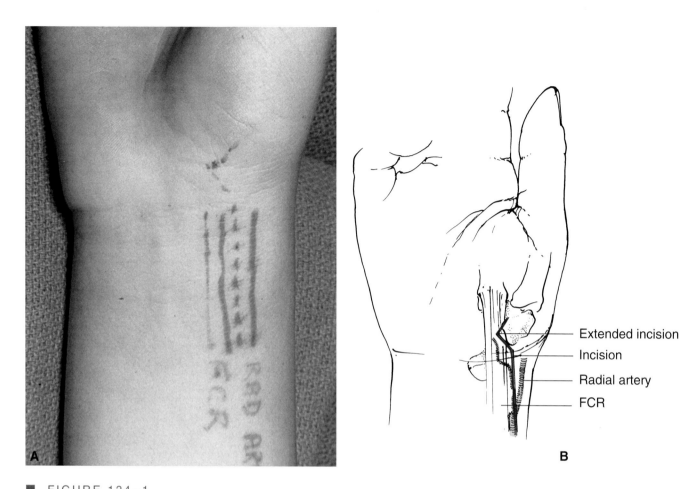

Extended incision

Incision

Radial artery

FCR

B

■ FIGURE 134–1
(A) Dotted line shows the recommended palmar skin incision between the flexor carpi radialis tendon and the radial artery. **(B)** The skin incision can be extended distal to the wrist flexor crease for greater exposure. FCR, flexor carpi radialis.

interval between the flexor carpi radialis tendon and the radial artery (Fig. 134–1). The flexor carpi radialis tendon is readily identified by palpation. The incision can be angulated across the wrist flexor crease if additional exposure is needed. The small branches of the radial artery are cauterized. This relatively avascular plane is used to proceed to the radiocarpal joint. The joint capsule and palmar radioscaphoid ligaments are incised. At this point, a self-retaining retractor is inserted for better exposure of the bone and joint. The nonunion site in the middle third of the scaphoid is usually noted in the center of the field (Fig. 134–2). Radial and ulnar deviation of the wrist will readily demonstrate motion at the nonunion site and will provide improved visualization of the entire scaphoid. A small Chandler retractor placed between the scaphoid and the articular surface of the radius will also assist in visualizing the operative area. In addition, this will allow evaluation of the integrity of the articular cartilage of the radius.

A small segment of cortical bone is removed from the palmar side of the proximal and distal halves of the scaphoid (Fig. 134–3). This cortical window can be made with small osteotomes or a rongeur. This will allow introduction of instruments to clean out the scar and sclerotic bone from the cavity of the scaphoid. The detritus is conservatively removed with a low-speed burr, and then, as bleeding bone is noted, a curette is used to excavate the cavity further and prevent damage to the viable bone. Usually the distal half of the scaphoid requires less debridement than the proximal side. In proximal-third nonunions, the debridement may have to extend to subchondral bone when the proximal fragment

■ FIGURE 134–2
(A) After opening the wrist capsule, the nonunion of the wrist and the scaphoid is usually in the center of the wound. FCR, flexor carpi radialis. **(B)** Extension of the wrist opens the nonunion site.

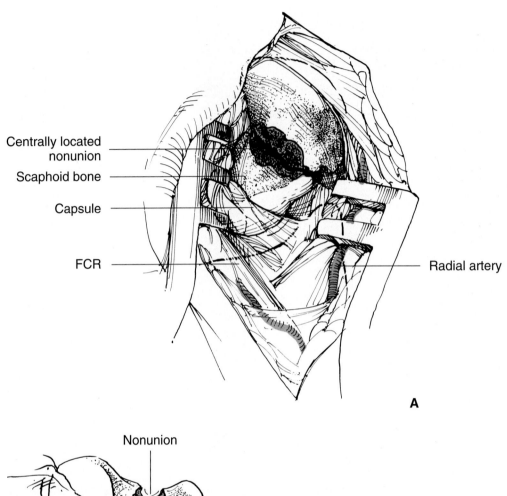

Centrally located nonunion

Scaphoid bone

Capsule

FCR

Radial artery

A

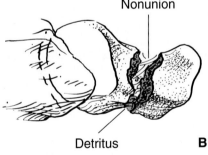

Nonunion

Detritus

B

is being curetted. This part of the operation is tedious and must be done very carefully to prevent perforation and injury to the articular cartilage.

After the debridement is completed, a Chandler retractor is used to reduce and approximate the cartilaginous edges of the dorsal and radial sides of the scaphoid. A smooth K-wire (0.9 or 1.1 mm) is inserted percutaneously into the scaphoid with power equipment. The wires are inserted distal to the radial styloid in the direction of the proximal end of the scaphoid (Fig. 134–4). Because there is no graft material in the cavity of the scaphoid, the position of the K-wires can be seen and adjusted as necessary. A second K-wire is then inserted, also under direct vision. After satisfactory positioning of the K-wires, both wires are backed out until the tips are just out of the cavity but still within the bone of the distal half of the scaphoid.

Bone graft from the iliac crest is preferred to bone from other sites. Cancellous bone graft is packed into both sides of the cavity in the scaphoid. Compressing the cancellous bone with a bone tamp provides additional stability. A small cortical strut of bone can be inserted just beneath the edges of the window in the proximal and distal parts of the scaphoid for greater stability at the nonunion site. Both K-wires are then advanced into

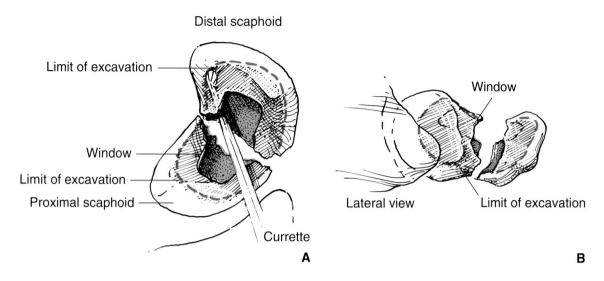

■ FIGURE 134–3

(A) A window is made in the bone and scar tissue is excised. **(B)** Cavities are created by removing dead bone until healthy bleeding bone is identified.

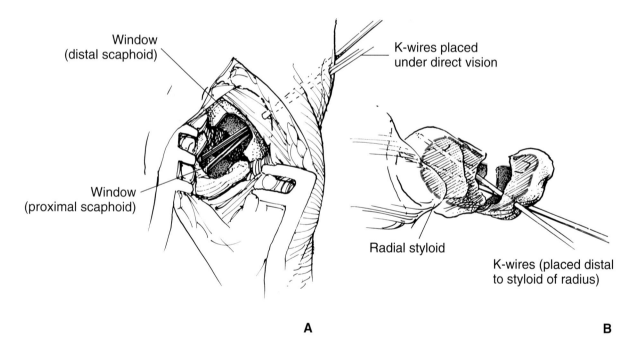

■ FIGURE 134–4

(A) K-wires are placed across the nonunion site of the scaphoid under direct vision. **(B)** A K-wire is placed so its point of entry into the proximal part of the scaphoid is satisfactory.

the subchondral bone of the proximal scaphoid (Fig. 134–5). It is preferable that the K-wires not be inserted into or across the radiocarpal joint. This is not always possible, however, especially in proximal-third nonunions. The K-wires are then trimmed so that the cut edges are present beneath the skin. The joint capsule is closed with absorbable suture and the skin incision is closed with fine nonabsorbable suture.

Initially, the thumb, hand, and wrist are immobilized in a palmar plaster splint that is extended to include the elbow. Ten days after the operation, an above-elbow thumb spica cast is applied. Six weeks after the operation, a below-elbow thumb spica cast is used.

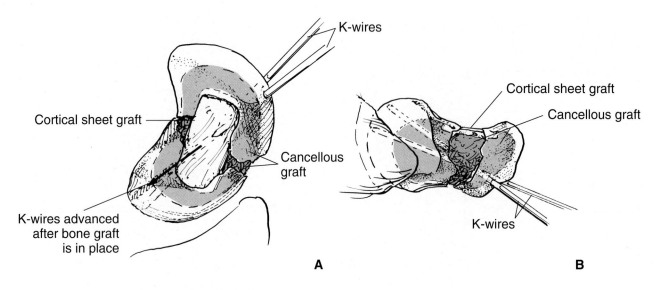

■ FIGURE 134–5
(A) After the cavities are packed with bone, the K-wires are advanced into the proximal scaphoid. **(B)** Bone graft material should not extend beyond the edges of the scaphoid.

The patient is then reevaluated with radiographs to determine when the scaphoid has united. If there is a question as to whether the scaphoid has completely united after a review of the radiographs, a CT scan can be used to determine more accurately if the bone has completely united. Healing of the nonunion of the scaphoid usually occurs in 3 to 4 months after the operation. As mentioned previously, proximal-third nonunions of the scaphoid usually take longer to heal than middle-third nonunions.

Once the scaphoid has united, the smooth K-wires are removed under local anesthesia. This can be done either in the office or in an outpatient surgery department.

■ TECHNICAL ALTERNATIVES

In my opinion, internal fixation of a scaphoid nonunion in conjunction with a bone graft is an integral part of doing the procedure. This provides stability to the nonunion site, which cannot be obtained by simply casting the extremity. Although I prefer to use smooth K-wires because of the ease and simplicity of insertion, other internal fixation methods have been recommended. The Herbert screw,[6,15] Enders plate,[3] and Power staples[13] all have their proponents.

Mild to moderate radioscaphoid arthritis restricted to the portion of the joint between the scaphoid and radial styloid can be treated by bone grafting of the scaphoid and at the same time doing a radial styloidectomy.

No operative technique is without problems and complications. The 1-mm smooth K-wires are preferred to the smaller sizes because the smaller ones can fatigue and fracture, especially in a large person. The K-wires can also back out before bone healing. This is especially true if poor technique is used, resulting in improper placement of the wires during the operation. If the cut ends of the K-wires are too long and they rest just beneath the skin, they can cause pain, skin irritation, and occasionally skin ulceration. This will often necessitate frequent cast changes and possibly premature removal of the K-wires. Irritation from the K-wires, however, rarely results in infection.

■ REHABILITATION

A rehabilitation program under the direction of a certified hand therapist is an important part of the recovery phase of the operation. The patient is instructed actively to exercise the fingers, elbow, and shoulder of the involved extremity during the period of cast immobilization.

The rehabilitation program is changed after the scaphoid has healed, the K-wires have been removed, and the patient has recovered from this second minor operation (usually

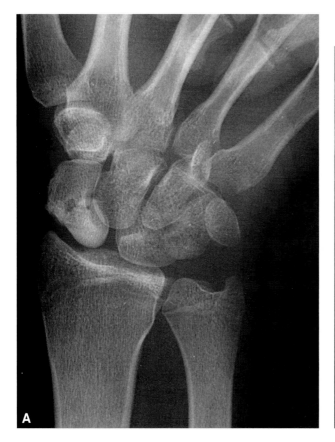
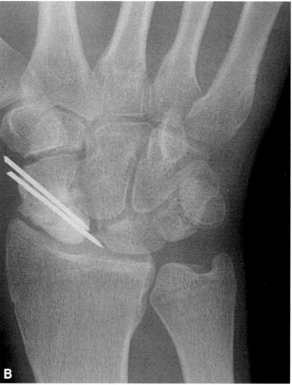

■ FIGURE 134–6

(A) A 17-year-old boy injured his right wrist while playing football. Evaluation 6 months later indicated the scaphoid was not united. **(B)** The bone is healed 3½ months after bone grafting and internal fixation.

about 7 to 10 days). At this time, the program is directed toward passive, active, and active assisted range of motion of the wrist and forearm. Once a reasonable range of motion of the wrist and forearm is obtained, strengthening exercises for the extremity are started. After about 2 to 3 months, the patient can be discharged to a home program. The patients are advised they should not return to rigorous physical activities for about 3 months after the scaphoid has united.

Under the guidance of a hand therapist, a greater degree of wrist motion and upper extremity strength will be recovered. Regardless of the rehabilitation program, the involved upper extremity will not be "normal." However, the patient is usually able to accommodate to any functional loss.

If the bone graft and internal fixation of the scaphoid nonunion is properly done and ■ OUTCOMES the patient is compliant with the postoperative immobilization of the upper extremity, a 97% union rate of the scaphoid can occur (Fig. 134–6).[14] Normal upper extremity strength and wrist motion will not be regained in spite of obtaining bony union of the scaphoid. In our experience, there was a postoperative grip strength increase of 30% in the involved extremity, but this represented an 18% grip loss compared to the uninjured extremity. Improvements in wrist motion were minimal compared to the preoperative motion, although the average total arc of postoperative motion (dorsiflexion and palmar flexion) averaged 117°.[14] However, pain relief and return to functional use of the extremity are very good after the procedure.[7,8,14] The development of radiocarpal arthritis seems to be slowed by union of the scaphoid;[14] however, a slow progression of radiocarpal degenerative changes seems to occur in spite of healing of the scaphoid nonunion.[7]

References

1. Adams JD, Leonard RD: Fracture of the carpal scaphoid. A new method of treatment with a report of one case. N Engl J Med, 1928; 198:401–404.
2. Cooney WP, Dobyns JH, Linscheid RL: Non-union of the scaphoid: Analysis of the results from bone grafting. J Hand Surg, 1980; 5:343–354.
3. Enders H: Plate fixation of scaphoid non-union. Presented at the American Society for Surgery of the Hand Annual Meeting, San Francisco, California, February, 1979.
4. Gelberman RH, Menon J: The vascularity of the scaphoid bone. J Hand Surg, 1980; 5:508–513.
5. Green DP: The effect of avascular necrosis on Russe bone grafting for scaphoid non-union. J Hand Surg, 1985; 10A:597–605.
6. Herbert TJ, Fisher WE: Management of the fractured scaphoid using a new bone screw. J Bone Joint Surg, 1984; 66B:114–123.
7. Hooning Van Duyvenbode JFF, Keijser LCM, Hauet EJ, Obermann WR, Rozing PM: Pseudarthrosis of the scaphoid treated by the Matti-Russe operation: A long-term review of 77 cases. J Bone Joint Surg, 1991; 73B:603–606.
8. Jiranek WA, Ruby LK, Millender LB, Bankoff MS, Newberg AH: Long-term results after Russe bone-grafting: The effect of malunion of the scaphoid. J Bone Joint Surg, 1992; 74A: 1217–1228.
9. Matti H: Technik und Resultate meiner Pseudo Arthrosenoperation. Zentralbl Chir, 1936; 63: 1442–1453.
10. Murray G: Bone graft for non-union of the carpal scaphoid. Br J Surg, 1934; 22:63–68.
11. Osterman AL, Mikulics M: Scaphoid non-union. Hand Clin, 1988; 14:437–455.
12. Russe O: Fracture of the carpal navicular: Diagnosis, non-operative treatment, and operative treatment. J Bone Joint Surg, 1960; 42A:759–768.
13. Shapiro JS: Power staple fixation in hand and wrist surgery: New applications of an old fixation device. J Hand Surg, 1987; 12A:218–227.
14. Stark HH, Rickard TA, Zemel NP, Ashworth CR: Treatment of ununited fractures of the scaphoid by iliac bone grafts and Kirschner-wire fixation. J Bone Joint Surg [Am], 1988; 70: 982–991.
15. Warhold LG, Osterman AL: Scaphoid fracture and non-union: Treatment by open reduction, bone graft, and a Herbert screw. Techniques in Orthopaedics, 1992; 7:7–18.
16. Zemel NP, Stark HH, Ashworth CR, Rickard TA, Anderson DR: Treatment of selected patients with an ununited fracture of the proximal part of the scaphoid by excision of the fragment and insertion of a carved silicone-rubber spacer. J Bone Joint Surg, 1984; 66A: 510–517.

135

Anterior Wedge Grafting for Scaphoid Nonunions

Nonunion of scaphoid waist fractures has a reported incidence that is between 5% and 50%.[5,9,15] These nonunions are sometimes asymptomatic but usually result in considerable clinical morbidity.[13,14] Many factors are responsible for the scaphoid's inability to heal its fractured surfaces. These include lack of patient compliance, missed diagnosis, inadequate extent and duration of immobilization, and vascular compromise. Newer theory focuses on the pathomechanics of the fracture and its overall effect on the stability of the carpus.[7,10,11,18] Classifications of scaphoid fractures in general are based on the presence of fracture displacement and a change in the spatial relationships of the carpal bones.[9,15] One millimeter or more of fracture surface offset as well as altered intercarpal angles indicate an unstable fracture and a high potential for scaphoid nonunion. Many clinicians are becoming more aggressive when indicating surgical treatment for unstable scaphoid fractures and nonunions. They recognize the poor results that can occur after conservative care of unstable scaphoid fractures, and usually recommend early operative intervention. Fisk emphasized the loss of scaphoid bone substance in the pathomechanics of carpal collapse and nonunion.[7] It appears that bone is not only lost at the time of injury, but also bone resorption can begin and progress as the fracture surfaces wear away because of abnormal pressure loads.[12]

Characteristically, the fracture collapses into a predictable deformity called "humpback." Some of these collapsed fractures unite but with malalignment, a condition that clinically has been shown to be suboptimal.[1,4] Surgical restoration of the collapsed scaphoid nonunions and malunions requires a thorough understanding of the displacement of the bony fragments, carpal collapse patterns, and the amount and configuration of scaphoid bone substance loss.

Our laboratory studied the injured and normal wrists in nine patients with scaphoid nonunions.[3] The technique that we previously reported used three-dimensional computer models of the scaphoid that were generated from computed tomography (CT) scans.[2] The models of the injured scaphoid were superimposed on the normal scaphoid templates from the contralateral wrist. Carpal surfaces are virtually unique, and the data representing the proximal and distal fracture fragments are separate digital files that are easily locked into their contralateral counterpart (Fig. 135–1). This allowed visualization and calculation of the bone lost as a result of the injury and persistent nonunion. More important, the rotational matrices provided the orientation of the proximal and distal scaphoid fragments to each other in the anatomic reference of the wrist. Ten percent (average) bone loss was seen; the amount of loss did not correlate with the duration of the scaphoid nonunion.

The defect was constant and exhibited a prismatic shape in which the base was quadrilateral and faced palmarly. The ulnar proximodistal dimension of the base was longer than its radial proximodistal dimension, and both formed the base of two triangular surfaces of the prism that faced radially and ulnarly. The proximal and distal surfaces also were quadrilateral and extended from the palmar surface to a uniform dorsal edge. Most bone loss occurred on the palmar and ulnar surfaces of the fractured scaphoid. More important, the proximal scaphoid fragment was extended, radially deviated, and supinated in relation to the distal scaphoid fragment. The distal scaphoid fragment was flexed, ulnarly deviated, and pronated in relation to the proximal fragment. These analyses improved our basic

■ HISTORY OF THE TECHNIQUE

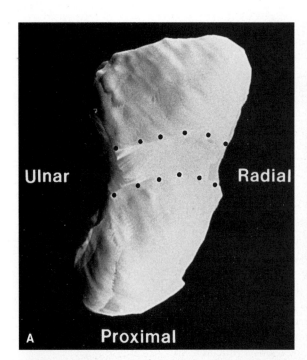
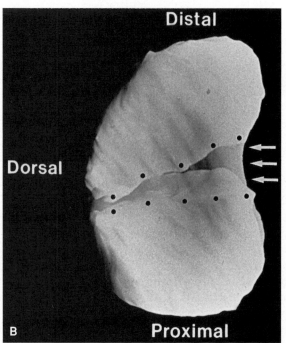
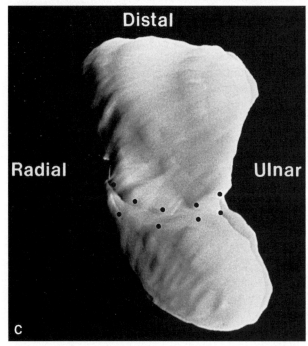
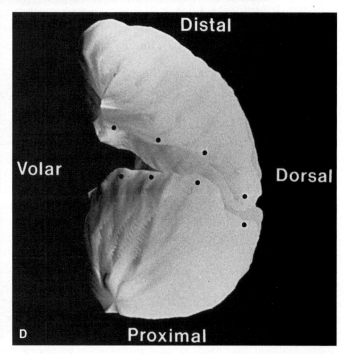

■ FIGURE 135–1

Photographs of the three-dimensional models generated from CT scans. The proximal and distal fracture fragments have been mapped onto the surfaces of the bone from the contralateral normal wrist (dots indicate configuration of normal bone). **(A)** Palmar view. **(B)** Ulnar view; arrows outline boundary of the contralateral normal scaphoid. **(C)** Dorsal view. **(D)** Radial view.

understanding of the injury and the anatomic characteristics of the nonunited scaphoid bone.

■ INDICATIONS AND CONTRAINDICATIONS

Our computer studies have helped develop surgical techniques that are applicable to unstable scaphoid fractures and nonunions as well as symptomatic and functionally limiting scaphoid malunions.

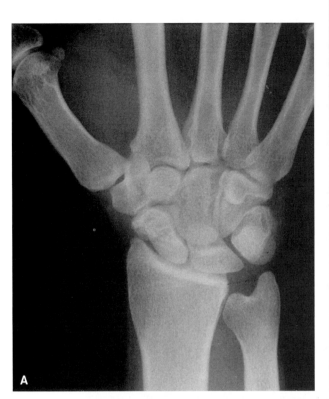
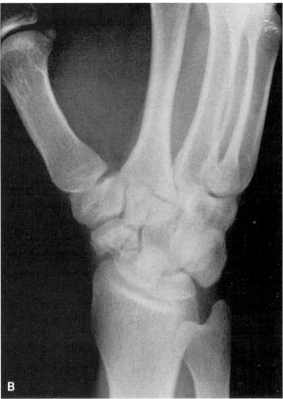
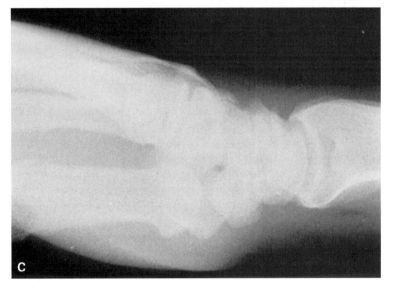

■ FIGURE 135–2

(A) Posteroanterior, (B) oblique, and (C) lateral radiographs of long-standing scaphoid non-union. Note the radiocarpal arthritis at the styloid interface (A), fracture displacement (B), and the DISI deformity (C).

This type of surgical reconstruction is indicated for acute scaphoid fractures if there are radiographic signs of fracture displacement (>1 mm) or carpal instability with abnormal scapholunate and capitolunate angles (Fig. 135–2). These fractures usually will not heal and will eventually be associated with degenerative arthritis of the wrist.

Surgical reconstruction of scaphoid nonunions is indicated in all cases after failed nonoperative treatment. Our techniques are applicable to those nonunions that are associated with carpal collapse, which is usually demonstrated radiographically by a dorsal intercalated segmental instability (DISI) deformity. Studies have shown that these wrists will develop scapholunate advanced collapse in a predictable sequence over time.[13,14] We emphasize that long-standing scaphoid waist nonunions (> 5 to 10 years) and waist fractures with proximal avascular changes can benefit from internal fixation and anterior wedge grafting. Complete restoration of scaphoid length and intercarpal alignment, however, are for the most part not possible.

Our operative techniques are applicable to the restoration of carpal alignment in the presence of scaphoid malunions, but this specific indication is not yet clearly defined. It is our opinion that nonunions are more frequent than malunions of the scaphoid. Also, we feel that truly symptomatic malunions are uncommon.

Our techniques are not applicable to scaphoid waist fractures and nonunions that are stable and can be appropriately treated with standard Russe techniques.[8,15] We do not recommend anterior wedge grafting for proximal pole fractures or proximal pole nonunions of the scaphoid, even though they are by definition also unstable.

■ SURGICAL TECHNIQUES

Our surgical technique is performed under general anesthesia because iliac bone graft is usually required. When radial styloidectomy is contemplated and enough bone graft can be obtained from this location, axillary anesthesia can be used. We emphasize to our anesthesia colleagues that adequate axillary anesthesia requires paralysis of the musculocutaneous nerve near its high takeoff from the lateral cord of the brachial plexus, because its termination as the lateral cutaneous nerve of the forearm is within the surgical field. Intravenous regional anesthesia is never used because we support releasing the tourniquet after the procedure to assess the possibility of injury to the radial artery and its branches.

A tourniquet is used and inflated 80 to 100 mm above the systolic blood pressure after exsanguination of the limb with an Ace bandage. Intravenous antibiotics are administered before the inflation of the tourniquet.

The two main surface anatomy landmarks are the volar tubercle of the scaphoid and the flexor carpi radialis (FCR) tendon. The tubercle is easily palpated at the base of the thenar eminence during radial and ulnar deviation of the wrist. The FCR tendon is palpable just ulnar to the tubercle.

The incision is 4 to 5 cm long and follows the radial edge of the FCR tendon to the distal wrist crease, and then proceeds more radially onto the thenar eminence. The latter extension makes access to the radial styloid process easier and provides good exposure to the distal fragment, which is rotated palmarly. The FCR is mobilized by incising its sheath and retracting the tendon ulnarly. We usually ligate the superficial branch of the radial artery. The capsule is divided in a longitudinal direction, and it is stripped from the volar lip of the radius ulnarly to expose adequately the proximal fragment and radially to expose adequately the fracture site and the radial styloid process. If the styloid is to be excised, the capsular stripping is carried around the dorsal radial edge of the radius by elevating the first dorsal compartment and its contents. This maneuver greatly enhances surgical exposure and protects the tendons during radial styloid resection. Capsular dissection is also carried distally and ulnarly to expose the capitatoscaphoid articulation. Usually, in long-standing scaphoid nonunions, debridement of capsular adhesions about the fracture site is required. Occasionally, the articular cartilage heals over the fracture site. In these cases, the nonunion site can usually be identified by moving the wrist side to side and probing the bone with a 25-gauge needle. Routinely, we mobilize both fragments using a small lamina spreader. On both sides of the bone defect we aggressively debride scar tissue using fine osteotomes, curettes, and rongeurs. At this time we determine the amount of bone graft that is needed. If DISI deformity of the lunate is noted on preoperative radiographs, we dissect more ulnarly to place a joystick or K-wire (K-wire; 0.045″) in the lunate and use it to correct the lunate's abnormal position. The wrist is extended to demonstrate the shape and size of the scaphoid defect. A bone block is obtained from the outer table of the iliac crest. It should be corticocancellous and measure approximately 15 mm on the cortical face and 12 mm on the four sides of the block. A small amount of cancellous bone is also removed to pack around the strut graft once it is inserted. In most

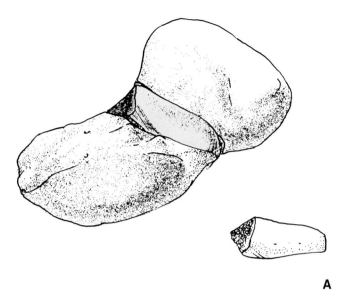

A

■ FIGURE 135–3
Diagrams of the shape of
the bone defect and graft
from palmar **(A)** and radial **(B)** surfaces.

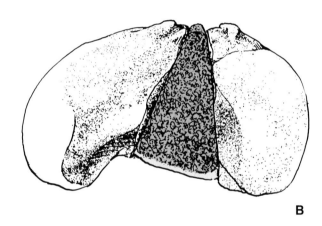

B

cases the palmar graft is 1 to 7 mm in the proximodistal direction. Using bone carpentry, we fashion the cortical face of the graft to fit the configuration of the defect obtained from our three-dimensional CT scans. The graft is made 2 to 3 mm longer on the ulnar palmar edge than the radial palmar edge. The graft is tapered to a thin dorsal ridge to conform to the prism shape previously defined (Fig. 135–3). Before its insertion, two 0.045″ K-wires are drilled retrograde through the distal fragment to exit the skin palmarly and radially on the thenar eminence. The bone graft is inserted and impacted. The K-wires are drilled across the graft into the dorsal aspect of the proximal scaphoid fragment (Fig. 135–4). We ensure that the pins do not enter the radiocarpal joint. The pins are cut off beneath the skin. Small defects are packed with cancellous graft, and the margins of the two fragments and palmar, ulnar, and radial surfaces of the graft are contoured. The capsular tissues are repaired and the skin is closed with everting sutures. A thumb spica short arm splint is applied.

Our technique is similar to that of Fernandez, but we think that measurements on plain radiographs of injured and uninjured scaphoids offer little advantage over direct visualization of the defect.[6] There are alternative surgical treatments for scaphoid waist nonunions. The major differences are related to bone grafting and fixation techniques. Other volar

■ TECHNICAL
ALTERNATIVES

■ FIGURE 135–4
Posteroanterior (A), oblique (B), and lateral (C) radiographs after surgical correction and bone grafting of scaphoid nonunion. Radial styloidectomy was performed. The DISI deformity usually cannot be totally corrected in long-standing cases. Arrows (B) outline the bone graft that restored scaphoid length and alignment.

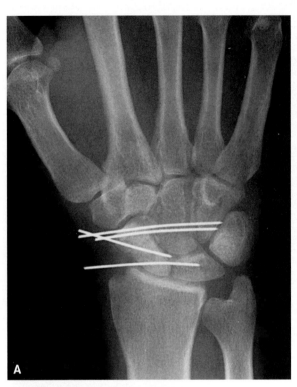
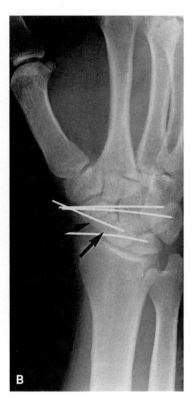
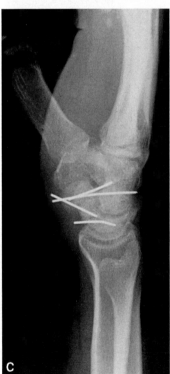

inlay grafting techniques are similar to that described by Russe[15] and popularized by Green.[8] Stark and co-authors[16] use a grafting technique similar to Russe's and supplement the procedure with K-wire fixation of the fractured scaphoid. Although the technique works well in stable fractures, its use in cases of unstable nonunions with loss of scaphoid length has limitations. Similarly, there is very limited application for dorsal peg and dorsoradial inlay bone grafting techniques, although we have inserted block and wedge grafts from the dorsal approach in a small number of unstable waist fractures. There are other methods of fracture fixation that can be applied to scaphoid waist nonunions with wedge bone graft supplementation. Herbert screws[9] and compression screws have been described with good success, but each requires more experience and more sophisticated equipment. These techniques have the advantage of lessening operative immobilization and returning the patient to activity sooner. But the major pitfall of these methods can be an emphasis on the fixation rather than the correction of the fracture displacement and the carpal instability. We have no experience with the use of power staples or compression blade plates in these injuries.

Skin sutures are removed in 7 to 10 days and immobilization is continued in a short arm thumb spica cast. New radiographs are obtained in 4 weeks and again in 8 weeks. Scaphoid views are not requested until wrist mobility is regained, usually after 8 weeks. After the second postoperative radiograph, a polyform removable thumb spica splint is fabricated and the patient is allowed to perform gripping exercises against sponge resistance in warm water or whirlpool. K-wires are removed in 8 weeks, at which time a more vigorous exercise program (active and active assisted wrist motion, gripping against increasing resistance) is started, unless radiographs show inadequate healing. In these cases we continue the removable thumb spica splint and resume the original gripping exercise program. For the most part, K-wires become loose between 8 and 12 weeks, and are usually removed. At this time, regardless of the radiographic appearance of the fracture, we increase the exercise program and decrease the immobilization. Use of a hand therapist is optional and depends on many factors, including compliance, patient location, and, more important, the ability of the patients to perform his or her own therapy program. Even though healing may be proceeding optimally, we do not allow the patient unrestricted activity or total discontinuance of the thumb and wrist splints for 3 months. At that point, a gradually increased activity level is permitted. We routinely do not allow return to golf, bowling, softball, tennis, and other athletic pursuits for 6 months after surgery, and then only in the presence of radiographic healing. Some patients demonstrate a persistent fracture line lucency that is small on radiographs, along with minimal clinical symptoms. These fractures should undergo CT or tomographic evaluation before increasing the patient's activity level. It is important to realize that the postoperative treatment for some nonunions of the scaphoid can be prolonged. Patients can reach a plateau and not gain from continuing an organized therapy program.

■ REHABILITATION

The literature concerning the clinical results after anterior wedge grafting for scaphoid nonunion is confusing. One major difficulty is that "scaphoid nonunion" has not been properly defined. Most investigators are using Herbert's classification to define a scaphoid fracture as a delayed union when it has not united radiographically in 6 weeks.[9] What constitutes "radiographic union" of the scaphoid is also controversial, and not the subject of this review.[9] More than one report shows a better union rate with the treatment of "delayed" versus "nonunion" of the carpal scaphoid.

Another factor that should be considered in comparing different treatment techniques is the use of and type of bone grafting. For the most part, unstable nonunions need bone supplementation. Warren-Smith and Barton abandoned standard Russe grafting techniques because a high percentage of their cases failed to achieve union.[17] They compared these cases to others in which they performed anterior wedge grafting and Herbert screw fixation, and found the latter technique had a higher success rate (82%) and resulted in better wrist movement. It should be noted that patients in this series were immobilized postoperatively an average of 12 weeks, in contradistinction to Herbert's original series in which similar union rates were achieved in fibrous (88%) and sclerotic (76%) nonunion with bone grafting and early wrist mobilization.[9,17] We have achieved radiographic union in 13 of 16 scaphoid nonunions (nonunited fractures > 4 months postinjury) in which anterior wedge grafting was used. Most of these nonunions were old and radial styloidec-

■ OUTCOMES

tomy was used in nine cases. All had DISI deformities that could be fully corrected in only two cases. None of the patients showed avascular necrosis of the proximal scaphoid segment. Long-term follow-up is not available, but the early clinical results indicate that the scaphoid fractures and nonunions that are treated by wedge grafting 6 months or sooner after the injury achieve better wrist motion. It is important to distinguish between the injury that produced the fracture and an injury that makes an existing nonunion symptomatic, because many scaphoid nonunions can be relatively painless until a subsequent injury occurs. In these wrists, there may be irreversible changes in the intercarpal relationships that will influence not only the procedure but the result.

References

1. Amadio PC, Berquist TH, Smith DK, Ilstrup DM, Cooney WB, Linscheid RL: Scaphoid malunion. J Hand Surg, 1989; 14A:679–687.
2. Belsole RJ, Hilbelink DR, Llewellyn JA, Stenzler S, Greene TL, Dale M: Mathematical analysis of computed carpal models. J Orthop Res, 1988; 6:116–122.
3. Belsole RJ, Hilbelink DR, Llewellyn JA, Dale M, Greene TL, Rayhack JM: Computed analyses of the pathomechanics of scaphoid waist non-unions. J Hand Surg, 1991; 16A:899–906.
4. Burgess RC: The effect of a simulated scaphoid malunion on wrist motion. J Hand Surg, 1987; 12A:774–776.
5. Dias JJ, Brenkel JJ, Finlay DBL: Patterns of union in fractures of the waist of the scaphoid. J Bone Joint Surg, 1989; 71B:307–310.
6. Fernandez DL: A technique for anterior wedge-shaped grafts for scaphoid nonunions with carpal instability. J Hand Surg, 1984; 9A:733–737.
7. Fisk GR: Carpal instability and the fractured scaphoid. Ann R Coll Surg Engl, 1970; 46:63–76.
8. Green DP: The effect of avascular necrosis on Russe bone grafting for scaphoid nonunion. J Hand Surg, 1985; 10A:597–605.
9. Herbert TJ, Fisher WE: Management of the fractured scaphoid using a new bone screw. J Bone Joint Surg, 1984; 66B:114–123.
10. Linscheid RL, Dobyns JB, Beabout JW, Bryan RS: Traumatic instability of the wrist: Diagnosis classification and pathomechanics. J Bone Joint Surg, 1972; 54:1612–1632.
11. Linscheid RL, Dobyns JB, Cooney WP: Volar wedge grafting of the carpal scaphoid in non-union associated with dorsal instability patterns. J Bone Joint Surg, 1982; 64B:632–633.
12. Linscheid RL, Dobyns JB, Cooney WP: Pathogenesis of carpal scaphoid in nonunion and malunion with biomechanical analysis. Orthop Trans, 1983; 7:482.
13. Mack GR, Bossee MJ, Gelberman RH, Yu E: The natural history of scaphoid nonunion. J Bone Joint Surg, 1984; 66A:504–509.
14. Ruby LK, Stinson J, Belsky MR: The natural history of scaphoid nonunion: A review of fifty-five cases. J Bone Joint Surg, 1985; 67A:428–432.
15. Russe O: Fracture of the carpal navicular: Diagnosis, non-operative treatment, and operative treatment. J Bone Joint Surg, 1960; 42A:759–768.
16. Stark HH, Richard TA, Zemel NP, Ashworth CR: Treatment of ununited fractures of the scaphoid by iliac bone grafts and Kirschner wire fixation. J Bone Joint Surg, 1988; 70A:982–991.
17. Warren-Smith CD, Barton NJ: Nonunion of the scaphoid: Russe graft vs Herbert screw. J Hand Surg, 1988; 13B:83–86.
18. Weber ER: Biomechanical implications of scaphoid waist fractures. Clin Orthop, 1980; 149:83–89.

136

EDWARD E.
ALMQUIST

Capitate Shortening Osteotomy

Kienböck[9] described the condition of lunate malacia in 1910, shortly after the use of radiography was introduced. Since then, a variety of surgical treatments for this condition have been devised. They fall into two general categories: removal of the lunate, and procedures to stimulate revascularization.

For advanced Kienböck disease, a complete removal of the lunate, replacing it with an interposition of either tendon or prosthetic material, has been a common and accepted treatment. More recently, the interposition arthroplasty has been accompanied by a limited arthrodesis. Other treatments in this category include limited arthrodeses including the lunate, such as radiolunate arthrodesis, when primarily one side of the joint is involved. In the second category are procedures whose purpose is restoration of viability and stability to the necrotic bone. They include curetting out necrotic bone, followed by bone grafting; placing vascular soft tissue stumps into the necrotic bone to stimulate healing; skeletal traction to decompress the forces across the lunate; and, most commonly, joint-leveling procedures.

Most of the compressive forces across the wrist pass through the lunate, so it is constantly under stress. The lunate has an extensive articular surface, and its blood supply, which radiates from volar or dorsal entry points, has limited access. As noted by Kashiwagi and co-authors,[8] Lee,[10] and Gelberman and co-authors,[6] a stress fracture may interrupt the vascular supply, resulting in segments of the lunate becoming devascularized. These segments weaken and secondary fracture lines may develop. The constant loading of the lunate with any hand activity stresses the fracture lines and may inhibit healing. Collapse may develop, with the lunate becoming further deformed; therefore, reducing the compressive forces across the lunate is a reasonable approach to enhance lunate revascularization, and is the basis for the joint-leveling procedures.

Capitate shortening with capitatohamate arthrodesis was devised by the author as a means of diminishing the forces across the lunate without increasing the relative length of the ulna and causing possible ulnar abutment. It was conceived as an extension of the capitatohamate arthrodesis as described by Chuinard and Zeman.[5] Hulten[7] noted the increased incidence of ulnar minus variance in patients with Kienböck disease, and Rossak[14] demonstrated increased shear stress on the lunate associated with the ulnar minus variance. Radial shortening and ulnar lengthening have been accepted as standard treatments, and patients who have early Kienböck disease and an ulnar minus variance, I believe, should be treated by radial shortening.[2,3] Some patients with Kienböck disease may have no ulnar minus variance, and in fact may have an ulnar plus variance. In these cases, shortening the radius or further elongating the ulna would produce significant length discrepancy, causing the ulna to protrude into the carpus. Palmer[13] showed that forces across the distal ulna are significantly increased with ulnar lengthening, and may clinically produce an impingement syndrome with damage to the triquetral articular cartilage, disruption of the lunotriquetral joint, and even erosion of the triquetrum and lunate adjacent to the ulna. Capitate shortening with capitatohamate fusion is thus a joint-leveling operation performed when there is no ulnar minus variance.

The specific indication for capitate shortening with capitatohamate arthrodesis is limited to Kienböck disease in the absence of ulnar minus variance and with a lunate with sufficient architectural congruity to allow revascularization (Fig. 136–1). Although there are

■ HISTORY OF THE TECHNIQUE

■ INDICATIONS AND CONTRAINDICATIONS

■ FIGURE 136–1
A posteroanterior radio-
graph of a 36-year-old
woman with Kienböck dis-
ease with neutral vari-
ance. The lunate has
cysts but no architectural
changes.

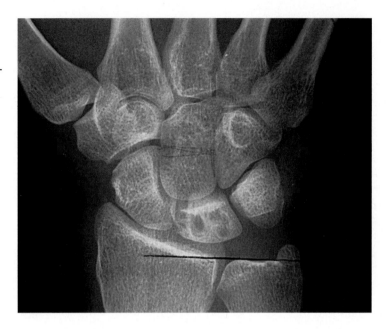

■ FIGURE 136–2
Diagram of a capitate-
shortening osteotomy with
a capitatohamate arthrod-
esis.

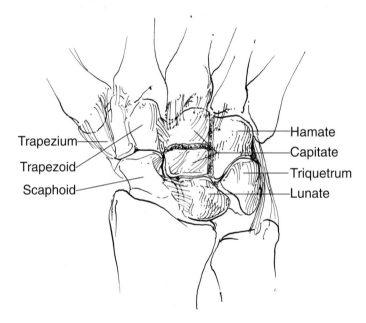

no clearly defined parameters, this procedure may be indicated for patients with stage I, II, or early stage III disease, as defined on the Lichtman scale.[11] In my experience, this degree of disease has only minor fragmentation, less than 1 mm of gapping between fragments, and no arthrosis between the lunate and the scaphoid.

This joint-leveling procedure is contraindicated if there is significant collapse of the convex surface of the lunate, marked narrowing of the lunate, or free fragments of necrotic bone within the body of the lunate. Arthritic changes between the radiolunate or lunato-capitate surfaces are specific contraindications to this procedure. Some patients with Kien-böck disease exhibit a dorsal intercalated segmental instability (DISI) pattern. This is usu-ally in an advanced stage of the disease, with considerable flattening or narrowing of the lunate, and they are not candidates for joint-leveling procedures.

■ SURGICAL
TECHNIQUES

The technique of capitate shortening with capitatohamate fusion is quite simple and straightforward (Fig. 136–2). Preoperative prophylactic antibiotics are given under axillary block or general anesthesia, and a dorsal, midline longitudinal approach is used. A curved incision seems to offer no advantage, and a transverse incision does not allow enough exposure. Flaps are elevated from the extensor retinaculum, which is then incised longitudinally between the fifth and sixth compartments, exposing the extensor digiti quinti tendon. The retinaculum is mobilized radially as a flap, so that the entire fourth compartment is exposed. The flap remains attached to the radius between the third and fourth compartments. This exposes the posterior interosseous nerve or the floor of the fourth compartment. Because the capsular incision would course through several branches of this nerve, I recommend resection of this nerve proximal to the radiocarpal joint. The small artery accompanying the nerve is cauterized and the joint is then opened. A longitudinal incision is made at the level of the capitate, proceeding across the lunate near the scapholunate border and into the radiolunate joint. To preserve blood supply, very little elevation of the capsule is done over the dorsum of the lunate. This gives adequate exposure of the convex surface of the lunate and provides direct visualization of the diseased bone.

Accurate grading of the disease can be done at this point. Because the structural changes observed on preoperative radiographs may not coincide with changes in the lunate that are seen on direct visualization, intraoperative inspection has a distinct advantage over imaging procedures. The patient must be informed before surgery that the surgeon's choice of an alternative procedure will ultimately depend on what is seen by direct visualization of the lunate. If the lunate is not too fragmented and the degree of malacia is mild, there is a good chance of revascularization, and a capitate-shortening procedure is elected. If the lunate is markedly fragmented or there are arthritic changes with cartilage loss on the surface of the lunate or on the adjacent surface of the radius, a joint-leveling procedure such as capitate shortening would be inadequate.[1]

If observations confirm that the operation is appropriate, capitate shortening proceeds by sharply dissecting the capsule from the more distal segments of the capitate and hamate, exposing the capitate and the capitatohamate joint. With a sharp, thin osteotome, a capitate osteotomy is performed just as the capitate curves more dorsally at the level of the distal dorsal articular surface of the scaphoid (Fig. 136–3). The initial cut is partial; a parallel cut, 2 to 4 mm, is made just proximal to the first cut. The usual shortening is 2 to 3 mm, but if there is a rather long capitate protruding considerably proximal to the proximal surface of the hamate, a 4-mm resection is performed. The parallel osteotomies are completed using a stepwise technique. The more proximal osteotomy is accomplished first. The capitate head is a very mobile segment once the osteotomy is completed, and it would be difficult to obtain enough stability to complete the osteotomy if the more distal segment were completed first. The volar capsule is visualized, but not disrupted. The bone segment can be removed with a small osteotome or curette, prying it up from the capsular surface. Most of the segment should come out in one section, leaving just the volar, cortical surface to be curetted free from the capsule. The mobile capitate head is easily compressed against the more distal segment with a curved blunt instrument without damaging the articular surface. Two crossing K-wires, usually 0.062 inches, are placed from the distal capitate, across the osteotomy, into the head of the capitate, but they should not penetrate the articular surface (Fig. 136–4). The articular surface is easily visualized, and if a K-wire should penetrate it, the wire can be withdrawn a few millimeters. The crossed wires give firm fixation. The adjacent surfaces between the capitate and the hamate are decorticated using a small osteotome and a small curette (Fig. 136–5). When this is completed, a compression clamp is placed against the hamate and capitate. Two parallel wires are inserted, one passing from the proximal hamate to the capitate head and the other from a more distal portion of the hamate to the body of the capitate (Fig. 136–6). A third parallel wire can be placed here as well. The wires are inserted percutaneously, but it is important to avoid the dorsal branch of the ulnar nerve, which can be seen through the elevated flaps. The position of the pins should be checked radiographically. When appropriate, small amounts of the bone resected from the capitate can be tamped into any remaining spaces between the capitate and hamate. Often, however, there is no room for bone graft.

■ FIGURE 136–3
The surgical procedure. An osteotomy is performed using a thin osteotome and avoiding penetration of the volar capsule. A 2- to 4-mm section in the waist of the capitate is removed.

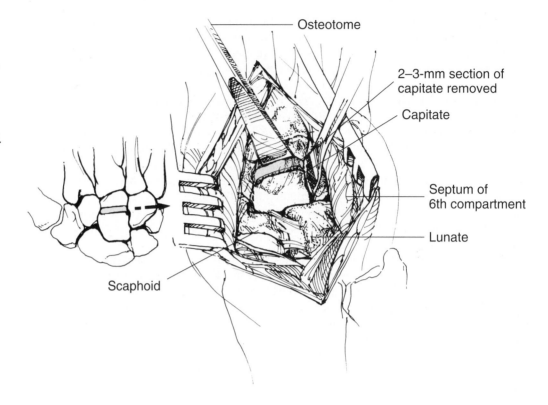

Osteotome

2–3-mm section of capitate removed

Capitate

Septum of 6th compartment

Lunate

Scaphoid

■ FIGURE 136–4
The surgical procedure. A blunt curved instrument compresses the head of the capitate (C) against the body while the K-wires are passed across the osteotomy site. MC III, third metacarpal.

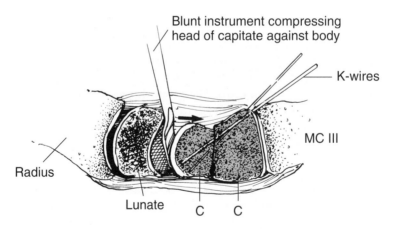

Blunt instrument compressing head of capitate against body

K-wires

MC III

Radius

Lunate   C   C

The pins are cut beneath the surface of the skin. The distal ends of the crossed K-wires in the capitate should be inserted so they are on the radial and ulnar sides of the common extensor tendons. The capsule is closed with interrupted heavy absorbable suture and the retinaculum is sutured back to the retinacular reflection between the fifth and sixth compartments with strong absorbable suture using mattress stitches. The tourniquet is released before closure of the subcutaneous tissues and hemostasis is obtained. Bupivacaine HCl 0.5% is infiltrated into the area for postoperative comfort, and a splint is applied to include the base of the thumb, leaving the fingers free. Prophylactic antibiotics are continued for 24 hours after surgery.

■ TECHNICAL ALTERNATIVES

Capitate shortening may also be done without the capitatohamate arthrodesis. Although clinical results are similar,[3] I believe the additional stability provided by the arthrodesis is desirable. The capitatohamate joint is almost immobile, providing only 5° of motion; benefits from the increased stability may outweigh the small loss of motion.

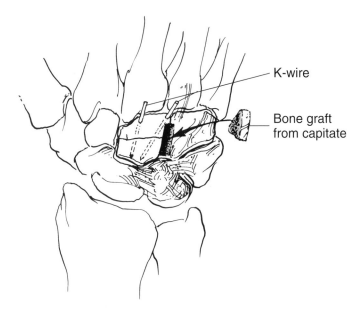

■ FIGURE 136–5
The surgical procedure.
The adjacent surfaces of
the capitate and hamate
are decorticated.

K-wire

Bone graft
from capitate

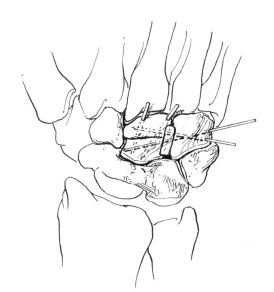

■ FIGURE 136–6
The surgical procedure.
Transverse K-wires fix
the hamate to each por-
tion of the capitate, and
bone graft is placed in
the crevice as needed.

Several technical difficulties may present during the capitate-shortening procedure. The greatest potential problem would be excessive or vigorous resection of bone from the waist of the capitate, resulting in devascularization of the capitate head. I use a sharp osteotome, not a power saw. This provides good control and avoids violating the capsule on the volar aspect of the capitate, which is essential to maintaining blood supply to the capitate head. The articular surface of the head of the capitate must not be compressed by clamping. Instead, a small, curved, blunt elevator must be used to compress the capitate head while inserting the wires. To preserve the blood supply to the dorsum of the lunate and the potential for revascularization, the lunate should be minimally dissected. The articular surfaces should be exposed just enough to stage the disease. The dorsal branch of the ulnar nerve must be identified so it can be avoided when inserting the transverse pins through the capitate and into the hamate. The extensor tendons, although usually more dorsal, should also be avoided.

Alternative procedures for advanced Kienböck disease exist. If only the radiolunate joint is affected, a radiolunate arthrodesis, with bone graft replacing the necrotic segments of the lunate, is an option. I also recommend fusing the scaphoid to the radius in this situation.[4] If both the lunatocapitate and radiolunate joints are affected, the best choices, in my experience, are complete wrist arthrodesis, or excision of the lunate with fascial arthroplasty combined with a scaphocapitate arthrodesis. The choice depends on the demands the patient places on the wrist, with heavy manual labor being an indication for wrist arthrodesis. If motion is the priority, lunate excision with a scaphocapitate arthrodesis can be successful. This limited wrist arthrodesis stabilizes the capitate to the scaphoid. I use a tendon graft in place of the lunate as described by Nahigian and co-authors.[12] I have not seen many good results after joint-decompressing procedures using scaphotrapezotrapezoid fusions. Finally, some patients with Kienböck disease exhibit a DISI pattern and require either an intercarpal or total wrist arthrodesis rather than a joint-leveling procedure.

■ REHABILITATION

Approximately 1 week after surgery, the short arm splint is changed to a short arm cast and skin sutures are removed. Light activity with the fingers and thumb is encouraged. The patient can drive a car and write with a large pen, but is asked to avoid heavy straining or lifting, which would cause forces across the joint. The cast is removed 8 weeks after surgery and radiographs are taken. If satisfactory healing of the osteotomy and fusion sites has occurred, the patient is placed in a short arm removable splint. Except in rare occasions, healing of the osteotomy and fusion has occurred within 8 weeks (Fig. 136–7). The patient is encouraged to continue light activities for the next month, including range of motion exercises, but heavy strain should be avoided. The pins are removed after healing has occurred, with care being taken to avoid the dorsal branch of the ulnar nerve when removing the transverse pins. Pin irritation of the dorsal branch of the ulnar nerve, resolving after pin removal, and erosion of the extensor tendon of the small finger by the pin, requiring surgical repair, have been the only complications noted.

After pin removal the patient is encouraged to increase activity level and range of motion, but continues to wear a protective splint to limit strain on the wrist until the lunate is revascularized. This may take up to a year. When revascularization is determined to

■ FIGURE 136–7
Postoperative radiograph shows capitate shortening with a capitatohamate arthrodesis.

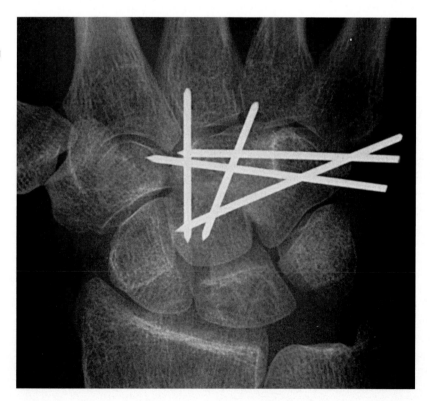

be present, the patient may perform more strenuous activities and may begin heavy strengthening exercises, such as with a work-simulating apparatus. Radiographic evaluation, including tomography, is used to determine lunate revascularization. This method may be imprecise, however, and magnetic resonance imaging, if affordable, would be more conclusive. Heavy or strenuous work activities are not advisable at any time with Kienböck disease, but patients often do not follow this advice.

The results of any treatment of Kienböck disease should be evaluated using two criteria: the functional condition of the patient, and the structural condition of the lunate. This operative procedure provides prompt, often dramatic pain relief that does not correlate with the revascularization of the lunate. This presumably relates to diminished forces acting across the lunate, and the resolution of synovitis. Improvement in symptoms may also result from partial denervation from resection of the distal branches of the posterior interosseous nerve. Most of these patients had been immobilized in a cast before the surgical treatment, and did not obtain relief simply from immobilization. Patients can be expected to have long-lasting pain relief, and most have discomfort only during strenuous activity.

Range of motion, which before surgery varied from day to day depending on the degree of synovial inflammation, increased only slightly after surgery. Grip strength measured about 80% of the opposite side. Most patients returned to their usual work or activity level, although I do not recommend heavy or strenuous activities. Patient satisfaction was very high. The goal of the procedure is revascularization of the lunate, and the results on radiographic evaluation have been satisfactory (Fig. 136–8). Eighty-three percent of the patients in our series revascularized and healed their fragmented lunate.[3] Should fragmentation and vascularity of the lunate persist, however, results eventually will be poor, even though patients may do well for a few years. Aseptic necrosis of the head of the capitate has not been observed. I was particularly concerned about this issue when this procedure was initially developed.

In summary, capitate-shortening osteotomy, with or without a capitatohamate arthrodesis, is an effective operation for treating patients with the earlier stages of Kienböck disease, when they have radiographically ulnar neutral or plus wrists.

■ OUTCOMES

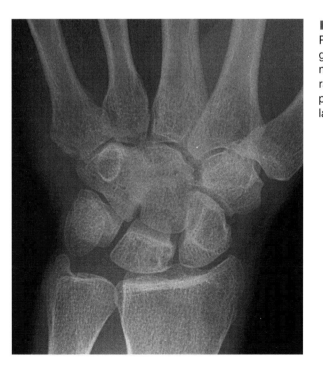

■ FIGURE 136–8
Posteroanterior radiograph at 13 postoperative months, with near-normal range of motion, good pain relief, and revascularization of the lunate.

References

1. Almquist EE: Kienböck's disease. Hand Clin, 1987; 3:141–148.
2. Almquist EE, Burns JF: Radial shortening for the treatment of Kienböck's disease. J Hand Surg, 1982; 7:348–352.
3. Almquist EE, Osterman AL, Carr C, Bach AW: Capitate shortening as a treatment for early Kienböck's disease. J Hand Surg, (in press).
4. Bach AW, Almquist EE, Newman DM: Proximal row fusion as solution for radiocarpal arthritis. J Hand Surg [Am], 1991; 16:424–431.
5. Chuinard RG, Zeman SC: Kienböck's disease: An analysis and rationale for treatment by capitate–hamate fusion. J Hand Surg, 1980; 5:290.
6. Gelberman RH, Bauman TD, Menon J, Akeson WH: The vascularity of the lunate bone and Kienböck's disease. J Hand Surg, 1980; 5:272–278.
7. Hultén O: Uber anatomische Variationen der Handgelenkknochen: Ein Beitrag zur Kenntnis der Genese zwei verschiedener Mondbeinveranderungen. Acta Radiol, 1928; 9:155–168.
8. Kashiwagi D, Fujiwara A, Inoue T, Liang FH, Iwamoto Y: An experimental and clinical study on lunatomalacia. Orthop Trans, 1977; 1:7.
9. Kienböck R: Uber traumatische Malazie des Mondbeins und ihre Folgezustande: Entartungsformen und Kompressionfrakturen. Fortschr Geb Rontgenstr, 1910–1911; 16: 77–103.
10. Lee M: The intraosseous arterial pattern of the carpal lunate bone and its relation to avascular necrosis. Acta Orthop Scand, 1963; 33:43–55.
11. Lichtman DM, Mack GR, Macdonald RI, Gunther SF, Wilson JN: Kienböck's disease: The role of silicone replacement arthroplasty. J Bone Joint Surg, 1977; 59A:899–908.
12. Nahigian SH, Li CS, Richey DG, Shaw DT: The dorsal flap arthroplasty in the treatment of Kienböck's disease. J Bone Joint Surg, 1970; 52A:245–252.
13. Palmer AK: Symposium on distal ulna injuries. Contemp Orthop, 1983; 7:81.
14. Rossak K: Druckverhaltnisse am Handgelenk unter besonderer Berucksichtigung von Fraktur-Mechanismen. Verhandlung der Deutschen Orthopädischen Gesellschaft, 1966; 296–299.

MICHAEL E. RETTIG
RONALD L.
LINSCHEID

137

Ulnar Lengthening Osteotomy

Adjustment of the length of the radius or the ulna by shortening or lengthening is commonly performed for disorders of the distal radioulnar joint or of the carpus. Ulnar lengthening is an accepted procedure for Kienböck disease, and this approach is sometimes required for treatment of nondissociative carpal instability or scapholunate dissociation.[5]

The rationale for lengthening the ulna to treat Kienböck disease is based on the observed association of the disease with the condition known as the ulnar minus variant.[1] Hultén introduced the observation that individuals with an ulna that was shorter than the radial articular surface at the lunate fossa measured perpendicular to the longitudinal axis of the forearm were at greater risk for development Kienböck avascular necrosis of the lunate.[4] In his original review, 74% of the wrists with necrosis of the lunate had this variation, whereas only 26% of 400 otherwise healthy wrists had it. No patient with Kienböck disease had an ulnar plus wrist. The short ulna allows for a concentration of forces on the most proximal radial aspect of the lunate. The ulnar aspect of the proximal articular surface of the lunate is often uninvolved.

Perrson initially described ulnar lengthening as a therapeutic alternative in Kienböck disease.[7] After the ulna is lengthened to a neutral or slightly positive variance, the ulnar head can provide sufficient support to neutralize the gradation of compliance between the lunate fossa of the radius and the softer triangular fibrocartilage. Perrson originally described an oblique osteotomy of the ulna fixed with a cerclage wire. Subsequent modification of this technique includes interposition bone graft and compression plates to allow more precise control of the fragments and to hasten bony healing.

Lengthening of the ulna decompresses and reduces the forces concentrated on the lunate, facilitating lunate healing and revascularization.[3] If the ulna is elongated, the triangular fibrocartilage is compressed and acts to support the ulnar aspect of the lunate and the articular facet of the triquetrum. However, this also induces a mild radial deviation that increases the joint-compressive force at the radioscaphoid articulation.[5]

Patients with Kienböck disease are considered candidates for ulnar lengthening if an ulnar minus or ulnar neutral variant is present and there is not yet severe carpal collapse or pancarpal arthritis. Kienböck disease is often staged as I through IV, with the latter representing carpal collapse and degenerative changes. Even the latter will occasionally respond with a decrease in painful symptoms. Staging on posteroanterior views of the wrist alone is prone to inaccuracy, with frequent underestimation of the degree of lunate involvement. Preoperative evaluation includes standard views of the wrist to determine ulnar variance and trispiral tomography to assess the severity of lunate involvement. The standard posteroanterior view is obtained with the elbow and shoulder at 90° and the wrist in neutral deviation, while the tube is directly perpendicular over the carpus. The amount of ulnar variance is measured and the size of the iliac bone graft necessary to obtain a plus 1 mm (+1 mm) ulnar variance[6] is determined. Trispiral tomography is an excellent method to evaluate the severity of lunate involvement. It also allows planning for open reduction and internal fixation of lunate fractures, if this appears possible. The tomograms can also be used to assess the articular surface of the radiocarpal joint and the capitolunate joint. Early degenerative changes in either of these two joints would preclude attempts at salvage of the lunate, and other reconstructive procedures, such as proximal row carpectomy or lunate excision with selected intercarpal fusion, would be

■ HISTORY OF THE TECHNIQUE

■ INDICATIONS AND CONTRAINDICATIONS

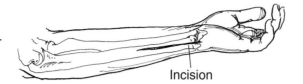

■ FIGURE 137–1
The ulna is exposed through a distal, longitudinal skin incision.

Incision

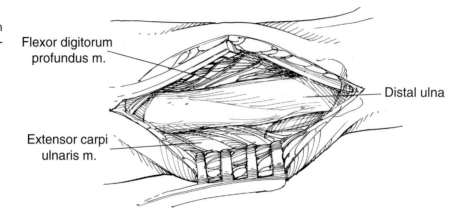

■ FIGURE 137–2
A subperiosteal dissection is used to expose the distal diaphysis of the ulna.

Flexor digitorum profundus m.

Distal ulna

Extensor carpi ulnaris m.

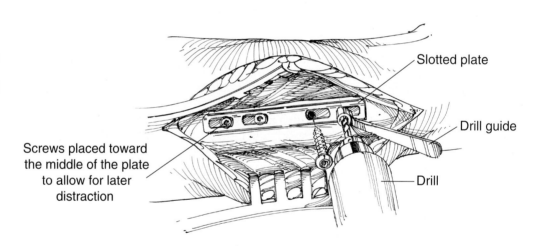

■ FIGURE 137–3
Affix a four-hole slotted plate, with each screw at the end of its respective slot nearest the center of the plate.

Slotted plate

Drill guide

Screws placed toward the middle of the plate to allow for later distraction

Drill

indicated. Ulnar lengthening can be combined with open reduction and internal fixation of a lunate fracture or vascularized bone grafting of the lunate. Because external fixator distraction is usually used with vascular pedicle grafting, ulnar lengthening allows the radius to be used for insertion of the fixator pins, which would tend to distract a radius-shortening osteotomy.

■ SURGICAL TECHNIQUES

After general endotracheal anesthesia or axillary block, the upper extremity and the opposite iliac crest are prepared for surgery. Intraoperative radiographs should be available for assessment of the amount of lengthening of the ulna.

The incision is made along the distal subcutaneous border of the ulna and over the ulnar head with the forearm in neutral rotation (Fig. 137–1). The extensor carpi ulnaris and the extensor carpi radialis are reflected, and the distal third of the ulna is exposed (Fig. 137–2). The location of the osteotomy is planned so that the distal screw holes of a four- or six-hole slotted plate can fit comfortably on the distal fragment. A slotted four- or six-hole plate is clamped to the ulna shaft, with the osteotomy centered in the middle of the plate. The screw holes are drilled and the screws inserted. The screws are inserted so that each lies at the end of its respective slot nearest the center of the plate (Fig. 137–3).

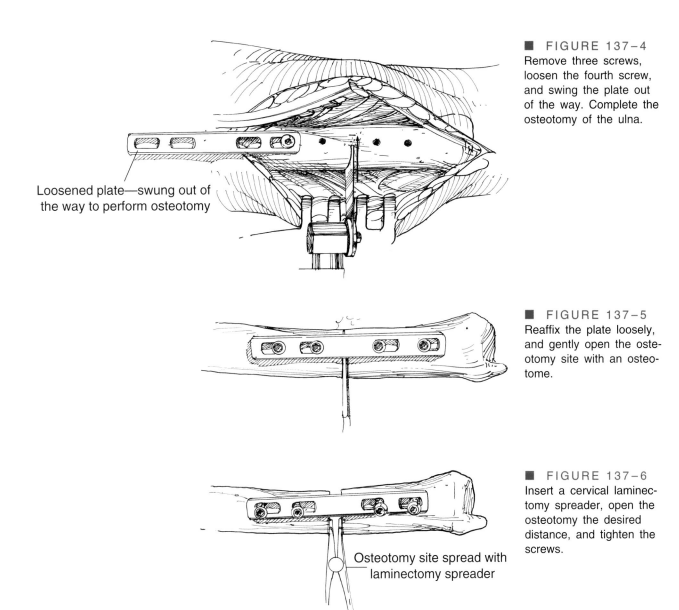

■ FIGURE 137–4
Remove three screws, loosen the fourth screw, and swing the plate out of the way. Complete the osteotomy of the ulna.

Loosened plate—swung out of the way to perform osteotomy

■ FIGURE 137–5
Reaffix the plate loosely, and gently open the osteotomy site with an osteotome.

■ FIGURE 137–6
Insert a cervical laminectomy spreader, open the osteotomy the desired distance, and tighten the screws.

Osteotomy site spread with laminectomy spreader

Insertion of the screws in this fashion will later allow distraction at the osteotomy site. Three screws are removed, the fourth is loosened, and the plate is swung out of the way (Fig. 137–4). Inserting the screws before completion of the osteotomy controls rotation and angulation of the two fragments. The osteotomy is then completed. The ulna is separated with an osteotome (Fig. 137–5) and then distracted with a cervical laminectomy spreader (Fig. 137–6). The correct amount of distraction, determined from the preoperative radiographs, is equal to the negative ulnar variance plus 1 or 2 mm. All of the screws are tightened to maintain distraction. The laminectomy spreader is then removed. Bicortical iliac crest bone graft is then obtained to maintain the osteotomy gap (Fig. 137–7). The graft is carefully sculpted and inserted. The cancellous aspect of the graft is placed toward the radius. The screws in the proximal or the distal fragment are loosened to allow the surrounding elastic tissues to apply compression across the graft. All of the screws are then tightened. Redundant projecting graft is trimmed and placed around the osteotomy site. Radiographs are then taken to check the new ulnar variance, the alignment of the ulna, and the length of the screws. A suction drain is inserted and the wound closed. The patient is placed into a well padded short arm splint.

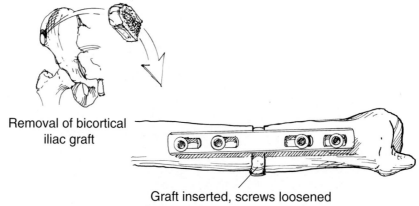

Removal of bicortical
iliac graft

Graft inserted, screws loosened
to allow for compression, then retightened

■ TECHNICAL
ALTERNATIVES

Ulnar lengthening is but one method of performing a joint-leveling procedure. Radial shortening provides a similar result without the necessity of obtaining a bone graft. Scaphotrapezotrapezoid arthrodesis, capitate recession, and capitolunate fusions are also used. It is possible to do an ulnar lengthening with an oblique or step-cut osteotomy. The fixation can also be altered to use dynamic compression plates or nonslotted plates if the planning is carried out meticulously. An interfragmentary screw may be used to fix the lengthening accurately at the expense of a narrowed waist at the osteotomy site, unless an oblique graft is also inserted.

■ REHABILITATION

Several days after surgery, a well padded short arm cast is applied. The cast is removed at 6 weeks and radiographs are taken. A thermoplastic ulnar gutter splint is worn until there is callus formation at both ends of the graft, and signs of early trabeculation extending across the cuts at each end of the graft. Radiographs are taken at 1-month intervals; this rarely exceeds 10 weeks' time. The patient can begin gentle active assisted exercises of the wrist at 6 weeks. Progressive resistive strengthening is started after healing of the osteotomy is assured. The goal of therapy is a moderate range of painless motion. Therapy is usually of value for 4 to 6 weeks.

■ OUTCOMES

Follow-up studies to date suggest that 80 to 85% of patients have significant relief of pain, improved grip strength, and increased range of motion, except for ulnar deviation. Healing of the lunate may occur if displacement and fragmentation is minimal; however, the lunate is always flattened. Ulnocarpal impingement may provide late discomfort. Results at 10 years and beyond almost always show moderate degenerative changes. Good results early tend to persist.

Ulnar lengthening has been tried for carpal instability, nondissociative (CIND), and scapholunate dissociation if there is an associated ulnar minus variance. The rationale is to provide adequate support under the lunate to modify the ulnar translation tendency of the lunate under compressive load.

The major complications include nonunion or delayed union of the osteotomy, malalignment, and overlengthening or underlengthening. The use of a slotted plate applied before the completion of the osteotomy, along with careful measurement of the preoperative radiographs to determine the size of the graft, can minimize these problems.[6] Intraoperative radiographs also aid in prevention of these difficulties. Ulnocarpal impaction, chondromalacia of the articular surface of the seat of the ulnar head, and radioscaphoid degenerative arthritis are other potential complications.

Nonunion after ulnar-lengthening osteotomy and bone grafting is rare.[1,8] In a recent review of ulnar-lengthening osteotomy, no ulnar nonunions were reported in 20 patients, though two delayed unions were present.[8] Ulnar nonunion can be treated with compression plating across the osteotomy site with additional cancellous bone grafting. A trial of electrical stimulation also could be considered before resorting to another operative procedure.

Ulnar lengthening as a component of vascularized bone grafting and restoration of lunate height has an advantage over radial shortening in that a distracting external fixator can be more easily inserted on the radius. Iliac cancellous bone is easily obtained at the same time as wafer graft.

Ulnar lengthening to a markedly positive ulnar variance will limit ulnar deviation owing to impingement between the distal ulna and the triquetrum. In one series, an approximate 10% average reduction of ulnar deviation compared to normal values was reported.[1] Excessive lengthening will restrict ulnar deviation even more, and possibly result in ulnar carpal pain secondary to the ulnar impaction syndrome that is now more frequently recognized in ulnar positive wrists. Predisposition to development of a degenerative tear of the triangular fibrocartilage is another potential problem with the excessively lengthened ulna.

Chondromalacia of the articular surface of the ulnar head may develop secondary to the often different anatomy of the distal radioulnar joint in the ulnar minus wrist. The slope of the sigmoid notch and ulnar head is most commonly at an angle with the longitudinal axis, which averages 20°.[2] In wrists with a marked ulnar minus variant, this angle may be even greater.[6] When the ulna is lengthened, the articular surface of the ulnar head is forced into the sigmoid notch, and pain with chondromalacic changes can result.[2] Radial shortening should be considered in those patients with Kienböck disease and an increased slope at the sigmoid notch to prevent this impingement.

The decompression of the lunate with ulnar lengthening shifts some pressure toward the proximal pole of the scaphoid and its articulation with the radius.[6] Radioscaphoid arthritis, which may already be present secondary to a palmar-flexed scaphoid, may be worsened.

References

1. Armistead RB, Linscheid RL, Dobyns JH, Beckenbaugh RD: Ulnar lengthening in the treatment of Kienböck's disease. J Bone Joint Surg, 1982; 64A:170–177.
2. Ekenstam FW: The distal radio ulnar joint: An anatomic experimental and clinical study with special reference to malunited fractures of the distal radius. Thesis, Uppsala University, Uppsala, Sweden, 1984.
3. Horii E, Garcia-Elias M, An KA, and co-authors: Effect of force transmission across the carpus in procedures used to treat Kienböck's disease. J Hand Surg, 1990; 15A:393–400.
4. Hultén O: Uber anatomische Variationen der Handgelenkknochen: Ein Beitrag zur Kenntnis der Genese zwei verschiedener Mondbeinveranderungen. Acta Radiol, 1928; 9:155–168.
5. Linscheid RL: Ulnar lengthening and shortening. Hand Clin, 1987; 3(2):69–79.
6. Linscheid RL: Ulnar lengthening. In: Neviaser R (ed): Controversies in Hand Surgery. New York: Churchill-Livingstone, 1990:159–166.
7. Perrson M: Pathogenese und Behandlung der Kienbockschen Lunatummmalazia: Der Frakturtheorie im Lichte der Effolge Operativer Radiusverkurzung (Hultén) und einer neuen Operationsmethode—Ulnaverlangerung. Acta Chir Scand, 1945; 92(Suppl 98).
8. Sundberg SB, Linscheid RL: Kienböck's disease: Results of treatment with ulnar lengthening. Clin Orthop, 1984; 187:43–51.

EDWARD A. STOKEL
THOMAS E. TRUMBLE

138

Distal Radial Shortening Osteotomy

■ HISTORY OF THE TECHNIQUE

Osteotomy to shorten the distal radius evolved from the treatment of Kienböck disease. Kienböck disease is usually associated with a negative ulnar variance.[5,7] Avascular necrosis of the lunate is thought to occur after repetitive trauma selectively loads the lunate, resulting in subclinical compression fracture and segmental disruption of the intraosseous blood supply.[4] Hultén is credited with initiating radial shortening osteotomy as a primary form of treatment.[1,13] Subsequent clinical experience was reported primarily in the European literature, with generally good results. Since Almquist reported his results in 1982, the technique has been well received and numerous clinical studies have supported the concept of shortening the radius to level the radiocarpal joint and minimize the compressive loads across the lunate.[1,3,8–10,13,14,16] Biomechanical studies have confirmed that joint-leveling procedures will decompress the lunate in patients with negative ulnar variance.[6,15] Controversy still exists regarding ulnar lengthening as an alternative method of joint leveling.[12,14] However, our experience and the experience of others supports shortening of the radius as a straightforward procedure with few complications.

■ INDICATIONS AND CONTRAINDICATIONS

Radial shortening osteotomy is indicated in a select group of patients with Kienböck disease. Patients who are ulna negative without significant collapse and fragmentation of the lunate, with no significant degenerative changes at the radiocarpal or midcarpal joint, are candidates for the procedure.[1,3,8,13] Even when early degenerative changes are evident, patients may benefit from radial shortening osteotomy.[9,13] In patients who are ulna neutral or ulna positive, the benefits are not as clear. In these patients, radial shortening osteotomy may be a relative indication provided no degenerative changes are present.[9] Contraindications to radial shortening include collapse and fragmentation of the lunate, or advanced degenerative arthrosis of the radiocarpal or midcarpal joints.

■ SURGICAL TECHNIQUES

Shortening of the radius is performed through a dorsal approach. The operation is performed under axillary block or general anesthesia, with tourniquet control. The patient is placed supine on the operating table, with the arm in a fully pronated position on the arm board. A longitudinal incision is made on the dorsal aspect of the distal forearm, beginning 2 cm distal to Lister's tubercle and extending proximally for 8 to 10 cm (Fig. 138–1). Large superficial veins are identified and protected. Smaller veins are coagulated. The superficial branches of the radial nerve are identified, protected, and retracted out of the field. Sharp dissection is continued to the level of the deep fascia, and the extensor retinaculum is identified. The interval between the extensor pollicis longus and extensor digitorum communis is identified at the distal margin of the extensor retinaculum. The roof of the third compartment is divided, allowing the extensor pollicis longus tendon to be retracted out of the field (Fig. 138–2). The septa between the third and fourth compartments is sharply divided. The proximal half of the extensor retinaculum, including the tendons in their compartments, is subperiosteally dissected in a radial and ulnar direction. The dissection can be continued distally, if necessary, to allow complete exposure of the distal radius. In general, however, the distal half of the extensor retinaculum can be left attached to the distal radius. It is important to maintain the integrity of the fourth compartment to avoid adhesions and bowstringing of the tendons. The interval between the exten-

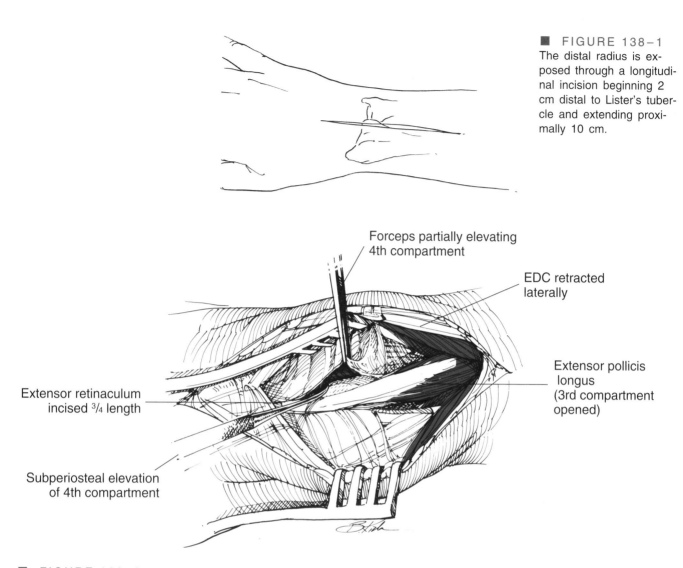

Forceps partially elevating 4th compartment

EDC retracted laterally

Extensor pollicis longus (3rd compartment opened)

Extensor retinaculum incised ¾ length

Subperiosteal elevation of 4th compartment

■ FIGURE 138–2
The extensor retinaculum is divided over the third compartment, allowing retraction of the extensor pollicis longus tendon. EDC, extensor digitorum communis.

sor carpi radialis brevis and the extensor digitorum communis is developed proximally, in a subperiosteal fashion, to expose the dorsal aspect of the distal radius. The extensor pollicis longus and abductor pollicis longus muscles are retracted out of the field as the dissection is carried proximally. Two Penrose drains may be looped around the tendons and clamped volarly to provide additional retraction.

The osteotomy site is selected at the metaphyseal–diaphyseal junction. The bone is scored longitudinally across the osteotomy site for later assessment of rotational alignment. A 3.5-mm T-plate is selected, and contoured to the dorsal aspect of the radius. Removal of Lister's tubercle may be necessary to accommodate the plate. The plate is temporarily positioned and secured with plate-holding clamps. The distal holes are then drilled and tapped in neutral fashion to accommodate 3.5-mm cortical screw fixation. The plate is removed and the parallel osteotomy lines are marked on the dorsal radius (Fig. 138–3). The osteotomy is performed with an oscillating saw. Two parallel transverse cuts are made, removing 2 to 4 mm of bone, including the width of the saw blade. The distal cut is performed first because it is easier to stabilize the proximal forearm when making the second cut (Fig. 138–4). If necessary, the distal cut may be angled slightly distally from ulnarly to radially, to decrease the radial inclination. The proximal and distal sections of

■ FIGURE 138–3
After predrilling and tapping of the distal screw holes for the T-plate, parallel osteotomy lines are marked on the radius. EPL, extensor pollicis longus.

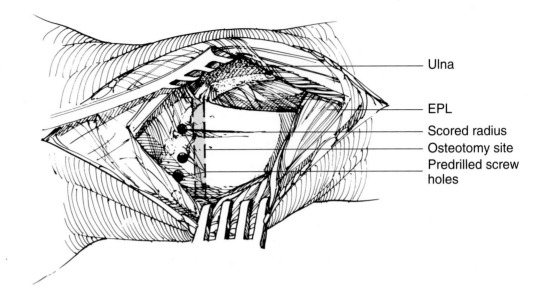

Ulna

EPL

Scored radius
Osteotomy site
Predrilled screw holes

■ FIGURE 138–4
First the distal and then the proximal osteotomy cuts are completed.

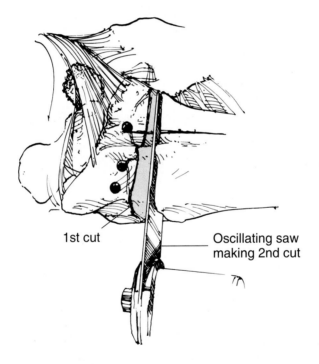

1st cut

Oscillating saw making 2nd cut

the radius are then approximated, and the parallel contact of the surface is verified. The plate is applied distally using the previously drilled holes. Rotation is verified using the previous longitudinal scoring. The proximal holes are then drilled sequentially and 3.5-mm cortical screws are eccentrically placed to provide compression (Fig. 138–5). Intraoperative anteroposterior and lateral radiographs are obtained to confirm plate placement and screw length.

The extensor retinaculum of the fourth dorsal compartment is secured to the periosteum around Lister's tubercle using permanent sutures, allowing the extensor pollicis longus tendon to pass superficially to the extensor retinaculum. The subcuticular structures are closed in layers using interrupted absorbable sutures. The skin is approximated using interrupted nylon sutures. Drains are used only if necessary. A sterile dressing is applied, followed by a volar plaster splint holding the wrist is slight extension. The patient is admitted overnight for pain management and elevation of the extremity.

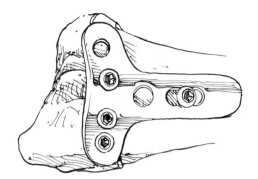

The proximal screws are then inserted, securing the plate and fixing the radius.

The dorsal approach avoids major neurovascular structures, involves a minimum of soft tissue dissection, and provides excellent exposure of the distal radius. The dorsal surface, however, is convex and irregular, and Lister's tubercle may need to be removed to contour the plate. The plate occupies a subcutaneous position and may irritate extensor tendons. Proximal dissection is somewhat limited because the extensor pollicis longus and abductor pollicis longus muscles cross the operative field. Postoperative scarring near the dorsal capsule may limit palmar flexion.

The volar approach to the distal radius is an alternative surgical approach.[1] The volar surface of the distal radius is flat and easily accommodates a contoured plate. The overlying pronator quadratus and flexor pollicis longus muscles protect the long flexor tendons from plate irritation. The dissection can easily be extended proximally. However, the volar approach involves more dissection, and the radial artery, palmar cutaneous branches of the median nerve, and superficial branches of the radial nerve are at risk for injury. Because the dissection involves deeper structures, the osteotomy is cumbersome, especially if changes in the radial inclination are desired.

A six-hole, 3.5-mm dynamic compression plate may be used instead of a T-plate. It may be easier to fit on the dorsum of the radius because Lister's tubercle will not be involved, and provides excellent compression. However, the plate is thicker and may occupy a more subcutaneous position, resulting in tendon irritation.

The amount of radial shortening necessary to decompress the lunate is currently unknown. Excessive shortening may produce excessive ulnocarpal loading, degeneration of the triangular fibrocartilage complex, and ulnar impingement.[11] Some authors recommend shortening equivalent to the preoperative ulnar variance.[2,8,13] Other authors advocate removal of a fixed length of bone.[4,11,12,16] Trumble et al, in a biomechanical study, used strain gauges to monitor lunate loading.[15] Their study concluded that 2 mm of radial shortening resulted in optimal lunate decompression, and that greater than 4 mm of shortening increased the risk of distal radioulnar joint disorders and ulnar impingement. This value has been corroborated by clinical studies.[9,16] If ulnar impingement does occur, symptoms usually resolve with ulnar shortening.[2,16]

■ TECHNICAL ALTERNATIVES

Active digital motion is encouraged immediately. Sutures are removed at 14 days and a removable wrist splint is applied. Active motion of the wrist and strengthening exercises are begun, preferably supervised by a physical therapist. The splint is worn for all activities until there is radiographic evidence of union, usually about 6 to 10 weeks. The patient may then decrease use of the splint and gradually increase activities. Strenuous activities should be avoided until there is clinical and radiographic evidence of complete union at approximately 16 weeks.

■ REHABILITATION

The outcomes from radial shortening are relatively favorable and predictable. Good clinical results after radial shortening osteotomy are reported in 70 to 100% of patients.[1,3,8–10,13,14,16] Pain relief is good to excellent in 90% of patients.[1,3,8–10,13,14,16] Flexion and extension usually improve 15°.[1,9,13,16] No loss of pronation or supination has been

■ OUTCOMES

noted after surgery.[1,13] Distal radioulnar joint instability has not been a problem.[13] Grip strength never returns to normal values, but improves to 70 to 80% of the opposite side.[1,3,9,13,14,16] Radiographically, the lunate will not regain its normal anatomy, but will show evidence of revascularization.[1,3,8,9] Progression of the disease, both clinically and radiographically, has been noted. This is rare, however, and usually occurs in patients in the advanced stages of collapse.[9,13]

Complications after radial shortening are rare. Persson reported three cases of nonunion and instead proposed ulnar lengthening.[12] Nonunion has only rarely been reported by other authors. Schattenkerk and co-authors reported 1 nonunion in 20 cases, and Weiss and co-authors reported 1 nonunion in 30 cases.[14,16] Other authors have reported no nonunions.[2,3,9,13] Tendonitis and irritation from retained plates are also possible.[1] Clinically, however, this is rarely a problem, and routine removal of the plates is unnecessary.

Radial shortening has been a reliable and successful method to treat Kienböck disease, and is readily accomplished using our surgical technique.

References

1. Almquist EE, Burns JF: Radial shortening for the treatment of Kienböck's disease: A 5- to 10-year follow-up. J Hand Surg, 1982; 7:348–352.
2. Almquist EE. Kienböck's disease. Hand Clin, 1987; 3:141–148.
3. Eiken O, Nicchajev I: Radius shortening in malacia of the lunate. Scand J Plast Reconstr Surg, 1980; 14:191–196.
4. Gelberman RH, Bauman TD, Menon J, Akeson WH: The vascularity of the lunate bone in Kienböck's disease. J Hand Surg, 1980; 5:272–278.
5. Gelberman RH, Salamon PB, Jurist JM, Posch JL: Ulnar variance in Kienböck's disease. J Bone Joint Surg, 1975; 57A:674–676.
6. Horii E, Garcia-Elias M, An KN, et al: Effect of force transmission across the carpus in procedures used to treat Kienböck's disease. J Hand Surg, 1990; 15A:393–400.
7. Hultén O: Uber anatomische Variationen der Handgelenkknochen: Ein Beitrag zur Kenntnis der Genese zwei verschiedener Mondbeinveranderungen. Acta Radiol, 1928; 9:155–168.
8. Kinnard P, Tricoire JL, Basora J: Radial shortening for Kienböck's disease. Can J Surg, 1983; 26:261–262.
9. Nakamura R, Imaeda T, Miura T: Radial shortening for Kienböck's disease: Factors affecting the operative result. J Hand Surg, 1990; 15B:40–45.
10. Ovesen J: Shortening of the radius in the treatment of lunatomalacia. J Bone Joint Surg, 1981; 63B:231–232.
11. Palmer AK, Glisson RR, Werner FW: Ulnar variance determination. J Hand Surg, 1982; 7:376–379.
12. Persson M: Causal treatment of lunatomalacia: Further experiences of operative ulna lengthening. Acta Chir Scand, 1950; 100:531–534.
13. Rock MG, Roth JH, Martin L: Radial shortening osteotomy for treatment of Kienböck's disease. J Hand Surg, 1991; 16A:454–458.
14. Schattenkerk ME, Nollen A, van Hussen F: The treatment of lunatomalacia: Radial shortening or ulna lengthening? Acta Orthop Scand, 1987; 58:652–654.
15. Trumble T, Glisson RR, Seaber AV, Urbaniak JR: A biomechanical comparison of the methods for treating Kienböck's disease. J Hand Surg, 1986; 11A:88–93.
16. Weiss APC, Weiland AJ, Moore JR, Wilgis EFS: Radial shortening for Kienböck's disease. J Bone Joint Surg [Am], 1991; 73:384–390.

139

Osteotomy for Malunion of the Distal Radius

A review of the relevant literature on radial osteotomies reveals that the earliest reports of surgical correction of the malunited fracture of the distal end of the radius were published in the 1930s. In 1932, Ghormley and Mroz[15] described 4 radial osteotomies in a study of 176 fractures of the wrist. These authors concluded that an osteotomy with or without a bone graft could improve the external appearance of a deformed wrist.

Durman in 1935[7] devised an ingenious opening wedge osteotomy with an interposed trapezoidal graft that was cut longitudinally from the distal end of the proximal radial fragment. The author found that additional distal ulnar resection was unnecessary to produce a good cosmetic result. In 1937, Campbell[4] published a technique in which the radius is osteotomized transversely about an inch above the radiocarpal joint through a radial approach between the brachioradialis and extensor pollicis brevis tendons. The graft, taken from the prominent medial border of the ulna with preservation of the distal radioulnar joint, was then inserted in the dorsoradial defect of the opening wedge osteotomy. Eleven of 19 cases treated with this technique had better functional and cosmetic results than those after simple osteotomy without graft interposition, which corrected only the backward angulation of the articular surface of the radius.

In 1945, Merle D'Aubigné and Joussement[23] proposed a multiple-facet, curved osteotomy in the sagittal plane (ostéotomie à facettes), designed to restore radial length without the need for a graft. However, by virtue of its form, this osteotomy produces a slight palmar displacement of the distal fragment with respect to the shaft of the radius, and permits no correction in the frontal plane.

In the 1970s, plate fixation of distal radial osteotomies to guarantee rigid fixation and early joint rehabilitation was advocated by various authors.[9,16,24,28] Other authors use similar techniques, but prefer fixation with percutaneous pins and cast immobilization[2,6,27,29,32] to avoid a second operation for hardware removal. In the past decade, further refinements of the technique, including the concomitant treatment of radioulnar problems, have been reported.[8,10–13,18]

■ HISTORY OF THE TECHNIQUE

The indication for surgical correction of the malunited radius depends on several factors. Wrist deformity after fracture may or may not produce symptoms, so that a basic differentiation between symptomatic and asymptomatic malunion is imperative in deciding whether treatment is necessary. Acceptable wrist function and absence of pain can be expected despite radiographic evidence of angular deformity, shortening, and degenerative changes. This is a common finding in elderly patients who no longer engage in strenuous manual activities and whose functional requirements at the wrist are therefore considerably reduced. Conversely, in younger, more active patients, especially those engaged in heavy manual work or who require a normal range of motion of the wrist, the deformity becomes symptomatic shortly after healing of the fracture. Malunion may be extra-articular, resulting in metaphyseal angulation and shortening, intra-articular with residual articular step-offs and incongruity at the radiocarpal or radioulnar joints, or combined (intra- and extra-articular). Although correction of extra-articular malunion may be safely delayed until the soft tissues offer an ideal surgical environment and maximal residual function of the wrist has been regained with physiotherapy, intra-articular deformity

■ INDICATIONS AND CONTRAINDICATIONS

should be dealt with as soon as possible before irreversible cartilage damage takes place. The surgical decision is based on limitation of joint motion, wrist disability, level of pain, degree of cosmetic deformity, and the radiographic findings.

A meticulous preoperative evaluation of wrist symptoms and their anatomic correlation with physical and radiographic findings is imperative to guarantee a good result. Exact localization of pain and tenderness at the radiocarpal, midcarpal, or radioulnar levels is important in deciding whether an additional operation at the distal radioulnar joint is necessary. Wrist arthroscopy, arthrograms, computed tomography (CT) scans, and magnetic resonance imaging are further valuable diagnostic measures to evaluate the condition of the articular cartilage, carpal ligaments, and radioulnar joint. Standardized plain radiographs of both wrists are usually sufficient to decide the surgical indication. Comparison of the uninjured side is particularly useful to analyze carpal malalignment, ulnar variance, and the inclination of the articular surface, which may vary anatomically. CT is useful to evaluate post-traumatic incongruence of the distal radioulnar joint, or subluxation or rotational malalignment of the distal radius.[19,25] The latter can be accurately measured by superimposing tracings of symmetric CT cuts of both forearms in neutral rotation. The proximal cut should include the bicipital tuberosity and the distal Lister's tubercle as bony references. The difference in rotation between the uninjured and the injured side represents the true bony rotational malalignment. CT scans may become necessary in cases where complex intra- and extra-articular corrections are planned with three-dimensional reconstruction imaging.[17]

I do not believe in fixed radiographic angles for determining whether correction is needed. Although a symptomatic dorsal or palmar shift of the flexion–extension arc of motion occurs when the articular surface is tilted more than 25° in the sagittal plane, patients with constitutional joint laxity may experience a painful midcarpal instability after a healed Colles fracture with a mild dorsal tilt (10 to 15°).[31] Furthermore, based on experimental evidence of radial overload of the articular cartilage,[26,30] a dorsal angulation between 20 and 30° should be considered a prearthritic condition. Radial shortening up to 10 to 12 mm without degenerative changes at the distal radioulnar joint can be corrected with the radial osteotomy alone.[9,10] However, in the presence of degenerative changes of the distal radioulnar joint with severe limitation of forearm rotation, an additional procedure on the ulnar side of the wrist is usually necessary to guarantee a successful result.[12,13]

In my experience, the indication for radial osteotomy is established by a symptomatic deformity with radiographic findings that suggest a poor prognosis for the future of the wrist. These are a prearthritic deformity, a mechanical imbalance of the carpus, and incongruence of the distal radioulnar joint. Contraindications for corrective osteotomy are advanced degenerative changes in the radiocarpal and intercarpal joints; fixed carpal malalignment or important trophic disturbances causing limited overall function of the wrist and fingers; or massive osteoporosis. I do not see an upper age limit for candidates for this operation, provided that there is adequate bone quality and impaired wrist function. Ideally, the osteotomy should be performed as soon as the soft tissues show no trophic disturbances, before radiographic evidence of advanced osteoporosis, and when the maximum possible motion of the wrist has been regained with physiotherapy. Whether an associated primary operation on the ulnar side of the wrist should be performed with an osteotomy of the distal radius depends on careful preoperative assessment of the distal radioulnar joint. I believe that partial ulnar head resection should be performed as a primary operation in combination with radial osteotomy when the patient's main symptom is painful limitation of forearm rotation due to post-traumatic osteoarthritis of the radioulnar joint. Instability and ulnocarpal impingement as a result of shortening, angulation, or malrotation of the distal end of the radius without degenerative arthritic changes can be corrected by restoration of the radial deformity alone in an effort to preserve the anatomic integrity of the distal radioulnar joint.

■ SURGICAL TECHNIQUES

Because radial shortening is a constant component of the deformity, an opening wedge osteotomy that is transverse in the frontal plane and oblique (parallel to the joint surface) in the sagittal plane, to provide lengthening, is recommended. The osteotomy should accomplish anatomic reorientation of the joint surface to guarantee normal load distribution, reestablish the mechanical balance of the midcarpal joint, and restore the anatomic relationships of the distal radioulnar joint. This osteotomy allows radial lengthening of as much as 10 to 12 mm and corrects (1) the volar tilt in the sagittal plane, (2) the radial inclination in the frontal plane, and (3) the rotational deformity in the horizontal plane. The bone defect that is created after displacement of the distal fragment is replaced with a corticocancellous bone graft taken from the iliac crest. If a partial or complete resection of the distal ulna is performed simultaneously, the resected ulnar head can be used to fill the radial defect.

Careful preoperative planning (Fig. 139–1) and the use of K-wires to mark the angle of deformity are mandatory to guarantee an accurate angular correction, simplify the procedure, and diminish the need of intraoperative radiographic control. Radiographs of the uninjured wrist are useful to determine the physiologic ulnar variance for each particular patient, and should be used to calculate restoration of radial length. For this procedure, general anesthesia is recommended because for most of the cases an iliac bone graft is used. In cases where the graft is taken from the resected distal ulna, regional anesthesia may be used.

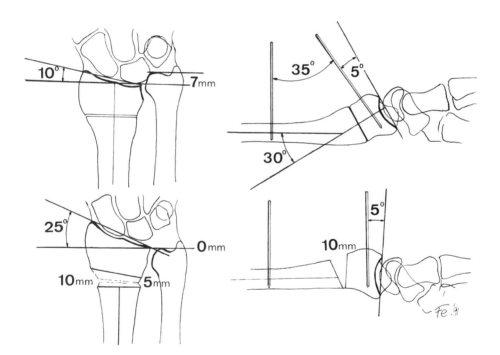

■ FIGURE 139-1

Preoperative planning of the osteotomy. *Top left:* For correction in the frontal plane, the amount of shortening (7 mm in this patient) is measured between the head of the ulna and the ulnar corner of the radius on the anteroposterior radiograph. The lines of the measurement are perpendicular to the long axis of the radius. The radial inclination is reduced to 10° in this patient. *Bottom left:* To restore the radial inclination to normal (average 25°), the osteotomy is opened more on the dorsoradial than on the dorsoulnar side. *Top right:* For correction in the sagittal plane, the dorsal tilt (30° in this patient) is measured between the line perpendicular to the joint surface and the long axis of the radius on the lateral radiograph. K-wires are introduced so that they subtend the angle that corresponds to the dorsal tilt plus 5° of volar tilt (30° + 5° = 35° in this patient). *Bottom right:* After opening the osteotomy by the correct amount, the K-wires lie parallel to each other. (From Fernandez D: Malunion of the distal radius current. In: Heckmann JD (ed): American Academy of Orthopaedic Surgeons, Instructional Course Lectures. January, 1993, pp 73–88.)

Technique for the mal-
united Colles fracture. **(A)**
Threaded wires subtend
the angle of correction in
the sagittal plane. **(B)**
The osteotomy is opened
dorsally and maintained
by applying a small fixa-
tor bar between the
threaded wires.

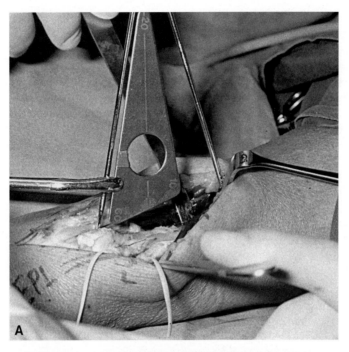

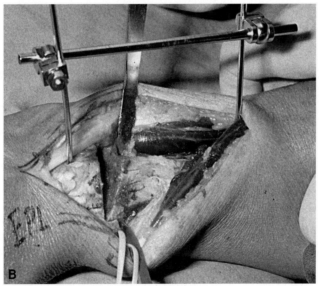

For *malunited Colles fractures,* a 7-cm longitudinal dorsoradial incision is used. It begins at a point 2 cm distal to Lister's tubercle and extends 5 cm proximally in the forearm (Fig. 139–2A). The extensor retinaculum is incised longitudinally between the third and fourth dorsal compartments. Next, the extensor pollicis longus tendon is dissected out of its groove and retracted with a rubber band. The distal part of the radius is exposed ulnarly by separating the extensor tendons of the fourth and fifth compartments with their fibrosy-novial sheaths. By raising these structures close to bone, the posterior interosseous nerve is automatically protected and displaced ulnarward. On the radial side, a periosteal eleva-tor is passed under the wrist extensor tendons. The tendons are separated from bone, placing two small Hohmann retractors on both sides of the future osteotomy site. Unless a combined intra- and extra-articular osteotomy is performed, dorsal wrist arthrotomy is not necessary. If T-plate fixation of the osteotomy is planned, Lister's tubercle should be removed with an osteotome to provide a flat surface on which to apply the plate. If K-

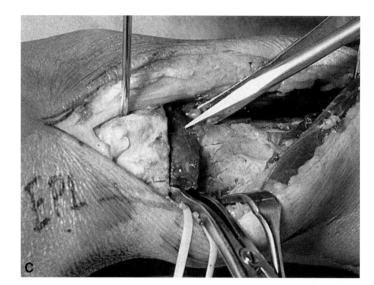

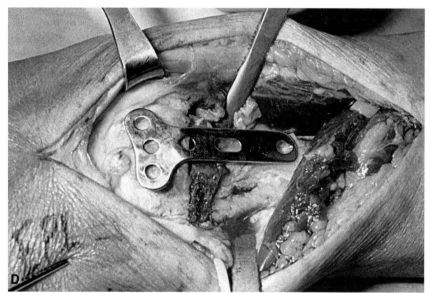

■ FIGURE 139–2
(continued)
(C) The osteotomy line is opened radially with a small spreader clamp, and the iliac bone graft is inserted into the dorsora-dial defect. **(D)** Provisional fixation is obtained with a K-wire through the radial styloid. The plate is positioned after removal of the external fixator.

wire or condylar plate fixation of the osteotomy is used, Lister's tubercle should be left in place, because it is a useful point of entry for dorsopalmar wire fixation, and does not interfere with the site of entry of the condylar plate blade. The osteotomy site is marked about 2.5 cm proximal to the wrist joint with an osteotome.

To ensure that the cut as seen in the sagittal plane is parallel to the joint surface, a fine K-wire is introduced through the dorsal part of the capsule into the radiocarpal joint and along the articular surface of the radius. According to the preoperative plan, two 2.5-mm K-wires with threaded tips are inserted, subtending the angle of correction in the sagittal plane on both sides of the future osteotomy (Fig. 139–2B). These wires not only serve to guide intraoperative angular correction, but to manipulate and maintain the distal fragment in the corrected position with a small external fixator bar until the graft is inserted in place. With careful protection of the volar soft tissues, the osteotomy is performed with the oscillating saw, taking care not to osteotomize completely the volar cortex (Fig. 139–2C). The osteotomy is then opened dorsally and radially by manipulating the wrist into flexion, by applying spreader clamps dorsally, or by using the 2.5-mm K-wires as joysticks. The osteotomy is opened until both wires are parallel in the sagittal plane. At this point, an external fixator bar with two clamps is placed between both K-wires to maintain the reduction of the distal fragment (Fig. 139–2D). Additional opening of the osteotomy on the radial side for correction of the ulnar tilt in the frontal plane is achieved with a small spreader clamp (Fig. 139–2C). The distal fragment rotates along the axis of the distal threaded K-wire. Complete tenotomy or Z-lengthening of the brachioradialis tendon is recommended to facilitate lengthening in malunions with severe radial deviation and shortening. For such cases, two additional K-wires with threaded tips may be used between both fragments, to which a distraction device can be applied temporarily on the radial side of the wrist. Next the iliac bone graft is shaped to conform to the dorsoradial bone defect and is inserted, making sure that there is a snug fit. The cortical portion of the graft should be oriented dorsally (Fig. 139–2C). At this point, a 1.6- or 2.0-mm K-wire is driven obliquely from the radial styloid across the graft into the proximal fragment, after which the threaded wires and the external fixator bar may be removed. With the elbow in 90° of flexion, intraoperative fluoroscopy may be advisable at this point to assess the quality of correction and radial lengthening before definitive internal fixation. For this, a second K-wire may be introduced across Lister's tubercle in an oblique dorsopalmar direction into the proximal fragment, as suggested by Rodriguez-Meythiaz and Chamay.[29] Rigid fixation with a T-plate or a titanium 2.7-mm condylar plate is another option that allows early unrestricted active motion of the wrist (Fig. 139–3). Plate fixation is recommended for cases with severe shortening, in which the opposite cortex has to be completely osteotomized to achieve full radial length. During wound closure, the extensor pollicis longus tendon can be relocated in its groove if Lister's tubercle is preserved during stabilization with K-wires; otherwise a proximal transverse retinacular flap should be interposed between the plate and the tendon to prevent attrition tendinitis. Deep suction drainage of the wound is advisable for 48 postoperative hours.

■ FIGURE 139–3
Internal fixation techniques for osteotomy of the distal radius. **(A)** With two 1.6-mm K-wires. One is inserted through the radial styloid, across the graft into the ulnar cortex of the proximal fragment; the other is inserted through Lister's tubercle across the graft into the volar cortex of the proximal fragment.[29] **(B)** With the A.O. 2.7-mm titanium condylar plate. **(C)** With the A.O. 3.5-mm, small-fragment T-plate.

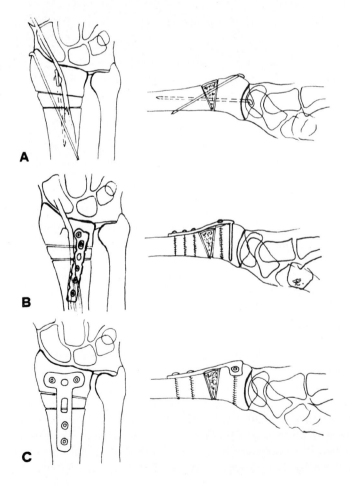

Malunited Smith fractures are exposed through a straight volar incision between the flexor carpi radialis tendon and the radial artery. The pronator quadratus muscle is detached radially and the flexor pollicis longus muscle is mobilized from the radial shaft. The malunion is approached subperiosteally by reflecting the pronator quadratus muscle to the ulnar side, and the soft tissues are protected with Hohmann retractors. The palmar opening wedge osteotomy, grafting, and plating are then carried out in a "reversed" manner—as in the Colles deformity, but from the volar side. However, care must be taken not to overcorrect the physiologic palmar tilt of 10° when manipulating the distal fragment into dorsiflexion. The application of a volar buttressing T-plate automatically derotates the pronated distal fragment by virtue of the flat surface of the plate. Plate fixation is therefore strongly recommended on the volar side because practically all malunited Smith fractures have a pronation deformity of the distal fragment and an apparent dorsal subluxation of the distal ulna. Dorsiflexion of the distal fragment and derotation as well as lengthening reorient the sigmoid notch of the radius with respect to the head of the ulna, thus restoring articular congruity of the radioulnar joint.

The most common pitfall with radial osteotomy is failure to achieve the desired anatomic correction (volar tilt and radial length) in spite of adequate preoperative planning. This is usually the result of faulty technique. If the cut in the sagittal plane is not perfectly parallel to the distal K-wire, correction in this plane will be insufficient. This can be compensated for by inserting a larger graft than planned. Disruption of the volar cortex may render the osteotomy unstable. If the volar gap opens during distraction, loss of volar tilt may occur. To avoid loss of correction until definitive plate fixation, temporary use of a wrist fixator between both fragments is advisable. Failure to restore complete length up to an ulnar plus variance of 2 to 3 mm is usually compatible with free forearm rotation (Fig. 139–4). Otherwise, in my experience, it is better to perform a simultaneous ulnar shortening rather than distracting the radius to full length.

■ TECHNICAL ALTERNATIVES

If adequate stability of the internal fixation cannot be achieved owing to preoperative underestimation of bone quality, the osteotomy should be protected in a forearm cast for 6 to 8 weeks. Occasional "settling" of the osteotomy with temporary graft resorption and slight loss of initial radial length may be observed if the bone is osteoporotic. Cast-free postoperative treatment in such cases is dangerous, with a high chance of implant loosening and nonunion. Attrition tendinitis of the extensor tendons is possible if there is direct contact with a metal plate, especially if the tendon is denuded of its sheath. If screw loosening occurs, tendon ruptures can occur where the tendon contacts the threads of the screw.

The wrist is immobilized in a volar plaster splint until the soft tissues have healed, which is usually by 2 weeks after the operation. Early wrist motion is permitted after suture removal in cases where rigid internal fixation can be achieved with plate fixation and there is good bone quality, without osteoporosis. In cases where K-wire fixation is used, a forearm cast for 4 weeks after suture removal is recommended. Heavy manual work is allowed between 6 to 8 weeks after radiographically confirmed union of the osteotomy. Dorsal plates are usually removed between 3 and 6 months after surgery to prevent attrition tendinitis of the extensor pollicis longus tendon. Volar plates, on the other hand, may be left in place.

■ REHABILITATION

Review of our series[10–13] showed that a satisfactory outcome without pain can be expected in malunions after extra-articular fractures when the preoperative range of motion of the wrist is more than 70% of normal, the wrist joint is free of degenerative changes both at the radiocarpal and intercarpal level, and there is no fixed carpal malalignment. Under these circumstances, and when shortening does not exceed 10 mm, restoration of the normal anatomy of the distal end of the radius and its relationships to the ulna offers highly satisfactory long-term results.

In a more recent review of subsequent patients treated in the past 10 years, an additional

■ OUTCOMES

■ FIGURE 139–4
(A) Radiographs (*top*) of a malunited Colles fracture with 32° of dorsal tilt and 11 mm of radial shortening. Immediate postoperative films (*bottom*) show anatomic correction of the distal fragment and restoration of radial length.

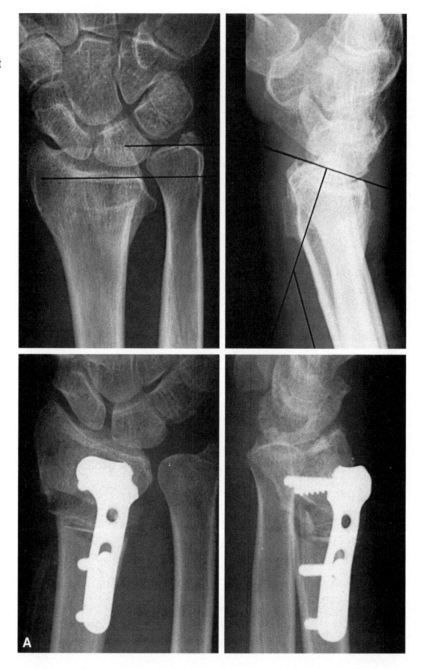

operation on the ulnar side of the wrist had to be performed in about 50% of a total of 80 radial osteotomies. This is the result of having extended the indications for operative treatment of malunions to include those that occur after intra-articular Colles fractures, malunions after comminuted fractures with severe shortening, and Smith fractures with subluxation of the distal radioulnar joint. Careful preoperative routine assessment of the radioulnar joint with CT scans has anticipated the need for an associated procedure at this level. However, we firmly believe that excisional arthroplasty of the distal ulna should be performed as a primary operation with radial osteotomy only in the presence of osteo-arthritic changes of the radioulnar joint. Ulnar plus variance, instability, and ulnocarpal impingement depending on radial shortening, metaphyseal angulation, or rotational malalignment without degenerative changes, usually can be corrected with restoration of radial anatomy alone, in an effort to preserve the anatomic integrity of the distal radioulnar joint.

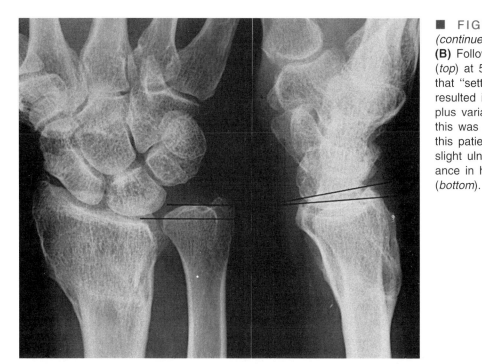

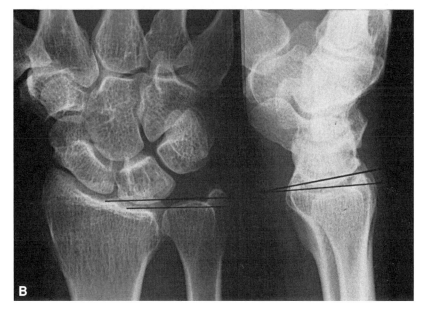

■ FIGURE 139–4
(continued)
(B) Follow-up radiographs (*top*) at 5 years show that "settling" of the graft resulted in 3 mm of ulnar plus variance. However, this was physiologic for this patient, who had a slight ulnar positive variance in his opposite wrist (*bottom*).

Our results have shown that partial resection of the ulnar head is a valuable adjuvant procedure in radial malunion and ulnar-sided wrist pain with degenerative changes of the radioulnar joint. In 15 consecutive patients in whom both operations were combined,[12] the remaining deficit of pronation was 12% and supination 14%, compared to preoperative deficits of 47 and 77%, respectively. Lengthening of the radius by osteotomy in turn corrects the ulnar variance, which is necessary to prevent painful stylocarpal impingement after hemiresection arthroplasty. If radial length cannot be obtained with radial osteotomy alone, an additional shortening osteotomy of the ulna has to be performed at the same time.

The overall results of our series of radial osteotomies are comparable to those of other authors who use similar techniques.[2,8,18,20,29,32] Our results have shown that with careful patient selection, correct indication, and refinements of the surgical technique, over 80%

excellent and good results can be expected. Initial complications and failures were caused either by technical errors, or by the improper selection of patients who had degenerative changes in the radiocarpal joint after intra-articular fracture or fixed dorsal–carpal malalignment that could not be corrected with the osteotomy.

Despite the substantially improved anatomic results of distal radial fractures with operative measures,[1,3,14,21] malunion still remains the most common complication of closed reduction and plaster fixation[5,22] for extra-articular fractures. Although deformity can be prevented with proper conservative treatment, if symptomatic malunion occurs, radial osteotomy offers better function, improves the external appearance, and normalizes the kinematics of the wrist. A successful outcome depends, however, on careful patient selection, precise angular correction, and the simultaneous assessment and treatment of associated radioulnar disorders.

References

1. Axelrod TJ, McMurtry RY: Open reduction and internal fixation of comminuted intra-articular fractures of the distal radius. J Hand Surg, 1990; 15A:1–11.
2. Bora FW, Ostermann AL, Zielinksi CJ: Osteotomy of the distal radius with a biplanar iliac bone graft for malunion. Bull Hosp Joint Dis Orthop Inst, 1984; 44:122.
3. Bradway JK, Amadio PC, Cooney WP: Open reduction and internal fixation of displaced comminuted intra-articular fractures of the distal end of the radius. J Bone Joint Surg, 1989; 71A:839–847.
4. Campbell WC: Malunited Colles' fractures. JAMA, 1937; 109:1105–1108.
5. Cooney MP, Dobyns JH, Linscheid RL: Complications of Colles fractures. J Bone Joint Surg, 1980; 62A:613–619.
6. Duparc U, Pacault JY, Valtin B: Traitement des cals vicieux du poignet par ostéotomie d'ouverture avec greffe osseuse. Ann Chir, 1977; 31:307.
7. Durman CD: An operation for correction of deformities of the wrist following fracture. J Bone Joint Surg, 1935; 17:1014–1016.
8. Ekenstam F, Hagert CG, Engkvist O, et al: Corrective osteotomy of malunited fractures of the distal end of the radius. Scand J Plast Reconstr Surg, 1985; 19:175.
9. Fernandez DL, Albrecht HU, Saxer U: Die Korrekturosteotomie am distalen Radius bei posttraumatischer Fehlstellung. Archiv für Orthopädische und Unfallchirurgie, 1977; 90:199.
10. Fernandez DL: Correction of posttraumatic wrist deformity in adults by osteotomy, bone-grafting, and internal fixation. J Bone Joint Surg, 1982; 64A:1164-1178.
11. Fernandez DL: Osteotomías del antebrazo distal: Indicación, técnica y resultados. Acta Ortopedica Latinoamericana, 1984; 11:55.
12. Fernandez DL: Radial osteotomy and Bowers arthroplasty for malunited fractures of the distal end of the radius. J. Bone Joint Surg, 1988; 70A:1538–1551.
13. Fernandez DL, Geissler WB: Korrektureingriffe bei Fehlstellungen am distalen Radius. Z Unfallchir Versicherungsmed Berufskr, 1989; 82:34.
14. Fernandez DL, Geissler WB: Treatment of displaced articular fractures of the radius. J Hand Surg, 1991; 16A:375–384.
15. Ghromley RK, Mroz RJ: Fractures of the wrist: A review of 176 cases. Surg Gynecol Obstet, 1932; 55:377–381.
16. Heim U: Stabilisation des ostéotomies de l'extrémité inférieure du radius par petite plaque en T. Ann Chir, 1977; 31:313.
17. Jupiter JB, Ruder J: Computer-generated bone models in the planning of osteotomy of multidirectional distal radius malunions. J Hand Surg, 1992; 17A:406–415.
18. Kerboul B, Le Saout J, Plossu JP, et al: Correction des cals vicieux de l'extrémité inférieure du radius par ostéotomie d'ouverture. Acta Orthop Belg, 1986; 52:134.
19. King GJ, McMurtry RY, Rubenstein JD, et al: Computerized tomography of the distal radioulnar joint: A correlation with ligamentous pathology in a cadaveric model. J Hand Surg, 1986; 11A:711–717.
20. Lehner M, Sennwald G: Korrekturosteotomie am distalen Vorderarm. Z Unfallchir Versicherungsmed Berufskr, 1989; 82:45.
21. Leung KS, Tsang HK, Chiu KH, et al: An effective treatment of comminuted fractures of the distal radius. J Hand Surg, 1990; 15A:11–17.

22. Meine J: Die Früh- und Spätkomplikationen der Radiusfraktur loco classico. Z Unfallchir Versicherungsmed Berufskr, 1989; 82:25.
23. Merle D'Aubigné R, Joussement: A propos du traitement des cals vicieux de l'extrémité inférieure du radius. Mém Acad Chir, 1945; 71:153.
24. Müller-Färber J, Griedel W: Der sekundäre Korrektureingriff am distalen Radius bei posttraumatischer Fehlstellung. Monatsschrift Unfallheilkunde, 1979; 82:23.
25. Myno DE, Palmer AK, Levinsohn M: The role of radiography and computerized tomography in the diagnosis of subluxation and dislocation of the distal radioulnar joint. J Hand Surg, 1983; 8A:23–31.
26. Pogue DS, Viegas SF, Patterson RM, Peterson PD, Jenkins DK, Sweo TD, Hokanson JA: Effects of distal radius fracture malunion on wrist joint mechanics. J Hand Surg, 1990; 15A: 721–727.
27. Posner MA, Ambrose L: Malunited Colles' fracture: Correction with a biplanar closing wedge osteotomy. J Hand Surg, 1991; 16A:1017–1026.
28. Renné J, Schmelzeiser H: Zur operativen Korrektur unter Verkürzung und in Fehlstellung verheilter typischer Radiusfracturen in Hadgelenksnähe. Monatsschrift Unfallheilkunde, 1974; 77:111.
29. Rodriguez-Meythiaz AM, Chamay A: Traitement des cals vicieux extra-articulaires du radius distal par ostéotomie d'ouverture avec interposition d'une greffe. Med et Hyg, 1988; 46: 27–57.
30. Short WH, Palmer AK, Werner FW, Murphy DJ: A biomechanical study of distal radial fractures. J Hand Surg, 1987; 12A:529–534.
31. Taleisnik J, Watson HK: Midcarpal instability caused by malunited fractures of the distal radius. J Hand Surg, 1984; 9A:350–357.
32. Watson HK, Castle TH: Trapezoidal osteotomy of the distal radius for unacceptable articular angulation after Colles' fracture. J Hand Surg, 1988; 13A:837–843.

PART

XI

Congenital Anomalies

140

Syndactyly Reconstruction

Syndactyly results from a failure of separation of digits during normal hand development.[14] Syndactyly is classified descriptively on the basis of the degree of skin bridging and the presence or absence of bony fusion. Complete syndactyly refers to a skin bridge extending to the tip of the digit, sometimes accompanied by a common nail plate, whereas incomplete indicates a shorter web. Simple syndactyly indicates the presence of a soft tissue bridge alone, whereas complex refers to the presence of bony fusion, usually involving the distal phalanges. Syndactyly may be an isolated condition, associated with other congenital anomalies, or a component of a syndrome.[7] The incidence of isolated syndactyly is 1 in every 2000 to 3000 births. Although most isolated cases are not inherited, when familial, the inheritance pattern is autosomal dominant with variable penetrance.[3,7] Males are affected more often than females, and whites more often than blacks.[7] The web between the long and ring fingers is most commonly involved, followed by the small–ring, index–long, and thumb–index, in order of decreasing frequency.[7]

The history of syndactyly surgery dates from the early 1800s and is fascinating to review.[6] The pitfalls of early procedures have been integral to the development of current techniques.[1,5,6] Although current operative designs vary, the principles of syndactyly reconstruction are well established.[1,5] The goal is to create independent digits with a more normal web. The normal web forms an oblique slope from proximal–dorsal to distal–palmar, and has a tetrahedral shape that extends to the middle of the proximal phalanx. In a reconstruction, a local flap must be used to create a new web of sufficient breadth and depth to allow abduction between digits.[1,3,6–8] Several flap designs have been advocated to reconstruct the new web.[1,4,6,9] A dorsal flap provides thin, compliant skin that matches the color of the dorsum of the hand.[1,7,9] In addition, a broad flap can be raised dorsally and will create the natural, sloping contour of the web.[1,7]

Although syndactyly is often described as webbed fingers, the amount of locally available skin is always insufficient for separation of a complete syndactyly.[7] Skin graft should be used liberally, because closing the wound prevents complete correction and does not provide sufficient skin for digit growth. Full-thickness skin grafts are preferable because they contract less than split-thickness grafts.

Longitudinal incisions on the digits will invariably cause scar contractures.[5,6] To avoid this complication, zig-zag incisions are used to create wound closures with interdigitating flaps after digit separation.[5] To avoid vascular compromise, only one side of the digit is released at a time. Therefore, multiple digit involvement requires planning of staged procedures based on hand function and deformity.[7]

Proper timing of surgery is often difficult to determine. Several factors must be considered, including the digits involved, the type of syndactyly, and the age of the patient.[2,3,10] Syndactyly involving digits of unequal length and many complex syndactylies progressively deform during growth owing to a tethering effect between the digits. These digits should be released during the first to second year of life.[8] An independent thumb should be established by 3 to 6 months of age to allow normal functional development. Simple syndactyly of the ring and middle fingers is better tolerated (Fig. 140–1); however, correction is usually performed by age 3 years. Unfortunately, the results of reconstruction at an early age are less predictable, primarily because of a higher incidence of scar contractures.[3,7,12] Thus, the timing of surgery is based on optimizing the development of hand function, prevention of progressive deformity, and technical considerations of surgery.

■ HISTORY OF THE TECHNIQUE

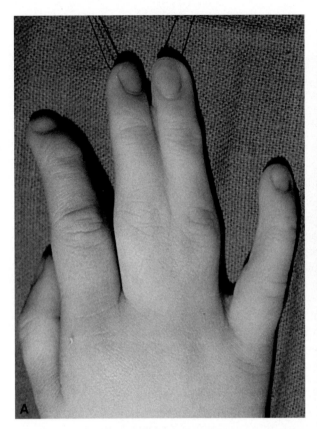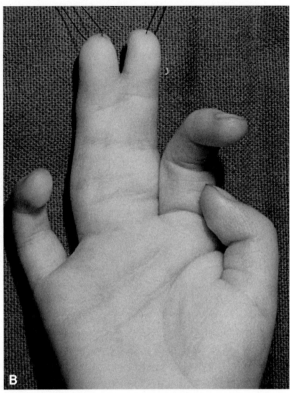

■ FIGURE 140–1
Dorsal **(A)** and palmar **(B)** intraoperative photographs of a 2½-year-old child with a simple, incomplete syndactyly of the long and ring fingers, before marking the skin incisions.

■ INDICATIONS AND CONTRAINDICATIONS

In some cases, such as incomplete long–ring finger syndactyly, the deformity causes minimal impairment, but is an obvious physical abnormality that can be corrected for cosmetic and social reasons. In other cases, such as thumb–index syndactyly, the syndactyly severely restricts hand function and causes rapidly progressive deformity.[2,7] When multiple digits are involved, the border digits will develop greater deformity and therefore should be released first to obviate further deformity.[7]

Syndactyly associated with other complicated hand deformities presents a significant reconstructive challenge. Although cosmetic considerations are important, improvement of function is more important than improvement of appearance. Even potential functional improvement must be weighed against the risks of surgery.[2] Attempts to make five independent digits may result in weak, unstable, poorly functional digits because of severe and possibly unrecognized hand dysplasia.[11] In some cases, hypoplastic digits are better left untreated or a digit ablated to create better function in the remaining digits.[7] Surgery may not be indicated for children with severe mental retardation, poor life expectancy, or multiple physical handicaps. The surgeon must have a thorough understanding of the risks and benefits of surgery before recommending operative treatment for a patient who may be able to adapt to the deformity.

■ SURGICAL TECHNIQUES

A comprehensive presentation of reconstructive techniques used in the treatment of the numerous variations of congenital syndactyly is beyond the scope of this chapter. A description of a release between the long and ring fingers illustrates the principles as well as many of the important details of syndactyly reconstruction.

General anesthesia is required for all syndactyly repairs during childhood. Documentation of the preoperative deformity should include radiographs, photographs, and an as-

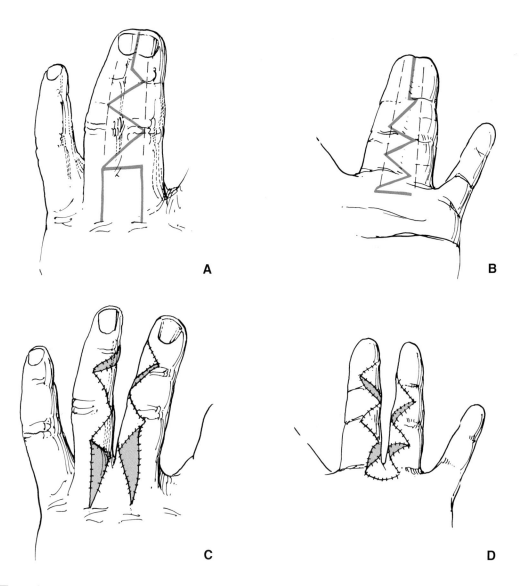

■ FIGURE 140–2

(A) Reconstruction of a complete, simple syndactyly of the long–ring fingers. A dorsal rectangular flap is outlined proximally and triangular flaps are outlined distally. **(B)** On the palmar surface, a proximal transverse incision is made halfway between the distal palmar crease and the proximal interphalangeal joint crease. Interdigitating triangular flaps are outlined in a zig-zag manner between the reference lines drawn on the midpalmar and mid-dorsal aspect of each digit. **(C)** A dorsal view after finger separation. Large skin grafts are required to cover the dorsal and proximal aspect of each finger. **(D)** A palmar view after finger separation. Again note that additional small grafts are necessary to avoid undue wound tension.

sessment of digit range of motion and joint stability. In some cases, these evaluations are best completed under anesthesia. Careful planning and drawing of incision lines is integral to the success of this operation (Fig. 140–2). Delay exsanguination and tourniquet elevation until all lines are drawn to maximize surgical time. Draw interrupted palmar and dorsal lines down the midline of each digit to serve as reference lines for the outlining of flaps. Mark the centers of the metacarpophalangeal (MP) and proximal interphalangeal (PIP) joints. A dorsal rectangular flap is preferred for web reconstruction for the reasons outlined earlier (Fig. 140–2A). The flap is based proximally and begins at the marks made over the MP joints. The sides proceed down the reference lines, with the distal edge of the flap made at the junction of the middle and distal thirds of the proximal phalanx. Interdigital triangular flaps are then outlined in a zig-zag fashion. Draw the first flap beginning at the distal corner of the rectangular flap on the shorter digit to the center of the PIP joint of the opposite finger. The remaining flaps vary depending on the length of the fingers. On shorter fingers, the next flap outline proceeds back across the web to the center of the opposite distal interphalangeal (DIP) joint. On longer fingers, two flaps should be planned between the PIP and DIP joints so that flap tip angles are approximately 60°, but not less than 45°. The final triangular flap extends from the DIP joint to the midline of the web at the level of the nail matrix. Division of the distal fingertips on the dorsal aspect is down the midline of the web or the common nail.

On the palmar surface, a proximal transverse incision is planned to join with the dorsal rectangular flap to form the new web (Fig. 140–2B). The incision is outlined to be equal in length to the distal edge of the dorsal flap and located midway between the distal palmar crease and the PIP joint flexion crease. The palmar triangular flaps are designed to interdigitate with the dorsal flaps during closure. To help design the flaps, it can be useful to draw circumferential lines extending from the tips of the dorsal flaps to the palmar reference lines of the same digit. The intersection points of these lines should bisect the bases of the palmar flaps. On the palmar surface opposite the dorsal rectangular flap, outline two additional triangular flaps. A palmar midline division can be used at the fingertip when the nails are separate. If a common nail is present, part of the distal palmar fingertip skin is used to create perionychial folds (Fig. 140–3). These long flaps are designed with sufficient lengths to reach the eponychium after finger separation. Although the flaps are narrow, they should not include the hyponychium of either finger. Rarely, a broad common nail and fingertip can be treated by skin closure with short triangular flaps made from the excess skin created by excision of the central portion of the nail, pulp, and bone.

After the tourniquet is inflated, carefully raise the skin flaps with atraumatic surgical technique to avoid crushing the delicate skin. Bipolar electrocoagulation should be used to limit tissue necrosis. Placing nylon traction sutures through the distal nail plates will allow gentle manipulation of the digits during dissection. Partial removal of subcutaneous fat will help with later closure and better skin graft take; however, venous drainage should not be unduly compromised. Begin the deeper dissection from the dorsum of the fingers. A variable amount of interconnecting fibrous tissue will be encountered between the digits. The thickest component of this tissue bridges Cleland's ligaments, which lie dorsal to the neurovascular bundles. Divide this fibrous tissue and excise larger portions, taking care to protect the neurovascular structures. Divide a common nail in the midline. A broad common nail and fingertip is narrowed by removing a strip of nail and nail bed along with excess pulp tissue from each finger. In complex syndactyly involving the distal phalanx, begin the separation at the PIP joint level and proceed distally to provide better visualization and to avoid injury to the fingertip skin during bony division. The bone can usually be cut with a scalpel. After identifying the neurovascular structures, continue the separation proximally until the common digital nerve or artery bifurcation is reached. If the nerve divides distally or forms a ring around a vessel, split the nerve proximally by

■ FIGURE 140–3
(A) Syndactyly with a common nail requires special distal flap design to reconstruct the perionychium. This technique provides full-thickness coverage without skin grafts. Long triangular flaps must be lifted very carefully to avoid flap necrosis. **(B)** Flaps are rotated to form the perionychium of each finger.

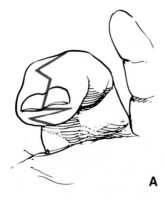

A

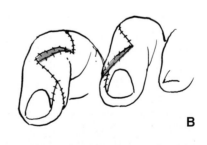

B

teasing the two branches apart with microforceps. Although distal bifurcation of the artery occurs occasionally, rarely is ligation of one branch necessary to construct the proper web. The transverse intermetacarpal ligament is not divided in typical cases with fingers of adequate length.

When finger separation is complete, suture the flaps into position, beginning with the dorsal rectangular flap, with 6-0 absorbable suture (Fig. 140–2C,D). Then sew the triangular interdigitating flaps with the finger in full extension. Although obvious skin defects are created on the dorsoproximal aspect of each digit, avoid the temptation to close completely the remaining wounds. Small skin grafts are almost universally required between portions of the triangular flaps. Release the tourniquet at this point, obtain good hemostasis, and ensure adequate vascularity to all flaps. Make patterns of the skin defects remaining on the two fingers. Obtain full-thickness skin grafts from the groin lateral to the femoral artery to avoid skin that will later grow hair. The graft should reproduce exactly the pattern of the defects. Although the procedure is tedious, the grafts must be securely sewn in place with multiple sutures. Meticulous technique creates well shaped fingers and a normal-appearing web space (Fig. 140–4).

Application of the postoperative dressing should be meticulous to ensure take of the skin grafts. Apply a petrolatum gauze to the wounds, followed by a gentle packing of Dacron batting or cotton gauze between the slightly abducted fingers to obtain gentle compression. The fingers are placed in near full extension at all joints and the bandage protected by a long arm cast with the elbow flexed to 90°. The fingers are left visible at the end of the cast for circulation checks. The parents are encouraged to limit the child's activity and attempt hand elevation for several days. Trapping the extremity between two shirts (the cast is put through the sleeve of the first shirt but not the second) will help protect the hand.

Numerous variations of flap design have been described.[2,4,6] These variations are most useful for incomplete syndactyly or difficult cases of complex syndactyly associated with

■ TECHNICAL ALTERNATIVES

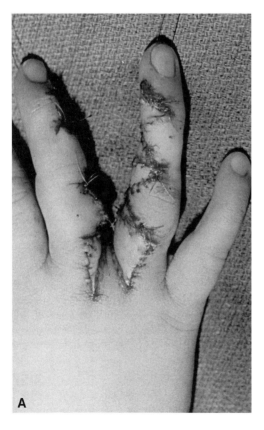
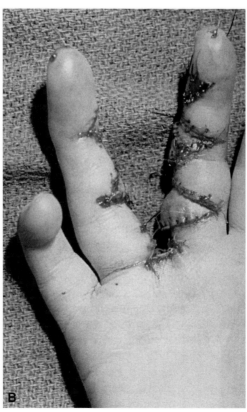

■ FIGURE 140–4
Dorsal **(A)** and palmar **(B)** postoperative photographs of the same 2½-year-old child after separation, flap rotation, and full-thickness skin grafting.

other hand deformities. Reconstruction of an incomplete syndactyly with a relatively short web can be accomplished without skin grafts using a variety of local flaps. The butterfly flap is an example of a double opposing Z-plasty that creates a natural-appearing web.[11] For local flaps to work effectively, the web must not extend to the level of the PIP joint.

When multiple digits are involved, alternating the proximal flaps used for web reconstruction between the volar and dorsal surfaces of adjacent webs helps prevent excessive scar formation on a single digit.[2] Multiple digit involvement associated with complicated hand deformities requires a thorough understanding of available variations in technique; these should be reviewed before embarking on difficult syndactyly reconstructions.[2,4,7]

Although a perfect result is difficult to achieve, several pitfalls and complications can be avoided. Improper flap design and excessive scarring are the key factors limiting a successful result.[3,8–10,12] Early distal migration of the new web results from a web flap that is too narrow or short. The flap is bordered by skin grafts and thus must have some excess breadth to allow for tethering from graft shrinkage. A longitudinal scar on the digit will invariably cause flexion and angulatory finger deformities that can become quite severe during growth. Triangular flaps should be designed to avoid creation of a gently undulating wound closure. This is accomplished by making acute zig-zag incisions with the proper tip angle and extending each incision to the digit midline; excessively sharp tip angles can cause tip necrosis and scarring.

Failure to use full-thickness skin grafts liberally and in the appropriate size is a common mistake.[3,10,12] Numerous small grafts are often required, and suturing is tedious in an infant digit. Nevertheless, flap closure under tension results in flap tip necrosis and development of contractures, and risks vascular compromise from postoperative swelling.[13] If skin graft loss occurs during healing, early regrafting must be done to avoid hypertrophic scars and contractures. Complete hemostasis and meticulous dressing application reduces graft loss.

■ REHABILITATION

The cast and dressing are usually removed after 2 to 3 weeks; however, some surgeons prefer to leave the original operative dressing on for 4 to 6 weeks. Some loss of the superficial layer of the skin grafts is often seen at the first dressing change. These wounds should be protected for an additional 2 weeks to avoid wound irritation with subsequent scar formation; a dressing and cast similar to the original is preferable. If areas of complete skin necrosis or graft loss are seen, the patient should be scheduled for a regrafting operation. After complete wound healing, no further dressings or splints usually are indicated, and the child may resume full activities and normal bathing. Occasionally, a custom scar pad can be used at night to help reduce scar hypertrophy. Formal therapy is indicated primarily for patients who had concurrent reconstructive procedures for other hand deformities.

■ OUTCOMES

A perfect cosmetic and functional outcome is difficult to achieve in syndactyly reconstruction, especially in the eyes of parents who often believe the healed wounds and skin graft areas are aesthetically displeasing. When complex hand deformities are present, the functional result is often related to the other anomalies. The parents must be cautioned that finger separation does not necessarily improve hand dexterity. A thorough preoperative discussion of the expectations and limitations of the surgical procedure will help parents prepare for the probable outcome. They must also understand that long-term follow-up is necessary, and that the initial result may not be permanent and therefore revision surgery may be needed.[13] One third of patients with simple syndactyly and two thirds of those with complex syndactyly require additional surgery.[3,10,12] Unfortunately, the earlier the initial surgery, especially in children younger than 18 months of age, the more likely it is that further surgery will be necessary.[3,7,12] Conversely, a delay in reconstruction may lead to skeletal deformities that are extremely hard to correct.[13]

The most common reasons for revision surgery are web recurrence and scar contractures.[3,6,10] Distal migration of the web is a common occurrence during rapid growth spurts, with an incidence of up to 60%.[9,10] Although total prevention of this problem is not possible, careful adherence to the principles of web reconstruction reduces the severity of recurrence. Longitudinal scar contractures in a growing child pose the greatest danger for recurrent deformity and functional impairment. Skeletal deformity can develop rapidly from scar contracture, and require revision with corrective osteotomy to realign the digit.[13] Approximately one third of patients require correction of scar contractures.[3,10,12] Whenever possible, revision surgery should be delayed until after the adolescent growth spurt to reduce the need for multiple revisions. However, skeletal deformity, joint contractures, and repetitive skin breakdown should not be allowed to occur. Under these circumstances, the benefits of early revision surgery far outweigh the risks and inconvenience of multiple operations.

References

1. Bauer TB, Tondra JM, Trusler HM: Technical modification in repair of syndactylism. Plast Reconstr Surg, 1956; 17:385–392.
2. Blauth W, Schneider-Sickert F: Syndactylies. In: Blauth W, Schneider-Sickert F (eds): Congenital Deformities of the Hand. Berlin: Springer-Verlag, 1981:10–71.
3. Brown PM: Syndactyly: A review and long term results. Hand, 1977; 9(1):16–27.
4. Buck-Gramcko, D: Congenital malformations: Syndactyly and related deformities. In: Nigst H, Buck-Gramcko D, Millesi H, Lister GD (eds): Hand Surgery. New York: Thieme, 1988; 12.12.
5. Cronin TD: Syndactylism: Results of zig-zag incision to prevent post-operative contracture. Plast Reconstr Surg, 1956; 18:460–468.
6. Davis JS, German WJ: Syndactylism. Arch Surg, 1930;21:32–75.
7. Flatt AE: Webbed Fingers. In: Flatt A (ed): The Care of Congenital Hand Anomalies, 2nd ed. St. Louis: Quality Medical Publishing, Inc., 1994:228–275.
8. Keret D, Ger E: Evaluation of a uniform operative technique to treat syndactyly. J Hand Surg, 1987; 12A:727–729.
9. Moss ALH, Foucher G: Syndactyly: Can web creep be avoided? J Hand Surg, 1990; 15B:193–200.
10. Percival NJ, Sykes PJ: Syndactyly: A review of the factors which influence surgical treatment. J Hand Surg, 1989; 14B:196–200.
11. Shaw DT, Li CS, Rickey DC, et al: Interdigital butterfly flap in the hand (double opposing Z-plasty). J Bone Joint Surg, 1973; 55A:1677–1679.
12. Toledo LC, Ger E: Evaluation of the operative treatment of syndactyly. J Hand Surg, 1979; 4A:556–564.
13. Wood VE: Congenital anomalies: Syndactyly. In: Boswick JA (ed): Complications in Hand Surgery. Philadelphia: WB Saunders, 1986:225–346.
14. Zaleske DJ: Development of the upper limb. Hand Clin, 1985; 1:383–390.

141

Constriction Ring Reconstruction

■ HISTORY OF THE
TECHNIQUE

Constriction ring syndrome has been managed by amputation of the part at or proximal to the ring, staged subcutaneous excision of the edematous tissues distal to the ring, excision of the ring either by single or staged procedures, Y–V-plasties, W-plasties, and single- or multiple-stage Z-plasties.[8,9,11,15] Amputation of an edematous yet potentially useful part of a limb or digit was abandoned after success with less drastic methods such as the Z-plasty. Similarly, excision of the ring and subcutaneous excision of the edematous tissues distal to the ring were abandoned because of the uniform failure of these techniques.[9,14] Only the Y–V-plasty, W-plasty, and Z-plasty procedures have survived as useful surgical alternatives, with the Z-plasty, owing to its tissue-sparing characteristics, being the most commonly used.[8,9,11,15] Ombrédanne, in 1937, described a surgical technique that he used for the correction of a congenital constriction ring of the lower extremity.[11] His technique is best described as a W-plasty, and included excision of the constriction ring along with opposing triangles of skin on each side, followed by subsequent interdigitation of the remaining triangles (Fig. 141–1). Miura, in 1984, described a modification of this technique that is a Y–V-and W-plasty combined.[8] He used this method to treat constriction rings in patients with severe lymphedema that jeopardized circulation (Fig. 141–2).

Although Borges[3] credits Berger[1] with the original description of a true double-flap transposition Z-plasty in 1904, it was Stevenson,[13] in 1946, who described its use for the correction of congenital constriction rings. The Z-plasty technique has remained as the most popular surgical treatment for constriction ring syndrome.[2,4,6,7,9,10,12–16]

■ INDICATIONS AND
CONTRAINDICATIONS

Deep constriction rings that produce significant lymphedema distal to the ring require surgical treatment both for cosmetic and functional purposes. Surgical correction is also advised when a noticeable construction ring is present without lymphedema.[15] Congenital constriction rings ideally should be reconstructed when the infant is between 6 to 12 months of age. Some cases with very deep and complete constriction rings are associated with severe venous and lymphatic congestion of the part distal to the band. Such cases are most often seen in the newborn nursery. Treatment is by observation only because these severely compromised parts will usually autoamputate. Simple, shallow grooves, especially incomplete rings without venous or lymphatic blockage, may not require treatment. With absorption of the infant's subcutaneous fat, the shallow groves often become less noticeable and cosmetically more acceptable.[14] However, if a cosmetically significant ring constriction remains, it may be corrected at a later date. In deep and complete rings in which the part distal to the ring is flail and without sensation, there is no potential for reconstruction and amputation is the procedure of choice. In cases of constriction rings with acrosyndactyly, the terminal syndactyly is usually corrected first, followed by treatment of the constriction ring when tissue homeostasis has been achieved, which is usually 3 to 4 months later. Constriction ring syndrome that is manifested by distal autoamputation may require revision of redundant terminal soft tissues or web deepening to improve function or cosmetic appearance.

The surgeon who treats this syndrome must know that (1) shallow rings have some subcutaneous fat and dorsal veins, in contrast to deep rings, in which there is no soft tissue between the ring and the underlying bone;[15] (2) in some deep rings even the extensor and flexor tendons and nerves are absent beneath the ring;[16,17] (3) in digits the dorsal deformity is the most prominent, in contrast to the palmar side, where the ring is not as

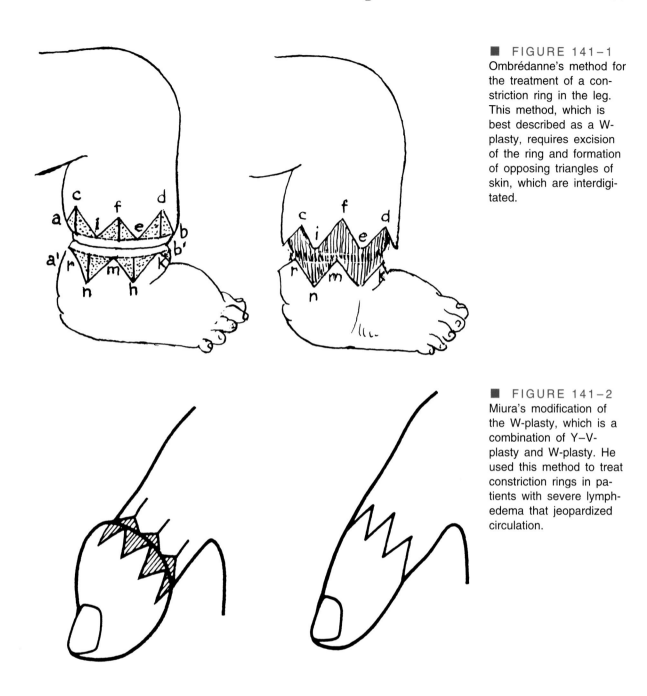

■ FIGURE 141–1
Ombrédanne's method for
the treatment of a con-
striction ring in the leg.
This method, which is
best described as a W-
plasty, requires excision
of the ring and formation
of opposing triangles of
skin, which are interdigi-
tated.

■ FIGURE 141–2
Miura's modification of
the W-plasty, which is a
combination of Y–V-
plasty and W-plasty. He
used this method to treat
constriction rings in pa-
tients with severe lymph-
edema that jeopardized
circulation.

deep and there is not as much redundant tissue; and (4) in some deep digital ring deformities the only venous drainage of the digit is through the venae comitantes of the digital
arteries, and these vascular structures must be preserved during surgical reconstruction.

Under tourniquet control, general anesthesia, and loupe magnification, the ring with
skin and subcutaneous tissue is excised down to the underlying tendons. Dorsal veins, if
present, are identified and dissected free from the surrounding subcutaneous tissues.
Loupe magnification will aid in preservation of dorsal veins, arteries, and venae comitantes. Redundant skin is usually present on each side of the ring, but most especially on
the distal side, and in digits is most prominent on the dorsal side. To obtain a tension-
free closure, not all of the redundant skin is excised. After excision of the ring, the skin and
subcutaneous tissues are mobilized as a composite layer. Next, a series of interconnected or
continuous 60° Z-plasties are marked out on the adjacent skin surfaces (Fig. 141–3). The

■ SURGICAL
TECHNIQUES

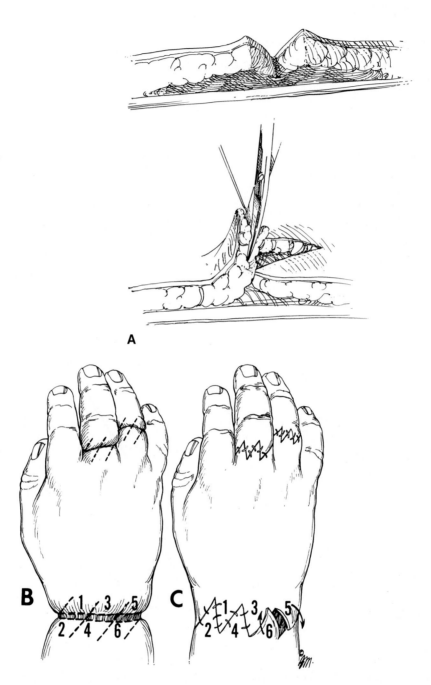

■ FIGURE 141–3
The standard 60° angle Z-plasty technique for constriction ring reconstruction. **(A)** The ring is excised down to the level between the fat and underlying vital structures. Redundant subcutaneous tissue is excised from the deep side of the mobilized flap to achieve an appropriate contour. **(B)** Sixty-degree interconnected Z-plasties are then laid out. Major arteries, venae comitantes, and nerves should be identified and preserved. Usually no more than one half of the circumference of the ring is corrected at the first operation. **(C)** The flaps of the Z-plasty are rotated and sutured with 5-0 or 6-0 chromic cat gut.

length of each limb of the Z-plasty should be one third to one half the diameter of the extremity or digit. The Z-plasty flaps are then developed with a generous layer of fat, and the flap tips are handled with fine skin hooks to avoid compromise of the tips. If the temporarily transposed flaps result in a bulge or raised band at the site of surgery, the flaps are thinned by removing fat from the deeper portions of the subcutaneous tissue. I have found this technique to be better than advancing the flaps, which may produce unwanted tension. All Z-plasties are closed with 5-0 or 6-0 chromic cat gut as skin sutures. Nonadherent gauze dressings are applied over a thin film of antibiotic ointment at the suture lines. Saline-moistened sterile cotton sheeting is used to make a conforming dressing about 1 cm thick over the operative site. Sterile cast padding is applied and the tourniquet released, followed by a long arm splint with the tips of all digits exposed for circulation checks. The splint and the dressings are removed at 10 to 12 days and the patient allowed to soak the hand in warm, soapy bath water. This facilitates spontaneous removal of the sutures and the skin debris or other residue at the operative site.

In shallow digital rings, it is safe to correct the ring deformity in one stage. However, in deep rings with no dorsal veins, it is best to correct the condition in two stages 2 to 3 months apart. Two-stage correction is also advised for constriction ring deformities about the arm and forearm. In two-stage digital correction, the dorsal half is corrected first because this is usually the deepest part of the ring. In some cases no other correction will be required.

Di Meo and others[4,7,10,16] have stated that complete single-stage excision of a circumferential constriction ring does not interfere with distal blood supply. They noted that although dorsal veins may be obstructed, the distal portion of the extremity can adapt and rely on venae comitantes alone for venous drainage. Hall and co-authors observed that the deep arterial system was the most important element for the nourishment of the overlying tissue via perforating vessels, and that this deep arterial system was not usually involved by the constriction ring.[7] However, most authors[2,5,6,8,9,12,14] agree with Stevenson[13] that staged Z-plasty is the accepted method of treatment.

■ TECHNICAL ALTERNATIVES

Both the W-plasty and Z-plasty performed in one or more stages have been used for correction of this condition.[2,8,11,15] The Z-plasty is favored over the W-plasty because it uses all available skin and avoids the potential for excessive skin tension at the repair site.[3–6,15] In most instances the ring is excised, except for those rings that are quite superficial.

Upton and Tan compared a series of constriction ring patients treated by traditional Z-plasties or W-plasties of skin with a comparable series treated by subcutaneous fat and fascial flaps and Z-plasties.[15] They reported significant long-term improvement in contour, with less recurrent skin indentation as well as less frequent complications with the subcutaneous flaps and Z-plasty technique. The W-plasty patients often had loss of the necessarily small tips of the flaps, which resulted in a very conspicuous saw-tooth deformity. All of their patients with deep rings who were treated with simple Z-plasties without contour correction (subcutaneous flaps) demonstrated some degree of recurrence of the deformity with growth. Upton and Tan stated that they solved this problem by advancing a layer of fat over the site of the ring to contour and fill in the defect before performing skin Z-plasty.

Upton and Tan's technique for dorsal digital deformities includes excision of all redundant skin, the sidewalls of the constriction ring, and excess dorsal adipose tissue. Some idea of the amount of soft tissue that needs to be excised can be determined by marking one sidewall of the constriction ring with marking ink and then pressing it against the opposing surface.[15] Subcutaneous flaps are mobilized and advanced to recontour the deformity as needed. Ideally, skin and subcutaneous closures are staggered and the Z-plasties are positioned along the midaxial side of the digit, which results in a transverse closure dorsally (Fig. 141–4). These modifications, as proposed by Upton and Tan,[15] are most suitable in the digit where most of the deformity is dorsal. However, with complete and deep bands in the wrist or forearm, the standard series of multiple Z-plasties using composite skin and subcutaneous tissue flaps of appropriate thickness is best.

Pitfalls with Z-plasty technique include (1) making the Z-plasty flaps too thick or too thin; (2) making the Z-plasty flaps too small or too large; (3) failure to preserve available dorsal veins and, in severe and deep rings, the vena comitantes that accompany the arteries; (4) inadequate excision of redundant soft tissue; and (5) one-stage correction of very deep and severe rings in digits or extremities that have two rings in tandem.

Flaps that are too thick may result in a bulky band about the repair site. Flaps that are too thin may indent or scar owing to an insufficient layer of fat, or become necrotic from insufficient blood supply. Z-plasty flaps that are too small may result in a composite annular scar that may mimic the original ring. Flaps that are too large are often cosmetically unacceptable. Failure to preserve dorsal veins when present or vena comitantes around

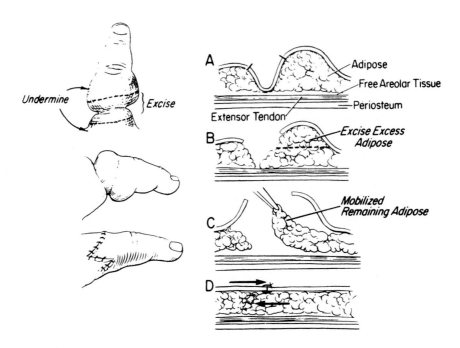

■ FIGURE 141–4
Upton and Tan's modification.[15] **(A,B)** Portions of the skin are excised from the side walls of the ring. Marking ink may be placed on one side of the wall and the two walls pressed together to indicate the amount of skin to be excised. Excess fat is removed, especially on the distal side of the ring. **(C)** Subcutaneous advancement flaps are mobilized to fill the defect. **(D)** Skin and subcutaneous closures are staggered if possible, and a standard 60° Z-plasty is completed on each midaxial side of the digit. This results in a nearly straight-line transverse closure dorsally.

the digital or forearm arteries may result in undesirable postoperative edema. Failure to excise sufficient amounts of redundant edematous tissue, especially distally, may make it difficult to obtain a smooth and balanced contour between the proximal and distal transposed flaps, and may result in a repair site that is raised and bulky. Attempting a one-stage correction of a deep ring in a digit or extremity with two rings in tandem can result in significant vascular compromise, and in such instances staged correction should be performed.

■ REHABILITATION

A formal physical therapy program is seldom required because most patients will spontaneously use the operated extremity and rapidly achieve satisfactory function. If postoperative edema is a problem, it may be controlled by elastic bandage wraps or custom-made elastic support sleeves.

■ OUTCOMES

Correction of a constriction ring usually results in improved cosmetic appearance, lessening or disappearance of edema in the part distal to the ring, and improved long-term function of the affected part. In my experience, the families of these patients have been uniformly pleased with the results of the surgical correction of these significant defects. Although necrosis of the tips of the rotated Z-plasty flaps may occur, this has not required any specific treatment and has not altered the usually satisfactory results. Even though the Z-plasty scars may be prominent in some instances, they are an acceptable alternative to the significant preoperative ring deformity. The dramatic improvement in contour of the extremity seen after Z-plasty correction has always justified the residual scars, in my opinion and in the opinion of the families of these patients.

References

1. Berger P: Autoplastie par dedoublement de la palmure et échange de la lambeaux. In Berger P, Mazet S (eds): Chirugie Orthopédique. Paris: G Ste inheil, 1904.
2. Bora FW Jr: Congenital constriction bands. In: Bora FW Jr (ed): Pediatric Upper Extremity Diagnosis and Management. Philadelphia: WB Saunders, 1986:61–62.
3. Borges AF: Historical review of Z-plastic techniques. Clin Plast Surg, 1977; 4:207–216.
4. Di Meo L, Mercer DH: Single-stage correction of constriction ring syndrome. Ann Plast Surg, 1987; 19:469–474.
5. Dobyns JH: Problems and complications in the management of upper limb anomalies. Hand Clin, 1986; 2:373–381.
6. Dobyns JH: Congenital ring syndrome (congenital constriction band syndrome). In: Green DP (ed): Operative Hand Surgery, 3rd Ed. New York: Churchill Livingstone, 1993:509–515.
7. Hall EJ, Johnson-Giebink R, Vasconez LO: Management of the ring constriction syndrome: A reappraisal. Plast Reconstr Surg, 1982; 69:532–536.
8. Miura T: Congenital constriction band syndrome. J Hand Surg, 1984; 9A:82–88.
9. Moses JM, Flatt AE, Cooper RR: Annular constricting bands. J Bone Joint Surg, 1979; 61A:562–565.
10. Muguti, GI: The amniotic band syndrome: Single stage correction. J Plast Surg, 1990; 43:706–708.
11. Ombrédanne L: Maladie amniotique. In: Ombrédanne L, Mathieu P (eds): Traité de Chururgie Orthopédique, Vol 1. Paris: Masson et Cie, 1937:44.
12. Patterson TJS: Congenital ring constrictions. Br J Plast Surg, 1961; 14:1–31.
13. Stevenson TW: Release of circular constricting scars by Z-flaps. Plast Reconstr Surg, 1946, 1:39–42.
14. Tachdjian MO: Constriction ring syndrome. In: Tachdjian MO (ed): Pediatric Orthopedics, 2nd Ed. Philadelphia: WB Saunders, 1990:291–297.
15. Upton J, Tan C: Correction of constriction rings. J Hand Surg, 1991; 16A:947–953.
16. Vusythikosol V, Hompuem T: Constriction band syndrome. Ann Plast Surg, 1988; 21:489–495.
17. Weeks PM: Radial, median and ulnar nerve dysfunction associated with congenital constricting band of the arm. Plast Reconstr Surg, 1982; 69:333–336.

142

Trigger Thumb Release

■ HISTORY OF THE
TECHNIQUE

Kelikian indicates that Nota provided the first description of congenital trigger thumb in 1850.[10] Several case reports and small series subsequently appeared in the literature of the first half of the twentieth century.[2,5,8,12,16,17] Most of these authors advocated surgical treatment using a transverse skin incision, longitudinal incision of the tendon sheath, and early postoperative motion. All reported excellent results. More recently, Dinham and Meggitt, Ger and co-authors, and Skov and co-authors reported their results after observation and surgical treatment of this condition in three large groups of patients.[3,7,13]

■ INDICATIONS AND
CONTRAINDICATIONS

Surgical release is indicated for the definitive treatment of any child with an established diagnosis of trigger thumb, provided that the child's age and overall health do not present a substantial risk to general anesthesia. These children typically present with an abnormal posture of the thumb. Usually the interphalangeal (IP) joint is fixed in a position of 20 to 75° of flexion[6,9] (Fig. 142–1), although occasionally it is locked in extension. Unlike adults, children rarely present with asynchronous motion or snapping at the IP joint. When the IP joint is fixed in flexion, any attempt to passively extend this joint will cause the metacarpophalangeal (MP) joint to hyperextend. A thickening or nodule ("Nota's node") is nearly always palpable on the palmar surface of the MP joint (Fig. 142–2). The remainder of the hand examination is negative. Both hands of the affected child should be examined because bilateral occurrence has been reported in 20 to 58% of patients with this condition.[3,7,11] The differential diagnosis includes all causes of flexion posture of the thumb, including cerebral palsy, arthrogryposis, isolated hypoplasia of thumb extensors, and thumb hypoplasia.[4] Trigger thumb may also occur in association with trisomy 13.[4]

Spontaneous resolution may occur and is most commonly noted if the diagnosis has been made at birth.[3] Spontaneous resolution after the age of 1 year is extremely unlikely and surgery is almost always required for these children. Surgical treatment is best completed before the age of 3 years. Although there are several reports in the literature that document complete resolution of symptoms after surgery regardless of age, delay in treatment beyond the age of 3 years may prolong recovery and result in residual deformity.[2,3,5,7,9,12,13,16]

■ SURGICAL
TECHNIQUES

After the induction of satisfactory general anesthesia, the patient is placed in the supine position on the operating table and a pneumatic tourniquet is applied about the proximal arm. The entire extremity is prepared and draped, the limb is exsanguinated, and the tourniquet is inflated. An assistant positions the forearm in full supination, the thumb in radial abduction and the thumb MP joint in the neutral position. Care is taken to avoid MP joint hyperextension. If the IP joint is locked in flexion, no attempt is made to manipulate it into extension at this time. The MP joint flexion crease is identified and the longitudinal axis of the proximal phalanx and metacarpal is visualized. A transverse skin incision is made immediately adjacent to but not in the MP joint flexion crease.[12] This incision should be bisected by the longitudinal axis of the proximal phalanx and metacarpal, and should extend only through the dermis. After completing the skin incision, a small skin hook is placed on each side of the wound. The assistant controls the distal skin hook and the patients' thumb with one hand and the proximal hook with the other hand. The assistant should retract and lift the skin edges. Lifting the skin edges elevates the skin flaps away from the digital nerves as the dissection proceeds. This facilitates exposure and reduces

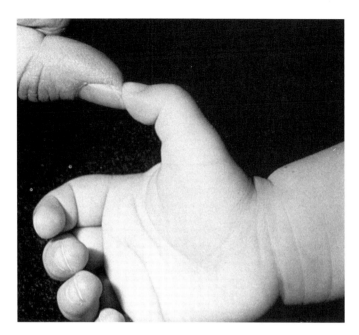

■ FIGURE 142-1
Interphalangeal joint locked in approximately 50° of flexion in a 15-month-old child.

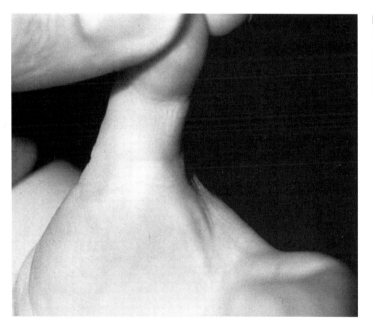

■ FIGURE 142-2
Visible and palpable thickening over the palmar surface of the metacarpophalangeal joint ("Nota's node").

the risk of iatrogenic injury to these structures. A blunt-tipped scissors is inserted into the center of the wound and used to separate the wound margins by spreading in a direction parallel to the flexor pollicis longus (FPL) tendon and digital nerves. Small strands of digital fascia are often encountered in the midline immediately below dermis. These are identified, isolated, and divided. The radial and ulnar margins of the wound are separated in a similar fashion, and the radial and ulnar proper digital nerves are identified (Fig. 142-3). Blunt dissection is continued in the midline in the areolar plane between the flexor tendon sheath and the subcutaneous tissues. This dissection should expose the entire A1 pulley and the proximal margin of the C1 pulley. The skin hooks are now replaced with small, blunt, right-angle retractors (e.g., Ragnells), and the pulley system and FPL are inspected. If the IP joint is locked in flexion, the FPL tendon usually presents with a fusiform enlargement just proximal to the A1 pulley (Fig. 142-4). The A1 pulley is now

■ FIGURE 142-3
Radial and ulnar proper
digital nerves isolated
and displayed.

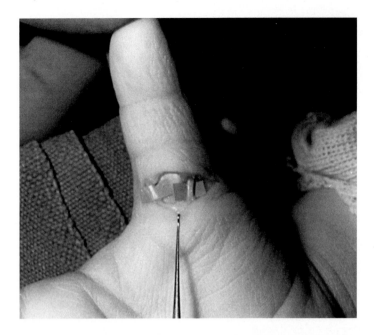

■ FIGURE 142-4
After release of the A1
pulley, fusiform thickening
of the flexor pollicis longus tendon is clearly visible.

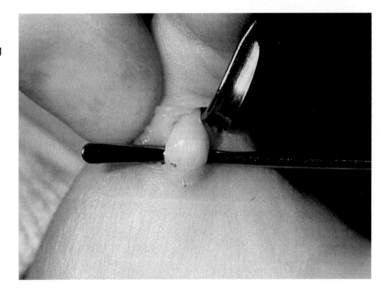

incised along its radial margin with a knife. The surgeon must be absolutely certain of
the location of the radial proper digital nerve during this portion of the procedure. The
incision begins at the proximal margin of the A1 pulley and proceeds distally until the
entire pulley is incised. The surgeon now passively extends the IP joint while holding the
MP joint in neutral and the thumb metacarpal in extension. FPL excursion is observed
and resistance, if any, is noted to IP joint extension. If tendon excursion is limited and
passive IP extension is restricted, then the tendon sheath incision is continued distally.
This extension should continue along the radial border of the sheath between the distal
edge of the A1 pulley and the distal attachment of the C1 pulley. The C1 pulley is not
incised. The wound is then irrigated and the skin closed using fine, absorbable sutures.
The skin edges should be carefully everted. A nonadherent gauze strip is applied to the
wound and covered with a 2 × 2-inch gauze sponge, and a 2-inch gauze wrap which is
extended to the wrist to prevent the dressing from slipping off in the immediate postoperative period. The tourniquet is then deflated.

The most significant potential pitfall associated with this procedure is laceration of a digital nerve. Although this complication has not been reported in children, Carrozella and co-authors reported four cases of radial digital nerve transection in adults, all of whom had a transverse skin incision.[1] They noted that the radial proper digital nerve is located 1.15 mm directly anterior to the radial sesamoid and only 2.19 mm beneath the dermis at the level of the MP joint flexion crease. Because there is no subcutaneous fat beneath the flexion crease, a transverse incision located in the MP joint flexion crease places the radial proper digital nerve at significant risk for injury. Despite these considerations, many authors have recommended a transverse incision in the MP joint flexion crease.[6,10] Alternative recommendations include a radially based "V"-shaped flap, a radial midlateral incision, and a longitudinal midline incision across the flexion crease.[1,2,7] Ger and co-authors contend that the longitudinal incision is safer because it more closely parallels the course of the radial proper digital nerve, and that it does not cause a problem with postoperative scarring or contracture.[7]

Additional technical alternatives reported in the literature include excision rather than incision of a portion of the flexor sheath, a reduction tenoplasty of the FPL, and subcutaneous division of the A1 pulley.[2,5,10,14] However, the authors of the largest reported series of patients did not use these techniques and reported excellent results.[3,7] Excision of the sheath and reduction tenoplasty both may expose the patient to the risk of tendon adherence and limited tendon excursion. Tanaka and co-authors reported their results with a subcutaneous technique completed under local anesthesia in a large group of patients who ranged in age from 5 to 80 years.[14] They concluded that this procedure was not indicated in children because it was too difficult for the young patient to provide sufficient cooperation for successful and safe completion of the procedure.

White and Jensen recommended thumb splinting in the postoperative period "for a couple of weeks," and reported excellent results in nine cases.[16] Most authors, however, recommend early motion and no postoperative splinting, and the results in all series with no splinting have been uniformly excellent.

Treatment alternatives other than surgery have been recommended by Dinham and Meggitt as well as Tsuyuguchi and co-authors.[3,15] Dinham and Meggitt recommended that only children who are older than 3 years of age at the time of presentation are indicated for surgery, and that all other children should undergo surgery only if spontaneous resolution does not occur after an appropriate period of observation. They observed spontaneous resolution within 1 year in 30% of children in whom the diagnosis was made at birth, and within 6 months in 12% in children who were 6 to 30 months of age at the time of diagnosis. Spontaneous resolution did not occur in any child older then 3 years at the time of presentation. However, more recent reports have failed to support these observations. Ger and co-authors and Skov and co-authors did not observe spontaneous resolution in any patients in their two series regardless of age at time of presentation.[7,13]

Tsuyuguchi and co-authors recommended that all children should be placed into a "coil spring splint" as primary treatment.[15] However, 25% of their patients had persistent symptoms after an average of 9.4 months of continuous splint wear.

The child's parents are instructed to keep the dressing clean and dry for 48 to 72 hours after surgery. The dressing is then removed by the parents and a bandaid is applied until the sutures are absorbed. Directed exercises and physical therapy are unnecessary. Unrestricted activity is encouraged after the dressing is removed.

Outcomes after release of congenital trigger thumb are uniformly excellent. Full IP joint range of motion is usually achieved within days to weeks. Although Dinham and Meggitt reported a 50% incidence of residual IP joint flexion contractures of 15° when surgical release was delayed until the child was more than 3 years old, no other reports have confirmed these observations.[3] Ger and co-authors reported that all 41 patients in their series had a full range of motion 1 year after surgery regardless of age.[7] They did note, however, that patients who had surgery after age 3 years recovered their motion much

■ TECHNICAL ALTERNATIVES

■ REHABILITATION

■ OUTCOMES

more slowly than those who had surgery at a younger age. Compere reported no postoperative motion deficits in a 20-year-old patient whose bilateral trigger thumbs had been untreated since age 3 years, and Skov and co-authors reported that all 37 patients in their series recovered a full postoperative range of motion regardless of their age at surgery.[2,13]

No reports have indicated any clinical problems with tendon bowstringing or adherence.[12] The surgical incision is inconspicuous, and wound healing complications have not been reported. Surgical release of a trigger thumb in an otherwise healthy child provides a predictable and satisfactory result and is the preferred method of treatment for this condition.

References

1. Carrozella J, Stern PJ, VonKuster LC: Transection of radial digital nerve of the thumb during trigger release. J Hand Surg [Am], 1989; 14A:198–200.
2. Compere FL: Bilateral snapping thumbs. Ann Surg, 1933; 97:773.
3. Dinham JM, Meggitt BF: Trigger thumbs in children: A review of the natural history and indications for treatment in 105 patients. J Bone Joint Surg, 1974; 56B:153–155.
4. Dobyns JH: Trigger digits. In: Green DP, Hotchkiss RN (eds): Operative Hand Surgery. New York: Churchill Livingstone, 1993:374–378.
5. Fahey JJ, Bollinger JA: Trigger fingers in adults and children. J Bone Joint Surg, 1954; 36A:1200–1218.
6. Flatt AE: The Care of Congenital Hand Anomalies. St. Louis: Quality Medical Publishing, 1994:90–92.
7. Ger E, Kupcha P, Ger D: The management of trigger thumb in children. J Hand Surg, 1991; 16A:944–946.
8. Hudson HW: Snapping thumb in childhood: Report of eight cases. N Engl J Med, 1935; 210:854–857.
9. Jahs SA: Trigger finger in children. JAMA, 1936; 107:1463.
10. Kelikian H: Congenital Deformities of The Hand and Forearm. Philadelphia: WB Saunders, 1974:558–565.
11. Rodgers WB, Waters PM: Incidence of trigger digits in newborns. J Hand Surg, 1994; 19A:364–368.
12. Sprecher EE: Trigger fingers in infants. J Bone Joint Surg, 1949; 31A:672–674.
13. Skov O, Bach A, Hammer A: Trigger thumbs in children: A follow-up study of thirty-seven children below fifteen years of age. J Hand Surg, 1990; 15B:466–467.
14. Tanaka J, Muraji M, Negoro H, Yamashita H, Nakano T, Nakano K: Subcutaneous release of trigger thumb and fingers in 210 fingers. J Hand Surg, 1990; 15B:463–465.
15. Tsuyuguchi Y, Tada K, Kawaii H: Splint therapy for trigger finger in children. Arch Phys Med Rehabil, 1983; 64:75–76.
16. White JW, Jensen WE: Trigger thumbs in infants. Am J Dis Child, 1953; 85:141–145.
17. Zadek I: Stenosing tenosynovitis of the thumb in infants. J Bone Joint Surg, 1942; 24:326–328.

143

Bifid Thumb Reconstruction

Since its first description by Digby in 1645, the bifid thumb has been extensively reported in the hand literature. Kanavel's[10] early recommendations of simple ablation of one of the duplicate thumbs led to universally poor results, and in the evolving desire to achieve Lister's[18] six qualities of a normal thumb, including length, stability, sensibility, mobility, dexterity, and power, newer reconstructive principles have been adopted. Attention to thenar muscle advancement, collateral ligament stability, recentralization of flexor and extensor tendons,[2] along with reconstructive osteotomies of the bony units all have yielded improved results. Even with strict adherence to these principles, complications and pitfalls do exist, and Miura[22] has warned of an approximate 25% need for revision. This chapter will review the bifid thumb reconstruction, its indications and contraindications, surgical techniques, complications, and postoperative rehabilitation and outcomes.

The infant born with a bifid thumb usually represents, by definition, an indication for surgical reconstruction. This condition, seen in approximately 0.8 per 1,000 births, with equal representation in both blacks and whites, but slightly more common in Native Americans and Asians, falls into the category of *duplication* as recommended by the International Federation of Societies for Surgery of the Hand. Although different presentations do exist with the bifid thumb, all to some degree will interfere with prehensile activity and require reconstruction. Classifications developed by Marks and Bayne,[20] Wassel,[27] and others have accurately described the different presentations of the duplicate thumb. The Wassel IV presentation, which involves the single but widened metacarpal and duplication of the proximal and distal phalanges distally (Figs. 143-1 and 143-2), is the most common presentation, seen in approximately 50% of all cases. Other presentations definitely exist in this classification and do necessitate modifications in the treatment plan, but overall goals remain the same. Specifically, they are to ablate the more hypoplastic of the two thumbs, but to combine structures from both to create a stable metacarpophalangeal (MP) joint; to align all bony units and centralize tendinous structures; to optimize range of motion of the reconstructed thumb; and to create a healthy sensate pulp for pinch and prehensile activity.

Absolute contraindications to surgical reconstruction exist, but usually are the result of the presence of more generalized systemic abnormalities possibly seen in this condition, than due to the duplicate thumb itself. Although such conditions as Holt-Oram, Diamond-Blackfan, and Fanconi's anemia usually are associated with hypoplastic thumbs, they can occur with duplicate thumbs, especially if it involves a triphalangeal component. To avoid potential intraoperative catastrophic events, hematologic indices, along with appropriate pediatric consultation, should be sought.

The development of prehensile activity follows a normal progression, and knowledge of this helps to pinpoint the optimum time for operation. Gross grasp and grip are usually seen at approximately 6 months of age, with thumb and index finger function at close to 1 year of age. Voluntary release is seen at approximately 18 months of age, with a functional pattern established between 2 to 3 years of age. There is usually no definite need to reconstruct before the infant is 1 year of age, and as pulmonary structures will mature greatly during this time, waiting will afford a much better anesthetic risk. Splinting the bifid thumb during this time has been supported in the Japanese literature to make the

■ FIGURE 143–1
Preoperative photograph
of the more common
Wassel Type IV bifid
thumb.

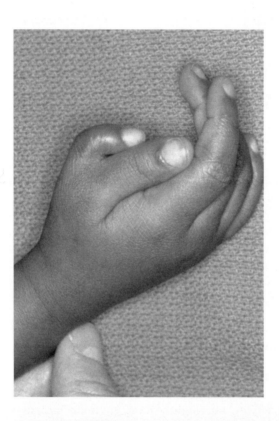

■ FIGURE 143–2
Preoperative radiograph
of the same patient. No-
tice the more hypoplastic
radial bifid component.

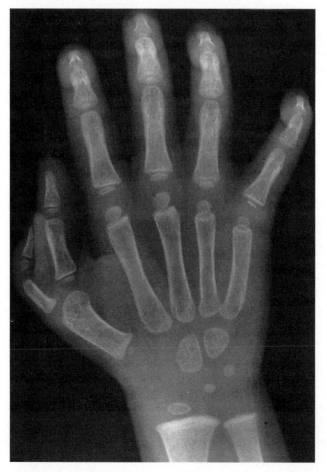

surgical reconstruction less complex. However, the splint usually is cumbersome for the child, difficult to keep in place, and usually not beneficial on a long-term basis.

Therefore, surgical reconstruction is optimum between 1 to 2 years of age. With continued growth, the neurovascular and tendinous structures will be larger, and postoperative casting will be easier to apply and maintain.

Although meticulous surgical technique is instrumental in obtaining a good result with bifid thumb reconstruction, equally as important is the preoperative planning. Hematologic indices, including complete blood count with differential, platelet count, along with PT and PTT, should be checked preoperatively to rule out thrombocytopenia or coagulopathy. Genetic counseling along with extensive discussion with the parents is important to explain that even though their child has a duplicate thumb, removal of the more hypoplastic one and reconstruction will still probably leave the child with a thumb that will be smaller than the contralateral normal one. Referring to the duplicate thumb as a "split thumb" as Ezaki[5] has stressed will help to further reinforce this with the parents. It also is vital to establish with the parents that even after optimum reconstruction, interphalangeal motion will remain limited, averaging between 0° to 30°. Postoperative sequelae such as the zigzag deformity, resulting from progressive angular deformity, should be discussed with the parents along with the approximate 25% need for revision. All of these factors, if well discussed preoperatively, hopefully will avoid any misconceptions that may arise and are instrumental in preoperative planning. Frequent physical examination of the child in the first year of life, along with periodic radiographic examination, is important in planning the proposed surgical procedure. Simple ablation of one of the thumbs has usually failed. The best results are obtained by ablating the hypoplastic thumb, centralizing flexor and extensor tendons, aligning bony units with osteotomies, reconstructing the MP collateral ligament, and judicious use of skin incisions providing adequate skin coverage. Observing the child while at play, or examining for skin creases on the bifid thumb, will usually reveal the radial component to be hypoplastic and better suited for removal. Palpation of the flexor and extensor tendons can give further information about their contribution to angular deformity, as they commonly will be displaced in a radial direction and need centralization. Lister along with Tupper and others have described the *pollex abductus*, an abnormal insertion of the flexor tendon into the radial aspect of the extensor apparatus that potentiates a possible angular deformity and needs to be evaluated both pre- and intraoperatively.[18,27] Periodic radiographic examination will give information on the bony units. Very commonly, a wide metacarpal head will be seen, that requires an intraoperative reduction osteotomy (Wassel IV). Collateral ligament instability needs to be assessed. Most commonly, the radiocollateral ligament to the MP joint is underdeveloped and requires reconstruction. The thenar muscle function should be evaluated, as its usual insertion is into the more radial thumb, and will require takedown and transfer to the reconstructed component at time of repair.

The surgery is performed under general anesthesia with the patient in the supine position and the upper extremity on a hand table. A tourniquet is placed high on the arm to prevent breakthrough intraosseous bleeding, and after exsanguination inflated to approximately 100 mm above systolic blood pressure.

The initial skin incision can either be longitudinal with later closure with a Z-plasty, or made in a zigzag fashion beginning just distal to the carpometacarpal joint, based on the radial aspect of the hand, and encircling the radial hypoplastic thumb, continuing distally to join the ulnar thumb. It is important to avoid the longitudinal scar as this can contribute to postoperative angular deformity. The skin flaps should be developed and retracted to allow exposure of all tissues until the actual deep anatomic structures have been defined. The presence of anomalous tendons along with neurovascular structures innervating the duplicate thumb should be identified and protected. Once the determination is made to remove the more hypoplastic thumb, the neurovascular structures can be safely ligated. The tendons should be dissected back to their bifurcation with attention to retaining these important structures for possible augmentation in the reconstructed thumb.

■ SURGICAL TECHNIQUES

The thenar muscles are identified, dissected from the surrounding tissue, and released from their insertion into the more radial hypoplastic thumb, which will be removed. Although the radial component is usually the hypoplastic one, the thenar muscles do attach to this, and it is instrumental to detach them for later readvancement to the remaining ulnar thumb. This should be tagged at its tendinous portion with a suture and retracted proximally to give better exposure to the usually widened metacarpal head.

At this point, a 10-mm wide strip of tissue, including periosteum from the proximal phalanx and capsule from the MP joint, along with the proximally based periosteum of the metacarpal, is developed and tagged for later distal and volar advancement to reconstruct the radial collateral ligament of the MP joint (Fig. 143–3). This dissection not only allows construction of the collateral ligament but also gives excellent access to the MP joint, where the widened metacarpal head, commonly even a dual faceted structure, is found (Wassel IV). This extra facet is shaved down with a no. 15 blade or no. 69 Beaver blade. If the metacarpal also is angulated in an ulnar direction, a closing wedge osteotomy based radially is now performed. Because the bony structures usually are small, a fine bone biter is usually all that is needed to create a closing wedge osteotomy based radially, leaving the ulnar cortex intact. It can then be closed down with manual pressure, straightening the thumb (Fig. 143–4). The osteotomy is fixed with a 0.028 or 0.035 Kirschner wire (Fig. 143–5). Osteotomies at the level of the proximal phalanx should be addressed at this point and, if needed, performed to confirm that all joint surfaces are aligned perpendicular to the longitudinal axis of the bone.

With the osteotomy aligned and fixed with the Kirschner wire, the reconstructed radial collateral ligament of the MP joint is sutured distal and volar to recreate its normal orientation (Fig. 143–6). The previously dissected thenar muscles are advanced and attached to the periosteum at the base of the proximal phalanx. The extensor pollicis longus and flexor pollicis longus tendons frequently need to be recentralized at this point. Also, abnormal insertions of the flexor pollicis longus (pollex abductus) need to be recognized and released to prevent potential angular deformity. Extratendinous structures from the ablated thumb can be used to augment or help centralize the retained tendinous structures, although in a majority of cases retained tendons are ample enough to motor the thumb. The incision is now closed with particular attention to using a zig-zag design to avoid development of

■ FIGURE 143–3
The 10-mm wide strip of periosteum and ligament is used to reconstruct the radial collateral ligament. (From: Morrissy RT: Atlas of Pediatric Orthopaedic Surgery. Philadelphia, JB Lippincott, 1992.)

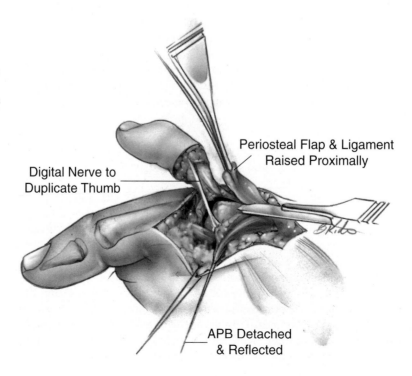

Periosteal Flap & Ligament
Raised Proximally

Digital Nerve to
Duplicate Thumb

APB Detached
& Reflected

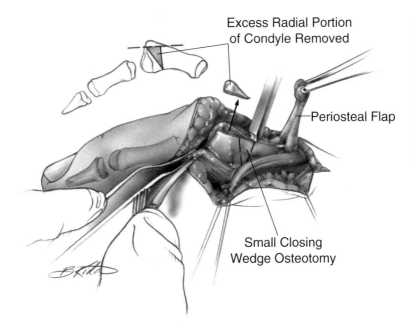

Excess Radial Portion of Condyle Removed

Periosteal Flap

Small Closing Wedge Osteotomy

■ FIGURE 143–4
The illustration showing the proposed reduction and closing wedge osteotomy with the reconstructed radial collateral ligament. (From: Morrissy RT: Atlas of Pediatric Orthopaedic Surgery. Philadelphia, JB Lippincott, 1992.)

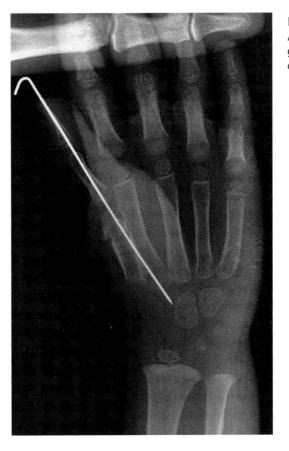

■ FIGURE 143–5
An intraoperative radiograph showing the osteotomy fixed with a K-wire.

a longitudinal contracted scar (Fig. 143–7). Final trimming of the skin flaps is better done at the end of the procedure, although shortage of skin is rarely a problem.

The pin is cut outside the skin, and the tourniquet let down before final application of the dressing to confirm satisfactory capillary refill. Intraoperative radiographs should be performed to check the pin and final position of the osteotomies. A long-arm splint is

■ FIGURE 143–6
The periosteal flap is sutured distal and volar to recreate the orientation of the radial collateral ligament. (From: Morrissy RT: Atlas of Pediatric Orthopaedic Surgery. Philadelphia, JB Lippincott, 1992.)

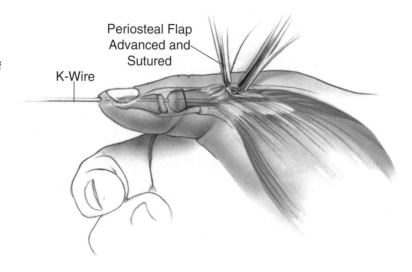

Periosteal Flap
Advanced and
Sutured

K-Wire

■ FIGURE 143–7
An intraoperative photograph of the reconstructed thumb.

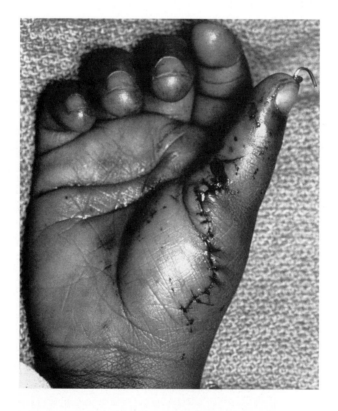

applied at this time, incorporating all the digits, including the thumb, in a boxing glove type fashion to optimize the chance of the dressing remaining on for the duration.

■ REHABILITATION

After surgery, patients, because of their young age, are usually kept overnight with the extremity elevated on 1 or 2 pillows. The patient usually is discharged the next day and a sling or sling-and-swathe type soft dressing is used to hold the dressing in place.

Usually the dressing is not changed for approximately 3 weeks, at which time radiographs are taken. If the osteotomies are healed, the pin is removed and the patient is placed into a resting thumb-spica splint out to the tip of the digit for an additional 2 to 3 weeks. The splint may be removed for bathing, and initiation of active range of motion is usually started at this time. At the end of this period, the splint can be reduced to nighttime and naptime wear, decreasing this to just nighttime wear for an additional 6 months.

The preceding discussion centered on the most common presentation of the bifid thumb, namely the Wassel IV type. Different presentations of the duplicate thumb will require alterations in the treatment plan, but overall goals as previously stated remain the same. For the more rare presentation of the Wassel II duplicate thumb, with a single proximal phalanx with a duplicate distal phalanx, the Bilhaut-Cloquet procedure with central excision of bone, soft tissue, and nail has been recommended, and the reader is provided references, although long-term follow-up has shown problems with the growth plate, nail growth, and decreased range of motion.

■ TECHNICAL ALTERNATIVES

Radiographs may sometimes reveal, as Bayne has described, a "mixed quality of duplication." This condition needs to be evaluated preoperatively as reconstruction will require removal of the radial component at the level of the metacarpal with transfer of the ulnar component to the base of the more radial metacarpal.

Potential problems with vascularity can exist. Although preoperative planning does not routinely call for the use of arteriography, Kitayama has studied the pattern of arterial distribution of the duplicate thumb and found that greater than 75% of the time there is a digital vessel to each component. However, 5% of the time there is only one digital vessel to the ulnar component, establishing possible ischemic consequences if the radial component is saved, although in actuality almost always the radial component is removed.[14]

Inadequate attention to proper skin closure to prevent longitudinal scar formation, thenar muscle advancement, radial collateral ligament reconstruction at the MP joint, realigning bony units perpendicular to joint surfaces, and centralizing tendinous structures can all separately and in combination contribute to progressive angular deformity. I again emphasize the importance of precise intraoperative attention to avoid these pitfalls and prevent an unsatisfactory result.

■ OUTCOMES

It is important in the early postoperative period to again discuss with the parents at length the long-term results after bifid thumb reconstruction. Reaffirming once more that the final appearance of the thumb will not be the same as the contralateral one is important. The interphalangeal (IP) joint motion will not increase greatly from the preoperative range and it is important to remind the parents that 0° to 30° of IP joint motion can be expected. Besides the limitations inherent in the surgical reconstruction, the normal continued growth of the child may further enhance the possibility of angular deformity, and reminding the parents of the reported 25% need for revision surgery is prudent at this point.[23] However, even with the reconstructed thumb being slightly smaller and slightly more stiff, the parents can expect their child to have a thumb that will remain very functional and of satisfactory appearance if the surgeon adheres to the recommended principles (Fig. 143–8).

Long-term follow-up by many authors has yielded similar results. Trombino, Blair and others, in more than 20 years of follow-up of 71 patients, found a 42% need for further revision, 20° of motion at the IP joint, with an 80% incidence of instability at the MP or IP joints when only simple excision of the bifid thumb component was performed, but much better results occurred with attention to careful surgical technique (William Blair, University of Iowa, personal communication). Other long-term studies, including those of Dobyns,[3] Goffin,[8] Miura,[22] and Bayne, all basically reaffirm these findings. In summarizing their complications, they usually include decreased motion, instability at the reconstructed MP joint, development of a longitudinal scar, incomplete correction, along with a characteristic angular deformity known as the zig-zag deformity. Decreased motion, especially at the IP joint, as stated, is common with some studies finding an average of 0° to 30° of motion. Repeat joint releases have not been successful and usually nothing is done for this, however, if the patient does have discomfort arthrodesis can be considered.

Instability at the reconstructed MP joint is usually the result of inadequate advancement

■ FIGURE 143–8
The same reconstructed thumb approximately 1 year after surgery.

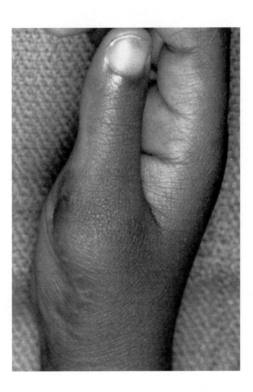

of the periosteal capsular flap and may need revision if this becomes problematic. Care must be taken in developing this periosteal capsular flap as retention of a bit of cartilage may later ossify and not only potentiate the instability but cause bony prominence at the metacarpal head. Frequently joint stiffness may result from secondary revision procedures, and again arthrodesis versus chondrodesis should remain viable options.

The most troublesome complication involves the development of a zig-zag deformity.[13] This is manifested by ulnar deviation at the proximal phalanx in combination with radial deviation of the distal phalanx, and has many causes including; (1) incompetent radial collateral ligament at the MP joint; (2) residual wide metacarpal head with under correction; (3) a longitudinal scar; and (4) radial displacement of the EPL and FPL. The infant's continual pinch mechanism accentuates this collapse pattern. This deformity can be further potentiated by the sometimes present pollex abductus which involves the aberrant attachment of the FPL to the EPL radially. The zig-zag deformity is unresponsive to conservative splinting and revision includes Z-plasty revision of the longitudinal scar, "slimming" down of the metacarpal head with possible reconstructive osteotomy, and many times removal of the radial half of the EPL tendon and reattachment of the FPL in a more centralized position.

References
1. Cheng JCY, Chan KN, Ma YFY: Polydactyly of the thumb: A surgical plan based on 95 cases. J Hand Surg, 1984; 9A:155–165.
2. Dobyns JH: Duplicate thumbs (split thumbs). In: Green DP (ed): Operative Hand Surgery, 3rd Ed, New York: Churchill Livingstone, 1993:440–450.
3. Dobyns JH, Lipscomb PR, et al: Management of thumb duplication. Clin Orthop, 1985;195: 26–44.
4. Evans D: Editorial: Polydactyly of the thumb. J Hand Surg, 1993; 18B:3–4.
5. Ezaki MB: Radial polydactyly. Hand Clin, 1990; 6:577–589.
6. Flatt A: Extra Thumbs. In: The Care of Congenital Hand Anomalies, 2nd Ed, St. Louis: Mosby, 1994:120–146.
7. Fujita S: Primary correction of clinoarthrotic deformity in thumb polydactyly. J Japan Soc Surg Hand, 1991; 8:171–177.

8. Goffin D, Leclercq C: Thumb duplication: Surgical treatment and analysis of sequels. Ann Hand Upper Limb Surg, 1990; 9:119–121.
9. Hartrampf CR, Vasconez LO, et al: Construction of one good thumb from both parts of a congenitally bifid thumb. Plast Reconstruct Surg, 1974; 54:149–151.
10. Kanavel AB: Congenital malformations of the hands. Arch Surg, 1932; 25:308–316.
11. Kawabata H, Masatomi K, et al: Treatment of residual instability and extensor lag in polydactyly of the thumb. J Hand Surg, 1983; 18B:5–8.
12. Kawabata H, Tada K, et al: Revision of residual deformities after operations for duplication of the thumb. J Bone Joint Surg, 1990; 72A:988–998.
13. Kitayama Y, Tsukade S: Patterns of arterial distribution in the duplicated thumb. Plast Reconstruct Surg, 1983; 72:535–541.
14. Kleinert HE, Greenburg AB, et al: Treatment of the reduplicated thumb. J Bone Joint Surg, 1973; 55A:874.
15. Landsmeer JMF: Studies in the anatomy of articulation. ACTA Anatomica, 1960, Supplement 288–303.
16. Light TR: Treatment of preaxial polydactyly. Hand Clin, 1992; 8:161–175.
17. Lister G: Pollex abductus in hypoplasia and duplication of the thumb. J Hand Surg, 1991; 16A:626–633.
18. Lister G: The choice of procedure following thumb amputation. Clin Orthop, 1985; 195:45–51.
19. Manske PR: Treatment of duplicated thumb using a ligamentous periosteal flap. J Hand Surg, 1898; 14A:728–733.
20. Marks TW, Bayne LG: Polydactyly of the thumb: Abnormal anatomy and treatment. J Hand Surg, 1978; 3A:107–116.
21. Miura T: An appropriate treatment for postoperative Z-formed deformity of the duplicated thumb. J Hand Surg, 1977; 2A:380–386.
22. Miura T: Duplicated thumb. Plast Reconstruct Surg, 1982; 69:470–479.
23. Simmons BP: Polydactyly. Hand Clin, 1985; 1:545–577.
24. Tada K, Kagawa KY, et al: Duplication of the thumb. J Bone Joint Surg, 1983; 65A:584–598.
25. Temtamy SA, McKusick VA: Polydactyly as an isolated malformation. In: The Genetics of Hand Malformations, New York: A. R. Liss, 1978:372–392.
26. Tupper J: Pollex abductus due to congenital malposition of the flexor pollicis longus. J Bone Joint Surg, 1969; 51A:1285–1290.
27. Wassel HD: The results of surgery for polydactyly of the thumb. Clin Orthop, 1969; 64: 175–193.
28. Wood VE: Polydactyly in the triphalangeal thumb. J Hand Surg, 1978; 3A:436–451.
29. Yasuda M: Pathogenesis of preaxial polydactyly of the hand in human embryos. J Embryol Exper Morphol, 1975; 33:745–756.

144

Pollicization

"Pollicization" means a construction of a thumb. The term derives from the Latin word *pollex*, for thumb. The technique is applicable in congenital cases as well as in trauma cases with amputation of the thumb. In congenital cases, the index finger or the radial-most finger is used in almost all patients; in trauma cases, any finger can be transposed to the site of the thumb, especially if it is also damaged.

The technique was used initially only in trauma cases and was published more than 100 years ago. Early techniques did not result in the preservation of sensibility. The refined technique with preservation of full sensibility by digital transposition on a neurovascular pedicle was described simultaneously by several authors in different countries: Gosset in 1949 in France,[10] Hilgenfeldt in 1950 in Germany[13] (first transposition of the middle finger in July 1943), Bunnell in 1952, and Littler in 1952 and 1953 in the United States.[7,15,16] Different clinical trials of this method in congenital cases were published several years later by Riordan,[19] Harrison,[11,12] Edgerton and co-authors,[8] and White.[22,23] I developed my standardized technique over a period of more than 10 years, publishing it in 1971 and again in 1981.[4,6] This technique modified the incision recommended by Blauth.[1,2] Other detailed descriptions of the pollicization technique were given by Engloff and Verdan,[9] Kleinman,[14] Manske and McCarroll,[17,18] Strickland and Kleinman,[20] and others.

Pollicization of the index finger or another radial finger is indicated in the following conditions: aplasia of the thumb, grade 3 and 4 hypoplasia of the thumb, five-fingered hand, triphalangeal hypoplastic thumb, special cases of thumb duplication and triplication, mirror hand, and partial aplasia of the thumb.

Although in most of these malformations the indication is clear, there is some controversy about the removal of the hypoplastic thumb and pollicization of the index finger in grades 3 and 4 hypoplasia of the thumb. In some cultures, it is of extreme religious importance to have a hand with five digits. Therefore, Japanese authors in particular have described techniques for reconstruction of a high-grade hypoplastic thumb, with major surgical efforts in several stages. Although a thumb is retained, the results are considered unsatisfactory from some points of view. Only in cases of hypoplasia grade 3A, in which a carpometacarpal thumb is present although unstable, is it justified to improve the hypoplastic thumb by joint stabilization, tendon transpositions, and skin plasties.

The main contraindication is hypoplasia of the index finger, which may occur in some cases of radial club hand.

The first 2 or 3 years of life are the optimal age for performing a pollicization procedure. Experienced surgeons often prefer to do this operation as early as the second half of the first year of life, to enhance the integration of the pollicized index finger into thumb functions. Long-term results show that the adaptation of the bones and muscles to the new role of a thumb, including hypertrophy, is better the earlier in life the operation is performed, with a consequently longer postoperative growth period.

The operation is performed under general anesthesia with tourniquet control to provide a bloodless field. The incision encircles the index finger at the level of the basal third of the proximal phalanx. The incision forms a dorsal triangle, which is split by a longitudinal incision up to the level of the proximal interphalangeal joint. On the palmar aspect, an "S"-shaped incision is made near the radial border of the palm, ending at the wrist skin

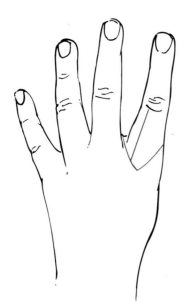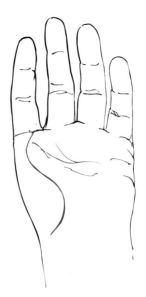

■ FIGURE 144–1
Skin incision for pollicization of the index finger.

crease (Fig. 144–1). This incision is quite different from the incision used in cases of traumatic amputation, where a palmar pedicled skin flap is usually used to cover the newly
formed web space. In congenital cases, the recession of the index ray reaches much more
proximally; the volume of the space comprising the proximal phalanx has been increased
by the reattachment of the interossei to this part of the former index finger, so that skin
has to be added to close this part. This can be done only by a skin flap with a dorsal
pedicle. In cases of syndactyly between a hypoplastic thumb and the index finger, the
incision is extended in a zig-zag form to the tip of the hypoplastic thumb.

The dissection starts with the identification of the neurovascular structures for the index
finger. In the radial neurovascular bundle, the artery can be much more radial than the
nerve in cases of a hypoplastic thumb (grade 3 or 4). In other cases, the artery on the
radial side of the index finger is completely missing. The ulnar neurovascular bundle has
to be separated from the middle finger by ligating the arterial branch to the radial side
of the middle finger and completing an interfascicular dissection of the common digital
nerves for 15 to 20 mm. Sometimes, the fascicles running to the middle finger form a ring
around the common digital artery. To prevent any kinking after transposition of the index
finger, this ring has to be widened by microsurgical dissection of the nerve. On the dorsal
aspect, at least one and preferably two of the veins have to be preserved together with
the two dorsal nerves.

The tendons of the extrinsic extensors and flexors are dissected. The A1 pulley and the
proximal aspect of the A2 pulley are divided. Sometimes, the superficial flexor has a
muscle belly in the palm; in other cases this muscle and tendon are absent. A lumbrical
muscle for the index finger is present in only about half of the cases; it forms the radial
slip of the dorsal aponeurosis, which inserts into the proximal phalanx. The ulnar slip is
formed by superficial parts of the first palmar interosseous, whereas its deeper part also
inserts onto the proximal phalanx. These insertions are detached. The lateral bands of
the dorsal aponeurosis are separated from the central band for later reattachment of the
interossei.

The metacarpal bone is divided at the level of the epiphyseal plate, which is deliberately
destroyed to prevent longitudinal growth of the metacarpal head remnant, after it assumes
the role of the trapezium. The metacarpal shaft is resected subperiosteally in a manner
that preserves the insertions of the radial wrist flexors and extensors. Usually, the proximal
osteotomy is performed at a level that preserves 4 to 6 mm of the base. Excision of the
metacarpal shaft provides better access to the two interossei. They are separated into their

proximal aspects, because they will now become antagonists. This dissection must be done very carefully so that the nerve supply to these muscles is not damaged.

At the end of this dissection, the index finger is pedicled only on its flexor and extensor tendons, the two palmar neurovascular bundles, and the dorsal veins and nerves.

Excision of most of the metacarpal bone has shortened the index finger, so that its length approximates that of a thumb. The fixation of the transposed index finger should be done in the correct position of a thumb. This means that the index finger is rotated 140 to 160° into pronation on the longitudinal axis and positioned in about 40° of abduction (Fig. 144–2). With regard to the wide range of motion in the metacarpophalangeal (MP) joint of a child, a hyperextension deformity would occur if the base of the metacarpal were fixed in its previous anatomic orientation. This hyperextension of the new thumb can be prevented by prefixing the index MP joint in full extension.[3–5] The metacarpal head is turned for about 70° into hyperextension and fixed with absorbable sutures to the base of the metacarpal (Fig. 144–3). The former technique of Kirschner wire fixation has been abandoned because it has become evident that it is necessary to achieve only fibrous rather than bony union.

For optimal function of the pollicized index finger, reestablishment of proper muscle balance is essential. Because the skeleton is shortened, the intrinsic as well as extrinsic muscles become relatively too long. They have to be shortened, with the exception of the flexor. The muscle belly will partially adapt to the new length by contracture, allowing a range of flexion that is sufficient for a thumb. The two interossei are reattached to the extensor aponeurosis, which is now at the level of the former proximal interphalangeal joint. The lateral bands are passed through the distal parts of the muscle bellies, and looped back onto themselves and sutured. The central part of the extensor aponeurosis is adapted to the new length by plication (Fig. 144–4). In cases of two or three extensor tendons, the most radial tendon can be reattached on the base of the new metacarpal (former proximal phalanx) as a new abductor pollicis longus.

With this procedure, the former index finger muscles and tendons will have the action of the following thumb muscles:

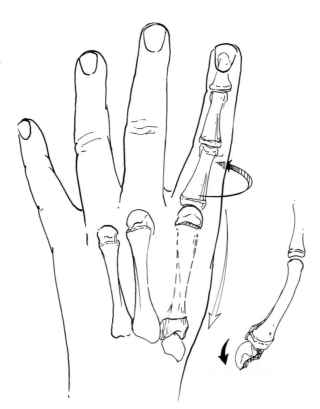

■ FIGURE 144–2
Most of the metacarpal bone is excised, the base is retained, and the digit is rotated into pronation and positioned in abduction.

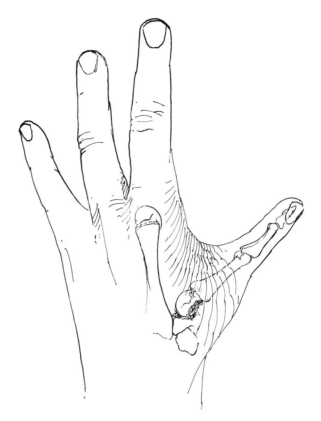

■ FIGURE 144–3
The metacarpal head is tilted about 70° into extension to prevent later hyperextension deformity, and is sutured in place.

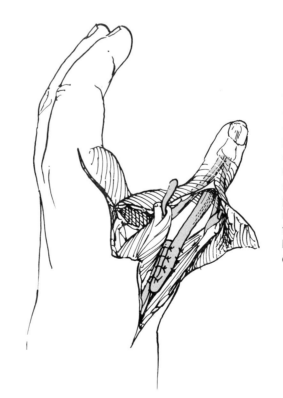

■ FIGURE 144–4
Muscular stabilization is achieved by reattachment of the two interossei to the lateral bands of the dorsal aponeurosis, shortening of the central band by plication, and fixation of the most radially located extensor tendon (mostly the index finger part of the extensor digitorum) as a new abductor pollicis longus to the base of the new metacarpal.

First dorsal interosseous—abductor pollicis brevis
First palmar interosseous—adductor pollicis
Extensor digitorum (part to the index)—abductor pollicis longus
Extensor indicis—extensor pollicis longus

The tension with which the tendons and muscles are sutured should be modest to avoid overpowering the flexor tendons, which are not shortened.

In the rare cases of absence of the first dorsal interosseous (also called the "abductor indicis" by some authors), active palmar abduction and opposition can be achieved by an immediate opponensplasty, with the flexor superficialis tendon of the digit to be transposed. This tendon is no longer used for the new thumb. This primary opponensplasty avoids secondary correction as reported by several authors, especially for a five-fingered hand.

After shortening and rotation of the index finger, the skin flaps will fall automatically into their new positions if the incision was placed correctly. The resulting suture line (Fig. 144–5) avoids any skin tension or even contracture. Suturing of the palmar wound margin contributes to maintaining the correct rotation of the new thumb. Usually, excess skin on the dorsoradial skin flap can be excised to fill the defect on the dorsum of the thumb at the new metacarpal level.

The appearance of the new thumb may be improved by further excision of a few millimeters of the skin on the palmar aspect of the former proximal phalanx. This will give the new thumb a more normal appearance by flattening the first web space.

The operation is finished by the application of an above-elbow plaster splint with inclusion of the new thumb.

■ TECHNICAL
ALTERNATIVES

Fortunately, the number of complications is quite small if both the operative details are carefully observed and the surgical technique is performed skillfully.[6] In my personal series of more than 500 pollicizations, marginal skin necrosis was seen in several cases but has not influenced the final outcome. I have seen one instance of complete necrosis of the pollicized digit. This was associated with unusual anomalies of the blood vessels, and was seen long before we were able to perform microvascular surgery. Three cases in which the radial digital artery was absent and the ulnar digital artery was accidentally divided were saved by microvascular arterial repair.

Another severe complication that can occur is division of the nerve supply to the first dorsal interosseous, which can result in a condition similar to a low median nerve palsy.

■ FIGURE 144–5
Suture line after transposition of the index finger to the site and position of a thumb.

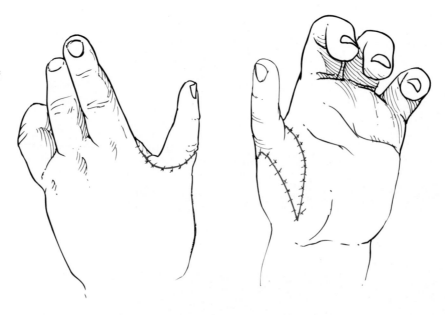

This happened in two cases in my series; in one the function of the thumb was improved by a secondary opponensplasty.

Aseptic necrosis of the metacarpal head was seen in 12 cases. It is a minor complication that has never caused either functional deficit or complaints. Ossification of the periosteal remnants at the base of the former second metacarpal bone was also seen in several cases, resulting in some limitation of the range of motion in the new carpometacarpal joint. In only one case was it necessary to improve mobility by excision of this new bone.

Although secondary procedures for improving the results were reported by several authors in a surprisingly high percentage of cases,[9,17,21] the indications for such an intervention were very limited in my own series of more than 500 pollicizations. A secondary opponensplasty was necessary on five occasions. In two patients a fusion of the new MP joint was done to correct a fixed flexion–adduction contracture. In two patients operated on early in my experience, an osteotomy was necessary to correct a hyperextension deformity, whereas two other patients underwent excision of excessive dorsal skin and subcutaneous tissue. Extensor tenolysis was indicated in three cases of pollicization in radial clubhand patients, and excision of periosteal ossification at the base of the new thumb was necessary in one patient. In four cases, it was necessary to shorten the remnants of the

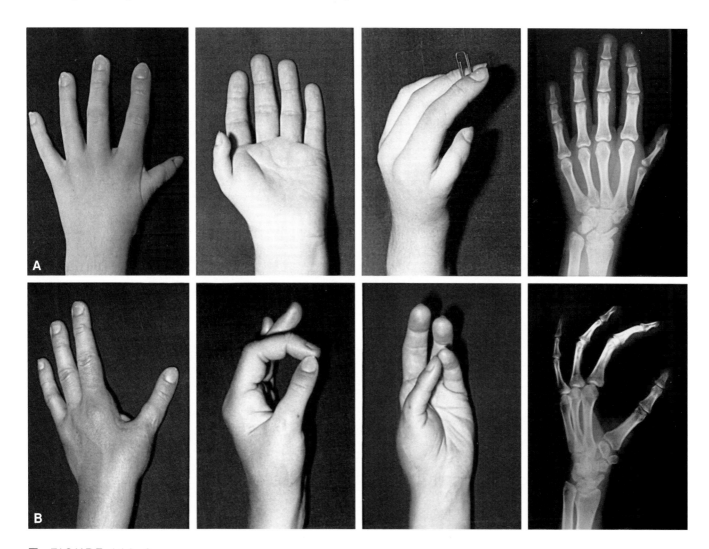

■ FIGURE 144–6

(A) Thumb hypoplasia grade 3B without a carpometacarpal joint in a 15-year-old girl; note the functional exclusion of the hypoplastic thumb. (B) Clinical and radiologic results 9 years after surgery.

former metacarpal, either because it was left too long primarily, or an abnormal basal epiphyseal plate produced too much length after several years of growth.

A carpal tunnel syndrome developed in five patients as a ''late complication'' many years after the primary operation. Some relationship to increased manual work was found in all of these cases.

■ REHABILITATION

The operated arm is elevated for the first 2 postoperative days. The necessary dressing changes are performed until the stitches can be removed. Immobilization is necessary for 3 weeks for complete healing of the tendons and muscle. After this period it is often necessary, especially in cases of considerable scar induration, to apply night bandages to maintain both thumb abduction and distal joint flexion. This should be done until the scar is softened.

A supervised program of postoperative exercises usually is not possible in infants and small children. The mother is instructed to perform simple activity-based exercises, using suitable toys and biscuits. This should be performed at intervals when the child is attentive. These opportunities are seldom available to physiotherapists.

After a few weeks, a key grip or tip pinch can usually be gained. Many months will be required before opposition to the little finger is achieved. Because the interphalangeal joint flexion depends on the spontaneous contracture of the flexor muscle belly, this motion usually occurs relatively late (several months).

■ OUTCOMES

The quality of the results depends mainly on the preoperative status of the different anatomic structures. If all structures of the index finger are present and normal, one can expect excellent results (Fig. 144–6).

Even under less ideal conditions, as in the radial club hand, the procedure is worthwhile, because a pinch grip is now possible and the cosmetic appearance of the hand is improved (Fig. 144–7). As a general rule, it can be said that patients with a radial club hand, a five-fingered hand, or a mirror hand have poorer results with regard to range of motion and stability. With the exception of a very few special cases, however, the postoperative condition is functionally and aesthetically satisfactory, and an improvement over the preoperative status.

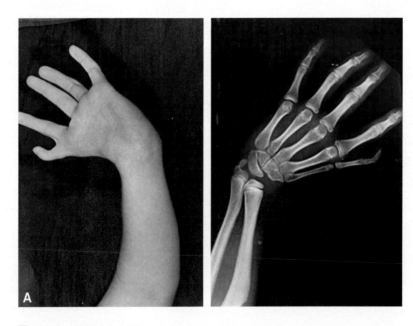

■ FIGURE 144–7

(A) Radial club hand with hypoplasia of the radius and hypoplastic triphalangeal thumb in an 11-year-old girl.

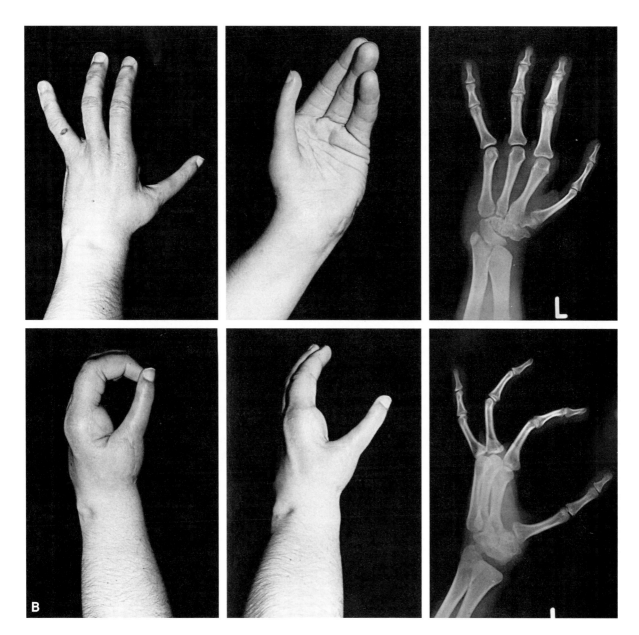

■ FIGURE 144–7

(continued)

(B) The clinical and radiologic results 6 years after surgery show satisfactory function and appearance.

References

1. Blauth W: Indikation und Technik des "Zeigefinger-Daumens" bei Daumenaplasien. Handchirurgie, 1969; 1:28–33.
2. Blauth W: Prinzipien der Pollizisation unter besonderer Berucksichtigung einer neuen Schnittfuhrung. Handchirurgie, 1970; 2:117–121.
3. Buck-Gramcko D: Pollicization of the index finger. J Bone Joint Surg, 1971; 53A:1605–1617.
4. Buck-Gramcko D: Thumb reconstruction by digital transposition. Orthop Clin North Am, 1977; 8:329–342.
5. Buck-Gramcko D: Angeborene Fehlbildungen der Hand/Congenital malformation of the hand. In: Nigst H, Buck-Gramcko D, Millesi H (eds): Handchirurgie/Hand Surgery, Vol. 1. Stuttgart: Thieme Verlag, 1981/1988 chap 12; 1–115.

6. Buck-Gramcko D: Complications and bad results in pollicization of the index finger (in congenital cases). Annals of Hand and Upper Limb Surgery, 1991; 10:506–512.

7. Bunnell S: Digit transfer by neurovascular pedicle. J Bone Joint Surg, 1952; 34A:772–774.

8. Edgerton MT, Snyder GB, Webb WL: Surgical treatment of congenital thumb deformities (including psychological impact of correction). J Bone Joint Surg, 1965; 47A:1453–1474.

9. Engloff DV, Verdan C: Pollicization of the index finger for reconstruction of the congenitally hypoplastic or absent thumb. J Hand Surg, 1983; 8:839–848.

10. Gosset J: La pollicisation de l'index (technique chirurgicale). J Chir, 1949; 65:403–411.

11. Harrison SH: Restoration of muscle balance in pollicization. Plast Reconstr Surg, 1964; 34:236–240.

12. Harrison SH: Pollicisation in cases of radial club hand. Br J Plast Surg, 1970; 23:192–200.

13. Hilgenfeldt O: Operativer Daumenersatz und Beseitigung von Greifstorungen bei Fingerverlusten. Stuttgart: Ferdinand Enke Verlag, 1950.

14. Kleinman WB: Management of thumb hypoplasia. Hand Clin, 1990; 6:617–641.

15. Littler JW: Subtotal reconstruction of the thumb. Plast Reconstr Surg, 1952; 10:215–226.

16. Littler JW: The neurovascular pedicle method of digital transposition for reconstruction of the thumb. Plast Reconstr Surg, 1953; 12:303–319.

17. Manske PR, McCarroll HR: Index finger pollicization for congenital absent or nonfunctioning thumb. J Hand Surg, 1985; 10A:606–613.

18. Manske PR, McCarroll HR: Reconstruction of the congenitally deficient thumb. Hand Clin, 1992; 8:177–196.

19. Riordan DC: Congenital absence of the radius. J Bone Joint Surg, 1955; 37A:1129–1140.

20. Strickland JW, Kleinman WB: Thumb reconstruction. In: Green DP (ed): Operative Hand Surgery, 3rd Ed. New York: Churchill Livingstone, 1993:2043–2156.

21. Sykes PJ, Chandraprakasam T, Percival NJ: Pollicization of the index finger in congenital anomalies: A retrospective analysis. J Hand Surg, 1991; 16B:144–147.

22. White WF: Pollicization for the missing thumb, traumatic or congenital. The Hand, 1969; 1:23–26.

23. White WF: Fundamental priorities in pollicization. J Bone Joint Surg, 1970; 52B:438–443.

145

Hypoplastic Thumb Reconstruction

Thumb hypoplasia has been classified into five types, as noted in Table 145–1, reflecting a progressive spectrum of thumb deficiencies. The classification system is useful in outlining treatment principles. At one end of the spectrum, type I deficiencies require no treatment; at the other end, types IV and V deficiencies cannot be reconstructed and pollicization is required; pollicization is discussed elsewhere and is not considered in this chapter. Types II and III hypoplasias have intermediate deficiencies and the potential for thumb reconstruction.

The basic four procedures used in the reconstruction of types II and III hypoplasias include: (1) deepening the thumb index web space, using transposition or rotation flaps (which are discussed in other chapters) (2) abductor digiti quinti (ADQ) opponensplasty, (3) stabilization of the metacarpophalangeal (MP) joint, and (4) correction of extrinsic tendon abnormalities.

Abductor Digiti Quinti Opponensplasty The ADQ opponensplasty is preferred over other opponensplasties in the treatment of the hypoplastic thumb for several reasons. As a musculotendinous unit on the ulnar aspect of the hand, it is reliably and predictably present in the radial-sided deficiencies. It is an expendable muscle, and there is no appreciable functional deficit after transfer. The muscle is the same length and is of equal strength to the abductor pollicis brevis (APB) and opponens pollicis (Opp P) muscles that it replaces. Pulley reconstruction is not required to alter the direction of pull. After transfer, the appearance of the thumb is improved by the added muscle mass in the deficient thenar area.

The transfer has been referred to as the "Huber opponensplasty," in recognition of the German surgeon who described the procedure in 1921 to restore opposition function after median nerve injuries. This inappropriately ignores the independent description of the procedure by Nicholaysen in the Scandinavian literature in the same year for treatment of poliomyelitis. The transfer received little subsequent attention until 1963, when Littler and Cooley[7] restored interest, reporting its use in four adult patients for median nerve paralysis. Riordan and co-authors first reported use of the transfer for congenital absence of the thenar muscles in 12 of 18 patients at the annual meeting of the American Society for Surgery of the Hand in 1975; although generally good results were noted, the authors never published the results of their study. In 1971, Wissenger and Singsen[15] reported success with the procedure in 14 patients for median nerve injuries or neurologic disorders, but one failure in a child with congenital absence of the thenar muscles. We[8] reported successful use of the ADQ opponensplasty in 20 of 21 hypoplastic thumb or postpollicization patients in 1978, and Oberlin and Gilbert[11] reported good results in 13 of 14 children with radial dysplasia.

Metacarpophalangeal Joint Stability Instability of the MP joint in type II hypoplastic thumbs has not always been recognized as a component part of types II and IIIA hypoplasia. When recognized, recommended treatment has been either soft tissue reconstruction or bony stabilization by arthrodesis. Soft tissue reconstruction is accomplished primarily by transverse division and pants-over-vest imbrication of the ulnar capsule.[8,14] The end

TABLE 145–1   THUMB HYPOPLASIA

Type I: Minimal Shortening and Narrowing

Type II: Moderate Underdevelopment
- Narrow thumb–index web space
- Intrinsic thenar muscle hypoplasia (APB/Opp P)
- MP joint instability

Type III: Extensive Underdevelopment
- Narrow thumb–index web space
- Intrinsic thenar muscle hypoplasia
- MP joint instability
- Extrinsic tendon abnormalities
- Metacarpal hypoplasia, CMC stable (IIIA)
- Proximal metacarpal aplasia, CMC unstable (IIIB)

Type IV: Pouce Flotant
- Rudimentary phalanges
- Thumb attached to hand by skin bridge containing vessels and nerves

Type V: Absent Thumb

APB, abductor pollicis brevis; CMC, carpometacarpal; MP, metacarpophalangeal; Opp P, opponens pollicis.

of the transferred opponensplasty tendon has also been used to supplement the imbricated capsule.[6,8,12,13]

Little has been written about arthrodesis of skeletally immature joints of the hand in children, because of concern for damaging the epiphyseal plate and causing growth abnormalities. Chondrodesis or fixation of two chondral joint surfaces after removing a thin layer of surface cartilage has usually been recommended in the skeletally immature hand; the incidence of "fusion" versus "fibrous" stability after this procedure is not known. Neviaser[10] obtained an ankylosis of the MP joint with approximately 20° radial instability in 10 hypoplastic thumbs by shaving the articular cartilage to expose the bony epiphysis, in association with Kirschner wire fixation. In 1988, we[5] reported successful epiphyseal arthrodesis in 94% of 47 digital joints of skeletally immature hands, including 6 of 6 MP joints in hypoplastic thumbs; there were no subsequent skeletal growth abnormalities.

Extrinsic Tendon Abnormalities   The observation that tendon abnormalities occur in association with hypoplastic thumbs and produce additional deformities was noted by Tupper[14] in four patients. The thumbs all had the typical features of type II hypoplasia, in addition to an aberrant extrinsic tendon (which ran from the volar forearm, along the radial side of the thumb, to insert both at the distal phalanx and as a conjoint tendon to the extensor mechanism, causing radial deviation of the thumb) and an absent flexor pollicis longus (FPL) tendon. He referred to this condition as pollex abductus. Similar reports of FPL and other extrinsic tendon abnormalities in hypoplastic thumbs have subsequently been reported;[1,2,4,6,9,12] these other extrinsic tendon abnormalities include absence of the extensor pollicis longus tendon, and a tendinous interconnection between the FPL and the extensor aponeurosis on the radial side of the thumb.

■ INDICATIONS AND CONTRAINDICATIONS

Type II hypoplasia includes three deficiencies (Fig. 145–1): (1) narrowed thumb–index web space, (2) hypoplasia of the intrinsic thenar muscles, primarily the APB and Opp P, and (3) instability of the MP joint, most frequently on the ulnar side. These thumbs should always be considered candidates for surgical reconstruction.

Type III hypoplasia is more extensive. It includes the previously noted type II deficiencies, plus extrinsic tendon abnormalities and metacarpal hypoplasia. If the metacarpal is hypoplastic but the basal carpometacarpal (CMC) joint is present and stable, we have

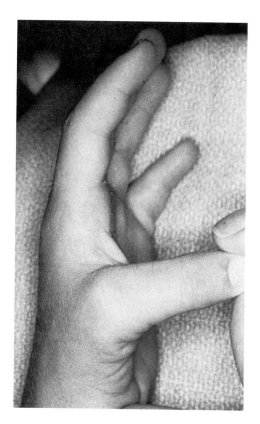

Type II hypoplastic thumb demonstrating muscle deficiency in the thenar eminence and ulnar collateral ligament instability.

identified these as type IIIA deficiencies;[9] type IIIA hypoplastic thumbs can usually be surgically reconstructed. If the proximal metacarpal is deficient and the basal thumb joint is unstable, we have identified these as a type IIIB deficiency; in contrast, these are not candidates for surgical reconstruction, and the preferred treatment is pollicization.

Type II   All patients with type II hypoplasia are candidates for surgical reconstruction. The clinical examination for the narrowed thumb–index web space includes observation of the adducted position of the first metacarpal; it forms an angle of less than 45° with the second metacarpal. Frequently, the web space skin margin extends distal to the thumb MP joint.

The clinical examination for hypoplastic superficial thenar muscles includes observation of flattening and underdevelopment of the thenar eminence, observation of thumb flexion rather than rotation (i.e., absence of opposition) during pinch activities, and palpation of weak superficial thenar musculature.

The clinical evaluation for MP instability is made by applying ulnar and radial stress to the joint, as well as observing the joint for an ulnar-collapsed pattern during pinch activities. The extent of MP instability does not necessarily correlate to the degree of first metacarpal adduction. All type II hypoplasias will have ulnar collateral ligament instability at a minimum;[8] severe hypoplasias with more global instability are infrequent, but do indicate the need for epiphyseal arthrodesis rather than soft tissue reconstruction. Epiphyseal arthrodesis[5] can be performed after an ossification center is apparent radiographically in the epiphysis of the proximal phalanx, generally by 2 to 4 years of age, depending on the extent of hypoplasia. In the case of global instability of a patient with an unossified epiphysis, the joint is stabilized by shaping the cartilage of the opposing joint surfaces and imbricating both the radial and ulnar capsular structures.

Type IIIA   Reconstruction of type IIIA hypoplastic thumbs can be considered if certain features are present on clinical and radiographic examination. The length of the thumb should extend at least to the midshaft of the proximal phalanx of the adjacent finger; even though this is shorter than the normal thumb, which reaches to the proximal interphalangeal joint, it will have sufficient length for functional activities. The thumb should have basal joint stability. Reconstruction of the CMC joint by free tissue transfer of a vascularized metatarsophalangeal joint converts a type IIIB thumb to a IIIA thumb.

The patient must be evaluated for tendon deficiencies in the flexion, extension, abduction (opposition), and adduction planes. Although tendon transfers can theoretically address all four deficiencies, we usually limit tendon transfer to produce active motion in only two directions, primarily opposition and extension. Fortunately, type IIIA hypoplastic thumbs frequently have flexion and adduction function, because the ulnar-innervated intrinsic muscles (adductor pollicis, deep portion of the flexor pollicis brevis [FPB]) are present. The surgeon may also consider transfer for an absent FPL to restore active flexion of the interphalangeal (IP) joint, but this may not be necessary for functional improvement.

The deformities produced by malpositioned or aberrant tendons are varied, but in general have the following characteristics. A tendinous interconnection between the flexor and extensor mechanisms (usually on the radial side of the thumb) restricts active IP flexion–extension, and is noted by absent skin creases at the IP joint. The thumb may be adducted at the unstable MP or at the IP joint, owing to an aberrant extrinsic radial tendon or to a radially malpositioned FPL; these malpositioned extrinsic tendons can usually be palpated on the radial aspect of the thumb during pinch activities.

Surgery is indicated to release the deforming tendons, or to replace deficient tendon function by tendon transfer.

■ SURGICAL
TECHNIQUES

General anesthesia is recommended. Children can be operated on at any age after 6 months, depending on the general physical condition; there is no upper-limit age restriction. There are several components to the operative procedure. These include (1) release of the thumb–index web space, (2) an ADQ opponensplasty, (3) MP joint stabilization, and (4) tendon releases and transfers. The components can be performed in any order, but usually are carried out as described.

Release of the thumb–index web space is usually accomplished by a various transpositional or rotational flaps, as discussed in other chapters.

The incision for the *ADQ opponensplasty* originates at the midulnar border of the proximal phalanx of the little finger, extending proximally along the midulnar axis of the palm. It curves radialward just distal to the pisiform, and then proximally at the base of the palm in the line of the fourth metacarpal, extending just to the wrist crease (Fig. 145–2). The thin membrane that envelopes the ADQ muscle is incised in the line of the incision. The muscle has dual tendon insertions. The distal insertion into the extensor hood is detached, retaining as much length as possible, including a portion of the extensor hood. The proximal insertion into the phalanx is intimately attached to the MP joint capsule, and care

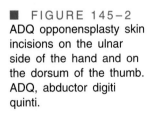

■ FIGURE 145–2
ADQ opponensplasty skin incisions on the ulnar side of the hand and on the dorsum of the thumb. ADQ, abductor digiti quinti.

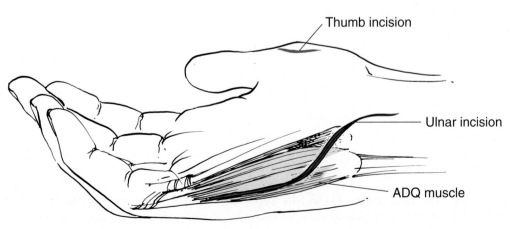

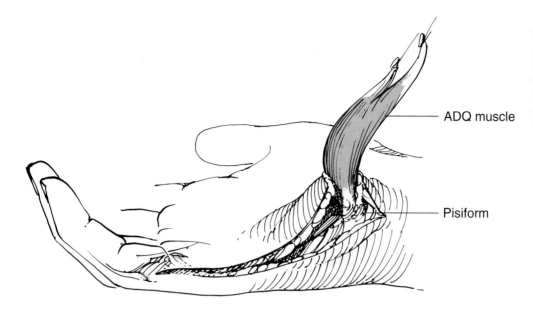

Elevation of the ADQ muscle by detachment of the two inserting tendons and dissection back to the origin on the pisiform. ADQ, abductor digiti quinti.

- ADQ muscle
- Pisiform

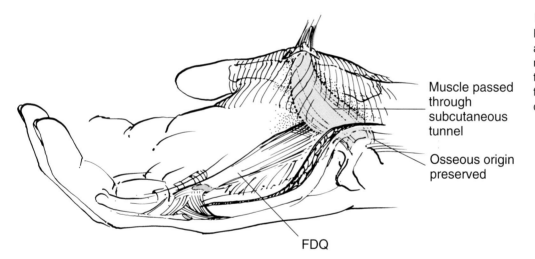

Passage of ADQ through a large subcutaneous tunnel from the pisiform to the MP joint of the thumb. FDQ, flexor digiti quinti.

- Muscle passed through subcutaneous tunnel
- Osseous origin preserved

FDQ

must be taken to preserve the capsular integrity as the tendon is detached from the capsule. Unfortunately, the proximal insertion may not be usable if it does not reach the MP joint of the thumb after transposition. The proper digital nerve is volar to the area of dissection and usually is not observed; however, the surgeon must be aware of its location and should dissect it out and protect it at this point if there is concern about its exact location. The ADQ muscle is dissected proximally to its origin on the pisiform (Fig. 145–3). Avoid dissection on the proximal radial side of the muscle origin where the neurovascular structures are known to enter. On occasion, the ADQ has a common origin with the flexor digiti quinti (FDQ), which the surgeon attempts to maintain, but it may be necessary to include some of the FDQ fibers with the transferred muscle. The ADQ muscle is not detached from its bony origin.

A second curved incision is made on the dorsoradial aspect of the thumb MP joint (Fig. 145–2), distinct from the incision to deepen the thumb–index web space. A large subcutaneous tunnel is made in the direction of the thenar eminence from the thumb incision to the pisiform, and the ADQ muscle is rotated radially approximately 75 to 90° to pass through the tunnel (Fig. 145–4). It is important that the muscle passes freely through the tunnel and is not constricted by soft tissue. On occasion, it is necessary to release a

■ FIGURE 145–5
Insertion of the two ADQ tendons into the radial MP capsule, as well as into the extensor hood mechanism. The distal insertion also reinforces the ulnar MP capsule after pants-over-vest imbrication. EPL, extensor pollicis longus; MP, metacarpophalangeal.

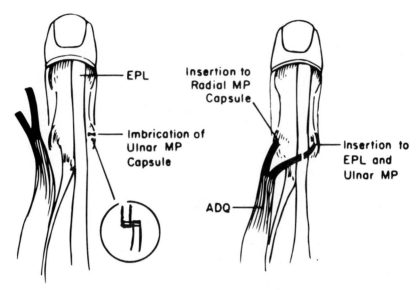

■ FIGURE 145–6
Epiphyseal arthrodesis is achieved at the MP joint by removing the articular cartilage, exposing the cancellous bone of the ossific nucleus of the proximal phalanx and the metacarpal head, and immobilizing with K-wires.

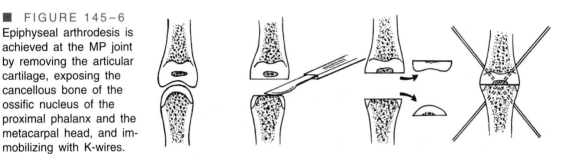

few of the originating muscle fibers on the ulnar side of the pisiform to obtain adequate length of the transferred muscle to reach the extensor hood at the MP joint, but the muscle should not be completely detached from its osseous origin. Experimental studies have determined that the attachment to the bony base is necessary to maintain adequate perfusion of the muscle.[3] The thumb is abducted, and the proximal tendon insertion is sutured to the radial capsule of the MP joint, as shown in Figure 145–5. The distal insertion is passed through and sutured to the extensor hood; the end of this tendon is then also sutured into the imbricated ulnar capsule (see later). If only a single tendon insertion is available, it is sutured to the extensor hood and the imbricated ulnar capsule.

Metacarpal phalangeal joint stabilization is accomplished by either ulnar capsule imbrication or epiphyseal arthrodesis. Ulnar capsular imbrication is preferred, particularly in very young patients before the development of an ossification center of the proximal phalangeal epiphysis; epiphyseal arthrodesis is necessary in the less frequently encountered presence of global instability of the MP joint. Ulnar capsular imbrication (Fig. 145–5) is performed through the dorsal thumb incision. The adductor tendon is incised transversely and retracted. The ulnar capsule is incised transversely and the joint inspected. The capsular tissues are imbricated in pants-over-vest fashion with multiple sutures, and the repair reinforced with the end of the distal tendon slip. The adductor tendon is repaired and the joint immobilized with a temporary longitudinal Kirschner wire for 4 weeks.

Epiphyseal arthrodesis (Fig. 145–6) is performed through the dorsal thumb incision before attaching the transferred ADQ tendons to the extensor hood. The collateral ligaments are detached and the joint is maximally flexed. Thin layers of articular cartilage surface are sequentially removed from the proximal phalanx with a sharp knife perpendicular to the shaft in the line of the anticipated plane of arthrodesis. The cuts progress deeper into the epiphysis until the center of ossification is reached, taking extreme caution not to proceed beyond this ossific nucleus into the physeal plate itself. A similar procedure is performed on the articular surface of the metacarpal head down to the bone, but it is not necessary to exercise as much caution in the absence of a physeal plate. The subchondral bone is denuded with a knife or fine curette and the cancellous surfaces are coapted and immobilized with longitudinal and crossed K-wires.

General principles guide the approach to *tendon releases and transfers*. Malpositioned FPL and other aberrant tendons, as well as interconnections between the flexor and extensor tendons, are released through a distal extension of the curved dorsoradial thumb incision. There is no routine inspection for malpositioned or aberrant tendons, but these abnormal structures should be looked for through the dorsal incision if there is concern. If the released muscles have adequate excursion, the tendons may be transferred to provide abduction or flexor function. The tendon releases are performed before MP joint stabilization, whereas tendon transfers to the thumb are performed after the stabilization.

The preferred opposition transfer is an ADQ opponensplasty, as described previously. In addition, an aberrant extrinsic tendon can supplement abductor function by transferring it to the base of the thumb metacarpal; this can be accomplished through a proximal extension of the dorsal thumb incision.

Thumb extension is obtained by transfer of the extensor indices proprius, or, alternatively, one of the slips of the common extensor tendon.

The deep FPB muscle is usually present and provides satisfactory thumb flexion. When the FPL is malpositioned along the radial side of the thumb, it can be used to facilitate flexion by releasing the soft tissues that tether it and placing it volarly. In the presence of full passive IP flexion and an absent FPL, the surgeon can consider a ring finger sublimis transfer and pulley reconstruction. These more extensive FPL procedures require an additional zig-zag incision on the volar surface of the thumb.

The absence of an adductor pollicis usually signals a markedly deficient hypoplastic thumb that is not satisfactory for reconstruction.

All wounds are closed with absorbable skin sutures and the thumb is immobilized in a supportive dressing, holding it extended at the MP joint and in a position of opposition. At 4 to 6 weeks (depending on the status of the epiphyseal arthrodesis), the dressing is removed and the thumb is placed in a position of opposition by a circumferential tape, crossing the thumb at the metacarpal head and based at the pisiform (Fig. 145–7).

■ TECHNICAL ALTERNATIVES

Littler and Cooley[7] detached the origin of the ADQ from the pisiform and based the transfer on the extended attachment to the flexor carpi ulnaris (FCU). We prefer to keep the muscle origin attached to the pisiform to serve as a stable base, enhance vascularization from the bone, and prevent undue tension on the neurovascular pedicle.[3] Littler and Cooley reported muscle fibrosis in one of four patients. We noted fibrosis in 1 of 21 children,[8] and in 1 of approximately 100 additional unreported patients. Oberlin and Gilbert[11] reported no fibrosis in the series of 14 children when the muscle was not detached.

Several reports have used a ring finger sublimis opponensplasty[6,12,13] because it is more substantial and potentially supplements the capsular imbrication more effectively. The shorter length of the ADQ tendon occasionally requires that the surgeon include a portion of the extensor hood as an extension to the tendon; however, this does not impair extension of the small finger MP joint.

In addition to imbricating the ulnar capsule, release of the radial MP capsule has been advocated in type IIIA hypoplasias when there is a fixed abduction deformity.[14] There is considerable concern that the additional MP capsular release will result in functional instability of the thumb; an epiphyseal arthrodesis is preferred by the author under these conditions.

An alternative to epiphyseal arthrodesis is "chondrodesis," which is the apposition of adjacent cartilaginous surfaces. This technique is more likely to result in pseudarthrosis with a potential for long-term instability, and carries with it the same potential risk to the growth plate. We prefer chondrodesis only when there is gross joint instability in conjunction with an epiphysis that is not yet ossified.

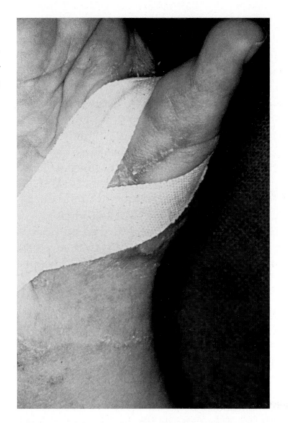

Potential errors in technique are possible, and require the careful attention of the surgeon to avoid them. These include damage to the proper ulnar digital nerve, injury to the primary neurovascular structures by dissecting on the radial side of the ADQ origin or at the pisiform, complete detachment of the ADQ muscle from the pisiform without retaining a stabilizing attachment to the FCU, passage of the ADQ muscle through a subcutaneous tunnel that is too narrow, and failure to stabilize adequately the ulnar side of the MP joint by capsular imbrication. Careful attention to surgical detail will avoid most of these technical problems. Failure to release a tendon interconnection or a malpositioned tendon may result in persistence of the restricted joint motion, but will not increase the deformity if there is adequate stability of the MP or IP joints.

■ REHABILITATION

After surgery, the thumb is maintained in a bulky opposition dressing for 4 to 6 weeks (depending on whether an arthrodesis is performed). The K-wires are removed at that time, and the thumb is taped in a position of opposition using 0.5-inch adhesive tape (Fig. 145–7) for an additional 6 weeks. The tape is looped from the pisiform circumferentially around the thumb at the level of the metacarpal head and back to the pisiform; it is important not to pass the tape at the level of the proximal phalanx, particularly if the ulnar collateral ligament has been imbricated. The child is allowed and encouraged to use the thumb for activities; it is changed on a daily basis as necessary by the parents. We have not found it necessary to use more rigid splinting, but would not hesitate to do so if the taping does not adequately hold the thumb or if the child resists wearing it. Formal rehabilitation training is not usually necessary.

■ OUTCOMES

The results of the ADQ plasty and stabilization of the MP joint have been most satisfactory. In 20 of 21 patients who were first reported in our series,[8] the transferred ADQ contracted and pulled the thumb into opposition, usually by 6 to 8 weeks. Pinch strength, dexterity, thumb function, and appearance were improved according to the subjective evaluation by the parents. It is our impression that the results have been similar in the subsequent patients (more than 100) on whom this procedure has been performed by us since 1978. Oberlin and Gilbert[11] reported 13 "good" or "very good" results in a series of 14 children.

The addition of extrinsic tendon transfers for the more complex IIIA hypoplastic thumbs adds to the complexity of the procedure. Nevertheless, the results have been satisfactory in that the thumb is more stable and better positioned for effective function than it was before surgery.[1,2,4,6,9,14]

References

1. Blair WF, Buckwalter JA: Congenital malposition of flexor pollicis longus: An anatomy note. J Hand Surg, 1983; 8:93–94.
2. Blair WF, Omer GE: Anomalous insertion of the flexor pollicis longus. J Hand Surg, 1981; 6: 241–244.
3. Dunlap J, Manske PR, McCarthy JA: Perfusion of the abductor digiti quinti after transfer on a neurovascular pedicle. J Hand Surg, 1989; 14A:992–995.
4. Fitch RD, Urbaniak JR, Ruderman RJ: Conjoined flexor and extensor pollicis longus tendons in the hypoplastic thumb. J Hand Surg, 1984; 9A:417–419.
5. Kowalski MF, Manske PR: Arthrodesis of digital joints in children. J Hand Surg, 1988; 13A: 874–879.
6. Lister G: Pollex abductus in hypoplasia and duplication of the thumb. J Hand Surg, 1991; 16A:626–633.
7. Littler JW, Cooley SGE: Opposition of the thumb and its restoration by abductor digiti quinti transfer. J Bone Joint Surg, 1963; 45A:1389–1396.
8. Manske PR, McCarroll HR Jr: Abductor digiti minimi opponensplasty in congenital radial dysplasia. J Hand Surg, 1978; 3:552–559.
9. Manske PR, McCarroll HR Jr: Reconstruction of the congenitally deficient thumb. Hand Clin, 1992; 8:177–196.
10. Neviaser RJ: Congenital hypoplasia of the thumb with absence of the extrinsic extensors, abductor pollicis longus, and thenar muscles. J Hand Surg, 1979; 4:301–303.
11. Oberlin C, Gilbert A: Transfer of the abductor digiti minimi (quinti) in radial deformities of the hand in children. Ann Chir Main, 1984; 3:215–220.
12. Strauch B, Spinner M: Congenital anomaly of the thumb: Absent intrinsics and flexor pollicis longus. J Bone Joint Surg, 1976; 58A:115–118.
13. Su CT, Hoopes JE, Daniel R: Congenital absence of the thenar muscles innervated by the median nerve. J Bone Joint Surg, 1972; 54A:1087–1090.
14. Tupper JW: Pollex abductus due to congenital malposition of the flexor pollicis longus. J Bone Joint Surg [Am], 1969; 51:1285–1290.
15. Wissinger HA, Singsen EG: Abductor digiti quinti opponensplasty. J Bone Joint Surg, 1977; 59A:895–898.

146

Centralization for Radial Dysplasia

The various operations described over the last century to treat radial club hands each have attempted to provide stable support of the hand.[14] Bardenheuer longitudinally split the distal ulna and wedged the carpus into the notch between the two halves of the ulna. Other attempts to buttress the carpus by placing tibial or fibular bone graft along the radial aspect of the ulna failed to provide satisfactory long-term results.

Sayre was the first to describe centralization of the carpus on the end of the ulna. He removed carpal bones (lunate and capitate) to achieve a stable reorientation of the limb. Lidge described centralization with preservation of the distal ulnar physis.[10] Most procedures have required carpal resection to lock the ulna into a carpal notch. Both Bayne and Watson have, however, advocated centralization without carpal resection to preserve wrist motion.[1,15]

Bayne has classified radial deficient limbs into four groups.[1] Type I limbs have a proximal and distal radial physis, but the radius is slightly shorter than the ulna because of diminished physeal growth. There is slight radial deviation of the hand. Type II limbs demonstrate a "radius in miniature." Growth is diminished at both proximal and distal physes. The ulna is thickened and bowed. Type III limbs demonstrate a partial absence of the radius. These limbs lack a true radial physis either proximally or distally. The hand is radially deviated. Type IV limbs have total absence of the radius. The unsupported hand is severely radially angulated.

The goals of centralization are to achieve a normal orientation of the hand relative to the forearm, to provide wrist stability, and to preserve wrist motion. A well-aligned limb possessing some wrist motion is achieved by placing the hand and carpus securely at the end of the ulna. This procedure eliminates excessive radial deviation and wrist flexion but does not provide forearm rotation because the hand is secured to the rotationally fixed ulna. Stabilization of the wrist also may provide more digital motion because digital tendon excursion results in digital motion rather than unintended wrist motion. Successful centralization improves the appearance of the limb, positions the hand so that more normal prehensile patterns develop, and increases the functional length of the limb.

Not all children with radial dysplasia are appropriate for centralization treatment. In Type I radial deficiency, the hand is well supported by the radius. The ulna is not bowed, and the hand–forearm alignment is usually satisfactory; centralization is rarely indicated. In contrast, types II, III, and IV limbs are usually appropriate for centralization.

The entire limb must be surveyed before deciding to centralize the wrist. If the elbow is stiff, the abnormal motion afforded at the untreated ulnocarpal junction may allow the child to reach his face and trunk. Because the abnormal wrist functionally substitutes for absent elbow motion, the mobility of these limbs should not be compromised by centralization. Elbow motion often improves with growth and may be enhanced by stretching or serial casts. If active elbow flexion is lacking, muscle transfer for elbow flexion should precede centralization. If elbow motion is not sufficient to allow the fingers to approximate the midline or reach the mouth after the centralization procedure, the operation is contraindicated. If centralization is carried out in an attempt to improve the appearance of a unilateral case with elbow stiffness, recurrence of radial deviation at the wrist is predictable unless a fixation pin crossing the wrist is retained until skeletal maturity.

The systemic health of the child also must be assessed before electing surgical intervention. Children with thrombocytopenia with an aplastic radius (TAR syndrome) often have low platelet counts early in life.[7] Hematologic consultation may be helpful in timing and planning surgery. These children should not undergo surgery until their platelet count is more than 75,000, usually at 3 or 4 years of age. Children with inevitably fatal conditions such as Fanconi's pancytopenia anemia probably should not be subjected to the rigors of centralization reconstruction.

Fixed radial deviation contracture, present at birth, is the result of both the lack of radial support of the carpus in utero and of the tethering effect of dysplastic soft tissue structures along the radial aspect of the forearm and wrist. If centralization is to be accomplished with maximal preservation of carpal and ulnar length, preliminary stretching of the soft tissues is essential. A stretching cast may be applied with the hand ulnarly deviated. The tight soft tissues along the radial aspect of the hand are stretched, bringing the hand distally and out of a radial deviation posture as the cast is molded. Alternatively, thermoplastic splints may be fabricated that tether the hand in an ulnar direction by applying three points of pressure to the limb. Parents also are taught to stretch the soft tissues toward a corrected posture with sessions lasting approximately 5 to 10 minutes, 4 or 5 times a day. Once the hand can be passively brought to a neutral position, surgical centralization can be done. This is usually performed when the child is between 4 and 12 months of age.

If the soft tissues do not respond to nonoperative stretching, or if the patient is first seen for treatment after 3 years of age, considerable ulnar diaphyseal shortening will be necessary to achieve centralization. The preliminary use of a skeletal lengthening device (such as the Ilizarov or Orthofix device) gradually stretches skin and soft tissues before centralization and thereby preserves maximal length in an already short limb.[8] The fixator is fixed to the ulna proximally and to multiple metacarpals distally. Distraction stretches the soft tissues along the radial aspect and distracts the hand and carpus from the ulna. Once sufficient soft tissue laxity has been achieved, the fixator is removed and centralization is performed. Soft tissue distraction lengthening is not routinely necessary in children who have undergone casting or splinting since birth; single stage centralization is usually possible in these children.

SURGICAL TECHNIQUES

Successful surgery depends on an understanding of the variations in pathologic anatomy and on an appreciation for the potential effect of growth on realignment of the limb.

In the untreated radius deficient forearm, the hand usually assumes a posture that is 90° to the longitudinal axis of the forearm. The carpal bones do not lie at the end of the ulna but rather abut the radial aspect of the ulna proximal to the distal articular surface.

Soft tissue abnormalities occur in muscles, tendons, and nerves.[6,13] Muscles along the radial aspect of the forearm often are ill defined with fusion of the extensor carpi radialis longus, extensor carpi radialis brevis, and brachioradialis muscles into a single poorly differentiated muscle mass. The median and radial nerves often merge superficially along the radial aspect of the forearm. An anlage of fibrous tissue representing the primitive radius may insert along the radial aspect of the carpus and also may tether the hand in a radially deviated position.

General anesthesia is used. The upper limb is prepared and draped in a fashion that allows a sterile tourniquet to be applied to the arm. This permits visualization of the entire limb during the surgical procedure and allows easy access to the tip of the olecranon, where the longitudinal stabilizing pin will exit.

When the hand is held in a corrected alignment, the skin and subcutaneous tissue is redundant along the ulnar aspect of the wrist. An L-shaped incision allows optimal exposure of underlying structures and flap contouring. The longitudinal limb of the incision is made over the dorsoradial aspect of the radially deviated hand and forearm. The transverse incision begins over the palmar ulnar aspect of the distal wrist crease and is carried

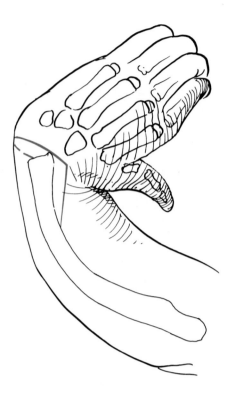

The skin incision runs longitudinally, parallel to the ulna, and transversely about the ulnar aspect of the wrist at the level of the distal wrist crease.

around the wrist dorsally to the level of the longitudinal incision. The dorsoulnar skin flap is mobilized (Fig. 146–1).

The extensor tendons are defined distal to the extensor retinaculum using careful surgical dissection. A vascular loop is placed around each tendon group. The extensor retinaculum is elevated, working from distally to proximally and from radially to ulnarly so that an ulnarly based retinacular flap is created. The extensor tendons are then reflected.

The hand is distracted radially and distally so that the articulation between the ulna and the carpus may be sharply defined. Care must be taken when incising the ulnocarpal capsule to preserve both the distal ulnar and the proximal carpal articular surfaces. The distal ulna is defined, preserving a rim of pericapsular tissue for later suturing to the carpus. Excessive mobilization or stripping of the distal ulna is avoided to prevent distal ulnar ischemia and resultant physeal arrest.

Each of the structures passing along the radial aspect of the ulnocarpal region is carefully defined. The location of the median nerve is extremely variable, but it must be identified and preserved. The tendons of the brachioradialis, extensor carpi radialis longus, and extensor carpi radialis brevis muscle group are identified and incised at their insertion onto the carpus or hand. If a fibrous anlage is present, it is excised. The flexor carpi radialis tendon is identified. It may be merged with the mobile wad muscles or may be a separate discreet structure.

If it is possible to easily reduce the carpus onto the end of the ulna, pin placement is accomplished next. If the hand cannot be readily placed onto the end of the ulna, a further search is made for tight volar or radial tethering structures. In some instances, the flexor superficialis muscles are extremely tight, and the fingers are severely flexed with the carpus reduced on the ulna. If the fingers are clenched into a fist when the carpus is reduced on the ulna, then either proximal row carpectomy or ulnar shortening may be elected. If osteotomy of the ulna is required to correct angulation, additional shortening may be carried out through the osteotomy site (Fig. 146–2). If ulnar osteotomy is not planned, proximal row carpectomy should excise the proximal scaphoid, the lunate, and triquetrum. The retained portion of the scaphoid may be contoured to help ensure ulnar deviation of the hand on the ulna.

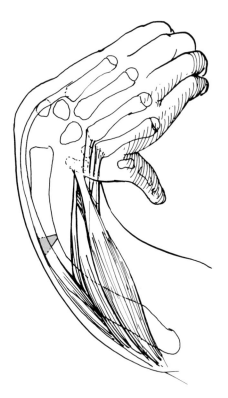

Pathologic anatomy is addressed by ulnar osteotomy, anlage excision, muscle releases, and extensor carpi ulnaris plication.

The articular surface of the ulna is examined. In children younger than 3 years of age, no contouring is needed. In older children, it may be necessary to contour or flatten the distal ulnar surface to provide a satisfactory platform for supporting the carpus. This may be accomplished by carefully shaving off the articular cartilage with a sharp knife.

A pin is selected to secure the carpus on the end of the ulna. Usually this is between a 0.062 C-wire and a 9/64-inch diameter Steinmann pin, depending on the age of the child and the size of the ulna. A pin track is drilled from the articular surface of the ulna out the tip of the olecranon. It may be difficult to pass this pin within the medullary canal because of curvature of the ulna and tapering of the medullary canal.

The carpus is predrilled with a similarly sized pin. The pin is drilled into the scaphoid and index metacarpal. The hand is positioned in slight ulnar deviation so that the pin exits through the radial border of the mid-diaphysis of the index metacarpal. When the hand is reduced on the ulna, it will assume the "radialization" position of ulnar displacement and angulation described by Buck-Gramcko[4] (Fig. 146-3). Buck-Gramcko suggested that when the hand is placed in this position the tendon forces are shifted ulnarward to create a more balanced wrist. If the hand is not placed in this position, the majority of muscle forces continue to lie radial to the ulnocarpal center of rotation and, therefore, recurrence is to be expected.

If the ulna is excessively curved, it will not be possible to pass a longitudinal pin down the shaft of the ulna. An ulnar closing wedge osteotomy will facilitate pin passage and will also improve the appearance of the limb. A transverse skin incision is made at the level at which the pin exits from the ulna. The ulna is exposed subperiosteally. The pin is withdrawn distally and a closing wedge osteotomy accomplished at the level of pin penetration. If additional shortening is required to relieve soft tissue tension and facilitate carpal reduction on the ulna, additional bone is removed at the osteotomy site. The osteotomy is closed and the pin is driven into the proximal diaphysis. This secures the osteotomy. The periosteum is repaired with interrupted sutures. The pin is advanced out the tip of the olecranon. The hand is then reduced onto the end of the ulna. The pin is driven antegrade into the predrilled hole in the carpus, exiting along the radial aspect of the index metacarpal. Intraoperative anteroposterior and lateral radiographs are required to

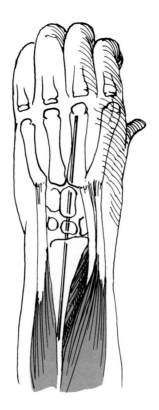 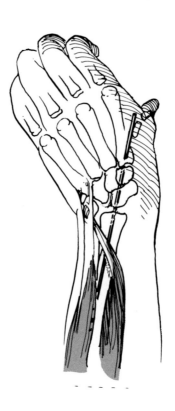

confirm appropriate pin position. If difficulty is encountered in placing a single pin that will secure the osteotomy as well as the ulnocarpal junction, two separate pins may be used.

The previously developed distally based ulnar capsular flap is advanced proximally and attached with nonabsorbable sutures to the periosteum along the ulnar aspect of the forearm. The proximally based dorsal capsular cuff is sutured to the distally based wrist capsule. Redundant capsule, if present, is excised distally to avoid dissection about the periphery of the distal ulna physis. The course of the extensor tendons is evaluated and a retinacular sling sutured to the dorsal wrist capsule so that the extensor tendons course over the center of the ulna. Because the relocated extensor carpi ulnaris tendon is often redundant, it is either advanced distally on the little finger metacarpal or is shortened by plicating. Pins are trimmed beneath the skin level. Pins should be superficial enough that they may be readily retrieved but deep enough so that skin irritation is avoided.

The excursion of the extensor carpi radialis longus and extensor carpi radialis brevis tendons should be evaluated. If the muscle is mobile, its tendon may be sutured into the extensor carpi ulnaris tendon. If excursion is poor, the tendon is simply allowed to retract after division.

The tourniquet is deflated. Vascularity of the skin flap is confirmed. The proximal ulnar flap is advanced distally and radially. The skin flap is trimmed along both its radial and distal borders to decrease the bulk of the soft tissues along the ulnar aspect of the wrist (Fig. 146-4). This final flap contouring will substantially improve the aesthetic appearance of the limb. The skin is closed with interrupted absorbable sutures.

The limb is placed in a bulky dressing incorporating plaster splints. A few days later the dressings are changed and a long arm cast or thermoplastic splint is applied. Care is taken to avoid pressure from cast or splint over the pin sites.

■ REHABILITATION

After 12 weeks, a radiograph is obtained to confirm osteotomy healing. The pin or pins are removed. The forearm is splinted until bony remodeling of the distal ulnar epiphysis is judged sufficient to support the carpus. This often requires full-time splinting for 2 or

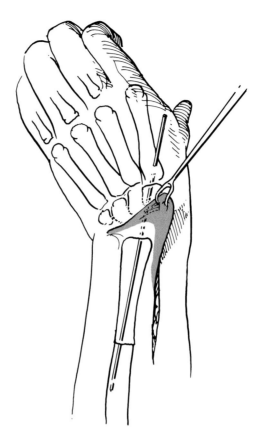

■ FIGURE 146–4
The skin flap is trimmed
along the distal and ulnar
margins.

3 years. Night splinting is continued until the wrist is stable, without a tendency to recurrent radial deviation.

Manske and co-authors[11] have described an elliptical ulnar-sided excision of skin to expose the wrist. They also advocate excision of a central block of carpal bones to create a notch or slot for the distal ulna. This maneuver provides enough shortening to relax the radial soft tissues and creates a stable pseudarthrosis. The surgeon does not have to expose the median nerve, correction is stable and well maintained, and redundant soft tissues along the ulnar border of the wrist are easily excised to provide a more satisfactory contour. However, wrist motion is severely limited or absent after this procedure, and access to the radial side of the wrist is limited.

■ TECHNICAL ALTERNATIVES

Watson and co-authors[15] have described an approach that combines z-plasties along the radial and ulnar aspects of the wrist. This approach provides direct visualization of the median nerve and all other soft tissue tethers along the radial side of the wrist and shifts redundant skin and subcutaneous tissue from the ulnar to the radial side of the wrist. However, this approach limits access to the dorsal and palmar aspects of the carpus and limits the ability of the surgeon to relocate or balance the digital extensors.

If the soft tissues do not respond to stretching, or if the patient first presents for treatment after 3 years of age with a severe or uncorrected deformity, consideration may be given to the preliminary use of an Ilizarov or other type of limb lengthening device to gradually stretch skin and soft tissues before centralization.[8] The fixator is fixed to the ulna proximally and to multiple metacarpals distally. Distraction stretches the soft tissues along the radial aspect and distracts the hand and carpus from the ulna. Once sufficient soft tissue laxity has been achieved, the fixator is removed and centralization is performed.

Numerous pitfalls may lead to early recurrence of deformity and an unsatisfactory result. The surgeon must clearly understand the anatomy of the articulation between the distal ulna and the carpus. Failure to understand this relationship will lead the surgeon to inadvertently enter the midcarpal joint rather than the ulnocarpal articulation. This may occur at the time of the initial capsulotomy or as the dissection proceeds across this joint from ulnar to radial. The median nerve should be the first structure identified on the radial aspect of the wrist in order to avoid injury to this critical structure. Resection and release of all radial and volar structures that tether the carpus must be thorough and aggressive to assure a complete correction. Accurate pin placement in the carpus and hand is critical since the position of the pin will determine the final position of the hand relative to the forearm. Intraoperative radiographs are essential to confirm that the pin is properly located in the hand as well as the ulna. Relocation and imbrication of tendons to rebalance the forces across the ulnocarpal articulation is an essential portion of the procedure. Failure to pay sufficient attention to this phase of the operation will lead to recurrent deformity. Postoperative immobilization must be of an adequate duration as well and should include night time splinting until skeletal maturity.

■ OUTCOMES

The distal ulnar physis will respond to the greater than "normal" physiologic stress of axial loading carrying the entire carpal load. With time the ulna broadens to provide greater support for the carpus and hand. In many cases the remodeled distal ulna will actually resemble a radius (Fig. 146–5).

The untreated ulna will usually grow to between 50% and 65% of the length of the contralateral normal ulna.[9] Therefore, even if centralization preserves the longitudinal growth potential of the distal ulna, the centralized limb will be substantially shorter than normal. If the distal ulna suffers an iatrogenic distal ulnar physeal arrest, the limb will be exceedingly short. Distraction lengthening of the ulna may be helpful in addressing this problem.[5]

Bayne and Klug's review of 51 surgically treated limbs followed for a minimum of at least 36 months demonstrated good results in 21 (41%) limbs, satisfactory results in 20 (39%) limbs, and unsatisfactory results in 10 (20%) limbs.[1] Good results were defined as a centralized hand with improved function, a hand–forearm angle of less than 30°, and more than 40° of wrist motion. Satisfactory results demonstrated improved function and cosmesis (by patient or parent questionnaire), a forearm–hand angle of less than 30°, but less than 40° of wrist motion. Limbs were considered unsatisfactory if the hand–forearm angle was more than 30°, or if family appraisal of the procedure was negative. The quality of the result was better when children were operated before 3 years of age, the soft tissues

■ FIGURE 146–5
This Type II radial deficient limb was treated by centralization. The remarkable ability of the distal ulna to broaden after centralization is illustrated on the left side. The right wrist is normal.

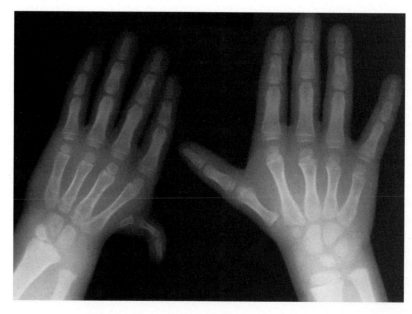

were supple from preoperative splinting, the carpal bones were surgically preserved, and diligent postoperative splinting was performed.

Watson and co-authors' review of 12 cases demonstrated that wrist motion could be achieved if carpal bones were retained but noted recurrence of radial deviation (increased forearm–hand angle) in many patients.[15]

Lamb carefully documented and contrasted growth in untreated and in centralized radial deficient limbs. The radial deficient limb is 40 to 50 mm long at birth and by age 12 ceases growth at between 100 to 140 mm of length. In 3 of 15 centralized limbs, growth was less than projected from untreated limb data.[9]

Bora and co-authors[2,3] studied a group of patients 10 to 25 years after centralization and observed little change in wrist position, or in wrist and elbow motion from comparable measurements in the same patients ten years previously. A mild increase in ulnar bowing was noted and a moderate increase in forearm–hand angle was observed. The authors strongly favored secondary tendon transfer of the flexor superficialis from the central digits around the ulnar border of the ulna, sutured into the dorsum of the metacarpals to diminish the tendency of recurrent radial deviation.

The most frequent problem noted in long-term follow-up is recurrence of deformity, characterized by residual or recurrent radial deviation and wrist flexion. If the wrist is stiff and angulated at skeletal maturity, wrist fusion will correct alignment.[12]

References

1. Bayne LG, Klug MS: Long-term review of the treatment of radial deficiencies. J Hand Surg, 1987; 12A:169–179.
2. Bora FW Jr, Nicholson JT, Cheema HM: Radial meromelia: The deformity and its treatment. J Bone Joint Surg, 1970; 52A:966–979.
3. Bora FW, Osterman AL, Kaneda RR, Esterhai J: Radial clubhand deformity. Long-term follow-up. J Bone Joint Surg, 1981; 63A:741–745.
4. Buck-Gramcko D: Radialization as a new treatment for radial club hand. J Hand Surg, 1985; 10A:964–968.
5. Dick HM, Petzoldt RL, Bowers WR: Lengthening of the ulna in radial agenesis: A preliminary report. J Hand Surg, 1977; 2:175–178.
6. Heikel HVA: Aplasia and hypoplasia of the radius. Acta Orthop Scand, 1959;Suppl 39:1–155.
7. Jones KL: Smith's Recognizable Patterns of Human Malformation, Fourth Ed, Philadelphia: W. B. Saunders Co, 1988:276.
8. Kessler I: Centralization of the radial club hand by gradual distraction. J Hand Surg, 1989; 14B:37–42.
9. Lamb D: Radial club hand. A continuing study of sixty eight patients with one hundred and seventeen club hands. J Bone Joint Surg, 1977; 59A:1–13.
10. Lidge RT: Congenital radial deficient club hand. J Bone Joint Surg, 1969; 51A:1041–1042.
11. Manske PR, McCarroll HR Jr, Swanson K: Centralization of the radial club hand—an ulnar surgical approach. J Hand Surg, 1981; 6:423–433.
12. Rayan GM: Ulnocarpal arthrodesis for recurrent radial club hand deformity in adolescents. J Hand Surg, 1992: 17A:–24-27.
13. Skerik SK, Flatt AE: The anatomy of congenital radial dysplasia. Clin Orthop Rel Res, 1969; 66:125–143.
14. Urban MA, Osterman AL: Management of radial dysplasia. Hand Clinics, 1990; 6:589–605.
15. Watson HK, Beebe RD, Cruz NI: A centralization procedure for radial clubhand. J Hand Surg, 1984; 9A:541–547.

PART

XII

Vessels

147

Venous Grafts for Ulnar Artery Thrombosis

Thrombosis of the ulnar artery at the wrist may be insignificant, or it may precipitate severe pain, cold intolerance, and neural dysfunction. In extreme cases, it may lead to the loss of one or more digits. From 1937 until 1964, surgical options were limited to regional sympathectomy, using the Leriche principle of surgical excision of the thrombosed segment and ligation of the artery,[15] or to proximal cervicothoracic sympathectomy. Thereafter, arterial reconstruction using microsurgical technique for end-to-end repair or for interposition reverse grafting became the primary method of revascularization,[4-6,12-14,18,19] and was first described by Trevaskis and co-authors in 1964,[19] then by Kleinert and Volianitis in 1965.[6]

In 1978, Koman and Urbaniak presented a treatment algorithm that included indications for reversed interposition vein grafts and emphasized the need for proper patient selection and technical proficiency to avoid thrombosis after revascularization and to obtain optimal treatment results.[12,13] However, historically, arterial reconstruction has not been necessary in all patients, and more recent reports have concentrated on methods to identify those patients in whom arterial reconstruction is necessary.[14,18-20] In many patients with ulnar artery thrombosis, environmental and behavioral modifications (such as the discontinuation of smoking), the use of oral medications or biofeedback, or simple surgical resection provides sufficient palliation of symptoms for patients to return to work.

There is still a group of patients, however, in whom arterial reconstruction is necessary. In these patients, failure to restore arterial integrity will result in necrosis or debilitating symptoms. Although, occasionally, end-to-end repair may be possible, it often is technically difficult, and therefore autogenous vein-grafting techniques adapted from lower extremity surgery have become the primary treatment when arterial reconstruction is needed.[6,19]

■ HISTORY OF THE TECHNIQUE

Reconstruction of a thrombosed ulnar artery is indicated when there is insufficient collateral flow to provide pulsatile digital perfusion capable of responding appropriately to stress.[8] When thrombosed segments are shorter than 1.5 cm or unusually long, or when tortuous vessels (often associated with aneurysms) are present, reconstruction by end-to-end repair is possible. In general, however, vessel damage is extensive and extends proximally and distally to the thrombosed arterial segment, and an interposition vein graft is necessary for reconstruction.

The goal of treatment is a *symptom-free, functional extremity*. The presence of pulsatile digital flow that responds appropriately to stress best correlates with this goal. The three major subgroups of extremities with thrombosis of the ulnar artery are shown in Table 147–1. In groups I and II, arterial occlusion occurs, but sufficient collateral circulation is present and the symptoms are related, in part, to sympathetic tone, which, when abnormal, prevents the response of pulsatile flow to metabolic demands.[9] Despite the presence of thrombosis, these patients have few symptoms because sympathetic tone is normal (group I); increased sympathetic tone in group II patients causes symptoms, but often they will respond to alternative treatment strategies (Table 147–2).

In group II patients who have undergone surgical exploration and Leriche-type periph-

■ INDICATIONS AND CONTRAINDICATIONS

TABLE 147–1. SUBGROUPS OF ULNAR ARTERY THROMBOSIS

Group I. Arterial occlusion, adequate collateral flow, normal sympathetic tone

Group II. Arterial occlusion, adequate collateral flow, increased sympathetic tone

Group III. Arterial occlusion, inadequate collateral flow, normal or increased sympathetic tone

---

TABLE 147–2. TREATMENT OPTIONS FOR SYMPTOMATIC ULNAR ARTERY THROMBOSIS

Increase collateral flow
1. Ruduce vasoconstrictor tone
   a. Eliminate nicotine
   b. Biofeedback
   c. Pharmacologic blockade with oral medications
2. Increase nutritional blood flow
   a. Calcium channel blockers, etc.
3. Sympathectomy
   a. Chemical
      1. Intra-arterial guanethidine, tolazoline, reserpine
      2. α,β-Blocking agents
      3. Epidural or brachial plexus sustained blockade
   b. Surgical
      1. Resection of thrombosed segment and ligation
      2. Periarterial sympathectomy
      3. Cervicothoracic sympathectomy
      4. Mechanical (surgical)
         a. Resection and ligation (Leriche type)
         b. Adventitial stripping

Restore circulation
1. Resection and end-to-end repair
2. Thrombectomy
3. Resection and vein graft
4. Periadventitial stripping[2]

---

eral sympathectomy (resection of the thrombosed segment and proximal and distal ligation), long-term functional and symptomatic results have been excellent.[12,14]

Surgical intervention is indicated in group II patients who do not respond to nonoperative modalities. Evaluation of extremity perfusion, including an assessment of vascular distribution into appropriate nutritional and thermoregulatory channels, is necessary to understand the pathophysiology of extremity symptoms. Peripheral ischemia may be the result of inadequate arterial inflow or the result of inappropriate arteriovenous shunting. Abnormal sympathetic hyperactivity—in theory precipitated by the thrombotic event—may cause arteriovenous shunting proximal to nutritional capillary beds, resulting in relative ischemia and resultant symptoms. The extent of sympathetic abnormality and the responsiveness of the microcirculation to repeated stress may be evaluated by temperature, laser Doppler flux, or plethysmography. The inability of the microcirculation to respond appropriately to stress mandates further evaluation or intervention. For example, after cold stress, microcirculatory flow should increase (increase in digital temperature and laser Doppler flux).[13]

Before considering surgical exploration, detailed anatomic information should be obtained from Doppler mapping,[3,8] Doppler flow studies,[1] real-time ultrasonography,[9] or arteriography. The current gold standard for anatomic information remains the contrast arteriogram. This evaluation of the vascular anatomy should provide an accurate estimate of: (1) the extent of the thrombosis; (2) the degree of proximal and distal intimal damage; (3) the location and the size of collateral vessels; (4) the presence of reconstituted distal flow; and (5) the presence or absence of embolic or occlusive "skip" lesions in the vascular tree. This information allows a preoperative prediction of the feasibility of arterial reconstruction and an estimation of whether autogenous vein grafting will be necessary. Arterial reconstruction is indicated in patients with ulnar artery thrombosis and inadequate collateral flow (group III). In general, autogenous vein grafts are necessary for arterial reconstruction. Although end-to-end repair may be possible technically, caution is advised because damage to the internal elastic and media arterial layers may be difficult to appreciate clinically. In my experience with over 40 arterial reconstructions, only one end-to-end repair has been possible.

To determine if arterial reconstruction is necessary, not only the arterial anatomy but also the physiologic capability of the symptomatic extremity must be understood. Preoperative testing or an intraoperative evaluation is designed to determine the ability of the collateral circulation to provide pulsatile flow to the digits and hand. The major contraindications to arterial reconstruction are vascular lesions with good collateral flow and absent symptoms, and inadequate distal vessels (i.e., absence of adequate outflow, or "runoff"). Relative contraindications include refusal of the patient to stop smoking, presence of polycythemia, inability or refusal of the patient to modify repetitive hand trauma, and the inability of the surgical team to reconstruct a thrombosed segment without damaging vital collateral flow to other digits or areas. Structurally, "adequate" collateral vessels (groups I and II) from the radial artery, deep palmar arch, or median artery (1) must be 1.5 mm or greater in diameter; (2) must be anastomosed distal to any thrombotic or embolic occlusive areas; and (3) must have the capability of providing distal pulsatile flow. Arteriography or real-time ultrasonography provide direct anatomic detail and define the presence or absence of adequately sized collaterals. However, stress data are necessary to evaluate functional capacity of these vessels. If symptoms persist in spite of nonoperative interventions, the following "anatomic" findings and observations in the presence of distal "runoff" indicate the need for arterial reconstruction: (1) thrombosis extending beyond the origin of one or more common digital arteries; (2) embolic occlusion distal to collateral inflow; (3) absence of the radial artery; (4) absence of the deep palmar arch; (5) absence of collateral vessels 1.5 mm or greater in diameter entering the arterial tree distal to the extent of the thrombus; or (6) distal embolic disease. In the presence of these findings, resection of the thrombosed segment and ligation with or without additional periarterial sympathectomy is contraindicated without intraoperative confirmation of adequate collateral flow.[7,10,11]

Intraoperative verification of the adequacy of collateral flow may be obtained subjectively by observations of stump distal backflow characteristics, or objectively by direct measurements of the distal stump pressure,[13] calculation of the digital brachial index (DBI),[20] or digital plethysmography.[18] Stump pressures or a DBI greater than 0.7 and "normal" plethysmographic wave patterns support adequate distal perfusion. Conversely, low pressure ratios and abnormal waveforms support the need for arterial reconstruction, if technically feasible and appropriate.[20]

■ SURGICAL TECHNIQUES

If the operation is performed with a vein graft obtained from the lower extremity, general anesthesia is preferable; if the vein graft is obtained from the upper extremity, an axillary block is adequate. Intravenous lidocaine HCl (Bier block), in general, does not provide adequate duration of anesthesia.

The extent and location of the thrombosed arterial segments can be delineated by adequate preoperative evaluation. The zone of injury will extend proximally and distally; therefore, the incision must be extensile, and variations of extensile carpal tunnel incisions are appropriate. I make an incision in the hypothenar crease from the wrist crease to the distal palmar crease. The distal extension is a zig-zag, and the proximal extension is parallel to the flexor carpi ulnaris tendon and midway between that tendon and the palmaris longus. Tourniquet control is important, and dissection under magnification is suggested.

The ulnar artery is identified proximal to the wrist crease and a rubberized loop is placed around it. The ulnar nerve is located and a loop of a different color is placed around it. The ulnar artery and superficial arch are then dissected through Guyon's canal into the palm. Major branches are not divided at this time. The carpal canal may be released to visualize terminal branches of the median nerve, to identify a median artery, and to minimize median nerve compression from edema or hemorrhage. Proper dissection will allow direct visualization of the distal ulnar artery, the entire superficial arch, and the origins of the common digital vessels.

The ulnar artery and its branches are inspected. The surgeon should observe the shape, color, and resilience of all vessels and note any obviously thrombosed or aneurysmal areas to define the extent of resection that will be required.

The abnormal vessel should be resected in its entirety. The extent of the resection is determined by removing the obviously thrombosed portion and then inspecting the interior of the vessel for fibrin clot and fibrous reaction. Serial sections are then made until normal vessels are seen under the operating microscope. Partial reconstruction of the lumen (recanalization) may be encountered, and should not be confused with undamaged vessel. An asymmetric lumen with loose-appearing intima and thickened media still within the zone of damage represents recanalization of a thrombotic area (Fig. 147–1). The intima should be inspected carefully for asymmetry, tears, redundancy, or exposed media. Damaged or exposed media proximal or distal to the arterial reconstruction will compromise patency. Resecting patent but compromised vessels involving proximal or distal collateral inflow or the origin of a common digital artery *commits the surgeon to arterial reconstruction*, and excessive dissection should not be performed unless the surgeon has the capability and the commitment to revascularize the hand. "Resection to normal" under the operating microscope is important and must be done if maximal patency rates

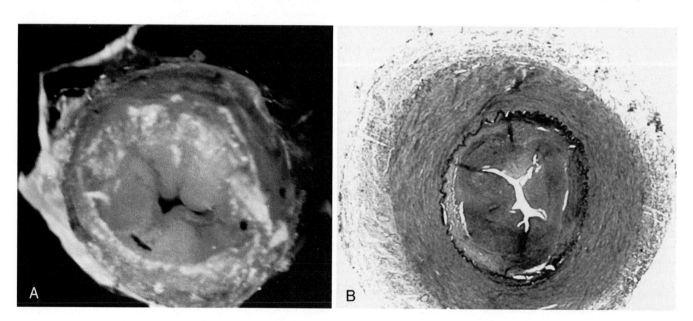

■ FIGURE 147–1

(A) Gross specimen of a thrombosed ulnar artery. Note the asymmetry of the lumen and the thickness of the vessel wall. **(B)** A cross-section (Verhoff stain; initial magnification × 10) confirms the abnormal intima, media, and adventitia. Note the disruption of the internal elastic lamina (black line). (Reproduced from Koman LA, Urbaniak JR: Ulnar artery thrombosis. Hand Clin, 1985; 1:311–325, with permission from WB Saunders Company.)

are to be obtained. If possible, it is preferable to resect proximally and distally until there is a patent branch within the specimen. Once all damaged vessels are resected, distal outflow may be assessed by observing "back-flow," measuring digital brachial pressure, and measuring back pressure by a catheter or digital plethysmograph after deflating the tourniquet (see Indications). The size of the defect and the number of anastomoses necessary are then determined.

A vein graft of appropriate length may be obtained from either the upper or the lower extremity. The distal cephalic or basilic vein may be obtained from the forearm, and the greater or lesser saphenous veins obtained from the foot and ankle are suitable graft material. Satisfactory results have been reported with both upper and lower extremity harvest sites.[13,16] Vessels may be harvested through multiple transverse incisions, through two transverse incisions aided by a vein stripper, or through extensile longitudinal exposure. Bleeding from venous branches must be prevented by ligation, vascular clips, or bipolar cauterization. During harvest and transport of the graft, it is important to maintain its proper orientation and length.

I prefer to harvest the saphenous vein through a single longitudinal incision under tourniquet control. The skin is marked over prominent veins and the leg exsanguinated with an Esmarch bandage, and the tourniquet inflated. Under loupe magnification, the saphenous vein is identified at the medial malleolar level and a vessel loop passed. The saphenous nerve is identified immediately adjacent to the greater saphenous vein, and its injury or transection is avoided if possible. If the vein is suitable in size and consistency, the incision is extended proximally and distally, the vessel is dissected free, and all branches are identified. On occasion, proximal branching is appropriate for a distal "Y" anastomosis. These valve-free proximal branches, when available, simplify reconstruction of multiple common branches of the superficial arch. Large and medium branches are ligated with 4-0 polyglycolic acid suture and small branches are coagulated with a bipolar cautery. Silver clips are used infrequently for controlling hemostasis from branches because they frequently slip off. Often a 5- to 7-cm area with few branches is found immediately above the medial malleolus.

The entire vessel is mobilized in situ and measured with a ruler. It is helpful to dissect most of the loose areolar tissue, exposing the adventitia, before the vein is removed. After adequate length is ensured (take 20 to 30% more than your wildest estimates would suggest), the proximal vessel is ligated with a 4-0 suture, clamped with a small hemostat, and transected between the ligature and the hemostat. To maintain proper orientation of the vessel, the hemostat is left in place and is not removed until the vascular repair is initiated. The distal vessel is then ligated and transected, and the graft is harvested. This portion, which will become the proximal artery, is never clamped. A consistent pattern of clamping decreases the likelihood that the proximal–distal orientation will be lost.

A blunt cannula is then inserted into the open distal vein and the vein is distended with heparinized saline to expose any leaks or injuries; these must be repaired. Leaks from branches may be tied either with 8-0 nylon circular suture or suture ligature. The latter is achieved by passing the needle through the stump of the branch and then tying the suture circumferentially. The use of silver clips and bipolar cautery are avoided, because they are associated with a higher failure rate unless the branches are longer than 3 mm. Small lacerations in the vessel may be repaired, but if the vessel is compromised seriously, it should be discarded and another obtained.

The length of the vein required and the number of distal anastomoses is determined before the vein is harvested. The vein graft may be sized on the basis of the in vivo measurement, but often it is wise to trim the graft to the proper length after inflow has been established. The vein graft must be reversed and its anatomically distal portion anastomosed to a normal segment of ulnar artery. In general, the proximal end-to-end anastomosis is performed first and its patency checked before the distal repair is performed. If the distal configuration of the graft is complex or if satisfactory exposure is difficult to achieve, the distal segment may be anastomosed first. Size discrepancies usually are not significant, but when they are significant, they may be managed by a less than

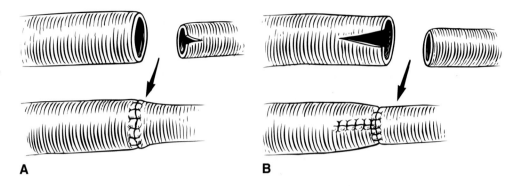

■ FIGURE 147–2
Techniques to manage
size discrepancies. **(A)**
"Opening V" in smaller
segment. **(B)** "Closing V"
in larger segment.

A   **B**

30° oblique cut in the artery, an "opening V" in the artery (Fig. 147–2A), or a "closing V" in the vein graft (Fig. 147–2B). Nylon 8-0 or 9-0 on a 100- to 135-μm needle is the suture of choice. Stay sutures are placed at 120°, and front and back segments are then repaired with interrupted sutures. Vascular approximating clamps are useful for vessel alignment and hemostasis. It is crucial to place all sutures through the intima, to avoid back or sidewall tethering, and to recognize and repair any vessel injury.

In short-segment grafts involving the ulnar artery and superficial arch, both end-to-end repairs may be done before the tourniquet is deflated. In larger or more complex grafts, deflating the tourniquet briefly for an earlier confirmation of flow through the vein graft is often beneficial. All repairs are performed with an operating microscope.

After the proximal repair is achieved, the distal anastomosis(es) is performed. The graft is trimmed to size (10% longer than the defect) and placed in its new bed in the wrist or palm. *Avoid twisting the graft.* Distal repairs are performed with 8-0 or 9-0 nylon suture on 100- to 135-μm needles. Size discrepancies are managed in a manner similar to that used in the proximal repair. Large differences in size may be handled best by creating a blind pouch (ligation of the end on the vessel) and an end-to-side repair (Fig. 147–3A); if two or more distal anastomoses are necessary, variables involving end-to-end and end-to-side repairs can be achieved in series (Fig. 147–3B). Complex reconstructions are necessary on occasion, and may include end-to-side anastomoses proximally and distally (Fig. 147–4) and "Y" grafts (Fig. 147–5).

Intraoperative heparin is given as one or two 2000- to 5000-unit boluses immediately before the tourniquet is released. Infusion of Dextran, 40 at 20 ml/hour, also is initiated in the operating room. I have not found postoperative heparin to be necessary; however, if the anastomosis is compromised by abnormal distal vessels and marginal run-off, systemic anticoagulation should be considered.

After all anastomoses are complete, the tourniquet is deflated and the repair(s) checked for patency or leaks. All bleeding is controlled and the wound is closed in a single layer from wrist to digit(s) using simple and/or vertical mattress and/or horizontal mattress sutures of 4-0 nylon. Subcutaneous sutures may be used proximal to the wrist, but the fascia is not repaired. A single Silastic 7-French drain is placed along the vein graft.

A large bulky hand and forearm dressing with dorsal plaster is applied from fingertips to above the elbow. The hand is in a functional position. The drain is left 12 to 24 hours. Circulation is assessed every hour for 6 hours, then every other hour for 24 hours. No smoking or chocolate or caffeine consumption is allowed. Dextran 40 infusion is continued at 20 ml/hour for 2 to 5 days, and salicylate 125 mg/day is administered. If sedation is necessary, chlorpromazine (25 mg p.o. tid) is used. Narcotic analgesia may be used as necessary.

■ TECHNICAL
ALTERNATIVES

The need for a patient-oriented approach cannot be overstated. Arterial reconstruction in an extremity that can be managed by a more forgiving technique can be harmful. The patient must be willing to play an active, cooperative role in the perioperative period.

During vein graft harvesting, pitfalls include: (1) selection of a vein graft that is too

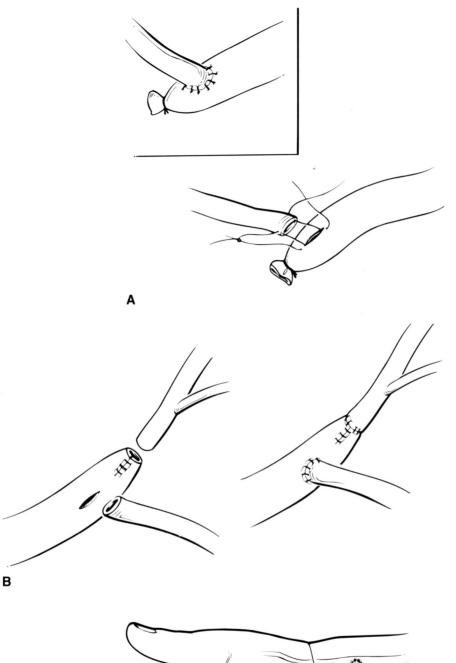

A

B

■ **FIGURE 147-3**
(A) End-to-side anastomoses after ligation of distal stump. **(B)** End-to-end anastomoses into the superficial arch and end-to-side anastomoses of a common digital artery to the vein graft.

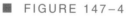

■ **FIGURE 147-4**
Schematic of arterial reconstruction using 14-cm reversed vein graft. The ulnar artery was not suitable to the midforearm level; therefore, an end-to-side anastomosis to the radial artery was performed. Because of the significant size discrepancy, the distal vein was ligated and three end-to-side repairs were performed.

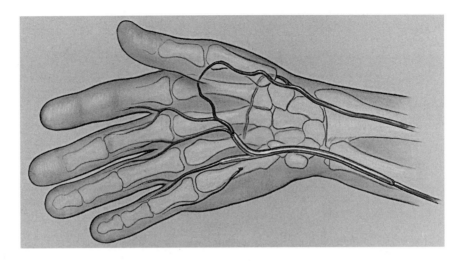

■ FIGURE 147–5

Schematic of an arterial reconstruction using an 18-cm reversed interposition vein graft from the contralateral saphenous vein. The proximal anastomosis was end-to-end to the ulnar artery. Distally a natural "Y"-fork allowed end-to-end anastomosis to the common digital artery to the ring and little fingers, and to the superficial arch. (Reproduced with permission from Koman LA, Urbaniak JR: Ulnar artery thrombosis. Hand Clin, 1985; 1:311–325, with permission from WB Saunders Company.)

small; (2) damage to the graft during dissection; (3) inadequate graft length; (4) injury to saphenous or other sensory nerves; and (5) loss of hemostasis at branches. Inadequate or iatrogenically compromised vessels should be discarded. Extensile exposure, attention to detail, and careful hemostasis are necessary. Postoperative wound appearance may be enhanced by appropriate drainage, careful hemostasis, and subcuticular closure of vein donor sites. The use of Steristrips (3M Surgical Supplies, Wallingford, Conn.) for 6 to 12 weeks and sunscreen will minimize scar spread and disfigurement.

Technical errors during anastomoses can be minimized by adequate exposure; the microscopic portion of the procedure should be "easy." One pitfall is failure to maintain the graft in the proper orientation when placing it, because twisting the graft more than 60° will compromise patency rates.[17] The role of intussusception anastomoses or mechanical couplers has yet to be delineated in arterial reconstruction with vein grafts. The surgeon must be honest when appraising the anastomosis, and if it is compromised, it must be redone.

■ REHABILITATION

Extensive rehabilitation is seldom necessary after vein grafting in ulnar artery thrombosis. After the completion of the surgical procedure, the hand is placed in a bulky compressive dressing with dorsal splints. This dressing allows the fingers freedom to move, and active range of motion is recommended. If the patient has difficulty with range of motion, then occupational therapy is added. A soft dressing is left in place for 2 weeks, at the end of which time the sutures are removed. The foot is dressed with a compressive dressing, which is removed at 5 days. A support stocking is recommended for 6 to 8 weeks and, if the main portion of the saphenous vein has been harvested, the patient is advised that there will be some swelling of the foot, which will diminish over time. At the time of discharge, the patient is instructed to take 125 mg of salicylates every morning and 200 mg of ibuprofen twice daily. At 2 weeks, if the wounds are healing, the patient is allowed increased use of the hand, but is not allowed to return to unrestricted activities for 6 to 8 weeks. Specific strengthening exercises are given only if the patient has pain or stiffness. The patient is instructed to avoid using the hand inappropriately, as a hammer, for example, and cautioned to avoid direct injury to the hand itself.

With the use of the above guidelines, and assuming a modicum of technical proficiency, patency rates of 70 to 85% are possible.[4,14,16,20] With patent vein grafts, ulcerations should heal and symptoms should improve. However, complete elimination of pain, cold intolerance, and neural dysfunction is uncommon. Improvement, not cure, is the rule, and the patient should understand that before proceeding with the operation. Vein graft occlusion in group I or group II extremities in which collateral vessels were not compromised by the resection will respond in a manner similar to that of extremities having undergone a "Leriche sympathectomy."[18] In group III extremities with true arterial insufficiency and inadequate collateral flow, escalation of symptoms, including further tissue necrosis, is likely if the graft becomes compromised or occluded.

■ OUTCOMES

References

1. Berger AC, Kleinert JM: Noninvasive vascular studies: A comparison with arteriography and surgical findings in the upper extremity. J Hand Surg, 1992; 17A:206–210.
2. Cho KO: Entrapment occlusion of the ulnar artery in the hand: A case report. J Bone Joint Surg, 1978; 60A:841–843.
3. Di Benedetto MR, Nappi JF, Ruff ME, Lubbers LM: Doppler mapping in hypothenar hammer syndrome: An alternate to arteriography. J Hand Surg, 1989; 14A:244–246.
4. Given KG, Puckett CL, Kleinert HE: Ulnar artery thrombosis. Plast Reconstr Surg, 1978; 61:405–411.
5. Goldner R, Koman LA: Microsurgery. In: Goldsmith HS (ed): Practice of Surgery. Philadelphia: Harper & Row, 1984:1–14.
6. Kleinert HE, Volianitis GJ: Thrombosis of the palmar arterial arch and its tributaries: Etiology and new concepts in treatment. J Trauma, 1965; 5:447–457.
7. Koman LA: Current status of noninvasive techniques in the diagnosis of upper extremity disorders. American Academy of Orthopaedic Surgeons Instructional Course Lectures, 1983; 32:61–76.
8. Koman LA: Diagnostic study of vascular lesions. Hand Clin, 1985; 1:217–231.
9. Koman LA, Bond GM, Carter RE, Poehling GG: Evaluation of upper extremity vasculature with high-resolution ultrasound. J Hand Surg, 1985; 10:249–255.
10. Koman LA, Nunley JA, Goldner JL, Seaber AV, Urbaniak JR: Isolated cold stress testing in the assessment of symptoms in the upper extremity: preliminary communication. J Hand Surg, 1984; 9:305–311.
11. Koman LA, Nunley JA, Wilkinson RH Jr, Urbaniak JR, Coleman RE: Dynamic radionuclide imaging as a means of evaluating vascular perfusion of the upper extremity: A preliminary report. J Hand Surg, 1983; 8:424–434.
12. Koman LA, Urbaniak JR: Thrombosis of ulnar artery at the wrist. In: American Academy of Orthopaedic Surgeons: Symposium on Microsurgery: Practical Use in Orthopaedics, St. Louis: CV Mosby, 1979, 119–132.
13. Koman LA, Urbaniak JR: Ulnar artery insufficiency: A guide to treatment. J Hand Surg, 1981; 6:16–24.
14. Koman LA, Urbaniak JR: Ulnar artery thrombosis. Hand Clin, 1985; 1:311–325.
15. Leriche R, Fontaine R, Dupertuis SM: Arterectomy: With followup studies on 78 operations. Surg Gynecol Obstet, 1937; 64:149–155.
16. Mehlhoff TL, Wood MB: Ulnar artery thrombosis and the role of interposition vein grafting: Patency with microsurgical technique. J Hand Surg, 1991; 16A:274–278.
17. Monsivais JJ, Espejo S: The influence of rotation of the pedicle on the patency of tissue transfer. Journal of the Southern Orthopedic Association, (in press).
18. Rothkopf DM, Bryan DJ, Cuadros CL, May JW Jr: Surgical management of ulnar artery aneurysms. J Hand Surg, 1990; 15A:891–897.
19. Trevaskis AE, Marcks KM, Rennisi VM, Berg EM. Thrombosis of the ulnar artery in the hand. Plast Reconstr Surg, 1964; 33:73–76.
20. Zimmerman NB, Zimmerman SI, McClinton MA, Wilgis EFS, Koontz CL, Buehner JW: Long-term recovery following surgical treatment for ulnar artery occlusion. J Hand Surg, 1994; 19A:17–21.

148

Digital Periarterial Symphathectomy

Over the years, patients presenting with chronic digital ischemia manifested by severe cold intolerance and pain, with or without tip ulcerations, have been treated with various techniques. Pharmacologically, vasodilators have been used for the treatment of these patients. Surgical techniques have included cervicothoracic sympathectomy and amputation. All of these techniques have resulted in outcomes that were generally discouraging. Flatt, in 1980, described digital artery sympathectomy.[2] He based this operation on the fact that the proximal sympathectomy on an anatomic basis did not denervate the distal digital blood vessels. He proposed a more distal sympathectomy based on the various anatomic considerations of the sympathetics. It was his reasoning that if the objective of the operation was to relieve the symptoms in the digit, it seemed logical that the sympathectomy should be performed as far distally as was practical. He reported eight patients who had a periarterial sympathectomy in the palm with beneficial results. In 1981, we elucidated the anatomical structures of the digital sympathetic nerves as they emerged from the digital nerve and their course to the arteries.[3] We suggested isolation and division of at least four of these branches and periarterial adventitial stripping distally in the finger as far as the proximal interphalangeal joint. Essentially, we took Flatt's concept and advanced it more distally in the finger. The feeling was that this was a segmental operation and that denervation of a segment of the artery with resultant additional blood flow would be more effective the closer it were done to the problem. For example, if the tips were ulcerated and the tips were cold, then the closer the denervation could be accomplished to the tips, the more blood would be supplied to the affected area. We chose the proximal segment of the digit because, anatomically, there were four distinct sympathetic branches, three from the proper digital nerve and one from the dorsal branch, that directly innervate the artery. This area also appeared to be safer to us as far as wound healing was concerned. We feared that if we ventured distal to the proximal interphalangeal joint, problems with wound healing would ensue closer to the ischemic area.

The sympathetic nerve fibers arise from the stellate and from the second and third thoracic sympathetic ganglia. They then join the peripheral nerves by many circuitous routes (Fig. 148–1). Other sympathetic nerves bypass the sympathetic chains and enter the brachial plexus through the cervical plexus or the nerve of Kuntz.[4] The sympathetic fibers travel within the substance of the major peripheral nerves to their destination in the forearm, wrist, and hand. They are located in the periphery of the median nerve and branch off into the palmar arch and digital arteries (Fig. 148–2). The ulnar artery is supplied in the forearm by a special nerve called the nerve of Henley, or the arterial branch of the ulnar nerve. It arises high in the forearm from the ulnar nerve and follows the ulnar artery in several filaments down to the palm of the hand. This nerve easily can be found running longitudinally along the course of the ulnar artery of the wrist.

In the hand, the palmar arterial arches are supplied by the median nerve primarily and, to a lesser extent, by the ulnar nerve. The superficial arch is, to a large extent, supplied by the nerves from the median nerve. In the digits, the sympathetic nerves travel within the digital nerve and exit to supply the sympathetic tone to the arterial muscle. From the level of the interdigital web to the midportion of the middle phalanx, there are approximately four large identifiable sympathetic branches traveling from the digital nerve to the

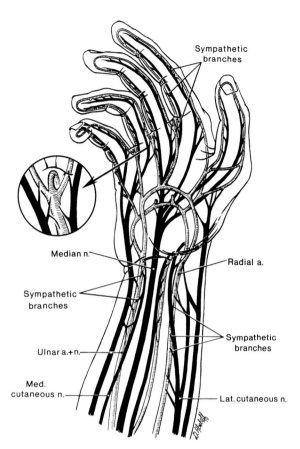

■ FIGURE 148-1
The sympathetic nervous
innervation in the fore-
arm, wrist and hand.

Sympathetic
branches

Median n.

Radial a.

Sympathetic
branches

Sympathetic
branches

Ulnar a.+n.

Med.
cutaneous n.

Lat. cutaneous n.

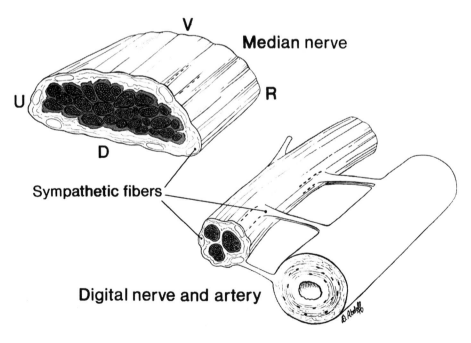

■ FIGURE 148-2
The location of the sym-
pathetic fibers within the
median nerve and the
cross-connections be-
tween the nerve and the
artery.

V

Median nerve

U

R

D

Sympathetic fibers

Digital nerve and artery

digital artery. The sympathetic nerves emerge from the digital nerve and travel to the
adventitia of the artery. (Fig. 148–3).[6]

It is based on this anatomic rationale that the operation of digital periarterial sympathectomy is devised. If one can effectively denervate a 2-cm section of artery in the proximal
segment of the finger, more blood can be delivered to the ischemic fingertip.

■ FIGURE 148–3
An anatomic dissection of the proximal segment of a digit, indicating the cross-connections between the nerve and the artery. The artery has a suture in the lumen.

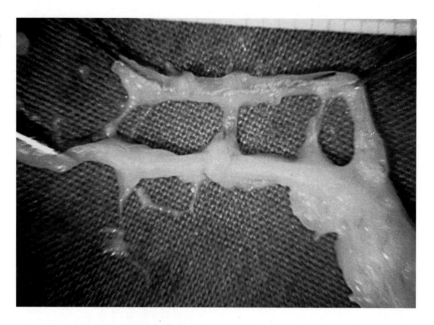

■ INDICATIONS AND CONTRAINDICATIONS

Digital periarterial sympathectomy is indicated in patients with disabling pain, cold intolerance, or tip ulcerations, provided they have no evidence of proximal causes of peripheral ischemia, have failed to respond to medical therapy, and have demonstrated a satisfactory response to cold stress testing.

Proximal vessel disease is ruled out by using noninvasive techniques or by digital subtraction angiography of the aortic arch and subclavian and brachial vessels. An aneurysm or constriction of the subclavian vessels can give rise to peripheral embolization and cause chronic digital ischemia. Correction of the proximal disease is absolutely necessary before any local treatment in the hand.[8]

Many patients experience a positive response to calcium channel blockers. Several studies have indicated that approximately 60% of patients with disabling chronic digital ischemia of a vasospastic nature will experience improvement with calcium channel blockers such as nifedipine.

Pulse volume recordings and digital perfusion pressures measured in the resting state and then under cold stress constitute the principal evaluation. Cold stress involves immersing the hand in water at 12°C. Normally, the resting pulse volume is altered significantly by cold stress and rebounds to normal or even better than normal by 5 minutes after the removal of the cold stress. The critical measurement is the digital brachial index, which is the ratio of the digital pressure to the brachial pressure. A normal digital brachial index is 0.9 to 1.0. If, after the cold stress, tracings do not show that the perfusion pressure has returned to the normal state, this is considered an abnormal test result.

The next step is to block the peripheral sympathetic nerve by injection of 2 ml of 0.5% lidocaine HCl around the proper digital nerves in the distal palm. This effectively stops the conduction of the digital nerves and their sympathetic contributions to the digital vessels. The patient is then subjected again to resting pulse volume recordings, cold stress, and then, 5 minutes after cold stress, repeat pulse volume recordings. A positive test is defined as improvement in both the cold stress and the postcold stress tracing after digital blockade, and indicates that the circulation of the digits should be improved by surgical sympathectomy. This type of patient is indicated for a periarterial sympathectomy. However, there must be a significant improvement in the cold stress and return after digital blockade of the sympathetic nerves for the patients to be considered candidates for surgery.

Surgery is contraindicated in those patients who have failed the preoperative testing. Cessation of smoking is mandatory for a satisfactory result, and therefore is a relative contraindication to this procedure. However, this procedure can be done if there is impending tissue loss with the agreement that the patient will stop smoking after surgery.

Periarterial digital sympathectomy is done with the aid of the operating microscope. If done on one finger, the procedure can be performed under local anesthesia as an outpatient surgery under tourniquet control. If the procedure is done on more than one digit, the necessity for regional anesthesia for tourniquet pain must be considered.

Digital sympathectomy includes isolation of the terminal branches of the sympathetic nerves that travel with the peripheral nerves, division of these terminal branches, and stripping of the adventitia from the common digital and proper digital arteries.

When reaching the adventitia of the artery, the sympathetic nerves divide and ascend or descend in a segmental fashion to form a network of sympathetic fibers surrounding the digital artery. The location of the sympathetic nerves has been studied by Morgan and co-authors[3] by examining catecholamine histofluorescence in the median, ulnar, and digital nerves. With the catecholamine histofluorescence technique, they showed that there were small, localized areas of fluorescence at the wrist level only in the external perimeter of the epineurium of the median nerve. The median nerve contained six to eight of these fluorescent areas around its perimeter, whereas the ulnar nerve contained only three to four groups. The digital nerves showed several areas of intense fluorescence only around the perimeter of the nerve within the epineurium. Branching could be seen associated with the fluorescent areas. The digital arteries had consistent, intense fluorescence only within the adventitia. The digital nerves, from the median nerve distribution, revealed more intense fluorescence and a greater number of sympathetic rich fluorescent areas than the ulnar digital nerves from the same specimens. This confirmed the fact that the sympathetic axons traveled within the peripheral nerves and sent frequent branches to arteries throughout their course.

Using a volar zig-zag incision, the neurovascular bundles are exposed from the distal palm and the interdigital web to the proximal interphalangeal joint (Fig. 148–4). The digital nerve is identified and gently retracted from the digital artery. As the digital nerve and digital artery are separated, the communication between these two structures can be seen. All connections between the nerve and the vessel are severed by sharp dissection. We always identify four sympathetic branches traveling from the digital nerve to the vessel and remove these branches. There is usually one branch arising from the posterior branch of the digital nerve, supplying the dorsal aspect of the digital artery.

With the aid of the operative microscope, using jeweler's forceps, and with some sharp dissection, the loose adventitia surrounding the common digital artery and proper digital artery is removed in a circumferential fashion for an area of 2 cm. This effectively removes all the terminal sympathetic branches, including those traveling in a longitudinal fashion along the vessel. The vessel must not be damaged and the media and intima must be left untouched; otherwise, thrombosis will occur. If a thrombosis is encountered distal to the proximal interphalangeal joint, the digital artery should be resected, as reported by Zook and Kleinert.[9] In two cases, local thrombectomy of the proper digital artery has been done.

Many times, there is not an immediate response to the strong circulating humeral component of norepinephrine that may still be present; however, a response is observable several hours after the operation. By the following day, the finger is usually warm and there is a temperature difference between the treated and untreated digits of as much as 60°C. There is often some numbness and tingling reported in the digit, which we believe is the result of a temporary neurapraxia of the digital nerve caused by surgical manipulation. Ulcers usually heal and pain is improved within 2 weeks.

In our experience, the distal proper digital neurovascular bundle should be addressed. The one branch from the posterior branch of the digital nerve also should be removed. Alternatively, Flatt[2] concentrates the dissection at a more proximal level at the common digital artery and digital nerve level in the palm.

During the adventitial stripping, one potential pitfall is for the surgeon to become too aggressive and actually injure the media of the artery. The important thing is to remove the loose nerve structure that runs longitudinally between the branches. This is usually located in the loose adventitial structures, and not in the deeper adventitial structures.

■ FIGURE 148-4
(A) The typical zig-zag
volar incision. (B) The
area of operative expo-
sure.

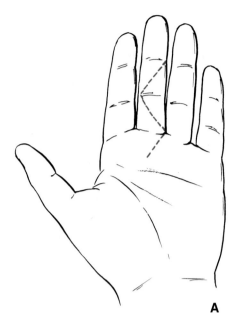

A

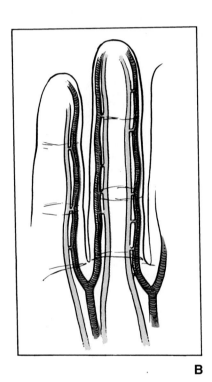

B

Care should be taken not to injure the digital vessel. Another potential problem is the rupture of branches of the artery, particularly that lateral branch going to the proximal interphalangeal joint and the flexor sheath. This usually is a substantial branch, and should be protected.

One potential advantage of the adventitial stripping in those patients with chronic vasculitis is that the adventitia can thicken and act as a constricting element about the vessel. If one opens this and allows the vessel to expand, there sometimes can be improvement in those patients.

■ REHABILITATION

There are no specific rehabilitation protocols for the care of these patients other than wound care and beginning motion. These patients usually require dressing for approximately 7 to 10 days and then suture removal, followed by beginning motion of the hand. Depending on the wound, the finger can be moved. If tip ulceration is a part of the patient's presentation, the tip can be gently debrided in the whirlpool during the postoperative phase. The patient will usually continue to experience some numbness, so there is very little pain in this period. Rehabilitation should continue until the patient gains full motion of the digit and has complete healing. Usually patients with desk jobs can work during this phase; those patients with manual jobs are generally off work until healing is complete. In our series, all patients have returned to their previous work environment.

Patients with scleroderma have had the poorest response, whereas young patients with vasculitis and primary vasospastic disorders have had the best response.[1] The postfrostbite patients have had excellent response. In a report by Reisman[5] of 51 digital sympathectomies in 42 patients, 49 digits showed complete improvement subjectively. Thirty-nine patients demonstrated marked improvement and had no recurrence of their symptoms. In our series of 50 patients, similar results have been obtained.[7] Those patients who have passed the rigorous preoperative testing—those who demonstrate a marked response to the chemical sympathectomy brought on by digital block—will predictably have an excellent result with surgical digital sympathectomy. Those patients with a moderately minor improvement will show only moderately minor improvement in the clinical situation as well. There is one patient with terminal scleroderma with an infected tip ulceration in which the procedure caused the complication of a finger amputation due to infection.

■ OUTCOMES

References

1. Eglof DV, Mifsud RP, Verdan C: Superselective digital sympathectomy in Raynaud's phenomenon. Hand, 1982; 15:110–114.
2. Flatt AE: Digital artery sympathectomy. J Hand Surg, 1980; 5:550–556.
3. Morgan R, Reisman N, Wilgis EFS: Anatomic localization of sympathetic nerves in the hand. J Hand Surg, 1983; 8:283–288.
4. Pick J: The Autonomic Nervous System. Philadelphia: JB Lippincott, 1970.
5. Reisman R: Surgical management of Raynaud's phenomenon. Texas Med, 1984; 80:44.
6. Spinner M: Kaplan's Functional and Surgical Anatomy of the Hand. Philadelphia: JB Lippincott, 1984.
7. Wilgis EFS: The evaluation and treatment of chronic digital ischemia. Ann Surg, 1981; 193:693.
8. Wilgis EFS: Vascular Injuries and Diseases of the Upper Limb. Boston: Little, Brown & Co., 1983.
9. Zook EG, Kleinert H, Von Beek A: Treatment of the ischemic finger secondary to digital artery occlusion. PRS, 1978; 62, 229.

■ INDEX

Page numbers in *italics* refer to illustrations; numbers followed by t indicate tables.